The Pharmacist's Expanded Role in Critical Care Medicine

Yasir Alzaidi • Mohamed Abdelzaher Gebily
Editors

The Pharmacist's Expanded Role in Critical Care Medicine

A Comprehensive Guide for Practitioners and Trainees

Volume II

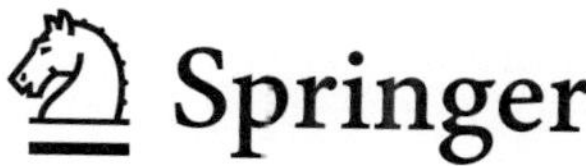 Springer

Editors
Yasir Alzaidi
Department of Pharmacy
Al Hada Armed Forces Hospital
Taif, Saudi Arabia

Mohamed Abdelzaher Gebily
Department of Intensive Care
Al Hada Armed Forces Hospital
Taif, Saudi Arabia

ISBN 978-3-031-77337-2   ISBN 978-3-031-77335-8   (eBook)
https://doi.org/10.1007/978-3-031-77335-8

© The Editor(s) (if applicable) and The Author(s), under exclusive license to Springer Nature Switzerland AG 2025

This work is subject to copyright. All rights are solely and exclusively licensed by the Publisher, whether the whole or part of the material is concerned, specifically the rights of translation, reprinting, reuse of illustrations, recitation, broadcasting, reproduction on microfilms or in any other physical way, and transmission or information storage and retrieval, electronic adaptation, computer software, or by similar or dissimilar methodology now known or hereafter developed.
The use of general descriptive names, registered names, trademarks, service marks, etc. in this publication does not imply, even in the absence of a specific statement, that such names are exempt from the relevant protective laws and regulations and therefore free for general use.
The publisher, the authors and the editors are safe to assume that the advice and information in this book are believed to be true and accurate at the date of publication. Neither the publisher nor the authors or the editors give a warranty, expressed or implied, with respect to the material contained herein or for any errors or omissions that may have been made. The publisher remains neutral with regard to jurisdictional claims in published maps and institutional affiliations.

This Springer imprint is published by the registered company Springer Nature Switzerland AG
The registered company address is: Gewerbestrasse 11, 6330 Cham, Switzerland

If disposing of this product, please recycle the paper.

Foreword

The role of the pharmacist in critical care medicine has become increasingly important and multifaceted in recent years. Critically ill patients are highly heterogeneous in terms of age, underlying comorbidities, prehospital medication usage, admission diagnoses, allergies, concurrent organ replacement therapies, and so on. The acute nature of their illness means that their condition and hence management can change rapidly during their stay, and the disease severity means that many will require multiple medications during, and after, their ICU stay. As integral members of the critical care team, ICU pharmacists have the essential training and knowledge to ensure that prescriptions are individualized such that each patient receives the best drug for them, at the optimal dose, with minimal adverse effects throughout their ICU and hospital stays. ICU pharmacists are also pivotal to successful antimicrobial stewardship programs and accurate interpretation of therapeutic drug monitoring, and their involvement in the diagnostic process and in identifying diagnostic, as well as medication, errors is increasingly encouraged.

Despite their increased presence on our ICUs and involvement in patient management, there are few textbooks aimed specifically at critical care pharmacists, particularly in terms of their potential role in diagnosis. Recognizing this important gap, the editors of this comprehensive book have gathered together 55 chapters that provide an overview of core aspects of critical care patient management from the pharmacist's perspective. The chapters, written by an international team of more than 100 experts, provide an important update on the physiological and pathological mechanisms of key areas of critical illness and the diagnostic and therapeutic approaches to these conditions for the pharmacist. There are chapters focusing on specific diseases or conditions, including shock, acute liver failure, acute kidney injury, delirium, and acute pulmonary embolism; chapters on interpretation of diagnostic tests, such as radiology and electrocardiography; chapters on therapeutic interventions, including mechanical ventilation, intravenous fluids, renal replacement therapy, ECMO, nutrition, and blood transfusion; and chapters on specific groups of ICU patients, including obstetric, oncology, transplant, and burn patients. Two of the chapters, on the approach to clinical reasoning in critical care and sustainable pharmacy practice in the ICU, are unique chapters to pharmacy education and training.

Providing an up-to-date overview of topics related to critical care and emphasizing the importance of correct diagnosis in providing appropriate and optimal treatment, this collection will help prepare ICU pharmacists for their multifaceted responsibilities as members of the ICU team, including an expanded role in limiting misdiagnosis. This book will serve as a useful resource for all pharmacists involved in the management of critically ill patients, whatever their level of experience and training, and I congratulate the editors on their achievement.

Université Libre de Bruxelles   Jean-Louis Vincent
Brussels, Belgium
Department of Intensive Care
Erasme University Hospital
Brussels, Belgium

Foreword

The critical care environment, encompassing the intensive care unit as well as critical care outreach to intermediate care units and the general ward in the form of rapid response systems and medical emergency teams, is tremendously challenging clinically and in terms of patient safety and quality. Pharmacists have a crucial and central role in ensuring the best quality of clinical care and promoting patient safety. Medication errors in these high-stress environments and situations are one of the most common patient safety and quality concerns, and pharmacists are the experts that intensivists, nurses, and respiratory therapists turn to for help in avoiding these types of medical errors. In addition, critically ill patients often receive a large number of medications and have deranged physiology and pharmacodynamics and pharmacokinetics that create a complicated milieu that needs to be carefully balanced to avoid complications and optimize outcome. Pharmacists enhance the quality of care by using their knowledge and education to guide the care team in making the best pharmacological choices for each patient. They also assist prescribers in making the most cost-effective choices, something that is crucial in the current healthcare environment where costs are a major concern. Their role, however, goes well beyond optimization of drug therapy and prevention of medication errors. In the ICU, pharmacists' role is increasingly underscored in ensuring precise diagnoses, a cornerstone for effective drug therapy. Notably, diagnostic errors in the ICU pose substantial concerns, as evidenced by a systematic review led by Winters et al. (2012), revealing alarming rates of errors, including those with lethal implications. Actively engaging in diagnostic deliberations, pharmacists leverage their extensive knowledge in pharmacotherapy to offer invaluable insights that either corroborate or challenge diagnoses. This interdisciplinary synergy is pivotal in aligning treatments with accurate diagnoses, thereby elevating the caliber of patient care.

This book aims to foster interdisciplinary team collaboration that cultivates a culture of safety and precision in patient care, essential for averting diagnostic pitfalls and ensuring therapeutic efficacy. The book contains chapters that enhance diagnostic reasoning and prevent diagnostic errors. In addition, the book provides a comprehensive state-of-the-art review of all topics related to critical care authored by experts from prestigious institutions. I congratulate Dr. Alzaidi on this achievement, and I hope that this book will inform administrators and providers as to the financial, safety, and quality benefits that pharmacists provide in the critical care environment and spur hospitals to make the central role of the pharmacist in the management of critically ill patients a universal reality that all intensive care units and their patients can enjoy and benefit from.

Department of Anesthesiology and Critical   Bradford D. Winters
Care Medicine, Co-Director of the
Johns Hopkins Hospital Surgical ICUs
and the Bayview Medical Center Surgical
and Burn ICUs, Core Faculty Armstrong Institute
for Patient Safety and Quality
The Johns Hopkins University School
of Medicine,
Baltimore, MD, USA

Foreword

The history of critical care pharmacists extends beyond 50 years, but the growth of services, personnel, research, and magnitude of impact has been exponential. Early in my critical care practice, the focus was on the recognition of our contributions and justification of our roles. While we created a ripple initially, the effect has magnified into a tidal wave of highly trained and engaged pharmacists providing comprehensive medication management for patients in a myriad of settings and with complex clinical problems and management programs.

Key milestones in the development of critical care pharmacists include organization as sections within professional organizations, description of our practice and services, Board Certification in 2012, expansion of critical care residency training programs, guideline and position paper authorship, leadership in influential multiprofessional organizations with active participation in committees, and ongoing documentation of our clinical and economic impact. While individuals are sometimes recognized, it is the influence of the whole that continues to build to tsunami levels.

This text provides a comprehensive view into the broad and expanding world of critical care pharmacy and pharmacologic challenges. I am consistently impressed and amazed by the dedication, knowledge, and creativity of my colleagues worldwide. We have come a long way from gentamicin dosing as a primary focus! The author list of this text includes an amazing group of contributors, and I congratulate them and the editors for comprehensive topics that illustrate current and future roles.

Importantly, the scope of contributions illustrates that we always have new areas to explore, new services to provide, and new growth opportunities. We will be challenged with tools like artificial intelligence or other new technologies, but I have faith that they will be harnessed to improve efficiency and processes. The ultimate reward will be the steadily improving care we provide, in conjunction with our critical care colleagues and teams.

At the same time, I feel that the million little things we do as pharmacists—consistently, every day (or night)—are the most important drivers for optimal patient outcomes (rather than the new and flashy). Additionally, the ability to admit when we are wrong (like my initial resistance to assuming responsibility for a valid medication history) is an important component of our growth as individuals and a professional.

Another important consideration is that while critical care pharmacists excel as entrepreneurs and love to develop new skills and services, a significant opportunity remains to ensure a consistent and standardized scope of practice that describes our foundation and commonalities of practice as a team of pharmacists. We need to ensure that other practitioners can understand and expect specific services, at a minimum. Other standardized tools that allow us to measure outcomes based on the severity of illness or complexity of therapeutics and care will strengthen our ability to document our impact as essential critical care team members.

The roles are limitless, and the tide is moving forward quickly.

Lebanon, IN, USA   Judith Jacobi

Contents of Volume II

Contents of Volume I

Contributors

Max W. Adelman Division of Infectious Diseases, Department of Medicine, Houston Methodist Hospital, Houston, TX, USA
Division of Pulmonary, Critical Care, and Sleep Medicine, Department of Medicine, Houston Methodist Hospital, Houston, TX, USA

Kathleen M. Akgün Yale University School of Medicine, Veterans Administration Connecticut Healthcare System, West Haven, CT, USA

Kaitlin M. Alexander University of Florida College of Pharmacy, Gainesville, FL, USA

Sajjadh M. J. Ali Beth Israel Deaconess Medical Center, Boston, MA, USA

Teresa A. Allison Department of Pharmacy, Memorial Hermann—Texas Medical Center, Houston, TX, USA

Yasir Alzaidi Department of Pharmacy, Al Hada Armed Forces Hospital, Taif, Saudi Arabia

Adrián Baranchuk Division of Cardiology, Queen's University, Kingston, ON, Canada

Nicholas Barker Cardiovascular Intensive Care Unit, Emory Saint Joseph's Hospital, Atlanta, GA, USA

Brooke Barlow Memorial Hermann-The Woodlands Medical Center, Houston, TX, USA

Erin F. Barreto Department of Pharmacy, Mayo Clinic Hospital—Rochester, Rochester, MN, USA

Christopher Bell Department of Pharmacy, Massachusetts General Hospital, Boston, MA, USA

Scott Benken Department of Pharmacy Practice, University of Illinois Chicago College of Pharmacy, Chicago, IL, USA

Karen Berger Nova Southeastern University, Fort Lauderdale, FL, USA
Broward Health Medical Center, Fort Lauderdale, FL, USA

Mauro Bernardi Department of Medical and Surgical Sciences, Alma Mater Studiorum—University of Bologna, Bologna, Italy

Sarah Bova University of Maryland Medical Center, Baltimore, MD, USA

Lauren R. Calnan Hillcrest Hospital South, Tulsa, OK, USA

Ryan Chaffee Department of Pharmacy, Massachusetts General Hospital, Boston, MA, USA

Cherylee W. J. Chang Department of Neurology, Duke University School of Medicine, Durham, NC, USA
Department of Neurosurgery, Duke University School of Medicine, Durham, NC, USA
Department of Medicine Division of Pulmonary, Allergy and Critical Care, Duke University School of Medicine, Durham, NC, USA

Lingye Chen Division of Pulmonary, Allergy, and Critical Care Medicine, Duke University School of Medicine, Durham, NC, USA

Michael Chen Anesthesiology, Perioperative and Pain Medicine, Stanford Hospital, Stanford, CA, USA

Sanjiv Chopra Beth Israel Deaconess Medical Center, Boston, MA, USA
Harvard Medical School, Boston, MA, USA

Aulina Chowdhury Boston Children's Hospital, Boston, MA, USA

Alana Ciolek New York-Presbyterian Hospital/Weill Cornell Medical Center, New York, NY, USA

Kevin G. Correa Division of Pulmonary, Allergy, and Critical Care Medicine, Stanford University, Palo Alto, CA, USA

Yuhamy Curbelo-Pena New York-Presbyterian Hospital, Columbia University Irving Medical Center, New York, NY, USA

Stephanie Davis Cardiovascular Surgical ICU and Clinical Nutrition, The Johns Hopkins Hospital, Baltimore, MD, USA

Michael A. DiCesare Department of Pharmacy, Hospital of the University of Pennsylvania, Philadelphia, PA, USA

Atul Dilawri Cardiothoracic Intensive Care, NewYork-Presbyterian Hospital, Columbia University Irving Medical Center, New York, NY, USA

Zachary Drabick Department of Pharmacy, University of Florida Health, Jacksonville, FL, USA

Amy L. Dzierba Department of Medicine, New York University Langone Health, New York, NY, USA

Lauren E. Eggert Division of Pulmonary, Allergy, and Critical Care Medicine, Stanford University, Palo Alto, CA, USA

Omar Elnaggar Anesthesiology, Perioperative and Pain Medicine, Stanford Hospital, Stanford, CA, USA

Annette Esper Division of Pulmonary, Allergy, Critical Care, and Sleep Medicine, Emory University School of Medicine, Atlanta, GA, USA

Alyson M. Esteves Dartmouth Hitchcock Medical Center, Lebanon, NH, USA

Hassan Farhan Anesthesiology, Perioperative and Pain Medicine, Stanford Hospital, Stanford, CA, USA

Juan M. Farina Division of Cardiothoracic Surgery, Mayo Clinic, Phoenix, AZ, USA

Nicholas Farina Michigan Medicine, Ann Arbor, MI, USA
College of Pharmacy, University of Michigan, Ann Arbor, MI, USA

Fionna Feller Division of Infectious Diseases, Vanderbilt University, Nashville, TN, USA

Fiorenza Ferrari Anestesia e Terapia Intensiva Adulti, Fondazione IRCCS Ca' Granda—Ospedale Maggiore Policlinico, Milan, Italy
International Renal research Institute of Vicenza (IRRIV), Vicenza, Italy

Jonathan Friedman Barnes Jewish Hospital, St. Louis, MO, USA

Lisa M. Gangarosa Division of Gastroenterology and Hepatology, Department of Medicine, UNC Chapel Hill School of Medicine, Chapel Hill, NC, USA

Sebastián Garcia-Zamora Coronary Care Unit, Delta Clinic, Rosario, Argentina

Ethan Garrigan Department of Anesthesiology, Duke University Medical Center, Durham, NC, USA

Jennifer A. Gass Ardent Health Services, Brentwood, TN, USA

Mohamed Abdelzaher Gebily, MD Consultant Intensivist, Director of Intensive Care Unit, Al Hada Armed Forces Hospital, Taif, Saudi Arabia
Former Director of ECMO program, KAMC, Jeddah, Saudi Arabia
Former Director of Critical Care Medicine Residency Program, KAMC, Jeddah, Saudi Arabia
Lecturer of Critical Care Medicine, Faculty of Medicine, Cairo University, Egypt

Gabrielle Gibson Barnes-Jewish Hospital Plaza, St Louis, MO, USA

Brian Gilbert Department of Pharmacy, Wesley Medical Center, Wichita, KS, USA

Neil Glassford Department of Intensive Care Medicine, Victorian Heart Hospital, Monash Health, Clayton, VIC, Australia
Department of Intensive Care Medicine, Monash Medical Centre, Monash Health, Clayton, VIC, Australia
Division of Acute and Critical Care, School of Public Health and Preventive Medicine, Monash University, Monash Health, Melbourne, VIC, Australia
School of Clinical Sciences, Monash University, Clayton, VIC, Australia

Lucas R. Goss Division of Pulmonary, Allergy, Critical Care, and Sleep Medicine, Emory University School of Medicine, Atlanta, GA, USA

Megan Grammatico Department of Internal Medicine, Yale School of Medicine, New Haven, CT, USA

Giacomo Grasselli Anestesia e Terapia Intensiva Adulti, Fondazione IRCCS Ca' Granda—Ospedale Maggiore Policlinico, Milan, Italy
Department of Pathophysiology and Transplantation, University of Milan, Milan, Italy

Traci M. Grucz Department of Pharmacy, The Johns Hopkins Hospital, Baltimore, MD, USA

Shyla Gupta Faculty of Medicine, University of Ottawa, Ottawa, ON, Canada

Kathleen M. Gura Department of Pharmacy, Division of Gastroenterology, Hepatology, and Nutrition, Boston Children's Hospital, Boston, MA, USA

Hala Halawi Houston Methodist Hospital, Houston, TX, USA

Brandy N. Hernandez Department of Pharmacy, Mayo Clinic Hospital—Rochester, Rochester, MN, USA

Lauren Kolodziej Barnes-Jewish Hospital Plaza, St Louis, MO, USA

Beth Hochman General Surgery & Critical Care Medicine, New York-Presbyterian Hospital, Columbia University Irving Medical Center, New York, NY, USA
Acute Care Surgery & Surgical Critical Care, NYU Langone Health, NYU Grossman School of Medicine, New York, NY, USA

GwangYee J. Hu Ernest Mario School of Pharmacy, Rutgers, the State University of New Jersey, Piscataway, NJ, USA
Robert Wood Johnson University Somerset, Somerville, NJ, USA

Nicole G. M. Hunfeld Department of Intensive Care Adults and Department of Hospital Pharmacy, Erasmus University Medical Center, Rotterdam, The Netherlands

Lauren A. Igneri Clinical Pharmacy Specialist, Critical Care, Department of Pharmacy, Cooper University Health Care, Camden, NJ, USA

Emaad J. Iqbal New York-Presbyterian Hospital, Columbia University Irving Medical Center, New York, NY, USA

Christine S. Ji Department of Pharmacy, Beth Israel Deaconess Medical Center, Boston, MA, USA

Heather Johnson University of Pittsburgh Medical Center, Pittsburgh, PA, USA University of Pittsburgh, Pittsburgh, PA, USA

Lesly V. Jurado Hernández Department of Pharmacy, Novant Health New Hanover Regional Medical Center, Wilmington, NC, USA

Ada Selina Jutba, PharmD, BCCCP Department of Pharmacy, Memorial Hermann Memorial City Medical Center, Houston, TX, USA

Nidhi Kataria Department of Laboratory Medicine and Pathology, Mayo Clinic, Rochester, MN, USA

Michael T. Kenes Michigan Medicine, Ann Arbor, MI, USA College of Pharmacy, University of Michigan, Ann Arbor, MI, USA

Soyoung Kristi Kim Clinical Pharmacy Specialist, Critical Care, Department of Pharmacy, Cooper University Health Care, Camden, NJ, USA

Bryan D. Kraft Division of Pulmonary, Allergy, and Critical Care Medicine, Duke University School of Medicine, Durham, NC, USA Division of Pulmonary and Critical Care Medicine, Washington University School of Medicine, Saint Louis, MO, USA

Justin Kreuter Department of Laboratory Medicine and Pathology, Mayo Clinic, Rochester, MN, USA

Caitlin E. Kulig Ernest Mario School of Pharmacy, Rutgers the State University of New Jersey, Piscataway New Jersey and St. Joseph's University Medical Center, Paterson, NJ, USA

Giovanna Landi Department of Cardio-Thoracic Surgery, Maastricht University Medical Centre (MUMNC+), Maastricht, The Netherlands

Grace Lee Los Angeles Medical Center, Kaiser Permanente, Los Angeles, CA, USA

Steven M. Lemieux Veterans Administration Connecticut Healthcare System, West Haven, CT, USA

Fanny Li Departments of Clinical Pharmacy and Pharmaceutical Services, University of California, San Francisco Health, San Francisco, CA, USA

Dusty Lisi Heart Failure, Emory Saint Joseph's Hospital, Atlanta, GA, USA

Natasha D. Lopez Department of Pharmacy, Massachusetts General Hospital, Boston, MA, USA

Uvette Lou Department of Pharmacy, Massachusetts General Hospital, Boston, MA, USA

Samantha Luk Department of Pharmacy, Massachusetts General Hospital, Boston, MA, USA

Fabio Macori Ospedale Santo Spirito Rome, Rome, RM, Italy

Kristin Madenci Brigham and Women's Hospital, Harvard Medical School, Boston, MA, USA

Ahmed A. Mahmoud Houston Methodist Hospital, Houston, TX, USA

Manu L. N. G. Malbrain First Department of Anaesthesiology and Intensive Therapy, Medical University Lublin, Lublin, Poland
Medical Data Management, Medaman, Geel, Belgium
International Fluid Academy, Lovenjoel, Belgium

Maricar Malinis Section of Infectious Diseases, Yale University School of Medicine, New Haven, CT, USA

Patrick Mazi Washington University in St. Louis, Barnes Jewish Hospital, St. Louis, MO, USA

Sharon L. McCartney Department of Anesthesiology, Pain, and Perioperative Medicine, University of Kansas, Kansas City, USA

Laura C. McNamara Department of Medicine, Beth Israel Deaconess Medical Center, Boston, MA, USA

Sachin Mehta Department of Anesthesiology, Pain, and Perioperative Medicine, University of Kansas, Kansas City, USA

Andres F. Miranda-Arboleda Brigham and Women's Hospital, Harvard Medical School, Boston, MA, USA

Alicia H. Muratore Division of Gastroenterology and Hepatology, Department of Medicine, UNC Chapel Hill School of Medicine, Chapel Hill, NC, USA

Andrea M. Nei Department of Pharmacy, Mayo Clinic Hospital—Rochester, Rochester, MN, USA

Haven Nisly Department of Medicine, Duke University School of Medicine, Durham, NC, USA

Cavan O'Kane Ernest Mario School of Pharmacy, Rutgers, the State University of New Jersey, Piscataway, NJ, USA
Penn Medicine Princeton Medical Center, Plainsboro Township, NJ, USA

Robert Olver Department of Intensive Care Medicine, Victorian Heart Hospital, Monash Health, Clayton, VIC, Australia
Department of Intensive Care Medicine, Monash Medical Centre, Monash Health, Clayton, VIC, Australia

Alejandro Narváez Orozco University of Antioquia, Medellín, Colombia

Alex Panuccio Los Angeles Medical Center, Kaiser Permanente, Los Angeles, CA, USA

Mona K. Patel Pulmonary, Critical Care & Sleep Medicine, NYU Langone Health, NYU Grossman School of Medicine, New York, USA

Tyler Peck Beth Israel Deaconess Medical Center, Harvard Medical School, Boston, MA, USA

Camille R. Petri Division of Pulmonary and Critical Care, Department of Medicine, Beth Israel Deaconess Medical Center, Harvard Medical School, Boston, MA, USA

Kayla Popova University of Michigan Health—Michigan Medicine, Ann Arbor, MI, USA

Andrew Posen Department of Pharmacy Practice, University of Illinois Chicago College of Pharmacy, Chicago, IL, USA

Leandro Luis Pozzer Section of Cardiac Electrophysiology, Buenos Aires Cardiovascular Institute, Buenos Aires, Argentina

Elias H. Pratt Division of Pulmonary Allergy, and Critical Care Medicine, Duke University School of Medicine, Durham, NC, USA

Malerie Pratt Brigham and Women's Hospital, Boston, MA, USA

Craig R. Rackley Division of Pulmonary Allergy, and Critical Care Medicine, Duke University School of Medicine, Durham, NC, USA

Lance Ray Department of Pharmacy, Denver Health Medical Center, Denver, CO, USA

Erin Reichert Department of Pharmacy, The Ohio State University, Wexner Medical Center, Columbus, OH, USA

Alyse Reichheld Department of Medicine, Beth Israel Deaconess Medical Center, Boston, MA, USA

Danilo Weir Restrepo Internal Medicine Resident, CES University, Medellín, Colombia

Adele Robbins Advanced Heart Failure and Transplant, Piedmont Hospital, Atlanta, GA, USA

Francisco Machiavello Roman Section of Infectious Diseases, Yale University School of Medicine, New Haven, CT, USA

Claudio Ronco International Renal research Institute of Vicenza (IRRIV), Vicenza, Italy

Mahmoud M. Sabawi Houston Methodist Hospital, Houston, TX, USA

Mehrnaz Sadrolashrafi Beth Israel Deaconess Medical Center, Boston, MA, USA

Ruben Santiago Department of Pharmacy, Jackson Memorial Hospital, Miami, FL, USA

Cina Sasannejad Department of Neurology, Duke University School of Medicine, Durham, NC, USA

Richard M. Schwartzstein Beth Israel Deaconess Medical Center, Harvard Medical School, Boston, MA, USA

Kristine N. Schwietz Department of Pharmacy, Massachusetts General Hospital, Boston, MA, USA

Yahya Shehabi Department of Intensive Care Medicine, Victorian Heart Hospital, Monash Health, Clayton, VIC, Australia
School of Clinical Sciences, Monash University, Clayton, VIC, Australia
Prince of Wales Clinical School of Medicine, University of New South Wales, Randwick, Sydney, NSW, Australia

Sheela V. Shenoi Yale University School of Medicine, Veterans Administration Connecticut Healthcare System, West Haven, CT, USA

Bethany R. Shoulders University of Florida College of Pharmacy, Gainesville, FL, USA

Sarah Matuszak Barnes-Jewish Hospital Plaza, St Louis, MO, USA

Chelsey Song University of Maryland Medical Center, Baltimore, MD, USA

Andrej Spec Washington University in St. Louis, Barnes Jewish Hospital, St. Louis, MO, USA

Katherine Spezzano University of Kentucky HealthCare, Lexington, KY, USA

Joanna L. Stollings Department of Pharmaceutical Services, Vanderbilt University Medical Center, Nashville, TN, USA
Critical Illness, Brain Dysfunction, and Survivorship (CIBS) Center, Vanderbilt University Medical Center, Nashville, TN, USA

David Sugrue Department of Pharmacy, UW Health, Madison, WI, USA

Lauren Sutton Barnes-Jewish Hospital Plaza, St Louis, MO, USA

Poornima Lakshmi Tamma New York-Presbyterian Hospital, Columbia University Irving Medical Center, New York, NY, USA

Erica Tavares Department of Pharmacy, Massachusetts General Hospital, Boston, MA, USA

Fernanda Tavares-Da-Silva Drug Safety, Organon BV, Brussels, Belgium

Seema S. Tekwani Division of Pulmonary, Allergy, Critical Care, and Sleep Medicine, Emory University School of Medicine, Atlanta, GA, USA

Hailey A. Thompson Department of Pharmacy, UW Health, Madison, WI, USA

Beverly Tomita Carle Illinois College of Medicine, University of Illinois, Urbana, IL, USA

Morgan Trammel Department of Pharmacy, Duke University Hospital, Durham, USA

Miguel H. Vicco Drug Safety Lead, Organon BV, Brussels, Belgium

Sybil E. Watkins Department of Internal Medicine, Vanderbilt University Medical Center, Nashville, TN, USA

Andrew J. Webb Massachusetts General Hospital, Boston, MA, USA

Dexter Wimer Departments of Clinical Pharmacy and Pharmaceutical Services, University of California, San Francisco Health, San Francisco, CA, USA

Adrian Wong Beth Israel Deaconess Medical Center, Boston, MA, USA

Nikitha Yagnala Department of Pharmacy, Hospital of University of Pennsylvania, Philadelphia, PA, USA

Giacomo Zaccherini Department of Medical and Surgical Sciences, Alma Mater Studiorum—University of Bologna, Bologna, Italy

Alberto Zanella Anestesia e Terapia Intensiva Adulti, Fondazione IRCCS Ca' Granda—Ospedale Maggiore Policlinico, Milan, Italy
Department of Pathophysiology and Transplantation, University of Milan, Milan, Italy

Part VII
Critical Care Infectious Diseases

Chapter 29
Common Infections in the Intensive Care Unit

Ahmed A. Mahmoud, Hala Halawi, Mahmoud M. Sabawi, and Max W. Adelman

29.1 Fever in the ICU

29.1.1 Background

In the 1800s, Carl Wunderlich, a German physician, defined average body temperature as 37.0 °C (98.6 °F); this temperature is commonly accepted, at least among laypeople, as "normal" [1]. Modern studies however have indicated that mean body temperature is closer to 98.0 °F and is decreasing over time, perhaps due to slower basal metabolic rates [2–5]. Further complicating accurate assessment of "normal" are physiologic diurnal temperature variation and differences between body sites [3, 6].

A fever is an elevated temperature outside of the normal range. Clinicians and patients often vigilantly monitor for fever as it may indicate pathology. There is no single definition of fever; however, a single temperature of ≥38.0 °C (100.4 °F) is a generally accepted standard [6, 7]. Despite this, the Society of Critical Care Medicine (SCCM) and Infectious Diseases Society of America (IDSA) guidelines define a fever in the ICU as a single temperature reading of ≥38.3 °C [8]. On the other hand, several temperature measurements above "normal" but below 38.0 °C may constitute a fever in certain populations [9]. Not yet mentioned, but important to note, is that fever is a symptom and not a disease in and of itself. Changing the

A. A. Mahmoud · H. Halawi · M. M. Sabawi
Houston Methodist Hospital, Houston, TX, USA

M. W. Adelman (✉)
Division of Infectious Diseases, Department of Medicine, Houston Methodist Hospital, Houston, TX, USA

Division of Pulmonary, Critical Care, and Sleep Medicine, Department of Medicine, Houston Methodist Hospital, Houston, TX, USA
e-mail: mwadelman@houstonmethodist.org

© The Author(s), under exclusive license to Springer Nature Switzerland AG 2025

Y. Alzaidi, M. A. Gebily (eds.), *The Pharmacist's Expanded Role in Critical Care Medicine*, https://doi.org/10.1007/978-3-031-77335-8_29

threshold to define "fever" will change sensitivity and specificity for fever as a tool to diagnose infection. For example, patients, especially elderly patients, may have an infection without fever, and lack of fever portends a worse prognosis [10, 11]. Interventions that expose a significant amount of blood to ambient air temperature, such as continuous renal replacement therapy and extracorporeal membrane oxygenation (ECMO), may "mask" fever, although specific data on this is limited. Similarly, anti-inflammatory medications may reduce temperature, although the effect is generally small and may be clinically insignificant [12, 13]. Inversely, patients with fever may have noninfectious causes for their elevated temperature.

Core temperature monitoring (using pulmonary artery or bladder catheters or an esophageal probe) is the gold standard for temperature detection, but these devices are rarely used [8, 14, 15]. Oral or rectal temperature is commonly monitored in practice, although these may vary by substantial amounts—as much as over 1 °C—compared to core temperature and differences are accentuated in patients with fever or hypothermia [16]. Other noninvasive temperature detection methods including tympanic infrared monitors appear to be even less accurate and should not be used [8, 17].

29.1.2 Causes of Fever in the ICU

29.1.2.1 Infections

Given the high prevalence of infections in the ICU and their significant associated morbidity and mortality [18–20], infection is commonly the first diagnostic consideration in an ICU patient with fever. Further, promptly treating severe infections with antibiotics and timely source control (if necessary) improves outcomes, and thus clinicians often first evaluate for infection before considering other potential causes of fever [21–23]. Potential causes of fever in the ICU are listed in Table 29.1.

Several common ICU interventions increase the risk for developing subsequent infections. Endotracheal intubation places patients at risk for ventilator-associated pneumonia (VAP), which occurs in 10–25% of intubated patients [24–26]. VAP diagnosis is notoriously difficult as signs and symptoms are nonspecific. However, clinicians should evaluate changes in oxygenation, character and frequency of secretions, and imaging to determine the likelihood of VAP and assess for associated complications including para-pneumonic effusions and pulmonary abscesses [27]. Vascular catheters may be a nidus for bloodstream infection; patients with indwelling central lines and fever should have peripheral blood cultures drawn to evaluate for catheter-related bloodstream infection (CRBSI) prior to antibiotic initiation [28]. While IDSA guidelines recommend semiquantitative catheter tip cultures to diagnose CRBSI when catheters are removed, in practice this is not commonly performed, and CRBSI diagnosis relies on ruling out other potential sources of bloodstream infection [28]. Other indwelling devices, including external ventricular drains, urinary catheters, nasogastric tubes (NGT), and even peripheral

Table 29.1 Potential causes of fever in the critically ill patient

Infections	Noninfectious syndromes
Associated with indwelling devices	*Potentially life-threatening*
Ventilator-associated pneumonia	Pulmonary embolism
Central line-related bloodstream infection	Myocardial infarction
Healthcare-associated meningitis/ventriculitis	Aspiration
Urinary tract infection	Pancreatitis
Sinusitis	Acute hemolytic transfusion reaction
	Adrenal insufficiency
	Hypo- or hyperthyroidism
	Cytokine storm
	Differentiation syndrome
	Intracranial hemorrhage
	Alcohol or benzodiazepine withdrawal
Not associated with indwelling devices	*Less likely to be life-threatening*
Clostridioides difficile infection	Postoperative inflammation
Postoperative infections	Deep venous thrombosis
Wound infection	Drug fever
Acalculous cholecystitis	Intramuscular hematoma
	Atelectasis
	Gout
	Cancer
	Mesenteric ischemia

intravenous catheters, may be a source for infection; management of fever should include evaluation of these sites (or sinuses in the case of prolonged NGT insertion), with potential device removal depending on the specific clinical situation [29–31].

In addition to indwelling devices, several other ICU-related interventions place patients at risk of infection. Postoperative surgical site infections are common and occur in over 10% of patients with gastrointestinal resections [32]. Although post-surgical fever due to inflammation is common, if the fever persists or occurs in a critically ill patient, cross-sectional imaging of the surgical site should be performed to determine the need for source control [8]. Antibiotics are administered to approximately 70% of ICU patients on any given day and are the most salient risk factor for *Clostridioides difficile* infection (CDI), the most common healthcare-associated infection [20, 33]. Patients with new-onset diarrhea in the ICU and without recent exposure to laxatives should be tested for CDI, regardless of antibiotic exposure [34]. Patients with prolonged critical illness are at risk for decubitus ulcers or other wounds that may become infected. Evaluation should include a careful clinical exam to assess for local signs of a skin and soft tissue infection, which may range from cellulitis to abscess and necrotizing fasciitis. Acalculous cholecystitis is associated with multiple conditions common in the ICU, including hypotension and total parenteral nutrition, that predispose to gallbladder hypokinesis and ischemia [35]. While acalculous cholecystitis may not be initiated by infection, secondary infection commonly occurs, and distinguishing infection from noninfection is difficult. This diagnosis should be considered in an ICU patient with fever and right upper quadrant abdominal pain or abnormalities in liver function testing [8].

29.1.2.2 Noninfectious Causes of Fever

Between 26% and 88% of ICU patients develop fever at some point during their ICU admission, and up to half of these febrile episodes are due to noninfectious causes [36, 37]. Ultimately, attributing a fever to a noninfectious cause requires that common infections are ruled out as noninfectious syndromes may occur concurrently with infections. Generally, the degree and pattern of fever are not helpful in narrowing the differential diagnosis [38].

While rare, several syndromes may cause fever and severe illness, including shock. Pulmonary embolism and myocardial infarction may occasionally present with fever; however, these pathologies are usually evident based on other findings [39–41]. Deep venous thromboses can cause fever [42], and some clinicians routinely perform upper and lower extremity venous Doppler for patients without an obvious cause of their fever. Adrenal crisis, acute hemolytic transfusion reaction, and severe hyper- or hypothyroidism may cause fever and should also be considered in the differential diagnosis of septic shock [43, 44]. Patients who have received chimeric antigen receptor (CAR) T-cell therapy may develop cytokine release syndrome; several other noninfectious diseases (including autoimmune and genetic disorders), as well as treatment for some hematologic malignancies, may cause a similar "cytokine storm" characterized by fever and possible progression to shock and multiorgan failure [45, 46].

While each of these syndromes can cause a wide spectrum of diseases, several noninfectious causes of fever do not generally cause severe illness. For example, while neuroleptic malignant syndrome and serotonin syndrome (resultant from exposure to antipsychotics and serotonergic agents, respectively) may cause significant hyperthermia and altered mental status, drug fever typically presents with few symptoms aside from fever and is difficult to diagnose. While drug fever usually occurs within days of starting an offending medication, presentation may be delayed in some cases [47]. Laboratory clues including abnormal liver enzymes and peripheral eosinophilia are variably present [48], and exam may or may not reveal a rash. Diagnosis of drug fever involves ruling out other causes of fever and temporal improvement of fever after discontinuation of the suspected offending agent. Commonly associated medications include antibiotics (especially beta-lactams) and anti-epileptics, but other drugs frequently used in the ICU, including heparin, may be implicated [49, 50].

In the neurologic ICU, fever is frequently due to subarachnoid hemorrhage or other central nervous system insults, including other intracranial hemorrhage subtypes [51, 52]. Hematomas at other sites, such as intramuscular, can also cause fever [53]. Similarly, fever can occur with ischemia or noninfectious inflammation of nearly any organ, including mesenteric ischemia and pancreatitis [8]. Cancer can cause fever, although patients with malignancy are additionally at high risk for infection and adverse outcomes if infection is not treated promptly [54, 55].

29.1.3 *Evaluation and Management*

Evaluation should focus on clues in the patient's history as well as signs and symptoms that allow the clinician to determine a likely source of fever, with subsequent diagnostic testing directed at the likely cause of fever. Most patients in the ICU should have at least a chest X-ray and blood cultures (two sets from different anatomic sites), with additional workup depending on specific diagnostic clues and suspected site of infection or noninfectious cause of fever [8]. Given the wide differential diagnosis for fever in the ICU, the list of potential diagnostic tests is long, and tempo of evaluation will depend on the severity of illness and diagnostic certainty. For example, a critically ill patient with fever and suspected septic shock without obvious source may require urgent cross-sectional imaging of the chest, abdomen, and pelvis. Other patients with isolated fever may not require extensive urgent evaluation.

Patients may rarely have prolonged fever without a clear diagnosis. These patients are a particular challenge. The SCCM/IDSA guidelines make a weak recommendation for performing positron emission tomography/computed tomography (PET/CT) in ICU patients with cryptic fever [8]. Limited data suggests that PET/CT may be sensitive in identifying a diagnosis [56, 57]; however, cost, availability, and need to transport a critically ill patient for a long diagnostic test may limit use. The guidelines recommend against white blood cell scans or routine abdominal ultrasounds [8]. Unfortunately, biomarkers including procalcitonin, white blood cell count, and C-reactive protein are not sufficiently sensitive or specific to rule in or out infection in critically ill patients with fever, but normal results of these tests may decrease the probability of infection when clinical suspicion is already low [8]. Several studies have evaluated the use of procalcitonin, for example, in other syndromes (such as sepsis and lower respiratory tract infection) with conflicting results [58–60].

Management is directed at the causative etiology of fever. Before a definitive cause for fever is determined, clinicians will often need to decide whether empiric antibiotics are indicated to treat potential infection. We discuss the role of empiric antibiotics further in the "Sepsis" section; however in general, the need for empiric antibiotics is based on the acuity of illness and likelihood of infection [61]. Empiric antibiotics are rarely required for isolated fever in an otherwise stable patient without an established diagnosis of infection; prescribing antibiotics in these settings may confound diagnosis and lead to adverse side effects, including CDI. Anti-inflammatories including acetaminophen and nonsteroidal anti-inflammatory medications may lead to minimal temperature reduction but do not improve other outcomes [12]. They are not routinely recommended but can be used for symptomatic treatment [8].

29.2 Sepsis

29.2.1 Background

Sepsis is a syndrome defined by life-threatening organ dysfunction caused by a dysregulated host response to infection [62]. Sepsis is a major contributor to morbidity and mortality worldwide: It is present in approximately 6% of adult hospitalizations and is associated with approximately 7% of all deaths in the United States and up to 20% of deaths worldwide [63–65]. Specific to the ICU, nearly one in five ICU admissions is due to sepsis, and an additional one in ten patients will develop sepsis during their ICU admission [66].

29.2.2 Diagnosis

Sepsis diagnosis is challenging as there is no gold standard for diagnosis, and signs and symptoms overlap significantly with several causes of noninfectious critical illness [67, 68]. Often, a definitive diagnosis of sepsis is made only retrospectively after ruling out other potential causes of clinical deterioration. Sepsis may manifest as nonspecific signs and symptoms (including fever, hypothermia, tachycardia, tachypnea, hypotension, hypoxia, and altered mental status) and organ dysfunction (including heart failure, shock liver, acute kidney injury, delirium, acute lung injury, and disseminated intravascular coagulation) [10, 62, 69].

Given the high morbidity and mortality associated with sepsis and the difficulty in diagnosis, it is both important and difficult to properly screen patients with potential sepsis. Available screening tools include the systemic inflammatory response syndrome (SIRS) criteria, sequential organ failure (SOFA) and quick sequential organ failure (qSOFA) scores, national early warning score (NEWS), and modified early warning score (MEWS) [61, 62, 70, 71]. The Surviving Sepsis Campaign (SSC) 2021 guidelines recommend against using qSOFA as a single screening tool for sepsis compared with SIRS, NEWS, or MEWS [61]. Several large retrospective studies of non-ICU patients have shown that NEWS and MEWS outperform qSOFA and SIRS in predicting in-hospital mortality and ICU transfer [72, 73]. Unfortunately, each of these tools may miss an unacceptably high proportion of patients with sepsis, and ultimately clinical judgment is required to make a presumptive diagnosis of sepsis [11, 74].

Several commonly assayed biomarkers are associated with sepsis but also lack specificity and sensitivity for diagnosis. For example, WBC count is frequently relied on as a potential signal of infection; however, its sensitivity may be as low as 50% [75]. Elevated CRP may be sensitive for sepsis but is also elevated in several noninfectious sepsis mimics [76, 77]. Similarly, procalcitonin may be up to 80% sensitive depending on the specific clinical scenario; however, there is significant heterogeneity including in immunocompromised and critically ill patients [78, 79].

Based on procalcitonin's variable sensitivity, the SSC guidelines recommend against using procalcitonin for antimicrobial initiation [61]. Several gene expression-based biomarkers are in clinical development, but none is currently ready for routine clinical use [80, 81]. Ultimately, presumptive diagnosis of sepsis requires careful integration of factors from the patient's history, combined with objective markers including laboratory testing and imaging. Critically, the diagnosis must be continuously evaluated, as a large proportion of patients admitted to the ICU with a diagnosis of sepsis are ultimately found to have noninfectious illness [82].

29.2.3 Management

Management is largely dictated by the likelihood of sepsis and degree of illness (Table 29.2). In situations where sepsis is likely, or where sepsis is possible and the patient has shock (hypotension with end-organ dysfunction), then early administration of empiric antibiotics is critical [61]. A landmark 2006 study demonstrated that survival decreases by 8% for every hour antibiotics are delayed in septic shock [21]. Since then, several studies have found similar results. A retrospective study of sepsis and septic shock patients in nearly 150 New York hospitals found that patients who received antibiotics 3–12 h after ED arrival had a 14% increased mortality compared to patients who received antibiotics less than 3 h from ED arrival [83]. Another retrospective study of sepsis patients across 21 Northern California EDs found a hospital mortality ratio of 1.09/h from ED presentation to antibiotic administration [84]. Importantly, the benefit from early antibiotics seems to be largely driven by patients with septic shock (and not sepsis alone) [22, 55, 85], which prompted the SSC's recommendation for expedited workup (and not immediate antibiotic administration) in patients with low likelihood of sepsis and shock absent [61]. Other patient groups, including patients with malignancy, may benefit from early antibiotics [55].

In addition to antibiotics, a prompt search for a source of sepsis is key, as delays in source control procedures are also associated with increased mortality [23]. This benefit is most pronounced in patients with gastrointestinal or skin and soft tissue infections requiring source control (e.g., perforated diverticulitis or necrotizing fasciitis, respectively) [23]. A diagnostic workup for potential sources of infection will depend on presenting signs and symptoms but will commonly include cross-sectional

Table 29.2 Antibiotic timing in suspected sepsis (adapted from Ref. [61])

	Shock present?		
		Yes	No
Likelihood of sepsis	Medium to high	Give antibiotics within 1 h	Give antibiotics within 1 h
	Low	Give antibiotics within 1 h	Expedited workup and continued clinical monitoring. Give antibiotics within 3 h if concern for sepsis persists

imaging if the initial source is not immediately clear or if required for operative planning. In addition to antibiotics, patients may benefit from fluids; a nuanced discussion of fluid administration in sepsis is outside the scope of this chapter.

After deciding to treat for sepsis, empiric antibiotics should be initiated promptly after drawing blood cultures. Empiric antibiotics are chosen to target likely pathogens before causative organisms are identified and are selected based on risk factors, patient history, and likely source of infection. The SSC 2021 guidelines recommend using empiric antimicrobials with methicillin-resistant *Staphylococcus aureus* (MRSA) coverage for sepsis patients at high risk of MRSA infections. Risk factors for MRSA include prior MRSA infection or colonization, recent IV antibiotics, recurrent skin infections or chronic wounds, presence of invasive devices, hemodialysis, recent hospital admission, and higher severity of illness [61].

Nearly all patients will additionally require empiric coverage that targets gram-negative organisms, for example with a third- or fourth-generation cephalosporin (e.g., ceftriaxone or cefepime, respectively) or a beta-lactam/beta-lactamase inhibitor combination (e.g., ampicillin/sulbactam or piperacillin/tazobactam). Most patients can be treated with a single agent (i.e., monotherapy) for gram-negative coverage, but certain factors may warrant dual gram-negative therapy to target resistant organisms, as adding an additional agent increases the likelihood of covering a resistant pathogen [61]. Patients who may benefit from dual coverage include those with recent healthcare-associated infections, antibiotic-resistant infections, or intravenous antibiotic use and patients with recent travel abroad, especially if they required hospitalization abroad, as several countries are endemic for highly resistant gram-negative pathogens [61, 86]. Similarly, patients with risk factors for extended-spectrum beta-lactamase (ESBL) and carbapenem-resistant Enterobacterales (CRE) may benefit from empiric treatment that targets these pathogens, for example carbapenems (in the case of ESBL) and novel beta-lactam/beta-lactamase inhibitor combinations such as ceftazidime/avibactam (in the case of CRE pathogens). Risk factors for ESBL/CRE infections include chronic kidney disease, previous colonization/infection with ESBL/CRE pathogens, urinary catheters, immunosuppression, and broad-spectrum antibiotic exposure [87–90]. The appropriate use of these agents in sepsis is not clearly defined, and several factors must be taken into account when deciding appropriate therapy, as both overly narrow and overly broad empiric therapy are associated with adverse patient outcomes [91]. Hopefully, future studies on rapid pathogen prediction or detection will allow for strategies to quickly select appropriate antibiotics to target causative microorganisms. For now, clinical judgment is often used, and antibiotics should be adjusted as appropriate based on culture results (once available) and the patient's clinical progression. Table 29.3 summarizes empiric antibiotic options in sepsis based on the site and type of infection; however, patient-specific factors should also be used to guide therapy [92].

Table 29.3 Potential empiric antibiotic choices based on suspected site of infection in septic patients. Society guidelines for specific infections are provided in the table as references

Site	Type	Common pathogens	Empiric
Pulmonary	Severe community-acquired pneumonia [93]	*Streptococcus pneumoniae, Haemophilus influenzae, Mycoplasma pneumoniae, Staphylococcus aureus, Legionella, Chlamydia pneumoniae, Moraxella catarrhalis, Pseudomonas aeruginosa*	Ceftriaxone, piperacillin-tazobactam, cefepime, ceftazidime, imipenem, meropenem, or aztreonam + azithromycin, clarithromycin, levofloxacin, or moxifloxacin + vancomycin or linezolid
	Healthcare-associated or ventilator-associated pneumonia [27]	GNRs including *Pseudomonas* and Enterobacterales, *Staphylococcus aureus*	Piperacillin-tazobactam, cefepime, ceftazidime, imipenem, meropenem, aztreonam, ciprofloxacin, levofloxacin, colistin, or polymyxin B + vancomycin or linezolid
Central nervous system	Healthcare-associated ventriculitis/meningitis [29]	*Staphylococcus aureus, Propionibacterium acnes, Streptococcus pneumoniae, Pseudomonas aeruginosa, Haemophilus influenzae,* Enterobacterales, *Acinetobacter baumannii*	Cefepime or meropenem + vancomycin, daptomycin, or linezolid
Skin and soft tissue	Necrotizing fasciitis [94]	*Staphylococcus, Streptococcus, Clostridium,* Enterobacterales	Piperacillin-tazobactam + vancomycin + clindamycin
	Severe non-purulent cellulitis [94]	*Staphylococcus, Streptococcus, Clostridium,* Enterobacterales	Piperacillin-tazobactam + vancomycin
	Severe purulent abscess [94]	*Staphylococcus aureus, Streptococcus*	Vancomycin, daptomycin, linezolid, or ceftaroline
	Moderate-severe diabetic foot infection [95]	GNRs including *Pseudomonas,* anaerobes, and *Staphylococcus aureus*	Piperacillin-tazobactam, meropenem, imipenem, or ceftazidime/cefepime/ciprofloxacin with metronidazole + vancomycin, linezolid, daptomycin, SMX-TMP, or doxycycline

(continued)

Table 29.3 (continued)

Site	Type	Common pathogens	Empiric
Intra-abdominal [96]	Severe extra-biliary community acquired	GNRs including *Pseudomonas*, anaerobes	Imipenem, meropenem, piperacillin-tazobactam, or ciprofloxacin/levofloxacin/ cefepime with metronidazole
	Severe acute community-acquired cholecystitis	GNRs including *Pseudomonas*, anaerobes	Imipenem, meropenem, piperacillin-tazobactam, or ciprofloxacin/levofloxacin/ cefepime with metronidazole
	Acute cholangitis	GNRs including *Pseudomonas*, anaerobes	Imipenem, meropenem, piperacillin-tazobactam, or ciprofloxacin/levofloxacin/ cefepime with metronidazole
	Healthcare-associated biliary	GNRs including *Pseudomonas*, anaerobes, *Staphylococcus aureus*, *Enterococcus*	Imipenem, meropenem, piperacillin-tazobactam, or ciprofloxacin/levofloxacin/ cefepime with metronidazole + vancomycin
Genitourinary	Acute pyelonephritis [97]	GNRs including Enterobacterales	Ceftriaxone or ciprofloxacin

GNR gram-negative rod, *SMX-TMP* sulfamethoxazole-trimethoprim

Although sepsis is commonly assumed to be caused by bacteria, a large proportion of cases may be caused by other pathogens including viruses and fungi. While there are generally no specific antiviral therapies empirically for sepsis, some patients may warrant empiric therapy against fungi, especially yeasts such as *Candida* spp. There have been several studies evaluating empiric anti-*Candida* treatment in ICU patients, which have shown mixed results [98, 99]. Decisions regarding empiric anti-*Candida* therapy are made on a case-by-case basis considering patient-specific risk factors. The SSC guidelines recommend basing the initiation of empiric antifungal therapy on risk factors such as those listed in Table 29.4 [61].

In sepsis, the method of administration of antimicrobials, particularly beta-lactams, is important. Beta-lactams exhibit increased bacterial killing by prolonging the time of drug above the bacterial minimum inhibitory concentration (MIC) [100]. A systematic review and meta-analysis on the effects of prolonged IV infusion of beta-lactam antibiotics compared to intermittent infusion in sepsis patients found that prolonged infusion was associated with lower 30-day all-cause mortality, hospital mortality, and ICU mortality and higher clinical cure [101]. Other pharmacokinetic (PK) and pharmacodynamic (PD) considerations should be made in the setting of sepsis [102]. Antibiotic administration via the intravenous route is preferred over enteral/oral route because blood is shunted away from the

Table 29.4 Risk factors/markers for fungal infections

Risk factors/markers for *Candida* infections
Candida colonization
Elevated serum beta-D-glucan assay
Neutropenia
Immunosuppression
Severity of illness
Longer intensive care unit length of stay
Central venous catheters and intravascular devices
IV drug use
Total parenteral nutrition
Broad-spectrum antibiotics
Gastrointestinal tract perforation
Emergency gastrointestinal or hepatobiliary surgery
Acute renal failure and hemodialysis
Severe thermal injury
Prior surgery
Risk factors/markers for endemic fungi (*Cryptococcus, Histoplasma, Blastomyces, Coccidioides*)
Antigen markers
Human immunodeficiency virus infection
Solid-organ transplant
High-dose corticosteroid therapy
Hematopoietic stem cell transplant
Diabetes mellitus
Risk factors/markers for invasive mold infections
Neutropenia
Serum/bronchial galactomannan assay
Solid-organ transplant
Hematopoietic stem cell transplant
High-dose corticosteroid therapy

gastrointestinal tract in septic shock [103]. Fluid resuscitation and the phenomenon of third spacing lead to greater volumes of distribution (V_d) for many antibiotics including beta-lactams, glycopeptides, and lipopeptides. Acute kidney injury secondary to shock leads to reduced clearance of renally eliminated antibiotics. The combination of higher V_d and lower clearance may require higher loading doses, but longer intervals between doses. Conversely, some patients have augmented renal function increasing drug clearance and increasing the risk of underdosing antibiotics [104]. In addition, many septic shock patients may undergo continuous renal replacement therapy, which may require dosing based on dialysate flow rate for many antibiotics [102].

29.3 Catheter-Related Bloodstream Infections

29.3.1 *Background*

Placement of central venous catheters (CVCs) is a common practice in hospitalized patients [105]. Indications for central venous access include need for parental nutrition, vasopressors, or chemotherapy; inability to place a peripheral venous catheter; and need for access for renal replacement therapy; each of these interventions and medications are common in the ICU. The most common sites for CVC placement are the femoral, internal jugular, and subclavian veins [106]. A major complication of CVC placement is catheter-related bloodstream infection (CRBSI). Despite significant reduction in CRBSI incidence, approximately 30,000 cases still occur in US hospitals annually, and these infections are associated with increased hospital costs and length of stay [107, 108].

29.3.2 *CRBSI Definition and Diagnosis*

CRBSI refers to bacteremia or fungemia in a patient who has an intravascular device and >1 positive blood culture obtained from a peripheral vein, clinical manifestations of infection, and no apparent source of bloodstream infection except for the catheter [28]. Intravascular devices include peripheral venous and arterial catheters, midline catheters, pulmonary arterial catheters, peripherally inserted central catheters, short- and long-term CVCs, and totally implantable devices. To diagnose infection, at least one of the following should be present [28]:

- Positive semiquantitative (>15 colony-forming units [CFUs] per catheter segment) or quantitative (>10^2 CFUs per catheter segment) catheter culture where the same organism is isolated from the catheter segment and a peripheral blood culture.
- Simultaneous quantitative cultures of blood with a ratio of greater than 3 to 1 CFU/mL of blood (catheter versus peripheral blood).
- Differential time to positivity (growth in a culture of blood obtained through catheter hub is detected by an automated blood culture system at least 2 h earlier than a culture of simultaneously drawn peripheral blood of equal volume).

Given the difficulty of the above diagnostic techniques, a clinical diagnosis of CRBSI is often made in patients with catheters after other sources of infection have been excluded [109]. Local signs and symptoms of infection, such as erythema, pain, and purulence at the catheter exit site, are possible but uncommonly reported [110].

29.3.3 CRBSI Risk Factors and Pathogenesis

The types of drugs administered through the catheter may increase the risk for CRBSI. For example, chemotherapy and total parenteral nutrition (TPN) have been identified as risk factors [111, 112]. The patient's immune status is important in relation to CRBSI; immunosuppression and hematopoietic stem cell transplantation (HSCT) are key risk factors [111, 113]. Aside from patient-specific factors, several factors related to the CVC itself affect the risk of infection. For example, longer implantation times are associated with higher risk [114]. Subclavian CVCs are associated with lower risk for infection than internal jugular or femoral CVCs, while internal jugular and femoral CVCs carry similar risk [115]. Non-tunneled catheters are associated with two to three times the risk for infection compared to tunneled catheters, and increasing number of lumens also increases CRBSI risk [111, 116].

Although gram-positive pathogens including *Staphylococcus aureus* and *Enterococcus* spp. are important CLABSI pathogens, *Candida* spp. are the most common cause of CRBSI in the ICU and are implicated in 27% of ICU-related CRBSIs [117]. Enterococci (17%), Enterobacterales (such as *E. coli* and *Klebsiella* spp., 16%), coagulase-negative staphylococci (14%), and *S. aureus* (9%) were the next most common causes in a National Healthcare Safety Report of CRBSIs from 2011 to 2017 [117]. Outside of the ICU, Enterobacterales and *S. aureus* were the most important pathogens. Importantly, *Candida* was the only organism type that increased in incidence over the study duration [117].

There are several potential mechanisms of CRBSI [118]. Most infections are assumed to occur with direct contamination of the catheter during insertion or with buildup of pathogenic microorganisms under sterile dressings over time. Several steps, including procedural checklists and routine skin preparation with chlorhexidine prior to catheter insertion, have been shown to decrease risk of CRBSI [119, 120]. Alternatively, catheters can become contaminated during manipulation of the catheter hub during medication infusion, leading to biofilm formation and eventual dissemination of organisms in the bloodstream [118]. Other mechanisms, including contamination of the infused medication and dissemination from a separate primary site, are less likely [118].

29.3.4 Management

If CRBSI is suspected, it is generally recommended to remove the catheter after drawing blood cultures, although urgency of catheter removal depends on several factors including the patient's clinical status and likelihood of CRBSI [28]. Initial empiric therapy for suspected CRBSIs should include empiric coverage for MRSA and gram-negative bacilli, generally an antipseudomonal beta-lactam such as cefepime or piperacillin-tazobactam [28, 121]. Empiric coverage for candidemia can be considered in patients with TPN, prolonged use of broad-spectrum antibiotics, hematologic malignancy, HSCT or SOT, femoral catheterization, or *Candida* colonization [28].

Specific recommendations for management and duration of therapy for CRBSIs depend on the pathogen isolated, and we have summarized these recommendations in Table 29.5. Coagulase-negative staphylococci (CoNS) uncomplicated CRBSIs (i.e., without associated metastatic infection or shock) are typically treated for 5–7 days after catheter removal; if the catheter is not removed, treatment is 10–14 days of systemic antibiotic therapy and antibiotic lock therapy. *S. lugdunensis* is a virulent CoNS species and should be managed like *S. aureus* [28].

Table 29.5 Antimicrobial treatment for catheter-related bloodstream infection depending on causative organism

Pathogen	Antimicrobial	Duration of therapy
Coagulase-negative staphylococci excluding *Staphylococcus lugdunensis*	Methicillin-resistant: vancomycin dose to target AUC over MIC >400 mg h/L or daptomycin 6–10 mg/kg IV daily Methicillin susceptible: cefazolin 2 g IV q8h, 2 g IV q4h, or oxacillin 2 g IV q4h	5–7 days if catheter removed 10–14 days if catheter retained along with antibiotic lock therapy
Staphylococcus aureus and *lugdunensis*	Methicillin resistant: vancomycin dose to target AUC over MIC >400 mg h/L or daptomycin 8–10 mg/kg IV daily Methicillin susceptible: cefazolin 2 g IV q8h, 2 g IV q4h, oxacillin 2 g IV q4h	14 days in uncomplicated infections 4–6 weeks in complicated infections
Enterococcus	Ampicillin susceptible: ampicillin 2 g IV q4h ± ceftriaxone 2 g IV q12h Ampicillin resistant, vancomycin susceptible: vancomycin dose to target AUC over MIC >400 mg h/L VRE: daptomycin 10 mg/kg IV q24h or linezolid 600 mg IV q12h	7–14 days in uncomplicated infections 4–6 weeks in complicated infections
Gram-negative bacilli	Cefepime 2 g IV q8h, ertapenem 1 g IV q24h, or meropenem 1 g IV q8h Narrow/targeting based on antibiotic susceptibilities and patient-specific factors	7–10 days after catheter removal
Candida	Anidulafungin 200 mg followed by 100 mg IV daily, caspofungin 70 mg followed by 50 mg daily, or micafungin 100 mg IV daily Fluconazole step-down oral therapy in selected patients	14 days for uncomplicated infection 4–6 weeks for complicated infection

VRE vancomycin-resistant *Enterococcus*

S. aureus infections typically require catheter removal followed by a 4–6-week course of treatment, although a 14-day course may be considered in patients with uncomplicated infection. For *S. aureus*, uncomplicated infections are defined as occurring in patients without diabetes, immunocompromise, prosthetic intravascular devices, endocarditis, thrombophlebitis, or metastatic infection, and fever and bacteremia must resolve promptly [28, 122]. It is recommended to obtain echocardiography at least 5–7 days after the onset of bacteremia to increase sensitivity in detecting valvular vegetations [28]. Vancomycin is the standard treatment for methicillin-resistant *S. aureus* (MRSA), and other options include linezolid and daptomycin [122, 123]. In a randomized controlled trial of linezolid compared to vancomycin, linezolid and vancomycin had similar microbiological success rates for treating MRSA BSIs [124]. In a systematic review of daptomycin compared to vancomycin for the treatment of MRSA BSI with or without endocarditis, daptomycin was associated with reduced risk of clinical failure and fewer treatment-limiting adverse effects, but no difference in mortality [125]. In another systematic review comparing daptomycin with vancomycin for MRSA BSIs with a vancomycin MIC greater than 1 mcg/mL, daptomycin was associated with lower mortality and higher treatment success [126]. However, vancomycin remains the standard treatment for MRSA due to clinical experience with this agent and concerns regarding heterogeneity and retrospective nature of the studies included in the mentioned meta-analyses: In a global survey, 53–97% of respondents use vancomycin as first-line therapy depending on the continent [123]. For methicillin-susceptible *S. aureus* (MSSA), anti-staphylococcal beta-lactams such as oxacillin, nafcillin, and cefazolin are first line, with patient-specific factors dictating antibiotic choice [127]. A retrospective multicenter study comparing beta-lactam to vancomycin therapy for MSSA BSIs found that definitive beta-lactam therapy was associated with a lower mortality compared to vancomycin [128].

It is recommended to remove short-term CVCs for CRBSI due to *Enterococcus*. Removal of long-term CVCs in enterococcal CRBSIs is recommended in the cases of insertion/pocket site infection, thrombophlebitis, sepsis, endocarditis, persistent bacteremia, or metastatic infection [28]. TEE is recommended for enterococcal CRBSIs in the presence of signs and symptoms of endocarditis, persistent bacteremia, or prosthetic valves [28]. Ampicillin is the drug of choice for ampicillin-susceptible *Enterococcus* species. Vancomycin is typically chosen for ampicillin-resistant, vancomycin-susceptible enterococci, while vancomycin-resistant enterococci (VRE) are treated with daptomycin or linezolid [28]. A retrospective study evaluating different doses of daptomycin (6, 8, 10 mg/kg) for enterococcal bacteremia found that 10 mg/kg was associated with a survival benefit and improved microbiological clearance [129]. A multicenter, prospective cohort study evaluating daptomycin versus linezolid for enterococcal bacteremia found high-dose daptomycin (≥9 mg/kg) and linezolid associated with a survival benefit compared to lower dose daptomycin (6–9 mg/kg). High-dose daptomycin and linezolid had similar survival benefits [130]. The duration of therapy is typically 7–14 days in uncomplicated infections and 4–6 weeks in complicated infections [28].

Removal of the catheter in gram-negative CRBSIs is associated with reduced relapse and mortality [131, 132]. After catheter removal, a 7–10-day course of therapy results in similar rates of clinical success, relapse, and mortality compared to longer courses [133]. Empiric therapy should target MDR gram-negative pathogens [121]. In a multicenter, randomized controlled trial, meropenem was associated with less microbiological failure compared to piperacillin-tazobactam for BSIs caused by AmpC-producing pathogens, and meropenem should also be used for ESBL-E CRBSIs [134, 135].

Candida CRBSIs also require catheter removal as catheter retention is associated with worse outcomes in multiple studies [28]. Empiric therapy with an echinocandin (anidulafungin, caspofungin, or micafungin) is recommended as initial therapy [136]. ICU patients with concern for CRBSI may be a particularly important group to treat empirically with antifungals as there is a high rate of *Candida* CRBSI in this population, although data on empiric antifungals are conflicting [98, 117]. Fluconazole can be considered in non-critically ill patients who are unlikely to have a fluconazole-resistant *Candida* species. Liposomal amphotericin B is an alternative to echinocandins and azoles in the setting of intolerance or resistance to those agents. Two weeks of therapy after blood culture clearance is recommended for uncomplicated infections, whereas longer courses (4–6 weeks) are recommended in cases of metastatic infection, osteomyelitis, endocarditis, or endophthalmitis [136].

29.4   Pneumonia

29.4.1   Background

Pneumonia, an infection of the pulmonary parenchyma, is the leading cause of hospitalization in the United States, one of the leading causes of deaths worldwide, and a common cause of sepsis and septic shock [65, 137]. There are a wide variety of pathogens that can cause pneumonia, and subtyping pneumonia can assist with workup and treatment aimed at the most likely pathogens. The ATS/IDSA guidelines stratify pneumonia into three subtypes depending on patient characteristics and location of acquisition: community-acquired pneumonia (CAP), hospital-acquired pneumonia (HAP), and ventilator-associated pneumonia (VAP) [27, 93]. For pneumonia to develop, generally the infecting pathogen must initially colonize the pharynx. The pathogen then reaches the lower respiratory tract via microaspiration and evades mechanical innate host defenses including mucociliary clearance and cough. This allows virulent microorganisms to reach the lung parenchyma, overcoming host defenses by high inoculum and virulence, resulting in clinical pneumonia. Other microorganisms are aerosolized and inhaled directly into the lungs [138]. In the case of HAP/VAP, additional factors such as gastric acid suppression, paralytic medications, and endotracheal intubation increase the risk of pneumonia [26, 139].

29.4.2   Community-Acquired Pneumonia

29.4.2.1   Overview

CAP is pneumonia acquired outside of the hospital and may commonly be treated in the outpatient setting. Despite this, CAP places a significant burden on the healthcare system. For example, there are as many as 35 CAP-related admissions per 1000 elderly patients annually [140]. Mortality from CAP ranges from 10% among hospitalized patients not requiring ICU-level care to 36% for patients admitted to the ICU [141]. In most cases, a causative microorganism is not identified, but in cases where a microorganism is detected, viral pathogens (including COVID-19, respiratory syncytial virus, and influenza) and *Streptococcus pneumoniae* are most common [142, 143]. Other bacterial pathogens such as *Haemophilus influenzae* and *Staphylococcus aureus*, as well as "atypical" organisms including *Moraxella catarrhalis* and *Legionella* species, are potential pathogens [93, 144].

CAP can be divided into two categories based on severity: mild/moderate CAP and severe CAP. Depending on the severity, mild/moderate CAP may be treated either in the outpatient or inpatient setting outside of an ICU [145, 146]. Severe CAP generally necessitates ICU admission and is defined by ATS/IDSA as having one major criterion (septic shock or mechanical ventilation) or three minor criteria (tachypnea, multi-lobar infiltrates, encephalopathy, uremia, leukopenia, thrombocytopenia, hypothermia, or hypotension) [93].

29.4.2.2   Diagnosis

A detailed and thorough clinical evaluation is crucial to diagnose pneumonia and assess for potential causative microorganisms. Several other syndromes including heart failure, pulmonary embolism, aspiration, etc. are commonly misdiagnosed as pneumonia, and no single test is sufficiently sensitive or specific to definitively diagnose pneumonia [147]. Patient history should include symptom onset, clinical setting, defects in host defenses, and exposures to specific pathogens [148, 149]. Specifically, patients with congestive heart failure, diabetes mellitus, alcohol use disorder, and chronic obstructive pulmonary disease are at an increased risk for pneumonia [142]. Imaging (chest radiography) combined with characteristic symptoms remains the gold standard in clinical diagnosis, and imaging can determine the extent of disease and presence of complications. Limitations to chest radiography include variable sensitivity (49–90%) and a low positive predictive value (16–42%) as there are several pneumonia mimics [150]. Chest computed tomography is more specific than chest X-ray and may aid in the detection of associated complications such as empyema and pulmonary abscess [151]. Lung ultrasound is a safe and rapid bedside examination with excellent sensitivity for pneumonia; however, limited experience with this modality has limited its uptake [152].

Sampling of the respiratory tract allows for several microbiologic tests to potentially identify a causative pathogen. The ATS/IDSA guidelines recommend sputum gram stain and culture for moderate-to-severe CAP; however, a recent meta-analysis demonstrated variable sensitivity (59–78%) and specificity (87–99%) of gram stain depending on the organism [93, 153]. For example, rates of false-negative gram stains were as high as 40% for *S. pneumoniae* [153]. For severely ill intubated patients, lower respiratory tract samples (for example, via bronchoscopy or mini-bronchoalveolar lavage) should be collected as the yield is superior to that of sputum culture [93]. Newer tests such as multiplex polymerase chain reaction (mPCR) may be more sensitive than culture and have a faster turnaround time to microorganism identification [154, 155]. While these tests may not be routinely available outside of high-income countries, they should likely be used in patients with severe CAP to assist with broadening or narrowing antibiotics [156]. Given the high prevalence of viral CAP, testing during respiratory illness season should additionally include influenza A and B, respiratory syncytial virus (RSV), and COVID-19 [93, 156, 157]. The IDSA recommends a reverse-transcription polymerase chain reaction (RT-PCR) for influenza detection and nucleic acid amplification testing (NAAT) for COVID-19 detection [158, 159]. For RSV, RT-PCR has replaced older methods of detection [160].

Several tests from non-respiratory tract specimens may additionally aid in microbiologic diagnosis and are recommended in patients with severe disease [93]. Blood cultures are rarely positive and are unlikely to change management but should nevertheless be collected in critically ill patients; a positive result may be informative although clinicians should be cautious of contaminants [93, 161]. Urine testing for pneumococcal and *Legionella* antigens is only recommended in patients with severe CAP or in cases with epidemiological risk factors, such as during *Legionella* outbreaks [93]. *Legionella* antigen testing should be coupled with either *Legionella*-specific culture or PCR testing on lower respiratory tract samples [93].

29.4.2.3 Treatment

In patients with non-severe CAP without risk factors for MRSA or *P. aeruginosa*, beta-lactam and macrolide combination therapy or respiratory fluoroquinolone monotherapy is recommended [93, 156, 162, 163]. Beta-lactams such as ampicillin-sulbactam or ceftriaxone are effective against streptococci and *Haemophilus influenzae*, whereas macrolides such as azithromycin act against atypical organisms including *Moraxella catarrhalis* and *Legionella* spp. Levofloxacin and moxifloxacin are fluoroquinolones which are broadly active against the above-listed pathogens, including atypical organisms. These treatment recommendations are largely based off a systematic review of 20 studies of patients with CAP in which beta-lactam and macrolide combination therapy was associated with lower mortality than beta-lactam monotherapy [93, 162]. Given the side-effect profile of fluoroquinolones and macrolides (including QTc prolongation and *C. difficile* infection), doxycycline is an alternative option; however, data on doxycycline efficacy is limited. Patients with non-severe CAP but with prior respiratory isolation of MRSA or *P. aeruginosa* should be empirically treated for these pathogens [93].

Patients with severe CAP should receive the same regimens as those listed above for non-severe CAP. The only recommended difference between patients with non-severe and severe CAP is that patients with severe CAP and risk factors for MRSA or *P. aeruginosa* should be initiated on treatments targeting MRSA (e.g., vancomycin or linezolid) or *Pseudomonas* (e.g., piperacillin-tazobactam or cefepime) as appropriate, with eventual de-escalation based on microbiologic testing [93]. Risk factors for MRSA or *P. aeruginosa* include hospitalization and parenteral antibiotic exposure in the last 90 days [93]. Although not specifically listed in ATS/IDSA guidelines, clinicians may consider specific patient characteristics including long-term care facility stay, recent antibiotic use, frequent COPD exacerbations, necrotizing pneumonia, empyema, and immunosuppression as placing patients at higher risk of MRSA or *P. aeruginosa* infection [164]. Finally, antibiotic therapy should be continued until the patient achieves clinical stability (resolution of vital sign abnormalities) and for no less than a total of 5 days [93].

Patients with witnessed or suspected aspiration do not need to be started on anaerobic coverage such as metronidazole or clindamycin [93]. Recent studies have demonstrated that rates of anaerobic pneumonia are much lower than previously thought and that anaerobes do not contribute significantly to pathogenesis [165]. Additionally, a recent meta-analysis found that the addition of anaerobic coverage in patients with suspected aspiration pneumonia does not improve mortality [166]. Nonetheless, if there is an anatomic disruption that creates a low-oxygen environment in the lungs (such as a lung abscess or empyema), anaerobic treatment is indicated [166, 167].

Oseltamivir, a neuraminidase inhibitor, should be given to any patient with pneumonia from influenza regardless of symptom duration, although early initiation is beneficial [93, 158, 168]. Currently, the only IDSA guideline-recommended antiviral treatment for COVID-19 in hospitalized patients is remdesivir, a prodrug causing a premature termination of the viral RNA transcription [169, 170]. The ACTT-1 Trial demonstrated a quicker time to recovery with remdesivir compared to placebo; however, the WHO SOLIDARITY trial did not show any improvement in hospital mortality with remdesivir in patients requiring mechanical ventilation [171, 172]. Nonetheless, remdesivir should be considered in high-risk or deteriorating patients while monitoring for bradycardia, liver injury, and QT prolongation [170, 173]. Remdesivir is safe in patients with chronic kidney disease [174].

The use and understanding of corticosteroids in CAP continue to evolve. Whereas antibiotics target the causative pathogen, corticosteroids reduce inflammation associated with a dysregulated immune response to the infection [175]. Although initial studies were inconclusive [176], the 2023 CAPE COD trial randomized over 800 patients with severe CAP to receive either 200 mg of hydrocortisone per day or placebo and demonstrated significant mortality reduction in the steroid arm (6.2% vs. 11.9%, $P = 0.006$) [175]. Largely because of the CAPE COD trial, the Society of Critical Care Medicine now recommends steroids in severe bacterial CAP [177]. On the other hand, corticosteroids should be avoided in influenza pneumonia as several studies have shown an association between corticosteroids and increased mortality [178].

Unlike in influenza, corticosteroids (dexamethasone 6 mg daily for 10 days) in COVID-19 pneumonia—as demonstrated initially in the RECOVERY trial and later in subsequent trials—reduce mortality and are a mainstay of therapy [179, 180]. The mortality benefit was shown in patients requiring supplemental oxygen, whereas increased mortality was observed in patients receiving steroids while not requiring oxygen [180, 181]. Steroid therapy in COVID-19 is not without risk. Prolonged use may increase the risk of delayed viral clearance (especially in immunosuppressed patients), adrenal suppression, and invasive infections such as pulmonary aspergillosis [182, 183]. Despite this, a large meta-analysis found no increased risk of serious adverse events in the patients receiving corticosteroids versus placebo [184]. The timing of corticosteroid initiation may additionally impact outcome, although this remains an area of debate. The RECOVERY trial found an increased risk of mortality in patients in which corticosteroid therapy was started more than 7 days after symptom onset, but this signal effect was not found in a large meta-analysis [180, 184].

29.4.3 HAP/VAP

29.4.3.1 Overview

HAP is pneumonia that occurs more than 48 h after hospital admission and is not associated with mechanical ventilation, whereas VAP occurs at least 48–72 h after endotracheal intubation [27]. These conditions are both associated with similar causative pathogens—including MRSA, *P. aeruginosa*, and other resistant gram negatives—and we will review them together here [27]. HAP may complicate approximately 1 in 200 hospital admissions and has a mortality rate of approximately 20% [185]. VAP continues to be one of the leading causes of ICU-acquired infections [186]. Up to 40% of intubated patients may acquire VAP, although rates vary based on the study, and the estimated attributable mortality rate from VAP is about 15% [26, 186, 187].

29.4.3.2 Diagnosis

HAP/VAP diagnosis requires a clinical suspicion of pneumonia with new or progressing radiographic infiltrates and positive microbiologic cultures (preferably from the lower respiratory tract in the case of VAP) [27, 186]. Similar to CAP, there are several HAP/VAP mimics, and a comprehensive clinical diagnosis remains the gold standard. Although the clinical pulmonary infection score (CPIS) may aid in diagnosis, controversy regarding its low specificity led it not to be recommended by the IDSA guidelines [93, 188]. In addition, the presence of fever, purulent secretions, leukocytosis or leukopenia, and increased respiratory rate with increased oxygen demand should be considered in the diagnosis [27]. As discussed above, chest X-rays have low sensitivity and specificity, and CT scan may be considered to assist with definitive diagnosis [27]. Ultrasound should be considered for patients presenting to the ICU for pneumonia as it is highly sensitive and specific in this population [189]. In addition to standard laboratory workup, the use of clinical biomarkers such as procalcitonin (PCT) and C-reactive protein (CRP) alongside clinical criteria to initiate antimicrobial therapy is not recommended [27]. Currently, evidence is lacking whether adding PCT or CRP to clinical criteria is sufficiently sensitive or specific to start or not start antibiotics. For example, one study showed that 16.5% and 16.8% of patients will have a missed diagnosis of HAP/VAP, whereas 8.5% and 18.7% will be incorrectly diagnosed as having HAP/VAP when utilizing PCT and CRP, respectively [27].

The current IDSA/ATS HAP/VAP guidelines recommend noninvasive sampling (e.g., endotracheal aspiration) with semiquantitative cultures in the initial workup rather than invasive sampling (e.g., bronchoscopy) with quantitative cultures [27]. As such, clinicians may consider endotracheal aspiration for VAP and spontaneous expectoration and/or sputum induction for HAP among non-intubated patients. The reasoning against routine invasive sampling is that this has not been shown to significantly impact important outcomes such as mortality, ICU length of stay, duration of mechanical ventilation, or antibiotic changes compared to the noninvasive approach [27]. In certain patient populations such as the immunocompromised and patients worsening despite empiric antibiotics, invasive sampling may be considered.

Additional diagnostics may help to target therapy after the empiric phase of treatment. For example, a recent meta-analysis showed that the MRSA nasal swab PCR was 70.9% sensitive and 90.3% specific and had a positive predictive value of 44.8% and negative predictive value of 96.5% for MRSA pneumonia [190]. Thus, a negative test will allow for safe discontinuation of anti-MRSA treatment. There is more data available regarding mPCR in HAP/VAP compared to CAP. As previously discussed, mPCR has a higher sensitivity than culture for pathogen detection [154]. With this high sensitivity, clinicians should take care in interpreting results, as these technologies do not differentiate between colonization and infection. For example, one study demonstrates a positive predictive value of only 52% for bacterial pneumonia [191]. This technology may have a specific role in the identification of virulent or MDR pathogens and assistance in antimicrobial optimization in the critically ill.

29.4.3.3   Treatment

Empiric treatment should include anti-*Staphylococcus aureus* and antipseudomonal agents [27]. Although guidelines recommend starting an agent targeting MRSA (vs. methicillin-susceptible *Staphylococcus aureus*) only in institutions (or units) where >10–20% of *S. aureus* is MRSA, in practice, empiric anti-MRSA agents are routinely started (at least in the United States, where MRSA prevalence is routinely higher than the proposed threshold) [27, 192]. Antibiotics targeting MRSA and *Pseudomonas* have been previously discussed (see "CAP"). Regarding antipseudomonal therapy, there is no data to support clear superiority of one agent, and clinicians should be aware of institutional resistance rates and antibiotic side-effect profiles to assist with choosing the most appropriate empiric regimen. The guidelines however highlight that aminoglycosides should not be used as monotherapy due to poor lung penetration and lack of studies evaluating aminoglycoside monotherapy [27]. Clinicians can consider combination therapy (generally including a beta-lactam and an aminoglycoside) in patients with septic shock or high risk for death due to *Pseudomonas* HAP/VAP, as the potential mortality benefit may outweigh possible side effects [27, 61, 193].

Patients with HAP and VAP are at risk of antibiotic-resistant pathogens such as carbapenem-resistant *Acinetobacter baumannii* (CRAB), *Stenotrophomonas maltophilia*, and carbapenem-resistant Enterobacterales (CRE) [194–196]. These organisms, especially CRAB and *S. maltophilia*, are common colonizers among critically ill patients and only require treatment if the patient has a clinical infection. If the decision is made to treat, then in the case of CRAB, a two-drug combination therapy is recommended [197]. An example of such is high-dose ampicillin-sulbactam with either minocycline, polymyxin, tigecycline, or cefiderocol [197]. In the case of *S. maltophilia*, a combination therapy of two antimicrobials with trimethoprim-sulfamethoxazole, minocycline/tigecycline, cefiderocol, or levofloxacin can be considered [197]. A detailed discussion of antimicrobials targeting CRE is beyond the scope of this chapter; however, clinicians should become familiar with regimens for these infections including ceftazidime/avibactam, ceftolozane/tazobactam, cefiderocol, and meropenem/vaborbactam.

Duration of therapy should not exceed 7 days if the patient improves. This is based on evidence that shorter durations of therapy reduced antibiotic exposure and recurrence of multidrug-resistant organisms with no impact on mortality, treatment failure, hospital length of stay, or duration of mechanical ventilation [27, 198, 199]. However, clinicians may extend treatment duration if the patient has not fully recovered or in the presence of complications such as parapneumonic effusion, empyema, or lung abscess.

29.5 Bacterial Meningitis

29.5.1 Background

Despite the use of effective therapies and availability of vaccines that target many common pathogens, meningitis remains an important and devastating global health disease with a fatality rate of 10–30% [200, 201]. Meningitis is characterized by inflammation of the brain and spinal cord and is often due to an infection, most commonly viral, bacterial (including tuberculous), or fungal. Other causes of meningitis include immune-mediated causes, chemical or medication-induced meningitis (e.g., intravenous immunoglobulin, trimethoprim-sulfamethoxazole, and nonsteroidal anti-inflammatory drugs), and neoplasm (e.g., leptomeningeal metastases).

Acute bacterial meningitis is a critical diagnosis, and delays in management are associated with increased morbidity and mortality [202]. This chapter primarily focuses on the diagnosis and management of acute bacterial meningitis, including both community-acquired and healthcare-associated meningitis. It is important to note, however, that viral meningoencephalitis, including due to herpes simplex virus (HSV), may present similarly [203]. Although we will not delve into the specifics of viral meningoencephalitis, clinicians should consider empiric antivirals while awaiting microbiology results.

29.5.2 Pathogenesis and Pathophysiology

Bacterial infections of the central nervous system occur via two routes of inoculation, either by hematogenous seeding or by direct contiguous spread from the cranial structures adjacent to the brain or foreign objects or during cerebral or spinal procedures [204]. Bacterial meningitis develops when pathogenic virulence factors overcome the host defense mechanisms. Most of the major meningeal pathogens possess the ability to evade several host defenses. These include *Streptococcus pneumoniae*, *Haemophilus influenzae*, *Neisseria meningitidis*, and *Escherichia coli*; these organisms utilize four processes to exert their pathogenesis: colonization of mucous membranes, invasion of the bloodstream, survival in the bloodstream, and finally penetration to the subarachnoid space [29]. Due to the lack of humoral immunity in the subarachnoid space, bacteria can multiply undisturbed [204]. Clinical meningitis is a result of the host inflammatory response to the inciting organism in the cerebrospinal fluid (CSF). A cascade of immune-mediated events leads to the release of pro-inflammatory mediators and further disruption of the blood-brain barrier, resulting in meningeal inflammation, brain edema, and neurologic damage [201, 204]. Another route of inoculation is direct spread from adjacent structures. In the setting of bacterial otitis media or sinusitis, bony defects (e.g., in the setting of mastoiditis) or thrombophlebitis can result in intracranial spread and bacterial meningitis [205, 206].

29.5.3 Clinical Features

The classic features of bacterial meningitis include fever, neck stiffness, headache, and altered mental status [207]. However, such symptoms occur in fewer than half of patients at presentation [208]. Additional signs of meningitis include the Kernig and Brudzinski signs. While those are highly specific for meningitis, their sensitivity is unfortunately poor [209, 210]. Other symptoms of meningitis include nausea, vomiting, photophobia, and less often altered mental status or seizures. The diagnosis of meningitis may be difficult but should be suspected in patients presenting with fever and headache. Table 29.6 displays some of the risk factors and characteristic features of common pathogenic causes of bacterial meningitis [29, 208, 211–214].

29.5.4 Diagnosis

The cornerstone of meningitis diagnosis involves CSF examination via a lumbar puncture (LP), and patients with potential meningitis should undergo an LP after an assessment of potential risks associated with this procedure, including risk for bleeding and herniation.

Table 29.6 Risk factors for and characteristic features of bacterial meningitis based on common pathogens

Pathogen	Clinical features and risk factors
Streptococcus pneumoniae	• Preceded by respiratory infection, otitis, sinusitis, or endocarditis • Alcohol use disorder • Asplenia • Elderly • Recurrent meningitis • Basilar skull fracture
Neisseria meningitidis	• Rapid evolution (stupor/delirium within hours) • Petechial or purpuric rash • Large ecchymoses • Circulatory shock • Local outbreaks • Congregate living (college students)
Haemophilus influenzae	• Upper respiratory tract infection or otitis in an unvaccinated child
Listeria monocytogenes	• Older adults and neonates • Pregnancy • Immunosuppression • Renal failure • Alcohol use disorder
Staphylococcus aureus	• Endocarditis • Neurosurgery or foreign body • Ventricular shunt or drain
Coagulase-negative staphylococci	• Neurosurgery or foreign body • Ventricular shunt or drain
Gram-negative bacilli[a]	• Neurosurgery • Ventricular drains • Advanced medical illnesses • Immunosuppression

[a] Includes *Escherichia coli*, *Enterobacter* species, *Pseudomonas aeruginosa*, *Klebsiella* species

29.5.4.1 Imaging

Complications from LP may occur, with the most feared being fatal herniation due to downward displacement of the cerebrum and brainstem resultant from a pressure gradient triggered by the LP. IDSA practice guidelines recommend obtaining brain computed tomography (CT) in patients at risk of herniation due to an elevated intracranial pressure or due to the presence of an intracranial mass lesion [29]. This guideline applies to patients with a history of CNS disease, immunocompromise, new-onset seizures, severe impairment of consciousness, focal neurological findings, or papilledema [215]. The decision to obtain a CT prior to performing an LP should not delay the administration of appropriate antibiotics if bacterial meningitis is suspected, and blood cultures should additionally be collected before antibiotics.

Although imaging is not routinely recommended in the diagnosis of meningitis, it may help to assess for associated complications including brain abscesses, mastoiditis, and venous thromboses. While both CT and magnetic resonance imaging (MRI) may be normal early in the course of disease, contrast-enhanced MRI, including with fluid-attenuated inversion recovery (FLAIR) sequencing, is highly sensitive for leptomeningeal enhancement [216, 217]. Negative results of neuroimaging, especially contrast-enhanced MRI, should prompt consideration of alternate diagnoses.

29.5.4.2 Spinal Fluid Examination

Examination of CSF in most cases of bacterial meningitis reveals a high opening pressure (20–50 cm of H_2O), elevated CSF white blood cell count (WBC) (>100 cells/mm^3) with neutrophilic predominance, low CSF-to-serum glucose ratio (less than 40%), and a high CSF protein content [29, 206]. In the event of a traumatic spinal tap, or in patients with intracerebral or subarachnoid hemorrhage, a false-positive elevation of CSF WBC count may be present; an elevated CSF red blood cell count may also be present in HSV meningoencephalitis [218]. To obtain a "corrected" CSF WBC count, the clinician can subtract one WBC for every 500–1000 red blood cells [219]. Some evidence suggests that CSF lactate can help differentiate between viral and bacterial meningitis and may outperform conventional testing to determine microbiologic etiology [220–222]. However, CSF lactate sensitivity is decreased in patients who received antimicrobial therapy prior to the LP [222].

In addition to blood cultures, a gram stain and culture of CSF should be obtained in all individuals presenting with suspected meningitis. CSF gram stain sensitivity ranges between 60% and 90% in adult patients with bacterial meningitis, with a specificity of nearly 100% [223, 224]. Gram stain and culture yield may be decreased in patients that receive antimicrobial therapy prior to the LP; however, the CSF profile may be less affected and can still aid in the differential diagnosis [223].

There are commercial multiplex meningitis/encephalitis polymerase chain reaction panels available to assess for several bacterial, viral, and fungal causes of meningitis. One panel, the FilmArray meningitis/encephalitis panel (Biofire Diagnostics,

Salt Lake City, UT, USA), is highly sensitive and specific for the tested viruses and bacteria, but less sensitive for *Cryptococcus* [225]. PCR may be most useful in patients who received antimicrobial therapy prior to LP and whose gram stain and cultures are negative and may also assist with rapid diagnosis as results are generally available within a few hours.

29.5.5 Treatment

General treatment principles include the following [29]:

1. Administration of empiric antimicrobial therapy promptly after performing an LP. If delays in LP are expected, then antimicrobial therapy should be administered shortly after obtaining blood cultures.
2. Use of bactericidal antimicrobials given the lack of CSF defenses and the possible presence of high bacterial inoculum.
3. Use of antimicrobials with adequate CSF penetration.
4. Use of intravenous antimicrobials; oral agents should be avoided due to concerns of lower tissue concentrations and less clinical experience with these agents in meningitis.
5. Duration of treatment is dependent on the causative pathogen, associated complications (e.g., cerebral abscess or metastatic infection), and timing of source control (e.g., ventricular drain removal).
6. Use of corticosteroids for suspected or proven pneumococcal meningitis in adults, and for *H. influenzae* in infants and children to reduce the risk of neurological complications:

    (a) Dosing: Dexamethasone 0.15 mg/kg every 6 h for 2–4 days.
    (b) Timing of administration: intravenous corticosteroids should be administered at the time of or prior to administering antibiotics.
    (c) Duration of therapy: 2–4 days.

The choice of empiric antimicrobials in patients with suspected bacterial meningitis is determined by the most likely bacteria dependent on the patient's age and risk factors (Fig. 29.1a, b) [29]. For community-acquired meningitis, third-generation cephalosporins (ceftriaxone or cefotaxime) are recommended to treat for *H. influenzae* (in children 1–23 months of age), *N. meningitidis*, and *S. pneumoniae*. Due to the high incidence of penicillin-resistant *S. pneumoniae*, vancomycin is recommended in addition to the third-generation cephalosporin agent until penicillin susceptibility is confirmed as these isolates are routinely susceptible to vancomycin. In addition to ceftriaxone/cefotaxime and vancomycin, ampicillin is recommended for *Listeria monocytogenes* coverage in neonates, adults above the age of 50 years, and immunocompromised patients. Once a pathogen is identified, therapy should be tailored based on susceptbilities. In patients that have received corticosteroids and in whom pneumococcal meningitis is suspected, the addition of rifampin to the

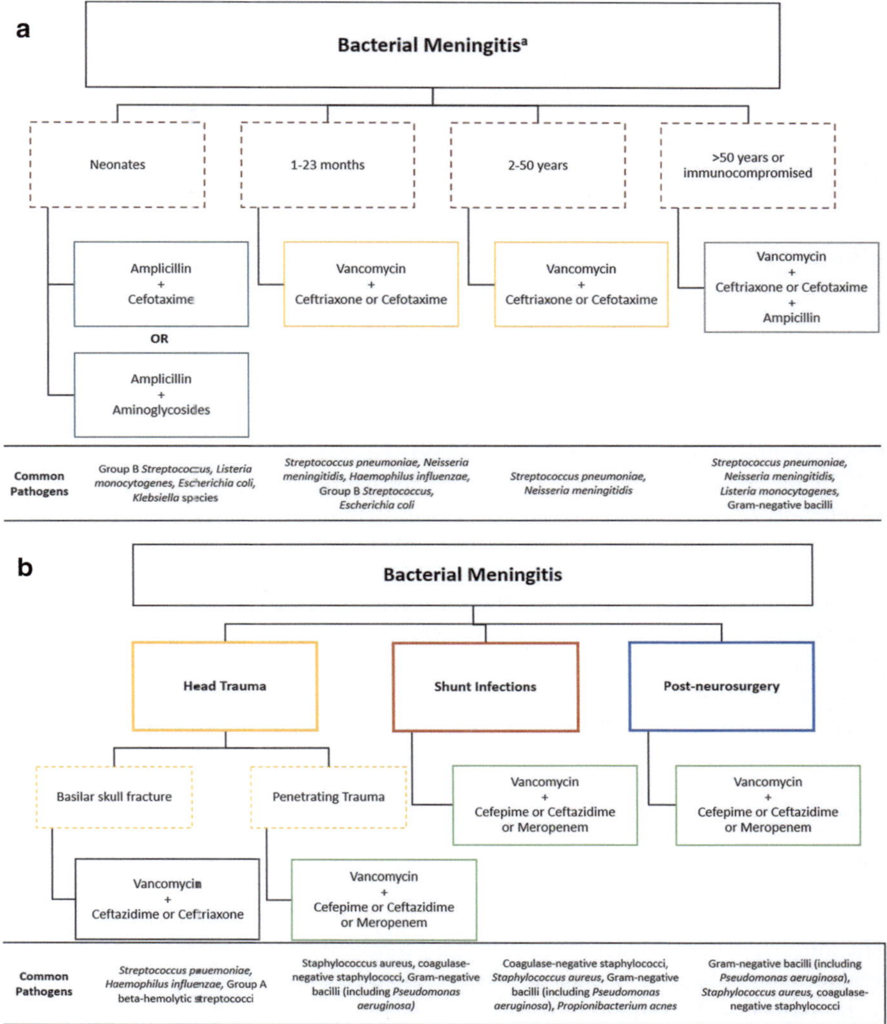

Fig. 29.1 (**a**) Suggested empirical antimicrobial therapy for bacterial meningitis based on patient age and risk factors. ªEmpiric antimicrobial therapy is guided by patient's age and other risk factors that may have predisposed the patient to meningitis. (**b**) Suggested empirical antimicrobial therapy for healthcare-associated meningitis and meningitis due to head trauma

empiric regimen can be considered. If pneumococcal meningitis is confirmed on cultures and the isolate shows intermediate susceptibility or resistance to ceftriaxone (minimum inhibitory concentration ≥ 1 mcg/mL), then rifampin may be continued along with the third-generation cephalosporin and vancomycin if the strain is rifampin susceptible. Similarly, in patients with staphylococcal meningitis/ventriculitis who still have intracranial catheter(s) in place, the addition of rifampin is suggested if the isolate is susceptible to rifampin. The duration of therapy is generally limited to 7 days for *N. meningitidis* and *H. influenzae*, at least 21 days for *Listeria*, and 14–21 days for all other pathogens [29, 226].

29.6 Intra-abdominal Infections

29.6.1 Background

Intra-abdominal infections (IAIs) are a broad group of disorders that include processes such as diverticulitis, peritonitis, cholangitis, and infected pancreatitis. This diverse set of diseases may result in contained foci of infection or peritoneal inflammation and purulence [227, 228]. The Surgical Infection Society categorizes IAIs as either complicated or uncomplicated [229]. Uncomplicated IAI (uIAI) involves intramural inflammation of the affected organ sparing any anatomic disruption and is generally treated conservatively. On the other hand, complicated IAI (cIAI) causes peritoneal inflammation with localized or diffuse peritonitis extending beyond the source organ [229, 230]. Separately, peritonitis occurs via separate mechanisms. Spontaneous bacterial (primary) peritonitis occurs via bacterial translocation through an intact gut wall [230]. Secondary peritonitis occurs from microbial contamination due to a laceration or perforation and is more likely to be polymicrobial [229]. Lastly, tertiary peritonitis is defined as recurrent or persistent infection despite treatment for primary or secondary peritonitis. Most commonly, this occurs in immunocompromised and critically ill patients with poor host defenses [230–232].

29.6.2 Pathophysiology

The intrinsic mucosal barrier is the primary mechanism for preventing bowel flora translocation. Mucosal breakdown from ischemia, surgery, or reperfusion injury (e.g.) may allow bacteria to cross this protective barrier, and the mucosal microbiome therefore dictates the infecting organism [229, 233]. Thus, clinicians should consider the anatomical source as well as patient risk factors such as previous surgeries and antibiotic exposure to determine optimal empiric antibiotic coverage before definitive microbiology is available. IAIs are generally polymicrobial and predominately involve gram-negative rods (GNRs) such as *Escherichia coli*, *Klebsiella*, and *Proteus* spp. [234]. Anaerobes such as *Bacteroides* and *Clostridium* spp. (11%) and gram-positive cocci (GPC) such as *Enterococcus* spp. (25%) and *Staphylococcus aureus* (10%) are also potential pathogens although less common [235, 236]. In addition to the above organisms, hospital-acquired IAI may involve other Enterobacterales species such as *Enterobacter* spp. and lactose non-fermenting negative GNR such as *Pseudomonas* and *Acinetobacter* spp. with potential for antibiotic resistance [237]. *Candida* spp. may be involved in hospital-acquired IAI specifically in patients with immunocompromise or prolonged antibiotic exposure, and infections arising from the esophagus or upper gastrointestinal tract [238].

29.6.3 Diagnosis

IAI diagnosis involves integrating patient subjective symptoms with objective information including physical exam and radiological and laboratory data, with a focus on the suspected anatomic site. Symptoms may include nausea, vomiting, and abdominal pain; in severe cases, symptoms of systemic illness including fevers and chills may indicate progression to sepsis [239]. Biomarkers such as C-reactive protein and procalcitonin may be of utility as indirect markers of inflammation and infection, respectively, but are not sufficiently sensitive or specific to rule in or out a diagnosis of IAI [240]. Ultimately, advances in ultrasound (US) and computed tomography (CT) have made these modalities indispensable for IAI diagnosis as well as guiding intervention and following response to therapy. Depending on the specific IAI, studies have demonstrated varying sensitivity and specificity of CT imaging. For example, CT sensitivity and specificity for the diagnosis of appendicitis in adults were 83% and 93%, respectively, whereas for acute cholecystitis, CT sensitivity was 94% and specificity was 59% [241–243]. Although MRI sensitivity and specificity are similar to those of CT, CT is generally the preferred initial imaging study due to ease, but MRIs may be recommended in pregnant patients [239].

29.6.4 Management

29.6.4.1 Source Control

The principal management of IAI is timely diagnosis with appropriate source control and antibiotic administration [244]. While "source control" generally refers to surgical or interventional procedures to decrease bacterial load, prompt administration of antibiotics based on suspected pathogens and immediate hemodynamic stabilization with fluids, vasopressors, and other supportive measures should be instituted to limit and reverse any impeding organ failure [229]. Further, the decision to pursue a source control procedure is complex and depends on the affected organ, operation required, and individual patient factors such as degree of acute illness and ability to withstand an operation. In general, a "step-up" approach to IAI management which involves initial conservative management is preferred when possible; this approach has been best described for infected pancreatitis [245, 246]. The complex medical decision-making regarding patient selection and procedure (invasive vs. noninvasive) is beyond the scope of this chapter. Further reading can be found in society guidelines [229, 244].

When required, source control procedures are crucial to reduce bacterial load and toxin production to allow host defenses and antibiotics to optimally clear infection [229]. The 2021 World Society of Emergency Surgery (WSES) guidelines recommend a multifaceted approach regarding the steps towards attaining source control. The guideline recommends a stepwise approach regarding the surgical approach of source control [244]. Initially, the operative goals are to remove any damaged tissues and foci of infection with a lavage of the intra-abdominal infection [244]. Depending on findings and ability to attain satisfactory source control, a repeat surgical intervention is either an on-demand or timed return to the operating room (OR) for further surgical control and "totalization" [244]. Importantly, source control procedures may allow for specimen collection to define the infecting organism and antibiotic susceptibility and facilitate antibiotic escalation or (more commonly) de-escalation.

29.6.4.2 Antibiotics

A multifaceted management approach includes administration of appropriate antibiotics, which encompasses antibiotic selection and pharmacokinetic optimization, determining duration of therapy, and continual assessment of patient response. Patient factors (complicated vs. uncomplicated IAI, community- vs. hospital-acquired IAI, previous antibiotic exposure, hospital length of stay, prior surgical interventions, and immunocompromised state) should be considered when selecting empiric antibiotics. Patients with mild-to-moderate disease severity admitted from the community with no risk factors for extended-spectrum beta-lactamase-producing Enterobacterales (ESBL-E) may be managed with regimens such as cephalosporins (e.g., ceftriaxone) combined with an anti-anaerobic agent [244] (e.g., metronidazole). Due to increasing resistance, fluoroquinolones should be avoided for empiric treatment [96]. Risk factors for ESBL-E include greater recent hospitalization, intravenous antibiotics, or ESBL infection/colonization [244]. Due to increasing resistance of community-acquired *E. coli* to ampicillin/sulbactam (up to 45%) and data demonstrating inferiority of this regimen compared to moxifloxacin, ampicillin/sulbactam is no longer recommended as empiric therapy [229, 247, 248]. However, de-escalation to this regimen for susceptible pathogens is appropriate once cultures are obtained [229, 249]. For community-acquired IAI, empiric coverage targeting enterococci and *Pseudomonas* is not usually necessary and should generally be avoided [250, 251].

For patients with HA-IAI or sepsis/septic shock, antibiotic coverage can be expanded to target *Pseudomonas*, enterococci, and ESBL-E [96]. Single drug regimens that target HA-IAI pathogens include beta-lactam/beta-lactamase inhibitors (e.g., piperacillin/tazobactam), while combination therapies that target both ESBL-E and anaerobes (e.g., cefepime and metronidazole) are reasonable options, especially for AmpC-producing organisms [197]. However, for critically ill patients with documented ESBL-E infection (i.e., not empiric therapy), carbapenems (e.g., meropenem and imipenem) are preferred [135, 197]. Ertapenem is an alternative carbapenem but lacks activity against *Pseudomonas* spp. Certain Enterobacterales, especially *Klebsiella pneumoniae*, may be resistant to carbapenems (i.e., carbapenem-resistant Enterobacterales [CRE]), and IAIs due to CRE are associated with increased mortality [252, 253]. Treatment of CRE infections depends on the specific mechanism of carbapenem resistance and should be made in conjunction with an infectious diseases specialist, but potential antibiotic options include ceftazidime-avibactam and meropenem-vaborbactam [197]. Lastly, empiric double coverage with aminoglycosides (in addition to one of the above agents) may be considered until attainment of culture results and de-escalation to definitive therapy [61]. Eravacycline, a recently approved agent, may be considered in patients with documented CRE [197]. The IGNITE4 trial demonstrated that eravacycline was non-inferior to meropenem in the treatment of ESBL-E organisms, noting that there was an under-representation of CRE [254, 255]. Like tigecycline, another tetracycline antibiotic, eravacycline lacks meaningful activity against *Pseudomonas* and *Proteus* spp. Tigecycline has been associated with increased mortality in bacteremia (which may result from IAI) and other serious infections [256]. It is unclear whether eravacycline similarly performs poorly in bacteremia, although there may be a class effect and caution should be exercised in bacteremia.

Empiric coverage for *Enterococcus* is not routinely indicated; however, patients with recent *Enterococcus* culture growth, or a positive rectal swab, can be covered for enterococci with vancomycin or ampicillin until culture results are available [257]. Empiric *Candida* coverage is not recommended except for patients with risk factors for candidiasis (such as solid-organ transplantation and other immunocompromise) [239, 244]. Additionally, patients with recent upper gastrointestinal surgery, anastomotic leak, or necrotizing pancreatitis who are not improving on empiric antibiotics may be considered for empiric antifungal therapy [136]. Fluconazole is an appropriate option unless the patient is severely ill or there is concern for a fluconazole-resistant isolate (for example, in patients receiving fluconazole prophylaxis or with recent isolation of fluconazole-resistant species such as *C. glabrata*). In these cases, an echinocandin such as micafungin should be used [229].

Anaerobic coverage should be instituted routinely as anaerobes—chiefly *Bacteroides* spp.—are present through the GI tract; however, upper GI infection may not necessarily require coverage [236]. The true incidence of anaerobic infection is difficult to determine as these organisms are difficult to culture and may not be isolated despite being present in a sample [229]. Despite this limitation, anaerobes are assumed to be present in most IAIs, and empiric therapy should include an agent with anti-anaerobe activity [229]. Single agents such as piperacillin/tazobactam or combination therapy including metronidazole are reasonable options. Clindamycin should be avoided due to increased clindamycin resistance among *Bacteroides*, risk of *Clostridioides difficile* infection, and superiority of metronidazole [229, 258, 259].

Determining duration of therapy is frequently a complex decision. Aside from the adequacy of source control, factors that influence duration include the causative agent and anatomic site. Once source control has been achieved, therapy should be limited to 4 days [239, 260]. This is based on the STOP-IT trial (Study to Optimize

Peritoneal Infection Therapy) in which patients with source control of complicated IAI randomized to a shorter course of antibiotics (4 ± 1 days) had no difference in a composite outcome (surgical site infection, recurrent IAI, or 30-day mortality) compared to patients who received up to 10 days of antibiotics [260]. There are certain circumstances that may necessitate a more prolonged duration including suboptimal source control, uncomplicated appendicitis, and ongoing percutaneous drainage [229, 239]. Frequently, serial imaging is needed to assess the adequacy of drainage. Lastly, for immunocompromised patients, duration of therapy should be individualized [229, 239].

29.7 Skin and Soft Tissue Infections (SSTIs)

29.7.1 Background

Skin and soft tissue infections (SSTIs) are common indications for emergency department evaluation [261]. SSTIs can be grouped into two categories: purulent (e.g., furuncles, carbuncles, or abscesses) and non-purulent (e.g., erysipelas, cellulitis, or necrotizing fasciitis) [94]. These infections are further classified by the severity of the infection: mild infections produce only local symptoms, whereas moderate-severe infections either (a) are accompanied by systemic signs of an infection, (b) have not responded to oral antibiotics or incision and drainage (in cases of a purulent SSTI), (c) occur in immunocompromised patients, or (d) have signs of a deeper infection [94]. SSTIs can be further grouped into necrotizing or non-necrotizing soft tissue infections. While most SSTIs are superficial and can be treated with supportive care or oral antibiotics, severe SSTIs are responsible for up to 11% of septic shock cases and have a case fatality rate of up to 10% [23, 262, 263]. In this chapter, we review the clinical presentation, diagnosis, and management of SSTIs, with an emphasis on infections encountered in the critical care setting: surgical site infections, infected pressure ulcers, and necrotizing skin infections, including necrotizing fasciitis, Fournier gangrene, clostridial myonecrosis or gas gangrene, and toxic shock syndrome.

29.7.2 Pathophysiology

The human skin is the first layer of protection against microbial infections. The low pH, sebaceous fluids, desquamation process, and presence of normal flora (including coagulase-negative staphylococci and *Corynebacterium* species) prevent the growth of pathogens [264–266]. Primary SSTI occurs when pathogens invade otherwise healthy skin; secondary SSTI occurs when microorganisms infect damaged skin following a breach in the skin barrier. Less commonly, SSTIs may result from

Table 29.7 Pathogenic causes of skin and soft tissue infections by exposure and comorbidities

Risk factor or exposure	Pathogen(s)
Fresh water [269, 270]	• *Aeromonas hydrophila* • *Plesiomonas shigelloides* • *Edwardsiella tarda* • *Pseudomonas aeruginosa* • *Shewanella* species
Salt water [269]	• *Vibrio vulnificus* • *Vibrio parahaemolyticus* • *Erysipelothrix rhusiopathiae*
Raw oyster ingestion [271]	• *Vibrio vulnificus* • *Vibrio parahaemolyticus*
Animal bite [272]	• *Pasteurella multocida* • *Capnocytophaga canimorsus* • Anaerobic bacteria
Human bite [273]	• *Eikenella corrodens* • Anaerobic bacteria • Viridans streptococci
Cirrhosis [274]	• *Klebsiella* species • *Escherichia coli* • *Vibrio vulnificus* and *Vibrio parahaemolyticus* following salt water or shellfish exposure • *Aeromonas* species following freshwater exposure
Immunocompromised or neutropenic individuals [275–277]	• Gram-negative bacilli, including *Pseudomonas aeruginosa* • *Clostridium* species • Invasive fungal infections

contiguous spread or hematogenous seeding [267]. SSTIs are most commonly caused by bacteria, and these SSTIs are referred to as acute bacterial skin and skin structure infections (ABSSSI). Isolation of a specific pathogen(s) is difficult and limited by current diagnostics [268]. Table 29.7 demonstrates some of the pathogenic causes of SSTIs based on exposure and/or patient comorbidities.

29.7.3   *Surgical Site Infections*

Surgical site infections (SSIs) can be divided into three categories: superficial incisional SSI, deep incisional SSI, or organ/space SSI [278]. Most surgical site infections occur >48–96 h after the surgical procedure. The mainstay of therapy involves suture removal along with incision and drainage. Antibiotics are indicated in patients' systemic signs of infection or with erythema and induration extending >5 cm from the wound. Empiric antibiotics should cover *S. aureus*, including MRSA in patients with risk factors such as nasal colonization or prior MRSA infection. Additionally, gram-negative and anaerobic coverage should be included empirically when treating surgical site infections of the axilla, gastrointestinal or genital tracts, and perineum. Therapy can then be tailored according to microbiology results [94].

29.7.4 *Infectious Complications of Skin and Soft Tissue Pressure Injuries*

Pressure injuries (PIs) are defined as a localized damage to the skin or underlying tissue resulting from pressure [279] and are associated with a significant morbidity [280]. PIs commonly affect areas with bony prominence, such as the sacrum, calcaneus, trochanters, or ischium [279]. Among hospitalized patients, PIs are most common among critically ill population [281], with a prevalence of 11–45% [282–284]. Since PIs may be colonized by a myriad of microorganisms, infected PIs are often polymicrobial [285]; however, the causative organism may not always be identical to that colonizing the ulcer. Commonly reported pathogens include *Enterobacter* species, Enterobacterales, *Pseudomonas aeruginosa*, *Staphylococcus* species (including MRSA), *Enterococcus faecalis*, and anaerobes [279, 285]. Importantly, bacterial colonization is routine and only requires treatment if there are local or systemic signs of infection.

Cellulitis associated with PI may present with warmth, erythema, tenderness, and induration. With deeper tissue involvement, symptoms often include necrosis, foul odor, and tissue discoloration. In some cases, patients may only present with systemic signs of an infection and minimal changes surrounding the soft tissue. Soft tissue infection may also progress to bacteremia [285]. Microbiological diagnosis of PI infection is challenging, since virtually all pressure ulcers are colonized with microorganisms. Superficial swab cultures should be avoided. Instead, a deep tissue biopsy during surgical debridement should be obtained for microbiologic evaluation [279].

The treatment approach for infection associated with a PI is determined by the extent of the infection and the presence of systemic signs of an infection. For superficial infections, management involves local wound care, nutritional support, pressure relief, and topical antiseptics [279]. For soft tissue infections associated with a PI, surgical debridement should be considered [279]. Considering the polymicrobial nature of infected PIs, empiric therapy should target aerobic and anaerobic gram-positive and gram-negative microorganisms. Evidence on the most optimal antimicrobial regimen for infected PIs is weak [286]. Once an organism(s) is identified, therapy should be tailored accordingly. The optimal duration of treatment is not well defined and is determined based on the rate of response to therapy, the area affected, and whether the infection is associated with bacteremia or osteomyelitis. Many patients have exposed bone underlying deep pressure ulcers, and the need for extended treatment for osteomyelitis is made on a case-by-case basis. Importantly, unless there is the possibility of wound healing and closure, antibiotics for osteomyelitis are generally not indicated [287].

29.7.5 *Necrotizing Soft Tissue Infection*

Necrotizing soft tissue infections (NSTIs) involve the deep tissues of the skin and can lead to widespread necrosis and systemic illness. The mortality rate associated with NSTIs remains high at 25–30% [288]. Therefore, rapid diagnosis and treatment with surgical debridement and broad-spectrum antibiotics are crucial [23]. NSTIs are especially fatal when associated with shock or other host factors including older age and immunocompromise [288].

NSTI may develop after a skin breach, leading to the introduction of organisms or spores into the soft tissue [289]. The proliferation of bacteria and release of toxins cause local tissue damage. Additionally, toxin release can result in platelet-leukocyte aggregates that occlude capillaries and cause damage to the vascular endothelium. As a result, fluid leakage, tissue swelling, and erythema ensue, leading to infection of the deeper tissue and ultimately occlusion of larger vessels with subsequent necrosis of all layers [288]. NSTI can also result from a nonpenetrating tissue injury (e.g., sprain, hematoma, or bacteremia), wherein cutaneous manifestations of the NSTI do not develop until late in the course of the infection and after ischemic destruction and necrosis have already occurred, which may lead to misdiagnosis [288].

While NSTIs can develop in any area of the body, they are mostly encountered in the extremities, genitalia, and perineum [290]. Several forms of NSTI exist, and any skin or soft tissue infection causing tissue necrosis can be labeled as an NSTI [290]. We will specifically discuss necrotizing fasciitis (NF), Fournier gangrene, and clostridial myonecrosis.

29.7.5.1 Necrotizing Fasciitis

Necrotizing fasciitis, the most common type of NSTI, involves the subcutaneous tissue and fascia [94]. NF can be classified based on microbiology [289]. Type I describes polymicrobial infections involving both aerobic and anaerobic microorganisms and is the most common type of NF. Risk factors for type I include diabetic or decubitus ulcers, rectal fissures, or infections after colonic, urologic, or gynecologic procedures [288, 289]. Fournier gangrene, a subset of type I NF, involves the perineal, perianal, and genital regions. It typically develops from a perianal infection that has spread along the facial planes to the genitalia, a urinary tract infection that has extended into the penis and scrotum, or trauma to the genital area providing a port of entry into the subcutaneous tissues [290]. Type II NF is monomicrobial, typically due to group A *Streptococcus* (GAS) or, less commonly, *S. aureus*. Type II NF is usually aggressive and may be initially missed as it spreads from the bloodstream, so characteristic lesions develop later in the disease course. When caused by GAS, type II NF can progress to streptococcal toxic shock syndrome (STSS). Other monomicrobial NFs include infections caused by gram-negative organisms, usually marine-related organisms such as *Vibrio vulnificus* or *Aeromonas* species; this is sometimes referred to as type III NF and is associated with a high mortality rate of 30–40% [291, 292]. Finally, NSTIs due to fungal organisms may be referred to as type IV NF and usually occur in immunocompromised patients or after trauma [288, 289].

Diagnosis

Early diagnosis of NF can be difficult. Patients presenting with NF may initially be misdiagnosed with cellulitis as NF can begin in the deep layers of the skin before manifesting with superficial erythema or edema. Importantly, patients with NF will often have a disproportionate level of pain compared to physical findings [293]. Any significant alteration in vital signs or inflammatory markers should prompt consideration of NF [289]. Clinical scores such as the Laboratory Risk Indicator for Necrotizing Fasciitis (LRINEC) lack sufficient sensitivity to definitively exclude NF [294, 295]. Therefore, patients presenting with an acute onset of severe pain in an extremity or SSTI with systemic signs of infection should be evaluated for severe NSTI or NF, even in the absence of an obvious port for microorganism entry or fever. Dermatological features of NF progress from erythema, tenderness, and warmth to development of bullae or blisters, and it ultimately results in crepitus, necrosis, and/or gangrene. Patients with NF can develop septic shock, toxic shock syndrome, and multiorgan failure [289].

Diagnostic imaging may delay definitive diagnosis and treatment of NF; physical exam and clinical judgment are the most essential aspects of initial diagnosis. Imaging may demonstrate gas in the soft tissues, but this finding may be absent in early disease or in type II NF. A definitive diagnosis of NF can be made during surgical exploration and tissue biopsy. During exploration, some findings that can support NF diagnosis include fascial or muscle necrosis and/or loss of fascial integrity or evidence of muscle involvement. Common findings include foul-smelling "dishwater" exudate, a dull gray appearance of the fascia, and a positive "finger test" in which there is lack of resistance to blunt dissection of the fascia with minimal bleeding [94, 288]. A definitive bacteriologic diagnosis can be made after obtaining culture and gram stain of the deep tissue involved or via positive blood cultures [94].

Treatment

Treatment of NF includes early surgical debridement and broad-spectrum antimicrobial therapy [94]. Surgical intervention is the most important therapy for NF and has been directly linked with an increased mortality if delayed or inadequately performed [23, 289]. In many cases, serial debridements are required for complete source control [94].

Definitive trials regarding antimicrobial therapy in NF are lacking. Generally, empiric treatment involves broad-spectrum antibiotics against aerobic and anaerobic gram-positive and gram-negative organisms, including MRSA. One approach is combining an agent active against MRSA, such as vancomycin, linezolid, or dapto-mycin, with a broad-spectrum beta-lactam or carbapenem (e.g., piperacillin-tazobactam or meropenem). Finally, clindamycin should be added for toxin inhibition in the event of a GAS or clostridial infection [94]. In vitro studies have also shown that linezolid reduces streptococcal toxin production. Given its concomitant MRSA coverage and rising clindamycin resistance among MRSA, linezolid may be an appropriate option [296]. However, due to the lack of robust clinical evidence, the latest 2014 IDSA guidelines do not include linezolid as an "antitoxin antibiotic" option in the management of GAS or clostridial NSTI [94]. The use of intravenous immunoglobulin (IVIG) for all forms of necrotizing fasciitis is controversial [297]. Previous studies were underpowered and inconclusive [298–300].

Once a microbial etiology has been confirmed, antimicrobial therapy should be modified accordingly. The duration of treatment is ill defined; current guidelines recommend continuation of antimicrobials until there are no further debridements required and the patient has clinically improved [94].

29.7.5.2   Clostridial Myonecrosis

Classification and Microbiology

Clostridial myonecrosis, also known as gas gangrene, is most commonly caused by *Clostridium perfringens*, *Clostridium novyi*, *Clostridium histolyticum*, and *Clostridium septicum*. *Clostridium* species are spore-forming aerotolerant to anaerobic bacilli commonly found in soil, marine sediments, and intestinal tracts of humans and animals. Clostridial myonecrosis is characterized by a progressive destruction of deep soft tissues and muscle. Traumatic gas gangrene is associated with *Clostridium perfringens*, whereas spontaneous gas gangrene is associated with *Clostridium septicum* [94].

Clinical Presentation

After trauma, muscle damage and decreased blood supply result in poor oxygenation creating an ideal environment for the growth of anaerobic clostridia. Initial symptoms include severe pain at the site of injury. As clostridia multiply and release endotoxins, tissue necrosis can ensue [94, 301]. While the skin initially appears pale, it quickly develops a reddish-blue color and crepitus. Untreated, the disease can progress to shock and multisystem organ failure. Bacteremia occurs in 15% of cases and can be associated with intravascular hemolysis due to clostridial toxins [94]. In contrast, spontaneous (i.e., nontraumatic) gas gangrene develops most commonly from the more aerotolerant *Clostridium septicum*. Risk factors include neutropenia or gastrointestinal malignancy. It results from bacteremia followed by hematogenous seeding of normal soft tissue. Spontaneous gangrene progresses rapidly, and diagnosis may not be considered until systemic signs appear [302].

Treatment

Like NF, treatment consists of emergent surgical debridement and appropriate antibiotic therapy. Initially, broad-spectrum antimicrobials should be administered since organisms other than *Clostridia* can result in myonecrosis. Once diagnosis is established by culture or gram stain, antimicrobials can be narrowed to a combination of high-dose penicillin and clindamycin. While clindamycin is active against *Clostridium* species, it is not recommended as monotherapy due to concerns for clindamycin resistance in *Clostridium perfringens* [94, 290]. Like the treatment of GAS, clindamycin is used for its inhibition of clostridial toxin production. Hyperbaric oxygen (HBO) has also been described as an adjunctive therapy for clostridial myonecrosis given its activity against *Clostridium perfringens* and suppression of clostridial alpha-toxin production [303]. However, due to the lack of high-quality data, its use is controversial.

29.7.5.3 Toxic Shock Syndrome

TSS is a rapidly progressive disease associated with shock, organ failure, and a high fatality rate. *Staphylococcus aureus* may result in classical TSS, whereas GAS (*Streptococcus pyogenes*) causes STSS; we will focus on STSS. While STSS can accompany an infection at any site, it most often complicates streptococcal SSTI.

Clinical Presentation

STSS is associated with rapid-onset shock and organ failure. Other symptoms include fever or hypothermia and altered mental status [304]. Symptoms of the underlying invasive GAS infection can be present and include localized warmth, swelling, and erythema followed by sloughing of the skin. Deep infections, including necrotizing fasciitis or myonecrosis, can quickly develop. Additionally, multiorgan dysfunction can develop, including renal failure, liver dysfunction, coagulopathy, acute respiratory distress syndrome, and disseminated intravascular coagulopathy. Toxin-mediated hemolysis can result in myoglobinuria and hemoglobinuria, which further exacerbate renal failure. Laboratory testing can reveal leukocytosis, hypoalbuminemia due to capillary leak syndrome, and an elevated serum creatinine kinase. Blood cultures are positive in around 60% of the cases [305].

Treatment

Management of STSS involves management of septic shock, surgical debridement of the site of infection (if applicable), antimicrobial therapy, and IVIG. Close and coordinated collaboration between teams is essential for the effective management of STSS [306]. After identification of GAS on culture, antimicrobial therapy should be tailored to include a beta-lactam agent, typically intravenous penicillin G to disrupt cell wall synthesis and clindamycin for protein synthesis inhibition [307]. Studies have demonstrated increased morbidity and mortality with penicillin mono-therapy [307, 308]. Beta-lactams are most effective against rapidly growing bacte-ria; therefore, their activity may diminish as the bacterial growth rate slows due to the reduced expression of penicillin-binding proteins [309]. The addition of clindamycin is essential for suppression of bacterial toxin production, and its activ-ity is unaffected by the stage of bacterial growth or inoculum size. Lastly, clindamy-cin may suppress the synthesis of PBPs and has a more prolonged post-antibiotic effect compared to beta-lactam antibiotics [310].

Studies have also evaluated the use of IVIG for STSS. A 2018 meta-analysis of five studies that included patients with STSS treated with clindamycin demonstrated a reduction in 30-day mortality with IVIG [311]. The proposed mechanism of IVIG against STSS includes antigen neutralization, and different batches of IVIG may possess different neutralizing activities. Therefore, more than one dose of IVIG should be administered. The following IVIG dosing has been previously described: 1 g/kg on day 1, followed by 0.5 g/kg on days 2 and 3 [298, 311].

29.8 *Clostridioides difficile* Infection

29.8.1 Background

Despite successful efforts to reduce the burden of *Clostridioides difficile* infection (CDI), it remains the most common healthcare-associated infection in the United States with an estimated 235,000 healthcare-associated cases annually [33, 312–314]. CDI is especially prevalent in the intensive care unit (ICU): 5–15% of patients hospitalized with CDI require ICU admission [315–317] and 2–5% of ICU patients develop CDI during their admission [318–320]. CDI severe enough to require ICU admission is associated with significant adverse effects, including mor-tality between 20% and 40% and readmission rate of up to 30% [318–322]. Treatment is based on disease severity and number of recurrences [34, 323]. In addi-tion to standard therapy, which includes either fidaxomicin or vancomycin, there are several adjunct therapies (including fecal microbiota transplantation [FMT]) that may be beneficial in select patients and are discussed further below.

29.8.2 Pathogenesis

Although 10–30% of ICU patients are "colonized" with *C. difficile* (i.e., have asymptomatic intestinal carriage) [324, 325], only a small proportion develop clini-cal disease [318, 325]. While clinical disease may be due to ICU acquisition of toxigenic strains, recent evidence indicates that the disease is frequently caused by strains that were initially colonizing asymptomatically and became pathogenic during ICU admission [325, 326]. The transition from asymptomatic carriage to disease is mediated by decreased "colonization resistance" of the normal gut microbiome to *C. difficile*. Under normal conditions, the gut microbiome protects against *C. difficile* overgrowth, toxin production, and clinical disease. However, when faced with selective pressure that alters the gut microbiome, *C. difficile* may be able to expand and produce toxins (especially toxin B), resulting in clinical disease [327, 328]. Therefore, medications that cause gut microbiome dysbiosis—particularly antibiotics—are key in CDI pathogenesis. While clindamycin and fluoroquinolones are commonly assumed to confer the highest risk of CDI, these associations were found in early studies and analyses of outpatients [329–331]. Among hospitalized patients, a large meta-analysis demonstrated that several commonly used antibiotics, including third- and fourth-generation cephalosporins, beta-lactam/beta-lactamase inhibitor combinations, and carbapenems, additionally confer high risk for subsequent CDI development [332]. Further, there is a direct association between the number of antibiotics prescribed and CDI risk [333].

Aside from antibiotics, other medications including steroids may be associated with increased risk [334]. Proton pump inhibitors (PPIs) have a Food and Drug Administration (FDA) warning for increasing the risk of CDI [335]; however, a meta-analysis of randomized controlled trials of gastric acid-suppressing medications in the ICU did not show an increase in CDI among patients prescribed gastric acid suppression [336]. Because CDI generally develops in otherwise sick patients, several factors associated with critical illness and gut microbiome dysbiosis including age, end-stage renal disease, inflammatory bowel disease, and malignancy confer increased risk of CDI development [320, 334]. After CDI develops, similar patient characteristics place patients at increased risk for severe disease and mortality [337, 338].

29.8.3 *Diagnosis*

CDI diagnosis is based on laboratory testing in appropriately selected patients. Crucially, patients without diarrhea should not be tested as testing may detect patients with asymptomatic colonization who do not require treatment. Patients should only be tested if they have ≥3 loose stools in a 24-h period without receipt of stool softeners or laxatives within the prior 48 h [34]. Additional CDI signs and symptoms, including leukocytosis, are neither sensitive nor specific for CDI diagnosis [339]; aside from not testing patients without diarrhea or with recent laxative use, further patient selection for CDI testing is left to individual clinicians. The 2017 Infectious Diseases Society of America (IDSA)/Society for Healthcare Epidemiology of America (SHEA) guidelines recommend a two-step algorithm for CDI testing [34]. In most clinical microbiology laboratories, stools are initially tested by polymerase chain reaction (PCR) to determine the presence of *C. difficile* gene encoding for toxin. Since PCR is sensitive but does not distinguish colonization from clinical disease—even if the toxin-encoding gene is present, it may not be "active"—positive PCR tests should be followed by a test for the toxin itself, which increases the positive predictive value [34]. Several other testing methods, including culture and testing for *C. difficile* antigens, are either cumbersome or expensive and therefore not routinely employed in clinical practice.

Patients with fulminant CDI and toxic megacolon may not be able to provide stool samples for testing. Perirectal swabs may be PCR positive for *C. difficile* [340], but test characteristics are not well defined in fulminant infection, and this test is not routinely conducted. In these patients, diagnosis is based on clinical suspicion, which can be heightened due to patient risk factors, recent receipt of antibiotics, and critical illness. Cross-sectional imaging, generally using computed tomography (CT) of the abdomen and pelvis, may be performed to assess for intestinal inflammation and associated complications such as perforation and abscesses. The absence of these findings on CT argues strongly against CDI [341].

29.8.4   Treatment

Treatment of an initial CDI episode is determined by the illness severity criteria established by the IDSA/SHEA guidelines [34, 323]. Initial episodes of non-severe CDI (white blood cell count ≤15,000 cells/mL and creatinine <1.5 mg/dL) and severe CDI (white blood cell count >15,000 cells/mL or creatinine >1.5 mg/dL without evidence of fulminant disease) should be treated with fidaxomicin 200 mg orally twice daily for 10 days. Vancomycin 125 mg orally four times daily for 10 days is an acceptable alternative [323]. This recommendation is based on several clinical trials that demonstrated improvement in clinical cure rates and decrease in recurrent episodes with fidaxomicin compared to vancomycin [342–344]. Fidaxomicin uptake may be limited by cost [345]. Although oral metronidazole used to be the standard of care [346], several clinical trials have demonstrated its inferiority compared to vancomycin [347, 348], and metronidazole is now only recommended as an alternative for non-severe CDI when alternate agents are unavailable [323].

Although IDSA/SHEA guidelines have recommended fidaxomicin since 2021 for the treatment of non-fulminant disease, first-line therapy for fulminant CDI—defined as CDI with hypotension or shock, ileus, or megacolon—remains vancomycin at a higher dose than that recommended for non-fulminant CDI (500 mg four times daily) [323]. While fidaxomicin appears to be superior to vancomycin in severe CDI, clinical familiarity with vancomycin and lack of comparative data in fulminant disease led the IDSA/SHEA guidelines to continue endorsing vancomycin as the first-line agent in these cases [323, 344].

In addition to oral vancomycin, patients with ileus and/or toxic megacolon can be treated with rectal instillation of vancomycin (500 mg vancomycin in 100 mL of normal saline). Although there are theoretical concerns of rectal perforation with retention enemas during colonic inflammation, several studies (totaling over 100 patients) have not demonstrated this outcome [349–352]. In addition, intravenous (IV) metronidazole (500 mg every 8 h) should be added based on a retrospective cohort study that demonstrated lower mortality with metronidazole and vancomycin compared to vancomycin alone, although a subsequent study did not corroborate these findings [353, 354]. The recommendation for both rectal vancomycin and IV metronidazole is based on a theoretical concern for decreased colonic delivery of oral vancomycin in the presence of ileus [34].

Other therapies are not specifically recommended in fulminant CDI but may be considered in selected patients. FMT prevents recurrence in over 90% of cases of multiply recurrent CDI and is recommended for patients with at least two recurrences [34, 355]. Several retrospective cohort studies have demonstrated improved outcomes with FMT (including decreased mortality and need for colectomy) when used in severe and fulminant CDI [356–360]. Since 2022, the FDA has approved two microbiome-based therapeutics for recurrent CDI [361, 362]; their place in the armamentarium has not been established for recurrent CDI let alone severe/fulminant CDI.

In addition to FMT, surgery (either total abdominal colectomy or loop ileostomy with antegrade vancomycin flushes) may be considered for refractory cases [34, 363]. Decisions regarding patient selection and timing of FMT or surgery, as well as technical decisions regarding specific procedures performed, are nuanced and outside the scope of this discussion; involving gastroenterologists and surgeons early for patients not responding to initial therapy is crucial. Bezlotoxumab is a monoclonal antibody against toxin B that decreases the risk of recurrence and is recommended in patients with recurrent CDI; patients with severe disease may benefit from this treatment given that they are at higher risk of recurrence [323, 364].

29.8.5 Prevention

Systematic measures to decrease CDI transmission include single-occupancy rooms for CDI patients and strict adherence to contact precautions and handwashing [34]. For individual patients, the mainstay of CDI prevention is discontinuing unnecessary antibiotics as even short courses of antibiotics have been associated with CDI development [365]. Primary and secondary prophylaxis with oral vancomycin may be beneficial for patients at high risk for CDI, especially those who require systemic antibiotics [366–368]. Duration of either treatment or prophylaxis after completion of systemic antibiotics is undefined, although it is probably reasonable to continue CDI therapy for 2–7 days after systemic antibiotics are completed. The American College of Gastroenterology recommends against probiotics for CDI prophylaxis (both primary and secondary) given little evidence of benefit and potential for harm, including probiotic-associated bloodstream infection [368, 369].

References

1. Wunderlich C. On the temperature in diseases: a manual of medical thermometry. 2nd ed. London: The New Sydenham Society; 1871.
2. Protsiv M, Ley C, Lankester J, Hastie T, Parsonnet J. Decreasing human body temperature in the United States since the industrial revolution. elife. 2020;9:9. https://doi.org/10.7554/eLife.49555.
3. Mackowiak PA, Wasserman SS, Levine MM. A critical appraisal of 98.6 degrees F, the upper limit of the normal body temperature, and other legacies of Carl Reinhold August Wunderlich. JAMA. 1992;268(12):1578–80.
4. Obermeyer Z, Samra JK, Mullainathan S. Individual differences in normal body temperature: longitudinal big data analysis of patient records. BMJ. 2017;359:j5468. https://doi.org/10.1136/bmj.j5468.
5. Geneva II, Cuzzo B, Fazili T, Javaid W. Normal body temperature: a systematic review. Open Forum Infect Dis. 2019;6(4):ofz032. https://doi.org/10.1093/ofid/ofz032.
6. Mackowiak PA, Chervenak FA, Grunebaum A. Defining fever. Open Forum Infect Dis. 2021;8(6):ofab161. https://doi.org/10.1093/ofid/ofab161.
7. Garner JS, Jarvis WR, Emori TG, Horan TC, Hughes JM. CDC definitions for nosocomial infections, 1988. Am J Infect Control. 1988;16(3):128–40. https://doi.org/10.1016/0196-6553(88)90053-3.
8. O'Grady NP, Alexander E, Alhazzani W, Alshamsi F, Cuellar-Rodriguez J, Jefferson BK, et al. Society of Critical Care Medicine and the Infectious Diseases Society of America guidelines for evaluating new fever in adult patients in the ICU. Crit Care Med. 2023;51(11):1570–86. https://doi.org/10.1097/CCM.0000000000006022.
9. High KP, Bradley SF, Gravenstein S, Mehr DR, Quagliarello VJ, Richards C, et al. Clinical practice guideline for the evaluation of fever and infection in older adult residents of long-term care facilities: 2008 update by the Infectious Diseases Society of America. Clin Infect Dis. 2009;48(2):149–71. https://doi.org/10.1086/595683.
10. Filbin MR, Lynch J, Gillingham TD, Thorsen JE, Pasakarnis CL, Nepal S, et al. Presenting symptoms independently predict mortality in septic shock: importance of a previously unmeasured confounder. Crit Care Med. 2018;46(10):1592–9. https://doi.org/10.1097/CCM.0000000000003260.
11. Kaukonen KM, Bailey M, Pilcher D, Cooper DJ, Bellomo R. Systemic inflammatory response syndrome criteria in defining severe sepsis. N Engl J Med. 2015;372(17):1629–38. https://doi.org/10.1056/NEJMoa1415236.
12. Sakkat A, Alquraini M, Aljazeeri J, Farooqi MAM, Alshamsi F, Alhazzani W. Temperature control in critically ill patients with fever: a meta-analysis of randomized controlled trials. J Crit Care. 2021;61:89–95. https://doi.org/10.1016/j.jcrc.2020.10.016.
13. Young P, Saxena M, Bellomo R, Freebairn R, Hammond N, van Haren F, et al. Acetaminophen for fever in critically ill patients with suspected infection. N Engl J Med. 2015;373(23):2215–24. https://doi.org/10.1056/NEJMoa1508375.
14. Erickson RS, Kirklin SK. Comparison of ear-based, bladder, oral, and axillary methods for core temperature measurement. Crit Care Med. 1993;21(10):1528–34. https://doi.org/10.1097/00003246-199310000-00022.
15. Schmitz T, Bair N, Falk M, Levine C. A comparison of five methods of temperature measurement in febrile intensive care patients. Am J Crit Care. 1995;4(4):286–92.
16. Niven DJ, Gaudet JE, Laupland KB, Mrklas KJ, Roberts DJ, Stelfox HT. Accuracy of peripheral thermometers for estimating temperature: a systematic review and meta-analysis. Ann Intern Med. 2015;163(10):768–77. https://doi.org/10.7326/M15-1150.
17. Cutuli SL, See EJ, Osawa EA, Ancona P, Marshall D, Eastwood GM, et al. Accuracy of non-invasive body temperature measurement methods in adult patients admitted to the intensive care unit: a systematic review and meta-analysis. Crit Care Resusc. 2021;23(1):6–13. https://doi.org/10.51893/2021.1.SR1.

18. Vincent JL, Bihari DJ, Suter PM, Bruining HA, White J, Nicolas-Chanoin MH, et al. The prevalence of nosocomial infection in intensive care units in Europe. Results of the European Prevalence of Infection in Intensive Care (EPIC) Study. EPIC International Advisory Committee. JAMA. 1995;274(8):639–44.

19. Vincent JL, Rello J, Marshall J, Silva E, Anzueto A, Martin CD, et al. International study of the prevalence and outcomes of infection in intensive care units. JAMA. 2009;302(21):2323–9. https://doi.org/10.1001/jama.2009.1754.

20. Vincent JL, Sakr Y, Singer M, Martin-Loeches I, Machado FR, Marshall JC, et al. Prevalence and outcomes of infection among patients in intensive care units in 2017. JAMA. 2020;323(15):1478–87. https://doi.org/10.1001/jama.2020.2717.

21. Kumar A, Roberts D, Wood KE, Light B, Parrillo JE, Sharma S, et al. Duration of hypotension before initiation of effective antimicrobial therapy is the critical determinant of survival in human septic shock. Crit Care Med. 2006;34(6):1589–96. https://doi.org/10.1097/01. CCM.0000217961.75225.E9.

22. Pak TR, Young J, McKenna CS, Agan A, DelloStritto L, Filbin MR, et al. Risk of misleading conclusions in observational studies of time-to-antibiotics and mortality in suspected sepsis. Clin Infect Dis. 2023;77(11):1534–43. https://doi.org/10.1093/cid/ciad450.

23. Reitz KM, Kennedy J, Li SR, Handzel R, Tonetti DA, Neal MD, et al. Association between time to source control in sepsis and 90-day mortality. JAMA Surg. 2022;157(9):817–26. https://doi.org/10.1001/jamasurg.2022.2761.

24. Metersky ML, Wang Y, Klompas M, Eckenrode S, Bakullari A, Eldridge N. Trend in ventilator-associated pneumonia rates between 2005 and 2013. JAMA. 2016;316(22):2427–9. https://doi.org/10.1001/jama.2016.16226.

25. Johnstone J, Muscedere J, Dionne J, Duan E, Rochwerg B, Centofanti J, et al. Definitions, rates and associated mortality of ICU-acquired pneumonia: a multicenter cohort study. J Crit Care. 2023;75:154284. https://doi.org/10.1016/j.jcrc.2023.154284.

26. Ehrmann S, Barbier F, Demiselle J, Quenot JP, Herbrecht JE, Roux D, et al. Inhaled amikacin to prevent ventilator-associated pneumonia. N Engl J Med. 2023;389(22):2052–62. https://doi.org/10.1056/NEJMoa2310307.

27. Kalil AC, Metersky ML, Klompas M, Muscedere J, Sweeney DA, Palmer LB, et al. Management of adults with hospital-acquired and ventilator-associated pneumonia: 2016 clinical practice guidelines by the Infectious Diseases Society of America and the American Thoracic Society. Clin Infect Dis. 2016;63(5):e61–111. https://doi.org/10.1093/cid/ciw353.

28. Mermel LA, Allon M, Bouza E, Craven DE, Flynn P, O'Grady NP, et al. Clinical practice guidelines for the diagnosis and management of intravascular catheter-related infection: 2009 update by the Infectious Diseases Society of America. Clin Infect Dis. 2009;49(1):1–45. https://doi.org/10.1086/599376.

29. Tunkel AR, Hasbun R, Bhimraj A, Byers K, Kaplan SL, Scheld WM, et al. 2017 Infectious Diseases Society of America's clinical practice guidelines for healthcare-associated ventriculitis and meningitis. Clin Infect Dis. 2017;64(6):e34–65. https://doi.org/10.1093/cid/ciw861.

30. Hooton TM, Bradley SF, Cardenas DD, Colgan R, Geerlings SE, Rice JC, et al. Diagnosis, prevention, and treatment of catheter-associated urinary tract infection in adults: 2009 international clinical practice guidelines from the Infectious Diseases Society of America. Clin Infect Dis. 2010;50(5):625–63. https://doi.org/10.1086/650482.

31. Marsh N, Larsen EN, Ullman AJ, Mihala G, Cooke M, Chopra V, et al. Peripheral intravenous catheter infection and failure: a systematic review and meta-analysis. Int J Nurs Stud. 2024;151:104673. https://doi.org/10.1016/j.ijnurstu.2023.104673.

32. GlobalSurg Collaborative. Surgical site infection after gastrointestinal surgery in high-income, middle-income, and low-income countries: a prospective, international, multicentre cohort study. Lancet Infect Dis. 2018;18(5):516–25. https://doi.org/10.1016/S1473-3099(18)30101-4.

33. Magill SS, O'Leary E, Janelle SJ, Thompson DL, Dumyati G, Nadle J, et al. Changes in prevalence of health care-associated infections in U.S. Hospitals. N Engl J Med. 2018;379(18):1732–44. https://doi.org/10.1056/NEJMoa1801550.

34. McDonald LC, Gerding DN, Johnson S, Bakken JS, Carroll KC, Coffin SE, et al. Clinical practice guidelines for Clostridium difficile infection in adults and children: 2017 update by the Infectious Diseases Society of America (IDSA) and Society for Healthcare Epidemiology of America (SHEA). Clin Infect Dis. 2018;66(7):e1–48. https://doi.org/10.1093/cid/cix1085.
35. Huffman JL, Schenker S. Acute acalculous cholecystitis: a review. Clin Gastroenterol Hepatol. 2010;8(1):15–22. https://doi.org/10.1016/j.cgh.2009.08.034.
36. Niven DJ, Laupland KB. Pyrexia: aetiology in the ICU. Crit Care. 2016;20(1):247. https://doi.org/10.1186/s13054-016-1406-2.
37. Kushimoto S, Yamanouchi S, Endo T, Sato T, Nomura R, Fujita M, et al. Body temperature abnormalities in non-neurological critically ill patients: a review of the literature. J Intensive Care. 2014;2(1):14. https://doi.org/10.1186/2052-0492-2-14.
38. Musher DM, Fainstein V, Young EJ, Pruett TL. Fever patterns. Their lack of clinical significance. Arch Intern Med. 1979;139(11):1225–8. https://doi.org/10.1001/archinte.139.11.1225.
39. Stein PD, Beemath A, Matta F, Weg JG, Yusen RD, Hales CA, et al. Clinical characteristics of patients with acute pulmonary embolism: data from PIOPED II. Am J Med. 2007;120(10):871–9. https://doi.org/10.1016/j.amjmed.2007.03.024.
40. Saad M, Shaikh DH, Mantri N, Alemam A, Zhang A, Adrish M. Fever is associated with higher morbidity and clot burden in patients with acute pulmonary embolism. BMJ Open Respir Res. 2018;5(1):e000327. https://doi.org/10.1136/bmjresp-2018-000327.
41. Lofmark R, Nordlander R, Orinius E. The temperature course in acute myocardial infarction. Am Heart J. 1978;96(2):153–6. https://doi.org/10.1016/0002-8703(78)90078-9.
42. Kazmers A, Groehn H, Meeker C. Do patients with acute deep vein thrombosis have fever? Am Surg. 2000;66(6):598–601.
43. Shenker Y, Skatrud JB. Adrenal insufficiency in critically ill patients. Am J Respir Crit Care Med. 2001;163(7):1520–3. https://doi.org/10.1164/ajrccm.163.7.2012022.
44. Bourcier S, Coutrot M, Ferre A, Van Grunderbeeck N, Charpentier J, Hraiech S, et al. Critically ill severe hypothyroidism: a retrospective multicenter cohort study. Ann Intensive Care. 2023;13(1):15. https://doi.org/10.1186/s13613-023-01112-1.
45. Fajgenbaum DC, June CH. Cytokine storm. N Engl J Med. 2020;383(23):2255–73. https://doi.org/10.1056/NEJMra2026131.
46. Sanz MA, Montesinos P. How we prevent and treat differentiation syndrome in patients with acute promyelocytic leukemia. Blood. 2014;123(18):2777–82. https://doi.org/10.1182/blood-2013-10-512640.
47. Grim SA, Romanelli F, Jennings PR, Ofotokun I. Late-onset drug fever associated with minocycline: case report and review of the literature. Pharmacotherapy. 2003;23(12):1659–62. https://doi.org/10.1592/phco.23.15.1659.31966.
48. Mackowiak PA, LeMaistre CF. Drug fever: a critical appraisal of conventional concepts. An analysis of 51 episodes in two Dallas hospitals and 97 episodes reported in the English literature. Ann Intern Med. 1987;106(5):728–33. https://doi.org/10.7326/0003-4819-106-5-728.
49. Oizumi K, Onuma K, Watanabe A, Motomiya M. Clinical study of drug fever induced by parenteral administration of antibiotics. Tohoku J Exp Med. 1989;159(1):45–56. https://doi.org/10.1620/tjem.159.45.
50. Hu Y, Han J, Gao L, Liu S, Wang H. Drug fever induced by antibiotics of beta-lactams in a patient after posterior cervical spine surgery-a case report and literature review. Front Surg. 2022;9:1065106. https://doi.org/10.3389/fsurg.2022.1065106.
51. Rabinstein AA, Sandhu K. Non-infectious fever in the neurological intensive care unit: incidence, causes and predictors. J Neurol Neurosurg Psychiatry. 2007;78(11):1278–80. https://doi.org/10.1136/jnnp.2006.112730.
52. Georgilis K, Plomaritoglou A, Dafni U, Bassiakos Y, Vemmos K. Aetiology of fever in patients with acute stroke. J Intern Med. 1999;246(2):203–9. https://doi.org/10.1046/j.1365-2796.1999.00539.x.
53. Adams SH, Myszewski J. Hematoma as a cause of a febrile and inflammatory response after tibial fractures. Proc (Bayl Univ Med Cent). 2020;33(4):677–8. https://doi.org/10.1080/08998280.2020.1783750.

54. Foggo V, Cavenagh J. Malignant causes of fever of unknown origin. Clin Med (Lond). 2015;15(3):292–4. https://doi.org/10.7861/clinmedicine.15-3-292.

55. Hechtman RK, Kipnis P, Cano J, Seelye S, Liu VX, Prescott HC. Heterogeneity of benefit from earlier time-to-antibiotics for sepsis. Am J Respir Crit Care Med. 2024;209:852. https://doi.org/10.1164/rccm.202310-1800OC.

56. Simons KS, Pickkers P, Bleeker-Rovers CP, Oyen WJ, van der Hoeven JG. F-18-fluorodeoxyglucose positron emission tomography combined with CT in critically ill patients with suspected infection. Intensive Care Med. 2010;36(3):504–11. https://doi.org/10.1007/s00134-009-1697-8.

57. Huang CK, Huang JY, Ruan SY, Chien KL. Diagnostic performance of FDG PET/CT in critically ill patients with suspected infection: a systematic review and meta-analysis. J Formos Med Assoc. 2020;119(5):941–9. https://doi.org/10.1016/j.jfma.2019.09.010.

58. Wirz Y, Meier MA, Bouadma L, Luyt CE, Wolff M, Chastre J, et al. Effect of procalcitonin-guided antibiotic treatment on clinical outcomes in intensive care unit patients with infection and sepsis patients: a patient-level meta-analysis of randomized trials. Crit Care. 2018;22(1):191. https://doi.org/10.1186/s13054-018-2125-7.

59. Huang DT, Yealy DM, Filbin MR, Brown AM, Chang CH, Doi Y, et al. Procalcitonin-guided use of antibiotics for lower respiratory tract infection. N Engl J Med. 2018;379(3):236–49. https://doi.org/10.1056/NEJMoa1802670.

60. Schuetz P, Wirz Y, Sager R, Christ-Crain M, Stolz D, Tamm M, et al. Effect of procalcitonin-guided antibiotic treatment on mortality in acute respiratory infections: a patient level meta-analysis. Lancet Infect Dis. 2018;18(1):95–107. https://doi.org/10.1016/S1473-3099(17)30592-3.

61. Evans L, Rhodes A, Alhazzani W, Antonelli M, Coopersmith CM, French C, et al. Surviving sepsis campaign: international guidelines for management of sepsis and septic shock 2021. Crit Care Med. 2021;49(11):e1063–143. https://doi.org/10.1097/CCM.0000000000005337.

62. Singer M, Deutschman CS, Seymour CW, Shankar-Hari M, Annane D, Bauer M, et al. The third international consensus definitions for sepsis and septic shock (sepsis-3). JAMA. 2016;315(8):801–10. https://doi.org/10.1001/jama.2016.0287.

63. Prest J, Nguyen T, Rajah T, Prest AB, Sathananthan M, Jeganathan N. Sepsis-related mortality rates and trends based on site of infection. Crit Care Explor. 2022;4(10):e0775. https://doi.org/10.1097/CCE.0000000000000775.

64. Rhee C, Dantes R, Epstein L, Murphy DJ, Seymour CW, Iwashyna TJ, et al. Incidence and trends of sepsis in US hospitals using clinical vs claims data, 2009-2014. JAMA. 2017;318(13):1241–9. https://doi.org/10.1001/jama.2017.13836.

65. Rudd KE, Johnson SC, Agesa KM, Shackelford KA, Tsoi D, Kievlan DR, et al. Global, regional, and national sepsis incidence and mortality, 1990-2017: analysis for the Global Burden of Disease Study. Lancet. 2020;395(10219):200–11. https://doi.org/10.1016/S0140-6736(19)32989-7.

66. Sakr Y, Jaschinski U, Wittebole X, Szakmany T, Lipman J, Namendys-Silva SA, et al. Sepsis in intensive care unit patients: worldwide data from the intensive care over nations audit. Open Forum Infect Dis. 2018;5(12):ofy313. https://doi.org/10.1093/ofid/ofy313.

67. Shappell CN, Klompas M, Ochoa A, Rhee C, CDC Prevention Epicenters Program. Likelihood of bacterial infection in patients treated with broad-spectrum IV antibiotics in the emergency department. Crit Care Med. 2021;49(11):e1144–50. https://doi.org/10.1097/CCM.0000000000005090.

68. Hooper GA, Klippel CJ, McLean SR, Stenehjem EA, Webb BJ, Murnin ER, et al. Concordance between initial presumptive and final adjudicated diagnoses of infection among patients meeting sepsis-3 criteria in the emergency department. Clin Infect Dis. 2023;76(12):2047–55. https://doi.org/10.1093/cid/ciad101.

69. Lelubre C, Vincent JL. Mechanisms and treatment of organ failure in sepsis. Nat Rev Nephrol. 2018;14(7):417–27. https://doi.org/10.1038/s41581-018-0005-7.

70. Bone RC, Balk RA, Cerra FB, Dellinger RP, Fein AM, Knaus WA, et al. Definitions for sepsis and organ failure and guidelines for the use of innovative therapies in sepsis. The ACCP/SCCM Consensus Conference Committee. American College of Chest Physicians/ Society of Critical Care Medicine. Chest. 1992;101(6):1644–55. https://doi.org/10.1378/chest.101.6.1644.
71. Subbe CP, Kruger M, Rutherford P, Gemmel L. Validation of a modified early warning score in medical admissions. QJM. 2001;94(10):521–6. https://doi.org/10.1093/qjmed/94.10.521.
72. Liu VX, Lu Y, Carey KA, Gilbert ER, Afshar M, Akel M, et al. Comparison of early warning scoring systems for hospitalized patients with and without infection at risk for in-hospital mortality and transfer to the intensive care unit. JAMA Netw Open. 2020;3(5):e205191. https://doi.org/10.1001/jamanetworkopen.2020.5191.
73. Churpek MM, Snyder A, Han X, Sokol S, Pettit N, Howell MD, et al. Quick sepsis-related organ failure assessment, systemic inflammatory response syndrome, and early warning scores for detecting clinical deterioration in infected patients outside the intensive care unit. Am J Respir Crit Care Med. 2017;195(7):906–11. https://doi.org/10.1164/rccm.201604-0854OC.
74. Qiu X, Lei YP, Zhou RX. SIRS, SOFA, qSOFA, and NEWS in the diagnosis of sepsis and prediction of adverse outcomes: a systematic review and meta-analysis. Expert Rev Anti-Infect Ther. 2023;21(8):891–900. https://doi.org/10.1080/14787210.2023.2237192.
75. Cavallazzi R, Bennin CL, Hirani A, Gilbert C, Marik PE. Is the band count useful in the diagnosis of infection? An accuracy study in critically ill patients. J Intensive Care Med. 2010;25(6):353–7. https://doi.org/10.1177/0885066610377980.
76. Buyuksirin M, Anar C, Polat G, Karadeniz G. Can the level of CRP in acute pulmonary embolism determine early mortality? Turk Thorac J. 2021;22(1):4–10. https://doi.org/10.5152/TurkThoracJ.2020.19048.
77. Povoa P, Coelho L, Almeida E, Fernandes A, Mealha R, Moreira P, et al. C-reactive protein as a marker of infection in critically ill patients. Clin Microbiol Infect. 2005;11(2):101–8. https://doi.org/10.1111/j.1469-0691.2004.01044.x.
78. Self WH, Balk RA, Grijalva CG, Williams DJ, Zhu Y, Anderson EJ, et al. Procalcitonin as a marker of etiology in adults hospitalized with community-acquired pneumonia. Clin Infect Dis. 2017;65(2):183–90. https://doi.org/10.1093/cid/cix317.
79. Hoeboer SH, van der Geest PJ, Nieboer D, Groeneveld AB. The diagnostic accuracy of procalcitonin for bacteraemia: a systematic review and meta-analysis. Clin Microbiol Infect. 2015;21(5):474–81. https://doi.org/10.1016/j.cmi.2014.12.026.
80. Miller RR 3rd, Lopansri BK, Burke JP, Levy M, Opal S, Rothman RE, et al. Validation of a host response assay, SeptiCyte LAB, for discriminating sepsis from systemic inflammatory response syndrome in the ICU. Am J Respir Crit Care Med. 2018;198(7):903–13. https://doi.org/10.1164/rccm.201712-2472OC.
81. Denny KJ, Lea RA, Lindell-Innes R, Haupt LM, Heffernan AJ, Harvey NR, et al. Diagnosing sepsis in the ICU: comparison of a gene expression signature to pre-existing biomarkers. J Crit Care. 2023;76:154286. https://doi.org/10.1016/j.jcrc.2023.154286.
82. Klein Klouwenberg PM, Cremer OL, van Vught LA, Ong DS, Frencken JF, Schultz MJ, et al. Likelihood of infection in patients with presumed sepsis at the time of intensive care unit admission: a cohort study. Crit Care. 2015;19(1):319. https://doi.org/10.1186/s13054-015-1035-1.
83. Seymour CW, Gesten F, Prescott HC, Friedrich ME, Iwashyna TJ, Phillips GS, et al. Time to treatment and mortality during mandated emergency care for sepsis. N Engl J Med. 2017;376(23):2235–44. https://doi.org/10.1056/NEJMoa1703058.
84. Liu VX, Fielding-Singh V, Greene JD, Baker JM, Iwashyna TJ, Bhattacharya J, et al. The timing of early antibiotics and hospital mortality in sepsis. Am J Respir Crit Care Med. 2017;196(7):856–63. https://doi.org/10.1164/rccm.201609-1848OC.
85. Taylor SP, Kowalkowski MA, Skewes S, Chou SH. Real-world implications of updated surviving sepsis campaign antibiotic timing recommendations. Crit Care Med. 2024;52:1002. https://doi.org/10.1097/CCM.0000000000006240.

86. Logan LK, Weinstein RA. The epidemiology of carbapenem-resistant enterobacteriaceae: the impact and evolution of a global menace. J Infect Dis. 2017;215(Suppl_1):S28–36. https://doi.org/10.1093/infdis/jiw282.

87. Perez-Galera S, Bravo-Ferrer JM, Paniagua M, Kostyanev T, de Kraker MEA, Feifel J, et al. Risk factors for infections caused by carbapenem-resistant Enterobacterales: an international matched case-control-control study (EURECA). EClinicalMedicine. 2023;57:101871. https://doi.org/10.1016/j.eclinm.2023.101871.

88. Vance MK, Cretella DA, Ward LM, Vijayvargiya P, Garrigos ZE, Wingler MJB. Risk factors for bloodstream infections due to ESBL-producing Escherichia coli, Klebsiella spp., and Proteus mirabilis. Pharmacy (Basel). 2023;11(2) https://doi.org/10.3390/pharmacy11020074.

89. Goyal D, Dean N, Neill S, Jones P, Dascomb K. Risk factors for community-acquired extended-spectrum beta-lactamase-producing enterobacteriaceae infections-a retrospective study of symptomatic urinary tract infections. Open Forum Infect Dis. 2019;6(2):ofy357. https://doi.org/10.1093/ofid/ofy357.

90. Tian X, Sun S, Jia X, Zou H, Li S, Zhang L. Epidemiology of and risk factors for infection with extended-spectrum beta-lactamase-producing carbapenem-resistant Enterobacteriaceae: results of a double case-control study. Infect Drug Resist. 2018;11:1339–46. https://doi.org/10.2147/IDR.S173456.

91. Rhee C, Kadri SS, Dekker JP, Danner RL, Chen HC, Fram D, et al. Prevalence of antibiotic-resistant pathogens in culture-proven sepsis and outcomes associated with inadequate and broad-spectrum empiric antibiotic use. JAMA Netw Open. 2020;3(4):e202899. https://doi.org/10.1001/jamanetworkopen.2020.2899.

92. Strich JR, Heil EL, Masur H. Considerations for empiric antimicrobial therapy in sepsis and septic shock in an era of antimicrobial resistance. J Infect Dis. 2020;222(Suppl 2):S119–31. https://doi.org/10.1093/infdis/jiaa221.

93. Metlay JP, Waterer GW, Long AC, Anzueto A, Brozek J, Crothers K, et al. Diagnosis and treatment of adults with community-acquired pneumonia. An official clinical practice guideline of the American Thoracic Society and Infectious Diseases Society of America. Am J Respir Crit Care Med. 2019;200(7):e45–67. https://doi.org/10.1164/rccm.201908-1581ST.

94. Stevens DL, Bisno AL, Chambers HF, Dellinger EP, Goldstein EJ, Gorbach SL, et al. Practice guidelines for the diagnosis and management of skin and soft tissue infections: 2014 update by the Infectious Diseases Society of America. Clin Infect Dis. 2014;59(2):e10–52. https://doi.org/10.1093/cid/ciu444.

95. Senneville E, Albalawi Z, van Asten SA, Abbas ZG, Allison G, Aragon-Sanchez J, et al. IWGDF/IDSA guidelines on the diagnosis and treatment of diabetes-related foot infections (IWGDF/IDSA 2023). Diabetes Metab Res Rev. 2023;40:e3687. https://doi.org/10.1002/dmrr.3687.

96. Solomkin JS, Mazuski JE, Bradley JS, Rodvold KA, Goldstein EJ, Baron EJ, et al. Diagnosis and management of complicated intra-abdominal infection in adults and children: guidelines by the Surgical Infection Society and the Infectious Diseases Society of America. Surg Infect. 2010;11(1):79–109. https://doi.org/10.1089/sur.2009.9930.

97. Gupta K, Hooton TM, Naber KG, Wullt B, Colgan R, Miller LG, et al. International clinical practice guidelines for the treatment of acute uncomplicated cystitis and pyelonephritis in women: a 2010 update by the Infectious Diseases Society of America and the European Society for Microbiology and Infectious Diseases. Clin Infect Dis. 2011;52(5):e103–20. https://doi.org/10.1093/cid/ciq257.

98. Timsit JF, Azoulay E, Schwebel C, Charles PE, Cornet M, Souweine B, et al. Empirical micafungin treatment and survival without invasive fungal infection in adults with ICU-acquired sepsis, Candida colonization, and multiple organ failure: the EMPIRICUS randomized clinical trial. JAMA. 2016;316(15):1555–64. https://doi.org/10.1001/jama.2016.14655.

99. Tang Y, Hu W, Jiang S, Xie M, Zhu W, Zhang L, et al. Effect of empirical antifungal treatment on mortality in non-neutropenic critically ill patients: a propensity-matched retrospective cohort study. Eur J Clin Microbiol Infect Dis. 2022;41(12):1421–32. https://doi.org/10.1007/s10096-022-04507-3.

100. Lodise TP, Lomaestro BM, Drusano GL, Society of Infectious Diseases Pharmacists. Application of antimicrobial pharmacodynamic concepts into clinical practice: focus on beta-lactam antibiotics: insights from the Society of Infectious Diseases Pharmacists. Pharmacotherapy. 2006;26(9):1320–32. https://doi.org/10.1592/phco.26.9.1320.
101. Li X, Long Y, Wu G, Li R, Zhou M, He A, et al. Prolonged vs intermittent intravenous infusion of beta-lactam antibiotics for patients with sepsis: a systematic review of randomized clinical trials with meta-analysis and trial sequential analysis. Ann Intensive Care. 2023;13(1):121. https://doi.org/10.1186/s13613-023-01222-w.
102. Phe K, Heil EL, Tam VH. Optimizing pharmacokinetics-pharmacodynamics of antimicrobial management in patients with sepsis: a review. J Infect Dis. 2020;222(Suppl 2):S132–41. https://doi.org/10.1093/infdis/jiaa118.
103. Fink MP. Adequacy of gut oxygenation in endotoxemia and sepsis. Crit Care Med. 1993;21(2 Suppl):S4–8. https://doi.org/10.1097/00003246-199302001-00002.
104. Chen IH, Nicolau DP. Augmented renal clearance and how to augment antibiotic dosing. Antibiotics (Basel). 2020;9(7) https://doi.org/10.3390/antibiotics9070393.
105. Climo M, Diekema D, Warren DK, Herwaldt LA, Perl TM, Peterson L, et al. Prevalence of the use of central venous access devices within and outside of the intensive care unit: results of a survey among hospitals in the prevention epicenter program of the Centers for Disease Control and Prevention. Infect Control Hosp Epidemiol. 2003;24(12):942–5. https://doi.org/10.1086/502163.
106. Kolikof J, Peterson K, Baker AM. Central venous catheter. Treasure Island, FL: StatPearls; 2024.
107. Warren DK, Quadir WW, Hollenbeak CS, Elward AM, Cox MJ, Fraser VJ. Attributable cost of catheter-associated bloodstream infections among intensive care patients in a nonteaching hospital. Crit Care Med. 2006;34(8):2084–9. https://doi.org/10.1097/01.CCM.0000227648.15804.2D.
108. NHSN. Bloodstream infection event (central line-associated bloodstream infection and non-central line associated bloodstream infection). 2024. https://www.cdc.gov/nhsn/pdfs/pscmanual/4psc_clabscurrent.pdf. Accessed 7 Mar 2024
109. Gahlot R, Nigam C, Kumar V, Yadav G, Anupurba S. Catheter-related bloodstream infections. Int J Crit Illn Inj Sci. 2014;4(2):162–7. https://doi.org/10.4103/2229-5151.134184.
110. Buetti N, Ruckly S, Lucet JC, Bouadma L, Garrouste-Orgeas M, Schwebel C, et al. Local signs at insertion site and catheter-related bloodstream infections: an observational post hoc analysis using individual data of four RCTs. Crit Care. 2020;24(1):694. https://doi.org/10.1186/s13054-020-03425-0.
111. Herc E, Patel P, Washer LL, Conlon A, Flanders SA, Chopra V. A model to predict central-line-associated bloodstream infection among patients with peripherally inserted central catheters: the MPC score. Infect Control Hosp Epidemiol. 2017;38(10):1155–66. https://doi.org/10.1017/ice.2017.167.
112. Ishizuka M, Nagata H, Takagi K, Kubota K. Total parenteral nutrition is a major risk factor for central venous catheter-related bloodstream infection in colorectal cancer patients receiving postoperative chemotherapy. Eur Surg Res. 2008;41(4):341–5. https://doi.org/10.1159/000160181.
113. Baxi SM, Shuman EK, Scipione CA, Chen B, Sharma A, Rasanathan JJ, et al. Impact of postplacement adjustment of peripherally inserted central catheters on the risk of bloodstream infection and venous thrombus formation. Infect Control Hosp Epidemiol. 2013;34(8):785–92. https://doi.org/10.1086/671266.
114. Hajjej Z, Nasri M, Sellami W, Gharsallah H, Labben I, Ferjani M. Incidence, risk factors and microbiology of central vascular catheter-related bloodstream infection in an intensive care unit. J Infect Chemother. 2014;20(3):163–8. https://doi.org/10.1016/j.jiac.2013.08.001.
115. Parienti JJ, Mongardon N, Megarbane B, Mira JP, Kalfon P, Gros A, et al. Intravascular complications of central venous catheterization by insertion site. N Engl J Med. 2015;373(13):1220–9. https://doi.org/10.1056/NEJMoa1500964.

116. Vats HS. Complications of catheters: tunneled and nontunneled. Adv Chronic Kidney Dis. 2012;19(3):188–94. https://doi.org/10.1053/j.ackd.2012.04.004.

117. Novosad SA, Fike L, Dudeck MA, Allen-Bridson K, Edwards JR, Edens C, et al. Pathogens causing central-line-associated bloodstream infections in acute-care hospitals-United States, 2011-2017. Infect Control Hosp Epidemiol. 2020;41(3):313–9. https://doi.org/10.1017/ice.2019.303.

118. O'Grady NP. Prevention of central line-associated bloodstream infections. N Engl J Med. 2023;389(12):1121–31. https://doi.org/10.1056/NEJMra2213296.

119. Wichmann D, Belmar Campos CE, Ehrhardt S, Kock T, Weber C, Rohde H, et al. Efficacy of introducing a checklist to reduce central venous line associated bloodstream infections in the ICU caring for adult patients. BMC Infect Dis. 2018;18(1):267. https://doi.org/10.1186/s12879-018-3178-6.

120. Yasuda H, Sanui M, Abe T, Shime N, Komuro T, Hatakeyama J, et al. Comparison of the efficacy of three topical antiseptic solutions for the prevention of catheter colonization: a multicenter randomized controlled study. Crit Care. 2017;21(1):320. https://doi.org/10.1186/s13054-017-1890-z.

121. Surapat B, Montakantikul P, Malathum K, Kiertiburanakul S, Santanirand P, Chindavijak B. Microbial epidemiology and risk factors for relapse in gram-negative bacteria catheter-related bloodstream infection with a pilot prospective study in patients with catheter removal receiving short-duration of antibiotic therapy. BMC Infect Dis. 2020;20(1):604. https://doi.org/10.1186/s12879-020-05312-z.

122. Liu C, Bayer A, Cosgrove SE, Daum RS, Fridkin SK, Gorwitz RJ, et al. Clinical practice guidelines by the Infectious Diseases Society of America for the treatment of methicillin-resistant Staphylococcus aureus infections in adults and children. Clin Infect Dis. 2011;52(3):e18–55. https://doi.org/10.1093/cid/ciq146.

123. Westgeest AC, Buis DTP, Sigaloff KCE, Ruffin F, Visser LG, Yu Y, et al. Global differences in the management of Staphylococcus aureus bacteremia: no international standard of care. Clin Infect Dis. 2023;77(8):1092–101. https://doi.org/10.1093/cid/ciad363.

124. Wilcox MH, Tack KJ, Bouza E, Herr DL, Ruf BR, Ijzerman MM, et al. Complicated skin and skin-structure infections and catheter-related bloodstream infections: noninferiority of linezolid in a phase 3 study. Clin Infect Dis. 2009;48(2):203–12. https://doi.org/10.1086/595686.

125. Maraolo AE, Giaccone A, Gentile I, Saracino A, Bavaro DF. Daptomycin versus vancomycin for the treatment of methicillin-resistant Staphylococcus aureus bloodstream infection with or without endocarditis: a systematic review and meta-analysis. Antibiotics (Basel). 2021;10(8) https://doi.org/10.3390/antibiotics10081014.

126. Samura M, Kitahiro Y, Tashiro S, Moriyama H, Hamamura Y, Takahata I, et al. Efficacy and safety of Daptomycin versus vancomycin for bacteremia caused by methicillin-resistant Staphylococcus aureus with vancomycin minimum inhibitory concentration >1 microg/mL: a systematic review and meta-analysis. Pharmaceutics. 2022;14(4) https://doi.org/10.3390/pharmaceutics14040714.

127. Lam JC, Stokes W. The Golden grapes of wrath—Staphylococcus aureus bacteremia: a clinical review. Am J Med. 2023;136(1):19–26. https://doi.org/10.1016/j.amjmed.2022.09.017.

128. McDanel JS, Perencevich EN, Diekema DJ, Herwaldt LA, Smith TC, Chrischilles EA, et al. Comparative effectiveness of beta-lactams versus vancomycin for treatment of methicillin-susceptible Staphylococcus aureus bloodstream infections among 122 hospitals. Clin Infect Dis. 2015;61(3):361–7. https://doi.org/10.1093/cid/civ308.

129. Britt NS, Potter EM, Patel N, Steed ME. Comparative effectiveness and safety of standard-, medium-, and high-dose daptomycin strategies for the treatment of vancomycin-resistant enterococcal bacteremia among veterans affairs patients. Clin Infect Dis. 2017;64(5):605–13. https://doi.org/10.1093/cid/ciw815.

130. Chuang YC, Lin HY, Chen PY, Lin CY, Wang JT, Chang SC. Daptomycin versus linezolid for the treatment of vancomycin-resistant enterococcal bacteraemia: implications of

daptomycin dose. Clin Microbiol Infect. 2016;22(10):890.e1–7. https://doi.org/10.1016/j.
cmi.2016.07.018.

131. Hanna H, Afif C, Alakech B, Boktour M, Tarrand J, Hachem R, et al. Central venous catheter-related bacteremia due to gram-negative bacilli: significance of catheter removal in preventing relapse. Infect Control Hosp Epidemiol. 2004;25(8):646–9. https://doi.org/10.1086/502455.

132. Lee YM, Moon C, Kim YJ, Lee HJ, Lee MS, Park KH. Clinical impact of delayed catheter removal for patients with central-venous-catheter-related Gram-negative bacteraemia. J Hosp Infect. 2018;99(1):106–13. https://doi.org/10.1016/j.jhin.2018.01.004.

133. San-Juan R, Ruiz-Ruigomez M, Aguado JM. How to manage central venous catheter-related bloodstream infections due to Gram-negative bacilli? Curr Opin Infect Dis. 2022;35(6):583–8. https://doi.org/10.1097/QCO.0000000000000855.

134. Stewart AG, Paterson DL, Young B, Lye DC, Davis JS, Schneider K, et al. Meropenem versus piperacillin-tazobactam for definitive treatment of bloodstream infections caused by AmpC beta-lactamase-producing Enterobacter spp, Citrobacter freundii, Morganella morganii, Providencia spp, or Serratia marcescens: a pilot multicenter randomized controlled trial (MERINO-2). Open Forum Infect Dis. 2021;8(8):ofab387. https://doi.org/10.1093/ofid/ofab387.

135. Harris PNA, Tambyah PA, Lye DC, Mo Y, Lee TH, Yilmaz M, et al. Effect of piperacillin-tazobactam vs meropenem on 30-day mortality for patients with E coli or Klebsiella pneumoniae bloodstream infection and ceftriaxone resistance: a randomized clinical trial. JAMA. 2018;320(10):984–94. https://doi.org/10.1001/jama.2018.12163.

136. Pappas PG, Kauffman CA, Andes DR, Clancy CJ, Marr KA, Ostrosky-Zeichner L, et al. Clinical practice guideline for the management of candidiasis: 2016 update by the Infectious Diseases Society of America. Clin Infect Dis. 2016;62(4):e1–50. https://doi.org/10.1093/cid/civ933.

137. ATS. Top 20 pneumonia facts—2019. 2019. https://www.thoracic.org/patients/patient-resources/resources/top-pneumonia-facts.pdf. Accessed 5 Mar 2024.

138. Sialer S, Difrancesco LF, Fabregas TF, Torres A. Community-acquired pneumonia. Metab Hum Dis. 2014;28:227–31.

139. Walaszek M, Kosiarska A, Gniadek A, Kolpa M, Wolak Z, Dobros W, et al. The risk factors for hospital-acquired pneumonia in the intensive care unit. Przegl Epidemiol. 2016;70(1):15–20, 107–10

140. McLaughlin JM, Khan FL, Thoburn EA, Isturiz RE, Swerdlow DL. Rates of hospitalization for community-acquired pneumonia among US adults: a systematic review. Vaccine. 2020;38(4):741–51. https://doi.org/10.1016/j.vaccine.2019.10.101.

141. Fine MJ, Smith MA, Carson CA, Mutha SS, Sankey SS, Weissfeld LA, et al. Prognosis and outcomes of patients with community-acquired pneumonia. A meta-analysis. JAMA. 1996;275(2):134–41.

142. Jain S, Self WH, Wunderink RG, Fakhran S, Balk R, Bramley AM, et al. Community-acquired pneumonia requiring hospitalization among U.S. adults. N Engl J Med. 2015;373(5):415–27. https://doi.org/10.1056/NEJMoa1500245.

143. Shoar S, Musher DM. Etiology of community-acquired pneumonia in adults: a systematic review. Pneumonia (Nathan). 2020;12:11. https://doi.org/10.1186/s41479-020-00074-3.

144. Johansson N, Kalin M, Tiveljung-Lindell A, Giske CG, Hedlund J. Etiology of community-acquired pneumonia: increased microbiological yield with new diagnostic methods. Clin Infect Dis. 2010;50(2):202–9. https://doi.org/10.1086/648678.

145. Lim WS, van der Eerden MM, Laing R, Boersma WG, Karalus N, Town GI, et al. Defining community acquired pneumonia severity on presentation to hospital: an international derivation and validation study. Thorax. 2003;58(5):377–82. https://doi.org/10.1136/thorax.58.5.377.

146. Fine MJ, Auble TE, Yealy DM, Hanusa BH, Weissfeld LA, Singer DE, et al. A prediction rule to identify low-risk patients with community-acquired pneumonia. N Engl J Med. 1997;336(4):243–50. https://doi.org/10.1056/NEJM199701233360402.

147. Metlay JP, Kapoor WN, Fine MJ. Does this patient have community-acquired pneumonia? Diagnosing pneumonia by history and physical examination. JAMA. 1997;278(17):1440–5.

148. Irwin RS, French CL, Chang AB, Altman KW, CHEST Expert Cough Panel. Classification of cough as a symptom in adults and management algorithms: CHEST guideline and expert panel report. Chest. 2018;153(1):196–209. https://doi.org/10.1016/j.chest.2017.10.016.

149. Gibson RL, Burns JL, Ramsey BW. Pathophysiology and management of pulmonary infections in cystic fibrosis. Am J Respir Crit Care Med. 2003;168(8):918–51. https://doi.org/10.1164/rccm.200304-505SO.

150. Lieberman D, Shvartzman P, Korsonsky I, Lieberman D. Diagnosis of ambulatory community-acquired pneumonia. Comparison of clinical assessment versus chest X-ray. Scand J Prim Health Care. 2003;21(1):57–60. https://doi.org/10.1080/02813430310000582.

151. Claessens YE, Debray MP, Tubach F, Brun AL, Rammaert B, Hausfater P, et al. Early chest computed tomography scan to assist diagnosis and guide treatment decision for suspected community-acquired pneumonia. Am J Respir Crit Care Med. 2015;192(8):974–82. https://doi.org/10.1164/rccm.201501-0017OC.

152. Javaudin F, Marjanovic N, de Carvalho H, Gaborit B, Le Bastard Q, Boucher E, et al. Contribution of lung ultrasound in diagnosis of community-acquired pneumonia in the emergency department: a prospective multicentre study. BMJ Open. 2021;11(9):e046849. https://doi.org/10.1136/bmjopen-2020-046849.

153. Del Rio-Pertuz G, Gutierrez JF, Triana AJ, Molinares JL, Robledo-Solano AB, Meza JL, et al. Usefulness of sputum gram stain for etiologic diagnosis in community-acquired pneumonia: a systematic review and meta-analysis. BMC Infect Dis. 2019;19(1):403. https://doi.org/10.1186/s12879-019-4048-6.

154. Murphy CN, Fowler R, Balada-Llasat JM, Carroll A, Stone H, Akerele O, et al. Multicenter evaluation of the BioFire FilmArray pneumonia/pneumonia plus panel for detection and quantification of agents of lower respiratory tract infection. J Clin Microbiol. 2020;58(7) https://doi.org/10.1128/JCM.00128-20.

155. Falsey AR, Branche AR, Croft DP, Formica MA, Peasley MR, Walsh EE. Real-life assessment of BioFire FilmArray pneumonia panel in adults hospitalized with respiratory illness. J Infect Dis. 2024;229(1):214–22. https://doi.org/10.1093/infdis/jiad221.

156. Martin-Loeches I, Torres A, Nagavci B, Aliberti S, Antonelli M, Bassetti M, et al. ERS/ESICM/ESCMID/ALAT guidelines for the management of severe community-acquired pneumonia. Intensive Care Med. 2023;49(6):615–32. https://doi.org/10.1007/s00134-023-07033-8.

157. Pagliano P, Sellitto C, Conti V, Ascione T, Esposito S. Characteristics of viral pneumonia in the COVID-19 era: an update. Infection. 2021;49(4):607–16. https://doi.org/10.1007/s15010-021-01603-y.

158. Uyeki TM, Bernstein HH, Bradley JS, Englund JA, File TM, Fry AM, et al. Clinical practice guidelines by the Infectious Diseases Society of America: 2018 update on diagnosis, treatment, chemoprophylaxis, and institutional outbreak management of seasonal influenzaa. Clin Infect Dis. 2019;68(6):e1–47. https://doi.org/10.1093/cid/ciy866.

159. Bhimraj A, Morgan RL, Shumaker AH, Lavergne V, Baden L, Cheng VC, et al. Infectious Diseases Society of America guidelines on the treatment and management of patients with COVID-19. Clin Infect Dis. 2020; https://doi.org/10.1093/cid/ciaa478.

160. Onwuchekwa C, Moreo LM, Menon S, Machado B, Curcio D, Kalina W, et al. Underascertainment of respiratory syncytial virus infection in adults due to diagnostic testing limitations: a systematic literature review and meta-analysis. J Infect Dis. 2023;228(2):173–84. https://doi.org/10.1093/infdis/jiad012.

161. Campbell SG, Marrie TJ, Anstey R, Dickinson G, Ackroyd-Stolarz S. The contribution of blood cultures to the clinical management of adult patients admitted to the hospital with community-acquired pneumonia: a prospective observational study. Chest. 2003;123(4):1142–50. https://doi.org/10.1378/chest.123.4.1142.

162. Lee JS, Giesler DL, Gellad WF, Fine MJ. Antibiotic therapy for adults hospitalized with community-acquired pneumonia: a systematic review. JAMA. 2016;315(6):593–602. https://doi.org/10.1001/jama.2016.0115.
163. Raz-Pasteur A, Shasha D, Paul M. Fluoroquinolones or macrolides alone versus combined with beta-lactams for adults with community-acquired pneumonia: systematic review and meta-analysis. Int J Antimicrob Agents. 2015;46(3):242–8. https://doi.org/10.1016/j.ijantimicag.2015.04.010.
164. Lewis PO. Risk factor evaluation for methicillin-resistant Staphylococcus aureus and Pseudomonas aeruginosa in community-acquired pneumonia. Ann Pharmacother. 2021;55(1):36–43. https://doi.org/10.1177/1060028020935106.
165. El-Solh AA, Pietrantoni C, Bhat A, Aquilina AT, Okada M, Grover V, et al. Microbiology of severe aspiration pneumonia in institutionalized elderly. Am J Respir Crit Care Med. 2003;167(12):1650–4. https://doi.org/10.1164/rccm.200212-1543OC.
166. Yoshimatsu Y, Aga M, Komiya K, Haranaga S, Numata Y, Miki M, et al. The clinical significance of anaerobic coverage in the antibiotic treatment of aspiration pneumonia: a systematic review and meta-analysis. J Clin Med. 2023;12(5) https://doi.org/10.3390/jcm12051992.
167. Rodriguez AE, Restrepo MI. New perspectives in aspiration community acquired pneumonia. Expert Rev Clin Pharmacol. 2019;12(10):991–1002. https://doi.org/10.1080/17512433.2019.1663730.
168. Moreno G, Rodriguez A, Sole-Violan J, Martin-Loeches I, Diaz E, Bodi M, et al. Early oseltamivir treatment improves survival in critically ill patients with influenza pneumonia. ERJ Open Res. 2021;7(1):00888. https://doi.org/10.1183/23120541.00888-2020.
169. Sheahan TP, Sims AC, Graham RL, Menachery VD, Gralinski LE, Case JB, et al. Broad-spectrum antiviral GS-5734 inhibits both epidemic and zoonotic coronaviruses. Sci Transl Med. 2017;9(396) https://doi.org/10.1126/scitranslmed.aal3653.
170. Bhimraj A, Morgan RL, Shumaker AH, Baden L, Cheng VCC, Edwards KM, et al. Infectious Diseases Society of America guidelines on the treatment and management of patients with COVID-19. Clin Infect Dis. 2022;78:e250. https://doi.org/10.1093/cid/ciac724.
171. Beigel JH, Tomashek KM, Dodd LE, Mehta AK, Zingman BS, Kalil AC, et al. Remdesivir for the treatment of Covid-19—final report. N Engl J Med. 2020;383(19):1813–26. https://doi.org/10.1056/NEJMoa2007764.
172. Consortium WHOST. Remdesivir and three other drugs for hospitalised patients with COVID-19: final results of the WHO solidarity randomised trial and updated meta-analyses. Lancet. 2022;399(10339):1941–53. https://doi.org/10.1016/S0140-6736(22)00519-0.
173. Kanagala SG, Dholiya H, Jhajj P, Patel MA, Gupta V, Gupta S, et al. Remdesivir-induced bradycardia. South Med J. 2023;116(3):317–20. https://doi.org/10.14423/SMJ.0000000000001519.
174. Stancampiano F, Jhawar N, Alsafi W, Valery J, Harris DM, Kempaiah P, et al. Use of remdesivir for COVID-19 pneumonia in patients with advanced kidney disease: a retrospective multi-center study. Clin Infect Pract. 2022;16:100207. https://doi.org/10.1016/j.clinpr.2022.100207.
175. Dequin PF, Meziani F, Quenot JP, Kamel T, Ricard JD, Badie J, et al. Hydrocortisone in severe community-acquired pneumonia. N Engl J Med. 2023;388(21):1931–41. https://doi.org/10.1056/NEJMoa2215145.
176. Saleem N, Kulkarni A, Snow TAC, Ambler G, Singer M, Arulkumaran N. Effect of corticosteroids on mortality and clinical cure in community-acquired pneumonia: a systematic review, meta-analysis, and meta-regression of randomized control trials. Chest. 2023;163(3):484–97. https://doi.org/10.1016/j.chest.2022.08.2229.
177. Chaudhuri D, Nei AM, Rochwerg B, Balk RA, Asehnoune K, Cadena R, et al. 2024 Focused update: guidelines on use of corticosteroids in sepsis, acute respiratory distress syndrome, and community-acquired pneumonia. Crit Care Med. 2024;52:e219. https://doi.org/10.1097/CCM.0000000000006172.

178. Zhou Y, Fu X, Liu X, Huang C, Tian G, Ding C, et al. Use of corticosteroids in influenza-associated acute respiratory distress syndrome and severe pneumonia: a systemic review and meta-analysis. Sci Rep. 2020;10(1):3044. https://doi.org/10.1038/s41598-020-59732-7.

179. van Paassen J, Vos JS, Hoekstra EM, Neumann KMI, Boot PC, Arbous SM. Corticosteroid use in COVID-19 patients: a systematic review and meta-analysis on clinical outcomes. Crit Care. 2020;24(1):696. https://doi.org/10.1186/s13054-020-03400-9.

180. RECOVERY Collaborative Group, Horby P, Lim WS, Emberson JR, Mafham M, Bell JL, et al. Dexamethasone in hospitalized patients with Covid-19. N Engl J Med. 2021;384(8):693–704. https://doi.org/10.1056/NEJMoa2021436.

181. Johns M, George S, Taburyanskaya M, Poon YK. A review of the evidence for corticosteroids in COVID-19. J Pharm Pract. 2022;35(4):626–37. https://doi.org/10.1177/0897190021998502.

182. Veeranki V, Prasad N, Meyyappan J, Bhadauria D, Behera MR, Kushwaha R, et al. The adverse effects of high-dose corticosteroid on infectious and non-infectious sequelae in renal transplant recipients with coronavirus disease-19 in India. Transpl Infect Dis. 2022;24(6):e13908. https://doi.org/10.1111/tid.13908.

183. Shah M, Reveles K, Moote R, Hand E, Kellogg D III, Attridge RL, et al. Risk of coronavirus disease 2019-associated pulmonary aspergillosis based on corticosteroid duration in intensive care patients. Open Forum Infect Dis. 2023;10(3):ofad062. https://doi.org/10.1093/ofid/ofad062.

184. WHO Rapid Evidence Appraisal for COVID-19 Therapies (REACT) Working Group, Sterne JAC, Murthy S, Diaz JV, Slutsky AS, Villar J, et al. Association between administration of systemic corticosteroids and mortality among critically ill patients with COVID-19: a meta-analysis. JAMA. 2020;324(13):1330–41. https://doi.org/10.1001/jama.2020.17023.

185. Jones BE, Sarvet AL, Ying J, Jin R, Nevers MR, Stern SE, et al. Incidence and outcomes of non-ventilator-associated hospital-acquired pneumonia in 284 US hospitals using electronic surveillance criteria. JAMA Netw Open. 2023;6(5):e2314185. https://doi.org/10.1001/jamanetworkopen.2023.14185.

186. Papazian L, Klompas M, Luyt CE. Ventilator-associated pneumonia in adults: a narrative review. Intensive Care Med. 2020;46(5):888–906. https://doi.org/10.1007/s00134-020-05980-0.

187. Melsen WG, Rovers MM, Groenwold RH, Bergmans DC, Camus C, Bauer TT, et al. Attributable mortality of ventilator-associated pneumonia: a meta-analysis of individual patient data from randomised prevention studies. Lancet Infect Dis. 2013;13(8):665–71. https://doi.org/10.1016/S1473-3099(13)70081-1.

188. Shan J, Chen HL, Zhu JH. Diagnostic accuracy of clinical pulmonary infection score for ventilator-associated pneumonia: a meta-analysis. Respir Care. 2011;56(8):1087–94. https://doi.org/10.4187/respcare.01097.

189. Lichtenstein DA, Meziere GA. Relevance of lung ultrasound in the diagnosis of acute respiratory failure: the BLUE protocol. Chest. 2008;134(1):117–25. https://doi.org/10.1378/chest.07-2800.

190. Parente DM, Cunha CB, Mylonakis E, Timbrook TT. The clinical utility of methicillin-resistant Staphylococcus aureus (MRSA) nasal screening to rule out MRSA pneumonia: a diagnostic meta-analysis with antimicrobial stewardship implications. Clin Infect Dis. 2018;67(1):1–7. https://doi.org/10.1093/cid/ciy024.

191. Maataoui N, Chemali L, Patrier J, Tran Dinh A, Le Fevre L, Lortat-Jacob B, et al. Impact of rapid multiplex PCR on management of antibiotic therapy in COVID-19-positive patients hospitalized in intensive care unit. Eur J Clin Microbiol Infect Dis. 2021;40(10):2227–34. https://doi.org/10.1007/s10096-021-04213-6.

192. Kourtis AP, Hatfield K, Baggs J, Mu Y, See I, Epson E, et al. Vital signs: epidemiology and recent trends in methicillin-resistant and in methicillin-susceptible Staphylococcus aureus bloodstream infections—United States. MMWR Morb Mortal Wkly Rep. 2019;68(9):214–9. https://doi.org/10.15585/mmwr.mm6809e1.

193. Tamma PD, Cosgrove SE, Maragakis LL. Combination therapy for treatment of infections with gram-negative bacteria. Clin Microbiol Rev. 2012;25(3):450–70. https://doi.org/10.1128/CMR.05041-11.
194. Wang N, Tang C, Wang L. Risk factors for acquired Stenotrophomonas maltophilia pneumonia in intensive care unit: a systematic review and meta-analysis. Front Med (Lausanne). 2021;8:808391. https://doi.org/10.3389/fmed.2021.808391.
195. Benaissa E, Belouad E, Maleb A, Elouennass M. Risk factors for acquiring Acinetobacter baumannii infection in the intensive care unit: experience from a Moroccan hospital. Access Microbiol. 2023;5(8) https://doi.org/10.1099/acmi.0.000637.v3.
196. Alnimr A. Antimicrobial resistance in ventilator-associated pneumonia: predictive microbiology and evidence-based therapy. Infect Dis Ther. 2023;12(6):1527–52. https://doi.org/10.1007/s40121-023-00820-2.
197. Tamma PD, Aitken SL, Bonomo RA, Mathers AJ, van Duin D, Clancy CJ. Infectious Diseases Society of America 2023 guidance on the treatment of antimicrobial resistant gram-negative infections. Clin Infect Dis. 2023 https://doi.org/10.1093/cid/ciad428.
198. Chastre J, Wolff M, Fagon JY, Chevret S, Thomas F, Wermert D, et al. Comparison of 8 vs 15 days of antibiotic therapy for ventilator-associated pneumonia in adults: a randomized trial. JAMA. 2003;290(19):2588–98. https://doi.org/10.1001/jama.290.19.2588.
199. Pugh R, Grant C, Cooke RP, Dempsey G. Short-course versus prolonged-course antibiotic therapy for hospital-acquired pneumonia in critically ill adults. Cochrane Database Syst Rev. 2015;2015(8):CD007577. https://doi.org/10.1002/14651858.CD007577.pub3.
200. Swartz MN. Bacterial meningitis—a view of the past 90 years. N Engl J Med. 2004;351(18):1826–8. https://doi.org/10.1056/NEJMp048246.
201. McGill F, Heyderman RS, Panagiotou S, Tunkel AR, Solomon T. Acute bacterial meningitis in adults. Lancet. 2016;388(10063):3036–47. https://doi.org/10.1016/S0140-6736(16)30654-7.
202. Auburtin M, Wolff M, Charpentier J, Varon E, Le Tulzo Y, Girault C, et al. Detrimental role of delayed antibiotic administration and penicillin-nonsusceptible strains in adult intensive care unit patients with pneumococcal meningitis: the PNEUMOREA prospective multicenter study. Crit Care Med. 2006;34(11):2758–65. https://doi.org/10.1097/01.CCM.0000239434.26669.65.
203. Bradshaw MJ, Venkatesan A. Herpes simplex virus-1 encephalitis in adults: pathophysiology, diagnosis, and management. Neurotherapeutics. 2016;13(3):493–508. https://doi.org/10.1007/s13311-016-0433-7.
204. Quagliarello V, Scheld WM. Bacterial meningitis: pathogenesis, pathophysiology, and progress. N Engl J Med. 1992;327(12):864–72. https://doi.org/10.1056/NEJM199209173271208.
205. Germiller JA, Monin DL, Sparano AM, Tom LW. Intracranial complications of sinusitis in children and adolescents and their outcomes. Arch Otolaryngol Head Neck Surg. 2006;132(9):969–76. https://doi.org/10.1001/archotol.132.9.969.
206. van de Beek D, Brouwer MC, Koedel U, Wall EC. Community-acquired bacterial meningitis. Lancet. 2021;398(10306):1171–83. https://doi.org/10.1016/S0140-6736(21)00883-7.
207. Hasbun R. Progress and challenges in bacterial meningitis: a review. JAMA. 2022;328(21):2147–54. https://doi.org/10.1001/jama.2022.20521.
208. van de Beek D, de Gans J, Spanjaard L, Weisfelt M, Reitsma JB, Vermeulen M. Clinical features and prognostic factors in adults with bacterial meningitis. N Engl J Med. 2004;351(18):1849–59. https://doi.org/10.1056/NEJMoa040845.
209. Akaishi T, Kobayashi J, Abe M, Ishizawa K, Nakashima I, Aoki M, et al. Sensitivity and specificity of meningeal signs in patients with meningitis. J Gen Fam Med. 2019;20(5):193–8. https://doi.org/10.1002/jgf2.268.
210. Thomas KE, Hasbun R, Jekel J, Quagliarello VJ. The diagnostic accuracy of Kernig's sign, Brudzinski's sign, and nuchal rigidity in adults with suspected meningitis. Clin Infect Dis. 2002;35(1):46–52. https://doi.org/10.1086/340979.

211. van Veen KE, Brouwer MC, van der Ende A, van de Beek D. Bacterial meningitis in alcoholic patients: a population-based prospective study. J Infect. 2017;74(4):352–7. https://doi.org/10.1016/j.jinf.2017.01.001.

212. Block N, Naucler P, Wagner P, Morfeldt E, Henriques-Normark B. Bacterial meningitis: aetiology, risk factors, disease trends and severe sequelae during 50 years in Sweden. J Intern Med. 2022;292(2):350–64. https://doi.org/10.1111/joim.13488.

213. Lucas MJ, Brouwer MC, van der Ende A, van de Beek D. Endocarditis in adults with bacterial meningitis. Circulation. 2013;127(20):2056–62. https://doi.org/10.1161/CIRCULATIONAHA.113.001545.

214. CDC. Meningococcal disease. 2022. https://www.cdc.gov/meningococcal/index.html. Accessed 29 Feb 2024.

215. Hasbun R, Abrahams J, Jekel J, Quagliarello VJ. Computed tomography of the head before lumbar puncture in adults with suspected meningitis. N Engl J Med. 2001;345(24):1727–33. https://doi.org/10.1056/NEJMoa010399.

216. Mahale A, Choudhary S, Ullal S, Fernandes M, Prabhu S. Postcontrast fluid-attenuated inversion recovery (FLAIR) sequence MR imaging in detecting intracranial pathology. Radiol Res Pract. 2020;2020:8853597. https://doi.org/10.1155/2020/8853597.

217. Duong MT, Rudie JD, Mohan S. Neuroimaging patterns of intracranial infections: meningitis, cerebritis, and their complications. Neuroimaging Clin N Am. 2023;33(1):11–41. https://doi.org/10.1016/j.nic.2022.07.001.

218. Poissy J, Champenois K, Dewilde A, Melliez H, Georges H, Senneville E, et al. Impact of Herpes simplex virus load and red blood cells in cerebrospinal fluid upon herpes simplex meningo-encephalitis outcome. BMC Infect Dis. 2012;12:356. https://doi.org/10.1186/1471-2334-12-356.

219. Seehusen DA, Reeves MM, Fomin DA. Cerebrospinal fluid analysis. Am Fam Physician. 2003;68(6):1103–8.

220. Huy NT, Thao NT, Diep DT, Kikuchi M, Zamora J, Hirayama K. Cerebrospinal fluid lactate concentration to distinguish bacterial from aseptic meningitis: a systemic review and meta-analysis. Crit Care. 2010;14(6):R240. https://doi.org/10.1186/cc9395.

221. Curtis GD, Slack MP, Tompkins DS. Cerebrospinal fluid lactate and the diagnosis of meningitis. J Infect. 1981;3(2):159–65. https://doi.org/10.1016/s0163-4453(81)91336-0.

222. Sakushima K, Hayashino Y, Kawaguchi T, Jackson JL, Fukuhara S. Diagnostic accuracy of cerebrospinal fluid lactate for differentiating bacterial meningitis from aseptic meningitis: a meta-analysis. J Infect. 2011;62(4):255–62. https://doi.org/10.1016/j.jinf.2011.02.010.

223. Tunkel AR, Hartman BJ, Kaplan SL, Kaufman BA, Roos KL, Scheld WM, et al. Practice guidelines for the management of bacterial meningitis. Clin Infect Dis. 2004;39(9):1267–84. https://doi.org/10.1086/425368.

224. Wu HM, Cordeiro SM, Harcourt BH, Carvalho M, Azevedo J, Oliveira TQ, et al. Accuracy of real-time PCR, Gram stain and culture for Streptococcus pneumoniae, Neisseria meningitidis and Haemophilus influenzae meningitis diagnosis. BMC Infect Dis. 2013;13:26. https://doi.org/10.1186/1471-2334-13-26.

225. Liesman RM, Strasburg AP, Heitman AK, Theel ES, Patel R, Binnicker MJ. Evaluation of a commercial multiplex molecular panel for diagnosis of infectious meningitis and encephalitis. J Clin Microbiol. 2018;56(4) https://doi.org/10.1128/JCM.01927-17.

226. van de Beek D, Drake JM, Tunkel AR. Nosocomial bacterial meningitis. N Engl J Med. 2010;362(2):146–54. https://doi.org/10.1056/NEJMra0804573.

227. Shirah GR, O'Neill PJ. Intra-abdominal infections. Surg Clin North Am. 2014;94(6):1319–33. https://doi.org/10.1016/j.suc.2014.08.005.

228. Wittmann DH, Schein M, Condon RE. Management of secondary peritonitis. Ann Surg. 1996;224(1):10–8. https://doi.org/10.1097/00000658-199607000-00003.

229. Mazuski JE, Tessier JM, May AK, Sawyer RG, Nadler EP, Rosengart MR, et al. The Surgical Infection Society revised guidelines on the management of intra-abdominal infection. Surg Infect (Larchmt). 2017;18(1):1–76. https://doi.org/10.1089/sur.2016.261.

230. Lopez N, Kobayashi L, Coimbra R. A comprehensive review of abdominal infections. World J Emerg Surg. 2011;6:7. https://doi.org/10.1186/1749-7922-6-7.

231. Blot S, De Waele JJ. Critical issues in the clinical management of complicated intra-abdominal infections. Drugs. 2005;65(12):1611–20. https://doi.org/10.2165/00003495-200565120-00002.

232. Calandra T, Cohen J, International Sepsis Forum Definition of Infection in the ICUCC. The international sepsis forum consensus conference on definitions of infection in the intensive care unit. Crit Care Med. 2005;33(7):1538–48. https://doi.org/10.1097/01.ccm.0000168253.91200.83.

233. Oldenburg WA, Lau LL, Rodenberg TJ, Edmonds HJ, Burger CD. Acute mesenteric ischemia: a clinical review. Arch Intern Med. 2004;164(10):1054–62. https://doi.org/10.1001/archinte.164.10.1054.

234. Blot S, Antonelli M, Arvaniti K, Blot K, Creagh-Brown B, de Lange D, et al. Epidemiology of intra-abdominal infection and sepsis in critically ill patients: "AbSeS", a multinational observational cohort study and ESICM Trials Group Project. Intensive Care Med. 2019;45(12):1703–17. https://doi.org/10.1007/s00134-019-05819-3.

235. Roehrborn A, Thomas L, Potreck O, Ebener C, Ohmann C, Goretzki PE, et al. The microbiology of postoperative peritonitis. Clin Infect Dis. 2001;33(9):1513–9. https://doi.org/10.1086/323333.

236. Montravers P, Lepape A, Dubreuil L, Gauzit R, Pean Y, Benchimol D, et al. Clinical and microbiological profiles of community-acquired and nosocomial intra-abdominal infections: results of the French prospective, observational EBIIA study. J Antimicrob Chemother. 2009;63(4):785–94. https://doi.org/10.1093/jac/dkp005.

237. Sartelli M, Catena F, Ansaloni L, Leppaniemi A, Taviloglu K, van Goor H, et al. Complicated intra-abdominal infections in Europe: a comprehensive review of the CIAO study. World J Emerg Surg. 2012;7(1):36. https://doi.org/10.1186/1749-7922-7-36.

238. Sartelli M, Weber DG, Ruppe E, Bassetti M, Wright BJ, Ansaloni L, et al. Antimicrobials: a global alliance for optimizing their rational use in intra-abdominal infections (AGORA). World J Emerg Surg. 2016;11:33. https://doi.org/10.1186/s13017-016-0089-y.

239. Sartelli M, Chichom-Mefire A, Labricciosa FM, Hardcastle T, Abu-Zidan FM, Adesunkanmi AK, et al. The management of intra-abdominal infections from a global perspective: 2017 WSES guidelines for management of intra-abdominal infections. World J Emerg Surg. 2017;12:29. https://doi.org/10.1186/s13017-017-0141-6.

240. Spoto S, Valeriani E, Caputo D, Cella E, Fogolari M, Pesce E, et al. The role of procalcitonin in the diagnosis of bacterial infection after major abdominal surgery: advantage from daily measurement. Medicine (Baltimore). 2018;97(3):e9496. https://doi.org/10.1097/MD.0000000000009496.

241. Doria AS, Moineddin R, Kellenberger CJ, Epelman M, Beyene J, Schuh S, et al. US or CT for diagnosis of appendicitis in children and adults? A meta-analysis. Radiology. 2006;241(1):83–94. https://doi.org/10.1148/radiol.2411050913.

242. Xiong B, Zhong B, Li Z, Zhou F, Hu R, Feng Z, et al. Diagnostic accuracy of noncontrast CT in detecting acute appendicitis: a meta-analysis of prospective studies. Am Surg. 2015;81(6):626–9.

243. Kiewiet JJ, Leeuwenburgh MM, Bipat S, Bossuyt PM, Stoker J, Boermeester MA. A systematic review and meta-analysis of diagnostic performance of imaging in acute cholecystitis. Radiology. 2012;264(3):708–20. https://doi.org/10.1148/radiol.12111561.

244. Sartelli M, Coccolini F, Kluger Y, Agastra E, Abu-Zidan FM, Abbas AES, et al. WSES/GAIS/SIS-E/WSIS/AAST global clinical pathways for patients with intra-abdominal infections. World J Emerg Surg. 2021;16(1):49. https://doi.org/10.1186/s13017-021-00387-8.

245. Sion MK, Davis KA. Step-up approach for the management of pancreatic necrosis: a review of the literature. Trauma Surg Acute Care Open. 2019;4(1):e000308. https://doi.org/10.1136/tsaco-2019-000308.

246. van Santvoort HC, Besselink MG, Bakker OJ, Hofker HS, Boermeester MA, Dejong CH, et al. A step-up approach or open necrosectomy for necrotizing pancreatitis. N Engl J Med. 2010;362(16):1491–502. https://doi.org/10.1056/NEJMoa0908821.

247. Solomkin JS, Mazuski JE, Bradley JS, Rodvold KA, Goldstein EJ, Baron EJ, et al. Diagnosis and management of complicated intra-abdominal infection in adults and children: guidelines by the Surgical Infection Society and the Infectious Diseases Society of America. Clin Infect Dis. 2010;50(2):133–64. https://doi.org/10.1086/649554.

248. Waltner-Toews RI, Paterson DL, Qureshi ZA, Sidjabat HE, Adams-Haduch JM, Shutt KA, et al. Clinical characteristics of bloodstream infections due to ampicillin-sulbactam-resistant, non-extended-spectrum-beta-lactamase-producing Escherichia coli and the role of TEM-1 hyperproduction. Antimicrob Agents Chemother. 2011;55(2):495–501. https://doi.org/10.1128/AAC.00797-10.

249. Chen CW, Ming CC, Ma CJ, Shan YS, Yeh YS, Wang JY. Prospective, randomized, study of ampicillin-sulbactam versus moxifloxacin monotherapy for the treatment of community-acquired complicated intra-abdominal infections. Surg Infect (Larchmt). 2013;14(4):389–96. https://doi.org/10.1089/sur.2012.017.

250. Harbarth S, Uckay I. Are there patients with peritonitis who require empiric therapy for enterococcus? Eur J Clin Microbiol Infect Dis. 2004;23(2):73–7. https://doi.org/10.1007/s10096-003-1078-0.

251. Worden LJ, Dumkow LE, VanLangen KM, Beuschel TS, Jameson AP. Antipseudomonal versus narrow-spectrum agents for the treatment of community-onset intra-abdominal infections. Open Forum Infect Dis. 2021;8(11):ofab514. https://doi.org/10.1093/ofid/ofab514.

252. Liu J, Zhang L, Pan J, Huang M, Li Y, Zhang H, et al. Risk factors and molecular epidemiology of complicated intra-abdominal infections with carbapenem-resistant enterobacteriaceae: a multicenter study in China. J Infect Dis. 2020;221(Suppl 2):S156–63. https://doi.org/10.1093/infdis/jiz574.

253. Adelman MW, Bower CW, Grass JE, Ansari UA, Soda EA, See I, et al. Distinctive features of ertapenem-mono-resistant carbapenem-resistant enterobacterales in the United States: a cohort study. Open Forum Infect Dis. 2022;9(1):ofab643. https://doi.org/10.1093/ofid/ofab643.

254. Solomkin JS, Gardovskis J, Lawrence K, Montravers P, Sway A, Evans D, et al. IGNITE4: results of a phase 3, randomized, multicenter, prospective trial of eravacycline vs meropenem in the treatment of complicated intraabdominal infections. Clin Infect Dis. 2019;69(6):921–9. https://doi.org/10.1093/cid/ciy1029.

255. Eljaaly K, Ortwine JK, Shaikhomer M, Almangour TA, Bassetti M. Efficacy and safety of eravacycline: a meta-analysis. J Glob Antimicrob Resist. 2021;24:424–8. https://doi.org/10.1016/j.jgar.2021.02.009.

256. FDA. FDA Drug Safety Communication: increased risk of death with Tygacil (tigecycline) compared to other antibiotics used to treat similar infections. 2010. https://www.fda.gov/drugs/drug-safety-and-availability/fda-drug-safety-communication-increased-risk-death-tygacil-tigecycline-compared-other-antibiotics. Accessed 1 Mar 2024.

257. Mehdorn M, Kolbe-Busch S, Lippmann N, Moulla Y, Scheuermann U, Jansen-Winkeln B, et al. Rectal colonization is predictive for surgical site infections with multidrug-resistant bacteria in abdominal surgery. Langenbecks Arch Surg. 2023;408(1):230. https://doi.org/10.1007/s00423-023-02961-x.

258. Boyanova L, Kolarov R, Mitov I. Recent evolution of antibiotic resistance in the anaerobes as compared to previous decades. Anaerobe. 2015;31:4–10. https://doi.org/10.1016/j.anaerobe.2014.05.004.

259. Jasemi S, Emaneini M, Ahmadinejad Z, Fazeli MS, Sechi LA, Sadeghpour Heravi F, et al. Antibiotic resistance pattern of Bacteroides fragilis isolated from clinical and colorectal specimens. Ann Clin Microbiol Antimicrob. 2021;20(1):27. https://doi.org/10.1186/s12941-021-00435-w.

260. Sawyer RG, Claridge JA, Nathens AB, Rotstein OD, Duane TM, Evans HL, et al. Trial of short-course antimicrobial therapy for intraabdominal infection. N Engl J Med. 2015;372(21):1996–2005. https://doi.org/10.1056/NEJMoa1411162.
261. Bouza E, Burillo A, Munoz P. How to manage skin and soft-tissue infections in the emergency department. Curr Opin Infect Dis. 2023;36(2):81–8. https://doi.org/10.1097/QCO.0000000000000906.
262. Shen HN, Lu CL. Skin and soft tissue infections in hospitalized and critically ill patients: a nationwide population-based study. BMC Infect Dis. 2010;10:151. https://doi.org/10.1186/1471-2334-10-151.
263. Novosad SA, Sapiano MR, Grigg C, Lake J, Robyn M, Dumyati G, et al. Vital signs: epidemiology of sepsis: prevalence of health care factors and opportunities for prevention. MMWR Morb Mortal Wkly Rep. 2016;65(33):864–9. https://doi.org/10.15585/mmwr.mm6533e1.
264. Korting HC, Hubner K, Greiner K, Hamm G, Braun-Falco O. Differences in the skin surface pH and bacterial microflora due to the long-term application of synthetic detergent preparations of pH 5.5 and pH 7.0. Results of a crossover trial in healthy volunteers. Acta Derm Venereol. 1990;70(5):429–31.
265. Roth RR, James WD. Microbial ecology of the skin. Ann Rev Microbiol. 1988;42:441–64. https://doi.org/10.1146/annurev.mi.42.100188.002301.
266. Gao Z, Tseng CH, Pei Z, Blaser MJ. Molecular analysis of human forearm superficial skin bacterial biota. Proc Natl Acad Sci USA. 2007;104(8):2927–32. https://doi.org/10.1073/pnas.0607077104.
267. Ki V, Rotstein C. Bacterial skin and soft tissue infections in adults: a review of their epidemiology, pathogenesis, diagnosis, treatment and site of care. Can J Infect Dis Med Microbiol. 2008;19(2):173–84. https://doi.org/10.1155/2008/846453.
268. Torres J, Avalos N, Echols L, Mongelluzzo J, Rodriguez RM. Low yield of blood and wound cultures in patients with skin and soft-tissue infections. Am J Emerg Med. 2017;35(8):1159–61. https://doi.org/10.1016/j.ajem.2017.05.039.
269. Diaz JH, Lopez FA. Skin, soft tissue and systemic bacterial infections following aquatic injuries and exposures. Am J Med Sci. 2015;349(3):269–75. https://doi.org/10.1097/MAJ.0000000000000366.
270. Pence MA. The brief case: wound infection with Plesiomonas shigelloides following a freshwater injury. J Clin Microbiol. 2016;54(5):1180–2. https://doi.org/10.1128/JCM.02651-15.
271. Cazorla C, Guigon A, Noel M, Quilici ML, Lacassin F. Fatal Vibrio vulnificus infection associated with eating raw oysters, New Caledonia. Emerg Infect Dis. 2011;17(1):136–7. https://doi.org/10.3201/eid1701.100603.
272. Abrahamian FM, Goldstein EJ. Microbiology of animal bite wound infections. Clin Microbiol Rev. 2011;24(2):231–46. https://doi.org/10.1128/CMR.00041-10.
273. Patil PD, Panchabhai TS, Galwankar SC. Managing human bites. J Emerg Trauma Shock. 2009;2(3):186–90. https://doi.org/10.4103/0974-2700.55331.
274. Hamza RE, Villyoth MP, Peter G, Joseph D, Govindaraju C, Tank DC, et al. Risk factors of cellulitis in cirrhosis and antibiotic prophylaxis in preventing recurrence. Ann Gastroenterol. 2014;27(4):374–9.
275. Fergie JE, Patrick CC, Lott L. Pseudomonas aeruginosa cellulitis and ecthyma gangrenosum in immunocompromised children. Pediatr Infect Dis J. 1991;10(7):496–500. https://doi.org/10.1097/00006454-199107000-00003.
276. Schade VL, Roukis TS, Haque M. Clostridium septicum necrotizing fasciitis of the forefoot secondary to adenocarcinoma of the colon: case report and review of the literature. J Foot Ankle Surg. 2010;49(2):159.e1–8. https://doi.org/10.1053/j.jfas.2009.06.007.
277. Paul J, Czech MM, Balijepally R, Brown JW. Diagnostic and therapeutic challenges of treating opportunistic fungal cellulitis: a case series. BMC Infect Dis. 2022;22(1):435. https://doi.org/10.1186/s12879-022-07365-8.
278. NHSN. Surgical Site Infection Event (SSI). 2024. https://www.cdc.gov/nhsn/pdfs/pscmanual/9pscssicurrent.pdf. Accessed 1 Mar 2024.

279. Kottner J, Cuddigan J, Carville K, Balzer K, Berlowitz D, Law S, et al. Prevention and treatment of pressure ulcers/injuries: the protocol for the second update of the international clinical practice guideline 2019. J Tissue Viability. 2019;28(2):51–8. https://doi.org/10.1016/j.jtv.2019.01.001.

280. Lyder CH, Wang Y, Metersky M, Curry M, Kliman R, Verzier NR, et al. Hospital-acquired pressure ulcers: results from the national Medicare Patient Safety Monitoring System study. J Am Geriatr Soc. 2012;60(9):1603–8. https://doi.org/10.1111/j.1532-5415.2012.04106.x.

281. Nowicki JL, Mullany D, Spooner A, Nowicki TA, McKay PM, Corley A, et al. Are pressure injuries related to skin failure in critically ill patients? Aust Crit Care. 2018;31(5):257–63. https://doi.org/10.1016/j.aucc.2017.07.004.

282. Cox J, Edsberg LE, Koloms K, VanGilder CA. Pressure injuries in critical care patients in US hospitals: results of the international pressure ulcer prevalence survey. J Wound Ostomy Continence Nurs. 2022;49(1):21–8. https://doi.org/10.1097/WON.0000000000000834.

283. Coyer F, Miles S, Gosley S, Fulbrook P, Sketcher-Baker K, Cook JL, et al. Pressure injury prevalence in intensive care versus non-intensive care patients: a state-wide comparison. Aust Crit Care. 2017;30(5):244–50. https://doi.org/10.1016/j.aucc.2016.12.003.

284. Zhao G, Hiltabidel E, Liu Y, Chen L, Liao Y. A cross-sectional descriptive study of pressure ulcer prevalence in a teaching hospital in China. Ostomy Wound Manage. 2010;56(2):38–42.

285. Livesley NJ, Chow AW. Infected pressure ulcers in elderly individuals. Clin Infect Dis. 2002;35(11):1390–6. https://doi.org/10.1086/344059.

286. Norman G, Dumville JC, Moore ZE, Tanner J, Christie J, Goto S. Antibiotics and antiseptics for pressure ulcers. Cochrane Database Syst Rev. 2016;4(4):CD011586. https://doi.org/10.1002/14651858.CD011586.pub2.

287. Wong D, Holtom P, Spellberg B. Osteomyelitis complicating sacral pressure ulcers: whether or not to treat with antibiotic therapy. Clin Infect Dis. 2019;68(2):338–42. https://doi.org/10.1093/cid/ciy559.

288. Bonne SL, Kadri SS. Evaluation and management of necrotizing soft tissue infections. Infect Dis Clin N Am. 2017;31(3):497–511. https://doi.org/10.1016/j.idc.2017.05.011.

289. Stevens DL, Bryant AE. Necrotizing soft-tissue infections. N Engl J Med. 2017;377(23):2253–65. https://doi.org/10.1056/NEJMra1600673.

290. Peetermans M, de Prost N, Eckmann C, Norrby-Teglund A, Skrede S, De Waele JJ. Necrotizing skin and soft-tissue infections in the intensive care unit. Clin Microbiol Infect. 2020;26(1):8–17. https://doi.org/10.1016/j.cmi.2019.06.031.

291. Tsai YH, Huang TY, Chen JL, Hsiao CT, Kuo LT, Huang KC. Bacteriology and mortality of necrotizing fasciitis in a tertiary coastal hospital with comparing risk indicators of methicillin-resistant Staphylococcus aureus and Vibrio vulnificus infections: a prospective study. BMC Infect Dis. 2021;21(1):771. https://doi.org/10.1186/s12879-021-06518-5.

292. Cheng NC, Cheng Y, Tai HC, Chien KL, Wang SH, Chen YH, et al. High mortality risk of type III monomicrobial gram-negative necrotizing fasciitis: the role of extraintestinal pathogenic Escherichia coli (ExPEC) and Klebsiella pneumoniae. Int J Infect Dis. 2023;132:64–71. https://doi.org/10.1016/j.ijid.2023.04.390.

293. Baiu I, Staudenmayer K. Necrotizing soft tissue infections. JAMA. 2019;321(17):1738. https://doi.org/10.1001/jama.2019.2007.

294. Neeki MM, Dong F, Au C, Toy J, Khoshab N, Lee C, et al. Evaluating the laboratory risk indicator to differentiate cellulitis from necrotizing fasciitis in the emergency department. West J Emerg Med. 2017;18(4):684–9. https://doi.org/10.5811/westjem.2017.3.33607.

295. Wong CH, Khin LW, Heng KS, Tan KC, Low CO. The LRINEC (Laboratory Risk Indicator for Necrotizing Fasciitis) score: a tool for distinguishing necrotizing fasciitis from other soft tissue infections. Crit Care Med. 2004;32(7):1535–41. https://doi.org/10.1097/01.ccm.0000129486.35458.7d.

296. Cortes-Penfield N, Ryder JH. Should linezolid replace clindamycin as the adjunctive antimicrobial of choice in group a streptococcal necrotizing soft tissue infection and toxic shock

syndrome? A focused debate. Clin Infect Dis. 2023;76(2):346–50. https://doi.org/10.1093/cid/ciac720.

297. Stevens DL, Bryant AE, Goldstein EJ. Necrotizing soft tissue infections. Infect Dis Clin N Am. 2021;35(1):135–55. https://doi.org/10.1016/j.idc.2020.10.004.

298. Darenberg J, Ihendyane N, Sjolin J, Aufwerber E, Haidl S, Follin P, et al. Intravenous immunoglobulin G therapy in streptococcal toxic shock syndrome: a European randomized, double-blind, placebo-controlled trial. Clin Infect Dis. 2003;37(3):333–40. https://doi.org/10.1086/376630.

299. Kadri SS, Swihart BJ, Bonne SL, Hohmann SF, Hennessy LV, Louras P, et al. Impact of intravenous immunoglobulin on survival in necrotizing fasciitis with vasopressor-dependent shock: a propensity score-matched analysis from 130 US hospitals. Clin Infect Dis. 2017;64(7):877–85. https://doi.org/10.1093/cid/ciw871.

300. Madsen MB, Hjortrup PB, Hansen MB, Lange T, Norrby-Teglund A, Hyldegaard O, et al. Immunoglobulin G for patients with necrotising soft tissue infection (INSTINCT): a randomised, blinded, placebo-controlled trial. Intensive Care Med. 2017;43(11):1585–93. https://doi.org/10.1007/s00134-017-4786-0.

301. Cline KA, Turnbull TL. Clostridial myonecrosis. Ann Emerg Med. 1985;14(5):459–66. https://doi.org/10.1016/s0196-0644(85)80292-4.

302. Srivastava I, Aldape MJ, Bryant AE, Stevens DL. Spontaneous C. septicum gas gangrene: a literature review. Anaerobe. 2017;48:165–71. https://doi.org/10.1016/j.anaerobe.2017.07.008.

303. Tibbles PM, Edelsberg JS. Hyperbaric-oxygen therapy. N Engl J Med. 1996;334(25):1642–8. https://doi.org/10.1056/NEJM199606203342506.

304. CDC. Streptococcal Toxic Shock Syndrome (STSS) (*Streptococcus pyogenes*). 2021. https://ndc.services.cdc.gov/case-definitions/streptococcal-toxic-shock-syndrome-2010/. Accessed 29 Feb 2024.

305. Stevens DL, Tanner MH, Winship J, Swarts R, Ries KM, Schlievert PM, et al. Severe group A streptococcal infections associated with a toxic shock-like syndrome and scarlet fever toxin A. N Engl J Med. 1989;321(1):1–7. https://doi.org/10.1056/NEJM198907063210101.

306. Schmitz M, Roux X, Huttner B, Pugin J. Streptococcal toxic shock syndrome in the intensive care unit. Ann Intensive Care. 2018;8(1):88. https://doi.org/10.1186/s13613-018-0438-y.

307. Babiker A, Li X, Lai YL, Strich JR, Warner S, Sarzynski S, et al. Effectiveness of adjunctive clindamycin in beta-lactam antibiotic-treated patients with invasive beta-haemolytic streptococcal infections in US hospitals: a retrospective multicentre cohort study. Lancet Infect Dis. 2021;21(5):697–710. https://doi.org/10.1016/S1473-3099(20)30523-5.

308. Zimbelman J, Palmer A, Todd J. Improved outcome of clindamycin compared with beta-lactam antibiotic treatment for invasive Streptococcus pyogenes infection. Pediatr Infect Dis J. 1999;18(12):1096–100. https://doi.org/10.1097/00006454-199912000-00014.

309. Stevens DL, Yan S, Bryant AE. Penicillin-binding protein expression at different growth stages determines penicillin efficacy in vitro and in vivo: an explanation for the inoculum effect. J Infect Dis. 1993;167(6):1401–5. https://doi.org/10.1093/infdis/167.6.1401.

310. Stevens DL, Maier KA, Mitten JE. Effect of antibiotics on toxin production and viability of Clostridium perfringens. Antimicrob Agents Chemother. 1987;31(2):213–8. https://doi.org/10.1128/AAC.31.2.213.

311. Parks T, Wilson C, Curtis N, Norrby-Teglund A, Sriskandan S. Polyspecific intravenous immunoglobulin in clindamycin-treated patients with streptococcal toxic shock syndrome: a systematic review and meta-analysis. Clin Infect Dis. 2018;67(9):1434–6. https://doi.org/10.1093/cid/ciy401.

312. CDC. Antibiotic resistance threats in the United States, 2019. 2019. cdc.gov/drugresistance/pdf/threats-report/2019-ar-threats-report-508.pdf. Accessed 24 Oct 2022.

313. Guh AY, Mu Y, Winston LG, Johnston H, Olson D, Farley MM, et al. Trends in U.S. burden of Clostridioides difficile infection and outcomes. N Engl J Med. 2020;382(14):1320–30. https://doi.org/10.1056/NEJMoa1910215.

314. Magill SS, Edwards JR, Bamberg W, Beldavs ZG, Dumyati G, Kainer MA, et al. Multistate point-prevalence survey of health care-associated infections. N Engl J Med. 2014;370(13):1198–208. https://doi.org/10.1056/NEJMoa1306801.

315. Bauer MP, Notermans DW, van Benthem BH, Brazier JS, Wilcox MH, Rupnik M, et al. Clostridium difficile infection in Europe: a hospital-based survey. Lancet. 2011;377(9759):63–73. https://doi.org/10.1016/S0140-6736(10)61266-4.

316. Chitnis AS, Holzbauer SM, Belflower RM, Winston LG, Bamberg WM, Lyons C, et al. Epidemiology of community-associated Clostridium difficile infection, 2009 through 2011. JAMA Intern Med. 2013;173(14):1359–67. https://doi.org/10.1001/jamainternmed.2013.7056.

317. Evans ME, Kralovic SM, Simbartl LA, Whitlock JL, Jain R, Roselle GA. Complications of hospital-onset healthcare facility-associated Clostridium difficile infections among veterans. Infect Control Hosp Epidemiol. 2016;37(6):717–9. https://doi.org/10.1017/ice.2016.33.

318. Karanika S, Paudel S, Zervou FN, Grigoras C, Zacharioudakis IM, Mylonakis E. Prevalence and clinical outcomes of Clostridium difficile infection in the intensive care unit: a systematic review and meta-analysis. Open Forum Infect Dis. 2016;3(1):ofv186. https://doi.org/10.1093/ofid/ofv186.

319. Micek ST, Schramm G, Morrow L, Frazee E, Personett H, Doherty JA, et al. Clostridium difficile infection: a multicenter study of epidemiology and outcomes in mechanically ventilated patients. Crit Care Med. 2013;41(8):1968–75. https://doi.org/10.1097/CCM.0b013e31828a40d5.

320. Zilberberg MD, Nathanson BH, Sadigov S, Higgins TL, Kollef MH, Shorr AF. Epidemiology and outcomes of clostridium difficile-associated disease among patients on prolonged acute mechanical ventilation. Chest. 2009;136(3):752–8. https://doi.org/10.1378/chest.09-0596.

321. Marra AR, Edmond MB, Wenzel RP, Bearman GM. Hospital-acquired Clostridium difficile-associated disease in the intensive care unit setting: epidemiology, clinical course and outcome. BMC Infect Dis. 2007;7:42. https://doi.org/10.1186/1471-2334-7-42.

322. Zilberberg MD, Shorr AF, Micek ST, Kollef MH. Clostridium difficile recurrence is a strong predictor of 30-day rehospitalization among patients in intensive care. Infect Control Hosp Epidemiol. 2015;36(3):273–9. https://doi.org/10.1017/ice.2014.47.

323. Johnson S, Lavergne V, Skinner AM, Gonzales-Luna AJ, Garey KW, Kelly CP, et al. Clinical practice guideline by the Infectious Diseases Society of America (IDSA) and Society for Healthcare Epidemiology of America (SHEA): 2021 focused update guidelines on management of Clostridioides difficile infection in adults. Clin Infect Dis. 2021;73(5):e1029–44. https://doi.org/10.1093/cid/ciab549.

324. Furuya-Kanamori L, Marquess J, Yakob L, Riley TV, Paterson DL, Foster NF, et al. Asymptomatic Clostridium difficile colonization: epidemiology and clinical implications. BMC Infect Dis. 2015;15:516. https://doi.org/10.1186/s12879-015-1258-4.

325. Miles-Jay A, Snitkin ES, Lin MY, Shimasaki T, Schoeny M, Fukuda C, et al. Longitudinal genomic surveillance of carriage and transmission of Clostridioides difficile in an intensive care unit. Nat Med. 2023;29(10):2526–34. https://doi.org/10.1038/s41591-023-02549-4.

326. Worley J, Delaney ML, Cummins CK, DuBois A, Klompas M, Bry L. Genomic determination of relative risks for Clostridioides difficile infection from asymptomatic carriage in intensive care unit patients. Clin Infect Dis. 2021;73(7):e1727–36. https://doi.org/10.1093/cid/ciaa894.

327. Lyras D, O'Connor JR, Howarth PM, Sambol SP, Carter GP, Phumoonna T, et al. Toxin B is essential for virulence of Clostridium difficile. Nature. 2009;458(7242):1176–9. https://doi.org/10.1038/nature07822.

328. Sehgal K, Khanna S. Gut microbiome and Clostridioides difficile infection: a closer look at the microscopic interface. Ther Adv Gastroenterol. 2021;14:1756284821994736. https://doi.org/10.1177/1756284821994736.

329. Tedesco FJ, Barton RW, Alpers DH. Clindamycin-associated colitis. A prospective study. Ann Intern Med. 1974;81(4):429–33. https://doi.org/10.7326/0003-4819-81-4-429.

330. Brown KA, Khanafer N, Daneman N, Fisman DN. Meta-analysis of antibiotics and the risk of community-associated Clostridium difficile infection. Antimicrob Agents Chemother. 2013;57(5):2326–32. https://doi.org/10.1128/AAC.02176-12.
331. Deshpande A, Pasupuleti V, Thota P, Pant C, Rolston DD, Sferra TJ, et al. Community-associated Clostridium difficile infection and antibiotics: a meta-analysis. J Antimicrob Chemother. 2013;68(9):1951–61. https://doi.org/10.1093/jac/dkt129.
332. Slimings C, Riley TV. Antibiotics and hospital-acquired Clostridium difficile infection: update of systematic review and meta-analysis. J Antimicrob Chemother. 2014;69(4):881–91. https://doi.org/10.1093/jac/dkt477.
333. Stevens V, Dumyati G, Fine LS, Fisher SG, van Wijngaarden E. Cumulative antibiotic exposures over time and the risk of Clostridium difficile infection. Clin Infect Dis. 2011;53(1):42–8. https://doi.org/10.1093/cid/cir301.
334. Furuya-Kanamori L, Stone JC, Clark J, McKenzie SJ, Yakob L, Paterson DL, et al. Comorbidities, exposure to medications, and the risk of community-acquired Clostridium difficile infection: a systematic review and meta-analysis. Infect Control Hosp Epidemiol. 2015;36(2):132–41. https://doi.org/10.1017/ice.2014.39.
335. US Food and Drug Administration. FDA Drug Safety Communication: Clostridium difficile associated diarrhea can be associated with stomach acid drugs known as proton pump inhibitors (PPIs). 2012. https://www.fda.gov/drugs/drug-safety-and-availability/fda-drug-safety-communication-clostridium-difficile-associated-diarrhea-can-be-associated-stomach. Accessed 2 Feb 2024.
336. Wang Y, Ye Z, Ge L, Siemieniuk RAC, Wang X, Wang Y, et al. Efficacy and safety of gastrointestinal bleeding prophylaxis in critically ill patients: systematic review and network meta-analysis. BMJ. 2020;368:l6744. https://doi.org/10.1136/bmj.l6744.
337. Abou Chakra CN, McGeer A, Labbe AC, Simor AE, Gold WL, Muller MP, et al. Factors associated with complications of Clostridium difficile infection in a multicenter prospective cohort. Clin Infect Dis. 2015;61(12):1781–8. https://doi.org/10.1093/cid/civ749.
338. Abou Chakra CN, Pepin J, Sirard S, Valiquette L. Risk factors for recurrence, complications and mortality in Clostridium difficile infection: a systematic review. PLoS One. 2014;9(6):e98400. https://doi.org/10.1371/journal.pone.0098400.
339. Bosch DE, Mathias PC, Krumm N, Bryan A, Fang FC, Greninger AL. Elevated white blood cell count does not predict Clostridium difficile nucleic acid testing results. Clin Infect Dis. 2021;73(4):699–705. https://doi.org/10.1093/cid/ciab106.
340. Kundrapu S, Sunkesula VC, Jury LA, Sethi AK, Donskey CJ. Utility of perirectal swab specimens for diagnosis of Clostridium difficile infection. Clin Infect Dis. 2012;55(11):1527–30. https://doi.org/10.1093/cid/cis707.
341. Sailhamer EA, Carson K, Chang Y, Zacharias N, Spaniolas K, Tabbara M, et al. Fulminant Clostridium difficile colitis: patterns of care and predictors of mortality. Arch Surg. 2009;144(5):433–9; discussion 9–40. https://doi.org/10.1001/archsurg.2009.51.
342. Louie TJ, Miller MA, Mullane KM, Weiss K, Lentnek A, Golan Y, et al. Fidaxomicin versus vancomycin for Clostridium difficile infection. N Engl J Med. 2011;364(5):422–31. https://doi.org/10.1056/NEJMoa0910812.
343. Guery B, Menichetti F, Anttila VJ, Adomakoh N, Aguado JM, Bisnauthsing K, et al. Extended-pulsed fidaxomicin versus vancomycin for Clostridium difficile infection in patients 60 years and older (EXTEND): a randomised, controlled, open-label, phase 3b/4 trial. Lancet Infect Dis. 2018;18(3):296–307. https://doi.org/10.1016/S1473-3099(17)30751-X.
344. Cornely OA, Vehreschild M, Adomakoh N, Georgopali A, Karas A, Kazeem G, et al. Extended-pulsed fidaxomicin versus vancomycin for Clostridium difficile infection: EXTEND study subgroup analyses. Eur J Clin Microbiol Infect Dis. 2019;38(6):1187–94. https://doi.org/10.1007/s10096-019-03525-y.
345. Patel D, Senecal J, Spellberg B, Morris AM, Saxinger L, Footer BW, et al. Fidaxomicin to prevent recurrent Clostridioides difficile: what will it cost in the USA and Canada? JAC Antimicrob Resist. 2023;5(1):dlac138. https://doi.org/10.1093/jacamr/dlac138.

346. Cohen SH, Gerding DN, Johnson S, Kelly CP, Loo VG, McDonald LC, et al. Clinical practice guidelines for Clostridium difficile infection in adults: 2010 update by the society for healthcare epidemiology of America (SHEA) and the infectious diseases society of America (IDSA). Infect Control Hosp Epidemiol. 2010;31(5):431–55. https://doi.org/10.1086/651706.

347. Zar FA, Bakkanagari SR, Moorthi KM, Davis MB. A comparison of vancomycin and metronidazole for the treatment of Clostridium difficile-associated diarrhea, stratified by disease severity. Clin Infect Dis. 2007;45(3):302–7. https://doi.org/10.1086/519265.

348. Stevens VW, Nelson RE, Schwab-Daugherty EM, Khader K, Jones MM, Brown KA, et al. Comparative effectiveness of vancomycin and metronidazole for the prevention of recurrence and death in patients with Clostridium difficile infection. JAMA Intern Med. 2017;177(4):546–53. https://doi.org/10.1001/jamainternmed.2016.9045.

349. Akamine CM, Ing MB, Jackson CS, Loo LK. The efficacy of intracolonic vancomycin for severe Clostridium difficile colitis: a case series. BMC Infect Dis. 2016;16:316. https://doi.org/10.1186/s12879-016-1657-1.

350. Apisarnthanarak A, Razavi B, Mundy LM. Adjunctive intracolonic vancomycin for severe Clostridium difficile colitis: case series and review of the literature. Clin Infect Dis. 2002;35(6):690–6. https://doi.org/10.1086/342334.

351. Kim PK, Huh HC, Cohen HW, Feinberg EJ, Ahmad S, Coyle C, et al. Intracolonic vancomycin for severe Clostridium difficile colitis. Surg Infect (Larchmt). 2013;14(6):532–9. https://doi.org/10.1089/sur.2012.158.

352. Malamood M, Nellis E, Ehrlich AC, Friedenberg FK. Vancomycin enemas as adjunctive therapy for Clostridium difficile infection. J Clin Med Res. 2015;7(6):422–7. https://doi.org/10.14740/jocmr2117w.

353. Rokas KE, Johnson JW, Beardsley JR, Ohl CA, Luther VP, Williamson JC. The addition of intravenous metronidazole to oral vancomycin is associated with improved mortality in critically ill patients with Clostridium difficile infection. Clin Infect Dis. 2015;61(6):934–41. https://doi.org/10.1093/cid/civ409.

354. Wang Y, Schluger A, Li J, Gomez-Simmonds A, Salmasian H, Freedberg DE. Does addition of intravenous metronidazole to oral vancomycin improve outcomes in Clostridioides difficile infection? Clin Infect Dis. 2020;71(9):2414–20. https://doi.org/10.1093/cid/ciz1115.

355. Kelly CR, Khoruts A, Staley C, Sadowsky MJ, Abd M, Alani M, et al. Effect of fecal microbiota transplantation on recurrence in multiply recurrent Clostridium difficile infection: a randomized trial. Ann Intern Med. 2016;165(9):609–16. https://doi.org/10.7326/M16-0271.

356. Cheng YW, Phelps E, Nemes S, Rogers N, Sagi S, Bohm M, et al. Fecal microbiota transplant decreases mortality in patients with refractory severe or fulminant Clostridioides difficile infection. Clin Gastroenterol Hepatol. 2020;18(10):2234–43.e1. https://doi.org/10.1016/j.cgh.2019.12.029.

357. Hocquart M, Lagier JC, Cassir N, Saidani N, Eldin C, Kerbaj J, et al. Early fecal microbiota transplantation improves survival in severe Clostridium difficile infections. Clin Infect Dis. 2018;66(5):645–50. https://doi.org/10.1093/cid/cix762.

358. Tixier EN, Verheyen E, Ungaro RC, Grinspan AM. Faecal microbiota transplant decreases mortality in severe and fulminant Clostridioides difficile infection in critically ill patients. Aliment Pharmacol Ther. 2019;50(10):1094–9. https://doi.org/10.1111/apt.15526.

359. Spartz EJ, Estafanos M, Mallick R, Gaertner W, Vakayil V, Jahansouz C, et al. Fecal microbiota transplantation for fulminant Clostridioides difficile infection: a combined medical and surgical case series. Cureus. 2023;15(2):e34998. https://doi.org/10.7759/cureus.34998.

360. Song YN, Yang DY, Veldhuyzen van Zanten S, Wong K, McArthur E, Song CZ, et al. Fecal microbiota transplantation for severe or fulminant Clostridioides difficile infection: systematic review and meta-analysis. J Can Assoc Gastroenterol. 2022;5(1):e1–11. https://doi.org/10.1093/jcag/gwab023.

361. US Food and Drug Administration. VOWST. 2023. https://www.fda.gov/vaccines-blood-biologics/vowst. Accessed 16 Feb 2024.

362. US Food and Drug Administration. REBYOTA. 2022. https://www.fda.gov/vaccines-blood-biologics/vaccines/rebyota. Accessed 16 Feb 2024.

363. Neal MD, Alverdy JC, Hall DE, Simmons RL, Zuckerbraun BS. Diverting loop ileostomy and colonic lavage: an alternative to total abdominal colectomy for the treatment of severe, complicated Clostridium difficile associated disease. Ann Surg. 2011;254(3):423–7; discussion 7–9. https://doi.org/10.1097/SLA.0b013e31822ade48.
364. Gerding DN, Kelly CP, Rahav G, Lee C, Dubberke ER, Kumar PN, et al. Bezlotoxumab for prevention of recurrent Clostridium difficile infection in patients at increased risk for recurrence. Clin Infect Dis. 2018;67(5):649–56. https://doi.org/10.1093/cid/ciy171.
365. Carignan A, Allard C, Pepin J, Cossette B, Nault V, Valiquette L. Risk of Clostridium difficile infection after perioperative antibacterial prophylaxis before and during an outbreak of infection due to a hypervirulent strain. Clin Infect Dis. 2008;46(12):1838–43. https://doi.org/10.1086/588291.
366. Carignan A, Poulin S, Martin P, Labbe AC, Valiquette L, Al-Bachari H, et al. Efficacy of secondary prophylaxis with vancomycin for preventing recurrent Clostridium difficile infections. Am J Gastroenterol. 2016;111(12):1834–40. https://doi.org/10.1038/ajg.2016.417.
367. Johnson SW, Brown SV, Priest DH. Effectiveness of oral vancomycin for prevention of healthcare facility-onset Clostridioides difficile infection in targeted patients during systemic antibiotic exposure. Clin Infect Dis. 2020;71(5):1133–9. https://doi.org/10.1093/cid/ciz966.
368. Kelly CR, Fischer M, Allegretti JR, LaPlante K, Stewart DB, Limketkai BN, et al. ACG clinical guidelines: prevention, diagnosis, and treatment of Clostridioides difficile infections. Am J Gastroenterol. 2021;116(6):1124–47. https://doi.org/10.14309/ajg.0000000000001278.
369. Mayer S, Bonhag C, Jenkins P, Cornett B, Watts P, Scherbak D. Probiotic-associated central venous catheter bloodstream infections lead to increased mortality in the ICU. Crit Care Med. 2023;51(11):1459–78. https://doi.org/10.1097/CCM.0000000000005953.

Chapter 30
Severe Infections Early After Solid-Organ Transplantation

Francisco Machiavello Roman, Maricar Malinis, and Fionna Feller

30.1 Introduction

Solid-organ transplant recipients (SOTrs) are at risk of severe infections that may rapidly progress to shock and end-organ damage, and they have a disproportionately high risk of infection by resistant organisms when compared to immunocompetent hosts. The assessment of the critically ill SOTr presenting with an infectious syndrome considers clinical and epidemiological variables related to the host and donor. The timing after transplantation and the type and intensity of immunosuppression define a patient's net state of immunosuppression, which predicts their risk of opportunistic infections. Latent endemic infections related to remote travel may become manifest after transplantation, and donor-derived infections, which may not have been recognized at the time of organ procurement, can present aggressively and lethally shortly after SOT.

Therapy is guided by two general principles: syndromic antimicrobial prescription (i.e., empiric therapy is directed against the expected pathogens of a specific infectious condition) and, in some situations, reduction of immunosuppression when feasible. Identification of the organisms colonizing the intestinal, genitourinary, and respiratory tracts of transplant candidates, particularly resistant species, can guide posttransplant empiric antimicrobial therapy in the intensive care setting. A careful review of drug-drug interactions between antimicrobials and antirejection agents, particularly calcineurin inhibitors and mTOR inhibitors, is essential.

This chapter provides an overview of common infections that may present in critically ill SOTr, with particular emphasis on infections occurring early after

F. Machiavello Roman · M. Malinis (✉)
Section of Infectious Diseases, Yale University School of Medicine, New Haven, CT, USA
e-mail: maricar.malinis@yale.edu

F. Feller
Division of Infectious Diseases, Vanderbilt University, Nashville, TN, USA

© The Author(s), under exclusive license to Springer Nature Switzerland AG 2025
Y. Alzaidi, M. A. Gebily (eds.), *The Pharmacist's Expanded Role in Critical Care Medicine*, https://doi.org/10.1007/978-3-031-77335-8_30

transplantation. We provide general recommendations about antimicrobial courses, but it is notable that randomized controlled trials are limited in the SOT population; hence, most of the evidence provided for these recommendations results from retrospective analysis or expert opinion.

30.2 Bloodstream Infections

Bloodstream infections (BSIs) are common among SOTrs. National surveillance studies estimate a 1-year bacteremia incidence of approximately 9%, with nearly 80% of infections occurring within the first year after transplantation [1]. Gram-negative bacilli cause most BSIs among SOTrs, responsible for over 75% of cases in kidney allograft recipients and over 50% of BSIs in lung, heart, and liver allograft recipients [2]. Rates of BSIs by *S. aureus* and *Enterococcus* spp. are overall stable or decreasing, mainly due to reduced endovascular catheter use after transplantation, but they remain associated with significant morbidity among SOTrs [3–5]. Candidemia is rare, only contributing to approximately 5% of BSI episodes, yet it is associated with significant rates of treatment failure and morbidity [6, 7].

BSIs occurring early after transplantation should always raise the possibility of a donor-derived infection. Eleven to fourteen percent of donors have bacteremia at the time of organ procurement. Despite this, an active donor bloodstream infection is not an absolute contraindication to organ donation, as prompt, effective antimicrobial therapy for at least 7 days after transplantation significantly reduces the risk of donor-derived infection [8]. When a donor-derived BSI is suspected, the organ procurement organization (OPO) should be contacted by the designated patient safety coordinator of the recipient's transplant center for additional information, such as antimicrobial susceptibilities of the pathogen and complications of bacteremia in the donor. Also, it is important for the OPO to inform other transplant centers that received organs from the same donor so they can appropriately investigate and manage their recipients.

Antimicrobial resistance is a significant concern when managing BSIs in SOTr, which are disproportionately affected by resistant pathogens [9]. This is in part explained by prolonged antimicrobial exposure and frequent contact with healthcare facilities (particularly intensive care units) before transplantation, but it has been established that SOTr status is an independent risk factor for infection by multidrug-resistant (MDR) bacteria [10–12]. Discordance between the resistance patterns of organisms isolated in SOTr and traditional hospital antibiograms has been noted, so caution is warranted when using this tool to guide empiric antimicrobial coverage [13]. When available, rapid genotypic (Biofire®, Luminex®, GenMark®) and phenotypic (Accelerate PhenoTest® BC Kit) antimicrobial resistance assays may be used to escalate or de-escalate antimicrobial therapy, but this recommendation is based on the consensus of expert opinion [14].

30.2.1 Gram-Negative BSIs

Escherichia coli and *Klebsiella pneumoniae* are the most frequent Gram-negative bacilli and Enterobacteriaceae implicated in BSIs [10]. *Pseudomonas aeruginosa* BSIs are more common among SOTrs than immunocompetent hosts, accounting for 8–15% of BSIs in a Spanish SOTr cohort [2]. The source of Gram-negative BSIs often correlates with the transplanted organ [2]. Rates of antibiotic resistance among Enterobacteriaceae vary between transplant centers, but they can be alarmingly high—as high as 40% of all isolates in a multicenter US cohort were found to produce extended-spectrum beta-lactamases (ESBLs), and 8% displayed carbapenem resistance [10, 11]. Colonization by an ESBL-producing or carbapenem-resistant organism in any body site within 1 year of transplantation is an independent risk factor for subsequent MDR BSIs, highlighting the importance of reviewing the antibiograms from prior infections when choosing empiric antimicrobial coverage [10, 11]. Counterintuitively, retrospective studies found that the rates of respiratory failure and septic shock among SOTrs were not higher when compared to non-SOTr with bacteremia, and the number of immunosuppressants inversely correlated with the risk of shock, challenging the notion that reduction of immunosuppression is imperative when managing sepsis and BSIs [2]. The optimal length of antimicrobial therapy has not been defined, but most providers prescribe courses of 7–14 days. Early retrospective data suggest that transition to oral antibiotics after 4 days of adequate treatment is equally effective and possibly safer than a full intravenous course when managing uncomplicated BSIs, i.e., those with adequate source control and no evidence of metastatic infections [15].

30.2.2 Gram-Positive BSIs

The cumulative incidence of bacteremia by Gram-positive cocci has been estimated at 2.8% during the first year after transplantation, half that of Gram-negative bacilli [1]. *Staphylococcus aureus* and *Enterococcus* spp. are the most common organisms of Gram-positive BSIs, with the latter being of particular concern among liver allograft recipients [4, 12]. Methicillin-resistant *Staphylococcus aureus* (MRSA) accounts for 26–100% of all *S. aureus* bloodstream isolates, and MRSA infections are associated with an overall 21% 30-day mortality among liver allograft recipients [16]. Endovascular infections are the most common source of *S. aureus* BSIs, and pretransplant colonization is a significant risk factor for subsequent infections. Compared to non-SOTr, retrospective studies found that SOTr experienced higher rates of shock and acute respiratory distress syndrome (ARDS), albeit with lower rates of metastatic infection [3]. Treatment recommendations are similar to those of immunocompetent hosts [5].

Enterococcus faecalis and *Enterococcus faecium* are common agents of BSIs. Vancomycin-resistant strains, most frequently seen with *E. faecium*, colonize 15%

of patients with chronic liver disease awaiting a transplant and liver transplant recipients [12] and may cause secondary bacteremia. Intra-abdominal infections are the most common source of BSIs. General treatment principles are similar to those of immunocompetent hosts. When treating vancomycin-resistant strains with daptomycin, it should be noted that treatment failure and increased 30-day mortality have been associated with doses under 10 mg/kg, assuming a normal renal function [12].

30.2.3 Candidemia

Candida species cause approximately 5% of all BSIs in SOTr. 3–5% of heart and lung allograft recipients experience candidemia, most frequently within 30 days of surgery [6, 17] and 1% of donors have candidemia at the time of organ procurement [8]. Despite their relative infrequency, episodes of candidemia are associated with a 60% mortality, and they can lead to injury of the graft vascular anastomosis through arteritis and mycotic aneurysms [6, 8]. *C. albicans* is the most common species implicated in BSIs, but fluconazole-resistant species like *C. glabrata* and *C. krusei* have become more prominent, possibly due to antimicrobial selection from azole prophylaxis. Special considerations when treating SOTr include drug-drug interactions of triazoles and calcineurin inhibitors (cyclosporine, tacrolimus) or mTOR inhibitors (sirolimus, everolimus), and low urinary concentrations of echinocandins and certain triazoles when the source of candidemia is a urinary tract infection.

30.3 Pneumonia and Other Respiratory Tract Infections

This section mainly addresses respiratory infections in lung transplant recipients who are at the highest risk of pulmonary infections. Compared to other SOTrs, the increased risk stems from donor pretransplant colonization by bacteria and fungi (often displaying antimicrobial resistance), more intense immunosuppression, ischemic airway injury after organ procurement, and an impaired cough mechanism [18]. Viral, bacterial, and fungal pulmonary infections in lung allograft recipients are significant causes of bronchiolitis obliterans syndrome (BOS) and chronic lung allograft dysfunction (CLAD), significantly impacting graft function and overall survival [19–21]. Conversely, infection risk is increased during the treatment of BOS due to increased immunosuppression.

30.3.1 Bacterial Infections

Bacterial pneumonia accounts for most early post-lung transplant infections and is most frequently seen within the first and third months after surgery [19, 22]. Risk factors for bacterial pneumonia include mechanical ventilation for more than 48 h after surgery, cardiovascular comorbidity, and a history of cystic fibrosis as the indication for lung transplantation [22, 23]. *Pseudomonas aeruginosa* and MRSA are the most encountered organisms, followed by *Acinetobacter* species and other Gram-negative bacilli [18, 19]. Empiric antimicrobial therapy should consider these organisms and those identified through recipient and donor pretransplant bronchoscopy. Infections by MDR *Pseudomonas aeruginosa*, *Burkholderia* species, and nontuberculous mycobacteria are of particular concern among lung transplant recipients with a history of cystic fibrosis and non-cystic bronchiectasis. Allograft colonization occurs frequently and quickly after surgery, with a median time to colonization as short as 23 days in some case series [24]. Hence, reviewing prior microbiological data and antibiograms is essential when deciding on an antimicrobial course. Atypical organisms are also important pathogens of pneumonia in lung allograft recipients. Among them, *Mycoplasma* and *Ureaplasma* species are especially relevant given their association with hyperammonemia syndrome, a condition characterized by encephalopathy, brain edema, and elevated serum ammonia levels that can lead to death through severe intracranial hypertension [25, 26]. When the syndrome is suspected, atypical coverage with a tetracycline, fluoroquinolone, or both should be started even before identifying these organisms (dual therapy is the preference of some experts; note that macrolides are not recommended as *Mycoplasma hominis* is universally resistant and *Ureaplasma* species display significant resistance to this antibiotic class) [27]. The length of antimicrobial therapy for bacterial pneumonia is usually 14 days for most bacterial pathogens, which may be prolonged in the event of slow recovery [18]. Local complications such as parapneumonic effusions or empyema occur in 3–5% of lung allograft recipients, and these should be explored when a patient appears to be failing antimicrobial therapy [18, 19].

30.3.2 Viral Infections

Community-acquired respiratory viruses (CARVs) follow bacteria as the most common organisms involved in pulmonary infections of SOTr and lung allograft recipients, particularly [22]. The incidence of viral respiratory infections among lung transplant recipients is 0.76–0.91/patient-year, and the risk of progression from a mild upper respiratory infection to a more severe lower respiratory infection varies between 6% and 40% [28]. SOTrs are at higher risk of respiratory failure, ICU admission, mechanical ventilation, and death compared to non-SOTrs despite similar incidences of viral respiratory infections between these groups [29]. The most frequently encountered CARVs in transplant recipients are influenza, parainfluenza, respiratory syncytial virus (RSV), human metapneumovirus, and coronaviruses, including SARS-CoV-2 [28, 30]. RSV infections are of special concern, given their association with acute and chronic lung allograft dysfunction [31, 32]. Antivirals are available for influenza A and B (neuraminidase inhibitors and baloxavir), RSV (ribavirin), adenovirus (cidofovir and brincidofovir), and SARS-CoV-2 (remdesivir, nirmatrelvir/ritonavir, molnupiravir); some experts also recommend using ribavirin in severe cases of parainfluenza and human metapneumovirus infections. A noteworthy difference with immunocompetent hosts is that the efficacy of antiviral agents likely persists for many days after infection as viral replication lasts longer in SOTr (i.e., it would be appropriate to treat a patient for influenza with neuraminidase inhibitors even if symptomatic for more than 2 days) [28, 29]. Rates of antiviral resistance are overall low, but this possibility should be entertained when high viral replication rates persist after completing a treatment course. Additional considerations when treating viral respiratory infections in SOTr include the possibility of using longer courses or higher doses of antivirals (e.g., prescribing 10 days of oseltamivir 150 mg twice daily for influenza, although data is limited for this practice) [28]; the importance of reducing or stopping antimetabolites (mycophenolate mofetil, azathioprine) while maintaining the doses of calcineurin inhibitors and steroids, particularly in SARS-CoV-2 infections [29]; and the probable benefit of adjuvant immunoglobulin in RSV and adenovirus lung infections [28, 33]. The treatment of RSV warrants special mention, as ongoing research efforts are dedicated to finding new treatment strategies. The benefit of ribavirin is mostly extrapolated from hematopoietic stem cell transplant recipients and neonates. There is a lack of high-quality data in the SOTr population and considerable variability in the practice standards between transplant centers [34]. Ribavirin is available in inhaled, oral, and intravenous formulations. Inhaled administration is falling out of favor due to concerns about its cost and the exposure of patients, visitors, and healthcare workers to its teratogenic effect. The oral presentation is often well tolerated, and side effects to monitor include hemolytic anemia, leukopenia, and neuropsychiatric symptoms [28, 33]. Some centers complement this antiviral with intravenous immunoglobulin (IVIg) or RSV-specific immunoglobulin and steroids. Of note, despite the well-established role of RSV in the appearance of CLAD, it is unclear if its incidence is reduced with antiviral treatment [31].

30.3.3 Fungal Infections

Although less frequent than bacterial and viral infections, fungal infections are associated with significant graft failure rates, morbidity, and mortality. *Aspergillus* and *Candida* species are the most common fungal organisms identified in pulmonary infections; *Candida albicans* is the predominant species, but non-*albicans* and fluconazole-resistant species are rising [18, 35]. Anti-mold prophylaxis with inhaled amphotericin B and/or a systemic triazole has reduced early invasive fungal infections [36], so invasive parenchymal disease is not a common phenomenon in the first months after transplantation. However, tracheobronchial anastomotic infections due to *Aspergillus* and *Candida* species (fungal tracheobronchitis) occur within the first 3 months after surgery in patients with prolonged airway ischemia. This is a severe condition with an estimated 23% mortality that may initially present asymptomatically, with later progression to purulence, ulceration, pseudomembranes, and necrosis of the airway anastomosis [18, 19, 35, 37, 38]. Treatment requires a combination of systemic therapy (triazole or echinocandin), inhaled amphotericin B, and surgical debridement. A second scenario of early invasive infections after transplantation is the occurrence of post-viral invasive fungal infections, which occur after 15% of episodes of respiratory viral infections [21]. *Aspergillus* species are most implicated in these infections, which occur in similar frequency after SARS-CoV-2, influenza, parainfluenza, human metapneumovirus, and respiratory syncytial virus (RSV) infections [21]. Invasive fungal infections occur shortly after respiratory viral infections, and they should be suspected when respiratory symptoms persist or progress after an initial viral respiratory illness.

30.4 Intra-abdominal Infections

Infections in recipients of intra-abdominal allografts (liver, kidney, pancreas, small bowel) are often the result of technical problems that arise during surgery [39]. These patients are at risk of common postsurgical complications, such as surgical site infections, and more severe, organ-specific infections. Unique challenges related to addressing intra-abdominal infections in SOTr include oligo-symptomatic presentations that are clinically indistinguishable from acute organ rejection, often delaying diagnosis and effective treatment, and the need for source control, which may occasionally lead to partial or complete allograft resection [39]. The principles of antimicrobial therapy are similar to those discussed for other infectious syndromes. Empiric coverage should be based on prior isolates of the recipient and donor and local antimicrobial susceptibilities. Although not a common intra-abdominal pathogen in immunocompetent hosts, *Pseudomonas aeruginosa* should always be included in the spectrum of SOTr's antimicrobial coverage [40]. Antifungals and antibiotics against vancomycin-resistant *Enterococcus* (VRE) are usually not necessary as first-line agents unless there is a concern for bowel perforation, known prior colonization by VRE, or severe sepsis that has failed to respond to common antimicrobials covering Gram-positive, Gram-negative, and anaerobic organisms [39, 41]. Early drainage of large collections is imperative, as it provides source control and allows for species identification and adjustment of antimicrobial therapy. Table 30.1 summarizes common organ-specific infections.

30.4.1 Liver-Specific Infections

Liver-specific infections include cholangitis, liver abscesses, infected bilomas, and infection of retained transjugular intrahepatic portosystemic shunt (TIPS) catheters. Empiric coverage should target Gram-negative, anaerobic, and enterococcal species; MRSA and VRE coverage is indicated in those known to be colonized by these organisms or those presenting in sepsis or shock [39, 41]. Length on therapy depends

Table 30.1 Common allograft-specific infections and their associated risk factors (adapted from Haidar and Green [39])

Allograft	Infection	Risk factors
Liver	Cholangitis	Hepatic artery thrombosis, biliary strictures, biliary leaks, Roux-en-Y biliary anastomosis
	Liver abscess	Hepatic artery thrombosis, allograft necrosis, Roux-en-Y biliary anastomosis, bloodstream infections, allograft biopsy
	Infected biloma	Biliary leak
	Endoptipsitis (infected transjugular intrahepatic portosystemic shunt catheter)	Retained TIPS catheter, recurrent bloodstream infections
Kidney	Renal/perinephric abscess	Surgical site infection, hematoma, urinary tract infection, ureteral leak
	Allograft candidiasis	*Candida* contamination of allograft preservation fluid
Pancreas	Pancreatic abscess, peritonitis	Leakage of donor duodenal content at anastomosis site
Intestine	Peritonitis	Arterial thrombosis/graft ischemia, anastomotic leaks

on the capacity to achieve source control and is highly individualized, driven by clinical progress and radiologic follow-up.

30.4.2 Kidney-Specific Infections

Allograft pyelonephritis and urinary tract infections are discussed in a separate section. Renal abscesses represent an uncommon complication after kidney transplantation, but they may be large and severe enough to prompt allograft nephrectomy. Empiric coverage should target Gram-negative bacilli, *Enterococcus* species, and possible donor-derived organisms [39]. *Candida* allograft infections are challenging, and they are often the result of contamination of the preservation fluid after organ procurement [42]. The disease spectrum includes abscesses, infected urinomas, and aneurysms of the graft anastomosis due to arteritis; the latter is a medical and surgical emergency that puts patients at risk of graft loss and death from aneurysmal rupture [39, 42]. Surgery (aneurysm repair or nephrectomy) and effective antifungals (fluconazole or amphotericin B deoxycholate for fluconazole-resistant strains) are the mainstay of therapy. There is some experience with using echinocandins and triazoles other than fluconazole, but given the low urinary penetration of these agents, their use should be individualized [39, 42].

30.4.3 Clostridioides difficile *Infection*

SOTrs are at increased risk of *C. difficile* infection (CDI) and severe disease manifestations compared to immunocompetent hosts. The frequency and timing of infection vary according to organ type. Lung and heart allograft recipients appear to have the highest incidence, whereas occurrence tends to be earlier in liver allograft recipients, as early as 1 month after transplantation [43, 44]. Up to 20% of SOTrs do not have antimicrobial exposure preceding a CDI episode; alternative factors such as intense immunosuppression, hypogammaglobulinemia, and enteritis secondary to antirejection medications (particularly mycophenolate) account for this observation [43]. There is a dearth of treatment recommendations specific to SOTr; the treatment principles are the same as those applied to immunocompetent hosts. Stopping antibiotics, when feasible, is the first therapeutic step. Severe disease is treated with high-dose oral or enteral vancomycin (500 mg every 6 h) and intravenous metronidazole. Even though standard vancomycin doses (125 mg every 6 h) achieve intraluminal concentrations significantly above the *C. difficile* minimum inhibitory concentration, these high doses are used to ensure sufficient distribution throughout the bowel [43, 45]. Early consideration for colectomy is warranted in patients without appropriate clinical response after 48 h of treatment. Fidaxomicin appears to be safe in SOTr. Its efficacy is similar to that of vancomycin in managing acute CDI [44]. Still, it may confer a decreased risk of recurrence and selection of vancomycin-resistant enterococci [43]. The benefit of IVIg is unclear, but some experts recommend its use in recurrent CDI episodes after confirming hypogammaglobulinemia [43–45]. The treatment duration of a first episode is 10 days, whereas recurrent episodes can be treated with prolonged vancomycin tapers over many weeks or a taper pulse fidaxomicin regime [43, 45]. Anecdotal evidence suggests that using bezlotoxumab, a fully human antibody that neutralizes *C. difficile* toxin B, is safe in SOTr and should be prescribed to patients treated for recurrence.

30.5 Urinary Tract Infections

This section addresses severe and complicated urinary tract infections (UTIs) in kidney transplant recipients, who are at the highest risk of UTIs among SOTrs. UTIs are associated with kidney allograft rejection and decline in function [46]. UTIs are reported to occur in 25% of all kidney transplant recipients (some series describe a prevalence of up to 80%, but cases of asymptomatic bacteriuria confound this estimate), and the highest incidence of infection occurs in the first 3–6 months after transplantation [46, 47]. Risk factors for severe disease (pyelonephritis or sepsis) in SOTr include the presence of a ureteral stent, vesicoureteral reflux, recent rejection, and induction with lymphocyte-depleting immunosuppression [47]. Common pathogens include Enterobacteriaceae and other Gram-negative bacilli such as *P. aeruginosa*. Rare cases of renal and perinephric abscesses due to *Mycoplasma* and *Ureaplasma* species have been described [46, 47]. Empiric coverage should be directed against common Gram-negative bacilli, including *P. aeruginosa*. Antibiograms from prior cultures should be used as a reference for possible colonization by ESBL-producing organisms, described in up to 25% of patients in some cohorts. The antimicrobial spectrum should be narrowed once microbiological data are available, and treatment length is usually 14 days, which may be prolonged if there are local complications such as a perinephric abscess. Reduction of immunosuppression should be strongly considered in patients with severe infection.

References

1. Neofytos D, Stampf S, Hoessly LD, D'Asaro M, Tang GN, Boggian K, Hirzel C, Khanna N, Manuel O, Mueller NJ, Van Delden C. Bacteremia during the first year after solid organ transplantation: an epidemiological update. Open Forum Infect Dis. 2023;10(6):ofad247. https://doi.org/10.1093/ofid/ofad247.
2. Eichenberger EM, Troy J, Ruffin F, Dagher M, Thaden JT, Ford ML, Fowler VG Jr. Gram-negative bacteremia in solid organ transplant recipients: clinical characteristics and outcomes as compared to immunocompetent non-transplant recipients. Transpl Infect Dis. 2022;24(6):e13969. https://doi.org/10.1111/tid.13969.
3. Eichenberger EM, Ruffin F, Sharma-Kuinkel B, Dagher M, Park L, Kohler C, Sinclair MR, Maskarinec SA, Fowler VG Jr. Bacterial genotype and clinical outcomes in solid organ transplant recipients with Staphylococcus aureus bacteremia. Transpl Infect Dis. 2021;23(6):e13730. https://doi.org/10.1111/tid.13730.
4. Inagaki K, Weinberg JB, Kaul DR. Risk of Staphylococcus aureus bacteremia before and after solid organ transplantation. Transplantation. 2023;107(8):1820–7. https://doi.org/10.1097/tp.0000000000004590.
5. Pereira MR, Rana MM. Methicillin-resistant Staphylococcus aureus in solid organ transplantation-guidelines from the American Society of Transplantation Infectious Diseases Community of Practice. Clin Transpl. 2019;33(9):e13611. https://doi.org/10.1111/ctr.13611.
6. Eichenberger EM, Satola S, Neujahr D, Fowler VG Jr, Gupta D, Ford M, Pouch SM. Candidemia in thoracic solid organ transplant recipients: characteristics and outcomes relative to matched uninfected and bacteremic thoracic organ transplant recipients. Clin Transpl. 2023;37(9):e15038. https://doi.org/10.1111/ctr.15038.
7. Fernández-Ruiz M, Cardozo C, Salavert M, Aguilar-Guisado M, Escolà-Vergé L, Muñoz P, Gioia F, Montejo M, Merino P, Cuervo G, García-Vidal C, Aguado JM. Candidemia in solid organ transplant recipients in Spain: epidemiological trends and determinants of outcome. Transpl Infect Dis. 2019;21(6):e13195. https://doi.org/10.1111/tid.13195.
8. Mehta SR, Logan C, Kotton CN, Kumar D, Aslam S. Use of organs from donors with bloodstream infection, pneumonia, and influenza: results of a survey of infectious diseases practitioners. Transpl Infect Dis. 2017;19(1) https://doi.org/10.1111/tid.12645.
9. So M, Walti L. Challenges of antimicrobial resistance and stewardship in solid organ transplant patients. Curr Infect Dis Rep. 2022;24(5):63–75. https://doi.org/10.1007/s11908-022-00778-1.
10. Anesi JA, Lautenbach E, Tamma PD, Thom KA, Blumberg EA, Alby K, Bilker WB, Werzen A, Tolomeo P, Omorogbe J, Pineles L, Han JH. Risk factors for extended-spectrum β-lactamase-producing enterobacterales bloodstream infection among solid-organ transplant recipients. Clin Infect Dis. 2021;72(6):953–60. https://doi.org/10.1093/cid/ciaa190.

11. Anesi JA, Lautenbach E, Thom KA, Tamma PD, Blumberg EA, Alby K, Bilker WB, Werzen A, Ammazzalorso A, Tolomeo P, Omorogbe J, Pineles L, Han JH. Clinical outcomes and risk factors for carbapenem-resistant enterobacterales bloodstream infection in solid organ transplant recipients. Transplantation. 2023;107(1):254–63. https://doi.org/10.1097/tp.0000000000004265.

12. Mercuro NJ, Gill CM, Kenney RM, Alangaden GJ, Davis SL. Treatment and outcomes of Enterococcus faecium bloodstream infections in solid organ transplant recipients. Transpl Infect Dis. 2020;22(2):e13251. https://doi.org/10.1111/tid.13251.

13. Rosa R, Simkins J, Camargo JF, Martinez O, Abbo LM. Solid organ transplant antibiograms: an opportunity for antimicrobial stewardship. Diagn Microbiol Infect Dis. 2016;86(4):460–3. https://doi.org/10.1016/j.diagmicrobio.2016.08.018.

14. Azar MM, Turbett S, Gaston D, Gitman M, Razonable R, Koo S, Hanson K, Kotton C, Silveira F, Banach DB, Basu SS, Bhaskaran A, Danziger-Isakov L, Bard JD, Gandhi R, Hanisch B, John TM, Odom John AR, Letourneau AR, et al. A consensus conference to define the utility of advanced infectious disease diagnostics in solid organ transplant recipients. Am J Transplant. 2022;22(12):3150–69. https://doi.org/10.1111/ajt.17147.

15. Nussbaum EZ, Koo S, Kotton CN. Oral Antibiotics for Treatment of Gram-Negative Bacteremia in Solid Organ Transplant Recipients: A Propensity Score Weighted Retrospective Observational Study. Clin Infect Dis. 2024;79(1):208–214.

16. Deppermann C, Peiseler M, Zindel J, Zbytnuik L, Lee WY, Pasini E, Baciu C, Matelski J, Lee Y, Kumar D, Humar A, Surewaard B, Kubes P, Bhat M. Tacrolimus impairs Kupffer cell capacity to control bacteremia: why transplant recipients are susceptible to infection. Hepatology. 2021;73(5):1967–84. https://doi.org/10.1002/hep.31499.

17. Fernández-Ruiz M, Cardozo C, Salavert M, Aguilar-Guisado M, Escolà-Vergé L, Muñoz P, Gioia F, Montejo M, Merino P, Cuervo G, García-Vidal C, Aguado JM; CANDIPOP Project, the CANDI-Bundle Group; GEIRASGEMICOMED (SEIMC)REIPI. Candidemia in solid organ transplant recipients in Spain: Epidemiological trends and determinants of outcome. Transpl Infect Dis. 2019;21(6):e13195.

18. Witt CA, Meyers BF, Hachem RR. Pulmonary infections following lung transplantation. Thorac Surg Clin. 2012;22(3):403–12. https://doi.org/10.1016/j.thorsurg.2012.04.006.

19. McCort M, MacKenzie E, Pursell K, Pitrak D. Bacterial infections in lung transplantation. J Thorac Dis. 2021;13(11):6654–72. https://doi.org/10.21037/jtd-2021-12.

20. Permpalung N, Bazemore K, Chiang TP, Mathew J, Barker L, Nematollahi S, Cochran W, Sait AS, Avery RK, Shah PD. Impact of COVID-19 on lung allograft and clinical outcomes in lung transplant recipients: a case-control study. Transplantation. 2021;105(9):2072–9. https://doi.org/10.1097/tp.0000000000003839.

21. Permpalung N, Liang T, Gopinath S, Bazemore K, Mathew J, Ostrander D, Durand CM, Shoham S, Zhang SX, Marr KA, Avery RK, Shah PD. Invasive fungal infections after respiratory viral infections in lung transplant recipients are associated with lung allograft failure and chronic lung allograft dysfunction within 1 year. J Heart Lung Transplant. 2023;42(7):953–63. https://doi.org/10.1016/j.healun.2023.02.005.

22. Fayyaz A, Raja M, Natori Y. Prevention and management of infections in lung transplant recipients. J Clin Med. 2023;13(1) https://doi.org/10.3390/jcm13010011.

23. Ruiz I, Gavaldà J, Monforte V, Len O, Román A, Bravo C, Ferrer A, Tenorio L, Román F, Maestre J, Molina I, Morell F, Pahissa A. Donor-to-host transmission of bacterial and fungal infections in lung transplantation. Am J Transplant. 2006;6(1):178–82. https://doi.org/10.1111/j.1600-6143.2005.01145.x.

24. Holm AE, Schultz HHL, Johansen HK, Pressler T, Lund TK, Iversen M, Perch M. Bacterial re-colonization occurs early after lung transplantation in cystic fibrosis patients. J Clin Med. 2021;10(6) https://doi.org/10.3390/jcm10061275.

25. Tam PCK, Hardie R, Alexander BD, Yarrington ME, Lee MJ, Polage CR, Messina JA, Maziarz EK, Saullo JL, Miller R, Wolfe CR, Arif S, Reynolds JM, Haney JC, Perfect JR, Baker AW. Risk factors, management, and clinical outcomes of invasive Mycoplasma and Ureaplasma infections after lung transplantation. Am J Transplant. 2023;24:641. https://doi.org/10.1016/j.ajt.2023.08.019.

26. Wigston C, Lavender M, Long R, Sankhesara D, Ching D, Weaire-Buchanan G, Mowlaboccus S, Coombs GW, Lam K, Wrobel J, Yaw MC, Musk M, Boan P. Mycoplasma and Ureaplasma donor-derived infection and hyperammonemia syndrome in 4 solid organ transplant recipients from a single donor. Open Forum Infect Dis. 2023;10(6):ofad263. https://doi.org/10.1093/ofid/ofad263.

27. Leger RF, Silverman MS, Hauck ES, Guvakova KD. Hyperammonemia post lung transplantation: a review. Clin Med Insights Circ Respir Pulm Med. 2020;14:1179548420966234. https://doi.org/10.1177/1179548420966234.

28. Bitterman R, Kumar D. Respiratory viruses in solid organ transplant recipients. Viruses. 2021;13(11) https://doi.org/10.3390/v13112146.

29. Munting A, Manuel O. Viral infections in lung transplantation. J Thorac Dis. 2021;13(11):6673–94. https://doi.org/10.21037/jtd-2021-24.

30. Bailey ES, Zemke JN, Choi JY, Gray GC. A mini-review of adverse lung transplant outcomes associated with respiratory viruses. Front Immunol. 2019;10:2861. https://doi.org/10.3389/fimmu.2019.02861.

31. de Zwart A, Riezebos-Brilman A, Lunter G, Vonk J, Glanville AR, Gottlieb J, Permpalung N, Kerstjens H, Alffenaar JW, Verschuuren E. Respiratory syncytial virus, human metapneumovirus, and parainfluenza virus infections in lung transplant recipients: a systematic review of outcomes and treatment strategies. Clin Infect Dis. 2022;74(12):2252–60. https://doi.org/10.1093/cid/ciab969.

32. Mahan LD, Points A, Mohanka MR, Bollineni S, Joerns J, Kaza V, La Hoz RM, Gao A, Zhang S, Torres F, Banga A. Characteristics and outcomes among lung transplant patients with respiratory syncytial virus infection. Transpl Infect Dis. 2021;23(4):e13661. https://doi.org/10.1111/tid.13661.

33. Marcelin JR, Wilson JW, Razonable RR. Oral ribavirin therapy for respiratory syncytial virus infections in moderately to severely immunocompromised patients. Transpl Infect Dis. 2014;16(2):242–50. https://doi.org/10.1111/tid.12194.

34. Gottlieb J, Torres F, Haddad T, Dhillon G, Dilling DF, Knoop C, Rampolla R, Walia R, Ahya V, Kessler R, Budev M, Neurohr C, Glanville AR, Jordan R, Porter D, McKevitt M, German P, Guo Y, Chien JW, et al. A randomized controlled trial of presatovir for respiratory syncytial virus after lung transplant. J Heart Lung Transplant. 2023;42(7):908–16. https://doi.org/10.1016/j.healun.2023.01.013.

35. Nosotti M, Tarsia P, Morlacchi LC. Infections after lung transplantation. J Thorac Dis. 2018;10(6):3849–68. https://doi.org/10.21037/jtd.2018.05.204.

36. De Mol W, Bos S, Beeckmans H, Lagrou K, Spriet I, Verleden GM, Vos R. Antifungal prophylaxis after lung transplantation: where are we now? Transplantation. 2021;105(12):2538–45. https://doi.org/10.1097/tp.0000000000003717.

37. Samanta P, Clancy CJ, Nguyen MH. Fungal infections in lung transplantation. J Thorac Dis. 2021;13(11):6695–707. https://doi.org/10.21037/jtd-2021-26.

38. Villalobos AP, Husain S. Infection prophylaxis and management of fungal infections in lung transplant. Ann Transl Med. 2020;8(6):414. https://doi.org/10.21037/atm.2020.03.102.

39. Haidar G, Green M. Intra-abdominal infections in solid organ transplant recipients: guidelines from the American Society of Transplantation Infectious Diseases Community of Practice. Clin Transpl. 2019;33(9):e13595. https://doi.org/10.1111/ctr.13595.

40. Taddei R, Riccardi N, Tiseo G, Galfo V, Biancofiore G. Early intra-abdominal bacterial infections after orthotopic liver transplantation: a narrative review for clinicians. Antibiotics (Basel). 2023;12(8) https://doi.org/10.3390/antibiotics12081316.

41. Kaviani A, Ince D, Axelrod DA. Management of antimicrobial agents in abdominal organ transplant patients in intensive care unit. Curr Transplant Rep. 2020;7(1):1–11. https://doi.org/10.1007/s40472-020-00268-0.

42. Albano L, Bretagne S, Mamzer-Bruneel MF, Kacso I, Desnos-Ollivier M, Guerrini P, Le Luong T, Cassuto E, Dromer F, Lortholary O, French Mycosis Study Group. Evidence that graft-site candidiasis after kidney transplantation is acquired during organ recovery: a multicenter study in France. Clin Infect Dis. 2009;48(2):194–202. https://doi.org/10.1086/595688.

43. Mullane KM, Dubberke ER, Practice AIC, o. Management of Clostridioides (formerly Clostridium) difficile infection (CDI) in solid organ transplant recipients: guidelines from the American Society of Transplantation Community of Practice. Clin Transpl. 2019;33(9):e13564. https://doi.org/10.1111/ctr.13564.
44. Nanayakkara D, Nanda N. Clostridium difficile infection in solid organ transplant recipients. Curr Opin Organ Transplant. 2017;22(4):314–9. https://doi.org/10.1097/MOT.0000000000000430.
45. Wong D, Nanda N. Clostridium difficile disease in solid organ transplant recipients: a recommended treatment paradigm. Curr Opin Organ Transplant. 2020;25(4):357–63. https://doi.org/10.1097/MCT.0000000000000778.
46. Bharati J, Anandh U, Kotton CN, Mueller T, Shingada AK, Ramachandran R. Diagnosis, prevention, and treatment of infections in kidney transplantation. Semin Nephrol. 2024:151486. https://doi.org/10.1016/j.semnephrol.2023.151486.
47. Goldman JD, Julian K. Urinary tract infections in solid organ transplant recipients: guidelines from the American Society of Transplantation Infectious Diseases Community of Practice. Clin Transpl. 2019;33(9):e13507. https://doi.org/10.1111/ctr.13507.

Chapter 31
Pulmonary Infections in People with HIV

Megan Grammatico, Sheela V. Shenoi, Steven M. Lemieux, and Kathleen M. Akgün

31.1 Aging with HIV

Persons living with HIV (PWH) with access to antiretroviral therapy (ART) are developing multiple chronic conditions associated with aging [1]. Chronic pulmonary conditions such as chronic obstructive pulmonary disease (COPD) and lung cancer are increasingly prevalent and may predispose to pulmonary-related infections for aging PWH [2].

For this chapter, we present the changing landscape of pulmonary infections among PWH. We specifically address epidemiology, risk factors including access to ART, and outcomes for bacterial pneumonia, fungal pneumonia in PWH including *Pneumocystis jirovecii* pneumonia (PJP; Table 31.1), tuberculosis and nontuberculous mycobacteria, and common respiratory virus infections (Table 31.2). We then address common chronic pulmonary conditions and how their prevalence could influence pulmonary infections in aging PWH. Finally, we consider the challenges frequently encountered while caring for aging PWH who are on ART and critically ill, focusing on barriers to medication administration, drug-drug interactions, and common as well as HIV-specific adverse drug events and cautions.

M. Grammatico
Department of Internal Medicine, Yale School of Medicine, New Haven, CT, USA

S. V. Shenoi (✉) · K. M. Akgün
Yale University School of Medicine, Veterans Administration Connecticut Healthcare System, West Haven, CT, USA
e-mail: Sheela.shenoi@yale.edu

S. M. Lemieux
Veterans Administration Connecticut Healthcare System, West Haven, CT, USA

© The Author(s), under exclusive license to Springer Nature Switzerland AG 2025

Y. Alzaidi, M. A. Gebily (eds.), *The Pharmacist's Expanded Role in Critical Care Medicine*, https://doi.org/10.1007/978-3-031-77335-8_31

Table 31.1 Overview of diagnosis and management of fungal pneumonia

Fungal species	CD4 threshold (cells/microL)	Diagnostics	Treatment
Pneumocystis	<200	CXR with GGO Sputum with cytopathology evaluation BAL PCR for PJP DNA 1–3-beta-D-glucan (nonspecific serum)	**Mild to moderate:** Trimethoprim-sulfamethoxazole 15–20 mg/kg/day (TMP) in 3 or 4 divided doses Or Clindamycin 450–600 mg PO every 6–8 h plus primaquine 30 mg (base) PO daily Or Atovaquone 750 mg PO every 12 h **Severe:** Trimethoprim-sulfamethoxazole 15–20 mg/kg/day (TMP) in 3 or 4 divided doses Or Pentamidine IV 4 mg/kg daily Or Clindamycin 600–900 mg IV every 6–8 h plus primaquine 30 mg (base) PO daily Plus Corticosteroids
Cryptococcus	<100	Crypto Ag on BAL ± serum BAL cytopathology	**Mild to moderate:** Fluconazole 400 mg PO daily for 6–12 months **Severe:** Amphotericin B deoxycholate 0.7–1 mg/kg IV daily plus flucytosine 25 mg/kg/dose 4 times daily for at least 2 weeks, then fluconazole 400–800 mg PO daily for 8 weeks, then fluconazole 200 mg PO daily for 1 year May use either liposomal amphotericin B (3–4 mg/kg IV daily) or amphotericin B lipid complex (5 mg/kg IV daily) in place of amphotericin B deoxycholate

(continued)

Table 31.1 (continued)

Fungal species	CD4 threshold (cells/ microL)	Diagnostics	Treatment
Aspergillus	No established threshold	Tissue invasion on path	Voriconazole 6 mg/kg IV every 12 h for two doses, then 4 mg/kg IV every 12 h for at least 6–12 weeks
Histoplasma	<150	CXR diffuse interstitial changes, LAD, miliary pattern Histo Ag	**Mild to moderate:** Itraconazole 200 mg PO every 8 h for 3 days, then itraconazole 200 mg PO every 12 h for at least 12 weeks **Severe:** Amphotericin B deoxycholate 0.7–1 mg/kg IV daily for 1–2 weeks, then itraconazole 200 mg PO every 8 h for 3 days, then itraconazole 200 mg PO every 12 h for at least 12 weeks May use either liposomal amphotericin B (3–5 mg/kg IV daily) or amphotericin B lipid complex (5 mg/kg IV daily) in place of amphotericin B deoxycholate
Coccidioides		Pulmonary opacities/cavitary nodules Culture from infected tissue	**Mild to moderate:** Fluconazole 400 mg PO daily[a] Or Itraconazole 200 mg PO every 12 h[a] **Severe:** Amphotericin B deoxycholate 0.5–1 mg/kg IV daily plus fluconazole 400–800 mg PO daily until the patient demonstrates clinical improvement, then fluconazole 400–800 mg PO daily for 12–24 weeks Or Amphotericin B deoxycholate 0.5–1 mg/kg IV daily plus itraconazole 200 mg PO every 12 h until the patient demonstrates clinical improvement, then itraconazole 200 mg PO every 12 h for 12–24 weeks May use either liposomal amphotericin B (3–5 mg/kg IV daily) or amphotericin B lipid complex (3–5 mg/kg IV daily) in place of amphotericin B deoxycholate

(continued)

Table 31.1 (continued)

Fungal species	CD4 threshold (cells/microL)	Diagnostics	Treatment
Blastomyces	<200	Culture from infected tissue	**Mild to moderate:** Itraconazole 200 mg PO every 8 h for 3 days, then itraconazole 200 mg PO every 12 h for 6–12 months **Severe:** Amphotericin B deoxycholate 0.7–1 mg/kg IV daily for 1–2 weeks, then itraconazole 200 mg PO every 8 h for 3 days, then itraconazole 200 mg PO every 12 h for 6–12 months May use either liposomal amphotericin B (3–5 mg/kg IV daily) or amphotericin B lipid complex (3–5 mg/kg IV daily) in place of amphotericin B deoxycholate
Paracoccidioides			**Mild to moderate:** Itraconazole 200 mg PO daily for 12 months **Severe:** Amphotericin B deoxycholate 0.7–1 mg/kg IV daily until the patient demonstrates clinical improvement, then itraconazole 200 mg PO daily for 12 months Or Trimethoprim-sulfamethoxazole 8–10 mg/kg (TMP) daily in 3 divided doses until the patient demonstrates clinical improvement, then itraconazole 200 mg PO daily for 12 months
Talaromyces			**Mild:** Itraconazole 200 mg PO every 8 h for 3 days, then itraconazole 200 mg PO every 12 h for 12 weeks **Moderate to severe:** Amphotericin B deoxycholate 0.7–1 mg/kg IV daily for 2 weeks, then itraconazole 200 mg PO every 8 h for 3 days, then itraconazole 200 mg PO every 12 h for 10 weeks May use liposomal amphotericin B (3–5 mg/kg IV daily) in place of amphotericin B deoxycholate

[a] Optimal duration of treatment is unclear

Table 31.2 Potential drug-drug interactions between antivirals and ART medications

Agent	Monitoring parameters	Antiretroviral medication
Oseltamivir	• Nausea • Vomiting • Headache Requires dose adjustment for renal dysfunction	No interactions
Baloxavir	• Nausea • Vomiting • Diarrhea	
Nirmatrelvir/ritonavir	• Diarrhea • Dysgeusia Strong CYP3A inhibitor. Temporarily discontinue medications that are inducers, inhibitors, and/or metabolized by CYP3A while taking nirmatrelvir/ritonavir; requires dose adjustment for renal dysfunction	
Molnupiravir	• Allergic dermatitis	
Remdesivir	• Bradycardia • Hepatotoxicity	

31.2 Bacterial Pneumonia

Respiratory failure is the most common reason for ICU admission in PWH [3]. Acute respiratory failure among PWH is most frequently associated with infections (both opportunistic and community acquired), including bacterial pneumonia [4–9]. The incidence of bacterial pneumonia has declined, from estimates of 13.2 cases/1000 person-years in 2008 to 6.8 cases/1000 person-years in 2018 in the Swiss cohort, with increased availability of ART [10, 11], though cases account for a substantial proportion of ICU admissions for respiratory failure [12–15].

Bacterial pneumonia (BP) can occur in patients with any CD4 count, but risk increases with lower CD4 counts, especially less than 50 cells per microliter. Among those with CD4 cell count <50 cells/microliter, the hazard ratio for BP was 7.68 [95% confidence interval 2.46–23.98] compared with those with CD4 count >500 cells/microliter in models adjusting for demographics, smoking, chronic pulmonary disease, prior pneumonia, and proton pump inhibitor use. Even PWH with CD4 counts between 350 and 499 cells/microliter had increased risk for BP relative to PWH whose CD4 counts are >500 cells/microliter [11]. These findings of persistently increased risk are hypothesized to result from subtle immunosuppression as a key risk factor for BP, even among PWH who have achieved viral suppression [11]. Other risk factors for BP among PWH are similar to uninfected persons, including age, use of intravenous drugs, proton pump inhibitors, and smoking status [11]. Of note, concomitant obstructive lung disease was associated with increased BP risk (adjusted hazard ratio = 4.82 [3.31–6.61]).

In addition to declines in overall pneumonia incidence over time, BP requiring hospitalization has decreased over time as well [14]. In a cohort of 3516 PWH compared with 328,738 uninfected patients from Denmark, hospitalization rates were

50.6/1000 person-years [42.9–59.7] in 1995–1996 among PWH hospitalized with BP and 19.7 hospitalizations/person-years in 2005–2007. While these declines are important among PWH, compared with uninfected, risk of hospitalization for pneumonia remained sixfold higher (incident rate ratio 5.9 [4.2–7.6]) for PWH compared to the general population.

Among PWH and BP, access to ART has a significant impact on outcomes. For PWH hospitalized for community-acquired pneumonia (though not necessarily admitted to the ICU), ART was associated with decreased 30-day mortality and shorter length of stay [16, 17]. The evidence supporting ART use for PWH experiencing critical illness has been less convincing. In fact, ART use is not consistently associated with improved outcomes, though there is evidence that it can decrease the risk of bacteremia in patients with BP. Additional areas of uncertainty persist surrounding ART initiation during critical illness. In PWH with CD4 count >500, immediate initiation of ART has been associated with 61% decrease of severe bacterial infection (of which pneumonia and tuberculosis were two of the four components in a composite endpoint) compared with delayed start of ART [18].

In ambulatory settings, ART use is likely associated with BP and respiratory infection rates that are similar to uninfected individuals. In a cohort study from 2015 to 2017 including 136 PWH (100% on ART with median CD4 = 686 cells/microliter (458–848) and 87% with VL <40 copies/ml at baseline) and 73 uninfected persons receiving care in London, UK, there was no difference in 1-year incidence of respiratory infections. However, PWH experienced worse symptoms and were more likely to seek care compared with uninfected patients in adjusted models [19].

People with HIV are uniquely susceptible to pneumonia due to *Streptococcus pneumoniae*. Other bacteria causing pneumonia include *Staphylococcus aureus*, *Haemophilus*, gram-negative rods including *Klebsiella* and *Pseudomonas*, as well as atypical organisms including *Moraxella*, *Legionella*, and *Mycoplasma*, though a great deal of this data is from the pre-ART era. Therapy depends on the etiologic bacterial organism. Adjunctive diagnostic tools including urine streptococcal antigen or urine legionella antigen can be useful. Until sputum culture results are available, or if not available at all, empiric therapy of community-acquired pneumonia can consist of ceftriaxone and doxycycline or ceftriaxone and azithromycin. For individuals who are frequently hospitalized, known to have been colonized with MRSA in the past, or in whom rapid MRSA screening is positive, empiric vancomycin or trimethoprim-sulfamethoxazole is warranted. For individuals who are frequently hospitalized and/or have a history of gram-negative infections including *Pseudomonas aeruginosa*, empiric therapy with third-generation cephalosporin with antipseudomonal coverage or piperacillin/tazobactam is appropriate. Globally, there are increasing reports of antimicrobial resistance that emphasize the need for laboratory testing to guide antibiotic therapy, as well as robust antimicrobial stewardship and infection control efforts in healthcare facilities [20]. Mortality among PWH with CAP ranges from 6% to 15% though it is low among those on ART and virologic control, similar to people without HIV [21].

31.3 PJP

P. jirovecii is an opportunistic fungal pathogen that causes severe pneumonia in immunocompromised hosts, especially PWH with CD4 counts less than 200 cells/microliter. ART has significantly reduced morbidity and mortality associated with HIV, but PJP remains an important cause of sepsis and respiratory failure in PWH in the ICU [22]. It is important to note that while HIV continues to confer the highest risk of PJP, increased numbers of ICU patients with predisposing immunosuppression make PJP more likely to be encountered in critically ill patients without HIV infection [23, 24].

The clinical presentation of PJP in PWH is nonspecific, and as such, making the diagnosis requires a high index of suspicion from treating clinicians. Patients classically present with fever, cough, subacute and progressive dyspnea, and marked hypoxemia. An elevated alveolar-arterial gradient may also be present. Elevated lactate dehydrogenase and 1,3-beta-D-glucan (1,3 BDG) may be elevated, but both lab tests lack the sensitivity and specificity to confirm the diagnosis alone. X-rays can be normal, but classic features include bilateral interstitial infiltrates. Chest CT will show dense ground-glass opacification. Factors associated with poor outcomes from PJP infection include increased age (especially age > 50), presence of respiratory failure (with need for mechanical ventilation or ICU admission serving as surrogate markers of same), hypoalbuminemia, severity of illness, and elevated alveolar-arterial gradient.

Pneumocystis jirovecii is extremely difficult to culture in vitro, and diagnosis has therefore traditionally relied on clinical symptoms, appropriate pretest probability, and confirmation with visualization of organisms on staining of either sputum or bronchoalveolar lavage (BAL) specimens. Unfortunately, these staining methods have been shown to have poor sensitivity for the detection of pneumocystis, especially when fungal burdens are low, such as when patients are taking PJP chemoprophylaxis. Newer molecular methods including PCR testing are increasingly relied upon [25]. Respiratory *Pneumocystis* PCR shows high sensitivity (100% in some studies) but relatively low specificity, especially with sputum samples rather than samples obtained from BAL fluid. Bronchoscopy with BAL should therefore be pursued whenever possible, though this remains challenging in resource-limited settings, and in patients with a classic presentation, empiric treatment should be strongly considered [22]. Concomitant positivity of serum 1,3-BDG and respiratory PCR increases the positive predictive value (compared to PCR alone) [26].

First-line therapy for PJP remains trimethoprim-sulfamethoxazole (TMP-SMX), generally divided into four intravenous doses daily for severe disease (Table 31.1). In patients with acute kidney injury or allergies to TMP-SMX, clindamycin with primaquine can be used as an alternative treatment. Use of primaquine requires testing for glucose-6-phosphate dehydrogenase (G6PD) deficiency. Adjuvant corticosteroids to reduce inflammation and associated lung injury should be used in HIV patients with partial pressure of arterial oxygen less than 70 mm Hg or with alveolar-arterial gradient greater than 35. Treatment should be for 21 days regardless of which regimen is used [27].

Side effects from TMP-SMX include hypersensitivity reactions, hepatitis, severe myelosuppression, and interstitial nephritis. PJP can still develop in patients on prophylaxis, though the risk is reduced. Prophylaxis in PWH should be given when CD4 count is <200 if the viral load is detectable and when CD4 count <100 cells/microliter regardless of VL, and secondary PCP prophylaxis should be initiated immediately upon successful completion of PCP therapy until CD4 counts increase to >200 cells/microliter or 3 months (as a result of ART).

Prior to widespread introduction of ART, in-hospital mortality of patients with PJP ranged from 13% to 25% [28, 29]. More recent studies report in-hospital PJP mortality to be around 10% [30], which has not changed much compared to the early ART era [28]. While this can seem discouraging, ICU mortality is difficult to compare across studies given institutional differences in the criteria for admission to an ICU. Survival at 5 years among those who survive PJP infection with pneumonia is correlated to ART adherence [31]. On the whole, PJP-related mortality seems to have decreased over time with access to ART, in part due to advances in critical care in addition to the direct impacts of ART [32].

31.4 Biomarkers for Diagnosis of PJP and Other Invasive Fungal Disease

While the majority of pulmonary infections among PWH are due to community-acquired pneumonia, fungal pneumonia remains of particular concern among patients experiencing profound immunosuppression (Table 31.1). In addition to the increased risk for *Pneumocystis jirovecii*, *Cryptococcus*, *Histoplasma*, and *Blastomyces* among PWH with CD4 counts below 200 cells/microliter, patients with structural lung diseases such as emphysema with blebs may be at risk for conditions such as *Aspergillus*. The dimorphic fungus, Emergomyces, formerly known as the *Emmonsia* sp., was first reported in South Africa among PWH with CD4 counts <50 cells/microliter and appears to be treated with azole antifungal medications and ART [33–35]. Finally, endemic fungi may cause pulmonary infection in immunocompetent PWH who are successfully on treatment.

The availability of minimally invasive serologic testing for fungal infections may promote broadening differential diagnoses and earlier treatment of invasive fungal pneumonias, particularly among patients in the ICU [36]. These tests may be especially efficient instead of waiting for cultures to result, which can take days to weeks, or may be less harmful than biopsies and invasive testing required for cytologic or pathologic evaluation to make a diagnosis. However, their increasingly widespread application in clinical practice has led to additional uncertainty over the frequency and severity of fungal pneumonias for PWH (Table 31.1). We describe commonly used biomarkers for fungal pneumonia, their performance from serum or from lower respiratory tract samples relative to tissue diagnosis, and whether they have been evaluated among PWH.

31.4.1 Galactomannan

Galactomannan is a polysaccharide of the outer cell wall layer of *Aspergillus* that is released during tissue invasion. Galactomannan can be used to guide diagnosis of *Aspergillus* infections. Sensitivity from serum samples is estimated between 60% and 80%, and specificity is estimated to be 80–95% [37, 38]. From BAL samples, the performance of galactomannan may reach sensitivity of 85–90% and specificity of 90–95%, including in patients who are immunocompromised in the ICU [39, 40]. However, evidence primarily including patients with hematologic diseases found less promising sensitivity and specificity of BAL galactomannan relative to serum samples [41, 42]. The role of galactomannan from BAL fluid for diagnosing aspergillosis in PWH has not been established.

31.4.2 1,3-Beta-D-Glucan

1,3-beta-D-glucan (BDG) is also found in the cell wall of pathogenic fungi, with the exception of *Mucor* and *Cryptococcus* [43]. 1,3-BDG may be particularly useful in the diagnosis of PJP with a sensitivity of 95% and specificity of 86% [44–46]. In a meta-analysis including five studies of PWH compared with five studies of those who were uninfected, there appeared to be no difference in BDG performance in identifying PJP or other invasive fungal infections by HIV status [45]. BDG use from BAL fluid has not been validated. The role of BDG testing alone for diagnosis of invasive *Candida* infections among critically ill patients is not supported, but there may be circumstances where it can be useful in conjunction with other testing modalities [47, 48].

While BDG testing can be an important tool for identifying opportunistic and invasive fungal infections using minimally invasive means, caution must be exercised as false positives are not uncommon, especially among patients receiving ICU care. False-positive results are more likely among patients receiving beta-lactam antibiotics, albumin, or immunoglobulin as well as patients with bacterial infections, all of which are not uncommon treatments or conditions in the ICU [43].

31.4.3 PCR, DFA, and Other Biomarkers

PCR may be helpful in diagnosing *Candida* infections with sensitivity estimated at 95% and specificity of 92% [47, 49]. Cryptococcal antigen (CrAg) is estimated to have greater than 95% sensitivity and specificity in CSF and blood samples among PWH [43, 50, 51]. CrAg does not perform as reliably among people without HIV infection. CrAg titers may be informative to estimate the burden of organisms and disease but should not be followed longitudinally.

Histoplasma antigen can be detected in the serum or urine with assays that have greater than 90% sensitivity and specificity, including among PWH [43, 52]. Decline in serum antigen levels occurs sooner than decline in urine samples although this might not be evident during the first 2 weeks of successful treatment among PWH [53].

31.4.4 Tuberculosis

31.4.4.1 Epidemiology

Tuberculosis (TB) disease is the leading cause of infectious death worldwide, aside from Covid-19. Global TB incidence is increasing, with an estimated 10.6 million new cases and 1.3 million deaths annually [54]. While the majority of cases of active tuberculosis disease occur in resource-limited settings, incidence in high-income countries (HICs) is increasing as well. In the United States, 5% or less of patients diagnosed with active TB have HIV coinfection, though in the rest of the world, the burden of TB and HIV coinfection is quite high. Further, TB is the leading cause of death among people with HIV. Drug-resistant TB, including both multiple drug-resistant TB (MDR TB) and extensively drug-resistant TB (XDR TB), also contributes to challenges in global TB control and in individual patient management [54]. PWH, due to impaired immune response, are at increased risk of developing active TB disease. In addition, PWH also infected with TB are at risk for poor outcomes due to challenges in diagnosis and biomedical and public health challenges in concurrent HIV/TB management [55].

The *Mycobacterium tuberculosis (MTB)* complex is comprised of *M. tuberculosis (Mtb*; the primary cause of human TB disease and focus in this chapter), *M. bovis, M. microti, M. canetti, and M. africanum.* The *Mtb* bacillus is an aerobic, weakly gram-positive rod that replicates approximately once every 24 h, requiring up to 8 weeks to grow in culture. This slow growth also contributes to lengthy treatment courses. Mtb is transmitted when an individual with active pulmonary TB disease coughs, sneezes, or speaks, emitting airborne droplet nuclei that are subsequently inhaled by a new host [56]. Droplets (5–10 μm in diameter) are able to reach the alveoli, where they are ingested by macrophages, triggering formation of granulomatous tubercles to respond to and contain Mtb, resulting in latent TB infection [57]. If the granulomatous response is impaired at the outset or if over time the cellular response becomes impaired, such as is the case in advanced HIV/AIDS but also with immunosenescence, corticosteroids, diabetes, alcohol use, and treatment with TNF-alpha inhibitors, Mtb can evade containment and travel through the lymphatics to the hilar lymph nodes, forming a Ghon complex, and subsequently travel throughout the body. Mtb most frequently (approximately 80% of cases) causes pulmonary TB disease manifesting in the upper lobes where oxygen concentration is high and lymphatic clearance is suboptimal; less frequently (~20% of cases), it is experienced as extrapulmonary (lymph nodes, central nervous system (CNS), joint, intra-abdominal, genitourinary) disease [57]. By entering the bloodstream, the mycobacterium can cause disseminated disease, often called "miliary TB" due to the appearance of millet seeds on chest imaging and on gross pathology. Traditionally, PWH with latent infection are considered noncommunicable, while those with disease are symptomatic and infectious. Increasingly, there is recognition of an intermediate stage of subclinical tuberculosis where patients do not have symptoms or signs of disease, yet there is clinical evidence of active and transmittable tuberculosis disease, though guidelines for detection and management continue to evolve [58].

31.4.4.2 Diagnosis

Diagnosis of TB is challenging due to its high prevalence worldwide, slow growth, and ability to be harbored as latent or active disease. Interferon gamma release assays (IGRAs) have been commonly used in the past but are limited in their inability to distinguish between latent and active tuberculosis. In a systematic review, the QuantiFERON-TB Gold In-Tube (QFT-GIT) had a pooled sensitivity of 69% and specificity of 52%, while the T-SPOT.TB had a pooled sensitivity of 83% and specificity of 61%; among PWH coinfected with TB, sensitivity decreased to 60% and 76%, respectively [35], leading the WHO to recommend that IGRAs not be used for diagnosis of active TB disease [36]. For screening among PWH, CRP $\geq$5 mg/L in addition to symptom screen has demonstrated value among hospitalized patients but does not take the place of specifically recommended diagnostic tools [59].

Though the traditional acid-fast bacilli (AFB) smear is widely available globally, it is approximately only 40–60% sensitive compared to culture [57]. PWH are more likely to have paucibacillary disease, i.e., fewer bacilli that are required to cause disease and fewer bacilli available, decreasing the sensitivity of AFB smear even further. These test attributes further limit the value of such a rapid test, particularly in PWH with extrapulmonary tuberculosis [60]. Culture of sputum or other fluid or tissue samples is encouraged but requires up to 6–8 weeks, though the time required may be halved using liquid culture. Among PWH, mycobacterial blood cultures may be useful adjunctively to detect disseminated disease [61]. However, due to the duration required for culture overall, the WHO has recommended that diagnosis, particularly among those with HIV [62], rely on rapid diagnostic technologies including PCR amplification platforms [63]. The primary rapid tool available in the

United States is GeneXpert, which uses the presence of rpoB gene and any gene mutations to provide a diagnosis within 2 h with concurrent identification of rifampin resistance. Overall sensitivity and specificity are 85% and 98%, respectively, among adults with pulmonary TB; among PWH, the performance was similar (81% and 98%, respectively). A revised GeneXpert platform, Xpert Ultra, increases sensitivity and specificity to 90% and 96% and among PWH, 88% and 95%, respectively [63]. Xpert diagnosis of non-sputum samples is feasible though not yet validated for use in the United States [64, 65]. Among PWH, in addition to Xpert, the WHO recommends Truenat MTB, nucleic acid amplification tests, loop-mediated isothermal amplification (TB-LAMP), molecular line probe assays, and urine lipoarabinomannan assay (LAM) which identifies a component of the mycobacterial cell wall [63]. Of these, the updated lateral flow urinary LAM (LF-LAM) has demonstrated distinctive value (sensitivity 52% (40–64%) and specificity 87% (78–93%)) as a point-of-care tool in hospitalized patients, particularly those with CD4 < 200 cells/microliter [63]. Whole-genome sequencing is increasingly being used for predicting drug resistance and will likely play a larger role in clinical practice in the near future [66].

31.4.4.3 Treatment

Empiric TB treatment can be initiated in patients with high clinical suspicion of active TB disease, though ideally specimens for laboratory confirmation should be simultaneously obtained. Initiation of TB treatment should be guided by data regarding previous exposure to antituberculosis agents and risk of exposure to drug-resistant TB, as well as comorbidities. PWH should receive ART integrated with TB treatment to improve overall outcomes. In the United States, guidelines state that PWH who have CD4 <50 cells/microliter should receive ART within 2 weeks; otherwise, ART can be initiated at 8 weeks to mitigate the potential for immune reconstitution inflammatory syndrome (IRIS)-related complications. IRIS can be managed with nonsteroidal anti-inflammatory drugs but more commonly with steroid taper over weeks; discontinuation of ART should be avoided. In the setting of critical illness, ART regimens might need to be revised for enteral feeding, mechanical ventilation, or gastrointestinal dysfunction [67].

Treatment of drug-sensitive TB requires a minimum of 6 months of multiple antituberculosis agents. In the 2-month induction phase, four drugs are initiated including isoniazid, rifampin, pyrazinamide, and ethambutol. Once sputum cultures are negative for 2 months, isoniazid and rifampin are given for the 4-month continuation phase. Daily dosing is preferred, though intermittent (two and three times per week) regimens are available with directly observed therapy for immunocompetent patients without cavitary disease. For those who do not convert to negative sputum culture within 2 months, the intensive phase is extended. Furthermore, treatment for extrapulmonary TB disease is generally extended to 6–9 months for bone or joint TB disease and 9–12 months for TB CNS disease/meningitis. The use of adjunctive steroids for CNS/TB meningitis has been debated though a recent study demonstrated no benefit among PWH [70]. There is no clear mortality benefit to corticosteroid use in pericardial TB [71]. A recent therapeutic advance is the development and approval of a 4-month regimen including daily isoniazid, rifapentine, pyrazinamide, and moxifloxacin for 2 months and then daily isoniazid, rifapentine, and moxifloxacin for another 2 months for those >40 kg and >12 years with drug-susceptible pulmonary TB disease [68]. Patients with extrapulmonary disease and prolonged QT or who are pregnant or breastfeeding are not eligible for the shortened regimen [69].

Drug interactions with antituberculosis agents abound, particularly with respect to rifamycin (Table 31.3). With respect to ART, the preferred regimen is the integrase inhibitor dolutegravir with two nucleoside/nucleotide reverse transcriptase inhibitors (NRTIs). Due to concerns about induction, dolutegravir 50 mg should be given twice daily in the context of rifampin use, though trials to determine the

Table 31.3 Potential drug-drug interactions and dosing in the care of pulmonary infections among people with HIV

Agent	Antiretroviral medications	Recommendation
Vancomycin	No interactions	15–20 mg/kg IV every 8–12 h Adjust dosing interval during instances of renal dysfunction
Piperacillin-tazobactam	No interactions	4.5 g IV every 6 h Adjust dosing interval during instances of renal dysfunction
Ceftriaxone	No interactions	1–2 g IV daily
Isoniazid[a]	No interactions	5 mg/kg (usual dose 300 mg) PO daily Use INH with pyridoxine 25–50 mg PO daily
Rifampin[a]	• NRTIs (use TAF with caution[b]) • EFV 600 mg • DTG, RAL (twice daily), (**Note:** Doses of these ARVs need to be adjusted when used with rifampin) • Ibalizumab	10 mg/kg (usual dose 600 mg) PO daily
	• DOR, ETR, EFV 400 mg, NVP, RPV (PO) • BIC, EVG/c, RAL (daily) • CAB/RPV (IM/PO) • Protease inhibitors • LEN (SC/PO)	Do not use
Ethambutol[a]	No interactions	**Weight-based dosing** • *40–55 kg*: 800 mg PO daily • *56–75 kg*: 1200 mg PO daily • *76–90 kg*: 1600 mg PO daily • *>90 kg*: 1600 mg PO daily[c]

(continued)

Table 31.3 (continued)

Agent	Antiretroviral medications	Recommendation
Pyrazinamide[a]	No interactions	**Weight-based dosing** • *40–55 kg*: 1000 mg PO daily • *56–75 kg*: 1500 mg PO daily • *76–90 kg*: 2000 mg PO daily • *>90 kg*: 2000 mg PO daily[c]
Bedaquiline	No interactions	400 mg PO daily for 2 weeks, then 200 mg PO three times weekly Do not use with rifamycin
Pretomanid	NNRTIs (EFV, ETR, NVP)	Do not use
Linezolid	No interactions	600 mg IV/PO BID. Consider use of TDM if taking rifampin concurrently
Moxifloxacin	No interactions	400 mg IV/PO daily for those >40 kg
Trimethoprim-sulfamethoxazole	No interactions	Mild to moderate PJP: 15–20 mg/kg/day (TMP) PO in 3 divided doses Moderate to severe PJP: 15–20 mg/kg/day (TMP) IV in 3 or 4 divided doses
Clindamycin	No interactions	Mild to moderate PJP: 450–600 mg PO every 6–8 h (in combination with primaquine) Severe PJP: 600 mg IV every 6 h or 900 mg IV every 8 h (in combination with primaquine)
Primaquine	No interactions	30 mg (base) PO daily (in combination with clindamycin) 30 mg base = 52.6 mg primaquine phosphate

[a] Adapted from US DHHS Guidelines [27]

[b] If TAF and rifamycins are coadministered, monitor for HIV treatment efficacy. Note that FDA labeling recommends not to coadminister

[c] Monitor for therapeutic response and consider TDM to assure dosage adequacy in patients weighing >90 kg

efficacy of once-daily dosing are in progress. Twice-daily dosing of dolutegravir should continue for 2 weeks after completing TB therapy. An alternative to dolutegravir is raltegravir, which should be used at 800 mg twice daily in the setting of rifampin. Given current data demonstrating reductions in serum concentrations of bictegravir and cabotegravir in the setting of rifampin, use of these integrase inhibitors is not currently recommended. Among NRTIs, rifampin is considered safe though there is less data with tenofovir alafenamide. Among non-nucleoside reverse transcriptase inhibitors (NNRTIs), efavirenz 600 mg has been shown to remain effective with rifampin though other NNRTIs should not be used. Protease inhibitors and cabotegravir/rilpivirine are not recommended with rifampin [27].

Treatment of drug-resistant TB, either multiple drug-resistant or extensively drug-resistant TB, can be initiated empirically based on suspected resistance due to prior exposure to antituberculosis medications, incomplete prior treatment, or epidemiological surveillance of the location where the TB disease was acquired. However, specimens for laboratory confirmation of resistance are critical to long-term treatment outcomes. Historically, a combination of at least five effective first- and second-line agents, usually including an injectable aminoglycoside for the initial 4–6-month intensive phase, were selected to construct a 24-month regimen. However, recent studies have determined that shorter course regimens can be effective. All oral 6-month regimens consisting of bedaquiline, pretomanid, and linezolid with or without moxifloxacin represent major breakthroughs in the management of drug-resistant TB [72–74], albeit with close monitoring for prolonged QTc, optic neuritis, peripheral neuropathy, and myelosuppression. The linezolid dosing of 1200 mg daily was associated with a high rate of adverse effects, leading to a subsequent study identifying a dose of 600 mg daily as preferable while maintaining treatment outcomes [73]. Furthermore, any induction of CYP3A4 can lead to drug-drug interactions. Integrated management of HIV coinfection is essential.

31.5 Noninfectious Chronic Pulmonary Conditions and Pulmonary Infections

31.5.1 COPD

PWH are at increased risk for multiple general medical conditions, including pulmonary conditions, compared with uninfected persons [75–78]. PWH who are aging have increased risk for developing chronic obstructive pulmonary disease (COPD). In a meta-analysis including 11 studies and 96,915 PWH compared with 230,949 uninfected, PWH had 14% higher prevalence of COPD compared with uninfected (pooled odds ratio = 1.14 [1.05–1.25]); findings persisted even after adjusting for tobacco use [77]. COPD has also been identified as the most prevalent general medical condition in one 10-year study, affecting 23.5% compared with 14.0% uninfected [79].

COPD prevalence varies with condition ascertainment (spirometry vs. self-report vs. diagnostic condition codes) [77, 80, 81]. Diagnostic codes are associated with the lowest prevalence (5.6% [4.6–6.7]), whereas spirometric measurements are associated with the highest prevalence (10.5–10.6%), regardless of using fixed ratio or lower limit of normal for defining airflow obstruction [77]. In addition, prevalence tends to be reported higher in North American and European cohorts compared with sub-Saharan African countries [77, 82–85]. Measuring airflow obstruction in 722 PWH in Uganda (mean age = 48 years, 90% on ART with median CD4 = 478 cells/microliter), 6.22% of participants had COPD [83]. Similar prevalence was identified in a SMART substudy including 1026 participants from 20 countries [85]. Another evaluation of PWH from Uganda estimated COPD among 3.1% ($n = 288$; median age 45 years, all but 1 on ART) [84]. TB has been identified as the strongest risk factor for COPD in these populations of PWH, although cigarette smoking and cooking fume exposures also convey a significant risk [83, 84].

31.5.2 Bronchiectasis

Bronchiectasis is a chronic airway disease marked by enlargement and destruction of the bronchioles with impaired ciliary clearance and closer approximation between the airways and its associated pulmonary artery. Bronchiectasis can develop as a result of repeated pulmonary infections (bacterial, TB, aspiration) [86]. Despite access to ART, radiographic and clinical bronchiectasis appears to be much more common among adolescents from sub-Saharan Africa with perinatally acquired HIV compared with U.S.-based observations, perhaps related to access to otherwise more favorable engagement and access to health care [87–89]. It remains unclear as to what extent HIV infection is an independent risk factor for the development of bronchiectasis [89–91].

While a result of chronic infections, bronchiectasis can also be exacerbated by bacterial overgrowth leading to excess mucus production, airway inflammation, and worsening airflow limitations. Similar to bronchiectasis in uninfected persons, without prompt attention with airway clearance therapy and effective antibiotics, PWH may experience bronchiectasis exacerbations that can lead to acute respiratory failure and hospitalization. Bronchiectasis exacerbations can also be accompanied by significant or massive hemoptysis requiring ICU admission. In such circumstances, airway clearance therapy and antibiotics are the mainstays of treatment for secretions, as well as support with supplemental oxygen for patients who are hypoxemic or even mechanical ventilation in more severe cases. Treatment of hemoptysis from bronchiectasis would be determined according to the standard of care, aiming to support the patient, identifying the likely culprit area of bleeding, ensuring airway protection, reversing coagulopathies, and pursuing advanced procedures to stop life-threatening hemoptysis, if indicated.

Living with chronic pulmonary conditions impacts the risk for subsequent pulmonary infection incidence, severity, and outcomes. As well, people with a history of bacterial pneumonia are at increased risk for developing obstructive lung diseases [92].

31.5.3 Other Pulmonary-Associated Conditions and Infection Risk

In addition to airway diseases, PWH continue to experience other chronic conditions associated with aging that can contribute to increased risk for ICU admission and associated infections. These include aspiration pneumonia, especially among people with cognitive impairments. Lung cancer is the leading cause of cancer death among PWH [93]. Identifying the additional risks for infection in addition to frank immunosuppression is imperative while managing PWH in the ICU.

31.5.4 Polypharmacy and Drug Interactions with Commonly Used Medications in the ICU

Polypharmacy increasingly affects persons aging with multiple chronic conditions. Polypharmacy may be of greater impact for PWH who are maintained on ART. Polypharmacy is associated with the risk for poor outcomes including falls, delirium, and death. In addition, polypharmacy can lead to otherwise unanticipated adverse drug events due to effects from metabolism of medications. While beyond the scope of this chapter to fully explicate common medication-related hazards for PWH admitted to the ICU, we will first identify commonly encountered ICU medications and ART interactions. We will then address the role of ART initiation or continuation in the ICU. However, it is important to recognize the changing landscape of aging with HIV and ART use. As such, clinicians should consult with HIV and pharmacy experts and consider resources such as http://www.hiv-druginteractions.org or http://www.hivinsite.com.

31.5.4.1 Drug Interactions Between ART and Common ICU Medications

Several medications used in the ICU can interact with ART and increase the risk for adverse drug events and medication toxicity (Table 31.3). The most common drug interactions tend to be related to metabolism through the CYP450 system. Protease inhibitors and co-administration of medications such as fentanyl, oxycodone, and hydrocodone may lead to higher-than-expected effects of opioids (Table 31.4) [22, 94]. Importantly, there do not appear to be dangerous drug interactions with dexmedetomidine or propofol and ART, so these agents may be preferred sedatives for use among PWH if no other contraindications are evident. Non-nucleoside reverse transcriptase inhibitors such as efavirenz or rilpivirine can lead to hepatotoxicity.

Among antimicrobial medications, commonly used antibiotics including beta-lactams, clindamycin, vancomycin, and linezolid do not typically have dangerous interactions with ART [94]. Quinolones should be used with caution due to QT

Table 31.4 Potential drug-drug interactions between sedatives and ART medications

Agent	Antiretroviral medication	Recommendation	Monitoring parameters
Propofol	No interactions	Nothing specific	• Hypotension • Hypertriglyceridemia leading to acute pancreatitis • Propofol infusion syndrome (PRIS) • Respiratory depression
Dexmedetomidine	No interactions	Nothing specific	• Bradycardia • Hypotension • Fever • Withdrawal
Fentanyl	Atazanavir Cobicistat Darunavir Lenacapavir Lopinavir Ritonavir	Monitor for increased effects of fentanyl due to CYP3A4 inhibition	• Chest wall rigidity • Constipation • Respiratory depression • Withdrawal
	Efavirenz Etravirine Nevirapine	Monitor for decreased effects of fentanyl due to CYP3A4 induction	
Morphine	No interactions	Nothing specific	• Constipation • Hypotension • Pruritus • Respiratory depression • Withdrawal • Use in renal dysfunction may lead to accumulation of active metabolites (morphine-3-glucuronide and morphine-6-glucuronide)
Hydromorphone	No interactions	Nothing specific	• Constipation • Pruritus • Respiratory depression • Withdrawal

(continued)

Table 31.4 (continued)

Agent	Antiretroviral medication	Recommendation	Monitoring parameters
Lorazepam	No interactions	Nothing specific	• Hypotension • Respiratory depression • Withdrawal • Propylene glycol toxicity when used at high doses as a continuous infusion
Diazepam	Atazanavir Cobicistat Darunavir Lenacapavir Lopinavir Ritonavir	Monitor for increased effects of diazepam due to CYP3A4 inhibition	• Hypotension • Respiratory depression • Withdrawal
	Efavirenz Etravirine Nevirapine	Monitor for decreased effects of diazepam due to CYP3A4 induction	
Midazolam	Atazanavir Cobicistat Darunavir Lenacapavir Lopinavir Ritonavir	Monitor for increased effects of midazolam due to CYP3A4 inhibition	• Hypotension • Respiratory depression • Withdrawal • Use in renal dysfunction may lead to accumulation of active metabolite (1-hydroxymidazolam)
	Efavirenz Etravirine Nevirapine	Monitor for decreased effects of midazolam due to CYP3A4 induction	
Ketamine	Atazanavir Cobicistat Darunavir Lenacapavir Lopinavir Ritonavir	Monitor for increased effects of ketamine due to CYP3A4 inhibition	• Tachycardia • Hypertension • Emergence delirium • Hypersalivation
	Efavirenz Etravirine Nevirapine	Monitor for decreased effects of ketamine due to CYP3A4 induction	

prolongation. Monitoring is required for patients receiving trimethoprim/sulfamethoxazole (either for PJP prophylaxis or treatment or other indications) and lamivudine as drug toxicities may occur. Azole medications are most problematic for PWH on ART as well as cause drug interactions with other commonly used ICU medications [22, 94].

31.5.4.2 ART Initiation or Continuation in the ICU

Ideally, treatment interruptions should be avoided among PWH unless there are concerns for ART-related adverse drug reactions [94]. ART may be especially important to initiate or continue for patients admitted to the ICU for AIDS-defining illnesses. While there is no established data on the timing of initiation of ART in the ICU, a meta-analysis including 12 studies with 1584 PWH admitted to an ICU suggested a short-term mortality benefit, defined as ICU and in-hospital deaths, for ART use in the ICU (odds ratio 0.53 [0.31–0.91]), although the studies were very heterogeneous [95]. ART administration in the ICU may be hampered due to limited or ineffective enteral access or absorption. As able, ICU clinicians should aim to minimize treatment interruptions (ideally no more than 2 days) but also assess for successful drug delivery through the gut. This may entail avoiding co-administration of medications that may alter ART absorption, such as gastric ulcer prophylaxis medications.

31.6 Conclusion

Access to ART has led to successful aging with HIV. While PWH are developing more chronic conditions including chronic pulmonary diseases, pulmonary infections continue to contribute to significant morbidity and mortality. ICU providers caring for PWH and pulmonary infections must remain vigilant, considering broad differentials for infectious etiologies and re-examining if multiple pathogens or processes could be co-occurring. ICU care for respiratory failure and sepsis and other ICU conditions primarily follows guideline-concordant ICU care, although adverse drug interactions with ART and dose adjustments should be guarded against.

References

1. Collini P, Mawson RL. A new era of HIV care for age-associated multimorbidity. Curr Opin Infect Dis. 2023;36(1):9–14. https://doi.org/10.1097/QCO.0000000000000890.
2. Leung JM. HIV and chronic lung disease. Curr Opin HIV AIDS. 2023;18(2):93–101. https://doi.org/10.1097/COH.0000000000000777.
3. Barbier F, Mer M, Szychowiak P, Miller RF, Mariotte E, Galicier L, et al. Management of HIV-infected patients in the intensive care unit. Intensive Care Med. 2020;46(2):329–42. https://doi.org/10.1007/s00134-020-05945-3. PubMed PMID: 32016535; PubMed Central PMCID: PMCPMC7095039.
4. De Palo VA, Millstein BH, Mayo PH, Salzman SH, Rosen MJ. Outcome of intensive care in patients with HIV infection. Chest. 1995;107(2):506–10. https://doi.org/10.1378/chest.107.2.506.
5. Akgun KM, Tate JP, Pisani M, Fried T, Butt AA, Gibert CL, et al. Medical ICU admission diagnoses and outcomes in human immunodeficiency virus-infected and virus-uninfected veterans in the combination antiretroviral era. Crit Care Med. 2013;41(6):1458–67. https://doi.

org/10.1097/CCM.0b013e31827caa46. PubMed PMID: 23507717; PubMed Central PMCID: PMC4283206.

6. Powell K, Davis JL, Morris AM, Chi A, Bensley MR, Huang L. Survival for patients with HIV admitted to the ICU continues to improve in the current era of combination antiretroviral therapy. Chest. 2009;135(1):11–7. https://doi.org/10.1378/chest.08-0980. PubMed PMID: 18719058; PubMed Central PMCID: PMC2742310.

7. Dickson SJ, Batson S, Copas AJ, Edwards SG, Singer M, Miller RF. Survival of HIV-infected patients in the intensive care unit in the era of highly active antiretroviral therapy. Thorax. 2007;62(11):964–8. https://doi.org/10.1136/thx.2006.072256. PubMed PMID: 17517829; PubMed Central PMCID: PMC2117109 Associate Editor (Statistics) of Sexually Transmitted Infections, part of the BMJ Publishing Group.

8. Chiang HH, Hung CC, Lee CM, Chen HY, Chen MY, Sheng WH, et al. Admissions to intensive care unit of HIV-infected patients in the era of highly active antiretroviral therapy: etiology and prognostic factors. Crit Care. 2011;15(4):R202. https://doi.org/10.1186/cc10419. PubMed PMID: 21871086; PubMed Central PMCID: PMC3387644.

9. van Lelyveld SF, Wind CM, Mudrikova T, van Leeuwen HJ, de Lange DW, Hoepelman AI. Short- and long-term outcome of HIV-infected patients admitted to the intensive care unit. Eur J Clin Microbiol Infect Dis. 2011;30(9):1085–93. https://doi.org/10.1007/s10096-011-1196-z.

10. Benito N, Moreno A, Miro JM, Torres A. Pulmonary infections in HIV-infected patients: an update in the 21st century. Eur Respir J. 2012;39(3):730–45. https://doi.org/10.1183/09031936.00200210.

11. Balakrishna S, Wolfensberger A, Kachalov V, Roth JA, Kusejko K, Scherrer AU, et al. Decreasing incidence and determinants of bacterial pneumonia in people with HIV: the Swiss HIV cohort study. J Infect Dis. 2022;225(9):1592–600. https://doi.org/10.1093/infdis/jiab573.

12. Afessa B, Green B. Bacterial pneumonia in hospitalized patients with HIV infection: the pulmonary complications, ICU support, and prognostic factors of hospitalized patients with HIV (PIP) study. Chest. 2000;117(4):1017–22. https://doi.org/10.1378/chest.117.4.1017.

13. Segal LN, Methe BA, Nolan A, Hoshino Y, Rom WN, Dawson R, et al. HIV-1 and bacterial pneumonia in the era of antiretroviral therapy. Proc Am Thorac Soc. 2011;8(3):282–7. https://doi.org/10.1513/pats.201006-044WR. PubMed PMID: 21653529; PubMed Central PMCID: PMC3132786.

14. Sogaard OS, Lohse N, Gerstoft J, Kronborg G, Ostergaard L, Pedersen C, et al. Hospitalization for pneumonia among individuals with and without HIV infection, 1995-2007: a Danish population-based, nationwide cohort study. Clin Infect Dis. 2008;47(10):1345–53. https://doi.org/10.1086/592692.

15. Sarkar P, Rasheed HF. Clinical review: respiratory failure in HIV-infected patients—a changing picture. Crit Care. 2013;17(3):228. https://doi.org/10.1186/cc12552. PubMed PMID: 23806117; PubMed Central PMCID: PMCPMC3706935.

16. Barakat LA, Juthani-Mehta M, Allore H, Trentalange M, Tate J, Rimland D, et al. Comparing clinical outcomes in HIV-infected and uninfected older men hospitalized with community-acquired pneumonia. HIV Med. 2015;16(7):421–30. https://doi.org/10.1111/hiv.12244. PubMed PMID: 25959543; PubMed Central PMCID: PMC5015437.

17. Madeddu G, Porqueddu EM, Cambosu F, Saba F, Fois AG, Pirina P, et al. Bacterial community acquired pneumonia in HIV-infected inpatients in the highly active antiretroviral therapy era. Infection. 2008;36(3):231–6. https://doi.org/10.1007/s15010-007-7162-0.

18. O'Connor J, Vjecha MJ, Phillips AN, Angus B, Cooper D, Grinsztejn B, et al. Effect of immediate initiation of antiretroviral therapy on risk of severe bacterial infections in HIV-positive people with CD4 cell counts of more than 500 cells per muL: secondary outcome results from a randomised controlled trial. Lancet HIV. 2017;4(3):e105–e12. https://doi.org/10.1016/S2352-3018(16)30216-8. PubMed PMID: 28063815; PubMed Central PMCID: PMCPMC5337625.

19. Brown J, Pickett E, Smith C, Sachikonye M, Brooks L, Mahungu T, et al. The effect of HIV status on the frequency and severity of acute respiratory illness. PLoS One. 2020;15(5):e0232977.

https://doi.org/10.1371/journal.pone.0232977. PubMed PMID: 32469981; PubMed Central PMCID: PMCPMC7259631.

20. Kumar V, Murali S, Goldberg J, Alonso B, Moretó-Planas L, Reid A, et al. Antibiotic susceptibility patterns of pathogens isolated from hospitalized patients with advanced HIV disease (AHD) in Bihar, India. JAC Antimicrob Resist. 2024;6(1):dlad151. https://doi.org/10.1093/jacamr/dlad151. PubMed PMID: 38170073; PubMed Central PMCID: PMCPMC10759003

21. Cillóniz C, García-Vidal C, Moreno A, Miro JM, Torres A. Community-acquired bacterial pneumonia in adult HIV-infected patients. Expert Rev Anti Infect Ther. 2018;16(7):579–88. https://doi.org/10.1080/14787210.2018.1495560.

22. Akgun KM, Miller RF. Critical care in human immunodeficiency virus-infected patients. Semin Respir Crit Care Med. 2016;37(2):303–17. https://doi.org/10.1055/s-0036-1572561.

23. Ko Y, Jeong BH, Park HY, Koh WJ, Suh GY, Chung MP, et al. Outcomes of Pneumocystis pneumonia with respiratory failure in HIV-negative patients. J Crit Care. 2014;29(3):356–61. https://doi.org/10.1016/j.jcrc.2013.12.005.

24. Li MC, Lee NY, Lee CC, Lee HC, Chang CM, Ko WC. Pneumocystis jirovecii pneumonia in immunocompromised patients: delayed diagnosis and poor outcomes in non-HIV-infected individuals. J Microbiol Immunol Infect. 2014;47(1):42–7. https://doi.org/10.1016/j.jmii.2012.08.024.

25. Bateman M, Oladele R, Kolls JK. Diagnosing Pneumocystis jirovecii pneumonia: a review of current methods and novel approaches. Med Mycol. 2020;58(8):1015–28. https://doi.org/10.1093/mmy/myaa024. PubMed PMID: 32400869; PubMed Central PMCID: PMC7657095.

26. Giacobbe DR, Dettori S, Di Pilato V, Asperges E, Ball L, Berti E, et al. Pneumocystis jirovecii pneumonia in intensive care units: a multicenter study by ESGCIP and EFISG. Crit Care. 2023;27(1):323. https://doi.org/10.1186/s13054-023-04608-1. PubMed PMID: 37620828; PubMed Central PMCID: PMC10464114

27. Services. DoHaH. Guidelines for the prevention and treatment of opportunistic infections in adults and adolescents with HIV. 2024.

28. Arozullah AM, Yarnold PR, Weinstein RA, Nwadiaro N, McIlraith TB, Chmiel JS, et al. A new preadmission staging system for predicting inpatient mortality from HIV-associated Pneumocystis carinii pneumonia in the early highly active antiretroviral therapy (HAART) era. Am J Respir Crit Care Med. 2000;161(4 Pt 1):1081–6. https://doi.org/10.1164/ajrccm.161.4.9906072.

29. Curtis JR, Greenberg DL, Hudson LD, Fisher LD, Krone MR, Collier AC. Changing use of intensive care for HIV-infected patients with Pneumocystis carinii pneumonia. Am J Respir Crit Care Med. 1994;150(5 Pt 1):1305–10. https://doi.org/10.1164/ajrccm.150.5.7952557.

30. Fei MW, Kim EJ, Sant CA, Jarlsberg LG, Davis JL, Swartzman A, et al. Predicting mortality from HIV-associated Pneumocystis pneumonia at illness presentation: an observational cohort study. Thorax. 2009;64(12):1070–6. https://doi.org/10.1136/thx.2009.117846. PubMed PMID: 19825785; PubMed Central PMCID: PMC2788120.

31. Lopez-Sanchez C, Falco V, Burgos J, Navarro J, Martin MT, Curran A, et al. Epidemiology and long-term survival in HIV-infected patients with Pneumocystis jirovecii pneumonia in the HAART era: experience in a university hospital and review of the literature. Medicine (Baltimore). 2015;94(12):e681. https://doi.org/10.1097/MD.0000000000000681. PubMed PMID: 25816039; PubMed Central PMCID: PMC4553998.

32. Miller RF, Allen E, Copas A, Singer M, Edwards SG. Improved survival for HIV infected patients with severe Pneumocystis jirovecii pneumonia is independent of highly active antiretroviral therapy. Thorax. 2006;61(8):716–21. https://doi.org/10.1136/thx.2005.055905. PubMed PMID: 16601092; PubMed Central PMCID: PMC2104703 Associate Editor of Sexually Transmitted Infections, part of the BMJ Publishing Group.

33. Kenyon C, Bonorchis K, Corcoran C, Meintjes G, Locketz M, Lehloenya R, et al. A dimorphic fungus causing disseminated infection in South Africa. N Engl J Med. 2013;369(15):1416–24. https://doi.org/10.1056/NEJMoa1215460.

34. Pierce J, Sayeed S, Doern CD, Bryson AL. Emergomyces pasteurianus in man returning to the United States from Liberia and review of the literature. Emerg Infect Dis. 2023;29(3):635–9. https://doi.org/10.3201/eid2903.221683. PubMed PMID: 36823688; PubMed Central PMCID: PMCPMC9973675.

35. Rofael M, Schwartz IS, Sigler L, Kong LK, Nelson N. Emmonsia helica infection in HIV-Infected Man, California, USA. Emerg Infect Dis. 2018;24(1):166–8. https://doi.org/10.3201/eid2401.170558. PubMed PMID: 29260669; PubMed Central PMCID: PMCPMC5749451.

36. Haydour Q, Hage CA, Carmona EM, Epelbaum O, Evans SE, Gabe LM, et al. Diagnosis of fungal infections. A systematic review and meta-analysis supporting American Thoracic Society practice guideline. Ann Am Thorac Soc. 2019;16(9):1179–88. https://doi.org/10.1513/AnnalsATS.201811-766OC.

37. Pfeiffer CD, Fine JP, Safdar N. Diagnosis of invasive aspergillosis using a galactomannan assay: a meta-analysis. Clin Infect Dis. 2006;42(10):1417–27. https://doi.org/10.1086/503427.

38. Maertens JA, Klont R, Masson C, Theunissen K, Meersseman W, Lagrou K, et al. Optimization of the cutoff value for the aspergillus double-sandwich enzyme immunoassay. Clin Infect Dis. 2007;44(10):1329–36. https://doi.org/10.1086/514349.

39. Guo YL, Chen YQ, Wang K, Qin SM, Wu C, Kong JL. Accuracy of BAL galactomannan in diagnosing invasive aspergillosis: a bivariate metaanalysis and systematic review. Chest. 2010;138(4):817–24. https://doi.org/10.1378/chest.10-0488.

40. Zou M, Tang L, Zhao S, Zhao Z, Chen L, Chen P, et al. Systematic review and meta-analysis of detecting galactomannan in bronchoalveolar lavage fluid for diagnosing invasive aspergillosis. PLoS One. 2012;7(8):e43347. https://doi.org/10.1371/journal.pone.0043347. PubMed PMID: 22905261; PubMed Central PMCID: PMCPMC3419176.

41. Racil Z, Kocmanova I, Toskova M, Buresova L, Weinbergerova B, Lengerova M, et al. Galactomannan detection in bronchoalveolar lavage fluid for the diagnosis of invasive aspergillosis in patients with hematological diseases-the role of factors affecting assay performance. Int J Infect Dis. 2011;15(12):e874–81. https://doi.org/10.1016/j.ijid.2011.09.011.

42. de Heer K, Gerritsen MG, Visser CE, Leeflang MM. Galactomannan detection in broncho-alveolar lavage fluid for invasive aspergillosis in immunocompromised patients. Cochrane Database Syst Rev. 2019;5(5):CD012399. https://doi.org/10.1002/14651858.CD012399.pub2. PubMed PMID: 31107543; PubMed Central PMCID: PMCPMC6526785 automation. Pfizer partly financed attendance to TIMM in Lisbon. None of the financial activities had any influence on the present work. KdH, ML, MG: No known conflicts of interest.

43. Thompson GR 3rd, Boulware DR, Bahr NC, Clancy CJ, Harrison TS, Kauffman CA, et al. Noninvasive testing and surrogate markers in invasive fungal diseases. Open Forum Infect Dis. 2022;9(6):ofac112. https://doi.org/10.1093/ofid/ofac112. PubMed PMID: 35611348; PubMed Central PMCID: PMCPMC9124589.

44. Karageorgopoulos DE, Qu JM, Korbila IP, Zhu YG, Vasileiou VA, Falagas ME. Accuracy of beta-D-glucan for the diagnosis of Pneumocystis jirovecii pneumonia: a meta-analysis. Clin Microbiol Infect. 2013;19(1):39–49. https://doi.org/10.1111/j.1469-0691.2011.03760.x.

45. Onishi A, Sugiyama D, Kogata Y, Saegusa J, Sugimoto T, Kawano S, et al. Diagnostic accuracy of serum 1,3-beta-D-glucan for pneumocystis jiroveci pneumonia, invasive candidiasis, and invasive aspergillosis: systematic review and meta-analysis. J Clin Microbiol. 2012;50(1):7–15. https://doi.org/10.1128/JCM.05267-11. PubMed PMID: 22075593; PubMed Central PMCID: PMCPMC3256688.

46. Son HJ, Sung H, Park SY, Kim T, Lee HJ, Kim SM, et al. Diagnostic performance of the (1–3)-beta-D-glucan assay in patients with Pneumocystis jirovecii compared with those with candidiasis, aspergillosis, mucormycosis, and tuberculosis, and healthy volunteers. PLoS One. 2017;12(11):e0188860. https://doi.org/10.1371/journal.pone.0188860. PubMed PMID: 29190812; PubMed Central PMCID: PMCPMC5708637

47. Hage CA, Carmona EM, Epelbaum O, Evans SE, Gabe LM, Haydour Q, et al. Microbiological laboratory testing in the diagnosis of fungal infections in pulmonary and critical care practice. An Official American Thoracic Society Clinical Practice Guideline. Am J Respir Crit Care

Med. 2019;200(5):535–50. https://doi.org/10.1164/rccm.201906-1185ST. PubMed PMID: 31469325; PubMed Central PMCID: PMCPMC6727169.

48. Hage CA, Carmona EM, Evans SE, Limper AH, Ruminjo J, Thomson CC. Summary for clinicians: microbiological laboratory testing in the diagnosis of fungal infections in pulmonary and critical care practice. Ann Am Thorac Soc. 2019;16(12):1473–7. https://doi.org/10.1513/AnnalsATS.201908-582CME.

49. Avni T, Leibovici L, Paul M. PCR diagnosis of invasive candidiasis: systematic review and meta-analysis. J Clin Microbiol. 2011;49(2):665–70. https://doi.org/10.1128/JCM.01602-10. PubMed PMID: 21106797; PubMed Central PMCID: PMCPMC3043518.

50. Hansen J, Slechta ES, Gates-Hollingsworth MA, Neary B, Barker AP, Bauman S, et al. Large-scale evaluation of the immuno-mycologics lateral flow and enzyme-linked immunoassays for detection of cryptococcal antigen in serum and cerebrospinal fluid. Clin Vaccine Immunol. 2013;20(1):52–5. https://doi.org/10.1128/CVI.00536-12. PubMed PMID: 23114703; PubMed Central PMCID: PMCPMC3535775.

51. Binnicker MJ, Jespersen DJ, Bestrom JE, Rollins LO. Comparison of four assays for the detection of cryptococcal antigen. Clin Vaccine Immunol. 2012;19(12):1988–90. https://doi.org/10.1128/CVI.00446-12. PubMed PMID: 23081814; PubMed Central PMCID: PMCPMC3535868

52. Martinez-Gamboa A, Niembro-Ortega MD, Torres-Gonzalez P, Santiago-Cruz J, Velazquez-Zavala NG, Rangel-Cordero A, et al. Diagnostic accuracy of antigen detection in urine and molecular assays testing in different clinical samples for the diagnosis of progressive disseminated histoplasmosis in patients living with HIV/AIDS: a prospective multicenter study in Mexico. PLoS Negl Trop Dis. 2021;15(3):e0009215. https://doi.org/10.1371/journal.pntd.0009215. PubMed PMID: 33684128; PubMed Central PMCID: PMCPMC7971897.

53. Hage CA, Kirsch EJ, Stump TE, Kauffman CA, Goldman M, Connolly P, et al. Histoplasma antigen clearance during treatment of histoplasmosis in patients with AIDS determined by a quantitative antigen enzyme immunoassay. Clin Vaccine Immunol. 2011;18(4):661–6. https://doi.org/10.1128/CVI.00389-10. PubMed PMID: 21307278; PubMed Central PMCID: PMCPMC3122570.

54. WHO. Global tuberculosis report. Geneva; 2023.

55. Gupta-Wright A. Tuberculosis diagnostics to reduce HIV-associated mortality: Barnett Christie lecture 2020. Clin Infect Pract. 2022;15:100152. https://doi.org/10.1016/j.clinpr.2022.100152.

56. Churchyard G, Kim P, Shah NS, Rustomjee R, Gandhi N, Mathema B, et al. What we know about tuberculosis transmission: an overview. J Infect Dis. 2017;216(6):S629–S35.

57. Lawn SD, Zumla AI. Tuberculosis. Lancet. 2011;378(9785):57–72. https://doi.org/10.1016/S0140-6736(10)62173-3.

58. Frascella B, Richards AS, Sossen B, Emery JC, Odone A, Law I, et al. Subclinical tuberculosis disease-a review and analysis of prevalence surveys to inform definitions, burden, associations, and screening methodology. Clin Infect Dis. 2021;73(3):e830–e41. https://doi.org/10.1093/cid/ciaa1402. PubMed PMID: 32936877; PubMed Central PMCID: PMCPMC8326537.

59. Dhana A, Hamada Y, Kengne AP, Kerkhoff AD, Rangaka MX, Kredo T, et al. Tuberculosis screening among HIV-positive inpatients: a systematic review and individual participant data meta-analysis. Lancet HIV. 2022;9(4):e233–e41. https://doi.org/10.1016/S2352-3018(22)00002-9.

60. Schluger NW. The acid-fast bacilli smear: hail and farewell. Am J Respir Crit Care Med. 2018;199(6):691–2. https://doi.org/10.1164/rccm.201809-1772ED.

61. Heysell SK, Thomas TA, Gandhi NR, Moll AP, Eksteen FJ, Coovadia Y, et al. Blood cultures for the diagnosis of multidrug-resistant and extensively drug-resistant tuberculosis among HIV-infected patients from rural South Africa: a cross-sectional study. BMC Infect Dis. 2010;10:344. https://doi.org/10.1186/1471-2334-10-344. PubMed PMID: 21134279; PubMed Central PMCID: PMCPMC3016377.

62. Dhana A, Hamada Y, Kengne AP, Kerkhoff AD, Rangaka MX, Kredo T, et al. Tuberculosis screening among ambulatory people living with HIV: a systematic review and individual

participant data meta-analysis. Lancet Infect Dis. 2022;22(4):507–18. https://doi.org/10.1016/S1473-3099(21)00387-X.

63. WHO. WHO consolidated guidelines on tuberculosis. Module 3: diagnosis—rapid diagnostics for tuberculosis detection, 2021 update. Geneva; 2021.

64. Boloko L, Schutz C, Sibiya N, Balfour A, Ward A, Shey M, et al. Xpert ultra testing of blood in severe HIV-associated tuberculosis to detect and measure Mycobacterium tuberculosis blood stream infection: a diagnostic and disease biomarker cohort study. Lancet Microbe. 2022;3(7):e521–e32. https://doi.org/10.1016/S2666-5247(22)00062-3.

65. Chen K, Malik AA, Nantasenamat C, Ahmed S, Chaudhary O, Sun C, et al. Clinical validation of urine-based Xpert® MTB/RIF assay for the diagnosis of urogenital tuberculosis: a systematic review and meta-analysis. Int J Infect Dis. 2020;95:15–21. https://doi.org/10.1016/j.ijid.2020.03.023.

66. Dookie N, Khan A, Padayatchi N, Naidoo K. Application of next generation sequencing for diagnosis and clinical management of drug-resistant tuberculosis: updates on recent developments in the field. Front Microbiol. 2022;13:775030. https://doi.org/10.3389/fmicb.2022.775030. PubMed PMID: 35401475; PubMed Central PMCID: PMCPMC8988194.

67. Richards GA, Zamparini J, Kalla I, Laher A, Murray LW, Shaddock EJ, et al. Critical illness due to infection in people living with HIV. Lancet HIV. 2024;11(6):e406–e18. https://doi.org/10.1016/S2352-3018(24)00096-1.

68. Dorman Susan E, Nahid P, Kurbatova Ekaterina V, Phillips Patrick PJ, Bryant K, Dooley Kelly E, et al. Four-month rifapentine regimens with or without moxifloxacin for tuberculosis. N Engl J Med. 2021;384(18):1705–18. https://doi.org/10.1056/NEJMoa2033400.

69. Carr WKE, Starks A, Goswami N, Allen L, Winston C. Interim guidance: 4-month rifapentine-moxifloxacin regimen for the treatment of drug-susceptible pulmonary tuberculosis—United States, 2022. MMWR Morb Mortal Wkly Rep. 2022;71:285–9.

70. Donovan J, Bang ND, Imran D, Nghia HDT, Burhan E, Huong DTT, et al. Adjunctive dexamethasone for tuberculous meningitis in HIV-positive adults. N Engl J Med. 2023;389(15):1357–67. https://doi.org/10.1056/NEJMoa2216218.

71. Mayosi BM, Ntsekhe M, Bosch J, Pandie S, Jung H, Gumedze F, et al. Prednisolone and Mycobacterium indicus pranii in tuberculous pericarditis. N Engl J Med. 2014;371(12):1121–30. https://doi.org/10.1056/NEJMoa1407380. PubMed PMID: 25178809; PubMed Central PMCID: PMCPMC4912834.

72. Nyang'wa B-T, Berry C, Kazounis E, Motta I, Parpieva N, Tigay Z, et al. A 24-week, all-oral regimen for rifampin-resistant tuberculosis. N Engl J Med. 2022;387(25):2331–43. https://doi.org/10.1056/NEJMoa2117166.

73. Conradie F, Bagdasaryan Tatevik R, Borisov S, Howell P, Mikiashvili L, Ngubane N, et al. Bedaquiline–pretomanid–linezolid regimens for drug-resistant tuberculosis. N Engl J Med. 2022;387(9):810–23. https://doi.org/10.1056/NEJMoa2119430.

74. Conradie F, Diacon Andreas H, Ngubane N, Howell P, Everitt D, Crook Angela M, et al. Treatment of highly drug-resistant pulmonary tuberculosis. N Engl J Med. 2020;382(10):893–902. https://doi.org/10.1056/NEJMoa1901814.

75. Crothers K, Huang L, Goulet JL, Goetz MB, Brown ST, Rodriguez-Barradas MC, et al. HIV infection and risk for incident pulmonary diseases in the combination antiretroviral therapy era. Am J Respir Crit Care Med. 2011;183(3):388–95. https://doi.org/10.1164/rccm.201006-0836OC. PubMed PMID: 20851926; PubMed Central PMCID: PMCPMC3266024.

76. Crothers K, Butt AA, Gibert CL, Rodriguez-Barradas MC, Crystal S, Justice AC, et al. Increased COPD among HIV-positive compared to HIV-negative veterans. Chest. 2006;130(5):1326–33. https://doi.org/10.1378/chest.130.5.1326.

77. Bigna JJ, Kenne AM, Asangbeh SL, Sibetcheu AT. Prevalence of chronic obstructive pulmonary disease in the global population with HIV: a systematic review and meta-analysis. Lancet Glob Health. 2018;6(2):e193–202. https://doi.org/10.1016/S2214-109X(17)30451-5.

78. Nanditha NGA, Paiero A, Tafessu HM, St-Jean M, McLinden T, Justice AC, et al. Excess burden of age-associated comorbidities among people living with HIV in British Columbia,

Canada: a population-based cohort study. BMJ Open. 2021;11(1):e041734. https://doi.org/10.1136/bmjopen-2020-041734. PubMed PMID: 33419911; PubMed Central PMCID: PMCPMC7799128.

79. Rowell-Cunsolo TL, Hu G, Bellerose M, Liu J. Trends in comorbidities among human immunodeficiency virus-infected hospital admissions in New York city from 2006–2016. Clin Infect Dis. 2021;73(7):e1957–e63. https://doi.org/10.1093/cid/ciaa1760. PubMed PMID: 33245318; PubMed Central PMCID: PMCPMC8678437.

80. Gingo MR, Balasubramani GK, Rice TB, Kingsley L, Kleerup EC, Detels R, et al. Pulmonary symptoms and diagnoses are associated with HIV in the MACS and WIHS cohorts. BMC Pulm Med. 2014;14:75. https://doi.org/10.1186/1471-2466-14-75. PubMed PMID: 24884738; PubMed Central PMCID: PMCPMC4021087.

81. Mugisha JO, Schatz EJ, Randell M, Kuteesa M, Kowal P, Negin J, et al. Chronic disease, risk factors and disability in adults aged 50 and above living with and without HIV: findings from the Wellbeing of Older People Study in Uganda. Glob Health Action. 2016;9:31098. https://doi.org/10.3402/gha.v9.31098. PubMed PMID: 27225792; PubMed Central PMCID: PMCPMC4880619.

82. Costiniuk CT, Nitulescu R, Saneei Z, Wasef N, Salahuddin S, Wasef D, et al. Prevalence and predictors of airflow obstruction in an HIV tertiary care clinic in Montreal, Canada: a cross-sectional study. HIV Med. 2019;20(3):192–201. https://doi.org/10.1111/hiv.12699. PubMed PMID: 30620136; PubMed Central PMCID: PMCPMC6590155.

83. Kayongo A, Wosu AC, Naz T, Nassali F, Kalyesubula R, Kirenga B, et al. Chronic obstructive pulmonary disease prevalence and associated factors in a setting of well-controlled HIV, a cross-sectional study. Copd. 2020;17(3):297–305. https://doi.org/10.1080/15412555.2020.1769583. PubMed PMID: 32462945; PubMed Central PMCID: PMCPMC8126339.

84. Ddungu A, Semitala FC, Castelnuovo B, Sekaggya-Wiltshire C, Worodria W, Kirenga BJ. Chronic obstructive pulmonary disease prevalence and associated factors in an urban HIV clinic in a low income country. PLoS ONE. 2021;16(8):e0256121. https://doi.org/10.1371/journal.pone.0256121. PubMed PMID: 34388209; PubMed Central PMCID: PMCPMC8362990.

85. Kunisaki KM, Niewoehner DE, Collins G, Nixon DE, Tedaldi E, Akolo C, et al. Pulmonary function in an international sample of HIV-positive, treatment-naive adults with CD4 counts >500 cells/muL: a substudy of the INSIGHT Strategic Timing of AntiRetroviral Treatment (START) trial. HIV Med. 2015;16 Suppl 1:119–28. https://doi.org/10.1111/hiv.12240. PubMed PMID: 25711330; PubMed Central PMCID: PMCPMC4341938

86. Milliron B, Henry TS, Veeraraghavan S, Little BP. Bronchiectasis: mechanisms and imaging clues of associated common and uncommon diseases. Radiographics. 2015;35(4):1011–30. https://doi.org/10.1148/rg.2015140214.

87. Ferrand RA, Desai SR, Hopkins C, Elston CM, Copley SJ, Nathoo K, et al. Chronic lung disease in adolescents with delayed diagnosis of vertically acquired HIV infection. Clin Infect Dis. 2012;55(1):145–52. https://doi.org/10.1093/cid/cis271. Epub 2012/04/05. PubMed PMID: 22474177; PubMed Central PMCID: PMCPMC3369563.

88. Mwalukomo T, Rylance SJ, Webb EL, Anderson S, O'Hare B, van Oosterhout JJ, et al. Clinical characteristics and lung function in older children vertically infected with human immunodeficiency virus in Malawi. J Pediatric Infect Dis Soc. 2016;5(2):161–9. https://doi.org/10.1093/jpids/piv045. PubMed PMID: 26407277; PubMed Central PMCID: PMCPMC5407134.

89. Goyal V, Grimwood K, Marchant J, Masters IB, Chang AB. Pediatric bronchiectasis: no longer an orphan disease. Pediatr Pulmonol. 2016;51(5):450–69. https://doi.org/10.1002/ppul.23380.

90. Masekela R, Anderson R, Moodley T, Kitchin OP, Risenga SM, Becker PJ, et al. HIV-related bronchiectasis in children: an emerging spectre in high tuberculosis burden areas. Int J Tuberc Lung Dis. 2012;16(1):114–9. https://doi.org/10.5588/ijtld.11.0244.

91. Berman DM, Mafut D, Djokic B, Scott G, Mitchell C. Risk factors for the development of bronchiectasis in HIV-infected children. Pediatr Pulmonol. 2007;42(10):871–5. https://doi.org/10.1002/ppul.20668.

92. Morris AM, Huang L, Bacchetti P, Turner J, Hopewell PC, Wallace JM, et al. Permanent declines in pulmonary function following pneumonia in human immunodeficiency virus-infected persons. The pulmonary complications of HIV infection study group. Am J Respir Crit Care Med. 2000;162(2 Pt 1):612–6. https://doi.org/10.1164/ajrccm.162.2.9912058.
93. Sigel K, Makinson A, Thaler J. Lung cancer in persons with HIV. Curr Opin HIV AIDS. 2017;12(1):31–8. https://doi.org/10.1097/COH.0000000000000326. PubMed PMID: 27607596; PubMed Central PMCID: PMCPMC5241551.
94. Walker CK, Shaw CM, Moss Perry MV, Claborn MK. Antiretroviral therapy management in adults with HIV during ICU admission. J Pharm Pract. 2022;35(6):952–62. https://doi.org/10.1177/08971900211000692.
95. Andrade HB, Shinotsuka CR, da Silva IRF, Donini CS, Yeh Li H, de Carvalho FB, et al. Highly active antiretroviral therapy for critically ill HIV patients: a systematic review and meta-analysis. PLoS One. 2017;12(10):e0186968. https://doi.org/10.1371/journal.pone.0186968. PubMed PMID: 29065165; PubMed Central PMCID: PMCPMC5655356.

Chapter 32
Invasive Fungal Infections in the Intensive Care Unit

Jonathan Friedman, Andrej Spec, and Patrick Mazi

32.1   Introduction

Fungi exist ubiquitously in the natural world. While the incidence of human infection peaked during the HIV epidemic of the late twentieth century, it has reemerged in recent years due to anthropogenic climate change and a growing population of immunosuppressed patients—a major risk factor for the development of invasive fungal infection (IFI). Additional factors associated with increase in IFI incidence include the use—and overuse—of broad-spectrum antibiotics and increased implantation of durable prosthetics (e.g., ventricular assist devices (VADs) and heart valves) (Table 32.1). Clinically significant fungi species can be divided into three groups—yeasts, dimorphic fungi, and monomorphic molds. While this classification does not accurately represent fungal phylogeny, it remains the most relevant structure for identification and diagnosis.

J. Friedman
Barnes Jewish Hospital, St. Louis, MO, USA

A. Spec (✉) · P. Mazi
Washington University in St. Louis, Barnes Jewish Hospital, St. Louis, MO, USA
e-mail: andrejspec@wustl.edu

© The Author(s), under exclusive license to Springer Nature Switzerland AG 2025
Y. Alzaidi, M. A. Gebily (eds.), *The Pharmacist's Expanded Role in Critical Care Medicine*, https://doi.org/10.1007/978-3-031-77335-8_32

Table 32.1 Risk factors for invasive fungal infections

Immune system dysfunction
Chemotherapy
Immunosuppressive biologics
Corticosteroids
Neutropenia
Transplant antirejection regimens
Advanced HIV
Central venous catheterization
Hemodialysis
Parenteral nutrition
Malignancy
Diabetes (especially when poorly controlled)
Surgery (especially abdominal procedures)
ICU admission
Critical illness (APACHE II score $\geq$20)
Broad-spectrum antibiotics

32.2 Yeasts

32.2.1 Candida spp.

Candida spp. are commensal fungi that inhabit the skin, gastrointestinal (GI) tract, and genitourinary (GU) tract. Isolation of *Candida* spp. from the airway, GI, or GU clinical samples is common and usually does not represent acute infection. Invasive candidiasis is evidenced by isolating *Candida* spp. from clinical samples collected outside of these expected sites—usually blood cultures. Colonization is a risk factor for invasive candidiasis, though it must be differentiated clinically from invasive disease. Invasive candidiasis is frequently the result of hematogenous spread or direct tissue penetration. It has an overall mortality of 40%.

There are numerous *Candida* spp.; however, the number of clinically relevant species is limited. *C. albicans* represents 44–79% of isolated species from clinical samples, though an epidemiologic shift to non-*albicans* species is occurring. Clinically relevant non-*albicans Candida* spp. includes *C. krusei*, *C. glabrata*, *C. parapsilosis*, *C. lusitaniae*, and *C. auris*. Recently, the taxonomic nomenclature of *Candida* spp. has been updated to reflect genomic phylogeny more accurately. Notable changes include *Pichia kudriavzevii* (formerly *C. krusei*) and *Nakaseomyces glabrata* (formerly *C. glabrata*). Healthcare providers should be aware of these changes and check for further updates to avoid misclassification of potential infections.

In the critical care setting, the most common clinical presentations of invasive candidiasis are candidemia (*Candida* bloodstream infection), endocarditis, and abdominal infections. *Candida* endocarditis is one of the most severe presentations of invasive candidiasis. It is the most common form of fungal endocarditis and carries a higher risk for thrombotic complications compared to bacterial endocarditis.

All cases of persistent candidemia should be investigated for *Candida* endocarditis with echocardiography. Vegetations observed on echocardiography due to *Candida* endocarditis are often larger compared to vegetations due to bacterial endocarditis, though vegetation size is not diagnostic. *Candida* endophthalmitis is a less uncommon but clinically relevant complication of candidemia. A patient complaint of visual disturbances or an inability to describe visual disturbances (i.e., an intubated patient or patient with altered mentation) in the setting of candidemia should prompt immediate consultation by an ophthalmology consultant and a dilated eye examination.

Obtaining species-level identification of these pathogenic fungi is crucial as they have significant empiric treatment implications. *C. krusei* is intrinsically fluconazole resistant. *C. glabrata* can develop resistance to azoles and echinocandins after exposure. *C. parapsilosis* isolates often have increased MICs to echinocandins. *C. lusitaniae* has intrinsic resistance to amphotericin B. *C. auris* is intrinsically resistant to many antifungals, with reported resistance to azoles and amphotericin B in up to 35% of clinical isolates. Once species-level identification is obtained, intrinsic resistance patterns of *Candida* spp. should be integrated into empiric antifungal selection until antifungal susceptibility can be obtained.

Biopsy of suspected sites of infection with histopathological analysis and/or isolation of *Candida* spp. from blood culture remains the diagnostic gold standard for invasive candidiasis. However, invasive sampling can be challenging to the point of infeasibility in the critically ill patient. In these cases, empiric antifungal treatment is recommended while awaiting clinical stability necessary to obtain tissue samples or while awaiting histopathologic results. Dedicated fungal isolator cultures are usually unnecessary for the detection of candidemia as *Candida* spp. routinely grow in standard blood cultures. Isolation of *Candida* spp. from blood culture should never be interpreted as a contaminant and warrants aggressive investigation and empiric antifungal therapy. Clinicians should promptly identify and remove any potential source of infection as able (e.g., removal of central venous catheters or other prosthetic materials). Clinical suspicion remains important as negative blood cultures can falsely reassure; the sensitivity of blood culture to detect candidemia is 50–70%. Many centers supplement the diagnostic evaluation for fungal pathogens with 1,3-β-D-glucan assays. 1,3-β-D-glucan is a highly evolutionary-conserved structural component of fungal cell walls. Current 1,3-β-D-glucan assays have a sensitivity of 75–100%. It is important to note that 1,3-β-D-glucan testing will detect many other fungi including *Aspergillus*, *Fusarium*, *Acremonium*, and *Saccharomyces* species. Subsequently, due to frequent *Candida* spp. colonization and cross-reactivity with other fungal pathogens, false positives are common and limit the clinical utility of 1,3-β-D-glucan assays.

Echinocandins are the preferred empiric antifungals for presumed invasive candidiasis and while awaiting antifungal susceptibility testing once a *Candida* spp. has been isolated from culture. Exceptions to this recommendation include *Candida* endophthalmitis, CNS infection, and urinary tract infections as the antifungal class has poor penetration into these tissues. Concern for or diagnosis of endophthalmitis typically requires treatment with an active azole and may be supplemented with

Table 32.2 Antifungal treatment dosing and dosing considerations (adult patients)

Antifungal	Dose	Dosing considerations
Fluconazole	400–800 mg q24h IV or PO 200 mg q24h can be used for consolidation/ maintenance therapy	Renal adjustment for CrCl <50 or RRT Multiple DDIs, careful medication reconciliation is recommended
Voriconazole	IV: 6 mg/kg q12h ×2 doses, then 3–4 mg/kg q12h PO: based on body weight ≥40 kg: 400 mg q12h ×2 doses, then 200 mg q12h <40 kg: 200 mg q12h ×2 doses, then 100 mg q12h	Avoid IV formulation if CrCl <50 due to vehicle Variable bioavailability and metabolism. TDM is recommended. Adjust dosing to target trough level of 1–5.5 µg/mL Multiple DDIs, careful medication reconciliation is recommended
Itraconazole	IV: not available in the USA Conventional capsules: 200 mg PO q8h ×3 days, then 200 mg po q12–24h Suba-itraconazole: 130 mg PO q8h ×3 days, then 130 mg PO q12–24h Oral solution: 100–200 mg PO q12–24h	Due to poor absorption, conventional capsules should be taken with food and an acidic beverage (e.g., cola) Oral solution should be administered in a fasting state TDM is recommended. Adjust dosing to target trough level of >2 µg/mL (itraconazole + hydroxyitraconazole) Multiple DDIs, careful medication reconciliation is recommended
Posaconazole	IV or tablet (delayed release): 300 mg q12h ×2 doses, then 300 mg q24h IR oral suspension: 200 mg q8h or 400 mg q12h	Delayed-release tablets are generally preferred to IR oral solution due to better absorption TDM is recommended. Adjust dosing to target trough level of >1–1.5 mg/L Multiple DDIs, careful medication reconciliation is recommended
Isavuconazole	372 mg IV/PO q8h ×6 doses, then 372 mg IV/PO q24h	TDM is recommended, though less commonly available compared to other azoles. Target trough ≥1 µg/mL Consider in patients with prolonged QTc. Associated with decreased QTc compared to prolonging effects of other azoles
Caspofungin	70 mg IV loading dose, then 50 mg q24h	Adjustment for hepatic dysfunction is no longer recommended
Anidulafungin	200 mg IV loading dose, then 100 mg q24h	Consider dose escalation for patient weight ≥140 kg
Micafungin	100 mg IV q24h	Consider dose escalation to 150 mg or 200 mg q24 for: – Patients on CRRT (not actually dialyzed, but binds to CRRT filters) – Patient weight ≥115 kg – Treatment of *Candida glabrata* – ECMO

(continued)

Table 32.2 (continued)

Antifungal	Dose	Dosing considerations
Amphotericin B deoxycholate	0.6–1.5 mg/kg q24h	Not recommended if liposomal formulations are available
Amphotericin B lipid formulations	3–5 mg/kg q24h Higher doses, up to 10 mg/kg q24h can be considered	Bolus infusion of crystalloid with dose to decrease nephrotoxicity Consider premedication with acetaminophen and diphenhydramine to decrease infusion reactions. May also consider corticosteroids in severe cases Monitor renal function and aggressively replete electrolytes
Flucytosine	50–100 mg/kg/day in four divided doses	Renal adjustment for CrCl <40 or hemodialysis Use ideal body weight

IV intravenous, *PO* by mouth, *CrCl* creatinine clearance, *RRT* renal replacement therapy, *TDM* therapeutic drug monitoring, *DDI* drug-drug interaction, *CRRT* continuous renal replacement therapy, *ECMO* extracorporeal membrane oxygenation

intravitreal antifungal injection as necessary, usually at the discretion of an ophthalmology consultant.

Uncomplicated candidemia requires 2 weeks of appropriate antifungal treatment. Most patients receive empiric echinocandin therapy and may be transitioned to an oral azole based on antifungal susceptibility testing (Table 32.2). In contrast, endophthalmitis and other complicated cases of invasive candidiasis should be treated for a minimum of 4 weeks. Additional treatment considerations for patients with immunocompromise or other complicating factors (e.g., need for total parenteral nutrition or inability to remove prosthetic material like VADs) should be made in conjunction with infectious disease consultation.

32.2.2 Cryptococcus *spp.*

Cryptococcosis is an invasive fungal infection most commonly due to infection with *Cryptococcus neoformans* and less frequently by *C. gattii*. Cryptococcosis is an opportunistic infection classically associated with advanced HIV infection though it may affect any immunocompromised patient. A diagnosis of cryptococcosis should prompt evaluation for immunocompromising conditions, including undiagnosed HIV. However, the incidence of cryptococcal infections in immunocompetent populations is increasing. The changing epidemiology is likely multifactorial, though increased thermotolerance and pathogenicity of *Cryptococcus* isolates resulting from anthropogenic climate change are leading hypotheses.

Infection begins with respiratory inoculation, which if not cleared can disseminate via hematogenous spread to the central nervous system (CNS), skin, and other melanin-rich sites. Localized cryptococcal infections can occur via direct tissue inoculation, though this clinical presentation is exceedingly rare. Isolation of *Cryptococcus* spp. from extrapulmonary sites should be considered disseminated disease prompting aggressive evaluation and treatment. Cryptococcal meningoencephalitis is a severe and common manifestation of cryptococcosis in the ICU. It commonly presents with headaches, fever, and nausea/vomiting. Patients with advanced immunosuppression may be unable to mount a sufficient immune and inflammatory response necessary to produce obvious symptoms. As a result, many immunocompromised patients experience delayed or missed diagnosis. Clinicians should maintain a high degree of suspicion for cryptococcal infection in the setting of mental status changes, such as personality shifts and cognitive decline in an immunocompromised patient. Late manifestations are caused by increased intracranial pressure (ICP) and can lead to seizures, papilledema, retinal hemorrhage, visual disturbances, and blindness and is associated with increased mortality.

The gold standard for diagnosis of cryptococcal meningitis is lumbar puncture with cerebrospinal fluid (CSF) analysis. Opening pressure, protein, glucose, and cell count should be routinely measured. CSF studies frequently will identify lymphocytic pleocytosis, elevated protein, and an elevated opening pressure, but abnormalities may be subtle or even absent in people living with HIV (PLWH) and other immunocompromised individuals. Cryptococcal antigen (CrAg) testing should be performed on collected CSF, as it has a >98% sensitivity and specificity for cryptococcosis. Serum CrAg performs similarly to CSF CrAG and can be used in PLWH that cannot undergo lumbar puncture. However, serum CrAg is only validated for use in PLWH; when it is used in other populations, it should be interpreted carefully. A positive serum CrAg supports a diagnosis of cryptococcosis, but a negative result is insufficient to definitively rule out infection in other patient populations. CrAg titers generally correlate with disease severity but should not be used to measure response to therapy as the titers can remain positive for months to years even in patients with clinical resolution of their infection.

The 90-day mortality from cryptococcal meningitis can reach as high as 32% even in resource-rich settings. Early aggressive management is paramount to improve patient outcomes. Mainstays of care include early diagnosis, serial lumbar punctures even in patients with normal opening pressures, initiation of antiretroviral therapy in PLWH, and aggressive antifungal therapy. There are several antifungal regimens and treatment considerations in specific patient populations; it is highly recommended to engage with infectious disease consultants for assistance treating patients with cryptococcosis. Typical treatment is 2 weeks of induction therapy with liposomal amphotericin B (LAmB) 3–5 mg/kg/day, flucytosine 25 mg/kg PO q6h, 10 weeks of consolidation therapy with fluconazole 400 mg PO q24h, followed by fluconazole 200 mg PO q24h as maintenance or secondary prophylaxis depending on the clinical situation. Based on recent clinical trial data, a novel treatment regimen can also be considered—induction therapy with a single 10 mg/kg dose of LAmB followed by 100 mg/kg/day of flucytosine and 1200 mg/day of fluconazole, 8–10 weeks of consolidation treatment with 800 mg/day of fluconazole, and then a minimum of 1 year of maintenance with 200 mg/day of fluconazole.

32.3 Dimorphic Fungal Infections

32.3.1 Histoplasmosis

Histoplasma capsulatum accounts for most infections caused by dimorphic fungi in North America. Though historically thought to be geographically restricted to the Ohio and Mississippi river valleys, recent research highlighted a more widespread distribution with cases occurring across North America. Residence in the historical hyperendemic regions should increase suspicion for histoplasmosis, though absence of this exposure does not sufficiently rule out this pathogen. Further, *Histoplasma* has now been isolated on every continent on the planet including Antarctica. Histoplasmosis is also a mimic of tuberculosis and should be considered in patients with similar clinical presentations, especially those from South America, Asia, Africa, and the Pacific Islands without a confirmed diagnosis of tuberculosis.

Typically, cases are minor and self-resolve without requiring medical care. However, others, especially among the immunocompromised individuals, can develop severe pulmonary or disseminated infection. Systemic infection commonly presents with fever, fatigue, respiratory symptoms, hepatosplenomegaly, unintentional weight loss, and cytopenia(s). Immunosuppressed patients may present with advanced disease manifesting as shock, respiratory failure, multi-organ failure, altered mental status, and coagulopathy. Disseminated histoplasmosis is also associated with secondary hemophagocytic lymphohistiocytosis (HLH). Because of this, clinicians should take care not to mistake histoplasmosis for bacterial sepsis or other sepsis mimics. Less commonly, histoplasmosis can infect the adrenal glands leading to adrenal insufficiency and subsequent shock that is refractory to fluids. High clinical suspicion is required to identify this manifestation and initiate treatment with corticosteroids.

Isolation of *Histoplasma* from cultures or histopathologic identification/confirmation in tissue sampling remain the diagnostic gold standards. However, culture results can take weeks, and obtaining tissue is often too invasive in an unstable ICU patient. Thus, urine antigen and blood *Histoplasma* antibody testing are frequently used to expedite putative diagnosis. Like most fungal diagnostic testing assays, *Histoplasma* antigen and antibody assays can cross-react with other fungal pathogens. CSF and bronchiolar lavage samples may also be used for antigen/antibody testing. Testing for histoplasmosis (and other dimorphic fungi) should be considered in patients with presumed community-acquired pneumonia (CAP), especially when the patient has failed appropriate antibacterial treatment. Lactate dehydrogenase (LDH), ferritin, alkaline phosphatase, and aspartate aminotransferase (AST)-to-alanine aminotransferase (ALT) ratios should be monitored. An AST-to-ALT ratio greater than 2 is suggestive of histoplasmosis in the absence of concurrent alcohol use.

Mortality rates can reach as high as 25% in resource-rich settings and up to 50% in resource-limited ones. Treatment of severe pulmonary or disseminated histoplasmosis should include supportive care combined with early and aggressive use of

LAmB. Consolidation therapy with an azole is recommended following amphotericin induction therapy. Itraconazole, posaconazole, and isavuconazole are preferred azoles, as fluconazole and voriconazole have been associated with worse outcomes (Table 32.3).

32.3.2   *Blastomycosis*

Blastomycosis develops following inhalation of aerosolized fungal spores, typically of the species *Blastomyces dermatitidis*, though *B. gilchristii*, *B. helicus*, and other cryptic species have also been implicated in infection. Like *Histoplasma*, *Blastomyces* was historically thought to be geographically restricted to the Ohio and Mississippi river valleys. However, recent research suggests a wider geographic distribution with additional studies identifying cryptic *Blastomyces* spp. implicated in infection in the western USA and Africa—areas not previously considered endemic for *Blastomyces*. There are reports of blastomycosis outbreaks associated with specific exposures such as the Wolf River in Wisconsin and the Billerud paper mill in Michigan, highlighting the importance of taking a thorough exposure history. While exposure to classically hyperendemic regions should prompt consideration of blastomycosis, lack of exposure is insufficient to exclude it as a diagnosis.

Like the other dimorphic fungi, blastomycosis is commonly misdiagnosed as CAP. Therefore, it should be considered in patients that fail to improve following appropriate antibacterial treatment or those that progress to respiratory failure with or without acute respiratory distress syndrome (ARDS). Unlike other dimorphic fungal infections, blastomycosis more frequently presents with extrapulmonary symptoms affecting the skin, bones, CNS, and genitourinary tracts. Disseminated disease leading to sepsis and multiorgan involvement is possible. In these cases, mortality can reach as high as 90%.

Diagnosis is confirmed through either visualization on histopathology (yeast forms with broad-based budding) or isolation culture. Antigen testing is available for more rapid testing, though cross-reactivity with other fungal pathogens is common. *Blastomyces* serologic testing is generally unhelpful due to low specificity. Treatment of blastomycosis is identical to the treatment of histoplasmosis.

Table 32.3 Half-life[a] of azole class antifungals

Fluconazole	20–50 h
Voriconazole	Variable, dose dependent
Itraconazole	35–40 h
Posaconazole	20–66 h
Isavuconazole	130 h

[a] Assumes normal renal function

32.3.3 *Coccidioidomycosis*

Coccidioides is hyperendemic to the deserts of the southwestern USA and Central and South America; anthropogenic climate change has disrupted these boundaries. As a result, *Coccidioides* and the other dimorphic fungi have been increasingly diagnosed outside of their usual locations and have been isolated from soil in Washington state.

Coccidioides commonly presents as a usually self-limiting CAP known as valley fever. Some cases can lead to hematogenous dissemination to the skin, meninges, and bones, especially in the immunocompromised patient. Therefore, an immunocompromised individual presenting with headaches and fevers after recent pneumonia should be evaluated for potential coccidioidomycosis meningitis. Patients are typically evaluated with serologic testing though many patients have delayed diagnoses due to late initiation of appropriate diagnostic testing.

Fluconazole is the preferred first-line therapy, though itraconazole may also be used. Severe cases may require more aggressive treatment with liposomal amphotericin B, especially in cases of respiratory compromise or meningitis.

32.4 Monomorphic Molds

Monomorphic molds are primarily responsible for superficial skin and soft tissue infection in the critical care setting, usually caused by dermatophytes like *Trichophyton*, *Microsporum*, and *Epidermophyton*. These organisms rarely cause serious infection; however, they can disrupt the skin barrier and allow other pathogens' entry. The classical clinical scenario is onychomycosis that can lead to disseminated *Fusarium* infection in a neutropenic patient.

Aspergillus spp., namely *A. fumigatus*, *A. flavus*, and *A. niger*, are the most common invasive molds. Others, such as *Fusarium* spp. *Scedosporium/Lomentospora*, and various mucormycetes (most commonly *Mucor* spp., *Rhizopus* spp., and *Rhizomucor* spp.), are also common and capable of causing a wide variety of infections.

Proven diagnosis of mold infection requires a patient/host risk factor (e.g., immunocompromise) and isolation of the pathogen from culture or histopathologic evidence. Isolation from culture is often unreliable, so histopathologic analysis is frequently required. Other tools such as matrix-assisted laser desorption ionization time of flight (MALDI-TOF) and polymerase chain reaction (PCR) assays have come to the forefront recently, though each test's clinical utility and cost-effectiveness remain debated. It is important to note that criteria for proven diagnosis were developed for use in clinical research. Clinical situation, patient characteristics/risk factors, and diagnostic testing can support a putative diagnosis and initiation of treatment (Table 32.4).

Table 32.4 Activity of antifungal agents

Fungal Pathogen	Polyenes		Azoles				Echinocandians			Other
	AMB	FLU	ITRA	VORI	POSA	ISA	ANID	CAS	MICA	5-FC
Candida albicans		C					E	E	E	
Candida tropicalis		C					E	E	E	
Candida parapsilosis		C					E	E	E	
Candida krusei			C	C	C		E	E	E	
Candida glabrata		C					E	E	E	
Candida auris		C					E	E	E	
Cryptococcus	*									X
Aspergillus fumigatus										
Aspergillus terres										
Mycormycetes	*									
Fusarium spp.	*			C	C	C				
Scedosporium										
Lomentospora										
Histoplasma	*		C							
Blastomyces	*		C							
Coccidioides	*	C								

* = Induction therapy for severe or disseminated infection

E = Empiric regimen until species identification and susceptibility testing is complete

C = Consolidation/step-down therapy

Note: green boxes indicate high level of antifungal activity and proven clinical benefit. Yellow boxes indicate high rates of antifungal resistance

AMB, amphotericin; FLU, fluconazole; ITRA, itraconazole; VORI, voriconazole; POSA, posaconazole; ISA, isavuconazole; ANID, anidulafungin; CAS, caspofungin; MICA, micafungin; 5-FC, flucytosine

32.4.1 Mucormycosis

While immunocompromise is the classic risk factor for all fungal infections, mucormycosis is commonly associated with neutropenia as well as poorly controlled diabetes mellitus. Trauma can also lead to direct inoculation of mucormycetes into wounds. Mucormycosis should be considered when breakthrough fungal infection occurs while a patient is receiving an antifungal with poor mucormycosis coverage, e.g., voriconazole or an echinocandin.

Rhinocerebral mucormycosis presents with fever, epistaxis, rhinorrhea, and headache. Progressive infection leads to periorbital edema, visual loss, diplopia, ptosis, ophthalmoplegia, proptosis, cavernous sinus thrombosis, and cerebral abscess. A black necrotic eschar may be present in the nasal mucosa. Mortality rates can reach as high as 60%. This is a surgical emergency, and otolaryngology (ENT) specialists should be rapidly consulted. Pulmonary mucormycosis occurs as a rapidly progressive pneumonia with similar radiological findings to other fungal pneumonia. Angioinvasion may lead to massive hemoptysis, requiring urgent intervention. Mucormycosis can also affect the gastrointestinal tract, CNS, and skin, though these are rare and often a result of intravenous drug use or direct inoculation via trauma or ingestion. Mortality rate for invasive disease is as high as 90%.

Diagnosis of mucormycosis relies on radiography findings as well as histopathology. Tissue culture is considered to have low sensitivity due to the organisms' fragility. Galactomannan and 1,3-β-D-glucan are absent or present in very low amounts in the agents of mucormycosis. A negative galactomannan or 1,3-β-D-glucan assay in the presence of a presumed fungal infection should raise clinical suspicion for mucormycosis.

Liposomal amphotericin B is the agent of choice for mucormycosis. Combination therapy with an echinocandin is a possibility, though its efficacy is unclear. Azoles like posaconazole or isavuconazole can be considered as a step-down or salvage therapy or for patients that do not tolerate amphotericin B. In cases of rhinocerebral mucormycosis, surgical evaluation and debridement are paramount to achieve source control and prevent further spread. Given the severity of disease and high mortality, we generally recommend higher doses of LAmB (e.g., 10 mg/kg) as a single initial dose followed by typical dosing when there is high suspicion for mucormycosis.

32.4.2 *Aspergillosis*

Aspergillus spp. commonly invade the respiratory system. Pulmonary aspergillosis can be divided into acute and chronic subtypes. Acute pulmonary and invasive aspergillosis is the most common form of encounter in ICUs. It classically presents with a triad of fever, pleurisy, and hemoptysis, though patients without the classical risk factors (e.g., immunocompromise) may present more subtle symptoms of generalized fatigue, fever, chest pain, dyspnea, and cough. Dissemination to the vasculature, CNS, eyes, skin, heart, GI tract, and kidneys is possible.

Chronic pulmonary aspergillosis (CPA) typically presents in patients with existing structural lung changes like chronic obstructive pulmonary disease (COPD), thoracic surgery, or cavitating infection like tuberculosis. There are four major clinical findings associated with CPA. Chronic cavitary pulmonary aspergillosis is the most common form, with multiple cavities found in the lungs and can progress to chronic fibrosing pulmonary aspergillosis if left untreated. Subacute invasive aspergillosis occurs in the mildly immunocompromised patient and presents similar to the chronic form but progresses more rapidly. Isolated *Aspergillus* nodules can also present with multiple small lesions <3 cm without cavitation and do not require treatment if asymptomatic. An aspergilloma is a fungal ball in the pulmonary cavity or pleura and can present with chronic cavitary pulmonary aspergillosis or subacute invasive aspergillosis.

Allergic bronchopulmonary aspergillosis (ABPA) is a hypersensitivity reaction to *Aspergillus* colonies in the airway in patients with existing pulmonary disease, e.g., asthma or cystic fibrosis. In addition to frequent asthma exacerbations, patients may report cough, fever, fatigue, and hemoptysis.

Diagnosis of acute pulmonary and invasive aspergillosis requires direct examination of tissue samples, respiratory cultures, and radiography. Serum *Aspergillus* galactomannan can be useful for making a putative diagnosis, though multiple infection and host factors affect the performance of this assay. Infectious disease or pulmonology consultation is recommended to assist with interpretation of testing results. Serum 1,3-β-D-glucans have limited use in this population and should not routinely be used for diagnosis. Chronic pulmonary aspergillosis is diagnosed similarly, although elevated serum *Aspergillus* IgG is supportive of the diagnosis. ABPA can only be diagnosed in the presence of asthma or cystic fibrosis, elevated *Aspergillus* IgE, and elevated total IgE. Two of the following must also be present: precipitating serum antibodies or elevated *Aspergillus* IgG, radiographic findings of ABPA, or eosinophilia in patients not receiving glucocorticoids.

Currently, voriconazole is recommended as the first-line treatment of acute pulmonary and invasive aspergillosis over amphotericin B. However, this recommendation is based on clinical trial data comparing voriconazole to amphotericin B deoxycholate, an amphotericin formulation now considered nearly obsolete. Newer liposomal formations of amphotericin B may also be considered as first-line treatment. Though aspergillosis is the most common invasive mold infection, LAmB is often preferred as empiric therapy while awaiting species identification because voriconazole has poor coverage for mucormycetes. Other triazoles may be considered in specific clinical situations (e.g., isavuconazole in patients with prolonged QTc). Antifungal combination therapy has not consistently shown benefit and is generally not recommended.

CPA is also treated by voriconazole, and triazoles may be used to tailor therapy or in progressive and/or symptomatic disease. Recommended duration can last up to 1 year with slow clinical response. ABPA treatment is centered around preventing further lung injury by limiting exacerbations and inflammation through prolonged corticosteroid taper. Itraconazole is usually recommended though other triazoles should be considered due to better tolerability and *Aspergillus* activity. Treatment usually lasts 16 weeks, though extended use up to 6 months may be considered in some patients. Cushing's syndrome may occur in concurrent steroid and triazole use due to triazoles' CYP450 inhibition. Though CPA and ABPA are not frequent causes of ICU admission, patients admitted to the ICU may have these conditions and be on antifungal therapy. Medication reconciliation is vital for recognizing potential drug-drug interactions (DDIs). Further, it is important to note the half-life of azoles as their effect on drug metabolism can persist for a prolonged period after discontinuation.

32.4.3 Fusariosis

Fusariosis is usually caused by either *Fusarium solani* or *Fusarium oxysporum* complexes. It can present as pneumonia, sinusitis, or local or disseminated cutaneous infection. Classically, fusariosis will present as new erythematous skin lesions with central necrosis in an immunocompromised patient, especially neutropenia. Any new-onset rash in this population should prompt rapid diagnostic evaluation and consideration of empiric antifungal treatment.

Like other mold infections, fusariosis diagnosis requires isolation from tissue culture or histopathologic identification. Notably, *Fusarium* spp. can sporulate in vivo making them the most common fungi to grow from blood culture. Thus, *Fusarium* spp. isolated from blood cultures are considered a definitive diagnosis. In contrast, *Aspergillus* isolated from blood culture nearly always represents a contaminated specimen. 1,3-β-D-glucan is a cell wall component of *Fusarium* spp., though 3-β-D-glucan assays are not specific for fusariosis and are not routinely recommended diagnostic testing. *Fusarium* spp. can also cross-react with *Aspergillus* galactomannan assays creating a false positive.

Invasive and/or disseminated infection is empirically managed with liposomal amphotericin B and a mold-active azole combination therapy. Once antifungal susceptibilities are determined, therapy can be consolidated to a mold-active triazole. Throughout treatment, it is important to reduce immune suppression therapy when possible and to avoid any further immune suppression, e.g., steroid use, unless critically necessary.

32.4.4 Scedosporiosis/Lomentosporiosis

Scedosporiosis and Lomentosporiosis are caused by *Scedosporium apiospermum* and *Lomentospora* (formerly *Scedosporium*) *prolificans*, respectively. The *S. apiospermum* complex contains several members, and susceptibility can vary from species to species. Both *S. apiospermum* and *L. prolificans* are found worldwide in soil and water. Incidence is low though it has been increasing in recent years.

Patients with chronic airway disease are commonly colonized with both species, though they are also implicated in invasive disease in immunocompromised patients. Infection usually presents nonspecifically, with fever, cough, fatigue, and chest pain. Endogenous and exogenous keratitis and endophthalmitis can also occur. Direct inoculation is one of the more common routes of infection, usually via trauma to the skin, soft tissue, and bone. Freshwater near-drowning accidents can lead to pulmonary *S. apiospermum* infections and in some cases can have hematogenous spread or direct entry through the nasal sinuses to the CNS. In contrast, *L. prolificans* is more commonly implicated in fungemia and endocarditis.

Diagnosis relies on culture and histopathology, though tissue cultures typically require longer incubation times. As a result, MALDI-TOF is a better choice for rapid species and susceptibility identification.

Scedosporiosis is treated with voriconazole due to amphotericin B resistance, while Lomentosporiosis is typically resistant to all antifungal therapies. Therefore, surgical intervention, immunosuppression reduction, and experimental combination therapy should all be utilized to maximize outcomes. Some novel antifungal agents like fosmanogepix, a fungal enzyme Gwt1 inhibitor, and olorofim, a fungal dihydroorotate dehydrogenase inhibitor, may have the potential for treating scedosporiosis/lomentosporiosis, but are not widely available.

32.4.5 Dermatophytosis

Dermatophytosis is most commonly caused by fungi of the genera *Trichophyton*, *Microsporum*, or *Epidermophyton*. These organisms live on the skin and metabolize keratin, causing infection of skin, nails, and hair. Nomenclature is based on infection location, e.g., tinea corporis (extremities/torso), tinea pedis (feet), tinea cruris (crural fold of the groin), tinea capitis (scalp), tinea barbae (beard), Majocchi's granuloma (hair other than beard or scalp), tinea manuum (hands), and tinea unguium (finger and toenails).

Diagnosis of these infections is usually clinical, with little reliance on laboratory testing. Samples can be treated with potassium hydroxide staining to facilitate identification. Additionally, skin or nail scrapings can be cultured, but this is rarely necessary and antifungal therapy can be initiated empirically. However, in cases of refractory or relapsed disease, culture may be useful to obtain susceptibilities. Topical over-the-counter antifungals like miconazole, clotrimazole, and terbinafine are usually sufficient for treatment. Systemic antifungal therapy utilizing terbinafine, fluconazole, and itraconazole may be required in cases of extensive or refractory disease.

Though superficial cutaneous fungal infections are uncommon reasons for ICU admission, they should be diagnosed and managed appropriately as they can cause skin barrier dysfunction and act as a portal of entry for other secondary infections.

Part VIII

Specific Emergencies in Critical Care

Chapter 33
Hypertensive Emergencies

Andrew Posen 🆔 and Scott Benken 🆔

33.1 Introduction

33.1.1 Definitions, Risk Factors, and Pathophysiology

Hypertensive crises encompass acute, severe elevations in blood pressure (BP). Hypertensive emergencies are often characterized by BP greater than 180/120 mmHg with target-organ dysfunction leading to a risk of significant morbidity and potential mortality [1–4]. Hypertensive urgencies, another facet of hypertensive crises, involve similar acute BP elevation but lack associated target-organ dysfunction. Despite their potential severity, hypertensive emergencies are relatively rare, occurring in only 1–2% of hypertensive patients over their lifetime [5]. Within hypertensive crises, emergencies constitute approximately one-fourth of presentations, with urgencies making up the remaining three-fourths [6]. Hypertensive emergencies generally require intensive care unit (ICU) level of care making them an important clinical presentation for critical care pharmacists to be involved with. Hospitalizations due to hypertensive emergencies have increased since 2000, possibly due to heightened awareness and improved diagnosis of these emergencies, but mortality remains low, with in-hospital mortality around 2.5%, and 1- and 10-year survival rates exceeding 90% and 70%, respectively [5, 7, 8].

There is significant debate about the utility of the above definitions and stratification as there is limited clinical trial evidence that cardiovascular outcomes are affected by acute management of elevations of BP outside of treating the underlying "compelling condition" [9]. Without clinical trial evidence for improved outcomes,

A. Posen · S. Benken (✉)
Department of Pharmacy Practice, University of Illinois Chicago College of Pharmacy, Chicago, IL, USA
e-mail: posen2@uic.edu; benken@uic.edu

© The Author(s), under exclusive license to Springer Nature Switzerland AG 2025
Y. Alzaidi, M. A. Gebily (eds.), *The Pharmacist's Expanded Role in Critical Care Medicine*, https://doi.org/10.1007/978-3-031-77335-8_33

there could be a misguided sense of urgency of care with isolated BP elevations, confusion over the goals and strategies to achieve BP control within the various underlying conditions, and limited diagnostic and therapeutic considerations when all conditions are cataloged together. As such, some proponents suggest retiring these definitions [9], but national and international guidelines have failed to do so [10].

Regardless of the debate surrounding definition, risk factors associated with hypertensive crises have been identified. Some include female sex, obesity, hypertensive or coronary heart disease, mental illness, and nonadherence to antihypertensive medications [11]. It is important to note that causes can vary nationally, regionally, and institutionally and could include underlying causes such as intoxications, nonadherence to antihypertensive regimens, withdrawal syndromes, stroke, drug interactions, spinal cord disorders, pheochromocytoma, pregnancy, and collagen vascular diseases [2, 12, 13]. Understanding the pathophysiology of hypertensive crises remains challenging, especially given the heterogeneity of presentations. At the foundation, however, is shared discordance between autoregulatory capacity and vascular response to the breakdown in autoregulation. Autoregulatory changes in vascular resistance respond to endogenous vasoconstrictors or vasodilators. During hypertensive emergencies, an acute BP elevation overwhelms autoregulation, leading to vascular wall stress, endothelial damage, and increased permeability. This permeability causes plasma leakage, activating platelets, initiating coagulation, and recruiting inflammatory mediators resulting in inappropriate vasoconstriction, microvascular thrombosis, hypoperfusion, and target-organ dysfunction [14–18].

33.2 Workup and Treatment Goals

33.2.1 Workup

While any target organ theoretically can be affected, certain organs are more commonly impacted than others due to differences in cardiac output, oxygen consumption, and autoregulatory capacity (Fig. 33.1) [6]. In patients with acute, severe BP elevations, comprehensive laboratory and diagnostic evaluations are crucial. The necessity of workup stems not from the need to establish an urgent diagnosis of primary hypertension but to detect other "compelling conditions" that have severe BP elevations as an accompaniment [9]. The specific tests ordered depend on the presenting symptoms and could include serum glucose, creatinine, electrolytes, completed blood count (CBC), liver function tests (LFTs), urine toxicology screen, fundoscopic examination, quantitative urinalysis (UA), chest radiography, electrocardiogram (ECG), echocardiography, urine or serum pregnancy screening, lactic dehydrogenase (LDH), haptoglobin, troponin, creatinine kinase (CK), peripheral blood smear, renal ultrasound, and/or head or chest CT [4, 19]. The diagnostic

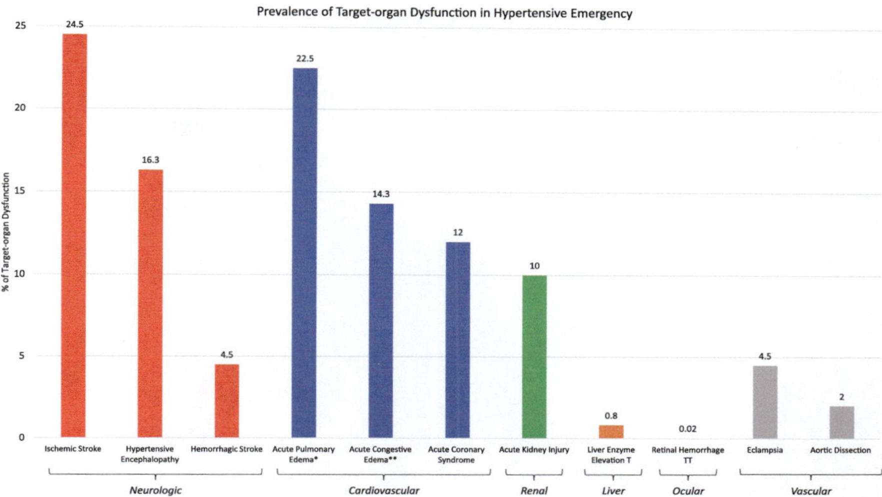

Fig. 33.1 Selected common target-organ dysfunction seen in hypertensive emergencies stratified by organ system. *Includes left ventricular failure. **Includes left and/or right ventricular failure. [T]Primarily seen in HELLP syndrome. [TT]Range of 0.01–0.02%. *HELLP* hemolysis, elevated liver enzymes, low platelet count. (Information from: Shantsila A, Dwivedi G, Shantsila E, et al. Persistent macrovascular and microvascular dysfunction in patients with malignant hypertension. Hypertension 2011;57:490–6; Vidaeff AC, Carroll MA, Ramin SM. Acute hypertensive emergencies in pregnancy. Crit Care Med 2005;33:S307–12; and Zampaglione B, Pascale C, Marchisio M, et al. Hypertensive urgencies and emergencies. Prevalence and clinical presentation. Hypertension 1996;27:144–7)

inquiry may result in findings that yield specific clinical presentations including malignant hypertension, hypertensive encephalopathy, or hypertensive thrombotic microangiopathy (TMA) [10]. Malignant hypertension is defined as severe BP elevation (often greater than 200/120 mmHg) associated with bilateral retinopathy as evidenced by hemorrhages, cotton wool spots, and/or papilledema. Hypertensive encephalopathy is defined by severe BP elevation associated with lethargy, seizures, cortical blindness, and/or coma in the absence of other explanations. Hypertensive TMA is defined by severe BP elevation associated with hemolysis (Coombs negative, elevated lactic dehydrogenase, unmeasurable haptoglobin, or schistocytes) and thrombocytopenia in the absence of other causes and improvement with BP-lowering therapy. Other presentations of hypertensive emergencies that are often termed "compelling conditions" include cerebral hemorrhage (Fig. 33.2a), ischemic stroke (AIS; Fig. 33.2b), acute coronary syndrome (ACS), acute pulmonary edema, aortic dissection, and eclampsia/preeclampsia/HELLP. The diagnostic significance of identifying these "compelling conditions" is that these subclassifications have distinct, individualized treatment goals and potentially unique therapeutic considerations (Table 33.1).

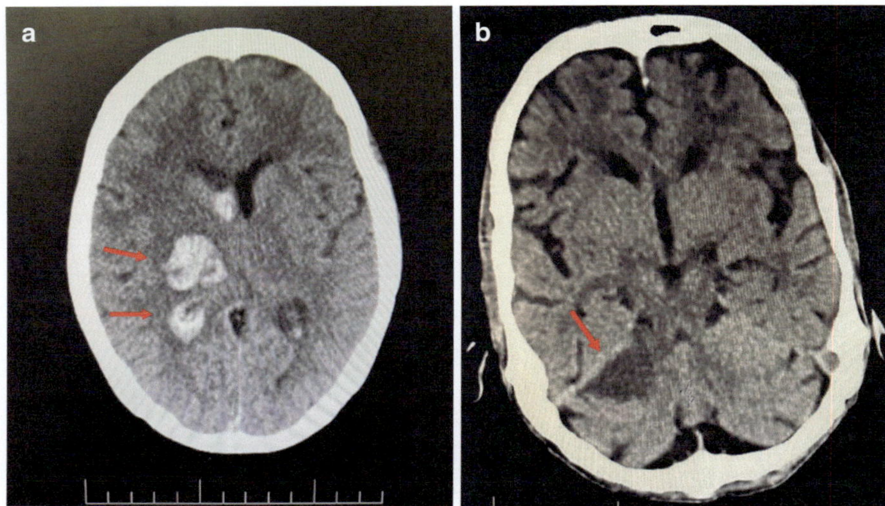

Fig. 33.2 Central nervous target-organ dysfunction in hypertensive emergency. Panel **a**: A non-contrast CT scan reveals acute intracerebral hemorrhage with surrounding edema in a patient with noncompliance with antihypertensive medications. Panel **b**: A non-contrast CT scan reveals acute ischemic stroke (AIS) in a patient with hypertensive emergency and history of drug abuse

33.2.2 *Treatment Goals*

Randomized controlled trials investigating various treatment approaches for the majority of hypertensive emergencies are lacking, with the exception being acute BP reduction in individuals with AIS or hemorrhagic stroke. The prevailing strategies and goals rely on consensus derived from clinical experience, observations, and assessments of intermediate outcomes, such as the time required to achieve predetermined BP goals and indicators of tissue perfusion. For hypertensive crises without target-organ dysfunction, there is general agreement that oral treatment is sufficient and an avoidance of overaggressive correction is warranted, though the concern for which agents to use or avoid is contested [25–27]. Treatment of patients with hypertensive emergencies is driven by the type of organ damage or what has been noted above as "compelling condition" (Table 33.1). Theoretically, the consistent, overarching treatment goal of any hypertensive emergency is to prevent and/or limit hypertensive damage by reducing significantly elevated BP. For those patients **without** "compelling conditions" it is reasonable to reduce MAP up to 25% over the first hour followed by a reduction to an SBP <160 mmHg and/or DBP <110 mg to be sustained over the following 24 h [4, 10]. After the first 24 h, it is reasonable to move the target BP goals to those of outpatient therapy (e.g., Joint National Committee [JNC] 8). Larger initial reductions in MAP (>50%) have been associated with negative neurologic complications and should be avoided [28–31]. For those with "compelling conditions," treatment goals are outlined in Table 33.1.

Table 33.1 Treatment goals for individual presentations of hypertensive emergency

Clinical presentation	Goal	Timeline
Acute coronary syndrome[a]	SBP <140 mmHg (while avoiding decreasing DBP by more than 60 mmHg)	As soon as able
Acute pulmonary edema[b]	SBP <140 mmHg (of particular importance in the non-intubated patient) *Note*: Often the goal is rapid preload reduction which may include loop diuresis, mechanical volume removal, and/or noninvasive positive-pressure ventilation. Afterload reduction may also be a goal.	As soon as able
Aortic dissection[c]	SBP <120 mmHg and heart rate <60 bpm	As soon as able
Eclampsia, severe preeclampsia, HELLP[b]	SBP <160 mmHg and DBP <105 mmHg *Note*: Additional treatment goals include seizure treatment/prevention with magnesium and fetal delivery as necessitated	As soon as able
Hemorrhagic stroke with SBP >180 mmHg[d]	SBP <140 or 160 mmHg (while keeping it above 110 mmHg and avoiding decreasing by more than 90 mmHg) *Note*: Greatest benefit was demonstrated with patients with hyperacute presentations (<6 h), small hematomas, and without ICP elevations.	As soon as able
	SBP <180 mmHg and/or MAP <130 mmHg in those with elevations in ICP or large hematomas	Over 24 h
Ischemic stroke with BP >220/120 mmHg who did not receive thrombolytic therapy or mechanical thrombectomy[e]	Reduce MAP by 15%	Within the first 24 h
Ischemic stroke eligible for thrombolytic therapy with BP greater than 185/110 mmHg[e]	<185/110 mmHg before administration of thrombolytic therapy <185/105 mmHg after thrombolytic therapy for the first 24 h	As soon as able Sustained through the first 24 h
Ischemic stroke with planned mechanical thrombectomy[e]	<185/110 mmHg before thrombectomy	As soon as able

BP blood pressure, *HELLP* hemolysis, elevated liver enzymes, and low platelets, *mmHg* millimeters of mercury

[a] van den Born et al. [19] and Rosendorff et al. [20]
[b] van den Born et al. [19]
[c] Hiratzka et al. [21]
[d] Hemphill et al. [22] and Sandset et al. [23]
[e] Powers et al. [24]

33.3 Treatment Approach

33.3.1 Preparation

The management of hypertensive emergency is time sensitive. If not already established, the medical team must promptly obtain intravenous (IV) access and implement intermittent BP monitoring. Each member of the medical team should be made aware of the decided treatment goal (*previous section*) and the desired time interval for achieving and maintaining target BP reduction. Medication orders should describe parameters coinciding with goals of therapy, including titration instructions for continuous infusions. Given the resources and attention demanded by hypertensive emergencies, patients should be managed in an ICU. Thus, for cases originating in the emergency department (ED), early contact with ICU teams is warranted.

Prior to initiating antihypertensive therapy, elements confounding the patient's BP should be addressed. A prime example is acute pulmonary edema, wherein the distressed, suffocating patient is swiftly disrobed by trauma shears and strongly encouraged to wear a mask akin to a fighter pilot (BiPAP). Recognizing the stress incurred by patients, whether related to the disease process or the medical team's management, anxiolysis with a low-dose benzodiazepine should be considered, contingent upon the perceived need for frequent and reliable mental status exams. In the previous example, 1 mg intravenous lorazepam will likely improve compliance with respiratory support and attenuate the exacerbating sympathetic surge [32]. Other examples of confounding elements include pain (e.g., acute aortic dissection, acute coronary syndrome), drug-induced hypertension, and alcohol or medication withdrawal (e.g., clonidine). Addressing these disturbances clarifies the progress of treatment and better informs treatment decisions.

33.3.2 The Ideal Antihypertensive

While pharmacotherapy may differ by the type of hypertensive emergency, there are ideal attributes shared among the preferred options. Fast onset of BP lowering appeals to time sensitivity. Reliable and predictable dose-dependent effects are desired for minimizing an emerging parameter of interest—blood pressure variability (BPV) (*discussed next*). A short effective half-life enables a fast offset if BP goals are surpassed and supports titratability. Lastly, drug-drug interactions, adverse drug reactions, and drug accumulation amidst organ dysfunction (i.e., renal dose adjustment) are important considerations when selecting treatments.

Most of the aforementioned properties are consistent with drugs administered via IV continuous infusion. Intravenous boluses are reasonable at times when patients require services outside the unit (e.g., computed tomography to rule out AIS); otherwise, IV continuous infusions are associated with better control of BPV

[33]. Blood pressure variability describes the extent of BP fluctuation over time [34]. For the purpose of hypertensive emergencies, short-term (<24 h) and very-short-term (beat-to-beat) deviations from average are most relevant. Methods for measuring BPV are still evolving, and real-time application to patient care is limited [35], but evidence connecting BPV minimization to improved clinical outcomes is growing [36–39]. The important takeaway for clinicians treating hypertensive emergencies is that smooth, controlled reduction of BP using an antihypertensive drug administered by IV continuous infusion is preferred.

33.3.3 Select Antihypertensive Review

Table 33.2 lists antihypertensive options and their clinical properties. Forewarning: due to the titration frequency associated with drugs administered as continuous IV infusions, invasive monitoring of BP by arterial line is recommended. The following paragraphs are dedicated to discussing key considerations in the use of each drug.

Table 33.2 Selective key characteristics of antihypertensive agents

Drug	IV dosing[a]	Preload	Afterload	Cardiac output[b]
Dihydropyridine calcium channel blockers				
Clevidipine • Onset: 2 min • Duration: 5–15 min	**CI**: Start 2–6 mg/h • Titrate q2min by 2 mg/h or by doubling the current infusion rate • Range: 1–32 mg/h	↔	↓	↑
Nicardipine • Onset: 5 min • Duration: 0.5–4 h[c]	**CI**: Start 5 mg/h • Titrate q5–10min by 2.5 mg/h consider dose reduction when response achieved • Range: 2.5–15 mg/h	↔	↓	↑
Vasodilators				
Nitroglycerin • Onset: 2 min • Duration: 10 min	**Bolus**[d] (optional): 400–1000 mcg over 1 min **CI (APE)**: Start 100–400 mcg/min • Titrate q3–5min by 25–50 mcg/min. If excessive BP reduction, dose reduce by 50% or discontinue • Range: 25–600 mcg/min **CI (AMI)**: Start 5–25 mcg/min • Titrate q5min by 5–25 mcg/min	↓	↓/↔	↔/↑
Sodium nitroprusside • Onset: Immediate • Duration: 3 min	**CI**: Start 0.25 mcg/kg/min • Titrate q5min by 0.5 mcg/kg/min • Range: 0.25–10 mcg/kg/min	↓	↓↓	↔/↑

(continued)

Table 33.2 (continued)

Drug	IV dosing[a]	Preload	Afterload	Cardiac output[b]
Hydralazine • Onset: 10 min • Duration: 2–12 h	**Bolus**: 5–20 mg over 1 min • May also be given IM: 10–40 mg[e]	↔	↓	↑
Adrenergic antagonists				
Labetalol • Onset: 5 min • Duration: 3 h	**Bolus**: 20 mg over 2 min • May repeat q10min as needed • Maximum studied 24-h dose: 300 mg **CI**: Start 2 mg/min • Titrate q10min by 1–2 mg/min. When BP goal achieved, dose reduce or discontinue • Range: 1–8 mg/min	↔	↓	↔/↓
Esmolol • Onset: 5 min • Duration: 15 min	**Bolus**[f] (optional): 500 mcg/kg over 1 min **CI**: Start 50 mcg/kg/min • Titrate q5min by 50 mcg/kg/min • Range: 25–300 mcg/kg/min	↔	↔	↓
Phentolamine • Onset: 2 min • Duration: 10 min	**Bolus**: 5 mg by rapid push • May repeat q10min as needed • Range: 5–15 mg/dose	↔	↓	↑
Others				
Enalaprilat • Onset: 10 min • Duration: 4–12 h	**Bolus**: 0.625–1.25 mg over 5 min • May repeat q6h • Usual individual dose maximum: 5 mg	↔/↓	↓	↔/↑
Fenoldopam • Onset: 5 min Duration: 30 min	**CI**: Start 0.1 mcg/kg/min • Titrate q15min by 0.05–0.1 mcg/kg/min • Range: 0.05–1.6 mcg/kg/min	↔/↓	↓	↔/↑

AMI acute myocardial infarction, *BP* blood pressure, *CI* continuous infusion, *APE* acute pulmonary edema, *IM* intramuscular

[a] Dosing recommendations were formed through compilation of FDA-approved listing, published evidence, and anecdotal experience. Dose and dosing range reflect usual practice but should not be construed as all-encompassing

[b] The effect of certain drugs on cardiac output can be specific to the clinical scenario. For example, whereas nitroglycerin is expected to increase cardiac output in patients affected by acute pulmonary edema with high systemic vascular resistance, other patients may not experience increased cardiac output

[c] Duration of effect will depend on duration of therapy, due to an intermediate elimination half-life of 45 min [40]

[d] Adjunctive nitroglycerin boluses given every 3–5 min may expedite clinical resolution [41, 42]

[e] Different pharmacokinetic/pharmacodynamic properties than IV administration

[f] Bolus can be given along with each up-titration in continuous infusion to more rapidly achieve therapeutic effect

Dihydropyridine calcium channel blockers (DHP-CCBs) selectively block voltage-dependent L-type calcium channels at vascular smooth muscle. As a result, they elicit arteriolar vasodilation with no effect on venous capacitance, thereby conferring reduced afterload, preserved preload, and increased cardiac output. DHP-CCBs are associated with favorable cerebral hemodynamics [43], and their side effect profile is consistent with vasodilation: headache, flushing, nausea, and vomiting.

Clevidipine is a water-insoluble DHP-CCB formulated as an oil-in-water emulsion (2 kcal/mL). Across its dosing range, clevidipine exhibits linear pharmacokinetics and pharmacodynamics, unaffected by treatment duration [44]. Its reliable dose-dependent effects are attributed to rapid metabolism by blood and extravascular esterases to an inactive metabolite [45]. Correspondingly, renal or hepatic impairment does not impact clevidipine's activity. Clevidipine emulsions are supplied with a concentration of 0.5 mg/mL, which translates to administering 2–4 mL/h at initiation. In practice, after accounting for the lumen volume interposed between the patient's bloodstream and clevidipine's port of entry, this could theoretically translate to a meaningful delay before the patient receives any drug. Such should be considered, especially with varying lengths of extension tubing.

Nicardipine is another useful DHP-CCB for the treatment of hypertensive emergency. Available for nearly two more decades than clevidipine, nicardipine has a denser compendium of supporting literature. For example, it is known to accumulate in ischemic tissues and therein ameliorate perfusion, due to increased protonation in more acidic environments, including the brain [40, 46]. Therefore, conditions involving myocardial or cerebral ischemia, such as vasospasm, angina, and stroke, may derive benefit with nicardipine treatment. Compared to clevidipine, however, it has a narrower dosing range, and its peak effects are delayed (~1 h), such that product labeling advises dose reduction once BP goals are achieved [47]. Due to poor water solubility, the fluid volume associated with prolonged nicardipine infusions may be excessive for some patients (e.g., heart failure, renal failure). Patients with hepatic or renal impairment may experience prolonged effects relative to healthy counterparts.

There are no head-to-head prospective trials comparing clevidipine to nicardipine for hypertensive emergencies. Systematic reviews including retrospective studies on acute neurovascular emergencies found no difference in time to BP control or BPV between agents [48, 49]. Nicardipine was the chosen antihypertensive in the ATACH-2 trial for BP reduction in patients with intracerebral hemorrhage [50]. Clevidipine has advantageous properties, but it is more expensive [51]. In general, DHP-CCBs are versatile options in treating hypertensive emergencies and are preferred in neurologic emergencies.

The next major group is the direct vasodilators. Nitroglycerin is a nitric oxide donor which positively affects distribution of myocardial blood flow and reduces preload via venodilation, at low doses [52]. At higher doses, nitroglycerin will reduce afterload by vasodilating arteries, making it useful to potentially improve cardiac output in cases of acute pulmonary edema [53, 54]. Hypertensive acute pulmonary edema is a dire phenomenon marked by significant respiratory distress and emission of frothy sputum [55]. In addition to noninvasive positive-pressure ventilation, high-dose IV nitroglycerin (>100 mcg/min) may hasten clinical resolution and stave off the need for endotracheal intubation [56, 57]. Some groups advocate for initial or intermittent boluses (600–2000 mcg) [41, 42, 57]. In practice, the treatment endpoint is clinical resolution of the acute episode, but teams should establish patient-specific BP thresholds to guide dose reduction or cessation of adjunctive nitroglycerin. Table 33.2 also describes gradual dosing of nitroglycerin for patients with acute myocardial infarction. Dose-limiting factors include headache, nausea, and vomiting [53]. Tachyphylaxis is expected to occur within 24 h of continuous use [58], which has been attributed to reduced bioconversion of nitroglycerin by sulfhydryl-dependent enzymatic processes [59].

Sodium nitroprusside (SNP), on the other hand, is a nitric oxide donor not prone to tachyphylaxis [60]. It possesses many ideal attributes, including fast onset, fast offset, and smooth, reliable, dose-dependent effects such that the infusion rate dictates the patient's BP [61]. It acts with incredible potency at both venous and arterial vasculature, reducing preload and afterload, while the change in cardiac output depends on the patient's left ventricular function. After nearly a century of use [62], having been extensively used in the operating theater and widely applied across the spectrum of hypertensive emergencies, SNP's popularity has since lessened [63–65]. Research in myocardial ischemia has identified "coronary steal," a phenomenon whereby infusion with SNP diverts myocardial blood flow away from ischemic regions [66, 67]. Studies monitoring cerebral blood flow have reported meaningful increases in intracranial pressure (ICP) following treatment with SNP, but the direct implications are not known [68, 69]. Therefore, it is theoretically advisable to avoid using SNP in hypertensive emergencies involving myocardial infarction or increased ICP (e.g., hemorrhagic stroke). Neither of these concerns have been definitively substantiated by outcome data in clinical trials [70–73].

A quick glance at SNP's molecular structure may arouse concern among chemistry enthusiasts. Following administration, SNP releases cyanide radicals with toxic potential [74], but to paraphrase Paracelsus, it is the dose that makes the poison [75]. Doses averaging ≤2 mcg/kg/min should not result in toxicity, even with prolonged administration [76, 77]. Higher doses release cyanide in excess of erythrocyte buffering capacity, which throughout the body is detoxified by transsulfuration into thiocyanate for urine elimination [78]. Normal stores of endogenous sulfur donors, however, will deplete after a 1-h infusion of 10 mcg/kg/min in an 80 kg patient [79, 80]. Thereafter, the rise of significant methemoglobinemia (>10%) would take another 16-h infusing at 10 mcg/kg/min [81]. Signs and symptoms of cyanide toxicity include headache, palpitations, tachypnea, lactic acidosis, labile BP, coma, and death. Trending acid-base status with serum lactate and arteriovenous blood gases (ABGs) can aid early recognition of toxicity [63]. The antidote for cyanide intoxication is hydroxocobalamin or combination sodium nitrite and sodium thiosulfate [82]. Thiocyanate, the natural metabolic byproduct of cyanide elimination, has significantly less toxic potential but will accumulate in renal dysfunction, to a relevant degree on the order of multiple days [80, 83]. Due to the risk of fetal cyanide poisoning, the European Society of Cardiology suggests reserving

SNP as a last-line option for controlling severe HTN in pregnancy [84]. With appropriate monitoring, clinicians can subdue cyanide-related fears and appreciate the historical antihypertensive effectiveness of SNP [63, 85].

The last direct vasodilator to discuss is hydralazine. Whereas the previous antihypertensives were administered by continuous IV infusion, hydralazine is given as an IV bolus. In addition to the negative implications of bolus administration on BPV, hydralazine has a characteristically unpredictable effect on BP [86]. Among proposed causes for the variable response [87], genetics may be most influential [88]. Hydralazine reduces afterload by affecting vascular calcium handling and possibly through generation of nitric oxide [89]. Whether by a sympathetically mediated baroreceptor reflex to vasodilation or by direct inotropic effects on the myocardium, hydralazine increases cardiac output [90, 91]. Because of this reflex, its use is not recommended in patients with coronary artery disease [20]. Hydralazine is no longer a first-line option for severe hypertension in pregnancy due to comparatively higher perinatal adverse effects [92]. It is listed as an essential medication to have in neurocritical care units and as an antihypertensive option for AIS [24, 93], with variable effects on ICP depending on autoregulatory capacity [83, 94].

Adrenergic antagonists inhibit catecholamine activity at alpha- and beta-receptors, wherein receptor selectivity determines their utility in hypertensive emergencies. Labetalol is perhaps the most versatile of the adrenergic antagonists and most common initial antihypertensive for hypertensive emergencies according to a US registry [95]. Contrary to experimental data and FDA-approved labeling for labetalol's relative potency at receptor sites [96–98], this "beta-blocker" is predominantly used for its alpha-1 antagonism to reduce afterload with minimal effects on heart rate [99]. Initially studied at bolus dosages between 0.5 and 2 mg/kg, it is now generally recommended to start with 10–20 mg IV before advancing to repeated boluses at 10-min intervals, as needed [24, 99, 100]. Continuous infusions may be used but are not ideal due to labetalol's 6-h half-life and risk for refractory hypotension [101]. Expected side effects include postural nausea and dizziness, and less commonly scalp tingling [99].

Esmolol is a short-acting, cardioselective beta-blocker administered by continuous IV infusion to rapidly reduce heart rate with insignificant effects on BP [102]. During medical management of acute aortic syndrome, anti-impulse therapy first employs esmolol to achieve the target heart rate (e.g., 60 bpm) and thereafter functions to oppose reflex tachycardia associated with vasodilator therapy [103]. With each up-titration of infusion rate, the original trials administered a bolus to expedite therapeutic effects associated with the new dose [104, 105], though this practice has been questioned given esmolol's rapid onset and short half-life [106, 107]. Doses greater than 200 mcg/kg/min have been associated with incident hypotension [102].

Phentolamine is a short-acting adrenergic antagonist whose alpha-1 activity reduces afterload and alpha-2 activity purportedly enhances endogenous norepinephrine-induced inotropy and chronotropy [108]. It is commonly listed as a preferred agent in hypertensive emergencies involving sympathetic or catecholaminergic excess, such as pheochromocytoma or stimulant intoxication [64, 65, 109]. Notable adverse effects include tachycardia and angina, so it should probably be avoided in patients with coronary artery disease or ACS [109]. Intramuscular administration is available, but generally is limited to diagnostic testing for pheochromocytoma. Due to delayed onset (>15 min) when given intramuscularly, its use in hypertensive emergency is inadvisable.

Enalaprilat would theoretically be the preferred option among patients with hyperreninemic forms of hypertensive emergencies because it is an IV angiotensin-converting enzyme (ACE) inhibitor [110, 111]. Due to potential delayed peak effects, unclear differences in incremental doses, and prolonged duration of action (12–24 h), it has limited utility in hypertensive emergency outside of adjunctive support [112, 113].

Last is fenoldopam, a selective agonist at dopamine-1 receptors (DA-1s). These receptors are most densely found in mesenteric and renal vasculature, where activation exerts a vasodilating effect that reduces afterload and preferentially enhances renal blood flow [114, 115]. Consequently, fenoldopam is primarily used for renal protection in the postoperative setting. It clearly has some benefit in that arena [116], but its purported natriuretic effects are variable and literature in hypertensive emergencies is dainty [117, 118]. Theoretically, it could be useful in hypertensive emergency [119], but nobody reports using it [95, 120].

33.4 Future Directions

Hypertensive emergency is a label applied to a diverse group of acute presentations associated with elevated BP. Optimal management, in terms of drug selection and goals of therapy, varies according to the underlying pathophysiology. Importantly, the hypertensive emergency label implies a shared theme: rapid and controlled BP reduction to minimize progression of target-organ damage. Translating this theme into specific treatment recommendations has room for improvement.

There is a deficiency of well-designed comparative trials to inform clinicians of the best approach to treatment. Increased opportunity for recruiting patients into hypertensive emergency research may stem from earlier recognition and diagnosis of hypertensive emergency. Such may then involve clarifying and unifying definitions of hypertensive emergency.

New antihypertensive drugs in the pipeline are primarily being investigated for treating chronic hypertension [121]. Nevertheless, their novel mechanisms may beckon development of an IV therapy with a role in hypertensive emergency. For example, mitigating the harmful effects of endogenous mediators like endothelin may help reduce progression of end-organ damage, independent of BP lowering [122].

The historic standard for measuring BP is the noninvasive upper-arm-cuff measurement. Unfortunately, this method is fraught with confounding variables, and its interpretation is limited by the frequency of measurement [123]. Continuous intra-arterial BP monitoring can nullify these outside influences and enables monitoring of real-time trends, making it a preferred modality in the management of hypertensive emergency. Under this scope, the possible next step for improving management of hypertensive emergency is real-time data on BPV. It is known that higher short-term BPV ($\leq$24 h) has prognostic significance in progressive end-organ damage [124, 125] and is acutely associated with worsened clinical outcomes [126–128], but standardized definitions of BPV and the means for translating BPV into real-time adjustments in clinical management are lacking [129]. Pending technological advancement and availability of prospective trials supporting sound methodology, our only recommendation in relation to BPV for hypertensive emergency is to aim for smooth BP reduction over time and favor the use of medications associated with lower BPV.

33.5 Conclusion

The critical care pharmacist clinician must quickly evaluate target-organ damage to distinguish between hypertensive emergency and hypertensive urgency. Additionally, the clinician should determine if the patient meets the criteria for a "compelling condition" of hypertensive emergency. Once the treatment objective is established, medication is chosen based on treatment goals, observed target-organ damage, pharmacokinetic and pharmacodynamic parameters of each drug, BPV profiles, and clinical data. Continuous monitoring for each patient is necessary to gauge progress toward target goal(s) and prevent inadvertent, excessively aggressive correction. The diagnosis and treatment of hypertensive emergency have significant room for improvement. Opportunities exist in standardizing definitions, expanding the repository of comparative data, and researching innovative technologies for real-time therapeutic monitoring.

References

1. Chobanian AV, Bakris GL, Black HR, Cushman WC, Green LA, Izzo JL, et al. The seventh report of the Joint National Committee on Prevention, Detection, Evaluation, and Treatment of High Blood Pressure: the JNC 7 report. JAMA. 2003;289:2560–72. https://doi.org/10.1001/jama.289.19.2560.
2. Johnson W, Le Nguyen M, Patel R. Hypertension crisis in the emergency department. Cardiol Clin. 2012;30:533–43. https://doi.org/10.1016/j.ccl.2012.07.011.
3. Mancia G, Kreutz R, Brunström M, Burnier M, Grassi G, Januszewicz A, et al. 2023 ESH guidelines for the management of arterial hypertension the task force for the management of arterial hypertension of the European Society of Hypertension: endorsed by the International Society of Hypertension (ISH) and the European Renal Association (ERA). J Hypertens. 2023;41:1874–2071. https://doi.org/10.1097/HJH.0000000000003480.
4. Muiesan ML, Salvetti M, Amadoro V, di Somma S, Perlini S, Semplicini A, et al. An update on hypertensive emergencies and urgencies. J Cardiovasc Med (Hagerstown). 2015;16:372–82. https://doi.org/10.2459/JCM.0000000000000223.
5. Deshmukh A, Kumar G, Kumar N, Nanchal R, Gobal F, Sakhuja A, et al. Effect of Joint National Committee VII report on hospitalizations for hypertensive emergencies in the United States. Am J Cardiol. 2011;108:1277–82. https://doi.org/10.1016/j.amjcard.2011.06.046.

6. Zampaglione B, Pascale C, Marchisio M, Cavallo-Perin P. Hypertensive urgencies and emergencies. Prevalence and clinical presentation. Hypertens (Dallas, Tex 1979). 1996;27:144–7. https://doi.org/10.1161/01.hyp.27.1.144.

7. Lane DA, Lip GYH, Beevers DG. Improving survival of malignant hypertension patients over 40 years. Am J Hypertens. 2009;22:1199–204. https://doi.org/10.1038/ajh.2009.153.

8. Webster J, Petrie JC, Jeffers TA, Lovell HG. Accelerated hypertension—patterns of mortality and clinical factors affecting outcome in treated patients. Q J Med. 1993;86:485–93. https://doi.org/10.1093/qjmed/86.8.485.

9. Fuchs FD, Gus M, Gonçalves SC, Fuchs SC. Is it time to retire the diagnosis "hypertensive emergency"? J Am Heart Assoc. 2023;12:e028494. https://doi.org/10.1161/JAHA.122.028494.

10. Unger T, Borghi C, Charchar F, Khan NA, Poulter NR, Prabhakaran D, et al. 2020 International society of hypertension global hypertension practice guidelines. Hypertension (Dallas, Tex 1979). 2020;75:1334–57. https://doi.org/10.1161/HYPERTENSIONAHA.120.15026.

11. Saguner AM, Dür S, Perrig M, Schiemann U, Stuck AE, Bürgi U, et al. Risk factors promoting hypertensive crises: evidence from a longitudinal study. Am J Hypertens. 2010;23:775–80. https://doi.org/10.1038/ajh.2010.71.

12. Aggarwal M, Khan IA. Hypertensive crisis: hypertensive emergencies and urgencies. Cardiol Clin. 2006;24:135–46. https://doi.org/10.1016/j.ccl.2005.09.002.

13. Shea S, Misra D, Ehrlich MH, Field L, Francis CK. Predisposing factors for severe, uncontrolled hypertension in an inner-city minority population. N Engl J Med. 1992;327:776–81. https://doi.org/10.1056/NEJM199209103271107.

14. Derhaschnig U, Testori C, Riedmueller E, Aschauer S, Wolzt M, Jilma B. Hypertensive emergencies are associated with elevated markers of inflammation, coagulation, platelet activation and fibrinolysis. J Hum Hypertens. 2013;27:368–73. https://doi.org/10.1038/jhh.2012.53.

15. Parrillo J, Dellinger R, editors. Critical care medicine principles of diagnosis and management in the adult. 3rd ed. Philadelphia: Mosby; 2008.

16. Shantsila A, Dwivedi G, Shantsila E, Butt M, Beevers DG, Lip GYH. Persistent macrovascular and microvascular dysfunction in patients with malignant hypertension. Hypertension (Dallas, Tex 1979). 2011;57:490–6. https://doi.org/10.1161/HYPERTENSIONAHA.110.166314.

17. van den Born B-JH, Löwenberg EC, van der Hoeven NV, de Laat B, Meijers JCM, Levi M, et al. Endothelial dysfunction, platelet activation, thrombogenesis and fibrinolysis in patients with hypertensive crisis. J Hypertens. 2011;29:922–7. https://doi.org/10.1097/HJH.0b013e328345023d.

18. Vaughan CJ, Delanty N. Hypertensive emergencies. Lancet (London, England). 2000;356:411–7. https://doi.org/10.1016/S0140-6736(00)02539-3.

19. van den Born B-JH, Lip GYH, Brguljan-Hitij J, Cremer A, Segura J, Morales E, et al. ESC Council on hypertension position document on the management of hypertensive emergencies. Eur Heart J Cardiovasc Pharmacother. 2019;5:37–46. https://doi.org/10.1093/ehjcvp/pvy032.

20. Rosendorff C, Lackland DT, Allison M, Aronow WS, Black HR, Blumenthal RS, et al. Treatment of hypertension in patients with coronary artery disease: a scientific statement from the American Heart Association, American College of Cardiology, and American Society of Hypertension. J Am Soc Hypertens. 2015;9:453–98. https://doi.org/10.1016/j.jash.2015.03.002.

21. Hiratzka LF, Bakris GL, Beckman JA, Bersin RM, Carr VF, Casey DE, et al. 2010 ACCF/AHA/AATS/ACR/ASA/SCA/SCAI/SIR/STS/SVM guidelines for the diagnosis and management of patients with thoracic aortic disease: a report of the American College of Cardiology Foundation/American Heart Association Task Force on Practice Guidelines, American Association for Thoracic Surgery, American College of Radiology, American Stroke Association, Society of Cardiovascular Anesthesiologists, Society for Cardiovascular Angiography and Interventions, Society of Interventional Radiology, Society of Thoracic Surgeons, and Society for Vascular Medicine. Circulation. 2010;121:e266–369. https://doi.org/10.1161/CIR.0b013e3181d4739e.

22. Hemphill JC, Greenberg SM, Anderson CS, Becker K, Bendok BR, Cushman M, et al. Guidelines for the management of spontaneous intracerebral hemorrhage: a guideline for healthcare professionals from the American Heart Association/American Stroke Association. Stroke. 2015;46:2032–60. https://doi.org/10.1161/STR.0000000000000069.
23. Sandset EC, Anderson CS, Bath PM, Christensen H, Fischer U, Gąsecki D, et al. European Stroke Organisation (ESO) guidelines on blood pressure management in acute ischaemic stroke and intracerebral haemorrhage. Eur Stroke J. 2021;6:XLVIII–LXXXIX. https://doi.org/10.1177/23969873211012133.
24. Powers WJ, Rabinstein AA, Ackerson T, Adeoye OM, Bambakidis NC, Becker K, et al. Guidelines for the early management of patients with acute ischemic stroke: 2019 update to the 2018 guidelines for the early management of acute ischemic stroke: a guideline for healthcare professionals from the American Heart Association/American stroke. Stroke. 2019;50:e344–418. https://doi.org/10.1161/STR.0000000000000211.
25. Grossman E, Messerli FH, Grodzicki T, Kowey P. Should a moratorium be placed on sublingual nifedipine capsules given for hypertensive emergencies and pseudoemergencies? JAMA. 1996;276:1328–31.
26. Just VL, Schrader BJ, Paloucek FP, Hoon TJ, Leikin JB, Bauman JL. Evaluation of drug therapy for treatment of hypertensive urgencies in the emergency department. Am J Emerg Med. 1991;9:107–11. https://doi.org/10.1016/0735-6757(91)90168-j.
27. Means L, Benken ST, Tesoro EP. Safety of immediate-release nifedipine. J Cardiovasc Pharmacol. 2016;68:395–9. https://doi.org/10.1097/FJC.0000000000000425.
28. Bannan LT, Beevers DG, Wright N. ABC of blood pressure reduction. Emergency reduction, hypertension in pregnancy, and hypertension in the elderly. Br Med J. 1980;281:1120–2. https://doi.org/10.1136/bmj.281.6248.1120.
29. Bertel O, Marx BE, Conen D. Effects of antihypertensive treatment on cerebral perfusion. Am J Med. 1987;82:29–36. https://doi.org/10.1016/0002-9343(87)90208-7.
30. Reed WG, Anderson RJ. Effects of rapid blood pressure reduction on cerebral blood flow. Am Heart J. 1986;111:226–8. https://doi.org/10.1016/0002-8703(86)90585-5.
31. Strandgaard S. Autoregulation of cerebral blood flow in hypertensive patients. The modifying influence of prolonged antihypertensive treatment on the tolerance to acute, drug-induced hypotension. Circulation. 1976;53:720–7. https://doi.org/10.1161/01.cir.53.4.720.
32. Khorsand MR, Enayatrad M, Yekesadat SM, Khodayar M, Noyani A. Comparison of midazolam versus captopril in patients with uncomplicated hypertensive urgency in emergency ward: double-blind randomized clinical trial. ARYA Atheroscler. 2022;18:1–8. https://doi.org/10.48305/arya.2022.26128.
33. Poyant JO, Kuper PJ, Mara KC, Dierkhising RA, Rabinstein AA, Wijdicks EFM, et al. Nicardipine reduces blood pressure variability after spontaneous intracerebral hemorrhage. Neurocrit Care. 2019;30:118–25. https://doi.org/10.1007/s12028-018-0582-0.
34. Parati G, Ochoa JE, Lombardi C, Bilo G. Assessment and management of blood-pressure variability. Nat Rev Cardiol. 2013;10:143–55. https://doi.org/10.1038/nrcardio.2013.1.
35. Parati G, Ochoa JE, Lombardi C, Bilo G. Blood pressure variability: assessment, predictive value, and potential as a therapeutic target. Curr Hypertens Rep. 2015;17:537. https://doi.org/10.1007/s11906-015-0537-1.
36. Hansen TW, Thijs L, Li Y, Boggia J, Kikuya M, Björklund-Bodegård K, et al. Prognostic value of reading-to-reading blood pressure variability over 24 hours in 8938 subjects from 11 populations. Hypertens (Dallas, Tex 1979). 2010;55:1049–57. https://doi.org/10.1161/HYPERTENSIONAHA.109.140798.
37. Manning L, Hirakawa Y, Arima H, Wang X, Chalmers J, Wang J, et al. Blood pressure variability and outcome after acute intracerebral haemorrhage: a post-hoc analysis of INTERACT2, a randomised controlled trial. Lancet Neurol. 2014;13:364–73. https://doi.org/10.1016/S1474-4422(14)70018-3.
38. Moullaali TJ, Wang X, Martin RH, Shipes VB, Robinson TG, Chalmers J, et al. Blood pressure control and clinical outcomes in acute intracerebral haemorrhage: a preplanned

pooled analysis of individual participant data. Lancet Neurol. 2019;18:857–64. https://doi. org/10.1016/S1474-4422(19)30196-6.

39. Tran QK, Najafali D, Tiffany L, Tanveer S, Andersen B, Dawson M, et al. Effect of blood pressure variability on outcomes in emergency patients with intracranial hemorrhage. West J Emerg Med. 2021;22:177–85. https://doi.org/10.5811/westjem.2020.9.48072.

40. Curran MP, Robinson DM, Keating GM. Intravenous nicardipine: its use in the short-term treatment of hypertension and various other indications. Drugs. 2006;66:1755–82. https:// doi.org/10.2165/00003495-200666130-00010.

41. Levy P, Compton S, Welch R, Delgado G, Jennett A, Penugonda N, et al. Treatment of severe decompensated heart failure with high-dose intravenous nitroglycerin: a feasibility and outcome analysis. Ann Emerg Med. 2007;50:144–52. https://doi.org/10.1016/j. annemergmed.2007.02.022.

42. Wilson SS, Kwiatkowski GM, Millis SR, Purakal JD, Mahajan AP, Levy PD. Use of nitroglycerin by bolus prevents intensive care unit admission in patients with acute hypertensive heart failure. Am J Emerg Med. 2017;35:126–31. https://doi.org/10.1016/j.ajem.2016.10.038.

43. Gaab MR, Czech T, Korn A. Intracranial effects of nicardipine. Br J Clin Pharmacol. 1985;20(Suppl 1):67S–74S. https://doi.org/10.1111/j.1365-2125.1985.tb05145.x.

44. Nordlander M, Sjöquist P-O, Ericsson H, Rydén L. Pharmacodynamic, pharmacokinetic and clinical effects of clevidipine, an ultrashort-acting calcium antagonist for rapid blood pressure control. Cardiovasc Drug Rev. 2004;22:227–50. https://doi.org/10.1111/j.1527-3466.2004.tb00143.x.

45. Ericsson H, Fakt C, Jolin-Mellgård A, Nordlander M, Sohtell L, Sunzel M, et al. Clinical and pharmacokinetic results with a new ultrashort-acting calcium antagonist, clevidipine, following gradually increasing intravenous doses to healthy volunteers. Br J Clin Pharmacol. 1999;47:531–8. https://doi.org/10.1046/j.1365-2125.1999.00933.x.

46. Sabbatini M, Strocchi P, Amenta F. Nicardipine and treatment of cerebrovascular diseases with particular reference to hypertension-related disorders. Clin Exp Hypertens. 1995;17:719–50. https://doi.org/10.3109/10641969509033632.

47. Cardene IV (nicardipine hydrochloride) [package insert]. Deerfield, IL: Baxter Healthcare Corporation; 2010

48. Brown CS, Oliveira JE, Silva L, Mattson AE, Cabrera D, Farrell K, Gerberi DJ, et al. Comparison of intravenous antihypertensives on blood pressure control in acute neurovascular emergencies: a systematic review. Neurocrit Care. 2022;37:435–46. https://doi. org/10.1007/s12028-021-01417-8.

49. Seifi A, Azari Jafari A, Mirmoeeni S, Shah M, Azari Jafari M, Nazari S, et al. Comparison between clevidipine and nicardipine in cerebrovascular diseases: a systematic review and meta-analysis. Clin Neurol Neurosurg. 2023;227:107644. https://doi.org/10.1016/j. clineuro.2023.107644.

50. Qureshi AI, Palesch YY, Barsan WG, Hanley DF, Hsu CY, Martin RL, et al. Intensive blood-pressure lowering in patients with acute cerebral hemorrhage. N Engl J Med. 2016;375:1033–43. https://doi.org/10.1056/NEJMoa1603460.

51. Saldana S, Breslin J, Hanify J, Heierman T, Larizadeh K, Sanchez M, et al. Comparison of clevidipine and nicardipine for acute blood pressure reduction in hemorrhagic stroke. Neurocrit Care. 2022;36:983–92. https://doi.org/10.1007/s12028-021-01407-w.

52. Nitroglycerin. Clinical pharmacology [database]. Elsevier. Accessed 12 Nov 2023.

53. Herling IM. Intravenous nitroglycerin: clinical pharmacology and therapeutic considerations. Am Heart J. 1984;108:141–9. https://doi.org/10.1016/0002-8703(84)90557-x.

54. Imhof PR, Ott B, Frankhauser P, Chu LC, Hodler J. Difference in nitroglycerin dose-response in the venous and arterial beds. Eur J Clin Pharmacol. 1980;18:455–60. https://doi. org/10.1007/BF00874655.

55. Luisada AA, Cardi L. Acute pulmonary edema; pathology, physiology and clinical management. Circulation. 1956;13:113–35. https://doi.org/10.1161/01.cir.13.1.113.

56. American College of Emergency Physicians Clinical Policies Subcommittee (Writing Committee) on Acute Heart Failure Syndromes. Clinical policy: critical issues in the evaluation and management of adult patients presenting to the emergency department with acute heart failure syndromes: approved by ACEP Board of Directors, June 23, 2022. Ann Emerg Med. 2022;80:e31–59. https://doi.org/10.1016/j.annemergmed.2022.05.027.

57. Mathew R, Kumar A, Sahu A, Wali S, Aggarwal P. High-dose nitroglycerin bolus for sympathetic crashing acute pulmonary edema: a prospective observational pilot study. J Emerg Med. 2021;61:271–7. https://doi.org/10.1016/j.jemermed.2021.05.011.

58. Larsen AI, Gøransson L, Aarsland T, Tamby JF, Dickstein K. Comparison of the degree of hemodynamic tolerance during intravenous infusion of nitroglycerin versus nicorandil in patients with congestive heart failure. Am Heart J. 1997;134:435–41. https://doi.org/10.1016/s0002-8703(97)70078-4.

59. Sage PR, de la Lande IS, Stafford I, Bennett CL, Phillipov G, Stubberfield J, et al. Nitroglycerin tolerance in human vessels: evidence for impaired nitroglycerin bioconversion. Circulation. 2000;102:2810–5. https://doi.org/10.1161/01.cir.102.23.2810.

60. Cottrell JE, Casthely P, Brodie JD, Patel K, Klein A, Turndorf H. Mechanism and prevention of tachyphylaxis and cyanide toxicosis after nitroprusside-induced hypotension. Surg Forum. 1978a;29:308–10.

61. Cohn JN, Burke LP. Nitroprusside. Ann Intern Med. 1979;91:752–7. https://doi.org/10.7326/0003-4819-91-5-752.

62. Johnson CC. Mechanism of actions and toxicity of nitroprusside. Exp Biol Med. 1928;26:102–3. https://doi.org/10.3181/00379727-26-4160.

63. Friederich JA, Butterworth JF. Sodium nitroprusside: twenty years and counting. Anesth Analg. 1995;81:152–62. https://doi.org/10.1097/00000539-199507000-00031.

64. Whelton PK, Carey RM, Aronow WS, Casey DE, Collins KJ, Dennison Himmelfarb C, et al. 2017 ACC/AHA/AAPA/ABC/ACPM/AGS/APhA/ASH/ASPC/NMA/PCNA guideline for the prevention, detection, evaluation, and management of high blood pressure in adults: executive summary: a report of the American College of Cardiology/American Heart Association Task Force. Circulation. 2018;138:e426–83. https://doi.org/10.1161/CIR.0000000000000597.

65. Williams B, Mancia G, Spiering W, Agabiti Rosei E, Azizi M, Burnier M, et al. 2018 ESC/ESH guidelines for the management of arterial hypertension. Eur Heart J. 2018;39:3021–104. https://doi.org/10.1093/eurheartj/ehy339.

66. Chiariello M, Gold HK, Leinbach RC, Davis MA, Maroko PR. Comparison between the effects of nitroprusside and nitroglycerin on ischemic injury during acute myocardial infarction. Circulation. 1976;54:766–73. https://doi.org/10.1161/01.cir.54.5.766.

67. Mann T, Cohn PF, Holman LB, Green LH, Markis JE, Phillips DA. Effect of nitroprusside on regional myocardial blood flow in coronary artery disease. Results in 25 patients and comparison with nitroglycerin. Circulation. 1978;57:732–8. https://doi.org/10.1161/01.cir.57.4.732.

68. Cottrell JE, Patel K, Turndorf H, Ransohoff J. Intracranial pressure changes induced by sodium nitroprusside in patients with intracranial mass lesions. J Neurosurg. 1978b;48:329–31. https://doi.org/10.3171/jns.1978.48.3.0329.

69. Turner JM, Powell D, Gibson RM, McDowall DG. Intracranial pressure changes in neurosurgical patients during hypotension induced with sodium nitroprusside or trimetaphan. Br J Anaesth. 1977;49:419–25. https://doi.org/10.1093/bja/49.5.419.

70. Passamani ER. Nitroprusside in myocardial infarction. N Engl J Med. 1982;306:1168–70. https://doi.org/10.1056/NEJM198205133061908.

71. Roitberg BZ, Hardman J, Urbaniak K, Merchant A, Mangubat EZ, Alaraj A, et al. Prospective randomized comparison of safety and efficacy of nicardipine and nitroprusside drip for control of hypertension in the neurosurgical intensive care unit. Neurosurgery. 2008;63:115–20; discussion 120–1. https://doi.org/10.1227/01.NEU.0000335078.62599.14.

72. Suri MFK, Vazquez G, Ezzeddine MA, Qureshi AI. A multicenter comparison of outcomes associated with intravenous nitroprusside and nicardipine treatment among patients

with intracerebral hemorrhage. Neurocrit Care. 2009;11:50–5. https://doi.org/10.1007/s12028-009-9192-1.

73. Yusuf S, Collins R, MacMahon S, Peto R. Effect of intravenous nitrates on mortality in acute myocardial infarction: an overview of the randomised trials. Lancet (London, England). 1988;1:1088–92. https://doi.org/10.1016/s0140-6736(88)91906-x.

74. Robin ED, McCauley R. Nitroprusside-related cyanide poisoning. Time (long past due) for urgent, effective interventions. Chest. 1992;102:1842–5. https://doi.org/10.1378/chest.102.6.1842.

75. Paracelsus T. Die dritte Defension von den newen Recepten. Basel: Labyrintus und Irrgang der vermeinten Artzet; 1574. p. 88.

76. Lipman J, Hesdorffer C, Fernandes Costa F, Roos CP, Eidelman J, Plit M. Vitamin B12 levels in the prolonged use of sodium nitroprusside. Crit Care Med. 1984;12:161–3. https://doi.org/10.1097/00003246-198403000-00002.

77. Pasch T, Schulz V, Hoppelshäuser G. Nitroprusside-induced formation of cyanide and its detoxication with thiosulfate during deliberate hypotension. J Cardiovasc Pharmacol. 1983;5:77–85. https://doi.org/10.1097/00005344-198301000-00012.

78. Hall VA, Guest JM. Sodium nitroprusside-induced cyanide intoxication and prevention with sodium thiosulfate prophylaxis. Am J Crit Care. 1992;1:19–25; quiz 26–7.

79. Ivankovich AD, Braverman B, Stephens TS, Shulman M, Heyman HJ. Sodium thiosulfate disposition in humans: relation to sodium nitroprusside toxicity. Anesthesiology. 1983;58:11–7. https://doi.org/10.1097/00000542-198301000-00003.

80. Schulz V. Clinical pharmacokinetics of nitroprusside, cyanide, thiosulphate and thiocyanate. Clin Pharmacokinet. 1984;9:239–51. https://doi.org/10.2165/00003088-198409030-00005.

81. MedicinesComplete: Sodium Nitroprusside. AHFS Drug Information. Accessed 19 Nov 2023.

82. Holstege C, Kirk M. Cyanide and hydrogen sulfide. In: Nelson L, Howland M, Lewin N, Smith S, Goldfrank L, Hoffman R, editors. Goldfrank's toxicologic emergencies. 11th ed. McGraw-Hill; 2019.

83. Rhoney DH, Liu-DeRyke X. Effect of vasoactive therapy on cerebral circulation. Crit Care Clin. 2006;22:221–43, vi. https://doi.org/10.1016/j.ccc.2006.02.009.

84. Regitz-Zagrosek V, Roos-Hesselink JW, Bauersachs J, Blomström-Lundqvist C, Cífková R, De Bonis M, et al. 2018 ESC guidelines for the management of cardiovascular diseases during pregnancy. Eur Heart J. 2018;39:3165–241. https://doi.org/10.1093/eurheartj/ehy340.

85. Hottinger DG, Beebe DS, Kozhimannil T, Prielipp RC, Belani KG. Sodium nitroprusside in 2014: a clinical concepts review. J Anaesthesiol Clin Pharmacol. 2014;30:462–71. https://doi.org/10.4103/0970-9185.142799.

86. Campbell P, Baker WL, Bendel SD, White WB. Intravenous hydralazine for blood pressure management in the hospitalized patient: its use is often unjustified. J Am Soc Hypertens. 2011;5:473–7. https://doi.org/10.1016/j.jash.2011.07.002.

87. Graves DA, Muir KT, Richards W, Steiger BW, Chang I, Patel B. Hydralazine dose-response curve analysis. J Pharmacokinet Biopharm. 1990;18:279–91. https://doi.org/10.1007/BF01062269.

88. Shepherd A, Lin MS, McNay J, Ludden T, Musgrave G. Determinants of response to intravenous hydralazine in hypertension. Clin Pharmacol Ther. 1981;30:773–81. https://doi.org/10.1038/clpt.1981.237.

89. Hydralazine. Clinical pharmacology [database]. Elsevier. Accessed 21 Nov 2023.

90. Azuma J, Sawamura A, Harada H, Awata N, Kishimoto S, Sperelakis N. Mechanism of direct cardiostimulating actions of hydralazine. Eur J Pharmacol. 1987;135:137–44. https://doi.org/10.1016/0014-2999(87)90605-4.

91. Leier CV, Desch CE, Magorien RD, Triffon DW, Unverferth DV, Boudoulas H, et al. Positive inotropic effects of hydralazine in human subjects: comparison with prazosin in the setting of congestive heart failure. Am J Cardiol. 1980;46:1039–44. https://doi.org/10.1016/0002-9149(80)90364-1.

92. Magee LA, Cham C, Waterman EJ, Ohlsson A, von Dadelszen P. Hydralazine for treatment of severe hypertension in pregnancy: meta-analysis. BMJ. 2003;327:955–60. https://doi.org/10.1136/bmj.327.7421.955.
93. Moheet AM, Livesay SL, Abdelhak T, Bleck TP, Human T, Karanjia N, et al. Standards for neurologic critical care units: a statement for healthcare professionals from the Neurocritical Care Society. Neurocrit Care. 2018;29:145–60. https://doi.org/10.1007/s12028-018-0601-1.
94. James DJ, Bedford RF. Hydralazine for controlled hypotension during neurosurgical operations. Anesth Analg. 1982;61:1016–9.
95. Katz JN, Gore JM, Amin A, Anderson FA, Dasta JF, Ferguson JJ, Kleinschmidt K, Mayer SA, Multz AS, Peacock WF, Peterson E, Pollack C, Sung GY, Shorr A, Varon J, Wyman A, Emery LA, Granger CB, et al. Practice patterns, outcomes, and end-organ dysfunction for patients with acute severe hypertension: the Studying the Treatment of Acute hyperTension (STAT) registry. Am Heart J. 2009;158:599–606.e1. https://doi.org/10.1016/j.ahj.2009.07.020.
96. Richards DA, Tuckman J, Prichard BN. Assessment of alpha- and beta-adrenoceptor blocking actions of labetalol. Br J Clin Pharmacol. 1976;3:849–55. https://doi.org/10.1111/j.1365-2125.1976.tb00637.x.
97. Richards DA, Prichard BN, Boakes AJ, Tuckman J, Knight EJ. Pharmacological basis for antihypertensive effects of intravenous labetalol. Br Heart J. 1977;39:99–106. https://doi.org/10.1136/hrt.39.1.99.
98. Trandate (labetalol hydrochloride) tablets [package insert]. San Diego, CA: Prometheus Laboratories Inc.; 2010.
99. MacCarthy EP, Bloomfield SS. Labetalol: a review of its pharmacology, pharmacokinetics, clinical uses and adverse effects. Pharmacotherapy. 1983;3:193–219. https://doi.org/10.1002/j.1875-9114.1983.tb03252.x.
100. Wilson DJ, Wallin JD, Vlachakis ND, Freis ED, Vidt DG, Michelson EL, et al. Intravenous labetalol in the treatment of severe hypertension and hypertensive emergencies. Am J Med. 1983;75:95–102. https://doi.org/10.1016/0002-9343(83)90141-9.
101. Fahed S, Grum DF, Papadimos TJ. Labetalol infusion for refractory hypertension causing severe hypotension and bradycardia: an issue of patient safety. Patient Saf Surg. 2008;2:13. https://doi.org/10.1186/1754-9493-2-13.
102. Turlapaty P, Laddu A, Murthy VS, Singh B, Lee R. Esmolol: a titratable short-acting intravenous beta blocker for acute critical care settings. Am Heart J. 1987;114:866–85. https://doi.org/10.1016/0002-8703(87)90797-6.
103. Carrel T, Sundt TM, von Kodolitsch Y, Czerny M. Acute aortic dissection. Lancet (London, England). 2023;401:773–88. https://doi.org/10.1016/S0140-6736(22)01970-5.
104. Reilly CS, Wood M, Koshakji RP, Wood AJ. Ultra-short-acting beta-blockade: a comparison with conventional beta-blockade. Clin Pharmacol Ther. 1985;38:579–85. https://doi.org/10.1038/clpt.1985.227.
105. Intravenous esmolol for the treatment of supraventricular tachyarrhythmia: results of a multicenter, baseline-controlled safety and efficacy study in 160 patients. The Esmolol Research Group. Am Heart J. 1986;112:498–505. https://doi.org/10.1016/0002-8703(86)90513-2.
106. Wiest D. Esmolol. A review of its therapeutic efficacy and pharmacokinetic characteristics. Clin Pharmacokinet. 1995;28:190–202. https://doi.org/10.2165/00003088-199528030-00002.
107. Wiest DB, Haney JS. Clinical pharmacokinetics and therapeutic efficacy of esmolol. Clin Pharmacokinet. 2012;51:347–56. https://doi.org/10.2165/11631590-000000000-00000.
108. Gould L, Reddy CV. Phentolamine. Am Heart J. 1976;92:397–402. https://doi.org/10.1016/s0002-8703(76)80121-4.
109. Grossman E, Ironi AN, Messerli FH. Comparative tolerability profile of hypertensive crisis treatments. Drug Saf. 1998;19:99–122. https://doi.org/10.2165/00002018-199819020-00003.
110. Hirschl MM, Binder M, Bur A, Herkner H, Woisetschläger C, Bieglmayer C, et al. Impact of the renin-angiotensin-aldosterone system on blood pressure response to intravenous enalaprilat in patients with hypertensive crises. J Hum Hypertens. 1997;11:177–83. https://doi.org/10.1038/sj.jhh.1000404.

111. Schmieder RE, Hilgers KF, Schlaich MP, Schmidt BMW. Renin-angiotensin system and cardiovascular risk. Lancet (London, England). 2007;369:1208–19. https://doi.org/10.1016/S0140-6736(07)60242-6.

112. DiPette DJ, Ferraro JC, Evans RR, Martin M. Enalaprilat, an intravenous angiotensin-converting enzyme inhibitor, in hypertensive crises. Clin Pharmacol Ther. 1985;38:199–204. https://doi.org/10.1038/clpt.1985.159.

113. Hirschl MM, Binder M, Bur A, Herkner H, Brunner M, Müllner M, et al. Clinical evaluation of different doses of intravenous enalaprilat in patients with hypertensive crises. Arch Intern Med. 1995;155:2217–23.

114. Holcslaw TL, Beck TR. Clinical experience with intravenous fenoldopam. Am J Hypertens. 1990;3:120S–5S. https://doi.org/10.1093/ajh/3.6.120s.

115. Nichols AJ, Ruffolo RR, Brooks DP. The pharmacology of fenoldopam. Am J Hypertens. 1990;3:116S–9S. https://doi.org/10.1093/ajh/3.6.116s.

116. Gillies MA, Kakar V, Parker RJ, Honoré PM, Ostermann M. Fenoldopam to prevent acute kidney injury after major surgery-a systematic review and meta-analysis. Crit Care. 2015;19:449. https://doi.org/10.1186/s13054-015-1166-4.

117. Bodmann KF, Tröster S, Clemens R, Schuster HP. Hemodynamic profile of intravenous fenoldopam in patients with hypertensive crisis. Clin Investig. 1993;72:60–4. https://doi.org/10.1007/BF00231120.

118. Patel JJ, Mitha AS, Sareli P, de Vaal JB. Intravenous fenoldopam infusion in severe heart failure. Cardiovasc Drugs Ther. 1993;7:97–101. https://doi.org/10.1007/BF00878316.

119. Brogden RN, Markham A. Fenoldopam: a review of its pharmacodynamic and pharmacokinetic properties and intravenous clinical potential in the management of hypertensive urgencies and emergencies. Drugs. 1997;54:634–50. https://doi.org/10.2165/00003495-199754040-00008.

120. Vuylsteke A, Vincent JL, de La Garanderie DP, Anderson FA, Emery L, Wyman A, et al. Characteristics, practice patterns, and outcomes in patients with acute hypertension: European registry for Studying the Treatment of Acute hyperTension (Euro-STAT). Crit Care. 2011;15:R271. https://doi.org/10.1186/cc10551.

121. Salvador VD, Bakris GL. Novel antihypertensive agents for resistant hypertension: what does the future hold? Hypertens Res. 2022;45:1918–28. https://doi.org/10.1038/s41440-022-01025-9.

122. Iglarz M, Clozel M. At the heart of tissue: endothelin system and end-organ damage. Clin Sci (Lond). 2010;119:453–63. https://doi.org/10.1042/CS20100222.

123. Schutte AE, Kollias A, Stergiou GS. Blood pressure and its variability: classic and novel measurement techniques. Nat Rev Cardiol. 2022;19:643–54. https://doi.org/10.1038/s41569-022-00690-0.

124. Frattola A, Parati G, Cuspidi C, Albini F, Mancia G. Prognostic value of 24-hour blood pressure variability. J Hypertens. 1993;11:1133–7. https://doi.org/10.1097/00004872-199310000-00019.

125. Parati G, Pomidossi G, Albini F, Malaspina D, Mancia G. Relationship of 24-hour blood pressure mean and variability to severity of target-organ damage in hypertension. J Hypertens. 1987;5:93–8. https://doi.org/10.1097/00004872-198702000-00013.

126. Chung P-W, Kim J-T, Sanossian N, Starkmann S, Hamilton S, Gornbein J, et al. Association between hyperacute stage blood pressure variability and outcome in patients with spontaneous intracerebral hemorrhage. Stroke. 2018;49:348–54. https://doi.org/10.1161/STROKEAHA.117.017701.

127. Manning LS, Rothwell PM, Potter JF, Robinson TG. Prognostic significance of short-term blood pressure variability in acute stroke: systematic review. Stroke. 2015;46:2482–90. https://doi.org/10.1161/STROKEAHA.115.010075.

128. Rodriguez-Luna D, Piñeiro S, Rubiera M, Ribo M, Coscojuela P, Pagola J, et al. Impact of blood pressure changes and course on hematoma growth in acute intracerebral hemorrhage. Eur J Neurol. 2013;20:1277–83. https://doi.org/10.1111/ene.12180.

129. Cucci MD, Benken ST. Blood pressure variability in the management of hypertensive emergency: a narrative review. J Clin Hypertens (Greenwich). 2019;21:1684–92. https://doi.org/10.1111/jch.13694.

Chapter 34
Diabetes Emergencies

Mehrnaz Sadrolashrafi

34.1 Diabetic Ketoacidosis (DKA)

34.1.1 Pathophysiology

DKA is the downstream effect of increased production of counterregulatory hormones (glucagon, catecholamines, cortisol, and growth hormone) due to absolute or relative insulin deficiency. This leads to increased gluconeogenesis, increased glycogenolysis, and decreased glucose utilization, resulting in hyperglycemia and osmotic diuresis. These processes, in turn, cause electrolyte abnormalities and the clinical dehydration state observed in DKA [1, 2]. Additionally, increased production of hormone-sensitive lipase leads to enhanced uptake of free fatty acids in the liver, stimulating the production of ketone bodies. This process results in metabolic acidosis and ketosis, which, together with hyperglycemia, form the classic triad of DKA [1, 2].

Euglycemic DKA (EDKA) is a subtype of DKA where the patient is experiencing ketoacidosis without significant hyperglycemia (typically serum glucose levels <250 mg/dL), which is the distinguishing factor between DKA and EDKA.

34.1.2 Causes

Identifying the precipitating factor leading to DKA is vital to reverse the current episode's underlying cause and prevent future events. The most common precipitating factor for DKA in adult patients is an infection followed by missed insulin doses

M. Sadrolashrafi (✉)
Beth Israel Deaconess Medical Center, Boston, MA, USA
e-mail: msadrola@bidmc.harvard.edu

© The Author(s), under exclusive license to Springer Nature Switzerland AG 2025
Y. Alzaidi, M. A. Gebily (eds.), *The Pharmacist's Expanded Role in Critical Care Medicine*, https://doi.org/10.1007/978-3-031-77335-8_34

857

(due to either a lack of adherence to insulin therapy, limited access to insulin, or a malfunction of the insulin pump). Other factors that can precipitate DKA include surgery, trauma, pregnancy, pancreatitis, acute myocardial infarction, cerebrovascular accident, a new diagnosis of type-1 diabetes, and certain medications [2].

This is a suggested list of medications associated with higher risk of inducing DKA/EDKA (not an inclusive list):

- Atypical antipsychotics [3]
- Calcineurin inhibitors (cyclosporine and tacrolimus) [4]
- Steroid [4]
- Protease inhibitors [5]
- PD-1 inhibitors (pembrolizumab, nivolumab, cemiplimab) [6]
- PD-L1 inhibitors (atezolizumab, avelumab, durvalumab) [6]
- CTLA-4 inhibitors (ipilimumab, tremelimumab) [6]
- SGLT2 inhibitors [7]

34.1.3 Clinical Presentation

Most patients diagnosed with DKA present with variable degrees of these classic symptoms based on the severity of the illness:

- Polyuria (increased urine output)
- Polydipsia (increased thirst)
- Gastrointestinal symptoms (nausea, vomiting, abdominal pain)
- Dry mucous membranes
- Tachycardia and hypotension due to dehydration
- Altered mental status, lethargy, stupor
- Kussmaul breathing (hyperventilation)
- The fruity smell of breath similar to the smell of acetone

34.1.4 Diagnostic Criteria

The American Diabetes Association (ADA) [8] and the Joint British Diabetes Society (JBDS) [9] are two of the leading organizations in publishing clinical recommendations for managing DKA and HHS. Based on the JBDS guidelines, the diagnosis of DKA is made if **all** of the following criteria are met:

1. Blood glucose concentration of >200 mg/dL or known diagnosis of diabetes
2. Blood ketone concentration of >3 mmol/L or significant ketonuria
3. Bicarbonate concentration of <15 mmol/L and/or venous pH <7.3

The ADA's definition incorporates the anion gap (>10 for mild versus >12 for moderate or severe DKA) to the above criteria similar to the JBDS guidelines to assess the severity of illness further. While certain hospitals in the USA may be using this severity category of mild, moderate, or severe DKA as a triage tool to discharge patients home versus admitting patients from the emergency department to general, intermediate, or intensive care units, there is lack of evidence whether this impacts patient-related outcomes. Additionally, this severity system has been utilized in some health systems as a triage tool for the utilization of subcutaneous vs intravenous forms of insulin for the management of patients with a diagnosis of DKA [10].

34.1.5 Treatment Approach

34.1.5.1 Fluid Resuscitation

The severity of hyperglycemia and elevated levels of beta-hydroxybutyrate can create an osmotic shift leading to the observed state of dehydration and hypovolemia in patients presenting with HHS (severe dehydration) and DKA. Hypovolemia can further decrease perfusion to the kidneys and impact their ability to excrete glucose. Hypoperfusion is another common cause of the pre-renal acute kidney injury observed in the majority of DKA and HHS cases, which are typically fluid-responsive. Dehydration can also be further exacerbated by some patients experiencing nausea or vomiting either related to the underlying infection or illness or as the progression of acidosis and dehydration related to DKA and HHS. The first step in managing DKA should focus on volume resuscitation. The choice of isotonic fluid of choice remains controversial. A study comparing 0.9% sodium chloride vs balanced crystaloid for the initial fluid replacement did not find any difference in time to resolution of DKA. In another study of subgroup analysis of two randomized controlled trials SALT-ED and SMART, treatment with balanced crystalloids resulted in more rapid resolution of DKA, suggesting that balanced crystalloids may be preferred over saline for acute management of adults with DKA [11]. The choice of fluid can be left to the discretion of the treating clinicians. However, depending on the total volume administered, the use of 0.9% sodium chloride may lead to non-anion gap metabolic acidosis due to hyperchloremia, potentially delaying the resolution of DKA.

Depending on the degree of dehydration, hypotension, and other systemic signs of low-volume status, patients may require 2–4 L of isotonic fluids during the first 2–4 hours of presentation. These suggested volumes may need to be adjusted based on factors such as a history of heart failure (which could be exacerbated by excess fluid administration), dialysis dependence, or anuric renal failure. Clinicians should routinely reassess volume status and administer fluid boluses as needed, balancing the risk of heart failure exacerbation and/or pulmonary edema from fluid overload. Once the initial resuscitation phase is complete, most patients can continue on maintenance fluids at 100–150 mL/h until euvolemia is achieved. Frequent physical exams should be considered to prevent volume overload, particularly in patients with a history of heart failure or those who are dialysis-dependent and anuric. The maintenance fluid infusion rate can be adjusted or discontinued based on exam findings once euvolemia is achieved. These patients may still require a dextrose infusion to accommodate insulin administration until ketosis is resolved and the resolution criteria, discussed later in the chapter, are met.

Intravenous sodium bicarbonate administration for treating metabolic acidosis in DKA has not been shown to improve outcomes in randomized controlled trials. Bicarbonate therapy should be reserved for cases with severe metabolic acidosis (pH <6.9) [12, 13].

34.1.5.2 Electrolyte Management

Decreased or lack of insulin availability in the blood can lead to a decrease in the shift of potassium intracellularly leading to hyperkalemia. As acidemia progresses due to the rise in beta-hydroxybutyrate and lactate concentrations in DKA, the bicarbonate level decreases as it buffers the increase in hydrogen ion concentration. Additionally, the intracellular shift of hydrogen ions leads to an extracellular shift of potassium as a buffering mechanism. This results in the hyperkalemia in the majority of cases, often observed before the initiation of volume resuscitation and insulin therapy. As osmotic diuresis progresses, aldosterone levels rise, leading to increased sodium reabsorption and further potassium excretion in the urine.

Hypokalemia

As discussed next in the chapter, insulin therapy causes an intracellular shift of potassium, which can lead to hypokalemia. Hypokalemia can become the rate-limiting factor in the continuation of insulin therapy and increase the risk of cardiac arrhythmias and life-threatening cardiac arrest in severe cases. Therefore, if the serum potassium level falls below 3–3.5 mmol/L, insulin therapy should be paused until potassium levels are replenished. The choice between intravenous, oral, or a combination of both therapies depends on the patient's ability to tolerate oral medications (considering potential nausea, vomiting, or altered mental status) and the availability of IV access (peripheral vs. central). In cases of refractory hypokalemia, it is important to ensure adequate magnesium repletion as well.

Hyperkalemia

It is not uncommon for patients with DKA to present with severe hyperkalemia and ECG changes, such as peaked T waves. While insulin therapy is considered first-line treatment for moderate to severe hyperkalemia, administering insulin without adequate fluid replacement can cause an intracellular shift, which may initially lower serum potassium levels. In DKA, there is often a total body potassium deficit despite elevated serum levels, due to acidosis and osmotic diuresis. Additionally, in the setting of DKA, there is a risk of intracellular potassium depletion. When insulin is administered before fluid resuscitation, it may enhance the intracellular shift of potassium, causing a rapid drop in serum potassium levels. This can exacerbate the relative hypokalemia and worsen the risk of cardiac arrhythmias, which can be fatal. In most DKA cases, observed hyperkalemia resolves with appropriate volume resuscitation. Once the patient is adequately volume-resuscitated, insulin therapy can be initiated if hyperkalemia persists. In cases of refractory hyperkalemia, other methods of shifting or excreting potassium may be required.

Hypomagnesemia

Hypomagnesemia can induce the kidneys' wasting of potassium. Especially in refractory hypokalemia cases, it is prudent to keep magnesium levels at the upper limit of normal levels to avoid further worsening of hypokalemia.

Hypophosphatemia

Insulin therapy causes an intracellular shift of phosphate, leading to hypophosphatemia. Additionally, phosphate excretion increases initially due to osmotic diuresis and later due to fluid administration in the management of DKA. Oral or intravenous phosphate supplementation may be used, depending on the patient's ability to tolerate oral medications, the severity of hypophosphatemia, and the availability of intravenous access.

34.1.5.3 Insulin Therapy

The primary problem in DKA is ketoacidosis rather than hyperglycemia. The primary goal of insulin therapy in DKA should be the resolution of ketoacidosis, rather than just correcting hyperglycemia. As insulin therapy progresses and glucose levels drop to <200–250 mg/dL, a dextrose infusion or dextrose containing maintenance fluids should be initiated. This helps maintain insulin infusion and prevent hypoglycemia while ensuring normoglycemia is sustained until the anion gap closes and ketoacidosis is resolved.

Both ADA and JBDS recommend initiation of insulin regular infusion at a weight-based fixed rate of 0.1 unit/kg/h capped at 15 units/h. Once glucose is less than 200 mg/dL (ADA) or 250 mg/dL (JBDS), dextrose-containing maintenance fluid is started and the insulin infusion rate is reduced by half to 0.05 unit/kg/h to maintain glucose less than 200 mg/dL (ADA) or 250 mg/dL (JBDS) while avoiding hypoglycemia until resolution of DKA.

A Bolus dose of insulin may not be needed upfront unless there is an anticipated delay in starting the infusion drip either due to IV access or access to compounding insulin drip.

There are other methods of titrating insulin infusion. The Yale Insulin Infusion Protocol, for example, uses a modifier to adjust the hourly insulin drip rate, aiming for a gradual rather than rapid decrease in glucose levels to ensure a controlled reduction.

The Glucommander method is a computerized algorithm used to titrate insulin infusion. It utilizes software that considers factors such as target blood glucose range, insulin sensitivity, correction factors, the current blood glucose level, the hourly rate of glucose change, and individual patient characteristics. Based on these inputs, the software calculates and suggests adjustments to the insulin infusion rate, aiming for a gradual and controlled reduction in blood glucose while minimizing the risk of hypoglycemia, based on a prespecified target glucose level [14].

Currently, there are no head-to-head comparisons of different insulin infusion titration strategies. Prospective studies comparing computer-based algorithms with fixed-rate algorithms are needed to determine if the cost of these software systems is justified by their clinical efficacy and safety outcomes.

In both DKA and EDKA, insulin therapy is the major step in breaking the cycle of ketoacidosis. However, differences in blood glucose levels upon presentation lead to variations in the management of insulin therapy between these two conditions.

Due to the marked elevation of glucose in traditional DKA, patients can be started on insulin therapy followed by continuous infusion of a dextrose-containing fluid once glucose falls below 200–250 mg/dL.

In EDKA, where blood glucose levels are near-normal or only mildly elevated despite the presence of ketoacidosis, insulin therapy is still required to address keto-acidosis. To prevent hyperglycemia, a dextrose infusion must be started concurrently with the insulin infusion. Due to the risk of volume overload, higher-concentration dextrose infusions (e.g., >10% Dextrose) may be needed.

DKA is considered to be resolved when serum bicarbonate is >15 mEq/L, pH >7.3, glucose is less than 200 mg/dL, and the anion gap is closed. The patient must be able to tolerate oral or enteral feeding. Once the resolution criteria are met, the patient can be transitioned from insulin infusion to subcutaneous form. The subcutaneous insulin dose can depend on various factors, such as whether the patient has type 1 or type 2 diabetes, age, body mass index (BMI), chronic kidney disease (CKD), and steroid use.

Calculating the maintenance subcutaneous insulin regimen after resolution of DKA/HHS:

1. Estimate total daily dose (TDD) of insulin at 0.4 unit/kg (total body weight)

    (a) If the patient is insulin naive, consider reducing TDD by 0.1 unit/kg
    (b) If BMI >30 kg/m^2, consider adding 0.1 unit/kg to the TDD
    (c) If age >70, recommend reducing TDD by 0.05 unit/kg
    (d) If CKD 4 or 5, recommend reducing TDD by an additional 0.1 unit/kg

2. Estimate correction factor for insulin sliding scale

   (a) Calculate correction factor (X) using the formula: $X = 1500/\text{TDD}$
   (b) Apply this factor: Administer one unit of insulin for every (X) mg/dL above the target glucose
   (c) Example: If TDD is estimated at 30, the correction factor is 50. Thus, administer approximately 1 unit of insulin for every 50 mg/dL above 150 mg/dL to bring blood glucose back to around 100 mg/dL

3. Prescribe long-acting insulin (~50% of TDD) and overlap with insulin infusion for 1–3 h to ensure absorption of subcutaneous insulin:

   • Prescribe about 50% of TDD as long-acting insulin (e.g., glargine)

4. Prescribe short-acting insulin (~50% of TDD) in three divided mealtime doses:

   • Prescribe approximately 50% of TDD in three divided doses of short-acting insulin (e.g., insulin lispro), with meals

Consider consulting an endocrinologist if there is a significant discrepancy—particularly in the basal insulin—where the calculated total daily dose exceeds the patient's home insulin regimen by more than 50%.

34.2 Hyperosmolar Hyperglycemic State (HHS)

34.2.1 Definition and Differences from DKA

The hyperglycemic hyperosmolar state is a less frequent hyperglycemic diabetes-related emergency. Although the incidence of HHS is less than DKA, it is associated with a higher mortality rate as high as 20% compared to DKA [8].

34.2.1.1 Pathophysiology [15]

HHS is driven by derangements in increased production of the counterregulatory hormones (glucagon, catecholamines, cortisol, and growth hormone) leading to increased gluconeogenesis and glycogenolysis without uptake of the excess glucose production by the cells. As the concentration of the glucose extracellularly increases, it creates an osmotic gradient that leads to a shift of water extracellularly, which in turn leads to osmotic diuresis and glucosuria to get rid of the excess glucose. This leads to hypovolemia secondary to excess osmotic diuresis and profound dehydration, which further exacerbates hyperglycemia. In contrast to diabetic ketoacidosis (DKA), the presence of insulin in the HHS prevents the body from resorting to anaerobic metabolism and subsequent production of ketone bodies. Therefore, patients with HHS do not experience ketoacidosis. It is though possible to have patients with HHS-DKA overlap syndrome, where features of both diagnoses are present at the same time.

34.2.1.2 Clinical Presentation

Clinical symptoms of HHS typically have a gradual onset from days to weeks. Patients diagnosed with HHS can have any combination of the following symptoms:

- Severe hyperglycemia
- Polyuria
- Altered mental status, confusion, lethargy, weakness
- Seizures, coma, or other focal neurological deficits
- Signs of dehydration and overall low-volume state

34.2.1.3 Diagnostic Criteria for HHS

The current U.S. guidelines define the diagnostic criteria for hyperosmolar hyperglycemic state (HHS) as a serum glucose level >600 mg/dL, serum osmolality >320 mOsm/kg, and the absence of beta-hydroxybutyrate [8].

The UK guidelines' diagnostic criteria for HHS has a slightly lower serum blood glucose cut-off of >540 mg/dL (30 mmol/L) [9].

34.2.1.4 Treatment Approach

Fluid Replacement

Fluid resuscitation is the most important step in managing HHS. Fluid replacement can reduce glucose concentrations and lower serum osmolality by promoting the shift of water into the intracellular space. Therefore, it is reasonable to delay initiation of insulin therapy until adequate volume resuscitation has been provided. The fluid shift can exacerbate hypernatremia, but this should not prompt the use of hypotonic fluids to correct it. Instead, hypernatremia and any further rise in sodium should raise concern if osmolality is not decreasing concurrently. If this occurs, additional volume resuscitation is warranted.

Data on the advantages and drawbacks of specific fluid replacement strategies in HHS are scarce.

Electrolyte Management

Electrolyte abnormalities similar to those discussed in the DKA section above are also observed in this condition.

Hypernatremia

As volume resuscitation with isotonic or balanced fluid is continued, serum sodium increases, serum glucose decreases, and serum osmolality decreases. The rise in serum sodium due to the intracellular fluid shift is not an indication for administering hypotonic fluids. Rather, hypernatremia is secondary to the unmasking of underlying hypertonicity and should be managed in the same way as chronic hypernatremia. There is a paucity of data on the rate of sodium correction in HHS. Based on data extrapolated from the management of hypernatremia in neonatal population, UK guidelines recommend that the rate of fall of serum sodium should not exceed 10 mmol/L in 24 h [16]. There is evolving data that faster correction of sodium >0.5 mmol/L/h can be safe without affecting neurological outcomes [17] and possibly shorter hospitalizations and significantly lower patient mortality without any signs of neurologic complications [18].

Insulin Therapy

Sodium and glucose are primary contributors to osmolality alterations. Swift changes in sodium and glucose levels can induce rapid fluid shifts, potentially resulting in severe neurological complications, such as cerebral edema and osmotic demyelination. Additionally, lowering glucose levels with early insulin use in HHS can abruptly decrease osmolality, increasing the risk of osmotic fluid shifts that may lead to hemodynamic instability. Monitoring the rate of change in osmolality is crucial when treating HHS.

In patients diagnosed with pure HHS, without DKA overlap, a weight-based fixed-rate intravenous insulin infusion should only be started once glucose concentration stops declining despite adequate fluid replacement. Due to the limited data, and to avoid rapid overcorrection of glucose and a swift drop in osmolality, the JBDS guidelines recommend a more conservative initial insulin infusion rate of 0.05 unit/kg/h for HHS. In contrast, the ADA recommends an initial rate of 0.1 unit/kg/h, with plans to reduce it to 0.02–0.05 unit/kg/h once glucose levels fall below 300 mg/dL.

For guidance on insulin dosage calculations for HHS, refer to the insulin section within the DKA management.

The resolution of HHS is defined by the normalization of serum osmolality and the resolution of altered mental status.

34.3 Management of Hypoglycemia

Treatment of hyperglycemia with diet and medications is the core treatment of diabetes. Glucose is the body's primary energy source, and a drop in glucose serum concentration can cause malfunctions at both cellular and organ levels. Hypoglycemia is defined as serum blood glucose less than 70 mg/dL. In mild cases, patients with hypoglycemia can experience headaches, sweating, shakiness, or increased heart rate [19]. In moderate to severe cases, these symptoms can progress to confusion, irritability, dizziness, blurred vision, and slurred speech. As blood glucose decreases to critically low levels, in severe cases of hypoglycemia one might experience seizures or coma.

Cortisol, catecholamines, glucagon, and insulin are key hormones that regulate glucose metabolism and transport in the body. While glucagon raises blood glucose levels, insulin works to lower them when levels are elevated. Disruptions in the production or function of these hormones can lead to dysglycemia [20].

Treatment of hypoglycemia varies depending on the patient's level of consciousness and their ability to take glucose or carbohydrates orally.

For conscious patients who can take oral intake, the ADA recommends the " 15-15 Rule," which involves consuming 15 g of simple carbohydrates and then rechecking blood glucose in 15 min. If blood glucose is still less than 70 mg/dL, another 15 g of carbohydrate is consumed, and glucose is rechecked after another 15 min. Carbohydrate sources high in protein should not be used to treat hypoglycemia, as they may increase insulin secretion.

In cases of severe hypoglycemia or when the patient has an altered mental status or is unable to take oral carbohydrates, IV dextrose, IV/IM/intranasal glucagon are viable treatment options, depending on IV access and drug availability [19].

It is vital to investigate the etiology of hypoglycemic events to address the underlying cause and treat these events as medical emergencies. Stressful clinical events such as trauma, critical illness, surgery, and infection can disrupt the balance between the production, metabolism, and action of cortisol, catecholamines, glucagon, and insulin [19]. In these situations, more frequent glucose monitoring may be necessary to assess the increased risk of hypoglycemia and prevent hypoglycemic events.

References

1. Umpierrez G, Korytkowski M. Diabetic emergencies—ketoacidosis, hyperglycaemic hyperosmolar state and hypoglycaemia. Nat Rev Endocrinol. 2016;12(4):222–32.
2. Dhatariya KK, Glaser NS, Codner E, Umpierrez GE. Diabetic ketoacidosis. Nat Rev Dis Primers. 2020;6(1):40.
3. Sugawara N, Yasui-Furukori N, Shimoda K. Risk evaluation of diabetic ketoacidosis associated with antipsychotics among patients with schizophrenia in the Japanese adverse event report database. J Psychosom Res. 2023;175:111533.
4. Yoshida EM, Buczkowski AK, Sirrs SM, et al. Post-transplant diabetic ketoacidosis—a possible consequence of immunosuppression with calcineurin inhibiting agents: a case series. Transpl Int. 2000;13(1):69–72.
5. Alavi IA. Steroid-induced diabetic ketoacidosis. Ann Intern Med. 1970;72(5):787.
6. Quandt Z, Young A, Anderson M. Immune checkpoint inhibitor diabetes mellitus: a novel form of autoimmune diabetes. Clin Exp Immunol. 2020;200(2):131–40.

7. Zhang L, Tamilia M. Euglycemic diabetic ketoacidosis associated with the use of a sodium-glucose cotransporter-2 inhibitor. CMAJ. 2018;190(25):E766–8.
8. Kitabchi AE, Umpierrez GE, Miles JM, Fisher JN. Hyperglycemic crises in adult patients with diabetes. Diabetes Care. 2009;32(7):1335–43.
9. Dhatariya KK, Joint British Diabetes Societies for Inpatient Care. The management of diabetic ketoacidosis in adults—an updated guideline from the Joint British Diabetes Society for Inpatient Care. Diabet Med. 2022;39(6):e14788.
10. Rao P, Jiang SF, Kipnis P, et al. Evaluation of outcomes following hospital-wide implementation of a subcutaneous insulin protocol for diabetic ketoacidosis. JAMA Netw Open. 2022;5(4):e226417.
11. Self WH, Evans CS, Jenkins CA, et al. Clinical effects of balanced crystalloids vs saline in adults with diabetic ketoacidosis: a subgroup analysis of cluster randomized clinical trials. JAMA Netw Open. 2020;3(11):e2024596.
12. Hale PJ, Crase J, Nattrass M. Metabolic effects of bicarbonate in the treatment of diabetic ketoacidosis. Br Med J (Clin Res Ed). 1984;289:1035–8.
13. Gamba G, Oseguera J, Castrejón M, et al. Bicarbonate therapy in severe diabetic ketoacidosis. A double-blind, randomized, placebo-controlled trial. Rev Investig Clin. 1991;43:234–8.
14. Ullal J, Aloi JA, Reyes-Umpierrez D, et al. Comparison of computer-guided versus standard insulin infusion regimens in patients with diabetic ketoacidosis. J Diabetes Sci Technol. 2018;12(1):39–46.
15. Pasquel FJ, Umpierrez GE. Hyperosmolar hyperglycemic state: a historic review of the clinical presentation, diagnosis, and treatment. Diabetes Care. 2014;37(11):3124–31.
16. Adrogue HJ, Madias NE. Hypernatremia. N Engl J Med. 2000;342:1493–9.
17. Muhsin SA, Mount DB. Diagnosis and treatment of hypernatremia. Best Pract Res Clin Endocrinol Metab. 2016;30(2):189–203. https://doi.org/10.1016/j.beem.2016.02.014.
18. Feigin E, Feigin L, Ingbir M, Ben-Bassat OK, Shepshelovich D. Rate of correction and all-cause mortality in patients with severe hypernatremia. JAMA Netw Open. 2023;6(9):e2335415.
19. American Diabetes Association Professional Practice Committee. 6. Glycemic goals and hypoglycemia: standards of care in diabetes—2024. Diabetes Care. 2024;47(Suppl_1):S111–25. https://doi.org/10.2337/dc24-S006.
20. Cryer PE, Davis SN, Shamoon H. Hypoglycemia in diabetes. Diabetes Care. 2003;26:1902–12.

Chapter 35
Oncologic Emergencies

Christopher Bell ⓘ, Ryan Chaffee ⓘ, Uvette Lou ⓘ, Samantha Luk ⓘ, and Erica Tavares ⓘ

35.1 Chimeric Antigen Receptor T-Cell (CAR-T)/Immune Effector Cell (IEC) Toxicities

35.1.1 Introduction

Chimeric antigen receptor T-cell (CAR-T) therapy, a type of immune effector cell (IEC) therapy, is a unique approach to immunotherapy in which a patient's T-cells are genetically modified ex vivo to create a subset of T-cells specifically targeted to a cancer marker [1–5]. These therapies [5] being living T-cells, endogenously expand in vivo without additional CAR-T/IEC infusions, recruit the patient's existing immune response for cancer cell kill, persist long term within the patient's immune system, and continue to surveille for the cancer markers post-infusion [1, 2, 4]. CAR-T/IEC therapies have improved outcomes for many cancers and the number of cancer markers targeted continues to increase [6]. However, there are significant toxicities associated with CAR-T/IEC therapy given their interaction with the patient's immune system [7].

35.1.2 Cytokine Release Syndrome (CRS)

One of the major and well-known CAR-T/IEC side effects is cytokine release syndrome (CRS), which is an acute, exaggerated inflammatory response to a stimulus (in this case, CAR-T/IEC therapy). CRS from these therapies is considered an

C. Bell · R. Chaffee · U. Lou (✉) · S. Luk · E. Tavares
Department of Pharmacy, Massachusetts General Hospital, Boston, MA, USA
e-mail: CSBELL@mgh.harvard.edu; rchaffee@mgh.harvard.edu; ulou@mgh.harvard.edu; soluk@mgh.harvard.edu; etavares@mgb.org

© The Author(s), under exclusive license to Springer Nature Switzerland AG 2025
Y. Alzaidi, M. A. Gebily (eds.), *The Pharmacist's Expanded Role in Critical Care Medicine*, https://doi.org/10.1007/978-3-031-77335-8_35

on-target, off-tumor toxicity, and thought to be due to activation of the endogenous immune system through T-cell activation [8].

CRS is characterized by fever, hypotension, rigors, tachycardia, hypoxia, respiratory failure, and capillary leak syndrome, which can proceed to multi-organ failure and death if not treated expediently. During CRS, multiple inflammatory markers are elevated, including C-reactive protein (CRP), interferon (INF)-gamma, tumor necrosis factor (TNF)-alpha, interleukin (IL)-2, IL-6, IL-10, IL-1-beta, ferritin, and lactate dehydrogenase (LDH), consistent with recruitment of the immune system and activation of the inflammatory cascade [9, 10]. The rates, peak, and duration of CRS vary based on the type of CAR-T/IEC therapy [8, 11]. In clinical trials, rates of any grade CRS were seen in a majority of patients, with grade 3 being observed in 1–48% depending on the cell product. However, it is important to note that methods of grading for CRS also vary across trials, making cross-trial comparisons difficult. The median onset of CRS occurs within 7 days of CAR-T administration for all CAR-T products and median durations vary from 4 to 10 days [12–17].

After CAR-T/IEC infusion, monitoring parameters for CRS include temperature, blood pressure, oxygenation, CRP, ferritin, LDH, and fibrinogen as indirect markers for inflammation [4, 11]. Some centers are also able to monitor IL-6 and IL-1 levels, which can assist with directing and evaluating response to therapy [9]. In addition, the absolute lymphocyte count (ALC) can be helpful as it may indirectly indicate CAR-T/IEC activity and expansion, seen as an increase in lymphocyte count [18]. Differentiating CAR-T/IEC CRS from CRS caused by other conditions, such as concurrent infection or sepsis, is important given the nonspecific presentation of CRS. Broad differential causes must be evaluated because treatment from CAR-T/IEC-associated CRS carry immunosuppressive, infectious, and other risks. Because sepsis and CRS presentation may be similar, clinicians should consider empirically treating patients for infection while concurrently evaluating/treating for CAR-T/IEC CRS [8, 11, 19].

35.1.2.1 CRS Grading Criteria

A multitude of CAR-T/IEC CRS grading criteria exist, but the 2019 ASTCT Consensus Grading Criteria is the most commonly used. These criteria unify multiple CAR-T/IEC CRS grading criteria into a single schema (Table 35.1) [11].

35.1.2.2 CRS Supportive Care and Treatment Options

Supportive care should be considered at all stages of CRS. Common CRS supportive care options include fluid resuscitation and potentially vasopressors for hypotension, oxygen for hypoxia, and antipyretics for fever. As CRS mimics other disease states, infectious workup as well as empiric, broad-spectrum antibiotics for febrile neutropenia or sepsis is also warranted as part of CRS supportive care [8, 11, 19].

Table 35.1 ASTCT consensus CRS grading criteria

CRS parameter	Grade 1	Grade 2	Grade 3	Grade 4
Fever (not attributable to any other cause)[a]	Temperature $\geq$ 38 °C	Temperature $\geq$ 38 °C With	Temperature $\geq$ 38 °C	Temperature $\geq$ 38 °C
Hypotension	None	Not requiring vasopressors	Requiring vasopressor with/ without vasopressin	Requiring multiple vasopressors (excluding vasopressin)
		And/Or[b]		
Hypoxia	None	Requiring low-flow[c] nasal cannula or blow-by	Requiring high-flow[d] nasal cannula, facemask, nonrebreather mask, or Venturi mask	Requiring positive pressure (CPAP, BiPAP, intubation and/ or mechanical ventilation)

[a] If patient receive antipyretics or anticytokine (tocilizumab, siltuximab, or anakinra) therapy, fever is no longer required to grade subsequent CRS and would be driven by hypotension and/or hypoxia
[b] CRS grade determined by the more severe CRS parameter
[c] High-flow nasal cannula is defined as oxygen delivered at >6 L/min
[d] Low-flow nasal cannula is defined as oxygen delivered at $\leq$6 L/min and includes blow-by oxygen

The FDA-recommended backbone of CRS treatment consists of tocilizumab and steroids [12–17]. Tocilizumab is an interleukin-6 (IL-6) receptor antagonist, targeting part of the inflammatory cascade, and is FDA-approved for use in rheumatoid arthritis [20]. Due to its mechanism of action, tocilizumab has found a niche for use in other inflammatory conditions like CRS. As part of the CAR-T/IEC therapy REMS programs, authorized hospitals are required to have two doses of tocilizumab available for every patient receiving CAR-T therapy, and doses must be available to be administered within 2 h. Tocilizumab is dosed at 8 mg/kg IV once with a weight cap of 100 kg (corresponding to a maximum dose of 800 mg given a minimum of 8 hours apart). Per the CAR-T/IEC package inserts, the maximum number of tocilizumab doses that may be given for CRS is four doses [12–17, 21]. No pre-medications are required prior to tocilizumab administration and the most common adverse event is infusion reactions, which can be managed by stopping the infusion and administering hypersensitivity medications, such as diphenhydramine and acetaminophen, as needed [20].

Studies have shown that tocilizumab administration can decrease CRS severity without affecting CAR-T/IEC efficacy [22, 23]. However, as tocilizumab only occupies the IL-6 receptors without addressing IL-6 itself, unbound IL-6 increases in peripheral circulation, causing a sharp rise in serum levels that do not necessarily indicate severity of CRS. This may cause unintended effects such as increasing the incidence of immune effector cell-associated neurotoxicity syndrome (ICANS), as the high IL-6 concentrations may increase diffusion of IL-6 across the blood-brain barrier [23]. As a result, tocilizumab should only be utilized to treat CRS without neurotoxicity and clinicians will need to weigh risks and benefits of tocilizumab in concurrent CRS and ICANS.

Corticosteroids are also routinely used to treat CRS, with dexamethasone being the most commonly used. The usual starting dose for dexamethasone is 10 mg orally or intravenously (IV). Depending on the severity of the CRS, dexamethasone can be escalated up to 10 mg every 6 h and then down titrated as the patient status improves [12–17]. In select, high-grade or refractory CRS cases, methylprednisolone 1 g IV is given once, or as a pulse dose daily for 2–4 days [12]. Given the myriad of corticosteroid-related side effects, it is expedient to taper steroids as guided by the patient's clinical status.

Unlike tocilizumab, steroids can also be used for CRS with concomitant ICANS as they have a global effect of decreasing the inflammatory cascade. Steroids can be used concurrently with tocilizumab. Studies have shown that short-term use of steroids can mitigate CRS with minimal effect on the efficacy of the CAR-T/IEC therapy [24]. Table 35.4 provides general guidance for treatment escalation based on CRS and ICANS grading. It is important to note that each cell product has a product-specific algorithm on its package insert, but institutions may choose to establish their own guidelines.

Aside from the standard tocilizumab and/or dexamethasone CRS treatment backbone, anakinra and siltuximab can also be considered in high-grade or refractory CRS. Anakinra is an IL-1 receptor antagonist [25] that can be used off-label for CAR-T toxicities at doses of 100 mg–200 mg daily up to every 6 h subcutaneously.

Like tocilizumab, anakinra inactivates a key component of the inflammatory cascade to decrease CRS. It can be used as an adjunctive medication to control CRS in addition to tocilizumab and/or steroids. Studies have demonstrated that anakinra can decrease CRS with minimal effect on CAR-T/IEC efficacy [26–30].

Siltuximab is an IL-6 antagonist that is dosed 11 mg/kg IV [31]. Unlike tocilizumab, siltuximab directly binds IL-6 and thus provides a slightly different mechanism for treating CRS. It can be used in tocilizumab-refractory CRS because it directly removes IL-6 from endogenous circulation rather than only displacing IL-6 from the receptor [29, 32, 33].

For the most severe and refractory cases of CRS, the benefits of halting CAR-T/IEC activity may surpass the benefits of treating the cancer with CAR-T/IEC due to CAR-T/IEC toxicity. In these cases, clinicians may choose to initiate an anti-T-cell therapy to kill actively dividing CAR-T/IECs, such as cyclophosphamide 1–2 g/m^2 IV for one dose [34, 35]. Data is limited in this area, and the benefits must be weighed against the risks of early stoppage of CAR-T/IEC activity and severe immunosuppression from aggressive anti-T-cell targeted therapies.

35.1.3 *Immune Effector Cell-Associated Neurotoxicity Syndrome (ICANS)*

Immune effector cell-associated neurotoxicity syndrome (ICANS) is another well-known side effect of CAR-T/IEC therapy. Although it can occur concurrently with CRS, ICANS can also be an independent process. Similar to CRS, the rates, peak, and duration of ICANS varies among CAR-T/IEC products [12–17].

ICANS is a grouping of various neurologic symptoms with stereotypical progression to a specific cluster of severe symptoms. The most common early manifestations of ICANS are tremor, dysgraphia, expressive aphasia, decreased attention, apraxia, lethargy, and headache. These symptoms can worsen to encephalopathy, obtundation, or coma [11]. Although the prior symptoms are the most common neurologic symptoms seen with ICANS, patients may also present with atypical neurologic symptoms, such as parkinsonism and movement disorders [36]. Unlike CRS, ICANS pathophysiology is less well understood. It is possible that ICANS is caused by multiple underlying etiologies such as increased interferon trafficking into the central nervous system (CNS) caused by increased systemic circulation of interferon, blood-brain barrier disruption, or activation of cytokines in the CNS [37].

35.1.3.1 ICANS Grading

During and post CAR-T/IEC, patients should be monitored for ICANS with routine neurological symptom assessment as well as the Immune Effector Cell-Associated Encephalopathy (ICE) score evaluations [11]. The ICE score is a modified version of the CARTOX-10 grading scale [8], which can also be used as a portion of the overall grading for ICANS. Both scales result in a number from 0 to 10 and points for both scales have equivalent scoring. An ICE or CARTOX-10 score of 0 indicates that the patient has no consciousness and has grade 4 ICANS. Those with a score of 1–2 are grade 3 ICANS, score of 3–6 are grade 2 ICANS, 7–9 are grade 1 ICANS, and a score of 10 is no ICANS [11]. A comparison of the two scales can be found in Table 35.2.

ICE scores are only a portion of the overall ASTCT Consensus Grading for ICANS in adults. The ASTCT Consensus Grading takes the ICE score, level of consciousness, seizure, motor findings, and any cerebral edema or elevated intracranial pressure into account when grading overall ICANS, giving us a better picture of all potential manifestations of ICANS that are not captured by the ICE or CARTOX-10 scores alone (Table 35.3).

35.1.3.2 ICANS Supportive Care and Treatment

As with CRS, ICANS symptoms are varied, and supportive care will be dependent on manifested symptoms. When patients have symptoms of ICANS, clinicians should investigate other causes for neurologic symptoms and mitigate or treat those causes if possible. For example, if a patient is on multiple sedating medications and has a decreased level of arousal, the clinician may choose to hold some of these medications to decrease confounding variables in assessing the patient's ICANS severity. Clinicians should also treat any ICANS symptoms that have direct treatments, such as giving antiepileptics for seizures [37]. In case of seizures, levetiracetam is the preferred antiepileptic agent in the CAR-T/IEC population due to its favorable safety profile and minimal drug-drug interactions [38]. It may be used at

Table 35.2 ICE and CARTOX grading scales

	ICE scale	ICE points	CARTOX-10 scale	CARTOX-10 points
Orientation	Year	1	Year	1
	Month	1	Month	1
	City	1	City	1
	Hospital	1	Hospital	1
	N/A	N/A	President/Prime minister of country	1
Naming	Name 3 objects	1 point per correct object	Name 3 objects	1 point per correct object
Following commands	Follow simple commands	1	N/A	N/A
Writing	Write a standard sentence	1	Write a standard sentence	1
Attention	Count backwards from 100 by 10	1	Count backwards from 100 by 10	1

Table 35.3 ASTCT consensus grading for ICANS in adults

Neurotoxicity feature	Grade 1	Grade 2	Grade 3	Grade 4
ICE score	7–9	3–6	0–2	0 (unarousable and does not perform ICE scores)
Depressed level of consciousness	Spontaneous awakening	Awakes to voice	Awakens only to tactile stimulus	Unarousable or requires vigorous or repetitive stimulation to arouse In a stupor or coma
Seizure	N/A	N/A	Any clinical seizure focal or generalized that resolves rapidly or nonconvulsive seizures on EEG that resolve with intervention	Life-threatening prolonged seizure (>5 min). Repetitive clinical or electrical seizures without return to baseline in between
Motor findings	N/A	N/A	N/A	Deep focal motor weakness (e.g., hemiparesis or paraparesis)
Elevated intracranial pressure or cerebral edema	N/A	N/A	Focal or local edema on imaging	Diffuse cerebral edema on neuroimaging or Decerebate or decorticate posturing or Cranial nerve VI palsy or Papilledema or Cushing's triad

a dose of 500 mg twice daily for seizure prophylaxis starting at the time of CAR-T/ IEC infusion and continuing until 30 days after infusion [39].

Corticosteroids are the mainstay of ICANS treatment. The corticosteroid dosing in ICANS is the same as CRS treatment dosing [12–17]. Tocilizumab should not be used to treat isolated ICANS as tocilizumab does not cross the blood-brain barrier and could potentially worsen ICANS by displacing systemic IL-6 to the central nervous system [4]. Table 35.4 contains general guidance on advancing treatment with increasing ICANS grading. Refer to the CAR-T/IEC product package inserts for product-specific guidance.

There is no consensus on treatment of steroid-refractory ICANS, but many treatments have been explored in small trials. As with CRS, anakinra and siltuximab can be considered. Anakinra has shown to be effective in steroid-refractory ICANS with decreased inflammatory markers and cytokine levels [26, 28, 40–43]. Off-label preparation of anakinra for IV administration may also be considered in cases of high-grade ICANS or concurrent CRS and ICANS. The IV administration allows for faster penetration and higher concentrations in the CNS to better treat ICANS [44]. The dosing is the same as the doses used for CRS.

Table 35.4 Management of CRS and ICANS

Toxicity grade	CRS	ICANS	CRS + ICANS
Grade 1[a]	Supportive care[b]	Supportive care Seizure prophylaxis if not started	Supportive care Seizure prophylaxis if not started
Grade 2	Tocilizumab 8 mg/kg[c] Consider dexamethasone 10 mg IV Q12–24H	Dexamethasone 10 mg IV Q6–12H	Tocilizumab[d] Dexamethasone 10 mg IV Q6H
Grade 3	Tocilizumab per grade 2 Dexamethasone 10 mg IV Q6–12H	Dexamethasone 10 mg IV Q6H	Tocilizumab Dexamethasone 10 mg IV Q6H
Grade 4[e]	Tocilizumab per grade 2 Methylprednisolone 1 g daily ×3 days	Methylprednisolone 1 g daily ×3 days	Tocilizumab Methylprednisolone 1 g daily ×3 days

[a] If persistent (>72 h) or refractory symptoms consider treating as Grade 2
[b] Supportive care should include antipyretics, antiemetics, analgesics and depending on the grade: fluids or pressors for hypotension, oxygen for hypoxia
[c] Tocilizumab Q8H for a maximum of four doses
[d] Consider benefits versus risks of tocilizumab for potential worsening of ICANS
[e] For refractory CRS or ICANS of any grade, consider alternative anticytokine such as anakinra or siltuximab, or anti-CAR-T/IEC therapies such as cyclophosphamide

Siltuximab, unlike tocilizumab, can be used for refractory ICANS by binding IL-6 directly and preventing it from entering the CNS. Siltuximab has been shown to improve not only ICANS, but also steroid-refractory ICANS [32, 45]. The siltuximab dose for ICANS is the same as CRS dose, 11 mg/kg. As with severe CRS, consider if treating ongoing ICANS takes precedence over treating the patient's underlying cancer, and if so, anti-CAR-T/IEC therapies may be considered [29].

35.1.4 Immune Effector Cell-Associated Hemophagocytic Lymphohistiocytosis-Like Syndrome (IEC-HS)

Immune effector cell-associated hemophagocytic lymphohistiocytosis-like syndrome (IEC-HS) is a hyperinflammatory syndrome with macrophage activation or hemophagocytic lymphohistiocytosis (HLH) features attributable to IEC/CAR-T therapy and is associated with progression or new onset of the following: cytopenias, hyperferritinemia, coagulopathy with hypofibrinogenemia, and/or transaminitis [11]. IEC-HS can occur either early or late post-IEC/CAR-T therapy, and some of the symptoms and manifestations may overlap with CRS. There has been increasing incidence of late IEC-HS that is independent of CRS peak and severity, which indicates that this is most likely a separate IEC/CAR-T complication from CRS. The incidence and rates of IEC-HS across the different IEC/CAR-T products are not yet well defined [11, 46, 47]. IEC-HS presentation is variable and can sometimes resolve spontaneously or may require additional treatment. Similar to

HLH, IEC-HS can progress to multi-organ failure and death if not caught and treated early [48].

35.1.4.1 IEC-HS Grading

As both CRS and IEC-HS are hyperinflammatory syndromes with very different treatment modalities, there are separate criteria for identifying IEC-HS with required, common, and other symptoms. The required IEC-HS criteria is an elevated ferritin (>2 × ULN or baseline from time of IEC/CAR-T infusion) and/ or rapidly rising ferritin per clinical assessment. The most common manifestations of IEC-HS include worsening inflammatory response after initial improvement with CRS-directed therapy, hepatic transaminase elevations (>5 × ULN or baseline from time of IEC/CAR-T infusion), hypofibrinogenemia (<150 mg/dL or <LLN), hemophagocytosis in bone marrow or other tissues, and cytopenias (new, worsening, or refractory to treatment). Other less common manifestations of IEC-HS include LDH elevations, coagulation abnormalities, increased direct bilirubin, new splenomegaly, new or persistent fever, neurotoxicity, pulmonary manifestations, new renal insufficiency, and hypertriglyceridemia [11].

Grading IEC-HS can be difficult given the overlap with other syndromes, but it is important to prevent IEC-HS progression into more substantial complications. Grading criteria from ASTCT [11] can be seen in Table 35.5.

35.1.4.2 IEC-HS Supportive Care and Treatment

IEC-HS supportive care consists of treating the symptoms if possible. Some examples of common symptoms that clinicians can support during IEC-HS include cytopenias, coagulopathies, organ dysfunction, and infections [11]. Cytopenias, which are common in IEC-HS, can be supported by transfusions, thrombopoietin, and/or other growth factors. Growth-colony stimulating factor (G-CSF) can be considered to alleviate neutropenia and decrease infectious risk in IEC-HS [11, 49]. However, some clinicians may exercise caution as there have been case reports of G-CSF and granulocyte macrophage-colony stimulating factor (GM-CSF) worsening HLH [50]. Coagulopathies can be treated with fibrinogen monitoring and replacement. Other organ dysfunctions can be treated as per standard of care. Infections in

Table 35.5 ASTCT IEC-HS grading

Grade	Definition
1	Asymptomatic or mild symptoms; requires observation and/or clinical and diagnostic evaluation. Intervention not indicated
2	Mild to moderate symptoms, with intervention indicated
3	Severe or medically significant but not immediately life-threatening
4	Life-threatening consequences: urgent intervention indicated

IEC-HS can be significant, especially in the setting of cytopenias and immunosuppressive IEC-HS treatments. Empiric and prophylactic antibiotic strategies should be implemented as needed [11]. In addition, as IEC-HS may mimic other clinical states, alternative diagnoses should continue to be considered as clinicians treat for IEC-HS.

First line treatment for IEC-HS is anakinra, plus or minus corticosteroids. Anakinra dosing for IEC-HS ranges from 100 to 200 mg every 6–12 h given either subcutaneously or IV [11]. Anakinra has been shown to have good effect in HLH patients [11, 51], and there are cases where anakinra has been successfully used for IEC-HS [52]. Corticosteroids have been a mainstay for HLH treatment [53] and IEC-HS is no exception. Steroids can be used as first line treatment or, if steroids were not used first-line, they can be added as second line to existing anakinra treatment. The corticosteroid of choice for treatment of IEC-HS is dexamethasone 10–40 mg IV daily, which is usually split into 10 mg doses throughout the day. The most common dose is dexamethasone 10 mg every 6 h [11]. Third line treatment consists of ruxolitinib 10 mg orally twice daily, which can be escalated to 20 mg twice daily if tolerated [11]. Ruxolitinib is a JAK1/JAK2 inhibitor, which causes downstream inhibition of key inflammatory cytokines [54], some of which are involved in IEC-HS processes. Ruxolitinib has been successfully used to treat HLH [55, 56] and should also alleviate IEC-HS. However, ruxolitinib can cause cytopenias and increases infection risk [54], which could limit the use of ruxolitinib if supportive care measures for the cytopenias and infections are not sufficient.

35.2 Febrile Neutropenia

35.2.1 Introduction

Antineoplastic treatment and certain hematologic cancers may cause myelosuppression, including the complication febrile neutropenia (FN) . Up to 15% of adult cancer patients are hospitalized for FN during their cancer diagnosis and treatment [57]. FN is an oncologic emergency where up to 30% of patients experience major complications, and in-hospital mortality is 9.5% [57]. The most commonly identified infectious sources include Gram-positive bacteria (such as *Staphylococcus, Streptococcus,* and *Enterococcus*), followed by Gram-negative Enterobacteriaciae (*Enterobacter* species, *Escherichia coli, Klebsiella* species, *Pseudomonas aeruginosa, Citrobacter* species, *Acinetobacter* species, and *Stenotrophomonas maltophilia*) [58].

35.2.2 Diagnosis

Febrile neutropenia consists of two components occurring simultaneously. The first component, fever, is defined as either a single orally taken temperature > 101 °F (38.3 °C), or 100.4 °F (38 °C) sustained for an hour or more [58–60]. Neutropenia is defined as an absolute neutrophil count (ANC) < 500 cells/mm^3 or an ANC expected to decrease to <500 cells/mm^3 within the next 48 h [58–60], with profound neutropenia defined as ANC < 100 cells/mm^3. Some patients with hematologic malignancies may also present with "functional neutropenia", which occurs when the ANC does not meet the predefined neutropenia threshold, but the circulating neutrophils are impaired or dysfunctional due to malignancy and patients are thus at high risk for infection, especially if they present with fever [58].

Early identification of patients who may be at risk for FN is key to prevent serious complications. Current guidelines suggest identifying any patients who present with fever and who have received chemotherapy within the past 6 weeks as at risk for FN [60], and triaging patients as FN with infectious cause until laboratory results confirm the ANC (Fig. 35.1).

Once the patient is designated as "at risk" for FN, clinicians should carry out all relevant workup to identify infectious source(s) within 15 min of triage, including but not limited to: conducting a history and physical, including reviewing for history of multidrug-resistant organisms (MDROs); drawing laboratory tests (complete blood count [CBC] with differential, serum electrolytes, renal function markers, liver function tests); obtaining imaging to diagnose source(s) of infection, such as chest X-rays in patients with respiratory symptoms; and obtaining blood cultures, as well as urine, respiratory, stool, wound, and/or cerebral spinal fluid as clinically indicated [58, 60]. When drawing blood cultures, at least 2 sets from different sites should be obtained, and if the patient has a central venous catheter (CVC), obtain one set from a peripheral site and another from the CVC [58, 60]. If patients present during respiratory virus season, or with flu-like/seasonal respiratory illness symptoms, performing a nasopharyngeal swab and subsequent respiratory viral panel is recommended [60]. Notably, the Infectious Diseases Society of America (IDSA) and American Society of Clinical Oncology (ASCO) FN guidelines predate the COVID-19 pandemic, so COVID-19 was not addressed in those guidelines; however, multiple national and international societies for cancer care released statements during the COVID-19 pandemic stating that patients presenting with possible FN should undergo rapid testing for COVID-19 [61].

35.2.3 Initial Antimicrobial Choice

A dose of empiric, IV, antipseudomonal β-lactam antibiotic monotherapy should be given within 1 h of FN patient triage [60]. Recommended antipseudomonal β-lactams include cefepime, meropenem, imipenem-cilastatin, and piperacillin-tazobactam [60]. If patients have true a β-lactam allergy, empirically treat with ciprofloxacin and clindamycin, or aztreonam and vancomycin combination [58]. Review patient history for Gram-negative MDROs, and escalate empiric antibiotics and use MDRO dosing if patient is colonized, previously infected with a MDRO, or the treatment center has high rates of MDROs [58, 60]. In patients with extended spectrum β-lactamases (ESBLs), consider upfront empiric carbapenems; for

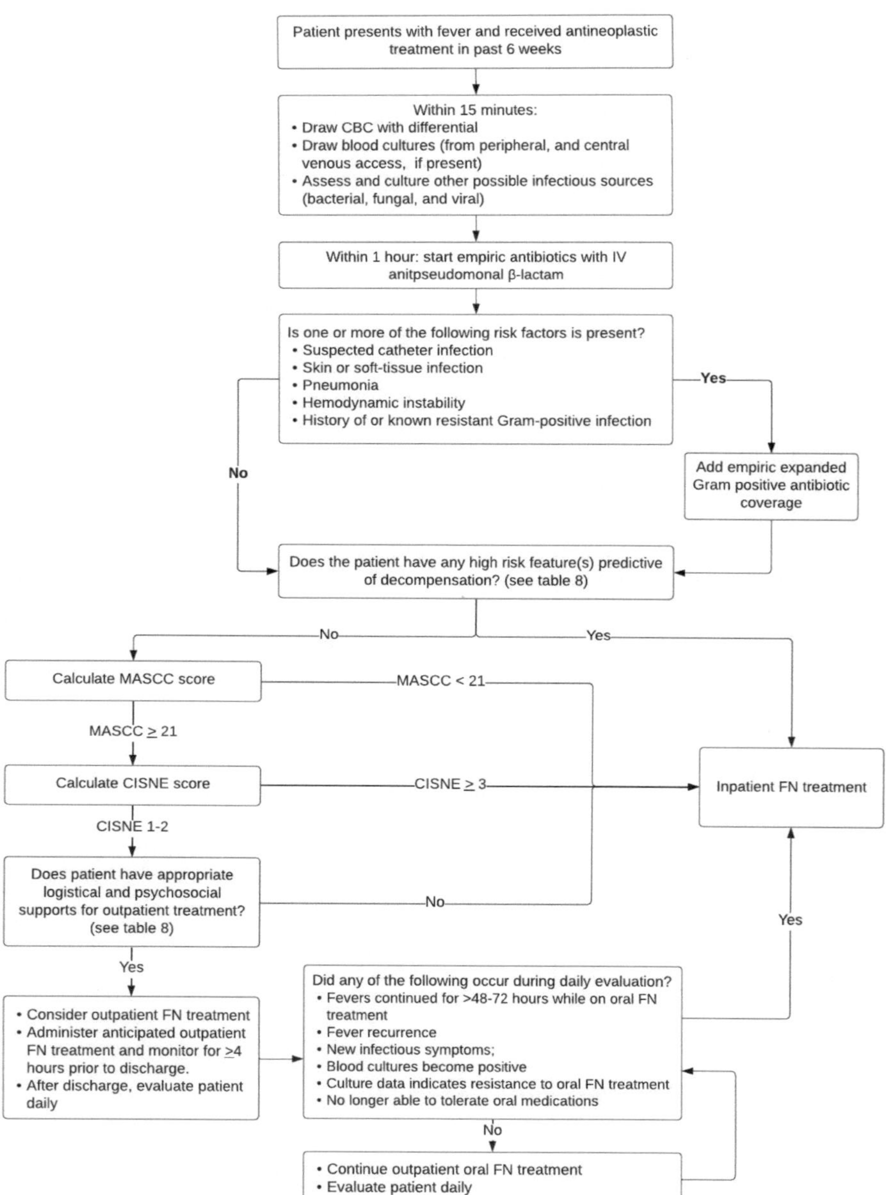

Fig. 35.1 Febrile neutropenia triage

Klebsiella pneumoniae carbapenemase (KPCs), meropenem-vaborbactam, ceftazidime-avibactam, imipenem-cilastatin-relebactam, cefiderocol, polymyxin-colistin or tigecycline can be considered [60, 62].

Adding extended Gram-positive organism coverage empirically is only recommended if the patient presents with one or more of the following: hemodynamic instability, suspected CVC or catheter infection, skin or soft-tissue infection, pneumonia on imaging, or prior infection/colonization/high treatment center rates of methicillin-resistant *Staphylococcus aureus* (MRSA) and/or vancomycin-resistant *Enterococcus* (VRE) [58, 60]. Utilize vancomycin, linezolid, or daptomycin for patients with MRSA (avoid daptomycin if patient is suspected to have pneumonia), and/or linezolid or daptomycin for patients with VRE [58, 60].

Upfront empiric antifungals are typically not recommended [58, 60], although if patients present with antifungal prophylaxis, they may continue their antifungal prophylaxis.

Generally, empiric antiviral treatment is not recommended in guidelines for empiric FN treatment in patients without a proven viral infection [60]. The exception is patients who present with flu-like symptoms after exposure or during an influenza outbreak, in which case neuraminidase inhibitor treatment should be given [60]. There are currently no national or international consensus guidelines addressing empiric COVID-19 treatment in FN patients and there is a lack of long-term follow-up and data in this area; therefore, empiric COVID-19 treatment should be based on national and/or institutional COVID-19 treatment standards, taking into consideration the patient's clinical status, likelihood of decompensation, and risks and benefits of giving steroids as they may cause further immunosuppression [61].

Growth factor for treating neutropenia in FN patient is not universally recommended due to inconsistent data about clinical benefit and lack of survival benefit [58].

35.2.4 Patient Risk Assessment and Treatment Locale

After timely FN patient triage and empiric antibiotic administration (see *Initial antibiotic choice*), clinicians should next assess the patient's risk level. Several risk stratification tools exist, but the primary purpose is to classify patients as low risk and high risk for infection and medical complications based on patient-specific characteristics and presenting symptoms [58, 60]. If patients qualify as low risk, they may have the option for possible antibiotic de-escalation and outpatient treatment, whereas high-risk patients will require hospitalization and IV antibiotic treatment [58, 60].

Initial risk stratification into low vs high risk involves Talcott's rule and the Multinational Association for Supportive Care in Cancer (MASCC) index [58, 60]. Talcott's rule groups patients into four groups (Table 35.8), where all patients except patients in group IV are considered to be high risk for developing FN-related complications and should receive inpatient treatment [58]. The MASCC score is then

Table 35.6 MASCC score calculation

Clinical feature	Points assigned
FN burden based on general clinical status (scores 3 and 5 are not cumulative)	• 5: no or mild symptoms • 3: moderate symptoms • 0: severe symptoms or moribund
No hypotension	• 5: SBP > 90 mmHg • 0: SBP < 90 mmHg
COPD (defined as active chronic bronchitis, emphysema, decrease in FEV, need for oxygen therapy and/or steroids and/or bronchodilators at FN presentation)	• 4: no COPD at FN presentation • 0: COPD at presentation
Tumor type	• 4: solid tumor • 4: hematologic malignancy with no prior fungal infection • 0: hematologic malignancy with prior fungal infection
Dehydration	• 3: no IV fluids required • 0: IV fluids required
Outpatient status	• 3: outpatient at FN presentation • 0: inpatient at FN presentation
Age (in years)	• 2: Age < 60 • 0: Age > 60

Low risk for complications: score ≥ 21
High risk for complications: score < 21

MASCC Multinational Association for Supportive Care in Cancer, *FN* febrile neutropenia, *SBP* systolic blood pressure, *COPD* chronic obstructive pulmonary disease, *FEV* forced expiratory volume

calculated as per Table 35.6, where patient-specific characteristics are totaled, and patients achieving a score ≥ 21 are considered to be low risk for complications, and score < 21 high risk [63].

Because analysis discovered that 7% of patients in Talcott group 4 and up to 11% of patients considered to be low risk per MASCC developed serious complications, an additional scoring tool, Clinical Index of Stable Febrile Neutropenia (CISNE) tool was created and validated to further aid in identifying low-risk FN patients [59]. Points for patient characteristics are assigned as per Table 35.7, then totaled, with scores of 0, 1–2, and 3 or higher considered to be low, intermediate, and high risk, respectively [59]. This score is applied to patients with solid tumors who appear clinically stable, have appropriate psychosocial supports, and access to 24-h care to further assess FN-related complication and mortality rates [59], and should be assessed *in addition to* Talcott and MASCC indices, if the patient is found to be Talcott group IV and MASCC low risk [60].

If the patient has any of the high-risk criteria listed in Table 35.8, then patient is considered high-risk and should receive inpatient FN treatment with IV antibiotics.

Table 35.7 CISNE score calculation

Clinical features	Points assigned
ECOG performance status >2	2
COPD	1
Chronic cardiovascular disease	1
Mucositis grade > 2 (per NCI Common toxicity criteria)	1
Monocytes <200 cells/mm^3	1
Stress-induced hyperglycemia	2

Low risk: score 0
Intermediate risk: score 1–2
High risk: score > 3

CISNE Clinical Index of Stable Febrile Neutropenia, *ECOG* Eastern Cooperative Oncology Group, *COPD* chronic obstructive pulmonary disease

Patients meeting all low-risk criteria in Table 35.8 can be considered for oral antibiotics and outpatient FN treatment if their fever responds to the empiric IV antibiotic, they are clinically stable, and they have the psychosocial supports and logistical considerations listed in Table 35.8 are in place [60]. Note that patients who were receiving fluoroquinolone prophylaxis or treatment prior to FN admission are not eligible for outpatient FN treatment even if they meet all low-risk criteria and must receive IV antipseudomonal β-lactam antibiotics [60].

Figure 35.1 reviews this triaging, diagnosis, and initial treatment process.

35.2.5 Pharmacologic Management, Continued

35.2.5.1 Outpatient Treatment

Oral FN treatment should consist of a fluoroquinolone (ciprofloxacin or levofloxacin) and amoxicillin/clavulanate [60]. Penicillin-allergic patients should receive fluoroquinolone with clindamycin [60]. Patients should receive the first dose of oral FN treatment in a monitored clinical setting to ensure tolerability and be observed for minimum 4 h prior to discharge to ensure clinical stability [60].

After discharge, if patients continue to fever for more than 48–72 h, have fever recurrence, develop new infectious symptoms, blood cultures become positive, culture data returns indicating resistance to oral FN treatment, or are no longer able to tolerate oral intake while receiving outpatient oral FN treatment should be re-evaluated and admitted for inpatient FN treatment (Fig. 35.1) [60].

Table 35.8 Risk stratification for patients presenting with FN. Low-risk patients may qualify for outpatient FN treatment if they have ALL of the listed low-risk factors; any patients with ANY high-risk features should be treated inpatient

Low-risk features	High-risk features	Criterion
Group IV: Outpatient with controlled cancer and without comorbidity	• Group I: Inpatient at time of fever onset • Group II: Outpatient with acute comorbidity where comorbidity requires hospitalization • Group III: Outpatient without comorbidity with uncontrolled cancer	Talcott
MASCC score > 21 indicating low risk for medical complications	MASCC score < 21 indicating high risk for medical complications	MASCC
CISNE score < 2	CISNE score > 3	CISNE
• No clinical factors listed in the column to the right • Fever and/or symptoms responded to initial IV antibiotic therapy • Neutropenia anticipated to last <7 days • Observed for at least 4 h • Able to take PO medications • Patient takes first dose of PO FN treatment and is observed • No allergies to FN treatment medication(s) Psychosocial and logistic requirements: • Live within 1 h or 30 miles (48 km) from clinic or hospital • Provider agrees to outpatient FN treatment • Ability to adhere to frequent follow-up visits • Caregiver at home at all times • Access to telephone and transportation at all times • No noncompliance or non-adherence history	Any of the following clinical criteria • Cardiovascular: syncope or presyncope; accelerated hypertension; new or worsening hypotension; uncontrolled heart failure, arrhythmias, or angina; clinically relevant bleeding; pericardial effusion • Hematologic: platelets <10,000/mm^3; Hgb <7 g/dL or Hct <21%; ANC <100/mm^3 with expected duration 7+ days; DVT or PE • Gastrointestinal: unable to swallow PO medications; new or worsening diarrhea; melena, hematochezia, or hematemesis; abdominal pain; ascites • Hepatic: LFTs >5× ULN or clinically relevant worsening LFTs; bilirubin >2 mg/dL or clinically worsening bilirubin • Infectious: clear site of infection based on symptoms, imaging, and/or culture data; severe sepsis; allergies to antimicrobials used for outpatient treatment; antibiotic use within 72 h of presentation; CVC infection • Neurologic: altered mental status; seizures; concern for or presence of CNS infection, noninfectious meningitis, or spinal cord compression; new or worsening neurologic deficit • Pulmonary: tachypnea; hypopnea; hypoxemia; hypercarbia; pneumothorax; pleural effusion; imaging suggestive of active intrathoracic process or with cavitary lung nodule • Renal: CrCl<30 mL/min; oliguria; clinically worsening renal function determined by treatment team; new hematuria; urinary obstruction; nephrolithiasis; clinically relevant dehydration; clinically relevant electrolyte abnormalities, acidosis or alkalosis requiring intervention • Other: major organ dysfunction; major comorbid condition; majorly abnormal or clinically worsening vital signs, symptoms, laboratory data, or imaging; physical or medical frailty; pregnancy or nursing; need for IV pain control; injuries; fractures; need for emergent radiation	IDSA and ASCO 2018 clinical factors disqualifying patient from outpatient FN care despite MASCC score, based on outpatient FN treatment clinical trial exclusion data

MASCC Multinational Association for Supportive Care in Cancer, *CISNE* Clinical Index of Stable Febrile Neutropenia, *FN* febrile neutropenia, *IDSA* Infectious Diseases Society of America, *ASCO* American Society of Clinical Oncology, *PO* oral, *IV* intravenous, *Hgb* hemoglobin, *Hct* hematocrit, *ANC* absolute neutrophil count, *DVT* deep vein thrombosis, *PE* pulmonary embolism, *CVC* central venous catheter, *CNS* central nervous system, *LFTs* liver function tests, *ULN* upper limit of normal, *CrCl* creatinine clearance

35.2.5.2 Inpatient Treatment

High-risk patients, or patients not otherwise qualifying for outpatient treatment, should be hospitalized for IV antibiotic therapy. Generally, the initially selected, empiric IV antipseudomonal antibiotic-based regimen can be continued, as well as any additional empiric coverage that was added based on patient-specific characteristics [58]. If infectious source is identified and/or culture data results, antibiotics and treatment duration should be adjusted based on those results [58]. However, only 20–30% of FN episodes will have sources identified [58].

35.2.5.3 Inpatient Treatment, Antibiotic Escalation

Generally, clinically stable patients on appropriate antipseudomonal β-lactam therapy who continue to fever despite empiric antibiotics do not generally require a change in antimicrobial coverage, unless an infectious source that is not covered by current antibiotic therapy is discovered [58]. If fevers continue, consider further infectious workup (such as further imaging, or obtaining cultures from other sites) for new sources of infection, particularly if the patient defervesced on initial empiric therapy and fever recurred afterwards [58]; in these patients, changing empiric antibiotic(s) can be considered. Noninfectious sources of fever should also be taken into consideration [58].

Patients who continue to be hemodynamically unstable or worsen after initial empiric antibiotics should have their antibiotics further expanded to include coverage for anaerobes, fungi, and Gram-negative, Gram-positive MDROs [58]. Empiric, dual β-lactam therapy should be avoided, and if additional Gram-negative coverage is required, escalating to a carbapenem, or adding an aminoglycoside, fluoroquinolone, aztreonam, or other non-β-lactam antimicrobial are options [58].

If high-risk patients continue to be febrile after 4–7 days of empiric antibiotics and are anticipated to be neutropenic for >10 days, conduct fungal workup [58]. At this point, clinicians can consider initiating empiric antifungal treatment with mold coverage, or, if the patient has no radiographic, serologic, or fungal culture data supporting fungal infection, empiric antifungals can be held until more signs of invasive fungal infection occur [58]. If empiric antifungals are started in patients who were already receiving antifungal prophylaxis, switch to a mold-active, IV antifungal in a different drug class than the prophylaxis [58]. Low-risk patients are generally not indicated for empiric antifungals [58].

35.2.5.4 Inpatient Treatment, Antibiotic De-escalation

For low-risk patients that are admitted to the hospital being treated for FN, initial empiric IV antibiotics can be de-escalated to oral antipseudomonal antibiotics if patients continue to be neutropenic, but are otherwise clinically stable and have adequate GI absorption [58]. Patients who were initially admitted but meet all low-risk criteria, have been afebrile and clinically stable for 3 days, and no identified infection, can be discharged to receive IV or oral antipseudomonal antibiotics as outpatient as long as there is daily follow-up until count recovery or until the infection is fully treated (whichever occurs last), can occur [58]. Suggested oral FN treatment is ciprofloxacin and amoxicillin-clavulanate [58].

In both low-risk and high-risk patients, if a patient's initial empiric antibiotic regimen included Gram-positive organism coverage with vancomycin or linezolid, and no Gram-positive infectious sources are identified after 48–72 h, then Gram-positive coverage can be discontinued [58].

If the infectious source is identified, empiric antibiotic coverage can be narrowed based on the culture and sensitivity data [58].

Please refer to Fig. 35.2 for a summary of FN antibiotic escalation and de-escalation.

35.2.5.5 Duration of Treatment

Generally, empiric FN treatment in low- and high-risk patients without an identified source is continued until ANC recovers to >500 cells/mm^3 with consistent upward increase [58].

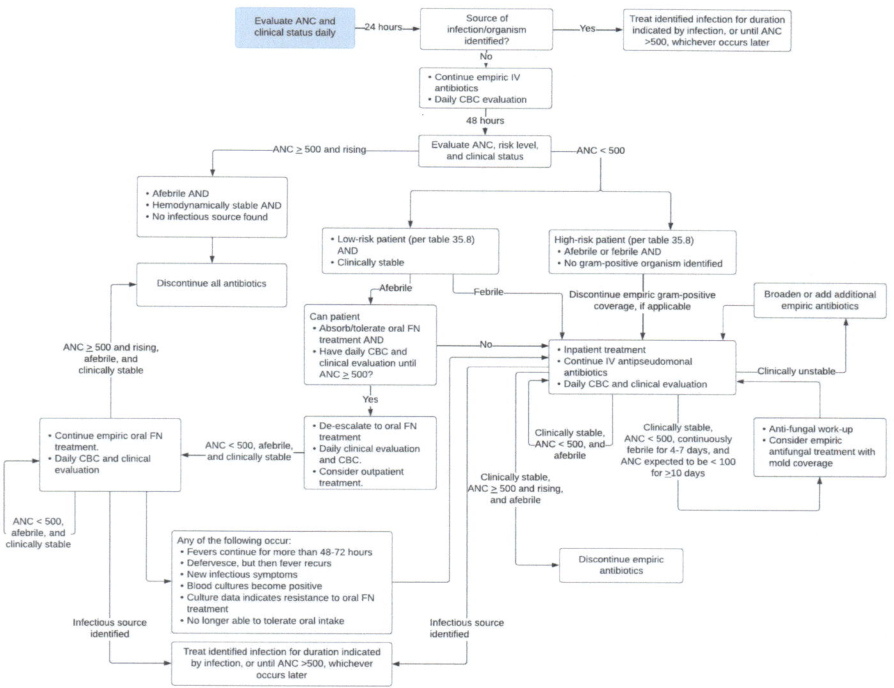

Fig. 35.2 Febrile neutropenia pharmacologic escalation and de-escalation pathway

In low-risk patients only, if cultures are negative for at least 48 h, and patients have been afebrile for 24 h, ceasing antibiotics prior to ANC reaching >500 cells/mm^3 can be considered [58]. Another approach for low-risk patients who have received at least 3 days of empiric antibiotics, defervesced, and demonstrate rising phagocyte, monocyte, reticulocyte, and/or neutrophil counts is to stop antibiotics even if ANC has not yet reached >500 cells/mm^3 since the rising counts demonstrate imminent bone marrow recovery [58].

Patients with an identified infectious source should be treated for the length of time appropriate for the identified source; if the duration of treatment is less than the duration of neutropenia, the targeted antibiotics should continue until ANC recovers to >500 cell/mm^3, or longer if clinically indicated [58]. Another option is to continue the targeted antibiotics for the normal duration of treatment, and if the patient is still neutropenic after treatment course is complete, they can be switched to oral fluoroquinolone prophylaxis until ANC >500 cells/mm^3 [58].

35.3 Hypercalcemia of Malignancy

35.3.1 Introduction

Hypercalcemia of malignancy (HCM) is a common oncologic emergency, affecting up to one third of cancer patients, predominantly the solid tumor and multiple myeloma populations [64]. Among solid malignancies, HCM is more commonly reported in non-small cell lung cancer, breast cancer, squamous-cell cancers of the head and neck, urothelial, and ovarian cancers [64]. HCM is a complication of advanced and metastatic malignancies, and a predictor of poor prognosis, with a median survival of 25–52 days after the onset of hypercalcemia, with better survival among those with hematologic malignancy or breast cancer. Stabilizing calcium levels along with administering cancer-targeted therapy is associated with longer survival rates [64].

35.3.2 Pathophysiology

One of the causes of hypercalcemia is irregularities in bone turnover, which is modulated by a balance of osteoblasts for bone formation and osteoclasts for bone resorption. A ligand for RANK (RANKL) on osteoblasts binds to nuclear factor-κB (RANK) surface receptors on osteoclasts, activating osteoclastic activity and stimulating bone turnover by regulating osteoclastogenesis. When mature osteoblasts secrete osteoprotegerin (OPG), OPG acts as a decoy and inhibits RANK/RANKL interaction, thus preventing osteoclast maturation and excessive skeletal resorption [65, 66]. Multiple myeloma in particular degrades OPG and releases RANKL, thereby increasing calcium [67].

Several other endogenous factors, including parathyroid hormone (PTH), 1,25-dihydroxy vitamin D, calcitonin, serum calcium, and phosphorous levels are responsible for calcium regulation. Osteoclasts can stimulate an increase in serum calcium and decrease in serum phosphorus by increasing renal calcium absorption and inhibiting renal phosphorus absorption, and by activating 1-α-hydroxylase in the kidney to convert 25-hydroxyvitamin D to active 1,25-hydroxyvitamin D. In response to hypercalcemia, parafollicular C cells in the thyroid gland secrete calcitonin, lowering serum calcium by inhibiting renal calcium and phosphorus reabsorption and suppressing bone resorption. The parathyroid gland secretes parathyroid hormone (PTH), which plays a major role in the regulation of calcium absorption and metabolism. PTH is responsible for activating 25-hydroxyvitamin D into 1,25-dihydroxyviamin D, stimulating calcium reabsorption in the distal part of the nephron and renal phosphorus excretion. Along with 1,25-dihydroxyvitamin D, PTH stimulates calcium mobilization from the bone to increase calcium concentrations in the plasma [65, 66, 68].

HCM is attributed to three main mechanisms. The most common mechanism, referred to as humoral hypercalcemia of malignancy (HHM), accounting for approximately 80% of cases, is mediated by parathyroid hormone-related peptide (PTHrP), [69]. PTHrP is structurally like PTH, acts on the same receptors, and is normally produced and secreted by various cells. Unregulated tumor secretion of PTHrP increases osteoclastic bone resorption and renal reabsorption of calcium by binding to PTH-PTHrP type 1 receptors in the bones and kidneys, while also enhancing the renal excretion of phosphorus [64, 65]. PTHrP does not seem to have the same influence on the production of 1,25-dihydroxyvitamin D as PTH, leading to variable 1,25-dihydroxyvitamin D serum levels among patients with HHM [64, 66]. PTHrP also acts on osteoblasts, leading to increased RANKL secretion, osteoclast maturation and resultant bone remodeling and calcium release into the plasma [66]. Malignancies most often associated with HHM include squamous-cell cancers of the head and neck, urothelial cancers, breast cancer, non-Hodgkin's lymphoma, and ovarian cancer [66]. HHM are not usually associated with bone metastases [64].

The second most common cause of HCM is local osteolytic hypercalcemia, which is usually associated with bone metastases and skeletal tumor burden. It accounts for approximately 20% of HCM cases, commonly occurring in multiple myeloma and metastatic breast cancer [65]. The production of local cytokines from the tumor enhances osteoclast activation and resorption, mainly through RANK/RANKL [65]. The calcium resorption from bone then exceeds the renal calcium excretion, leading to hypercalcemia [64].

Other less common causes of HCM are also humoral, resulting from the production of hormones involved in bone remodeling by the tumor [64]. Tumors that upregulate the extrarenal production of 1,25 dihydroxy vitamin D, causing increased intestinal absorption of calcium and osteolytic bone resorption account for roughly 1% of HCM cases, mostly Hodgkin's and non-Hodgkin's lymphoma [65]. Rare tumors can cause ectopic hyperparathyroidism by producing excess PTH. Parathyroid cancers also cause hypercalcemia from excess secretion of PTH [64]. Table 35.9 summarizes the characteristics of the different causes of HCM.

Table 35.9 Characteristics of hypercalcemia of malignancy types

	Humoral			Local osteolytic	
Primary factor	PTHrP	1,25 dihydroxy vitamin D	PTH	TNF, IL-6, IL-1, MIP, and others	PTHrP, TNF, IL-6, IL-1, and others
Malignancy	Lung, breast, renal, and others	Hematologic, T-cell lymphoma	Parathyroid cancer, neuroendocrine, ovarian, and others	Myeloma or lymphoma in bone	Breast, lung, kidney
Bone metastases, tumor in bone	None or few	None or few	None or few	Extensive	Extensive
PTH	Low	Low	High	Low	Low
PTHrP	High or normal	Low	Low	Low	Variable
1,25-dihydroxy vitamin D	Variable	High	High	Variable	Low
Phosphorous	Low	High	Low	Variable	Variable
Osteoclast activity	High	High	High	High	High

PTHrP parathyroid hormone-related peptide, *PTH* parathyroid hormone, *TNF* tumor necrosis factor, *IL-6* interleukin-6, *IL-1* interleukin-1, *MIP* macrophage inhibitory protein

35.3.3 *Diagnosis and Evaluation*

Total serum calcium (SCa), which measures both bound and unbound calcium, is the most readily available and widely used laboratory measurement for diagnosing hypercalcemia. Serum albumin is also important, as 40% of SCa is bound to calcium, and necessary for the interpretation of the serum calcium level in hypoalbuminemic patients. A corrected calcium level should be calculated for patients with abnormal albumin levels using the formula: 0.8 (4.0 − serum albumin) + SCa = total corrected calcium. Changes in pH can also alter the proportion of calcium that is bound to albumin). Ionized calcium (iCa) levels may be obtained if the total corrected calcium is believed to be inaccurate and repeat measurements of calcium levels should be performed to exclude any possible outliers.

HCM can be categorized as mild (SCa ULN − 12 mg/dL [ULN − 3 mmol/L] or iCa ULN − 1.75 mmol/L), moderate (Sca 12–14 mg/dL [3–3.5 mmol/L] or iCa 1.75–2 mmol/L), or severe (SCa >14 mg/dL [>3.5 mmol/L] or iCa > 2 mmol/L) [69]. Symptoms in mild hypercalcemia include fatigue, constipation, polyuria, and polydipsia [69]. Higher SCa levels and/or rapidly increasing elevated SCa levels (e.g., rate of >1 g/dL per 24 h) can cause cognitive dysfunction, renal failure, and arrhythmias [64, 69].

Serum phosphorus should also be measured as it may be significantly elevated or low in different classes of hypercalcemia. Upon confirming hypercalcemia, PTHrP can be measured as this is the most common mediator of HCM. Additional testing of 25-hydroxyvitamin D and 1,25-dihydroxyvitamin D levels may be drawn for evaluation of excess vitamin D production or supplementation. PTHrP, PTH, and vitamin D values can be useful in determining the cause of HCM [65]. HCM treatment can proceed without waiting for these levels to return since the some of these tests may take significant time to result, and knowing the type of HCM does not currently affect initial HCM treatment.

Serum creatinine and estimated glomerular filtration rate measurement should also be obtained to assess renal function.

Signs and symptoms of hypercalcemia include cognitive changes, gastrointestinal disturbances, renal impairment, and cardiac arrhythmias. Cognitive disturbances brought on by HCM include anxiety, mood changes, and a decline in cognitive functioning [66]. This can be seen in mild cases of HCM and may develop with higher SCa levels into altered mental status and in extreme cases posterior reversible leukoencephalopathy (PRES), and coma [66]. Gastrointestinal symptoms include abdominal pain, nausea, vomiting, poor appetite, and constipation. Extreme dehydration is a common side effect of HCM, caused by the anorexia, nausea, vomiting, and nephrogenic diabetes insipidus associated with elevated SCa levels, often leading to pre-renal acute kidney injury. This impairment in renal function decreases the ability of the kidney to excrete calcium, further worsening hypercalcemia [64]. Patients with hypercalcemia often present with shortened QT intervals during electrocardiogram (ECG) monitoring, with severe hypercalcemia mimicking ST-segment elevation [66]. Ventricular arrhythmias such as ventricular fibrillation may develop in severe hypercalcemia [66].

35.3.4 Treatment

Treating the underlying malignancy with cancer-directed therapy is the main goal in HCM. Mild, asymptomatic HCM may not require immediate treatment, and can be addressed after diagnostic workup of the malignancy has been completed and a plan for cancer-directed therapy is established [65]. Symptomatic, or moderate to severe HCM require interventions with the goal of temporizing SCa levels until cancer treatment can begin, especially if the HCM is associated with renal or neurologic, or cardiac injury. Immediate treatment is required for patients with corrected SCa levels >13 mg/dL, rapidly increasing elevated SCa levels, and/or altered mental status regardless of SCa levels [64]. Please refer to Fig. 35.3 for a suggested hypercalcemia treatment algorithm and to Table 35.10 for a summary of pharmacologic treatments for hypercalcemia of malignancy.

Interventions include correcting hypovolemia, enhancing renal excretion of calcium, and antiresorptive medications [69]. Review medications and discontinue any potential contributors to elevated SCa levels such as calcium and vitamin D supplementation, parenteral nutrition, thiazide diuretics, lithium, and theophylline [65].

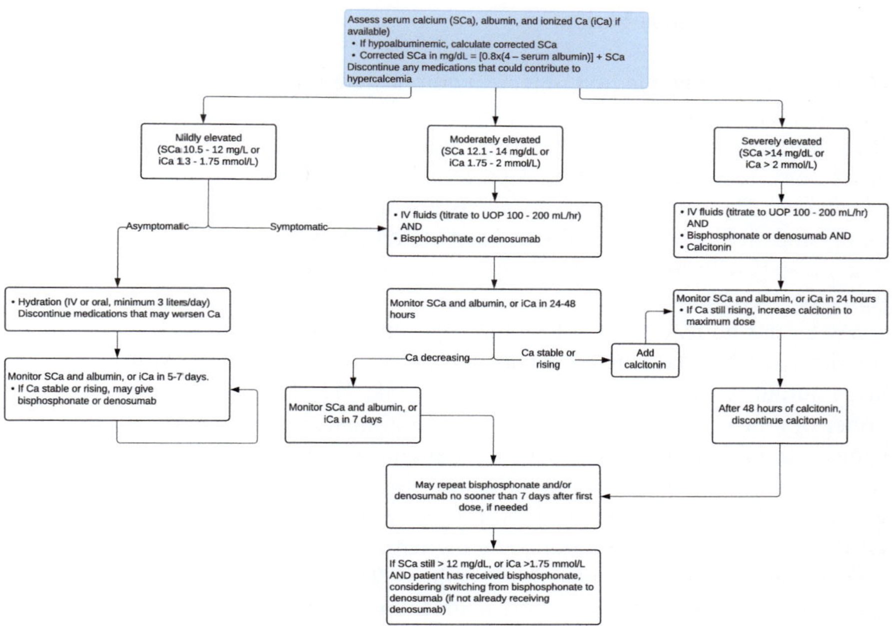

Fig. 35.3 Hypercalcemia of malignancy treatment algorithm

Table 35.10 Summary of pharmacologic therapies used to treat hypercalcemia of malignancy

Drug class	Drugs	Dose	Onset	Notes
IV fluid (isotonic)	Normal saline	1000–2000 mL bolus, followed by 150–300 mL/h infusion	Minutes to hours	Titrate to UOP 100–200 mL/h May require concomitant diuresis
Bisphosphonates	Pamidronate	60–90 mg IV infused over 2–24 h	Onset: 48–96 h Peak effect: 5–7 days	Maximum 1 dose every 7 days Use longer infusion times for patients with renal insufficiency or renal injury May be used in patients with SCr up to 4.5 mg/dL
	Zoledronic acid	4 mg IV infused over 15–60 min		
PTH antagonist	Calcitonin	4–8 unit/kg IM/SQ q6–12H	Onset: 1–4 h Peak effect: 4–6 h	Tachyphylaxis occurs in 48–72 h Intranasal route not recommended
RANKL inhibitor	Denosumab	60–120 mg SQ	Median 9 days to reach Ca < 11.5 mg/dL (range 5–19 days)	Studied in bisphosphonate refractory HCM

35.3.4.1 Intravenous Fluids

Hydration should be the first treatment administered. It enacts its rapid therapeutic effect by correcting volume depletion and enhancing renal calcium excretion [69]. Intravenous fluids, preferably isotonic saline, should be used to restore a euvolemic state. Isotonic saline is preferred to ringer's lactate due to its absence of calcium. The use of ringer's lactate is not advised in this setting due to its calcium content, albeit at physiological concentration, with an exception for patients who present with hyperchloremic metabolic acidosis or develop it with isotonic saline resuscitation [70].

An initial bolus of 1–2 L followed by a maintenance rate of 150–300 mL/h for the next 2–3 days may be required for volume repletion, titrating to goal urine output (UOP) of 100 to 200 mL/h [65, 68, 71]. Once euvolemia is reached, either oral or maintenance IV fluids are continued to maintain UOP until other agents used for HCM take effect [71]. Patients at high risk for volume overload, such as congestive heart failure or anuric renal failure will require smaller volumes and closer volume status monitoring. Using loop diuretics such as furosemide in conjunction with fluids to increase calcium excretion is limited in efficacy and may exacerbate renal injury. Therefore, loop diuretic therapy should be reserved for patients with heart failure or those requiring diuresis [71].

The onset of effect of hydration therapy for HCM is immediate, lowering SCa by 1-1.5 mg/dL; however, it is not long lasting and not effective monotherapy for moderate to severe HCM [68, 71].

35.3.4.2 Bisphosphonates

The bisphosphonates zoledronic acid and pamidronate inhibit osteoclast-mediated bone resorption, induce osteoclast apoptosis, and decrease osteoblast apoptosis [65, 66]. Both zoledronic acid and pamidronate have been used for HCM, with zoledronic acid being a more potent agent at lowering calcium as well as maintaining normocalcemia [72].

Bisphosphonates have been associated with nephrotoxicity, and many patients with HCM may also present with acute renal injury from HCM. Treating HCM with bisphosphonates may help improve serum creatinine (SCr) as SCa decreases, and patients with SCr up to 4.5 mg/dL have been included in HCM studies utilizing bisphosphonates [72]. Even in patients with renal dysfunction, zoledronic acid and pamidronate have similar rates of SCa lowering as patients without renal impairment [73]. Recommended strategies to mitigate bisphosphonate nephrotoxicity include adequate hydration prior to giving bisphosphonates, and prolonging the bisphosphonate infusion. Prolonging pamidronate infusions 2 h or longer for those with renal insufficiency is suggested, and zoledronic acid should be administered over 15–60 min [69].

If severe hypercalcemia persists, bisphosphonate retreatment may be given after a minimum of 7 days have passed since the first bisphosphonate dose was administered [74]. Adverse events in addition to kidney dysfunction include flu-like symptoms of fever, myalgias, and fatigue for the first 1–2 days after the infusion. Hypocalcemia, hypophosphatemia, ocular symptoms of uveitis and scleritis, and very rarely osteonecrosis of the jaw. Osteonecrosis of the jaw typically develops in patients who have received bisphosphonates for at least 4 months and have undergone dental procedures while on therapy [64, 66].

Onset of bisphosphonate effect can take up to approximately 2–4 days and should be administered within 48 h of diagnosis in combination with fluid resuscitation [65].

35.3.4.3 Denosumab

Denosumab is a human monoclonal antibody with affinity to RANKL, reducing osteoclast activity by preventing osteoclast formation from pre-osteoclasts [66, 69]. Bisphosphonates in contrast target mature osteoclasts to induce apoptosis [69]. Denosumab, given as 120 mg subcutaneously weekly for 3 weeks, then every 4 weeks thereafter, can be used to treat HCM refractory to bisphosphonates, defined as SCa that does not decline to 11.5 mg/dL or lower 7–30 days after treatment with an IV bisphosphonate [75, 76]. In clinical practice, denosumab is not typically given weekly as originally investigated for the treatment of HCM, and dosing frequency is instead determined by SCa level.

An advantage of denosumab compared to bisphosphonate in patients with underlying renal insufficiency is that denosumab is not renally eliminated [69]. The Endocrine Society clinical practice guideline recommends either the use of an IV bisphosphonate or denosumab in adult patients with HCM, with a preference for denosumab in those with underlying renal insufficiency [69]. Denosumab use in renal impairment has been found to cause greater and prolonged hypocalcemia however, and reduction of the dose to 60 mg or a weight-based dose of 0.3 mg/kg subcutaneously may be considered [77].

Side effects for denosumab include arthralgias, nausea, diarrhea, dyspnea, hypocalcemia, hypophosphatemia and a risk of osteonecrosis of the jaw with long-term use. Currently, denosumab is also significantly more costly than either IV zoledronic acid or pamidronate.

Denosumab has a slow onset, with a median time to response of 9 days (range 5–19 days) [75].

35.3.4.4 Calcitonin

Calcitonin has a rapid onset of action (within hours) in reducing SCa levels and is recommended for use as a bridging agent given within 48 h of diagnosis of HCM in combination with hydration and antiresorptive agents [69]. The reduction of SCa is low, about 1–2 mg/dL, and not sufficient in treating moderate to severe

HCM alone with IV fluid therapy. It is most useful when given concomitantly with antiresorptive agents in severe HCM to allow for initial lowering of SCa while awaiting the prolonged onset of action for IV bisphosphonates and denosumab [64]. Tachyphylaxis with calcitonin develops about 48–72 h after use due to the downregulation of the calcitonin receptors. Calcitonin is usually administered at a dose of 4–8 international units/kg subcutaneously or intramuscularly every 6–12 h, limited to 48–72 h [71]. Subcutaneous administration is recommended over intramuscular route to minimize injection site pain. The commercial form of calcitonin is derived of salmon origin, and caution is advised in patients with suspected hypersensitivity to calcitonin-salmon [78]. Calcitonin is also a cost prohibitive treatment and may be restricted to treatment of severe HCM in combination with antiresorptive medications [69]. Intranasal calcitonin is not recommended for the treatment of HCM, due to lack of efficacy.

35.3.4.5 Other Treatments

Glucocorticoids decrease calcium absorption in the gastrointestinal tract and inhibit the 1-α-hydroxylase enzyme, interfering with the conversion of 25-hydroxyvitamin D to calcitriol [69]. The use of glucocorticoids may be useful in the case of HCM caused by ectopic production of 1,25-dihydroxyitamin D, seen almost exclusively with lymphomas [69]. Dietary/supplemental calcium must also be restricted, and patients will often continue to have HCM despite glucocorticoid treatment. Patients usually require the addition of an IV bisphosphonate or denosumab. Glucocorticoids should also be discontinued if not helpful in reducing SCa levels following 10 days of administration [71].

Cinacalcet is approved for the treatment of HCM in adult patients with parathyroid carcinoma [69]. Cinacalcet is a calcimimetic agent that activates the calcium sensing receptor (CaSR), found on the surface of parathyroid glands and along the nephrons and other tissues for the regulation of PTH synthesis and secretion [71]. Activation of the CaSR increases its sensitivity to extracellular calcium, leading to a reduction in PTH and then SCa levels [71]. Intravenous bisphosphonates or denosumab may be used initially for severe HCM prior to the start of cinacalcet therapy due to their quicker onset of action and greater efficacy.

Patients presenting with severe HCM with acute renal injury with oliguria may require hemodialysis or peritoneal dialysis with low-calcium dialysate.

35.4 Malignant Spinal Cord Compression

Malignant or metastatic spinal cord compression (MSSC), if not recognized and treated immediately, can be a devastating complication of advanced cancer with high morbidity and mortality. Patients with MSCC may experience severe, immobilizing pain and significant neural damage. Prompt recognition of signs and symptoms of MSSC such as new or worsening back pain aid in a timely diagnosis and prevention of permanent disability [79].

MSCC occurs in about 2.5–5% of patients with advanced, metastatic cancer and is associated with a poor prognosis [79]. The majority of cancers associated with hospitalization for MSSC are lung, prostate, or breast cancer [79]. Spinal cord compression (SCC) is also the presenting symptom of systemic cancer in 20–34% of cancer patients [79].

35.4.1 Pathophysiology

Malignant cells spread to the vertebral body via a hematogenous route. The growing tumor mass within the vertebrae or spinal cord compresses the adjacent vertebral venous plexus, spinal artery, thecal sac, and spinal cord, causing inflammation, neurological damage, and pain. The malignant cells weaken the bone and may cause vertebral compression fractures. The bony fragments of the compression fracture may also damage the spinal cord. The thoracic spine is most commonly affected in MSCC, followed by lumbosacral and cervical spine [79]. If not emergently addressed, MSCC may result in irreversible neural necrosis and resultant permanent disability.

35.4.2 Diagnosis

Patients typically present with back pain, motor weakness, sensory deficits, and bowel or bladder incontinence. Signs and symptoms vary according to the position of the lesion and spinal location. Back pain is the most common symptom, occurring in 80–95% of patients, is typically constant, aching, and worse at night or early morning, and may be intensified by coughing, sneezing, Valsalva maneuvers, and lying flat. A large percentage of patients also present with motor deficits at time of diagnosis of MSCC, with a feeling of heaviness or clumsiness in the extremities [79]. Less commonly, patients may present with sensory changes and bowel or bladder dysfunction.

Spinal imaging should be performed urgently for oncology patients with known bone metastases or with malignancies that commonly metastasize to bone presenting with new-onset back pain and/or new neurological deficits [79]. Magnetic resonance imaging (MRI) of the entire spine is recommended in order to establish the extent of the injury [79]. Computed tomography myelography is performed only when MRI is contraindicated [79].

35.4.3 *Treatment*

Glucocorticoids, in particular dexamethasone, as first line therapy provide analgesia and preserve neurological function. Dexamethasone downregulates the production of vascular endothelial growth factor and prostaglandin E2, decreasing spinal cord edema and delaying neurological damage. A study comparing high-dose dexamethasone as an adjunct to radiotherapy in patients with MSCC to radiotherapy alone administered a dexamethasone IV bolus of 96 mg, followed by 96 mg orally for 3 days, followed by a 10 day taper [80]. Gait function was obtained in a larger percentage of dexamethasone patients (81%) compared to those not receiving steroid therapy (63%) [80]. While treatment with high-dose dexamethasone did not extend median survival, a larger proportion of patients treated with dexamethasone were still ambulatory after 6 months in comparison to the group with no treatment [80]. A pilot study comparing high-dose dexamethasone (96 mg for 3 days, then tapered) with moderate dose (16 mg for 3 days, then tapered) in patients with MSCC undergoing radiation therapy found no significant difference in functional outcomes at 1 month, but more serious adverse events in the high-dose group [81]. A Cochrane review comparing trials utilizing high-dose vs moderate or no-dose steroids for the treatment of MSCC similarly found serious side effects to be more frequent in the high-dose groups, including more significant adverse events such as perforated gastric ulcers, psychoses, and death due to infections [82]. Therefore, typical dexamethasone doses for MSCC are 10 mg IV bolus once, followed by 4–6 mg IV every 6 h. Patients can then be converted to oral dexamethasone and have their dose tapered as tolerated over a period of 2 weeks (usually after completing radiation therapy) [79].

Most patients also need opioid therapy for pain relief, including continuous IV opioid infusions or patient controlled analgesia for those with moderate to severe pain. Corticosteroids also aid with the treatment of neuropathic pain. Other neuropathic agents, including gabapentin, pregabalin, and tricyclic antidepressants, may also be used and provide some pain relief, although they have not been specifically evaluated in MSCC [79].

Bisphosphonates, nonsteroidal anti-inflammatory drugs (NSAIDs), and acetaminophen may also contribute to pain relief. Bisphosphonates improve pain over several weeks by decreasing bone breakdown, with a maximum effect occurring at 4 weeks, and prevent further skeletal-related events. Use caution when using NSAIDs in patients with renal and cardiac comorbidities, thrombocytopenia, and consider the added risk for gastrointestinal ulceration when using NSAIDs in combination with corticosteroids. [79]. Opioid therapy, limited mobility, and nerve injury place patients with MSCC at high risk for constipation. Prophylaxis with a stimulant and osmotic laxative is usually effective [79].

Non-pharmacologic interventions include surgery and radiation. Surgical intervention can result in immediate and sustained relief while also improving neurological damage. A typical procedure is surgical decompression with instrumented fusion. Deciding to pursue surgery prior to radiation involves patient-specific factors of spinal stability, neurologic deficits, and patient prognosis [79]. The Spinal Instability Neoplastic Score (SINS) may be used in determining need for intervention [83]; this scoring tool considers factors such as global spinal location of the tumor, type and presence of pain, bone lesion quality, and spinal alignment [84]. Pain caused by vertebral fractures can also be treated by percutaneous cement reinforcement (vertebroplasty or kyphoplasty) [83]. Vertebroplasty and kyphoplasty alone generally are not indicated for patients with evidence of neurological injury but may be useful for painful vertebral compression factors in patients without neurological deficits. Pain relief is typically seen within 1–3 days [83].

Radiation may also be used to treat MSCC when MSCC is caused by radiation-sensitive cancer. Radiation dose, number of fractions, and duration varies and is determined by prognosis and life expectancy [79].

35.5 Tumor Lysis Syndrome

35.5.1 Introduction

Tumor lysis syndrome (TLS) is the most common oncologic emergency in adult patients with a hematologic malignancy, occurring due to the acute and massive release of cellular contents from malignant cells when they lyse [85, 86]. TLS is most common in patients with acute leukemias or high-grade lymphomas, but can occur in other tumor types, particularly in patients with high tumor burden or in patients with tumor cells that are highly sensitive to chemotherapy [86, 87]. Patients at risk for TLS should undergo further risk assessment and may require prophylaxis or treatment. When patients with a malignancy require intensive care, the ICU pharmacist plays an important role in assessing risk for TLS, monitoring associated labs, and ensuring proper prophylaxis or interventions are initiated.

35.5.2 Pathophysiology

Understanding the pathophysiology of TLS can help the ICU pharmacist make recommendations for prophylaxis and treatment in patients at risk of experiencing TLS. When malignant cells undergo lysis spontaneously or due to treatment (cytotoxic chemotherapy, radiation, cytolytic antibody therapy, etc.), the intracellular components of the cell are rapidly released into the blood stream, overloading transport mechanisms in the kidneys and preventing adequate solute urinary excretion. These cellular components include potassium, phosphorus, nucleic acids from DNA, and cytokines. In particular, malignant cells can also contain higher levels of phosphorus compared to normal cells [88]. TLS occurs when the release of cellular contents into the bloodstream causes hyperkalemia, hyperuricemia, hyperphosphatemia, and/or hypocalcemia, which may subsequently lead to clinical sequelae, including renal injury, cardiac arrhythmias, and death [85].

Table 35.11 Tumor lysis syndrome risk factors

Malignancy	– Acute myeloid leukemia (AML) – Acute lymphoblastic leukemia (ALL) – Burkitt's lymphoma – Diffuse large-cell lymphomas – Solid tumors that are highly proliferative and/or are highly sensitive to chemotherapy
Tumor size or disease burden	– Tumor size >10 cm – LDH > 2 × upper limit of normal (ULN) – White blood cell count >25,000/μL
Renal function	– Preexisting renal failure or dysfunction – Oliguria
Uric acid	– Baseline serum uric acid >7.5 mg/dL (450 μmol/L)

Table 35.12 Laboratory values associated with tumor lysis syndrome

Electrolyte disturbance	Laboratory threshold
Hyperuricemia	Uric acid >8.0 mg/dL (475.8 μmol/L)
Hyperkalemia	Potassium >6.0 mmol/L
Hyperphosphatemia	Phosphorus >4.5 mg/dL (1.5 mmol/L)
Hypocalcemia	Corrected calcium <7.0 mg/dL (1.75 mmol/L) or Ionized calcium <4.5 mg/dL (1.12 mmol/L)

Hyperkalemia due to the rapid release of potassium into the bloodstream can lead to serious and potentially fatal arrhythmias, including ventricular fibrillation, ventricular tachycardia, and Torsades de Pointes [89].

Hyperphosphatemia may cause nausea, vomiting, diarrhea, and seizures. Additionally, it may lead to associated hypocalcemia, which may be asymptomatic but has the potential to cause seizure and dysrhythmia. Furthermore, the binding of phosphate to calcium may lead to precipitation of calcium phosphate crystals into organs, most notably the kidneys, resulting in possible acute kidney injury.

Hyperuricemia occurs due to the purine nucleic acids that are released into the bloodstream as DNA that are then catabolized to hypoxanthine and xanthine, and then to uric acid via xanthine oxidase [86]. Like calcium phosphate crystal-induced kidney injury, accumulation of uric acid, which has low solubility relative to xanthine, may also lead to crystal formation in renal tubules and subsequent kidney injury.

35.5.3　Risk Factors

The likelihood and severity of TLS depend on several factors related to the patient and characteristics of the malignancy (Table 35.11). These risk factors include the tumor mass or disease burden, the tendency of the tumor cell to lyse and its sensitivity to treatment, patient-specific factors such as preexisting renal dysfunction, and supportive care such as electrolyte repletion given to the patient [86]. The higher the tumor mass or extent of the malignancy, the more cells are available to lyse their contents into the bloodstream. Patients with hematological malignancies including acute leukemias and aggressive lymphomas are typically at the highest risk of significant cell lysis. It is important to note however that TLS can occur in any malignancy, including solid tumors, if disease burden is large, disease proliferation is high, and certain highly effective cancer-directed therapies are used, such as venetoclax [87, 90–92]. Assess TLS risk factors for patients with a malignancy and ensure they receive appropriate prophylaxis and treatment if necessary.

35.5.4   Classification and Definitions

The Cairo and Bishop classification system is a commonly used tool to define and classify TLS [85, 86]. In this system, TLS is classified as either laboratory or clinical [93]. Laboratory TLS is defined as at least two of the following metabolic abnormalities exceeding the specified thresholds in Table 35.12 or changing >25% from baseline within 3 days before or the 7 days after treatment is initiated: hyperkalemia, hyperuricemia, hyperphosphatemia, and hypocalcemia (Table 35.12).

Another system used to identify TLS is the Howard criteria [86]. The Howard criteria states that two TLS-associated electrolyte disturbances must occur simultaneously (i.e., within the same 24-h period), removes the 25% change from baseline threshold, and considers any symptomatic hypocalcemia. In this criteria, calcium should be corrected for hypoalbuminemia.

Clinical TLS occurs when laboratory TLS occurs at the same time as an acute kidney injury, seizures, cardiac arrhythmias, or death.

35.5.5   Prevention

Pharmacologic treatments to address and prevent tumor lysis syndrome are intended to prevent TLS-related morbidity and mortality related to renal failure and the need for dialysis [85].

35.5.6   Hydration, Output, and Prophylaxis

TLS prevention should begin as soon as a high-risk malignancy is suspected. For patients who present with spontaneous TLS, after treating the initial TLS, take measures to prevent further TLS. Whenever possible, start TLS prevention at least 48 h prior to giving antineoplastic treatment in order to optimize patient's clinical status before cancer-directed treatment [85]. The hyperuricemia section of Table 35.13 summarizes TLS prevention strategies.

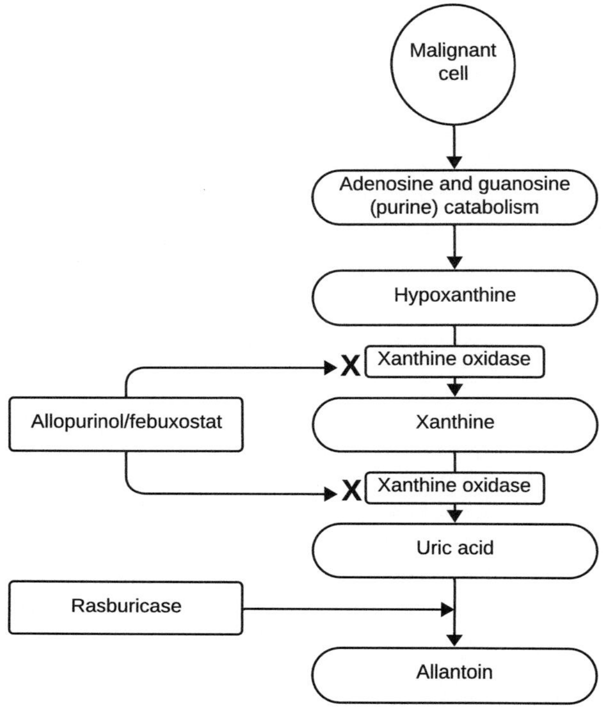

Fig. 35.4 Xanthine pathway

Patients that are at risk for TLS should receive aggressive IV hydration to promote renal perfusion and urine output, improve the clearance of uric acid and phosphorus, and help maintain glomerular filtration and renal blood flow. In patients that are at a high risk of experiencing TLS, IV fluids should be given at a target amount of 2500–3000 mL/m^2/day with a goal urine output of 2 mL/kg/h [85]. Preferably, hydration alone will be used to increase urine output. However, if urine output remains below goal despite adequate hydration, or fluid overload occurs, consider diuresis with a loop diuretic. Diuretics should be avoided in patients that are hypovolemic or if there is concern for obstructive uropathy.

One approach to prevent TLS-induced hyperuricemia is to block conversion of xanthine to uric acid. Allopurinol is an inhibitor of xanthine oxidase, which is the enzyme that converts hypoxanthine to xanthine and xanthine to uric acid [94]. Based on its mechanism (Fig. 35.4), allopurinol will not reduce existing uric acid; it will only prevent the formation of new uric acid after DNA is released from lysed cells. Allopurinol should be administered at a dose of 300 mg/m²/day or 10 mg/kg/day (max of 800 mg/day) given orally 2–3 divided doses [85]. For ease of dosing and administration, in practice patients may receive 300 mg twice daily. Allopurinol undergoes renal elimination and therefore should be dose-reduced 50% in patients with renal dysfunction or renal failure. In some situations, providers may be hesitant to utilize allopurinol in patients with renal dysfunction or an acute kidney injury (AKI); the ICU pharmacist can reassure the medical team that it is appropriate to still use allopurinol at a 50% dose reduction (i.e., 300 mg once daily). For patients unable to take allopurinol due to hypersensitivity, febuxostat, another xanthine oxidase inhibitor, may be given at a dose of 40–120 mg once daily [82, 95, 96]. Because xanthine oxidase inhibitors take 48–72 h to begin lowering uric acid, start xanthine oxidase inhibitor therapy as soon as TLS risk is identified.

Monitoring TLS labs and being proactive at addressing electrolyte abnormalities is a key component of managing TLS. In high-risk patients, TLS monitoring may be performed as frequently as every 4–6 h, and in lower risk patients, monitoring can occur every 12–24 h [85]. As TLS risk decreases, TLS monitoring frequency can also

Table 35.13 Managing hyperuricemia and electrolyte abnormalities

Abnormality	Intervention
Hyperuricemia	
Uric acid <9.0 mg/dL	Allopurinol 300 mg orally once or twice daily plus aggressive hydration (dose reduce allopurinol 50% for renal dysfunction)
Uric acid ≥9.0–12.0 mg/dL	Rasburicase 3 mg IV × 1 dose[a], allopurinol, and hydration
Uric acid >12.0 mg/dL	Rasburicase 6 mg IV × 1 dose[a], allopurinol, and hydration
Hyperkalemia	
Potassium 6.0–7.0 mg/dL and asymptomatic	Sodium zirconium cyclosilicate 10 g orally three times daily for up to 48 h
Potassium >7.0 mg/dL or symptomatic	Regular insulin 5–10 units IV bolus + dextrose 25–50 g IV and/or Calcium gluconate 1–2 g IV over 2–5 min and/or Sodium bicarbonate 1–2 mEq/kg IV push
Hyperphosphatemia	
Phosphorus >4.5 mg/dL	Sevelamer 800–1600 mg orally three times daily with meals
Hypocalcemia	
Corrected calcium <7.0 mg/dL or ionized calcium <4.5 mg/dL and asymptomatic	– No intervention recommended
Corrected calcium <7.0 mg/dL or ionized calcium <4.5 mg/dL and symptomatic	Calcium gluconate 1–2 g IV[b]

[a] May repeat rasburicase dose if uric acid not sufficiently reduced
[b] Consider renal consultation if calcium repletion is necessary and phosphate is also elevated

decrease. Because TLS is a phenomenon that occurs with high tumor burden, TLS monitoring and prevention is generally only necessary with newly diagnosed patients, prior and during the first cycle of antineoplastic treatment, or at disease relapse, when patients are beginning a different treatment for their malignancy. Once 3–7 days or more have passed after the last dose of chemotherapy and no further signs and symptoms of TLS are detected, TLS prophylaxis can be stopped [85].

35.5.7 *Treatment*

Although the goal is to prevent laboratory or clinical TLS from occurring, in some situations patients may initially present with TLS or may experience TLS after starting therapy despite preventive measures. Table 35.13 summarizes treatment modalities for each TLS-associated electrolyte abnormality.

35.5.7.1 Hyperkalemia

Hyperkalemia is the most acutely dangerous component of TLS, therefore, when it occurs, the goal is to remove or shift serum potassium out of the bloodstream as quickly as possible due to risk of fatal arrhythmias [86]. In patients with a serum potassium greater than 7.0 mEq/L or with EKG abnormalities (peaked T waves, QRS complex widening) immediate intervention is necessary [85]. In patients with a moderately elevated serum potassium (6.0–7.0 mEq/L) that are asymptomatic, less intensive intervention may be considered. In addition to recommending potential interventions for hyperkalemia, the ICU pharmacist should also ensure that potassium supplementation or products that contain potassium are avoided or used cautiously in patients at risk of TLS.

In patients with asymptomatic, moderate hyperkalemia, potassium binding agents including sodium zirconium cyclosilicate (SZC) or sodium polystyrene sulfonate (SPS) should be administered to reduce serum potassium and lower further potassium from being absorbed in the gastrointestinal lumen [85]. SZC is given at a dose of 10 g three times daily for up to 48 h; SPS is given at a dose of 15–30 g once [97, 98]. Historically, SPS was the primary potassium binder agent used for emergent hyperkalemia [86]. However, SZC was FDA-approved in 2018 and should be strongly considered over SPS as it has a quicker onset of action and does not have a risk of intestinal necrosis, which is a rare but serious risk of SPS [98–100].

For severe or symptomatic hyperkalemia, more intense intervention may be necessary. Regular insulin 5–10 units or 0.1 units/kg should be given as an IV bolus to temporarily shift serum potassium intracellularly [85, 101]. This should be given along with 25–50 g of dextrose IV to prevent insulin-induced hypoglycemia. Calcium gluconate should be given at dose of 1–2 g over 2–5 min or 100–200 mg/kg via slow IV infusion [85, 102]. Calcium gluconate does not affect serum potassium levels, but it does stabilize myocardial cell membranes which reduces the risk of dysrhythmia.

Sodium bicarbonate at a dose of 1–2 mEq/kg given via IV push may also be considered to cause an influx of potassium intracellularly [85]. Sodium bicarbonate and calcium gluconate should not be given via the same line as they are incompatible.

35.5.7.2   Hyperuricemia

Because xanthine oxidase inhibitors prevent uric acid from being formed but do not reduce existing serum uric acid levels, if patients present with or develop severe hyperuricemia, aggressive hydration and a xanthine oxidase inhibitor may not be sufficient and administering rasburicase may be necessary. Rasburicase is a recombinant urate-oxidase enzyme that catabolizes uric acid to allantoin (Fig. 35.4), a highly soluble metabolite of uric acid [103]. Rasburicase is FDA-approved to be given as a weight-based dose of 0.2 mg/kg/dose once daily for up to 5 days [104]. Although effective, rasburicase is costly. Various studies have evaluated one-time, flat doses of rasburicase for TLS-associated hyperuricemia, and have found that single doses of rasburicase 3 mg or 6 mg are often effective at adequately lowering uric acid [105–109]. Based on established literature, consider using flat dose rasburicase instead of weight-based dosing in adult patients.

When rasburicase is necessary, use a 3 mg dose if the uric acid level is ≤ 12 mg/dL, and 6 mg if uric acid is >12 mg/dL [108]. Rasburicase will begin to decrease uric acid levels within 4 h of administration and will continue to decrease uric acid for at least 24 h [110]. The onset of action and duration of effect should be taken into consideration when evaluating post-dose uric acid levels to determine if an additional dose of rasburicase is indicated. When measuring uric acid levels after giving rasburicase, uric acid lab samples should be kept on ice or in an ice water bath and be analyzed within 4 h of collection in order to ensure that rasburicase does not continue to significantly metabolize and reduce the serum uric acid contained in the sample [104, 111].

Rasburicase is contraindicated in patients with a known glucose-6-phosphate dehydrogenase (G6PD) deficiency due to risk of hemolysis [104]. Patients with a G6PD deficiency are unable to metabolize hydrogen peroxide, a breakdown product of the urate-oxidase reaction caused by rasburicase, which leads to the risk of hemolysis. Prior to administering rasburicase, the ICU pharmacist should check if the patient has a G6PD deficiency and recommend checking a G6PD level if the status is unknown. In practice, a patient's G6PD level is often unknown and the G6PD level will likely not be available before the rasburicase is needed. In those situations, patients requiring rasburicase should be screened for risk factors for G6PD deficiency based upon ancestry (African, African American, Mediterranean, Middle Eastern, or Southeast Asian decent) [112]. In those determined to be at risk for G6PD deficiency, it should be confirmed that the patient understands the risk of hemolysis and is willing to accept blood products prior to administering rasburicase (i.e., not opposed to accepting blood products due to religious beliefs).

Rasburicase administration does not preclude xanthine oxidase inhibitor use. Once rasburicase degrades existing uric acid, xanthine oxidase inhibitors and hydration should be started/continued in order to prevent further uric acid build-up and maximize uric acid lowering. Additionally, once patients progress to the point of needing renal replacement therapy (RRT), rasburicase is no longer needed because the goal of utilizing pharmacologic TLS prophylaxis/treatment is to prevent the need for dialysis and also because RRT removes uric acid.

35.5.7.3 Hyperphosphatemia

There are several strategies that may be used to reduce phosphate levels and risk of hyperphosphatemia-associated complications. Medications or IV solutions containing phosphate should be avoided if possible and patients should maintain adequate hydration to decrease the risk of phosphate calcium precipitation and promote elimination [85]. Oral phosphate binders may also be administered to reduce phosphate levels. Sevelamer 800–1600 mg orally three times daily or aluminum hydroxide 50–150 mg/kg/day orally or via alternate enteral routes every 6 h may be used. Calcium carbonate may be considered as a potential phosphate binding agent; however, it should be avoided in patients with normal or elevated calcium level due to risk of increasing calcium and leading to phosphate calcium precipitation.

35.5.7.4 Hypocalcemia

Patients with hypocalcemia that are asymptomatic should not typically receive any intervention with calcium supplementation due to increasing the risk of calcium phosphate precipitation if calcium becomes elevated [85]. In patients with hypoalbuminemia, the ICU pharmacist should consider calculating corrected calcium or recommending ionized calcium be checked to assess if a patient meets the criteria for hypocalcemia. If patients are symptomatic from hypocalcemia, calcium gluconate 1–2 g IV may be considered. If symptomatic patients requiring calcium repletion also have hyperphosphatemia, a renal consult should be considered given the further increased risk of calcium phosphate precipitation.

References

1. Locke FL, Neelapu SS, Bartlett NL, Siddiqi T, Chavez JC, Hosing CM, Ghobadi A, Budde LE, Bot A, Rossi JM, Jiang Y, Xue AX, Elias M, Aycock J, Wiezorek J, Go WY. Phase 1 results of ZUMA-1: a multicenter study of KTE-C19 anti-CD19 CAR T cell therapy in refractory aggressive lymphoma. Mol Ther. 2017;25(1):285–95. https://doi.org/10.1016/j.ymthe.2016.10.020.
2. Maude SL, Laetsch TW, Buechner J, Rives S, Boyer M, Bittencourt H, Bader P, Verneris MR, Stefanski HE, Myers GD, Qayed M, De Moerloose B, Hiramatsu H, Schlis K, Davis KL, Martin PL, Nemecek ER, Yanik GA, Peters C, Baruchel A, Boissel N, Mechinaud F, Balduzzi A, Krueger J, June CH, Levine BL, Wood P, Taran T, Leung M, Mueller KT, Zhang Y, Sen K, Lebwohl D, Pulsipher MA, Grupp SA. Tisagenlecleucel in children and Young adults with B-cell lymphoblastic leukemia. N Engl J Med. 2018;378(5):439–48. https://doi.org/10.1056/NEJMoa1709866.

3. Miliotou AN, Papadopoulou LC. CAR T-cell therapy: a new era in cancer immunotherapy. Curr Pharm Biotechnol. 2018;19(1):5–18. https://doi.org/10.2174/1389201019666180418095526.

4. Neelapu SS, Locke FL, Bartlett NL, Lekakis LJ, Miklos DB, Jacobson CA, Braunschweig I, Oluwole OO, Siddiqi T, Lin Y, Timmerman JM, Stiff PJ, Friedberg JW, Flinn IW, Goy A, Hill BT, Smith MR, Deol A, Farooq U, McSweeney P, Munoz J, Avivi I, Castro JE, Westin JR, Chavez JC, Ghobadi A, Komanduri KV, Levy R, Jacobsen ED, Witzig TE, Reagan P, Bot A, Rossi J, Navale L, Jiang Y, Aycock J, Elias M, Chang D, Wiezorek J, Go WY. Axicabtagene Ciloleucel CAR T-cell therapy in refractory large B-cell lymphoma. N Engl J Med. 2017;377(26) 2531–44. https://doi.org/10.1056/NEJMoa1707447.

5. Wei J, Han X, Bo J, Han W. Target selection for CAR-T therapy. J Hematol Oncol. 2019;12(1):62. https://doi.org/10.1186/s13045-019-0758-x.

6. Sermer D, Brentjens R. CAR T-cell therapy: full speed ahead. Hematol Oncol. 2019;37 (Suppl 1):95–100. https://doi.org/10.1002/hon.2591.

7. Sterner RC, Sterner RM. CAR-T cell therapy: current limitations and potential strategies. Blood Cancer J. 2021;11(4):69. https://doi.org/10.1038/s41408-021-00459-7.

8. Neelapu SS. Managing the toxicities of CAR T-cell therapy. Hematol Oncol. 2019;37(Suppl 1):48–52. https://doi.org/10.1002/hon.2595.

9. Giavridis T, van der Stegen SJC, Eyquem J, Hamieh M, Piersigilli A, Sadelain M. CAR T cell-induced cytokine release syndrome is mediated by macrophages and abated by IL-1 blockade. Nat Med. 2018;24(6):731–8. https://doi.org/10.1038/s41591-018-0041-7.

10. Wang Z, Han W. Biomarkers of cytokine release syndrome and neurotoxicity related to CAR-T cell therapy. Biomark Res. 2018;6:4. https://doi.org/10.1186/s40364-018-0116-0.

11. Lee DW, Santomasso BD, Locke FL, Ghobadi A, Turtle CJ, Brudno JN, Maus MV, Park JH, Mead E, Pavletic S, Go WY, Eldjerou L, Gardner RA, Frey N, Curran KJ, Peggs K, Pasquini M, DiPersio JF, van den Brink MRM, Komanduri KV, Grupp SA, Neelapu SS. ASTCT consensus grading for cytokine release syndrome and neurologic toxicity associated with immune effector cells. Biol Blood Marrow Transplant. 2019;25(4):625–38. https://doi.org/10.1016/j.bbmt.2018.12.758.

12. Abecma [package insert]. Celgene Corporation, a Bristol-Myers Squibb Company, Summit; 2024.

13. Breyanzi [package insert]. Juno Therapeutics, Inc., a Bristol-Myers Squibb Company, Bothell; 2024.

14. Carvykti [package insert]. Horsham: Janssen Biotech, Inc.; 2024.

15. Kymriah [package insert]. East Hanover: Novartis Pharmaceuticals Corporation; 2022.

16. Tecartus [package insert]. Santa Monica: Kite Pharma, Inc.; 2024.

17. Yescarta [package insert]. Santa Monica: Kite Pharma, Inc.; 2024.

18. Faude S, Wei J, Muralidharan K, Xu X, Wertheim G, Paessler M, Bhoj VG, Grupp SA, Maude SL, Rheingold SR, Pillai V. Absolute lymphocyte count proliferation kinetics after CAR T-cell infusion impact response and relapse. Blood Adv. 2021;5(8):2128–36. https://doi.org/10.1182/bloodadvances.2020004038.

19. Santomasso BD, Nastoupil LJ, Adkins S, Lacchetti C, Schneider BJ, Anadkat M, Atkins MB, Brassil KJ, Caterino JM, Chau I, Davies MJ, Ernstoff MS, Fecher L, Funchain P, Jaiyesimi I, Mammen JS, Naidoo J, Naing A, Phillips T, Porter LD, Reichner CA, Seigel C, Song JM, Spira A, Suarez-Almazor M, Swami U, Thompson JA, Vikas P, Wang Y, Weber JS, Bollin K, Ghosh M. Management of immune-related adverse events in patients treated with chimeric antigen receptor T-cell therapy: ASCO guideline. J Clin Oncol. 2021;39(35):3978–92. https://doi.org/10.1200/JCO.21.01992.

20. Actemra [package insert]. South San Francisco: Genentech, Inc.; 2022.

21. Le RQ, Li L, Yuan W, Shord SS, Nie L, Habtemariam BA, Przepiorka D, Farrell AT, Pazdur R. FDA approval summary: tocilizumab for treatment of chimeric antigen receptor T cell-induced severe or life-threatening cytokine release syndrome. Oncologist. 2018;23(8):943–7. https://doi.org/10.1634/theoncologist.2018-0028.

22. Cassanello G, Luttwak E, Devlin SM, Luna De Abia A, Corona M, Landego I, Parascondola A, Saldia A, Alarcon Tomas A, Dahi PB, Lin RJ, Palomba ML, Park JH, Salles G, Perales M-A, Scordo M, Shouval R, Shah GL. Evaluation of the impact of tocilizumab use in recipients of CAR T cells for non-Hodgkin lymphoma. Blood. 2023;142(Supplement 1):6898. https://doi.org/10.1182/blood-2023-190500.
23. Wang X, Zhang B, Zhang Q, Zhou H, Sun Q, Zhou Y, Li T, Zhou D, Shen Z, Zhang J, Li P, Liang A, Zhou K, Han L, Hu Y, Yang Y, Cao J, Li Z, Xu K, Sang W. Impact of tocilizumab on anti-CD19 chimeric antigen receptor T-cell therapy in B-cell acute lymphoblastic leukemia. Cancer. 2024;130:2660. https://doi.org/10.1002/cncr.35316.
24. Liu S, Deng B, Yin Z, Pan J, Lin Y, Ling Z, Wu T, Chen D, Chang AH, Gao Z. Corticosteroids do not influence the efficacy and kinetics of CAR-T cells for B-cell acute lymphoblastic leukemia. Blood Cancer J. 2020;10(2):15.
25. Kineret [package insert]. Stockholm: Swedish Orphan Biovitrum AB; 2020.
26. Frigault MJ, Gallagher KM, Wehrli M, Valles B, Casey K, Lindell K, Trailor M, Cho H, Brown JL, Horick NK. A phase II trial of anakinra for the prevention of CAR-T cell mediated neurotoxicity. Blood. 2021;138:2814.
27. Gazeau N, Liang EC, Voutsinas JM, Barba P, Iacoboni G, Kwon M, Ortega JLR, López-Corral L, Hernani R, Ortiz-Maldonado V. Anakinra for refractory cytokine release syndrome or immune effector cell-associated neurotoxicity syndrome after chimeric antigen receptor T cell therapy. Transplant Cell Ther. 2023;29(7):430–7.
28. Gazeau N, Liang EC, Wu QV, Voutsinas JM, Barba P, Iacoboni G, Kwon M, Ortega JLR, Lopez-Corral L, Hernani R, Ortiz-Maldonado V, Martinez-Cibrian N, Martinez AP, Maziarz RT, Williamson S, Nemecek ER, Shadman M, Cowan AJ, Green DJ, Kimble E, Hirayama AV, Maloney DG, Turtle CJ, Gauthier J. Anakinra for refractory cytokine release syndrome or immune effector cell-associated neurotoxicity syndrome after chimeric antigen receptor T cell therapy. Transplant Cell Ther. 2023;29(7):430–7. https://doi.org/10.1016/j.jtct.2023.04.001.
29. Jain MD, Smith M, Shah NN. How I treat refractory CRS and ICANS after CAR T-cell therapy. Blood. 2023;141(20):2430–42. https://doi.org/10.1182/blood.2022017414.
30. Park JH, Nath K, Devlin SM, Sauter CS, Palomba ML, Shah G, Dahi P, Lin RJ, Scordo M, Perales MA, Shouval R, Tomas AA, Cathcart E, Mead E, Santomasso B, Holodny A, Brentjens RJ, Riviere I, Sadelain M. CD19 CAR T-cell therapy and prophylactic anakinra in relapsed or refractory lymphoma: phase 2 trial interim results. Nat Med. 2023;29(7):1710–7. https://doi.org/10.1038/s41591-023-02404-6.
31. Sylvant [package insert]. Hertfordshire: EUSA Pharma (UK), Ltd.; 2019.
32. Bajwa AK, Zhao Q, Geer MJ, Mian A, Lin C, Frame D, Westholder J, Tossey J, Ghosh M, Galal A. Efficacy of Siltuximab for chimeric antigen receptor T-cell therapy toxicities-a multicenter retrospective analysis. Blood. 2023;142:4502.
33. Chen F, Teachey DT, Pequignot E, Frey N, Porter D, Maude SL, Grupp SA, June CH, Melenhorst JJ, Lacey SF. Measuring IL-6 and sIL-6R in serum from patients treated with tocilizumab and/or siltuximab following CAR T cell therapy. J Immunol Methods. 2016;434:1–8. https://doi.org/10.1016/j.jim.2016.03.005.
34. Garfall AL, Lancaster E, Stadtmauer EA, Lacey SF, Dengel K, Ambrose DE, Chen F, Gupta M, Kulikovskaya I, Vogl DT, Plesa G, Weiss BM, Ferthio R, Richardson C, Melenhorst JJ, Levine BL, June CH, Milone M, Cohen AD. Posterior reversible encephalopathy syndrome (PRES) after infusion of anti-Bcma CAR T cells (CART-BCMA) for multiple myeloma: successful treatment with cyclophosphamide. Blood. 2016;128(22):5702. https://doi.org/10.1182/blood.V128.22.5702.5702.
35. Graham CE, Lee WH, Wiggin HR, Supper VM, Leick MB, Birocchi F, Yee AJ, Petrichenko A, Everett J, Bushman FD, Sadrzadeh H, Rapalino O, Chiu D, Arrillaga-Romany I, Maus MV, Frigault MJ, Gallagher KME. Chemotherapy-induced reversal of ciltacabtagene autoleucel-associated movement and neurocognitive toxicity. Blood. 2023;142(14):1248–52. https://doi.org/10.1182/blood.2023021429.

36. Cohen AD, Parekh S, Santomasso BD, Gállego Pérez-Larraya J, van de Donk N, Arnulf B, Mateos MV, Lendvai N, Jackson CC, De Braganca KC, Schecter JM, Marquez L, Lee E, Cornax I, Zudaire E, Li C, Olyslager Y, Madduri D, Varsos H, Pacaud L, Akram M, Geng D, Jakubowiak A, Einsele H, Jagannath S. Incidence and management of CAR-T neurotoxicity in patients with multiple myeloma treated with ciltacabtagene autoleucel in CARTITUDE studies. Blood Cancer J. 2022;12(2):32. https://doi.org/10.1038/s41408-022-00629-1.

37. Schubert ML, Schmitt M, Wang L, Ramos CA, Jordan K, Muller-Tidow C, Dreger P. Side-effect management of chimeric antigen receptor (CAR) T-cell therapy. Ann Oncol. 2021;32(1):34–48. https://doi.org/10.1016/j.annonc.2020.10.478.

38. Levetiracetam injection [package insert]. Lake Forest: Hospira, Inc.; 2023.

39. Saw JL, Sidiqi MH, Ruff M, Hocker S, Alkhateeb H, Ansell SM, Bennani NN, Dingli D, Hayman SR, Johnston PB, Kapoor P, Kenderian SJ, Kourelis TV, Kumar SK, Paludo J, Shah MV, Siddiqui MA, Warsame R, Rosenthal A, Grill M, Castro JE, Siegel J, Abdel Rahman ZH, Kharfan-Dabaja MA, So E, Lin Y. Acute seizures and status epilepticus in immune effector cell associated neurotoxicity syndrome (ICANS). Blood Cancer J. 2022;12(4):62. https://doi.org/10.1038/s41408-022-00657-x.

40. Diorio C, Vatsayan A, Talleur AC, Annesley C, Jaroscak JJ, Shalabi H, Ombrello AK, Hudspeth M, Maude SL, Gardner RA. Anakinra utilization in refractory pediatric CAR T-cell associated toxicities. Blood Adv. 2022;6(11):3398–403.

41. Gazeau N, Barba P, Iacoboni G, Kwon M, Bailen R, Reguera JL, Corral LL, Hernani R, Ortiz-Maldonado V, Perez-Martinez A. Safety and efficacy of two anakinra dose regimens for refractory CRS or ICANS after CAR T-cell therapy. Blood. 2021;138:2816.

42. Strati P, Jallouk A, Deng Q, Li X, Feng L, Sun R, Adkins S, Johncy S, Cain T, Steiner RE. A phase 1 study of prophylactic anakinra to mitigate ICANS in patients with large B-cell lymphoma. Blood Adv. 2023;7(21):6785–9.

43. Wehrli M, Gallagher K, Chen YB, Leick MB, McAfee SL, El-Jawahri AR, DeFilipp Z, Horick N, O'Donnell P, Spitzer T, Dey B, Cook D, Trailor M, Lindell K, Maus MV, Frigault MJ. Single-center experience using anakinra for steroid-refractory immune effector cell-associated neurotoxicity syndrome (ICANS). J Immunother Cancer. 2022;10(1):e003847. https://doi.org/10.1136/jitc-2021-003847.

44. Galea J, Ogungbenro K, Hulme S, Greenhalgh A, Aarons L, Scarth S, Hutchinson P, Grainger S, King A, Hopkins SJ. Intravenous anakinra can achieve experimentally effective concentrations in the central nervous system within a therapeutic time window: results of a dose-ranging study. J Cereb Blood Flow Metab. 2011;31(2):439–47.

45. Patel S, Cenin D, Corrigan D, Hamilton BK, Kalaycio M, Sobecks RM, Anwer F, Khouri J, Dean RM, Winter A. Siltuximab for first-line treatment of cytokine release syndrome: a response to the national shortage of tocilizumab. Blood. 2022;140(Supplement 1):5073–4.

46. Hashmi H, Bachmeier C, Chavez JC, Song J, Hussaini M, Krivenko G, Nishihori T, Kotani H, Davila ML, Locke FL. Haemophagocytic lymphohistiocytosis has variable time to onset following CD19 chimeric antigen receptor T cell therapy. Br J Haematol. 2019;187(2):e35–8.

47. Lichtenstein DA, Schischlik F, Shao L, Steinberg SM, Yates B, Wang H-W, Wang Y, Inglefield J, Dulau-Florea A, Ceppi F. Characterization of HLH-like manifestations as a CRS variant in patients receiving CD22 CAR T cells. Blood. 2021;138(24):2469–84.

48. Fugere T, Baltz A, Mukherjee A, Gaddam M, Varma A, Veeraputhiran M, Gentille Sanchez CG. Immune effector cell-associated HLH-like syndrome: a review of the literature of an increasingly recognized entity. Cancers (Basel). 2023;15(21):5149.

49. Jain T, Olson TS, Locke FL. How I treat cytopenias after CAR T-cell therapy. Blood. 2023;141(20):2460–9.

50. Wang S, Degar BA, Zieske A, Shafi NQ, Rose MG. Hemophagocytosis exacerbated by G-CSF/GM-CSF treatment in a patient with myelodysplasia. Am J Hematol. 2004;77(4):391–6.

51. Mehta P, Cron RQ, Hartwell J, Manson JJ, Tattersall RS. Silencing the cytokine storm: the use of intravenous anakinra in haemophagocytic lymphohistiocytosis or macrophage activation syndrome. Lancet Rheumatol. 2020;2(6):e358–67.

52. Major A, Collins J, Craney C, Heitman AK, Bauer E, Zerante E, Stock W, Bishop MR, Jasielec J. Management of hemophagocytic lymphohistiocytosis (HLH) associated with chimeric antigen receptor T-cell (CAR-T) therapy using anti-cytokine therapy: an illustrative case and review of the literature. Leuk Lymphoma. 2021;62(7):1765–9.

53. La Rosée P. Treatment of hemophagocytic lymphohistiocytosis in adults. Hematology 2014, the American Society of Hematology Education Program Book. 2015;2015(1):190–196.

54. Jakafi [package insert]. Wilmington: Incyte corporation; 2023.

55. Keenan C, Nichols KE, Albeituni S. Use of the JAK inhibitor ruxolitinib in the treatment of hemophagocytic lymphohistiocytosis. Front Immunol. 2021;12:614704.

56. Zhao L, Yang H, Qu W-y, Lu Y-j, Feng Z. Case report: ruxolitinib plus dexamethasone as first-line therapy in haemophagocytic lymphohistiocytosis. Front Oncol. 2023;13:1054175.

57. Kuderer NM, Dale DC, Crawford J, Cosler LE, Lyman GH. Mortality, morbidity, and cost associated with febrile neutropenia in adult cancer patients. Cancer. 2006;106(10):2258–66. https://doi.org/10.1002/cncr.21847.

58. Freifeld AG, Bow EJ, Sepkowitz KA, Boeckh MJ, Ito JI, Mullen CA, Raad II, Rolston KV, Young J-AH, Wingard JR. Clinical practice guideline for the use of antimicrobial agents in neutropenic patients with cancer: 2010 update by the Infectious Diseases Society of America. Clin Infect Dis. 2011;52(4):e56–93. https://doi.org/10.1093/cid/cir073.

59. Carmona-Bayonas A, Jiménez-Fonseca P, Virizuela Echaburu J, Antonio M, Font C, Biosca M, Ramchandani A, Martínez J, Hernando Cubero J, Espinosa J, Martínez de Castro E, Ghanem I, Beato C, Blasco A, Garrido M, Bonilla Y, Mondéjar R, Arcusa Lanza M, Aragón Manrique I, Manzano A, Sevillano E, Castañón E, Cardona M, Gallardo Martín E, Pérez Armillas Q, Sánchez Lasheras F, Ayala de la Peña F. Prediction of serious complications in patients with seemingly stable febrile neutropenia: validation of the clinical index of stable febrile neutropenia in a prospective cohort of patients from the FINITE study. J Clin Oncol. 2015;33(5):465–71. https://doi.org/10.1200/jco.2014.57.2347.

60. Taplitz RA, Kennedy EB, Bow EJ, Crews J, Gleason C, Hawley DK, Langston AA, Nastoupil LJ, Rajotte M, Rolston K, Strasfeld L, Flowers CR. Outpatient management of fever and neutropenia in adults treated for malignancy: American Society of Clinical Oncology and Infectious Diseases Society of America clinical practice guideline update. J Clin Oncol. 2018;36(14):1443–53. https://doi.org/10.1200/jco.2017.77.6211.

61. Aapro M, Lyman GH, Bokemeyer C, Rapoport BL, Mathieson N, Koptelova N, Cornes P, Anderson R, Gascón P, Kuderer NM. Supportive care in patients with cancer during the COVID-19 pandemic. ESMO Open. 2021;6(1):100038. https://doi.org/10.1016/j.esmoop.2020.100038.

62. Tamma PD, Aitken SL, Bonomo RA, Mathers AJ, Van Duin D, Clancy CJ. Infectious Diseases Society of America 2023 guidance on the treatment of antimicrobial resistant gram-negative infections. Clin Infect Dis. 2023:ciad428. https://doi.org/10.1093/cid/ciad428.

63. Klastersky J, Paesmans M, Rubenstein EB, Boyer M, Elting L, Feld R, Gallagher J, Herrstedt J, Rapoport B, Rolston K, Talcott J. The Multinational Association for Supportive Care in cancer risk index: a multinational scoring system for identifying low-risk febrile neutropenic cancer patients. J Clin Oncol. 2000;18(16):3038–51. https://doi.org/10.1200/jco.2000.18.16.3038.

64. Guise TA, Wysolmerski JJ. Cancer-associated hypercalcemia. N Engl J Med. 2022;386(15):1443–51.

65. Goldner W. Cancer-related hypercalcemia. J Oncol Pract. 2016;12(5):426–32. https://doi.org/10.1200/jop.2016.011155.

66. Mirrakhimov AE. Hypercalcemia of malignancy: an update on pathogenesis and management. N Am J Med Sci. 2015;7(11):483.

67. Hofbauer LC, Schoppet M. Clinical implications of the osteoprotegerin/RANKL/RANK system for bone and vascular diseases. JAMA. 2004;292(4):490–5. https://doi.org/10.1001/jama.292.4.490.

68. Chakhtoura M, El-Hajj Fuleihan G. Treatment of hypercalcemia of malignancy. Endocrinol Metab Clin North Am. 2021;50(4):781–92. https://doi.org/10.1016/j.ecl.2021.08.002.
69. El-Hajj Fuleihan G, Clines GA, Hu MI, Marcocci C, Murad MH, Piggott T, Van Poznak C, Wu JY, Drake MT. Treatment of hypercalcemia of malignancy in adults: an Endocrine Society clinical practice guideline. J Clin Endocrinol Metab. 2023;108(3):507–28. https://doi.org/10.1210/clinem/dgac621.
70. Rajasekaran A, Bade N, Cutter GR, Rizk DV, Zarjou A. Lactated Ringer's solution and risk of hyperkalemia in patients with reduced kidney function. Am J Med Sci. 2022;364(4):433–43. https://doi.org/10.1016/j.amjms.2022.04.024.
71. Asonitis N, Angelousi A, Zafeiris C, Lambrou GI, Dontas I, Kassi E. Diagnosis, pathophysiology and management of hypercalcemia in malignancy: a review of the literature. Horm Metab Res. 2019;51(12):770–8. https://doi.org/10.1055/a-1049-0647.
72. Major P, Lortholary A, Hon J, Abdi E, Mills G, Menssen HD, Yunus F, Bell R, Body J, Quebe-Fehling E, Seaman J. Zoledronic acid is superior to pamidronate in the treatment of hypercalcemia of malignancy: a pooled analysis of two randomized, controlled clinical trials. J Clin Oncol. 2001;19(2):558–67. https://doi.org/10.1200/jco.2001.19.2.558.
73. Hsu EH, Ryan B. Safety and efficacy of intravenous bisphosphonates for the treatment of hypercalcemia in patients with cancer and baseline renal dysfunction. J Hematol Oncol Pharm. 2022;12(4):207–15.
74. Walker MD, Shane E. Hypercalcemia: a review. JAMA. 2022;328(16):1624–36. https://doi.org/10.1001/jama.2022.18331.
75. Hu MI, Glezerman IG, Leboulleux S, Insogna K, Gucalp R, Misiorowski W, Yu B, Zorsky P, Tosi D, Bessudo A, Jaccard A, Tonini G, Ying W, Braun A, Jain RK. Denosumab for treatment of hypercalcemia of malignancy. J Clin Endocrinol Metab. 2014;99(9):3144–52. https://doi.org/10.1210/jc.2014-1001.
76. Stopeck AT, Lipton A, Body JJ, Steger GG, Tonkin K, de Boer RH, Lichinitser M, Fujiwara Y, Yardley DA, Viniegra M, Fan M, Jiang Q, Dansey R, Jun S, Braun A. Denosumab compared with zoledronic acid for the treatment of bone metastases in patients with advanced breast cancer: a randomized, double-blind study. J Clin Oncol. 2010;28(35):5132–9. https://doi.org/10.1200/jco.2010.29.7101.
77. Cicci JD, Buie L, Bates J, van Deventer H. Denosumab for the management of hypercalcemia of malignancy in patients with multiple myeloma and renal dysfunction. Clin Lymphoma Myeloma Leuk. 2014;14(6):e207–11. https://doi.org/10.1016/j.clml.2014.07.005.
78. Miacalcin [package insert]. East Hanover: Novartis Pharmaceuticals Corporation; 2014.
79. Lawton AJ, Lee KA, Cheville AL, Ferrone ML, Rades D, Balboni TA, Abrahm JL. Assessment and management of patients with metastatic spinal cord compression: a multidisciplinary review. J Clin Oncol. 2019;37(1):61–71. https://doi.org/10.1200/jco.2018.78.1211.
80. Sørensen S, Helweg-Larsen S, Mouridsen H, Hansen HH. Effect of high-dose dexamethasone in carcinomatous metastatic spinal cord compression treated with radiotherapy: a randomised trial. Eur J Cancer. 1994;30A(1):22–7. https://doi.org/10.1016/s0959-8049(05)80011-5.
81. Graham PH, Capp A, Delaney G, Goozee G, Hickey B, Turner S, Browne L, Milross C, Wirth A. A pilot randomised comparison of dexamethasone 96 mg vs 16 mg per day for malignant spinal-cord compression treated by radiotherapy: TROG 01.05 Superdex study. Clin Oncol (R Coll Radiol). 2006;18(1):70–6. https://doi.org/10.1016/j.clon.2005.08.015.
82. George R, Jeba J, Ramkumar G, Chacko AG, Tharyan P. Interventions for the treatment of metastatic extradural spinal cord compression in adults. Cochrane Database Syst Rev. 2015;2015(9):CD006716. https://doi.org/10.1002/14651858.CD006716.pub3.
83. Coleman R, Hadji P, Body JJ, Santini D, Chow E, Terpos E, Oudard S, Bruland Ø, Flamen P, Kurth A, Van Poznak C, Aapro M, Jordan K. Bone health in cancer: ESMO clinical practice guidelines. Ann Oncol. 2020;31(12):1650–63. https://doi.org/10.1016/j.annonc.2020.07.019.
84. Fisher CG, DiPaola CP, Ryken TC, Bilsky MH, Shaffrey CI, Berven SH, Harrop JS, Fehlings MG, Boriani S, Chou D, Schmidt MH, Polly DW, Biagini R, Burch S, Dekutoski MB, Ganju A, Gerszten PC, Gokaslan ZL, Groff MW, Liebsch NJ, Mendel E, Okuno SH, Patel S, Rhines

LD, Rose PS, Sciubba DM, Sundaresan N, Tomita K, Varga PP, Vialle LR, Vrionis FD, Yamada Y, Fourney DR. A novel classification system for spinal instability in neoplastic disease: an evidence-based approach and expert consensus from the Spine Oncology Study Group. Spine (Phila Pa 1976). 2010;35(22):E1221–9. https://doi.org/10.1097/BRS.0b013e3181e16ae2.

85. Coiffier B, Altman A, Pui CH, Younes A, Cairo MS. Guidelines for the management of pediatric and adult tumor lysis syndrome: an evidence-based review. J Clin Oncol. 2008;26(16):2767–78. https://doi.org/10.1200/JCO.2007.15.0177.

86. Howard SC, Jones DP, Pui CH. The tumor lysis syndrome. N Engl J Med. 2011;364(19):1844–54. https://doi.org/10.1056/NEJMra0904569.

87. Baeksgaard L, Sorensen JB. Acute tumor lysis syndrome in solid tumors—a case report and review of the literature. Cancer Chemother Pharmacol. 2003;51(3):187–92. https://doi.org/10.1007/s00280-002-0556-x.

88. Arseneau JC, Canellos GP, Banks PM, Berard CW, Gralnick HR, DeVita VT Jr. American Burkitt's lymphoma: a clinicopathologic study of 30 cases. I. Clinical factors relating to prolonged survival. Am J Med. 1975;58(3):314–21. https://doi.org/10.1016/0002-9343(75)90597-5.

89. Cheson BD, Frame JN, Vena D, Quashu N, Sorensen JM. Tumor lysis syndrome: an uncommon complication of fludarabine therapy of chronic lymphocytic leukemia. J Clin Oncol. 1998;16(7):2313–20. https://doi.org/10.1200/JCO.1998.16.7.2313.

90. Godoy H, Kesterson JP, Lele S. Tumor lysis syndrome associated with carboplatin and paclitaxel in a woman with recurrent endometrial cancer. Int J Gynaecol Obstet. 2010;109(3):254. https://doi.org/10.1016/j.ijgo.2010.02.005.

91. Krishnan G, D'Silva K, Al-Janadi A. Cetuximab-related tumor lysis syndrome in metastatic colon carcinoma. J Clin Oncol. 2008;26(14):2406–8. https://doi.org/10.1200/JCO.2007.14.7603.

92. Noh GY, Choe DH, Kim CH, Lee JC. Fatal tumor lysis syndrome during radiotherapy for non-small-cell lung cancer. J Clin Oncol. 2008;26(36):6005–6. https://doi.org/10.1200/JCO.2008.19.4308.

93. Cairo MS, Bishop M. Tumour lysis syndrome: new therapeutic strategies and classification. Br J Haematol. 2004;127(1):3–11. https://doi.org/10.1111/j.1365-2141.2004.05094.x.

94. Krakoff IH, Meyer RL. Prevention of hyperuricemia in leukemia and lymphoma: use of Alopurinol, a xanthine oxidase inhibitor. JAMA. 1965;193:1–6. https://doi.org/10.1001/jama.1965.03090010007001.

95. Takai M, Yamauchi T, Ookura M, Matsuda Y, Tai K, Kishi S, Yoshida A, Iwasaki H, Nakamura T, Ueda T. Febuxostat for management of tumor lysis syndrome including its effects on levels of purine metabolites in patients with hematological malignancies—a single institution's, pharmacokinetic and pilot prospective study. Anticancer Res. 2014;34(12):7287–96.

96. Tamura K, Kawai Y, Kiguchi T, Okamoto M, Kaneko M, Maemondo M, Gemba K, Fujimaki K, Kirito K, Goto T, Fujisaki T, Takeda K, Nakajima A, Ueda T. Efficacy and safety of febuxostat for prevention of tumor lysis syndrome in patients with malignant tumors receiving chemotherapy: a phase III, randomized, multi-center trial comparing febuxostat and allopurinol. Int J Clin Oncol. 2016;21(5):996–1003. https://doi.org/10.1007/s10147-016-0971-3.

97. Batterink J, Lin J, Au-Yeung SH, Cessford T. Effectiveness of sodium polystyrene sulfonate for short-term treatment of hyperkalemia. Can J Hosp Pharm. 2015;68(4):296–303. https://doi.org/10.4212/cjhp.v68i4.1469.

98. Peacock WF, Rafique Z, Vishnevskiy K, Michelson E, Vishneva E, Zvereva T, Nahra R, Li D, Miller J. Emergency potassium normalization treatment including sodium zirconium cyclosilicate: a phase II, randomized, double-blind, placebo-controlled study (ENERGIZE). Acad Emerg Med. 2020;27(6):475–86. https://doi.org/10.1111/acem.13954.

99. Clase CM, Carrero JJ, Ellison DH, Grams ME, Hemmelgarn BR, Jardine MJ, Kovesdy CP, Kline GA, Lindner G, Obrador GT, Palmer BF, Cheung M, Wheeler DC, Winkelmayer WC, Pecoits-Filho R, Conference P. Potassium homeostasis and management of dyskalemia in kidney diseases: conclusions from a kidney disease: improving global outcomes (KDIGO)

controversies Conference. Kidney Int. 2020;97(1):42–61. https://doi.org/10.1016/j.kint.2019.09.018.

100. Kosiborod M, Peacock WF, Packham DK. Sodium zirconium cyclosilicate for urgent therapy of severe hyperkalemia. N Engl J Med. 2015;372(16):1577–8. https://doi.org/10.1056/NEJMc1500353.

101. Moussavi K, Fitter S, Gabrielson SW, Koyfman A, Long B. Management of hyperkalemia with insulin and glucose: pearls for the emergency clinician. J Emerg Med. 2019;57(1):36–42. https://doi.org/10.1016/j.jemermed.2019.03.043.

102. Panchal AR, Bartos JA, Cabanas JG, Donnino MW, Drennan IR, Hirsch KG, Kudenchuk PJ, Kurz MC, Lavonas EJ, Morley PT, O'Neil BJ, Peberdy MA, Rittenberger JC, Rodriguez AJ, Sawyer KN, Berg KM, Adult Basic and Advanced Life Support Writing Group. Part 3: Adult basic and advanced life support: 2020 American Heart Association guidelines for cardiopulmonary resuscitation and emergency cardiovascular care. Circulation. 2020;142(16_suppl_2):S366–468. https://doi.org/10.1161/CIR.0000000000000916.

103. Mahfooz K, Sohail H, Gvajaia A, Arif U, Grewal D, Muppidi MR, Vohra V, Tarique A, Vasavada A. Rasburicase in treating tumor lysis syndrome: an umbrella review. Cancer Pathog Ther. 2023;1(4):262–71. https://doi.org/10.1016/j.cpt.2023.07.001.

104. Elitek [package insert]. Bridgewater: Sanofi-Aventis U.S. LLC; 2022.

105. Feng X, Dong K, Pham D, Pence S, Inciardi J, Bhutada NS. Efficacy and cost of single-dose rasburicase in prevention and treatment of adult tumour lysis syndrome: a meta-analysis. J Clin Pharm Ther. 2013;38(4):301–8. https://doi.org/10.1111/jcpt.12061.

106. Hossain S, Naber M, Yacobucci MJ. A retrospective observational study of a low fixed-dose rasburicase protocol for the treatment of tumor lysis syndrome in adults. J Oncol Pharm Pract. 2022;28(6):1326–31. https://doi.org/10.1177/10781552211021147.

107. McDonnell AM, Lenz KL, Frei-Lahr DA, Hayslip J, Hall PD. Single-dose rasburicase 6 mg in the management of tumor lysis syndrome in adults. Pharmacotherapy. 2006;26(6):806–12. https://doi.org/10.1592/phco.26.6.806.

108. Trifilio SM, Pi J, Zook J, Golf M, Coyle K, Greenberg D, Newman D, Koslosky M, Mehta J. Effectiveness of a single 3-mg rasburicase dose for the management of hyperuricemia in patients with hematological malignancies. Bone Marrow Transplant. 2011;46(6):800–5. https://doi.org/10.1038/bmt.2010.212.

109. Yu X, Liu L, Nie X, Li J, Zhang J, Zhao L, Wang X. The optimal single-dose regimen of rasburicase for management of tumour lysis syndrome in children and adults: a systematic review and meta-analysis. J Clin Pharm Ther. 2017;42(1):18–26. https://doi.org/10.1111/jcpt.12479.

110. Pession A, Melchionda F, Castellini C. Pitfalls, prevention, and treatment of hyperuricemia during tumor lysis syndrome in the era of rasburicase (recombinant urate oxidase). Biologics. 2008;2(1):129–41. https://doi.org/10.2147/btt.s1522.

111. Lim E, Bennett P, Beilby J. Sample preparation in patients receiving uric acid oxidase (rasburicase) therapy. Clin Chem. 2003;49(8):1417–9. https://doi.org/10.1373/49.8.1417.

112. Alrahmany D, Omar AF, Al-Maqbali SRS, Harb G, Ghazi IM. Infections in G6PD-deficient hospitalized patients-prevalence, risk factors, and related mortality. Antibiotics (Basel). 2022;11(7):934. https://doi.org/10.3390/antibiotics11070934.

Chapter 36
Alcohol Withdrawal Syndrome

Adrian Wong

36.1 Introduction

Alcohol use disorder (AUD), estimated to occur in 10% of adults within the United States in 2021, is a growing clinical concern due to its associated morbidity and mortality, such as progression to liver damage or failure [1]. During the COVID-pandemic within the United States, the frequency of alcohol ingestion and heavy drinking increased significantly, especially in younger patients, females, and non-Hispanic White populations [2]. As the incidence of AUD grows, so will the number of patients who potentially develop alcohol withdrawal syndrome (AWS), which occurs due to a decrease in alcohol consumption (e.g., cessation) which the body has relied on to maintain homeostasis. Given the morbidity and mortality associated with AWS, it is important for the pharmacist to be aware of risk factors for AWS that predict severity, identify AWS in the critically ill, and understand the therapies that have been shown to be effective for management of AWS.

36.2 Epidemiology

The incidence of AWS within the inpatient setting is variable, ranging from 1 to 32%, which is dependent on the primary admission diagnosis and clinical setting (e.g., ward, intensive care unit [ICU]) [3, 4]. The development of AWS during hospitalization increases the risk of infectious complications (e.g., pneumonia), need for mechanical ventilation, and need for ICU admission, along with increased mortality [4]. It is challenging to identify AWS in the critically ill for multiple reasons,

A. Wong (✉)
Beth Israel Deaconess Medical Center, Boston, MA, USA
e-mail: awong7@bidmc.harvard.edu

© The Author(s), under exclusive license to Springer Nature Switzerland AG 2025

Y. Alzaidi, M. A. Gebily (eds.), *The Pharmacist's Expanded Role in Critical Care Medicine*, https://doi.org/10.1007/978-3-031-77335-8_36

including the inability to ask patients about their alcohol use and disease states that may mimic the presentation of AWS, such as ICU delirium.

36.2.1 Definitions

The epidemiology of AWS depends on the study's definition, which may also factor in severity of symptoms. In an effort to standardize research on AWS within the critically ill, the American Thoracic Society defines severe AWS (SAWS) as, "A progressive state of central nervous system hyperexcitation due to reduction or cessation of alcohol use resulting in severe signs and symptoms of hyperautonomia and hyperactive delirium" [5]. Other definitions that have been used to determine severity of AWS include score thresholds (e.g., Clinical Institute Withdrawal Assessment for Alcohol Scale Revised ≥15) or how much benzodiazepine (BZD) is needed to manage symptoms. Resistant alcohol withdrawal (RAW), defined as the requirement of at least 40 mg of diazepam equivalents in 1 h, has been proposed [6, 7]. Having a clear definition of AWS used within studies allows for improved generalizability and to understand the severity of AWS in a study population.

36.3 Pathophysiology

Neuroadaptations that occur from chronic alcohol use affect the balance of γ-aminobutyric acid (GABA) and glutamate. These adaptations allow for "normal" functioning despite abnormal number and function of these receptors. When alcohol intake is decreased in patients (e.g., access to alcohol, illness, hospital admission) who have had these neuroadaptations, this increases the risk of AWS, since homeostasis is now altered. The serum level of alcohol that a patient experiences initial signs of AWS will differ by the patient. The resultant decrease in alcohol leads to less inhibition via GABA agonism, causing an imbalance with excitatory glutamate and leading to the symptomatology of AWS. It is also suspected that repeated episodes of AWS leads to the phenomenon of "kindling," which increases future risk for AWS [8]. Kindling is the process where repeated insult leads to neuroadaptations that sensitize to future insults. Although largely supported by experimental models which have found that AWS leads to decreased seizure threshold, clinical data suggest that the incidence of AWS seizures were associated with prior withdrawal [9, 10].

Additional mechanisms of AWS that are being evaluated include chemokine ligand 2, corticotropin-releasing factor, and interleukin-6, which may serve as future therapeutic targets for management of AWS.

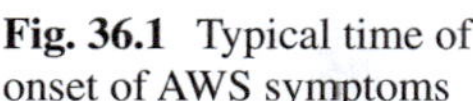

Fig. 36.1 Typical time of onset of AWS symptoms

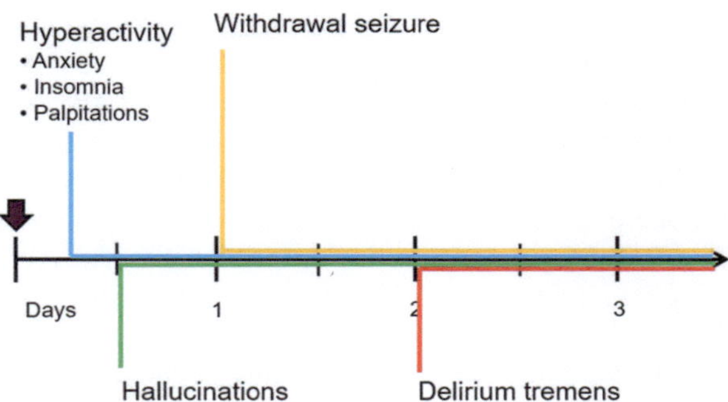

36.4 Symptoms

The symptomatology of AWS varies by patient, ranging from hemodynamic changes from autonomic symptoms, to delirium and seizures, and most severely delirium tremens. The typical time to onset is described in Fig. 36.1, with AWS typically resolving within 5–7 days of onset [11]. Therefore, it is important to determine a patient's last alcohol intake, when possible.

Data suggest that there are sex differences in symptomatology of AWS, with males more frequently exhibiting signs of seizures and delirium tremens (DTs) than females [12]. Patient who develop AWS seizures are associated with a 13-fold increase in mortality than a general patient population [13]. A history of DTs or AWS seizures, alcohol level on admission (>13 mg/dL), highest CIWA-Ar (>16.5) are associated with increased risk of need for ICU admission for management of AWS [14].

36.5 Diagnosis

The early diagnosis of AWS is needed to prevent further morbidity and mortality. Challenges, specifically in the critically ill include that patients may not be able to verbalize their alcohol intake and its symptomatology representing other commonly seen syndromes in the critically ill.

36.5.1 Predicting Severity of AWS

Within the ICU, multiple methods of evaluating risk for AWS have been used, including the potential severity of symptoms. Common risk factors include history of AWS including the spectrum of AWS symptoms, and laboratory markers indicating chronic liver disease (e.g., thrombocytopenia, elevated liver enzymes). There are growing data identifying risk factors for AWS, specifically more severe AWS, which is harder to manage than general AWS (Table 36.1).

One of the most recent tools that has been developed is the Prediction of Alcohol Withdrawal Severity (PAWSS) [15]. The PAWSS was developed using a systematic literature search and was subsequently refined in an internal medicine population. The PAWSS primarily relies on prior history of AWS as well as AUD, but also includes clinical data of blood alcohol level as well as signs of autonomic activity. This tool uses a score of four as a threshold to determine if a patient is at high risk for moderate to severe AWS. A subsequent study found that the sensitivity of the tool was 93%, while its specificity was 99.5% [17].

36.5.2　AWS Scoring Tools: CIWA-Ar, mMINDS, SEWS

There are multiple diagnostic tools that have been used for AWS, which include the most common, the Clinical Institute Withdrawal Assessment for Alcohol Scale Revised (CIWA-Ar), as well as the modified Minnesota Detoxification Scale (mMINDS) and the Severity of Ethanol Withdrawal Scale (SEWS) [18–20]. A study comparing these three tools in the ICU found that clinical correlations by nurses were similar although the mMINDS was considered the easiest to use [21]. Limitations of the three aforementioned diagnostic tools is its reliance on

Table 36.1 Summary of risk factors that predict severe AWS

PAWSS [15]
– Recent intoxication within past 30 days
– Prior AWS
– Prior withdrawal seizures
– Prior delirium tremens
– Prior alcohol rehabilitation treatment
– Prior alcohol-related blackout
– Concomitant use of "downers" within past 90 days (e.g., barbiturates, BZDs)
– Concomitant abuse of other substances within past 90 days
– Positive blood alcohol level (>200 mg/dL)
– Evidence of autonomic activity (e.g., HR >120, tremor, sweating, agitation, nausea)
Resistant alcohol withdrawal [16]
– Younger age
– Male sex
– Non-Hispanic White race
– History of psychiatric illness
– Higher serum ethanol concentration
– Alanine transaminase, aspartate transaminase above normal reference range
– Thrombocytopenia
– Hypochloremia
– Hypokalemia

PAWSS Prediction of Alcohol Withdrawal Severity

patient-reported symptoms, which may not be possible in ICU patients, the difficulty in differentiating AWS from other diagnoses that may be common in the ICU, such as ICU delirium, as well as reliance on vital signs, which may be affected by a patient's disease states, as well as medications. One alternative that has been proposed is the use of sedation scale scores, which are commonly used in patients who are mechanically ventilated [22]. This study found that CIWA-Ar was only performed in 56% of patients, while the Richmond Agitation Sedation Scale (RASS) score was performed in 94% of patients. They also found that both mechanically ventilated and Black patients were less likely to have a CIWA-Ar performed.

36.6 Prevention and Treatment

The management of AWS includes prevention (e.g., early identification of patients at risk), as well as treatment, which should involve medications that target underlying pathophysiology. Additionally, early identification of AWS is important to prevent progression to more severe manifestations, such as DTs. A large challenge within the critically ill is differentiating AWS symptoms from other syndromes that may mimic AWS, such as ICU delirium, metabolic encephalopathy, sepsis, or withdrawal from other substances. There is no specific test to evaluate if AWS is occurring but the framework in Fig. 36.2 may be helpful in identifying AWS compared to other mimics.

Some medications that have been evaluated for the prevention of issues associated with AUD such as AWS include baclofen [23]. This trial found that high-dose baclofen (dosed based on renal function) was associated with a decrease in agitation-related events in mechanically ventilated patients, compared to placebo. Despite this benefit, baclofen was associated with longer duration of mechanical ventilation and ICU length of stay, as well as increased risk of delayed awakening (defined as no eye opening at 72 h of cessation of sedation).

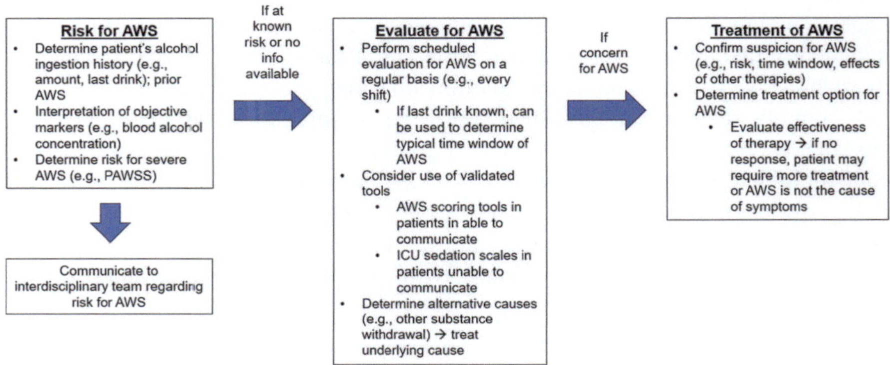

Fig. 36.2 Framework of identification of potential AWS in critically ill patients. *AWS* alcohol withdrawal syndrome, *ICU* intensive care unit, *PAWSS* Prediction of Alcohol Withdrawal

The management of AWS has been shown to be variable, including a multicenter cohort study evaluating treatment of RAW and a survey of critical care pharmacists [11, 24]. The multicenter cohort study found that 16 unique medications were identified in clinical documentation to have been used for AWS, with a total of 74 different combinations of medications used. The survey showed variation in institutional AWS guidelines, preferred first-line treatment, and when therapies were used, including phenobarbital and dexmedetomidine [24].

36.6.1 Medications Targeting Underlying Pathophysiology

The treatment of AWS relies on GABA agonists, with BZDs being a prominent first-line option. However, growing data suggest the use of other agents that may be more beneficial than BZDs in patients with severe AWS, such as phenobarbital and ketamine. A summary of non-BZD medications that target the underlying pathophysiology of AWS is detailed in Table 36.2, describing their mechanism, studied dosing, and treatment considerations based on published literature.

36.6.1.1 Benzodiazepines

BZDs are generally used as first-line therapy for management of AWS due to significant data supporting this practice [40]. The choice of BZD is dependent on considerations such as medication availability, route of administration, pharmacokinetics, and hepatic function, with diazepam and lorazepam the most frequently studied. Drug shortages are an increasing issue, which has affected BZDs, such as lorazepam. Certain BZDs (e.g., chlordiazepoxide) are only available enterally, which may be a limitation in patients who are altered from their AWS. BZDs have variable pharmacokinetics, including onset and duration of action, half-life, and hepatic metabolism. The BZDs of lorazepam, oxazepam, and temazepam are hepatically metabolized through glucuronidation rather than oxidation, which is more preserved with hepatic dysfunction that may exist in patients with AUD [41]. Finally, dosing strategies of BZDs differ by institution, although data suggest that a symptom-triggered strategy (e.g., based on CIWA), is associated with equivalent outcomes but decreased BZD doses, duration of therapy, and decreased risk of oversedation, compared to fixed-schedule regimens [42–44]. Overall, BZD as first-line therapy may be appropriate for patients without a history of AWS complications (e.g., delirium, seizure), with a symptom-triggered approach to prevent risk of oversedation.

Table 36.2 Non-BZD medications that target the underlying pathophysiology of AWS

Medication	Mechanism	Studied dosing	Comments
Ethanol [25–27]	– GABA$_A$ agonist – NMDA inhibitor	– 200 mL of 100% ethanol; titrated up to 600 mL – 10% ethanol infusion started at 50 mL/h; titrated to 30% ethanol for up to 48 h	– Generally not well tolerated, with risk of oversedation – Highly variable kinetics results in difficult dose titration – Studied primarily in prevention of AWS, not treatment
Ketamine [28–30]	– NMDA antagonist	– 0.3–1.6 mg/kg/h, with optional loading dose	– Low risk for respiratory depression; does not require mechanical ventilation – Effect on catecholamine reuptake leading to hypertension and tachycardia and mimic signs of AWS – Studied as adjunct therapy
Phenobarbital [6, 31–34]	– GABA$_A$ agonist – AMPA inhibitor	– Loading dose of 6–15 mg/kg IV – Escalating doses of 65 mg, 130 mg, 260 mg IV	– Targets glutamate receptors, allowing for targeting of multiple mechanisms of AWS – Synergistic effects with BZDs due to different effect (i.e., duration of chloride channel opening) on GABA$_A$ receptors – Considerations of drug interactions given CYP metabolism induction
Propofol [35–39]	– GABA$_A$ agonist – NMDA inhibitor	– 10–100 mcg/kg/min	– Fast onset and offset of action – Causes respiratory depression, requiring mechanical ventilation during use – Causes bradycardia and hypotension which may affect certain AWS scoring tools – Adverse effects include hypertriglyceridemia, propofol-related infusion syndrome

AMPA α-amino-3-hydroxy-5-methyl-4-isoxazolepropionic acid

36.6.1.2 Phenobarbital

A therapy that has seen increased interest for AWS is phenobarbital (PHB). Dosing strategies for PHB are quite variable, including the focus on a front-loaded dose compared to the use intermittent dosing. Data suggest benefit of the front-loaded strategy compared to lower dosing. A PHB taper has also been studied, although the long half-life of PHB may not require this strategy and prolong its effects, including its impact on induction of CYP drug metabolism [45]. Outcomes PHB has been studied to be beneficial in have included reduced need for ICU admission, need for mechanical ventilation, need for physical restraints, hospital length of stay, and rate of ED readmission within 3 days [6, 46–49]. Data is limited in its role in patients with neurologic injury due to their exclusion from existing studies, which may be due to its concern for oversedation, given its long half-life, as well as drug interactions such as nimodipine used in patients with subarachnoid hemorrhage. Additionally, given its hepatic metabolism, limited data exist regarding optimal dosing regimens for patients with chronic liver disease, which may require lower doses.

36.6.2   Medications Not Targeting Underlying Pathophysiology

Many medications have been evaluated for the management of AWS that do not target the underlying pathophysiology of AWS (i.e., GABA, glutamate) (see Table 36.3). The use of a BZD-sparing protocol using clonidine, dexmedetomidine, gabapentin, and valproic acid was associated with decreased need for BZDs, need for ICU admission, hospital mortality and length of stay, and need for 30-day readmission, with certain beneficial outcomes persisting even at 1-year post-protocol implementation [75].

The use of dexmedetomidine has been associated with decreased use of BZDs although data is inconsistent regarding the benefit. The retrospective EvADE study found that adjunct dexmedetomidine did not reduce CIWA-Ar from baseline and increased need for BZDs, ICU length of stay and need for physical restraints [76]. One issue with the use of dexmedetomidine, which has been studied as first-line therapy for AWS is its lack of GABA-agonist activity, which has been associated with risk of seizures since it does not target the underlying pathophysiology of AWS.

36.6.3   Pharmacogenomics

Although data are limited, one potential explanation for the variable effect of certain medications used for AWS (e.g., dexmedetomidine, diazepam) may be explained by pharmacogenomics. Studies evaluating the effect of CYP3A4 polymorphisms on diazepam response have found that polymorphisms affect therapeutic concentrations which lead to better efficacy or increased risk of adverse events [77, 78]. CYP2A6 polymorphisms have been associated with decreased metabolism, leading to increased plasma concentrations of dexmedetomidine and increasing the risk of adverse effects [79].

Table 36.3 Non-BZD medications that do not target the underlying pathophysiology of AWS

Medication	Mechanism	Studied dosing	Comments
Baclofen [23, 50]	– GABA$_B$ agonist	– 10 mg enterally three times daily	– Short duration of action – Only available in enteral form – Accumulates with renal dysfunction
Carbamazepine [51–53]	– Inhibition of voltage-sensitive Na and/or Ca channels → Stabilizes neuronal membranes	– 400–4725 mg/day – Sustained release form: 200 mg three times daily; 400 mg twice daily	– Limited data suggest similar efficacy to BZDs and barbiturates – Induction of CYP metabolism; self-inducer
Clonidine [54, 55]	– α_2-agonist	– Enteral: up to 0.6 mg daily – IV: 0.5–2.8 mcg/kg/h infusion	– Available in different formulations (dependent on country) – May be beneficial in patients withdrawing from other substances – May mask autonomic abnormalities without affecting underlying pathophysiology of AWS – Causes bradycardia and hypotension which may affect certain AWS scoring tools
Dexmedetomidine [35, 56–61]	– Selective α_2-agonist	– 0.2–1.5 mcg/kg/h (optional loading dose, although generally associated w/hemodynamic instability)	– Data suggest effective in ↓ BZD requirements, ↓ hospital and ICU length of stay – May be beneficial in patients withdrawing from other substances – May mask autonomic abnormalities without affecting underlying pathophysiology of AWS – Causes bradycardia and hypotension which may affect certain AWS scoring tools – Seizures reported in patients who have not received GABA agonists

(continued)

Table 36.3 (continued)

Medication	Mechanism	Studied dosing	Comments
Gabapentin [62–66]	– Inhibition of voltage-sensitive Ca channels → Stabilizes neuronal membranes	– 600 mg enterally every 8 h w/ optional load (800–1200 mg once); taper over 5 days	– Data suggest effective in ↓ BZD requirements, ↓ hospital and ICU length of stay – Only available in enteral form – Potential drug of abuse – Accumulates with renal dysfunction
Levetiracetam [67–69]	– Unclear (potentially indirect modulation of GABA signaling)	– 500 mg enterally twice daily	– Limited data to suggest benefit in AWS – Generally well-tolerated although may cause agitation that may mimic adrenergic signs of AWS
Oxcarbazepine [52, 70]	– Inhibition of voltage-sensitive Na and/or Ca channels → Stabilizes neuronal membranes	– 200 mg enterally three times daily ×72 h → 300 mg daily	– Only available in enteral form – Increased risk of hyponatremia than carbamazepine – Less drug interactions than carbamazepine
Pregabalin [71]	– Inhibition of voltage-sensitive Na and/or Ca channels → Stabilizes neuronal membranes	– 150 mg enterally twice daily ×48 h → taper 100 mg every other day	– Limited data to suggest benefit in AWS – Only available in enteral form – Not hepatically metabolized
Valproic acid [72–74]	– Inhibition of voltage-sensitive Na channels → Stabilizes neuronal membranes – Binding to presynaptic $GABA_B$ receptors → ↑ release of GABA – Activation of glutamic acid decarboxylase → ↑ GABA synthesis	– Immediate release: 400 mg enterally every 8 h – Sustained release: 300 mg enterally three to four times daily; 500 mg enterally three times daily	– Data suggest ↓ duration of AWS treatment and hospital length of stay – Hepatic metabolism – Adverse effects include hyperammonemia, thrombocytopenia, transaminase elevation

36.7 Adjunctive Therapies

36.7.1 Thiamine

The role of thiamine in patients with AUD is to treat deficiency to prevent the onset of Wernicke-Korsakoff syndrome, which may cause permanent memory impairment [80]. Multiple mechanisms may be responsible for this deficiency in patients with AUD, such as poor nutritional diet, impaired absorption or storage. Although thiamine deficiency in this population is well known and supplementation is recommended by guidelines, data suggest that approximately 40% of patients with alcohol withdrawal do not receive thiamine within a critically ill population [44, 81]. Data is inconsistent in regard to how thiamine should be given, including the route and dose [80].

One controversy is whether thiamine should be given before glucose in patients with concern for Wernicke-Korsakoff syndrome. The theoretical concern is that administration of glucose in a thiamine-deficient patient will lead to further depletion of thiamine, potentially exacerbating encephalopathy or developing lactate through anaerobic metabolism [82]. Data supporting this mechanism are limited, with data suggesting that this is not of clinical concern in a retrospective cohort study evaluating clinical outcomes such as Glasgow Coma Scale scores [83]. A delay in providing therapy for hypoglycemia, especially in patients who are symptomatic, may cause a more significant impact on patient outcomes, compared to waiting for thiamine to be administered first [82].

Limited data support an optimal route or dose of thiamine. Although historically believed that thiamine has poor bioavailability and has saturable absorption, one study found that oral thiamine at doses up to 1500 mg resulted in rapid absorption that was not saturable [84]. However, it should be noted that this was performed in healthy subjects, which limits the ability to extrapolate to critically ill patient populations which are more likely to have impaired organ function and pharmacokinetics. A commonly recommended dose of 500 mg three times daily is used but does not have much clinical basis in evaluating published literature. Data from a Cochrane review also were not able to determine an appropriate dose, route, frequency, or duration of therapy [80]. A randomized controlled trial evaluated patients for the prevention and treatment of Wernicke-Korsakoff syndrome in Australia, comparing multiple parenteral doses of thiamine for 5 days using standardized cognitive assessment tools [85]. The authors found no differences in cognitive assessments or neurological symptoms in either the prevention or treatment arms by dosing strategy. This trial illustrates the difficulties in determining the clinical effects of thiamine on this syndrome, with it being underpowered as a challenge in meeting its targeted sample size.

Overall, thiamine is a generally well-tolerated medication with small risk of harm, namely that of injection site reactions, which occur in <1% of patients even with doses as high as 500 mg administered via intravenous push [86]. However, parenteral thiamine shortages have occurred over time, which may limit availability.

Therefore, it is important for continued research to occur in this area to evaluate the most appropriate dose, route, frequency, and duration of therapy, which will likely be patient-specific.

36.7.2 Alcohol Use Disorder

Although this chapter is focused on the management of AWS, it is extremely important that patients with AUD are connected with therapy and resources to prevent further episodes of AWS. Data evaluating severity of AUD has also demonstrated associations of severe AUD with higher risk of AWS than those with mild-to-moderate AUD (68.3 vs. 4.2%) [87]. Data suggest that patients who develop AWS are often not started (<10%) on medications for AUD (MAUD) at hospital discharge [88, 89]. Data support the role of the pharmacist in initiating therapy for AUD. A recent systematic review and meta-analysis of clinical trials found that naltrexone (at a dose of 50 mg daily) and acamprosate were significantly associated with improved outcomes compared to placebo [90]. Available guidance for the management of AUD includes the Canadian 2023 guidelines [91].

36.8 Research Gaps

Despite the growing data on the management of AWS, many research gaps exist, some of which are discussed in the 2021 American Thoracic Society research statement on AWS. Some prime areas of future research include additional therapies for the management of AWS, focused on non-GABA and glutamate therapies. The role of PHB needs further research despite its growing interest, including dosing strategies dependent on patient-specific characteristics (e.g., risk of oversedation, liver or neurologic injury) and its impact on clinically relevant drug interactions. Limited data show how to best implement strategies to manage SAWS at population level, with the need to engaged key stakeholders. Additionally, use of trial networks, such as those that have been used for COVID-19, would be beneficial at studying more generalizable therapeutic strategies for AWS and AUD.

36.9 Role of the Pharmacist

The role of the pharmacist in the management of AWS is multifactorial. This includes identifying patients at risk of AWS, risk for severe AWS, determining appropriate therapies for AWS, and connecting patients with therapies and resources for AUD. Staying up-to-date on medication therapies for AWS is another important role, which also includes education of the medical teams on which therapies should be considered for a patient, based on patient-specific characteristics.

36.10 Conclusion

The management of AWS in the critically ill continues to have constant updates in literature, including risk factors and therapies for AWS. Pharmacists play a critical role in the management of AWS through their knowledge of medication therapies that are most appropriate for a patient.

References

1. Section 5 PE tables—Results from the 2021 National Survey on Drug Use and Health: detailed tables, SAMHSA, CBHSQ. https://www.samhsa.gov/data/sites/default/files/reports/rpt39441/NSDUHDetailedTabs2021/NSDUHDetailedTabs2021/NSDUHDetTabsSect5pe2021.htm#tab5.6b. Accessed 29 Oct 2023.
2. Pollard MS, Tucker JS, Green HD Jr. Changes in adult alcohol use and consequences during the COVID-19 pandemic in the US. JAMA Netw Open. 2020;3(9):e2022942. https://doi.org/10.1001/jamanetworkopen.2020.22942.
3. Ahmed N, Kuo Y. Risk of alcohol withdrawal syndrome in hospitalized trauma patients: a national data analysis. Injury. 2022;53(1):44–8. https://doi.org/10.1016/j.injury.2021.08.017.
4. Marti-Aguado D, Gougol A, Gomez-Medina C, et al. Prevalence and clinical impact of alcohol withdrawal syndrome in alcohol-associated hepatitis and the potential role of prophylaxis: a multinational, retrospective cohort study. EClinicalMedicine. 2023;61:102046. https://doi.org/10.1016/j.eclinm.2023.102046.
5. Steel TL, Afshar M, Edwards S, et al. Research needs for inpatient management of severe alcohol withdrawal syndrome: an official American Thoracic Society research statement. Am J Respir Crit Care Med. 2021;204(7):e61–87. https://doi.org/10.1164/rccm.202108-1845ST.
6. Gold JA, Rimal B, Nolan A, Nelson LS. A strategy of escalating doses of benzodiazepines and phenobarbital administration reduces the need for mechanical ventilation in delirium tremens*. Crit Care Med. 2007;35(3):724–30. https://doi.org/10.1097/01.CCM.0000256841.28351.80.
7. Hack JB, Hoffman RS, Nelson LS. Resistant alcohol withdrawal: does an unexpectedly large sedative requirement identify these patients early? J Med Toxicol. 2006;2(2):55–60. https://doi.org/10.1007/BF03161171.
8. Goddard GV. The kindling model of epilepsy. Trends Neurosci. 1983;6:275–9. https://doi.org/10.1016/0166-2236(83)90118-2.
9. Alberto GE, Klorig DC, Goldstein AT, Godwin DW. Alcohol withdrawal produces changes in excitability, population discharge probability, and seizure threshold. Alcohol Clin Exp Res. 2023;47(2):211–8. https://doi.org/10.1111/acer.15004.
10. Brown ME, Anton RF, Malcolm R, Ballenger JC. Alcohol detoxification and withdrawal seizures: clinical support for a kindling hypothesis. Biol Psychiatry. 1988;23(5):507–14. https://doi.org/10.1016/0006-3223(88)90023-6.
11. Wong A, Benedict NJ, Kane-Gill SL. Multicenter evaluation of pharmacologic management and outcomes associated with severe resistant alcohol withdrawal. J Crit Care. 2015;30(2):405–9. https://doi.org/10.1016/j.jcrc.2014.10.008.

12. Frontiers | Sex difference in alcohol withdrawal syndrome: a scoping review of clinical studies. https://www.frontiersin.org/articles/10.3389/fpsyt.2023.1266424/full. Accessed 8 Nov 2023.

13. Sansone G. Long-term outcome of alcohol withdrawal seizures. Eur J Neurol—Wiley Online Library. https://onlinelibrary.wiley.com/doi/10.1111/ene.16075. Accessed 8 Nov 2023.

14. Mohan G, Bhide P, Abu-Shanab A, et al. Predictors of escalation to intensive care unit level of care among admissions for alcohol withdrawal. J Community Hosp Intern Med Perspect. 2023;13(5):8. https://doi.org/10.55729/2000-9666.1241.

15. Maldonado JR, Sher Y, Ashouri JF, et al. The "prediction of alcohol withdrawal severity scale" (PAWSS): systematic literature review and pilot study of a new scale for the prediction of complicated alcohol withdrawal syndrome. Alcohol. 2014;48(4):375–90. https://doi.org/10.1016/j.alcohol.2014.01.004.

16. Benedict NJ, Wong A, Cassidy E, et al. Predictors of resistant alcohol withdrawal (RAW): a retrospective case-control study. Drug Alcohol Depend. 2018;192:303–8. https://doi.org/10.1016/j.drugalcdep.2018.08.017.

17. Maldonado JR, Sher Y, Das S, et al. Prospective validation study of the prediction of alcohol withdrawal severity scale (PAWSS) in medically ill inpatients: a new scale for the prediction of complicated alcohol withdrawal syndrome. Alcohol Alcohol. 2015;50(5):509–18. https://doi.org/10.1093/alcalc/agv043.

18. Sullivan JT, Sykora K, Schneiderman J, Naranjo CA, Sellers EM. Assessment of alcohol withdrawal: the revised clinical institute withdrawal assessment for alcohol scale (CIWA-Ar). Br J Addict. 1989;84(11):1353–7. https://doi.org/10.1111/j.1360-0443.1989.tb00737.x.

19. DeCarolis DD, Rice KL, Ho L, Willenbring ML, Cassaro S. Symptom-driven lorazepam protocol for treatment of severe alcohol withdrawal delirium in the intensive care unit. Pharmacother J Hum Pharmacol Drug Ther. 2007;27(4):510–8. https://doi.org/10.1592/phco.27.4.510.

20. Beresford T, Anderson M, Pitts B, et al. The severity of ethanol withdrawal scale in scale-driven alcohol withdrawal treatment: a quality assurance study. Alcohol Treat Q. 2017;35(3):232–42. https://doi.org/10.1080/07347324.2017.1322418.

21. Bradley M, Kiser TH, Mueller SW, Reynolds PM, MacLaren R. Correlation between and nursing satisfaction with CIWA-Ar, mMINDS, and SEWS scoring tools for the assessment of severe alcohol withdrawal syndrome in ICU patients. 2023. https://journals.sagepub.com/doi/1 0.1177/10600280221102562?url_ver=Z39.88-2003&rfr_id=ori:rid:crossref.org&rfr_dat=cr_ pub%20%200pubmed. Accessed 11 Oct 2023.

22. Steel TL, Giovanni SP, Katsandres SC, et al. Should the CIWA-Ar be the standard monitoring strategy for alcohol withdrawal syndrome in the intensive care unit? Addict Sci Clin Pract. 2021;16(1):21. https://doi.org/10.1186/s13722-021-00226-w.

23. Vourc'h M, Garret C, Gacouin A, et al. Effect of high-dose baclofen on agitation-related events among patients with unhealthy alcohol use receiving mechanical ventilation: a randomized clinical trial. JAMA. 2021;325(8):732–41. https://doi.org/10.1001/jama.2021.0658.

24. Cucci MD, Palm N, Vazquez D, Mullen C, Heavner MS. Survey of critical care practices for alcohol withdrawal syndrome in the intensive care unit. JACCP J Am Coll Clin Pharm. 2022;5(9):950–8. https://doi.org/10.1002/jac5.1674.

25. Fullwood JE, Mostaghimi Z, Granger CB, et al. Alcohol withdrawal prevention: a randomized evaluation of lorazepam and ethanol (AWARE) pilot study. Am J Crit Care. 2013;22(5):398–406. https://doi.org/10.4037/ajcc2013283.

26. Gipson G, Tran K, Hoang C, Treggiari M. Comparison of enteral ethanol and benzodiazepines for alcohol withdrawal in neurocritical care patients. J Clin Neurosci. 2016;31:88–91. https://doi.org/10.1016/j.jocn.2016.02.028.

27. Weinberg JA, Magnotti LJ, Fischer PE, et al. Comparison of intravenous ethanol versus diazepam for alcohol withdrawal prophylaxis in the trauma ICU: results of a randomized trial. J Trauma Acute Care Surg. 2008;64(1):99. https://doi.org/10.1097/TA.0b013e31815eb12a.

28. Wong A, Benedict NJ, Armahizer MJ, Kane-Gill SL. Evaluation of adjunctive ketamine to benzodiazepines for management of alcohol withdrawal syndrome. Ann Pharmacother. 2015;49(1):14–9. https://doi.org/10.1177/1060028014555859.

29. Pizon AF, Lynch MJ, Benedict NJ, et al. Adjunct ketamine use in the management of severe ethanol withdrawal. Crit Care Med. 2018;46(8):e768. https://doi.org/10.1097/CCM.0000000000003204.

30. Shah P, McDowell M, Ebisu R, Hanif T, Toerne T. Adjunctive use of ketamine for benzodiazepine-resistant severe alcohol withdrawal: a retrospective evaluation. J Med Toxicol. 2018;14(3):229–36. https://doi.org/10.1007/s13181-018-0662-8.

31. Rosenson J, Clements C, Simon B, et al. Phenobarbital for acute alcohol withdrawal: a prospective randomized double-blind placebo-controlled study. J Emerg Med. 2013;44(3):592–598. e2. https://doi.org/10.1016/j.jemermed.2012.07.056.

32. Oks M, Cleven KL, Healy L, Wei M, Narasimhan M, Mayo PH, Kohn N, Koenig S. The safety and utility of phenobarbital use for the treatment of severe alcohol withdrawal syndrome in the medical intensive care unit. 2020. https://journals.sagepub.com/doi/10.1177/0885066618783947?url_ver=Z39.88-2003&rfr_id=ori:rid:crossref.org&rfr_dat=cr_pub%20%200pubmed. Accessed 8 Nov 2023.

33. Nelson AC, Kehoe J, Sankoff J, Mintzer D, Taub J, Kaucher KA. Benzodiazepines vs barbiturates for alcohol withdrawal: analysis of 3 different treatment protocols. Am J Emerg Med. 2019;37(4):733–6. https://doi.org/10.1016/j.ajem.2019.01.002.

34. Tidwell WP, Thomas TL, Pouliot JD, Canonico AE, Webber AJ. Treatment of alcohol withdrawal syndrome: phenobarbital vs CIWA-Ar protocol. Am J Crit Care. 2018;27(6):454–60. https://doi.org/10.4037/ajcc2018745.

35. Lizotte RJ, Kappes JA, Bartel BJ, Hayes KM, Lesselyoung VL. Evaluating the effects of dexmedetomidine compared to propofol as adjunctive therapy in patients with alcohol withdrawal. Clin Pharmacol Adv Appl. 2014;6:171–7. https://doi.org/10.2147/CPAA.S70490.

36. Wong A, Benedict NJ, Lohr BR, Pizon AF, Kane-Gill SL. Management of benzodiazepine-resistant alcohol withdrawal across a healthcare system: benzodiazepine dose-escalation with or without propofol. Drug Alcohol Depend. 2015;154:296–9. https://doi.org/10.1016/j.drugalcdep.2015.07.005.

37. Ludtke KA, Stanley KS, Yount NL, Gerkin RD. Retrospective review of critically ill patients experiencing alcohol withdrawal: dexmedetomidine versus propofol and/or lorazepam continuous infusions. Hosp Pharm. 2015;50(3):208–13. https://doi.org/10.1310/hpj5003-208.

38. Sohraby R, Attridge RL, Hughes DW. Use of propofol-containing versus benzodiazepine regimens for alcohol withdrawal requiring mechanical ventilation. Ann Pharmacother. 2014;48(4):456–61. https://doi.org/10.1177/1060028013515846.

39. Use of propofol infusion in alcohol withdrawal-induced refractory delirium tremens | Ugeskriftet.dk. https://ugeskriftet.dk/dmj/use-propofol-infusion-alcohol-withdrawal-induced-refractory-delirium-tremens. Accessed 8 Nov 2023.

40. Benzodiazepines for alcohol withdrawal. https://doi.org/10.1002/14651858.CD005063.pub3.

41. Peppers MP. Benzodiazepines for alcohol withdrawal in the elderly and in patients with liver disease. Pharmacother J Hum Pharmacol Drug Ther. 1996;16(1):49–58. https://doi.org/10.1002/j.1875-9114.1996.tb02915.x.

42. Daeppen JB, Gache P, Landry U, et al. Symptom-triggered vs fixed-schedule doses of benzodiazepine for alcohol withdrawal: a randomized treatment trial. Arch Intern Med. 2002;162(10):1117–21. https://doi.org/10.1001/archinte.162.10.1117.

43. Holleck JL, Merchant N, Gunderson CG. Symptom-triggered therapy for alcohol withdrawal syndrome: a systematic review and meta-analysis of randomized controlled trials. J Gen Intern Med. 2019;34(6):1018–24. https://doi.org/10.1007/s11606-019-04899-7.

44. The ASAM clinical practice guideline on alcohol withdrawal management. J Addict Med. https://journals.lww.com/journaladdictionmedicine/fulltext/2020/06001/the_asam_clinical_practice_guideline_on_alcohol.1.aspx. Accessed 24 Oct 2023.

45. Thaller M, Wong A, Yankama T, Eche IM, Elsamadisi P. Evaluation of clinical outcomes associated with phenobarbital with taper compared to no taper for the management of alcohol withdrawal syndrome. 2024. https://journals.sagepub.com/doi/abs/10.1177/10600280241236412. Accessed 28 Mar 2024.

46. Lebin JA, Mudan A, Murphy CE, Wang RC, Smollin CG. Return encounters in emergency department patients treated with phenobarbital versus benzodiazepines for alcohol withdrawal. J Med Toxicol. 2022;18(1):4–10. https://doi.org/10.1007/s13181-021-00863-2.
47. Shah P, Stegner K, Rachid M, Hanif T, Dodd KW. Front-loaded phenobarbital dosing is associated with a lower incidence of mechanical ventilation in patients with severe alcohol withdrawal. In: B105. Critical care: counterparts—Non-pulmonary critical care and multi-organ failure. American Thoracic Society international conference abstracts. American Thoracic Society; 2019:A4144. https://doi.org/10.1164/ajrccm-conference.2019.199.1_MeetingAbstracts.A4144.
48. Bosch NA, Crable EL, Ackerbauer KA, et al. Implementation of a phenobarbital-based pathway for severe alcohol withdrawal: a mixed-method study. Ann Am Thorac Soc. 2021;18(10):1708–16. https://doi.org/10.1513/AnnalsATS.202102-121OC.
49. Bosch NA, Law AC, Walkey AJ. Phenobarbital for severe alcohol withdrawal syndrome: a multicenter retrospective cohort study. Am J Respir Crit Care Med. 2022;206(9):1171–4. https://doi.org/10.1164/rccm.202203-0466LE.
50. Lyon JE. Treating alcohol withdrawal with oral baclofen: a randomized, double-blind, placebo-controlled trial. J Hosp Med—Wiley Online Library. 2011. https://shmpublications.onlinelibrary.wiley.com/doi/10.1002/jhm.928. Accessed 8 Nov 2023.
51. Stuppaeck CH, Pycha R, Miller C, Whitworth AB, Oberbauer H, Fleischhacker WW. Carbamazepine versus oxazepam in the treatment of alcohol withdrawal: a double-blind study. Alcohol Alcohol. 1992;27(2):153–8. https://doi.org/10.1093/oxfordjournals.alcalc.a045214.
52. Schik G, Wedegaertner F, Liersch J, Hoy L, Emrich H, Schneider U. Oxcarbazepine versus carbamazepine in the treatment of alcohol withdrawal. Addict Biol. 2005;10(3):283–8. https://doi.org/10.1080/13556210500224015.
53. Eyer F, Schreckenberg M, Hecht D, et al. Carbamazepine and valproate as adjuncts in the treatment of alcohol withdrawal syndrome: a retrospective cohort study. Alcohol Alcohol. 2011;46(2):177–84. https://doi.org/10.1093/alcalc/agr005.
54. Baumgartner GR, Rowen RC. Clonidine vs chlordiazepoxide in the management of acute alcohol withdrawal syndrome. Arch Intern Med. 1987;147(7):1223–6. https://doi.org/10.1001/archinte.1987.00370070037005.
55. Sehnert W, Brecht H, Nowak F. High dose intravenous clonidine is superior to intravenous clomethiazole in severe alcohol withdrawal syndrome (delirium tremens). Crit Care. 1997;1(1):P133. https://doi.org/10.1186/cc100.
56. Crispo AL. Comparison of clinical outcomes in nonintubated patients with severe alcohol withdrawal syndrome treated with continuous-infusion sedatives: dexmedetomidine versus benzodiazepines. Pharmacotherapy—Wiley Online Library. 2014. https://accpjournals.onlinelibrary.wiley.com/doi/abs/10.1002/phar.1448. Accessed 8 Nov 2023.
57. Bielka K, Kuchyn I, Babych V, Martycshenko K, Inozemtsev O. Dexmedetomidine infusion as an analgesic adjuvant during laparoscopic cholecystectomy: a randomized controlled study. BMC Anesthesiol. 2018;18:44. https://doi.org/10.1186/s12871-018-0508-6.
58. VanderWeide LA, Foster CJ, MacLaren R, Kiser TH, Fish DN, Mueller SW. Evaluation of early dexmedetomidine addition to the standard of care for severe alcohol withdrawal in the ICU: a retrospective controlled cohort study. J Intensive Care Med. 2016;31(3):198–204. https://doi.org/10.1177/0885066614554908.
59. Mueller SW, Preslaski CR, Kiser TH, et al. A randomized, double-blind, placebo-controlled dose range study of dexmedetomidine as adjunctive therapy for alcohol withdrawal*. Crit Care Med. 2014;42(5):1131. https://doi.org/10.1097/CCM.0000000000000141.
60. Tolonen J, Rossinen J, Alho H, Harjola VP. Dexmedetomidine in addition to benzodiazepine-based sedation in patients with alcohol withdrawal delirium. Eur J Emerg Med. 2013;20(6):425. https://doi.org/10.1097/MEJ.0b013e32835c53b3.

61. Frazee EN, Personett HA, Leung JG, Nelson S, Dierkhising RA, Bauer PR. Influence of dexmedetomidine therapy on the management of severe alcohol withdrawal syndrome in critically ill patients. J Crit Care. 2014;29(2):298–302. https://doi.org/10.1016/j.jcrc.2013.11.016.

62. Mariani JJ, Rosenthal RN, Tross S, Singh P, Anand OP. A randomized, open-label, controlled trial of gabapentin and phenobarbital in the treatment of alcohol withdrawal. Am J Addict. 2006;15(1):76–84. https://doi.org/10.1080/10550490500419110.

63. Mariani JJ. Pilot randomized placebo-controlled clinical trial of high-dose gabapentin for alcohol use disorder. Alcohol Clin Exp Res—Wiley Online Library. 2021. https://onlinelibrary.wiley.com/doi/10.1111/acer.14648. Accessed 8 Nov 2023.

64. Anton RF, Latham P, Voronin K, et al. Efficacy of gabapentin for the treatment of alcohol use disorder in patients with alcohol withdrawal symptoms: a randomized clinical trial. JAMA Intern Med. 2020;180(5):728–36. https://doi.org/10.1001/jamainternmed.2020.0249.

65. Levine AR, Carrasquillo L, Mueller J, Nounou MI, Naut ER, Ibrahim D. High-dose gabapentin for the treatment of severe alcohol withdrawal syndrome: a retrospective cohort analysis. Pharmacother J Hum Pharmacol Drug Ther. 2019;39(9):881–8. https://doi.org/10.1002/phar.2309.

66. DeFoster RE, Morgan RJ, Leung JG, et al. Use of gabapentin for alcohol withdrawal syndrome in the hospital setting: a randomized open-label controlled trial. Subst Use Misuse. 2023;58(13):1643–50. https://doi.org/10.1080/10826084.2023.2236223.

67. Krebs M, Leopold K, Richter C, et al. Levetiracetam for the treatment of alcohol withdrawal syndrome: an open-label pilot trial. J Clin Psychopharmacol. 2006;26(3):347. https://doi.org/10.1097/01.jcp.0000219926.49799.89.

68. Richter C, Hinzpeter A, Schmidt F, et al. Levetiracetam for the treatment of alcohol withdrawal syndrome: a multicenter, prospective, randomized, placebo-controlled trial. J Clin Psychopharmacol. 2010;30(6):720. https://doi.org/10.1097/JCP.0b013e3181faf53e.

69. Youland KM, Miller RF, Mahoney LJ, Borgert AJ, Gundrum JD. Levetiracetam as adjunctive therapy for acute alcohol withdrawal syndrome in hospitalized patients. J Clin Psychopharmacol. 2014;34(6):704. https://doi.org/10.1097/JCP.0000000000000209.

70. Koethe D. Oxcarbazepine—Efficacy and tolerability during treatment of alcohol withdrawal: a double-blind, randomized, placebo-controlled multicenter pilot study. Alcohol Clin Exp Res—Wiley Online Library. 2007. https://onlinelibrary.wiley.com/doi/10.1111/j.1530-0277.2007.00419.x. Accessed 8 Nov 2023.

71. Förg A, Hein J, Volkmar K, et al. Efficacy and safety of Pregabalin in the treatment of alcohol withdrawal syndrome: a randomized placebo-controlled trial. Alcohol Alcohol. 2012;47(2):149–55. https://doi.org/10.1093/alcalc/agr153.

72. Rosenthal RN, Perkel C, Singh P, Anand O, Miner CR. A pilot open randomized trial of valproate and phenobarbital in the treatment of acute alcohol withdrawal. Am J Addict. 1998;7(3):189–97. https://doi.org/10.1111/j.1521-0391.1998.tb00336.x.

73. Longo LP, Campbell T, Hubatch S. Divalproex sodium (Depakote) for alcohol withdrawal and relapse prevention. J Addict Dis. 2002;21(2):55–64. https://doi.org/10.1300/J069v21n02_05.

74. Myrick H, Brady KT, Malcolm R. Divalproex in the treatment of alcohol withdrawal. Am J Drug Alcohol Abuse. 2000;26(1):155–60. https://doi.org/10.1081/ADA-100100597.

75. Smith JT, Sage M, Szeto H, et al. Outcomes after implementation of a benzodiazepine-sparing alcohol withdrawal order set in an integrated health care system. JAMA Netw Open. 2022;5(2):e220158. https://doi.org/10.1001/jamanetworkopen.2022.0158.

76. Collier TE, Farrell LB, Killian AD, Kataria VK. Effect of adjunctive dexmedetomidine in the treatment of alcohol withdrawal compared to benzodiazepine symptom-triggered therapy in critically ill patients: the EvADE study. J Pharm Pract. 2022;35(3):356–62. https://doi.org/10.1177/0897190020977755.

77. Skryabin VY, Zastrozhin M, Torrado M, et al. Effects of CYP2C19*17 genetic polymorphisms on the steady-state concentration of diazepam in patients with alcohol withdrawal syndrome. Hosp Pharm. 2021;56(5):592–6. https://doi.org/10.1177/0018578720931756.

78. Skryabin VY, Zastrozhin MS, Grishina EA, et al. Using the CYP3A activity evaluation to predict the efficacy and safety of diazepam in patients with alcohol withdrawal syndrome. J Pharm Pract. 2022;35(4):518–23. https://doi.org/10.1177/0897190021997000.

79. Fang C, Ouyang W, Zeng Y, et al. CYP2A6 and GABRA2 gene polymorphisms are associated with dexmedetomidine drug response. Front Pharmacol. 2022;13. https://www.frontiersin.org/articles/10.3389/fphar.2022.943200. Accessed 4 Oct 2023.

80. Day E. Thiamine for prevention and treatment of Wernicke-Korsakoff Syndrome in people who abuse alcohol | Cochrane Library. 2013. https://www.cochranelibrary.com/cdsr/doi/10.1002/14651858.CD004033.pub3/full. Accessed 24 Oct 2023.

81. Thiamine supplementation in patients with alcohol use disorder presenting with acute critical illness: a nationwide retrospective observational study. Ann Intern Med. 175(2). https://www.acpjournals.org/doi/10.7326/M21-2103. Accessed 11 Oct 2023.

82. Schabelman E, Kuo D. Glucose before thiamine for Wernicke encephalopathy: a literature review. J Emerg Med. 2012;42(4):488–94. https://doi.org/10.1016/j.jemermed.2011.05.076.

83. Merlin MA, Carluccio A, Raswant N, DosSantos F, Ohman-Strickland P, Lehrfeld DP. Comparison of prehospital glucose with or without IV thiamine. West J Emerg Med. 2012;13(5):406–9. https://doi.org/10.5811/westjem.2012.1.6760.

84. Smithline HA, Donnino M, Greenblatt DJ. Pharmacokinetics of high-dose oral thiamine hydrochloride in healthy subjects. BMC Clin Pharmacol. 2012;12(1):4. https://doi.org/10.1186/1472-6904-12-4.

85. Dingwall KM, Delima JF, Binks P, Batey R, Bowden SC. What is the optimum thiamine dose to treat or prevent Wernicke's encephalopathy or Wernicke–Korsakoff syndrome? Results of a randomized controlled trial. Alcohol Clin Exp Res. 2022;46(6):1133–47. https://doi.org/10.1111/acer.14843.

86. Aldhaeefi M, McLaughlin K, Goodberlet M, Szumita P. Evaluation of the safety of 500 mg intravenous push thiamine at a tertiary academic medical center. Sci Prog. 2022;105(2):00368504221096539. https://doi.org/10.1177/00368504221096539.

87. Diagnostic criteria for identifying individuals at high risk of progression from mild or moderate to severe alcohol use disorder | Critical Care Medicine | JAMA Network Open | JAMA Network. https://jamanetwork.com/journals/jamanetworkopen/fullarticle/2810438. Accessed 8 Nov 2023.

88. Krimpuri R, Youngs C, Emerman C. Initiation of medication for alcohol use disorder for inpatients with alcohol withdrawal syndromes. J Stud Alcohol Drugs. 2023;84(2):293–7. https://doi.org/10.15288/jsad.22-00219.

89. Chockalingam L, Burnham EL, Jolley SE. Medication prescribing for alcohol use disorders during alcohol-related encounters in a Colorado regional healthcare system. Alcohol Clin Exp Res. 2022;46(6):1094–102. https://doi.org/10.1111/acer.14837.

90. McPheeters M, O'Connor EA, Riley S, et al. Pharmacotherapy for alcohol use disorder: a systematic review and meta-analysis. JAMA. 2023;330(17):1653–65. https://doi.org/10.1001/jama.2023.19761.

91. Wood E, Bright J, Hsu K, et al. Canadian guideline for the clinical management of high-risk drinking and alcohol use disorder. CMAJ. 2023;195(40):E1364–79. https://doi.org/10.1503/cmaj.230715.

Chapter 37
Management of Drug Overdose and Intoxications in the ICU

Lauren R. Calnan and Jennifer A. Gass

37.1 Introduction

Drug overdoses and intoxications have grown in frequency and are becoming a common diagnosis within critical care units. Poison control centers reported 2.08 million human exposure calls with 75.5% reported as unintentional, 19.3% intentional, and 3.1% adverse reactions in the year 2021. Of the substances reported, 11.2% were related to analgesics, 7.5% from the sedative, hypnotic, or antipsychotic classes, 6.8% cardiovascular medications, 4.5% alcohols, and 3.2% stimulants or street drugs [1]. While it is no surprise that analgesics carry the highest percentage of overdoses and intoxications, the increase of opioid overdose deaths between 2019 and 2020 was 38%, with nearly 75% of overdose deaths in 2020 involving opioids [2]. As the opioid epidemic continues, we are seeing not only increasing numbers of illicit drug use, but more frequent potential for products laced with additional, unanticipated agents such as fentanyl. Not only is this increasing the difficulty and decreasing the success of resuscitation in event of a severe overdose, but also raises concerns for withdrawal of different agents and successful management to prevent adverse events. Establishing contact with poison control can be vital as poison control centers not only assist with treatment recommendations and status changes, but are able to generate data to guide population statistics and alert providers to emerging intoxicants. Whether intentional or accidental, identification of overdose or intoxication is vital and pharmacists can assist the team with rapid treatment. Pharmacists are trained in pharmacokinetics, pharmacodynamics, adverse reactions, and side effects of medications as well as knowledge of antidotes,

L. R. Calnan (✉)
Hillcrest Hospital South, Tulsa, OK, USA

J. A. Gass
Ardent Health Services, Brentwood, TN, USA

© The Author(s), under exclusive license to Springer Nature Switzerland AG 2025
Y. Alzaidi, M. A. Gebily (eds.), *The Pharmacist's Expanded Role in Critical Care Medicine*, https://doi.org/10.1007/978-3-031-77335-8_37

making them a vital team member to the treatment team. Understanding of common toxidromes, notification to poison control centers, management of common overdoses, as well as occurrences for false positive drug screens are essential for identification and treatment of overdoses and intoxications.

37.2 Initial Management

Initial assessment and management of any clinical emergency are key and can be easily broken down into what is referred to as ABCDE: Airway, Breathing, Circulation, Disability, Exposure [3]. Airway involves assessing if the patient has a patent airway, and this may be assessed by listening for sounds of obstructions such as changes in respiration, wheezing, or difficulty speaking. Breathing involves monitoring of respiratory rate and oxygen saturation. In the event a patient does not have a patent airway or is unable to adequately oxygenate, suctioning the airway and providing oxygenation by either high-flow oxygen therapy or intubation with mechanical ventilation can be necessary for airway protection or respiratory failure. Assessment of circulation includes monitoring the patient's heart rate, blood pressure, and obtaining an electrocardiogram as well as simple assessments such as skin color or paleness and capillary refill time. Obtaining intravenous access for fluid resuscitation or vasopressor support in the event that the patient is not circulating will be crucial in addition to allowing opportunity for obtaining labs such as routine labs, serum drug levels, or toxicology levels. Labs assessed at this time can also assist with assessment and treatment of disability. Disability addresses level of consciousness and can be assessed by the AVPU (alert, voice responsive, pain responsive, or unresponsive) assessment or evaluation of the Glasgow Coma Score. While the initial ABCs will be quickly determined and included in the disability assessment, labs and toxidrome assessment at this time can point to reversible causes of altered mental status such as rapid glucose administration for hypoglycemia or naloxone for opioid toxicity. Exposure assessment involves removal of clothing to assess for signs of trauma such as bleeding, bruising or broken bones, signs of drug abuse such as needle marks, and temperature assessment [3].

In the event the ABCDE assessment suggests occurrence of an overdose or ingestion, decontamination, enhanced drug elimination, antidote administration, and contact with poison control centers should occur after stabilization of the patient.

37.3 Toxidromes

One of the fundamental tenets in the identification and early treatment of intoxicating agents is the use of unique constellations of symptoms known as toxidromes. Using toxidromes, a basic patient physical exam can provide the necessary information to identify potential intoxicants and direct early management. Pharmacists are able to assist the medical team using key observations for early identification including mental status, vital signs, pupillary status, skin, and gastrointestinal status (Table 37.1), thus further assisting the medical team with the most likely intoxicant and treatment.

Anticholinergics are a common intoxication and one of the classic toxidromes [6]. Medical training about the classic picture of the anticholinergic toxidrome often includes the mnemonic "Hot as a Hare, Dry as a Bone, Blind as a Bat, Red as a Beet and Mad as a Hatter." The pneumonic refers to the extreme decrease in cholinergic tone resulting in hot, flushed, dry skin, dilated pupils, increased body temperature, and altered mental status including delirium and hallucinations. Although this overdose is infrequently fatal, it is a common toxicity that can occur either intentionally or unintentionally due to the wide number of medications with anticholinergic properties and the increased sensitivity to these in the elderly has placed many of these agents on the American Geriatrics Society Beers List [7]. Notable medications include first-generation antihistamines such as diphenhydramine, antidepressants including amitriptyline, and a variety of other agents including atropine, benztropine, promethazine, oxybutynin, and cyclobenzaprine. The list is extensive but thankfully the majority of cases only require supportive care [6]. Symptom management often begins with management of agitation utilizing benzodiazepines as

Table 37.1 Toxidrome summary [4, 5]

	Mental status	Vital signs	Pupillary status	Skin	Gastrointestinal status
Anticholinergic	Altered mental status Delirium Hallucinations Seizures	Tachycardia Hypertension Hyperthermia	Mydriasis	Anhidrosis Flushing	Hypoactive bowel sounds
Cholinergic	Confusion Muscle weakness	Bradycardia Hypertension	Miosis	Diaphoresis	Diarrhea Involuntary urination Emesis
Sympathomimetic	Delirium Agitation Myoclonus Seizures	Tachycardia Hypertension Hyperthermia	Normal	Diaphoresis	Normal
Sedative/ Hypnotic	Depressed	Decreased respiratory drive Bradycardia Hypotension	Normal	Normal	Hypoactive bowel sounds
Opioids	Sedated	Decreased respiratory drive Bradycardia Hypotension	Miosis	Normal	Hypoactive bowel sounds

first-line therapy and may require high doses. Cooling measures may be necessary in cases of severe hyperthermia, and fluids should be administered if rhabdomyolysis is suspected. Gastrointestinal motility can be severely slowed and can impair elimination, thus bowel regimens may be necessary; however, some agents may lead to the formation of a bezoar and result in obstruction so caution should be exercised [8].

The cholinergic toxidrome is defined by excess secretions, bradycardia, neuromuscular weakness and bronchoconstriction, vomiting, and gastrointestinal distress [9]. This constellation of symptoms is commonly taught utilizing the SLUDGE (Salivation, Lacrimation, Urinary frequency, Diaphoresis/Diarrhea, Gastrointestinal distress, Emesis) or DUMBBBELS (Diarrhea/Diaphoresis, Urinary frequency, Miosis, Bradycardia, Bronchorrhea, Bronchospasm, Emesis, Lacrimation, Salivation) pneumonic. Although there are notable medications that are associated with cholinergic activity such neostigmine, rivastigmine, and donepezil, true toxicity is most commonly associated with insecticide and organophosphate exposure [10]. These exposures may be through inhalation, direct contact, or incidental ingestion. Nerve agents, such as sarin gas, most commonly associated with warfare and acts of terrorism are also known for this form of toxicity [11]. Cholinergic toxicity is not a common medication-related toxicity but early intervention is the key to successful treatment as exposures are estimated to be common worldwide [10]. Identification of the toxidrome followed by swift utilization of safety equipment can prevent further contamination and harm to health care providers. Due to the environmental exposure nature of most of these toxicities, early contact with poison control is paramount to directing appropriate care.

Sympathomimetic agents activate our sympathetic nervous system resulting in heightened states of awareness and fully prepare for the flight or fight response [12]. Most commonly associated with stimulant agents, this toxicity will present with symptoms of delirium and agitation, hypertension, tachycardia, hyperthermia, and diaphoresis. Unlike anticholinergic and cholinergic toxicities that can often be the result of errors and inadvertent exposure, stimulant abuse is common place. Among prescription medications that may lead to sympathomimetic toxicity are stimulants used in the treatment of attention deficit disorder (ADD) and attention deficit hyperactivity disorder (ADHD). However, more commonly intoxication is the result of a wide range of illicit substances including cocaine, methamphetamine, mephedrone, and 3,4-methylenedioxy-N-methylamphetamine (MDMA). These agents do not have an antidote, and supportive care is the mainstay of therapy. Benzodiazepines are generally first line to manage agitation and prevent seizures. Additional symptoms may also need management including use of short-acting antihypertensives for blood pressure not resolved with agitation management, cooling for significant hyperthermia, and hydration if rhabdomyolysis is a concern. Many of these patients may suffer from addiction disorders and may ultimately benefit from intervention for their addiction.

Sedative and hypnotic toxicity is frequently the result of misuse of prescription medications and results in a depressed mental state along with decreased respiratory drive, hypotension, and bradycardia [13]. The presentation can be very similar to opioid-related intoxication but does not include a pupillary change. Commonly used medications displaying this toxicity include benzodiazepines and barbiturates, but may also include antidepressants, antipsychotics, anticonvulsant agents, and others. Toxicity may be the result of direct abuse, inappropriate dosing based on age or organ function, drug interactions, or coadministration with the other intoxicating agents such as alcohol. Treatment is varied depending on the offending agent, and substance abuse counseling may be warranted in many cases.

Opioid abuse and related toxicity have reached a crisis level across the United States, due, in part, to ever increasing availability. Prescription opioids such as oxycodone, hydrocodone, and morphine were originally the drug of choice, but later illicit production of heroin and now illicit fentanyl and derivatives have provided greater availability and potency of these highly addictive medications [14]. As with other toxidromes, opioid intoxication can occur incidentally due to polypharmacy or may be the result of abuse or intentional overdose [15]. Symptomatic patients experiencing opioid toxicity will have notable decreased respiratory drive, sedation, constricted pupils, and often constipation and hypoactive bowel sounds. In acute poisoning, decreased respiratory drive can progress to full apnea and death. Naloxone is a potent antidote for the neurologic and cardiopulmonary symptoms. However, consideration for the half-life of the causative agent must be considered because repeat naloxone doses may be required. Further, in patients with an abuse history, discharge with naloxone may prevent death in-route to a hospital in the future and substance abuse counseling should be provided.

37.4 Management of Common Drug Overdoses

37.4.1 Opioids

Increased access to opioids has contributed to this drug class becoming the leading drug of abuse and cause of drug overdoses. While illicit drug use has increased frequency of overdose occurrence, overdose can occur in newly prescribed opioid naïve patients as well as unintentional overdoses. Ingestion, inhalation, injection, intranasal, rectal, transdermal, and transmucosal routes may all lead to toxicity depending on the agent and in most instances small doses can have detrimental effects. Opioids act at the mu, kappa, and delta receptors for analgesic effect; however, each receptor gives way to symptoms of overdose (Table 37.2).

Table 37.2 Opioid receptor targets and effects [15, 16]

Receptor	Activity
Mu	Analgesia, bradycardia, euphoria, gastrointestinal dysmotility, respiratory depression, decrease in respiratory response to hypoxia and development of apnea
Kappa	Analgesia, diuresis, dysphoria, hallucinations, miosis
Delta	Analgesia, cough suppression, inhibition of dopamine release, mood modulation

Key signs and symptoms of opioid overdose include decreased respiratory drive, increased sedation, and pinpoint pupils or miosis. In severe cases, respiratory distress, bradycardia, and hypotension lead to respiratory failure and subsequent cardiac arrest. The mainstay of treatment for opioid overdose after stabilization of the patient is reversal with a mu-opioid receptor antagonist such as naloxone. Naloxone may be administered intravenously, intranasally, intramuscularly, and subcutaneously and is available in kits for the general public. Naloxone doses may need to be repeated with escalating doses every 2–3 min to illicit a response or reversal of symptoms. Due to its fast onset of action of 2–5 min, yet short duration of 30–120 min prompts close monitoring of patients and possible necessity of redosing [16, 17]. Patients experiencing toxicity from long-acting agents like methadone, extended-release products, formation of bezoar, or continue to require bolus dosing of naloxone to maintain stability may require continuous infusion naloxone with adjustment of dosing based on symptoms [18] (Table 37.4).

Special patient situations should be considered with the vast availability of opioids. Patients should be evaluated for fentanyl patches, and prompt removal is required if present. Opioid agonists such as methadone and loperamide may induce QT prolongation and require electrocardiogram monitoring for arrhythmias such as Torsades de pointes. Tramadol and meperidine overdose should also be monitored for serotonin syndrome or possible seizures from toxicity. With the increase in illicit drugs, evaluation for patients that could be potential body packers should be considered. Radiographic imaging is recommended, and close monitoring for signs and symptoms of opioid overdose are critical as packets may leak or burst leading to rapid systemic effects and toxicity. Gastric decontamination with activated charcoal or whole bowel irrigation may be considered, however should be limited to patients with a protected airway and do not show signs of bowel obstruction in order to reduce potential for bursting of drug packets [16].

37.5 Acetaminophen

With its wide availability in over-the-counter cough and cold remedies and presence in combination prescription pain medications, acetaminophen continues to be one of the most frequently encountered toxicities and a leading cause in liver failure. Therapeutic doses of acetaminophen 325–1000 mg three to four times a day are commonly utilized for analgesia and as an antipyretic with limited adverse effects in the majority of patients. Maximum daily doses of 3 g have been recommended on an outpatient basis with absolute maximum of 4 g per day to decrease risk of hepatotoxicity; however, unintentional overdoses remain common with the variety of dosages available and the use of combination products. Immediate release and extended-release products can also complicate treatment and evaluation of timelines in the event of overdose [59–61]. Acetaminophen is hepatically metabolized by UDP-glucuronosyltransferase (UGT), sulfotransferase (SULT), and cytochrome P450 enzyme CYP2E1, however when increased concentrations are introduced, development of toxic metabolites leads to accumulation and increased risk of hepatic injury.

Primary metabolites produced are sulfate and glucuronide conjugates with a highly toxic and reactive intermediate metabolite called N-acetyl-p-benzoquinone imine (NAPQI). At therapeutic doses, glutathione rapidly conjugates and detoxifies NAPQI to form the nontoxic compounds cysteine and mercapturate. While high-risk ingestions are considered those of at least 30 g of acetaminophen, symptoms of toxicity have been seen at doses of acetaminophen greater than 4 g per day [62–64]. Toxic doses lead to a saturation of phase II metabolizing enzymes resulting in depletion of glutathione and increase in NAPQI production. Without glutathione available for covalent binding to NAPQI, the formation of NAPQI-protein adducts leads to oxidative stress, hepatic necrosis, and hepatic cell death [59, 60, 62, 65].

Patients presenting within 24 h of overdose are commonly asymptomatic; however, they may present with nausea, vomiting, and lethargy (Table 37.3). Liver enzyme effects are typically seen after 24 h, however in massive overdoses, derangements can be seen as early as 12 h post-overdose. Due to a serum half-life of acetaminophen of 2–3 h in healthy patients, peak serum concentrations are typically seen within 4 h of overdose with immediate release products. Half-life may be prolonged to 5 h in patients with hepatic or renal insufficiency, and peak serum concentrations delayed in overdose with extended-release products or presence of co-ingestion. Liver derangements become evident between 24 and 48 h post-ingestion with a peak typically noted at 96 h with associated right upper quadrant pain, jaundice, coagulopathy, and encephalopathy leading to multiorgan effects such as oliguria, acute renal failure, and hepatorenal failure [59, 62].

After decontamination strategies, activated charcoal within 1–2 h after ingestion may be useful up to 4 h for extended-release products, N-acetylcysteine (NAC) remains the gold standard therapy for acetaminophen toxicity by repleting glutathione stores, thereby enhancing NAPQI conjugation to nontoxic metabolites [64]. Initiation of NAC therapy within 8–10 h post-ingestion has been recommended in

Table 37.3 Timeline of acetaminophen toxicity [59, 62]

Stage	Time from ingestion	Symptoms	Labs
Stage 1	24 h	Asymptomatic to nausea, vomiting, abdominal pain, malaise	ALT and AST may begin to rise as early as 12 h in massive overdose, however typically remain normal
Stage 2	24–48 h	Right upper quadrant pain/tenderness	ALT, AST, and total bilirubin increase, prolonged PT, increase in serum creatinine
Stage 3	72–96 h	Jaundice, coagulopathy, encephalopathy, oliguria, acute renal failure, hepatorenal failure, multiorgan failure	ALT and AST peak, hypoglycemia, prolonged prothrombin time, lactic acidosis
Stage 4	4 days–2 weeks	Recovery phase if patient survives	

ALT alanine aminotransferase, *AST* aspartate aminotransferase, *PT* prothrombin time patients with possible or probable risk for hepatotoxicity as determined by the Rumack–Matthew nomogram [66, 67]. Limitations to the use of the nomogram include unknown time of ingestion, ingestion of extended-release formulation, chronic ingestions, and acute overdoses presenting outside 24 h post-ingestion. The nomogram also has not been validated for acetaminophen levels drawn prior to 4 h post-ingestion or for patients who have a history of repeated overdose [62, 66]. In patients where nomogram plotting indicates possible hepatotoxicity or if criteria preclude nomogram usage with an elevated ALT or acetaminophen serum concentration of greater than 20 µg/mL, NAC therapy is recommended [59, 66]. NAC may be administered by intravenous or oral route; however, it is important to note oral therapy can be intolerable with common side effects such as nausea and vomiting. Due to side effects as well as longer duration of therapy, IV therapy is most utilized and up until recent years has been administered as a three-bag regimen over 21 h (Table 37.4). More recent studies of a two-bag versus three-bag regimen demonstrated shorter delays, less interruptions, less systemic reactions, and a non-inferior

Table 37.4 Common intoxication treatment doses

	Treatment and dosing regimens	
Opioids [18–21]	Naloxone IV, IM, SubQ: 0.04–2 mg with increasing dose every 2–3 min as needed	
	Naloxone intranasal: 2–8 mg with increasing dose every 2–5 min as needed	
	Naloxone endotracheal: 0.8–5 mg when no other route available	
	Naloxone continuous infusion: 2/3 initial effective bolus dose per hour	
Acetaminophen [22–24]	Oral NAC (72-h regimen)	Loading dose: 140 mg/kg; max 15 g/dose; followed by Maintenance dose: 70 mg/kg every 4 h for 17 doses; max 7.5 g/dose
	IV NAC 3-bag method (21-h regimen)	Bag 1: 150 mg/kg over 60 min; max 15 g/dose; followed by Bag 2: 50 mg/kg over 4 h; max 5 g/dose; followed by Bag 3: 100 mg/kg over 16 h; max 10 g/dose
	IV NAC 2-bag method (20-h regimen)	Bag 1: 200 mg/kg over 4 h; followed by Bag 2: 100 mg/kg over 16 h Max total dose: 30 g
Salicylates [25–27]	Sodium bicarbonate 8.4% 150 mL/dextrose 5% 1000 mL at a rate to induce urine output of 2–3 mL/kg/h	
	Sodium bicarbonate 50–100 mEq or 1–2 mEq/kg over 1–2 min, repeated as needed to goal urine pH	
	Sodium bicarbonate 8.4% 150 mL/dextrose 5% 1000 mL at rate of 150 mL/h	

(continued)

Table 37.4 (continued)

	Treatment and dosing regimens
Methanol [28, 29]	Loading dose: fomepizole 15 mg/kg IV; followed by Fomepizole 10 mg/kg every 12 h for 4 doses If additional doses: fomepizole 15 mg/kg every 12 h
Ethylene glycol [29–31]	Loading dose: fomepizole 15 mg/kg IV; followed by Fomepizole 10 mg/kg every 12 h for 4 doses If additional doses: fomepizole 15 mg/kg every 12 h
Organophosphates [32–36]	Atropine 1–5 mg IV bolus, doubled every 5 min until adequate response in secretions, heart rate, and blood pressure – Followed by atropine infusion titrated at 10–30% of the total dose required to stabilize the patient per hour, continued for 48–72 h
	Pralidoxime (2-PAM) 1–2 g IV over 30 min followed by 1 g every 6–12 h or 0.5–1 g/h infusion
	Pralidoxime (2-PAM) 30 mg/kg bolus over 20 min followed by 8 mg/kg/h or 30 mg/kg every 4 h
	Obidoxime (Toxigonin) 4 mg/kg over 20 min followed by 0.5 mg/kg/h or 2 mg/kg every 4 h
Serotonin syndrome [37]	Cyproheptadine oral 12 mg followed by 2 mg every 2 h if symptoms continue
	Maintenance dose of cyproheptadine oral 8 mg every 2 h
Tricyclic antidepressants [38–40]	Sodium bicarbonate 50–100 mEq bolus as needed to maintain goal pH 7.45–7.55
	Sodium bicarbonate 1–2 mEq/kg bolus as needed to maintain goal pH 7.45–7.55
	Sodium bicarbonate 1 mEq/kg bolus, followed by sodium bicarbonate 150 mEq/L dextrose 5% in water
	Sodium bicarbonate 1–2 mEq/kg bolus, followed by sodium bicarbonate 150 mEq/L dextrose 5% in water
Sulfonylureas [41–44]	Dextrose 50% (25 g) 50 mL IV bolus as needed for persistent hypoglycemia
	Dextrose 5% or dextrose 10% in water continuous IV infusion to maintain blood glucose >80 mg/dL
	Octreotide 50–100 µg subcutaneously or intravenously every 6–8 h as needed
Methemoglobinemia [45, 46]	Methylene blue 1–2 mg/kg over 5–10 min; max single dose 100 mg
	May repeat after 1 h if symptoms persist or methemoglobin concentration > 60%
Iron [47, 48]	Deferoxamine 15 mg/kg/h up to 24 h

(continued)

Table 37.4 (continued)

	Treatment and dosing regimens
Digoxin [49, 50]	Reported doses variable; for known ingestion amount or known digoxin levels see manufacturer online calculator
	Acute ingestion, unknown amount: Digoxin Immune Fab (DIGIFab®) 800 mg

	Acute ingestion, known amount:
	    Digoxin Immune Fab Calculation (number of 40 mg vials)
	    Amount ingested (mg) × 0.8/0.5 mg

	Chronic toxicity, unknown digoxin level: Digoxin Immune Fab 240 mg

	Chronic toxicity, known digoxin level:
	    Digoxin immune fab calculation (number of 40 mg vials)
	    Serum digoxin concentration (ng/mL) × weight (kg)/100

Beta-blockers [51–56]	Glucagon IV 50 µg/kg followed by 1–15 mg/h continuous infusion titrated to blood pressure and/or heart rate response
	Insulin 1 unit/kg bolus IV followed by 0.5–1 unit/kg/h continuous infusion Max: 10 units/kg/h In conjunction with dextrose 50% 25 g IV bolus followed by dextrose 10% IV infusion
Calcium channel blockers [55, 57, 58]	Calcium chloride 10% 10–20 mL every 10–20 min for 3–4 doses
	Insulin 1 unit/kg bolus IV followed by 0.5–1 unit/kg/h continuous infusion Max: 10 units/kg/h In conjunction with dextrose 50% 25 g IV bolus followed by dextrose 10% IV infusion
	20% lipid emulsion 1.5 mL/kg IV bolus followed by 0.25–0.5 mL/kg/min over 30 min

efficacy in preventing acute hepatic failure. These benefits have led to increased utilization of a two-bag regimen [22–24]. With variable regimens utilized, recent guidelines recommend a regimen which delivers at minimum NAC 300 mg/kg orally or IV during the first 20–24 h of therapy. Consultation with state poison control centers and health care facility protocols is recommended for determining which regimen to utilize and to avoid risk of under-dosing. In the event the patient weighs more than 100 kg, guidelines recommend utilizing the same dosing regimen for under 100 kg patients, except the calculation should be capped at 100 kg of body weight [64]. While recommended IV therapy is dosed at 20–21 h, in many instances NAC therapy may be continued at 100 mg/kg until patient meets the specified criteria: acetaminophen level decreased to less than 10 µg/mL demonstrating a clinical response, serum AST and ALT nearing normal or demonstrating clinical response defined by some as decrease of at least 50%, improvement of coagulopathy such as international normalized ratio (INR) less than 2 or normalized PT, and lack of clinical symptoms such as altered mental status or renal failure [64, 68–70].

In recent years, fomepizole has been used and recommended by some poison centers as an off-label adjunctive therapy in acetaminophen overdose. Known for its use in toxic alcohol poisonings, fomepizole may diminish NAPQI formation by CYP2E1 inhibition further eliminating formation of protein adducts and oxidative metabolites of acetaminophen toxicity [69, 71]. Case reports have demonstrated in patients with massive overdose improvement in ALT when used in conjunction with NAC at a dose of fomepizole 15 mg/kg infusion followed by fomepizole 10 mg/kg 12 h later [71–73]. While usage is increasing for this indication, comparative literature is still lacking outside of case reports.

37.6 Salicylates

Poison control data from 2018 found acetylsalicylic acid, commonly known as aspirin, to be involved in 17,380 cases of salicylate poisoning [74, 75].Salicylates are present as the bismuth subsalicylate oral formulation, methyl salicylate in topical and liquid formulations, available as rectal suppository formulation, and the most commonly prescribed, acetylsalicylic acid for antiplatelet and analgesia. Wide availability in over-the-counter oral and topical products, enteric coated and immediate release oral agents, and indications for antiplatelet, analgesia, anti-inflammatory, and antipyretic use make it a common agent in both intentional acute overdose and unintentional chronic overdoses. Identification of acute versus chronic ingestion and understanding metabolic processes affected are key in management, as well as the kinetic variations between formulations. Salicylate products are metabolized into salicylate, the primary metabolite responsible for toxicity.

Acetylsalicylic acid undergoes hydrolysis through esterases within the gastrointestinal mucosa, erythrocytes, and liver to form salicylic acid. Furthermore, salicylate is conjugated by glycine within the liver to inactive metabolites that are eliminated via renal excretion, however in overdoses, metabolic pathways become saturated. As the salicylate concentrations increase, protein binding decreases leading to an increase in volume of distribution. As hepatic metabolism becomes more saturated and protein binding decreased, the unbound fraction of salicylic acid increases leading to prolonged elimination via the kidneys [74, 76–78]. While with therapeutic doses salicylate is excreted unchanged in the urine at small amounts, this elimination route becomes integral in the treatment of overdose. Accumulation of salicylate within the serum concentration leads to acid-base derangements caused by uncoupling of mitochondrial oxidative phosphorylation as well as direct stimulation of cerebral medulla affecting respiratory drive (Table 37.5) [74, 77, 80].

Presentation may be more quickly identified in acute ingestions compared to chronic. Acute ingestions have been found to be more intentional in younger populations compared to chronic ingestions leading to unintentional overdose being in elderly populations with comorbid conditions. Acute ingestions may present with gastrointestinal irritation, tinnitus, and hyperventilation while chronic ingestions may appear more nonspecific due to underlying presence within tissue and serum concentrations (Table 37.6). Due to the presence of already saturated tissues and

Table 37.5 Pathophysiology [74, 77, 79]

Salicylate action	Pathophysiologic changes		Clinical effect
Mitochondrial oxidative phosphorylation	Anaerobic metabolism	• Pyruvate -> Lactate	• Lactic acidosis
		• Inability to buffer hydrogen ions -> lactate	• Lactic acidosis
		• Decrease in ATP, increase in catabolism	• Glycolysis, increased heat production, increased carbon dioxide
Stimulation of cerebral medulla	Hyperpnea	• Hyperventilation	• Respiratory alkalosis
		• Increase in pH	• Compensatory metabolic acidosis
COX-1 and 2 inhibitions	Decreased prostacyclin	• Gastric ulcer formation	• Gastrointestinal bleeding

ATP adenosine triphosphate, *COX* cyclooxygenase

Table 37.6 Salicylate toxicity symptoms [74, 76]

	Serum concentration	Symptoms
Acute ingestions	15–30 mg/dL	Therapeutic range, asymptomatic
	30–50 mg/dL	Tinnitus, vertigo, nausea, vomiting, hyperventilation
	50–70 mg/dL	Febrile, diaphoresis, dehydration, listless, incoordination
	>75 mg/dL	Hallucinations, seizures, noncardiogenic pulmonary edema, cerebral edema, coma, cardiovascular collapse
Chronic ingestions	Do not reliably correlate, but should be collected for baseline	Tinnitus, tremor, restlessness, confusion, altered mental status, slurred speech, hallucinations, hyperpyrexia, tachypnea, noncardiogenic pulmonary edema, metabolic acidosis, respiratory alkalosis, seizures, coma

metabolic pathways, serum concentration may not correlate with chronic ingestions as with acute, and may present as other disease states requiring in-depth assessment.

While there is no antidote for salicylate intoxication, supportive care is first priority in the form of establishing and maintaining an airway as well as attempting to reduce further absorption of the drug. In the event enteric-coated formulations were ingested, systemic effects may be delayed up to 12 h from ingestion and imaging to determine presence of bezoars is recommended as this can also affect rate of absorption [78]. Administration of activated charcoal within 2 h of ingestion may reduce absorption of salicylates; however, focus will be on volume, electrolyte, and acid-base status. Increased glycolysis and impaired gluconeogenesis leading to hypoglycemia as well as neurologic symptoms are common, in part, to central nervous system glucose being depleted relative to serum glucose. Dehydration risk should be managed with volume resuscitation in addition to monitoring, and potassium supplementation as potassium depletion can affect urine alkalinization [27, 77]. To minimize the risk of noncardiogenic pulmonary edema, monitoring of fluid overload should prompt appropriate adjustment of fluids [74]. Urinary excretion is utilized as a means to enhance salicylate clearance and is a mainstay of therapy. Sodium bicarbonate infusion has been the gold standard for urine alkalinization in salicylate overdoses as increasing urine pH and increasing glomerular filtration rates expedite renal excretion. The goal is to maintain urinary pH between 7.5 and 8.5 with bicarbonate therapy; however, patients may present with mixed acid-base disorders and it is reasonable to avoid elevating arterial pH to 7.5 especially in the presence of respiratory alkalosis (Table 37.4). Oral bicarbonate and acetazolamide therapy are not recommended as oral therapy can increase salicylate absorption by increasing gastrointestinal pH and acetazolamide can interfere with tubular salicylate secretion and increase plasma salicylate levels [74]. In severe overdoses displaying significant central nervous system abnormalities, salicylate levels nearing 100 mg/dL, clinical deterioration, evidence of end-organ damage, or refractory to urine alkalinization, hemodialysis is recommended (Table 37.7) [27, 77]. Due to saturation of protein binding and increased free fraction of salicylate, hemodialysis is able to remove as well as correct acid-base disturbances [27, 74].

Table 37.7 Dialyzability and half-life of common intoxicants

Intoxicant	Classification of dialyzability	T1/2
Acetaminophen [81–83]	Dialyzable	2–7 h CrCL <30: 2.0–5.3 h
Salicylates [82, 84, 85]	Dialyzable	Variable by agent and formulation
Toxic alcohols [28, 30, 82, 86–88]		
Isopropanol	Dialyzable	Variable[a]
Methanol	Dialyzable	Variable[a]
Diethylene glycol	Dialyzable	Variable[a]
Ethylene glycol	Dialyzable	Variable[a]
Propylene glycol	Dialyzable	Variable[a]
Antidepressants		
Tricyclic antidepressants [82, 89, 90]		
Amitriptyline	Not dialyzable	13–36 h
Doxepin	Not dialyzable	15 h Metabolite: 31–51 h
Nortriptyline	Not dialyzable	14–51 h Elderly: 23.5–79 h
Selective serotonin reuptake inhibitors (SSRIs) [82, 91]		
Citalopram	Not dialyzable	24–48 h Average: 35 h
Escitalopram	Not dialyzable	27–32 h

Fluoxetine	Not dialyzable	Parent drug:
		  Acute: 1–3 days
		  Chronic: 4–6 days
		  Cirrhosis: 7.6 days
		Metabolite: 9.3 days
		  Cirrhosis: 12 days

Paroxetine	Not dialyzable	IR: 21 h CR: 15–20 h

(continued)

Table 37.7 (continued)

Intoxicant	Classification of dialyzability	T1/2
Sertraline	Not dialyzable	26 h Metabolite: 62–104 h
Serotonin/norepinephrine reuptake inhibitors (SNRIs) [82, 92]		
Desvenlafaxine	Not dialyzable	10–11 h
Duloxetine	Not dialyzable	8–22 h
Venlafaxine	Not dialyzable	IR: 3–7 h Metabolite: 9–13 h ER: dependent on formulation
Dopamine/norepinephrine reuptake inhibitors [82, 93]		
Bupropion	Not dialyzable	21–30 h
Sulfonylureas [82, 94]		
Glimepiride	Not dialyzable	5–9 h
Glipizide	Not dialyzable	2–5 h
Glyburide	Not dialyzable	4–10 h
Iron [95]	Dialyzable	Variable by agent and formulation
Beta-blockers [82, 96–99]		
Acebutolol	Moderately dialyzable	Parent 3–4 h Metabolite 8–13 h
Atenolol	Dialyzable	6–7 h ESRD 15–35 h
Betaxolol	Not dialyzable	14–22 h ESRD: approx. doubled
Bisoprolol	Moderately dialyzable	9–12 h CrCl <40: 27–36 h Cirrhosis: 8–22 h
Carvedilol	Not dialyzable	7–10 h
Labetalol	Not dialyzable	6–8 h
Metoprolol	Slightly dialyzable	3–4 h
Nadolol	Dialyzable	20–24 h
Propranolol	Not dialyzable	IR: 3–6 h ER: 8–10 h
Sotalol	Dialyzable	12 h Anuric: up to 69 h
Timolol	Not dialyzable	2–2.7 h
Calcium channel blockers [82, 100, 101]		
Amlodipine	Not dialyzable	30–52 h
Diltiazem	Not dialyzable	IR: 3–4.5 h ER: 4–9.5 h
Nifedipine	Not dialyzable	2–5 h Cirrhosis: 7 h
Verapamil	Not dialyzable	IR: 2.8–12 h ER: 12 h
Drugs of abuse [82, 102–105]		
Amphetamines	Not dialyzable	Variable by agent and formulation
Barbiturate	Dialyzable	Variable by agent and formulation

(continued)

Table 37.7 (continued)

Intoxicant	Classification of dialyzability	T1/2
Benzodiazepines	Not dialyzable	Variable by agent and formulation
Cocaine	Not dialyzable	
Opioids		
Buprenorphine	Not dialyzable	Buccal film: 16–38 h ER injection: variable by formulation IV: 1.2–7.2 h Sublingual tablet: 37 h Patch: 26 h
Codeine	Not dialyzable	2.5–3.5 h
Fentanyl	Not dialyzable	IV: 2–4 h Patch: 20–27 h Nasal Spray: 15–25 h
Heroin	Not dialyzable	1.7–5.3 min Metabolites: 2–3 h
Hydrocodone	Not dialyzable	IR: 4 h ER: 7–12 h, variable by formulation
Hydromorphone	Dialyzable	IR: 2–3 h ER: 8–15 h
Meperidine	Slightly dialyzable	2.5–4 h Cirrhosis: 7–11 h Metabolite: 8–16 h
Methadone	Not dialyzable	9–87 h
Morphine	Moderately dialyzable	IR: 2–4 h ER: 11–24 h, variable by formulation
Oxycodone	Slightly dialyzable	IR: 3.2–4 h ER: 4.5–5.6 h, variable by formulation
Tramadol	Dialyzable	IR: 5–7 h Metabolite: 6–8 h ER: 7–10 h, variable by formulation Metabolite: 8–11 h, variable by formulation
Other		
Anticholinergics [106]	Not dialyzable	Variable by agent and formulation
Baclofen [107, 108]	Moderately dialyzable	2.7–4.7 h
Carbamazepine [109–111]	Dialyzable	IR: 25–65 h ER: 35–40 h Metabolite:34–43 h
Digoxin [82, 112, 113]	Not dialyzable	Parent: 8 h Metabolite: 3–12 h
Lithium [106, 114, 115]	Dialyzable	18–36 h
Metformin [106, 116, 117]	Dialyzable	Plasma: 4–9 h Blood: ~17 h
Phenytoin [106, 118, 119]	Dialyzable	7–42 h
Valproic acid [106, 120, 121]	Dialyzable	9–19 h

[a] Variables based on co-ingested agents and organ function, active metabolite half-lives can also vary significantly based on these and other factors [28, 30, 86]

37.7 Alcohols

Toxic alcohols are a group of alcohols most commonly including isopropanol, methanol, diethylene glycol, ethylene glycol, and propylene glycol. Poisoning with these alcohols can occur under a number of different conditions, and many are the result of intentional or unintentional ingestion of a wide variety of household and automotive chemicals [122, 123]. Some toxic alcohols can also be absorbed through inhalation or contact with the skin. However, the common thread between toxic alcohols is that the majority derives their toxicity from toxic metabolites, and they produce inebriating effects similar to ethanol. Due to the wide availability of some of these toxic alcohols in commonly available household products, accidental poisoning may occur with children and pets or may be the result of attempts to become inebriated [124]. Additionally, intentional self-harm is another cause of ingestion. In any case, the key to optimal outcomes is early recognition and treatment.

Toxic alcohols are typically rapidly absorbed within minutes of ingestion and start as a substrate for the enzyme, alcohol dehydrogenase which converts the alcohol to an aldehyde, or acetone in the case of isopropanol, via oxidation (Fig. 37.1) [125, 126]. The resulting aldehyde metabolites are oxidized via a second enzymatic conversion by aldehyde dehydrogenase. Isopropanol is directly toxic while the remainder of the alcohol exerts their toxic effects through the metabolites produced from the alcohol substrate.

Initial clinical symptoms of almost all toxic alcohols will be associated with an inebriated-like state but will later progress to a wide variety of organ dysfunctions. The timeline for symptomology can vary based on concomitant ingestion of ethanol as ethanol is a competitive substrate with high affinity for the alcohol

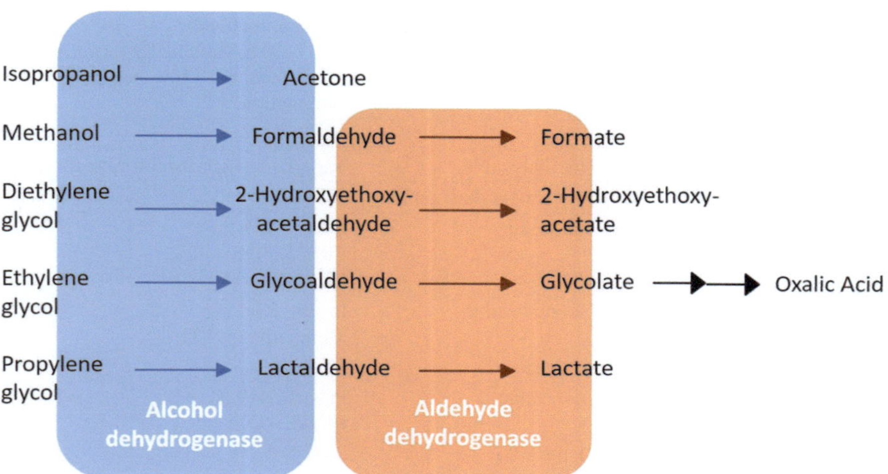

Fig. 37.1 Metabolism of toxic alcohols via alcohol dehydrogenase and aldehyde dehydrogenase

dehydrogenase enzyme and co-ingestion will slow the production of the various toxic metabolites.

Isopropyl alcohol (isopropanol) toxicity is unique as it is directly toxic and, although the exact mechanism of toxicity has not been fully elucidated, CNS depression, specifically brain stem depression, is thought to be the predominate component [124]. Typical symptoms following early inebriation include ketosis without acidosis, abdominal pain, vomiting, and nausea. Ultimately, this can progress to hemorrhagic gastritis [28, 124]. Other findings include loss of corneal and deep tendon reflexes, miosis and in the case of severe intoxications may be associated with hypotension [28]. Lethal doses are typically in the range of 2–4 mL/kg but these may vary.

Methanol does not typically result in an inebriating effect unlike the other alcohols discussed; however, methanol ingestion results in the formation of formic acid which leads to the development of an anion-gap acidosis [28]. Formic acid is also damaging to the retinal and optic nerve and is the reason methanol toxicity is commonly associated with diminished vision or full blindness [31, 127]. Other symptoms may include abdominal pain, respiratory symptoms, and neurologic symptoms including coma and a Parkinson-like presentation [128]. Ingestions between 30 and 240 mL (1 g) per kg are considered lethal but permanent damage to eyesight can occur with ingestions of as little as 30 mL of methanol.

Diethylene glycol toxicity will often present in three distinct phases [31]. Phase 1 is associated with a metabolic acidosis, inebriation, and gastrointestinal symptoms. Phase 2 can occur within a few days as acute kidney injury occurs which is often the cause of death. Phase 3 is the expression of neurologic involvement including nerve palsy, paralysis, coma, and death.

Ethylene glycol itself is generally considered nontoxic but is inebriating, osmotically active and the cause of increased osmolality with intoxication [30]. Glycolic acid is one of the toxic metabolites of ethylene glycol and the one believed to be primarily responsible for the associated anion-gap metabolic acidosis seen with ethylene glycol intoxication [30, 31]. The metabolite of ethylene glycol, oxalate, will deposit in the form of insoluble calcium oxalate crystals into a variety of tissues including the heart, lungs, and kidneys resulting in the observed organ dysfunction [129]. This deposition into the renal tubules is responsible for proximal tubular necrosis. Lethal doses of ethylene glycol are around 1500 mg/kg (1–2 mL/kg of 95% concentrated solution) [30].

Propylene glycol toxicity is often closely tied to benzodiazepine use, particularly high-dose prolonged infusions in the hospital as propylene glycol is a carrier in parenteral formulations of benzodiazepines used for sedation [130]. Patients experiencing propylene glycol toxicity will often have only an increased osmolal gap, but can progress to developing a lactic acidosis along with acute kidney injury, hypotension, dysrhythmias, seizures, and multi-system organ dysfunction [130, 131]. The risk of these symptoms increases with pre-existing hepatic and renal dysfunction.

The key to treatment of a toxic alcohol toxicity is early treatment [132, 133]. With isopropyl alcohol toxicity, supportive measures form the backbone of treatment [86]. Primarily this comes in the form of IV hydration. Since the alcohol itself is directly toxic, inhibition of metabolism via alcohol dehydrogenase serves no therapeutic purpose and results in delayed clearance of the isopropanol. As a result, alcohol dehydrogenase inhibitors should not be used [134]. In patients with very elevated serum isopropanol levels (>500 mg/dL) or in the presence of lactic acidosis or hypotension, hemodialysis may be indicated but would be very rare (Table 37.7) [86, 124]. The patient should continue to be monitored until they have achieved clinical sobriety [86]. Most patients will recover without any long-term sequelae, however, in those patients attempting self-harm or with ethanol dependency further medical and psychological management may be required.

Methanol intoxication should also include typical supportive care with fluids [28]. However, additional treatment modalities are available for methanol including fomepizole, ethanol, and potentially dialysis (Table 37.7) [28, 31]. Fomepizole, a competitive inhibitor of the alcohol dehydrogenase enzyme, prevents the conversion of the relatively nontoxic methanol to the toxic metabolite formate [29]. Fomepizole is FDA approved for the treatment of methanol toxicity or suspected ingestion and is typically started at a methanol concentration greater than 20 mg/dL. Patients without evidence of end-organ toxicity and without metabolic acidosis or only mild metabolic acidosis may be considered for treatment with fomepizole after reaching a higher methanol concentration of 32 mg/dL [28]. If methanol levels are delayed or unattainable, any evidence of retinal toxicity or a bicarbonate level below 15 mmol/L would be an indication to initiate fomepizole therapy (Table 37.4). Fomepizole is administered intravenously with a loading dose followed by four additional doses [28, 29]. If a methanol concentration below 20–32 mg/dL is not attained or the patient has not achieved normal acid-base status at the completion of the initial 4 doses, additional doses are needed and the dose must be increased due to an auto induction mechanism [28]. Alternatives include using ethanol as a competitive inhibitor; however, dosing is complicated, requires critical care oversight, results in intoxication and is a less preferred method versus fomepizole [28, 31]. Both methanol and formate, the toxic metabolites, are highly dialyzable and should be considered with toxic ingestions. Use of fomepizole stops the production of the metabolite, but dialysis allows the removal of the substrate (methanol) as well as this metabolite (formate) and can lead to a shorter length of stay (Table 37.7). Dialysis becomes absolutely indicated with metabolic acidosis accompanying new visual impairment. Dialysis should be considered relatively indicated in the presence of methanol concentrations greater than 50 mg/dL, renal failure, known ingestion of a lethal dose or metabolic acidosis non-responsive to resuscitation [28, 135]. During dialysis, fomepizole frequency will increase to every 4 h and returns to every 12 h after dialysis is completed [29].

Although fomepizole is not approved in the case of diethylene glycol intoxication, it has been used successfully [136, 137]. Considering that diethylene glycol is readily dialyzable and often associated with kidney injury, using both strategies seems reasonable and has been successful (Table 37.7) [138].

As with methanol, fomepizole is an FDA approved agent in the treatment of ethylene glycol intoxication with the same mechanism and effect as seen with methanol [29, 30]. With a few exceptions, initiation of fomepizole for ethylene glycol should follow the same guidance as previously discussed with methanol (Table 37.4) [30, 31]. The biggest difference occurs in those patients who do not exhibit or have mild metabolic acidosis and have no end-organ symptoms. In this case, fomepizole can be deferred unless the ethylene glycol concentration is 62 mg/dL or higher [30]. Ethanol remains a treatment alternative but with the same limitations previously mentioned [30, 31]. Dialysis is generally not needed with appropriate and timely administration of fomepizole outside of renal failure; however, severe metabolic acidosis, electrolyte derangements, and renal impairment should lead the practitioner to seriously consider dialysis (Table 37.7). Additional therapies may be considered based on symptomology. Sodium bicarbonate may be considered with acidosis and calcium with hypocalcemia but care should be taken as this may lead to increased production of calcium oxalate crystals, and benzodiazepines can be used to manage seizures. The addition of magnesium, vitamin B6, and thiamine may also help to move metabolism toward the nontoxic metabolites.

Propylene glycol is generally considered safe but intravenous administration at a high dose can lead to toxicity [131, 139, 140]. Treatment involves stopping the offending agent and in severe cases may include hemodialysis (Table 37.7).

37.8 Organophosphates

Nerve agents, such as organophosphates, have a history of being closely associated with chemical warfare during the twentieth century and in later years with terrorist attacks; however, their use as a pesticide is more widespread. Within the United States, organophosphate exposures are less common; however, these agents can be readily found and used in rural agricultural areas (Table 37.8). Developing countries tend to see higher rates of organophosphate exposures and self-poisonings due to being more agriculturally driven and therefore wider availability. Exposure and toxicity can occur via ingestion, inhalation, and dermal absorption with the most toxic route being inhalation [141].

Organophosphates exert their toxic effects by inhibiting acetylcholinesterase. Acetylcholine is a neurotransmitter which stimulates nicotinic and muscarinic receptors resulting in widespread systemic effects such as cardiovascular,

Table 37.8 [34, 141, 142]

Use	Organophosphate compound
Pesticides	Chlorpyrifos, dichlofenthion, dichlorvos, dimethoate, malaoxon, monocrotophos, paraoxon parathion, phorate, profenofos, prothiofos, quinalphos, tetraethyl pyrophosphate
Medicinal (lice treatment)	Malathion
Military nerve agents	Sarin, soman, tabun, VX, Novichok

Table 37.9 Organophosphate/cholinergic symptoms [33, 34, 142, 144–146]

Central nervous system	Muscarinic		Nicotinic
Loss of respiratory drive	Bronchospasm Bronchorrhea Pulmonary edema		Muscle weakness Flaccid paralysis
Loss of consciousness	Bradycardia Hypotension		Hypertension tachycardia
Ataxia Seizures	Miosis Blurred vision		Mydriasis
Headaches Coma	Diaphoresis Excessive excretions		Sweating Fasciculations
Emotional lability anxiety Confusion agitation Apathy Giddiness	Salivation Lacrimation Urination Defecation Gastric cramping Emesis	Defecation Urination Miosis Bradycardia Bronchospasm Bronchorrhea Emesis Lacrimation Salivation	

gastrointestinal, respiratory, and exocrine functions. The function of acetylcholinesterase is to degrade acetylcholine to prevent accumulation at synaptic junctions, thus preventing overstimulation and neurotransmission [143]. Table 37.9 lists key symptoms of cholinergic toxicity; however,s mortality is caused by respiratory compromise and subsequent failure.

Onset of symptoms can range from minutes to days depending on agent and route of exposure, with inhalation having the quickest systemic effects [33, 141]. Toxicity can present in up to three phases depending on the chemical structure of the agent and amount of exposure, the first being acute or initial cholinergic crisis where manifestations of muscarinic and nicotinic receptor overstimulation are seen within minutes to hours. Airway management becomes critical for patients to survive phase one as respiratory failure is leading cause of death in these poisonings. Some patients may experience phase two, or an "intermediate syndrome," which presents as muscle weakness and can occur 24–96 h after an exposure. "Intermediate syndrome" typically results in respiratory muscle weakness as well as limb and cranial nerve weaknesses and paralysis requiring mechanical ventilation or re-intubation which can last up to weeks. The final phase of organophosphate toxicity is delayed polyneuropathy which involves inhibition of neuropathy target esterase (NTE) within the nervous system. This third phase can present without other features of cholinergic toxicity and can occur weeks after acute ingestion with symptoms such as paresthesia in extremities, ataxia, and paralysis [34, 141, 142, 145].

Treatment strategies begin with decontamination. Personal protective equipment should be utilized by emergency personnel including, but not limited to, vapor and fluid impermeable gear as well as respirators to prevent further exposure. Clothing should be removed and sealed to prevent off-gassing, and patient should be washed as appropriately able with either soap and water or dry decontamination procedures [33, 142, 144, 146]. Gastric lavage and activated charcoal may be considered based on patient's cognitive and airway status in the event of pesticide ingestion within 1 h of presentation, however should not be prioritized over stabilization or supportive care and is likely to not provide additional benefit [33, 34, 141, 142]. In patients requiring rapid sequence intubation and mechanical ventilation, the use of nondepolarizing agents may be preferred due to prolonged paralysis with depolarizing agents such as succinylcholine [34, 147]. Benzodiazepines should be utilized for treatment of seizures [33, 34, 141, 142].

Of the agents indicated for treatment of organophosphate toxicity, it is important to note that there is no consensus on recommended dosing across the board, thus multiple dosing strategies may be considered. Inhibition of muscarinic receptor activity with atropine is first-line treatment (Table 37.4). While able to ameliorate muscarinic and cardiac side effects, atropine provides no action at nicotinic receptors. Atropine administration in the setting of organophosphates requires much larger dosages than other listed indications and is based on severity of poisoning. Atropine can be given as intravenous boluses in mild to moderate cases or intravenous boluses followed by infusion in severe symptoms and is indicated when pulmonary status is compromised [33, 34, 142]. Glycopyrrolate can be utilized in organophosphate toxicities where atropine is not readily available; however, it is not recommended as first line. Glycopyrrolate is not as effective as atropine due to its inability to cross the blood–brain barrier into the central nervous system [34, 144]. After atropine administration, oxime therapy is utilized to reactivate acetylcholinesterase, thus decreasing acetylcholine. Two oximes utilized are pralidoxime and obidoxime (Table 37.4); however, their efficacy is dependent on agent of toxicity and if the bond between organophosphate and acetylcholinesterase enzyme has "aged" or become irreversible. Oxime therapy has been noted to be most effective when initiated within the first 24 h [34, 141]. Atropine must be administered prior to oxime therapy in order to reduce muscarinic effects such as bronchopulmonary edema and secretions. Pralidoxime proves the most effective against nicotinic effects such as muscle weakness and paralysis, including respiratory muscle paralysis. An autoinjector of both atropine and pralidoxime is available for emergency personnel to be utilized for rapid response and administration in the event of organophosphate terrorist attacks [33, 34, 141, 142].

While not as commonly seen, carbamates such as neostigmine, physostigmine, and pyridostigmine can manifest in the same manner as organophosphate poisoning due to their mechanism of action being acetylcholinesterase inhibitors. The key difference with carbamates compared to true organophosphates is their reversible inhibition and shorter duration of activity compared to organophosphates which develop irreversible inhibition with aging. In patients presenting in carbamate overdose, supportive care, stabilization, and atropine are utilized, whereas oxime therapy is not [34, 148].

37.9 Antidepressants

Over the years, there has been an increased focus on mental health. In 2021, there was an estimated 57 million adults struggling with mental illness defined as a mental, behavioral, or emotional disorder [149]. With antidepressant drug classes having off-label indications outside of mental health like fibromyalgia, neuropathy, migraine prophylaxis, and smoking cessation, their prescribing and utilization has grown across the board. Medication classes such as selective serotonin reuptake inhibitors (SSRIs), serotonin/norepinephrine reuptake inhibitors (SNRIs), and dopamine/norepinephrine reuptake inhibitors (DNRI) have begun to replace formerly commonplace tricyclic antidepressants (TCA); however, all listed drug classes are still widely used and can present in intentional overdoses as well as severe adverse reactions or unintentional intoxications (Table 37.10).

As described in the drug class name, most of these drug classes inhibit reuptake of serotonin, norepinephrine, or dopamine leading to increased concentrations of these neurotransmitters. SSRIs, SNRIs, and DNRIs have varying activity at each site, but lack activity at the muscarinic and adrenergic receptors where the TCAs block muscarinic and adrenergic receptors, specifically H1-histamine and α-adrenergic receptors [150]. While initial supportive care is similar between these four classes, there are nuances that are key to the treatment of specific overdoses. Activated charcoal may be administered in the event patients present within 1–2 h of ingestion and are able to maintain a protected airway. In the event of modified-release formulation ingestion such as bupropion, activated charcoal may be administered later than the 2-h mark and whole bowl irrigation may be considered [40, 151, 152, 155, 156]. In patients who present or become hypotensive, crystalloid fluid administration is recommended first line followed by vasopressor support if there is an inadequate response. Norepinephrine is recommended in event of TCA overdose specifically due to alpha-adrenergic activity, but can be used in all classes of overdose [40]. Benzodiazepines can be utilized for seizure management, and phenobarbital has been used as an alternative for seizures in refractory cases [40, 150, 151].

Due to their mechanism of action, SSRIs and SNRIs carry the risk of serotonin syndrome by causing overstimulation of receptors within the peripheral and central nervous system. Serotonin syndrome can occur from overdose, drug interactions with other serotonergic agents such as meperidine and linezolid, and as a severe adverse effect outside of overdose situations with these drug classes. Symptoms may occur within hours to days of initiation of one of these medications or after dosage increase and can range from mild to severe. Hallmarks of serotonin syndrome include autonomic instability, altered mental status, hyperreflexia, and spontaneous, inducible, or ocular clonus [151]. While there have been varying criteria used to definitively diagnose serotonin syndrome, the most widely used in part to its ease of use is the Hunter Serotonin Criteria (Table 37.11). Diagnosis of serotonin syndrome must be in the presence of a serotonergic agent or recent use. Some literature references use within previous 5 weeks due to the long half-life of some SSRIs;

Table 37.10 Antidepressant classes (not all inclusive) [40, 150–154]

	SSRI	SNRI	NDRI	TCA
Common medications	Citalopram Escitalopram Fluoxetine Fluvoxamine Paroxetine Sertraline	Duloxetine Desvenlafaxine Venlafaxine	Bupropion	Amitriptyline Clomipramine Doxepin Imipramine Nortriptyline
Mechanism of action	– Selective serotonin reuptake inhibitor	– Serotonin and norepinephrine reuptake inhibitor	– Norepinephrine and dopamine reuptake inhibitor	– Norepinephrine and serotonin reuptake inhibitor – Varying blockade of muscarinic receptors – Varying blockade of H-1 receptors – Varying blockade of α-1 receptors
Symptoms of overdose	– Altered mentation – Sedation – Blurred vision – Tremor – Nausea/vomiting – Seizures – Hypotension – Tachycardia – QTc prolongation	– Altered mentation – Sedation – Blurred vision – Tremor – Nausea/vomiting – Seizures – Hypotension – Tachycardia – QTc prolongation (venlafaxine specific) – Cardiac sodium channel blockade (venlafaxine specific)	– Lethargy – Tremors – Nausea/vomiting – Sinus tachycardia – Hypertension – Bezoar formation of ER products – Seizures	– Altered mentation – Dry mouth and skin – Hyperthermia – Decreased bowel sounds – Seizures – Coma – Hypotension – Hypertension – Tachycardia – QRS prolongation leading to bradycardia and heart block – QTc prolongation

(continued)

Table 37.10 (continued)

	SSRI	SNRI	NDRI	TCA
Primary overdose concern	Serotonin syndrome	Serotonin syndrome	Seizures ER formulations	QRS prolongation
Observation in asymptomatic patients	Minimum 8 h	Minimum 8 h	Minimum 18 h or 24 h in ER formulation overdose	Minimum 6 h

SSRI selective serotonin reuptake inhibitor, *SNRI* serotonin/norepinephrine reuptake inhibitor, *NDRI* norepinephrine/dopamine reuptake inhibitor, *TCA* tricyclic antidepressant, *ER* extended-release

Table 37.11 Hunter serotonin toxicity criteria [157]

In the presence of a serotonergic agent
Spontaneous clonus
Inducible clonus plus agitation or diaphoresis
Ocular clonus plus agitation or diaphoresis
Tremor plus hyperreflexia
Hypertonia plus temperature > 38 °C plus ocular clonus or inducible clonus

however, patients who have recently been initiated on a serotonergic agent, had dose increased, a suspected intentional or unintentional overdose, or new drug interactions should be evaluated for signs and symptoms of serotonin syndrome [37, 151, 158].

Serotonin syndrome in most cases resolves within 24 h of treatment. First-line treatment requires removal of precipitating drug(s). Benzodiazepines can be utilized to manage agitation and muscle rigidity. Hyperthermia results from muscle rigidity, so rapidly abating muscle rigidity is key to prevent progression of rhabdomyolysis. Active cooling measures may also be utilized; however, antipyretic agents are not effective. In severe cases where temperature exceeds 105 °F or 41 °C, intubation followed by sedation and neuromuscular blockade can be seen to treat muscle rigidity and decrease core temperature [37, 151]. Hypertension should be treated with short-acting agents as vital signs may be labile and fluctuating, and hypotension treated with crystalloids or norepinephrine if fluid refractory. Administration of the serotonin agonist cyproheptadine (Table 37.4) is recommended for moderate to severe cases of serotonin syndrome and may be crushed and administered by nasogastric tube in intubated patients. There is not an intravenous formulation. Other agents that have been tested and recommended against include propranolol, bromocriptine, and dantrolene [37]. Case reports have illustrated the use of olanzapine for treatment; however, there is not enough data at this time to recommend its use [159]. Chlorpromazine, while available as intravenous formulation, has been used as an alternative to cyproheptadine; however, carries concerns for worsening hyperthermia as well as contributing to hypotension and lowering of the seizure threshold [37, 91].

Bupropion is the only dopamine and norepinephrine reuptake inhibitor on the market and has increased in usage over the years. While it lacks the risk of serotonin syndrome associated with SSRIs and decreased risk of cardiac complications compared to TCAs, bupropion carries an increased risk of seizures in the setting of overdose and can occur at differing timeframes depending on the formulation ingested. Bupropion is available as immediate release (IR), 12-h sustained-release (SR), and 24-h extended-release (ER) formulations, making it critical to be aware of which formulation a patient may have ingested. In the event of SR or ER formulations, gastrointestinal decontamination may be attempted and effective due to formation of bezoars; however, cognitive status should be closely assessed and prioritized [155, 156]. The extended-formulation produces the "ghost pill" phenomena where a tablet shell can be excreted in the stools and may assist with identification or confirmation of ingestion type [160]. Patients may present with sinus tachycardia, lethargy, agitation, and hallucinations in addition to seizures. In severe overdoses arrhythmias may occur, most commonly as sinus tachycardia but may progress to ventricular arrhythmias; however, most cardiac complications are tachycardic in nature. There have been reports of QRS widening that is refractory to sodium bicarbonate infusion, thus this could be an indication of possible massive bupropion ingestion in cases where the intoxicant is unknown [161, 162].

Seizure activity is the most common symptom of bupropion overdose with occurrence in up to roughly 31% of bupropion cases [152, 163]. Seizures risk increases as doses exceed 450 mg per day and should be anticipated for doses greater than 2500 mg. Onset of seizure activity can be delayed 4–8 h on IR formulations and up to 14–24 h on SR [150, 152, 164]. Tachycardia, agitation, hallucinations, and tremors have been found to occur more frequently in patients who experience seizure activity; however, patients without these symptoms should still be monitored for seizure [152, 164]. Benzodiazepines are recommended first line for seizure activity as well as in patients experiencing neurological symptoms.

Tricyclic antidepressant or TCA symptoms begin roughly 2–6 h post-ingestion and can become quite severe with cardiac complications [154, 165]. Anticholinergic effects such as hyperthermia, agitation, delirium, and blurred vision are common in addition to sinus tachycardia. Electrocardiography monitoring is recommended in TCA ingestions due to risk of cardiac abnormalities such as QRS prolongation (Fig. 37.2) caused by sodium channel blockade resulting in delayed depolarization. This sodium channel blockade can contribute to hypotension caused by decreased peripheral resistance secondary to α-receptor blockade [40, 167, 168].

Hypotension should be treated with norepinephrine in patients who are refractory to intravenous crystalloids. Patients may develop arrhythmias such as atrial fibrillation, ventricular tachycardia, ventricular fibrillation, and QT prolongation

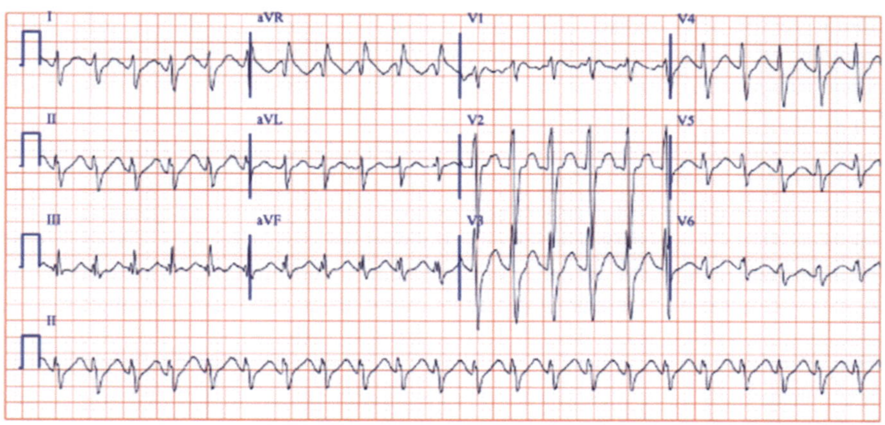

Fig. 37.2 TCA electrocardiogram [166]

leading to Torsades de pointes [168]. Ventricular arrhythmias that are refractory to sodium bicarbonate therapy or become life-threatening should be treated with Class Ib anti-arrhythmics such as lidocaine. Anti-arrhythmics from the other Vaughan Williams classes may potentiate toxicity by contributing to prolonged depolarization or QT intervals further increasing risk of arrhythmias. Magnesium therapy may also be considered in refractory cases and should be utilized in patients experiencing Torsades de pointes [40, 167].

Sodium bicarbonate is the treatment of choice for cardiac conduction abnormalities in the presence of TCA overdose. Criteria for alkalinization with sodium bicarbonate include QRS complex prolongation greater than 100 ms, impaired cardiac conduction including wide complex tachycardia, right bundle branch block, or refractory hypotension, and cardiac arrest. When utilized, the goal serum pH is 7.45–7.55. Therapy is recommended for treatment of impaired conduction but is not recommended as empiric or prophylactic therapy. While the exact mechanism is unknown, alkalinization of blood plasma results in reduced level of free drug as well as potentially increasing sodium concentration while decreasing potassium concentration to overcome sodium channel blockade [167, 169]. While there is not complete consensus on dosing of sodium bicarbonate, it may be administered as either a bolus or continuous infusion (Table 37.4).

Close monitoring and correction of electrolytes should be provided. Literature discusses the utilization of alkalinization and hyperventilation with controlled ventilation, and while ventilation management is outside the scope of pharmacy practice, it is important to note these techniques may be used in combination and management requires multi-disciplinary interaction and therapies. Monitoring for profound alkalosis will be critical due to association of increased mortality in the utilization of alkalinization via drug administration and respiratory management [167, 170]. Intralipid emulsion administration has been used off-label in patients with severe hemodynamic compromise and is still considered experimental in this setting [40, 167].

37.10 Sulfonylureas

Sulfonylureas have a long-standing history of use for glycemic control in type II diabetes mellitus and continue to be used due to low cost. Along with its well-established efficacy as an oral glycemic control agent, the hypoglycemic effects of this drug class are the leading adverse effect and symptom of toxicity. Sulfonylureas stimulate insulin secretion from the pancreas by depolarizing pancreatic β cells via potassium ion efflux reduction. Second-generation sulfonylureas like glipizide, glyburide, and glimepiride are the most commonly available agents within the United States and have peak plasma concentrations within 1–8 h with an onset of action of 1–3 h. Most agents have a listed duration of action of up to 24 h; however, the presence of renal or hepatic dysfunction can extend this up to 72 h due to prolonged half-lives [44, 171, 172]. Predisposing risk factors for sulfonylurea-induced hypoglycemia outside of intentional overdose in nondiabetics include advanced age, poor nutritional or calorie restricted status, sustained physical exercise, alcohol consumption, acute illness, drug interactions, and disease state interactions with disease states such as renal, hepatic, or cardiovascular disease [173]. Signs and symptoms of hypoglycemia such as confusion, dizziness, fatigue, shaking, diaphoresis as well as nausea, vomiting, and tachycardia are the most common clinical presentation, however as hypoglycemia persists more severe adverse effects such as hypotension, hemiparesis, seizures, cardiovascular collapse, and death are seen [44, 174].

For patients who are asymptomatic on presentation, monitoring should be continued a minimum of 8 h with continued glucose monitoring prior to decision to discharge [43]. In patients presenting within 1 h of ingestion, activated charcoal may be administered if patient is neurologically intact. Treatment and prevention of hypoglycemia defined as glucose <60 mg/dL are the focus of sulfonylurea toxicity management. Administration of oral glucose or intravenous dextrose is first line, pending neurologic status of patient and persistence of hypoglycemia (Table 37.4) and should typically be monitored every 15–60 min until stable [43, 44]. Rebound hypoglycemia can be seen in patient requiring continued boluses or infusion of dextrose due to dextrose stimulating endogenous insulin production, which appears to be more prominent in nondiabetic or non-insulin dependent patients [173, 175].

In patients with refractory or rebound hypoglycemia, octreotide has been utilized to restore glycemic control. Octreotide is a somatostatin analog which exerts its activity on pancreatic cell hyperpolarization by inhibiting calcium influx, thus reducing insulin secretion [172, 174]. Octreotide may be administered as a subcutaneous injection or intravenously (Table 37.4), and therapy may extend up to or more than 24 h post-ingestion due to extended half-life of sulfonylurea agents. During octreotide therapy, dextrose infusion may continue but should begin to be tapered off as glucose permits. Other therapies that have been utilized are glucagon and diazoxide, but are no longer recommended. Glucagon induces gluconeogenesis thus promoting insulin secretion which can further exacerbate hypoglycemia. Diazoxide carried a risk of hypotension and tachycardia and is reportedly no longer being manufactured [41, 44].

37.11 Methemoglobinemia

Hemoglobin is responsible for the transport of oxygen and carbon dioxide within the red blood cells. When hemoglobin is oxidized from a ferrous (Fe^{2+}) to ferric (Fe^{3+}) state, it becomes methemoglobin and becomes unable to transport oxygen and carbon dioxide [46, 176, 177]. Reductase pathways maintain normal physiologic methemoglobin below 1%. While methemoglobinemia can be hereditary or acquired, this chapter will not discuss hereditary causes or pathophysiology. Acquired cases can occur from exposure to medications or diet (Table 37.12) that lead to rapid oxidization and increased concentrations of methemoglobin compared to hemoglobin in the blood stream. This increase leads to methemoglobinemia resulting in tissue ischemia and progresses into tachypnea, vascular collapse, coma,

Table 37.12 Acquired methemoglobinemia agents [46, 177, 178]

Diet	Medications	Chemicals
Fava beans	Acetaminophen	Aniline dyes
Nitrate-rich foods Beets Carrots Meets cured in salts Spinach	Amyl nitrate Benzocaine Chloroquine Dapsone EMLA Metoclopramide	Chloramine
Well-water nitrates	Methylene blue	Copper sulfate
	Nitric oxide Nitroglycerin Nitroprusside Phenazopyridine	Fumes Wood Plastic Automobile exhaust
	Phenytoin Prilocaine Primaquine	Herbicides/pesticides Monolinuron Paraquat
	Rasburicase	Mothballs
	Silver nitrite	Nitroethane
	Sulfonamides	Petrol octane booster
	Zopiclone	

and death in severe cases. In 2021, the United States Food and Drug Administration (FDA) released a warning against ingesting "poppers," or energy shot beverages as well as novelty small bottle packages marketed as incense, deodorizers, and polish removers which contain amyl, butyl, isobutyl, or propyl nitrites [179]. Multiple case reports have demonstrated patients presenting to emergency departments after recreational inhalation or ingestion of "poppers" leading to cases of methemoglobinemia due to the presence of amyl, butyl, isobutyl, or propyl nitrites [180–182].

Patients presenting in methemoglobinemia crisis often present with nonspecific symptoms (Table 37.13). Signs of cyanosis such as pale skin or mucous membranes, shortness of breath, fatigue are present; however, patients remain refractory or exhibit minimal improvement to oxygen administration due to lack of oxygen carrying capabilities. The hallmark sign of methemoglobinemia is dark pigmentation of blood. Blood draws will have a dark chocolate brown color compared to redder de-oxygenated blood. Urine may also be darker in nature due to excretion of methemoglobin [46, 176].

Supportive care begins with removal of the offending agent, cardiac support if necessary, and establishing and maintaining an airway. The treatment drug of choice in acquired methemoglobinemia treatment is methylene blue. Through an oxidation-reduction pathway, methylene blue increases the rate of reduction of the iron moiety of methemoglobin to hemoglobin via nicotinamide adenine dinucleotide phosphate (NADPH), thus decreasing methemoglobin when methylene blue is administered at doses <4 mg/kg. At higher doses, methylene blue can have a paradoxical effect where it activates oxidation of Fe^{2+} to Fe^{3+}, thereby increasing methemoglobin concentrations as well as inducing hemolysis, and is considered toxic at doses of

Table 37.13 Methemoglobin concentration and symptoms [177, 178, 183]

Methemoglobin concentration	Symptoms
<20%	Anxiety, cyanosis, low pulse oximetry, often asymptomatic
20–50%	Headache, light-headed, dizziness. fatigue, confused, syncope, tachycardia, tachypnea, chest pain
50–70%	Arrhythmias, metabolic acidosis, seizures, delirium, coma
>70%	Severe hypoxemia, death

methylene blue >7 mg/kg [45, 46, 176, 177, 183]. Onset of action occurs within 30–60 min, however in cases with methemoglobin concentrations >60% or offending agents with long half-lives such as dapsone, repeat doses may be warranted and rebound concentrations can be seen (Table 37.4) [45, 46].

Patients with glucose-6-phsophate dehydrogenase (G6PD) deficiency should not receive methylene blue. The NADPH pathway requires G6PD; therefore, methylene blue will be ineffective at converting methemoglobin to hemoglobin and will increase the risk of increasing severity of methemoglobinemia and inducing hemolysis [45, 46, 177]. Methylene blue should also be used with caution in severe renal impairment and signs of methylene blue toxicity should be monitored. One side effect that can be noted and alarming to patients if not warned is the presence of blue-green urine and feces due to excretion via urine and feces. Blue discoloration of skin should warrant evaluation of the patient as this could indicate toxic levels of methylene blue and potential for worsening methemoglobinemia and hemolysis [45].

37.12 Iron

An essential mineral commonly found in many foods and dietary supplements, iron is necessary for the production of hemoglobin and oxygen transfer throughout the body [184]. Iron supports muscle and connective tissue health and is required for basic cellular function, growth, and neurological development. Throughout various stages of life and in those with specific medical conditions, iron intake or iron stores may be inadequate. This is most common in pregnant women, children, and infants, those with gastrointestinal disorders, cancer, and heart failure; along with frequent blood donors and women with heavy menstrual bleeding. In these cases, iron supplementation becomes necessary to support health. Iron supplementation comes in a variety of iron salts and dosing and is often found in multivitamins, children's and prenatal vitamins, all resulting in varied quantities of elemental iron. However, acute iron intoxication can occur and is a life-threatening condition [185, 186]. Although children are the most vulnerable to intoxication with iron, children's vitamins with a limited iron content are rarely the source [47]. Children often develop life-threatening toxicity when they unintentionally ingest adult preparations of multivitamins or prenatal vitamins [75, 187, 188].

Iron toxicity occurs as a result of direct injury to the gastrointestinal mucosa [47]. This is followed by fluid and blood loss, hemorrhagic necrosis of the gastric mucosa and ultimately perforation and peritonitis. Cellular level effects include disruption of cellular metabolism in the nervous system, heart, and liver, formation of free radicals and impaired oxidative phosphorylation resulting in cellular death.

Acute iron toxicity occurs in a multi-staged process. The stages of toxicity are outlined below (Table 37.14).

Notably patients may progress through each stage or may skip stages all together. Stages are better defined by the symptoms than the timeline [47, 189].

Peak serum iron levels below 350 mcg/dL are generally considered to be associated with minimal toxicity [190]. Moderate toxicity is most associated with levels between 350 and 500 mcg/dL. Severe toxicity and the need for antidote administration are associated with levels greater than 500 mcg/dL; however, patients can develop severe toxicity at any level. This may be, in part, related to the timing on levels relative to ingestion and the rapid disposition of iron into tissues.

Treatment of acute iron toxicity varies with the severity of symptoms. In those who remain asymptomatic for 4–6 h after ingestion, no treatment is necessary. In patients with rapidly resolving GI symptoms and normal vital signs, they should remain under observation and receive supportive care to ensure they are not in the second stage of toxicity. Aggressive care should be provided to any patients who are symptomatic or has any hemodynamic instability. Hypoperfusion and hypovolemia should be treated with an intravenous crystalloid infusion. Some iron formulations are radio-opaque, thus if abdominal X-ray indicates large quantities of visible pills in the stomach, gastric lavage may be considered but is not highly effective. Whole bowel irrigation can be used when started prior to full absorption [156]. Administration of polyethylene glycol solution at 250–500 mL/h in children and 1.5–2 L/h in adults via nasogastric tube will speed transit and decrease absorption. Activated charcoal binds poorly to iron and should not be utilized [189, 191]. In patients with systemic symptoms including shock, coma, metabolic acidosis, gross intestinal blood loss, or serum levels >350 mcg/dL, deferoxamine should be administered. Deferoxamine is a chelating agent which removes iron from tissues and

Table 37.14 Acute iron toxicity stages [47, 189]

Stage	Time frame	Symptoms
Stage 1	0.5–6 h post-ingestion	Initial GI symptoms: vomiting, diarrhea, abdominal pain, hematemesis, hematochezia
Stage 2	6–24 h post-ingestion	Recovery: gastrointestinal symptoms abate despite toxic ingestion
Stage 3	6–72 h post-ingestion	Recurrent GI symptoms: vomiting, diarrhea, abdominal pain, hematemesis, hematochezia, shock, metabolic acidosis, hepatic dysfunction, renal failure, cardiomyopathy, and coagulopathies
Stage 4	12–96 h post-ingestion	Liver failure: progression to hepatic failure with elevated aminotransferases
Stage 5	2–8 weeks	Healing gastrointestinal mucosa: pyloric and proximal bowel scaring and obstruction

plasma and is considered the antidote to acute iron toxicity (Table 37.4). Higher doses of deferoxamine have been reported; however, caution must be used to prevent deferoxamine-related hypotension [192]. Other notable side effects include anaphylaxis which has been reported rarely, tachycardia, hypotension, shock, urticaria and, when used for greater than 24 h, exacerbation and development of acute respiratory distress syndrome (ARDS).

37.13 Digoxin

Approved by the FDA in 1954, digoxin has been a commonly used cardiac glycoside for the last 70 years [193]. However, early descriptions of the use of foxglove, from which digitalis is derived, for medicinal purposes predate FDA approval by more 150 years [194]. Medicinal use of foxglove was described as early as 1785, but prior to the identification of its medicinal use, foxglove was clearly identified as a poisonous plant more than 400 years ago. This creates an ongoing challenge with the use of modern day digoxin which carries a narrow therapeutic window, multiple contraindications to use with a variety of co-morbidities and multiple medication interactions increasing the risk of toxicity with use [193]. Despite the obvious opportunities for toxicity and potential for malicious use in poisoning, these fatal cases of digoxin toxicity have remained relatively infrequent and appear to be in decline [50, 194–196]. However, 1% of patients receiving digoxin for heart failure develop some digoxin toxicity and of patients over the age of 40 who experience an adverse drug event, 1% of these are from the digoxin [195]. Pediatric poisoning is most commonly associated with ingestion of the foxglove plant or medication.

Digoxin exerts its therapeutic effects by increasing intracellular influx of calcium into cardiac myocytes resulting in increased cardiac contractility and cardiac output [193]. This occurs though inhibition of the sodium-potassium ATPase pump resulting in increased intracellular sodium, which in turn drives calcium influx. A secondary mechanism of action is the prolongation of the cardiac action potential because of a rise in the intracellular calcium levels which results in decreased rate of conduction through the atrioventricular node and resulting slowed ventricular response. This results in a medication that demonstrates efficacy in the treatment of heart failure and assisting in the rate control of atrial fibrillation. Toxicity results from extreme inhibition of the sodium-potassium ATPase pump which results in increased automaticity and inotropy which leads to potentially life-threatening arrhythmias (Cummings). Excessive atrioventricular node blockade leads to potentially life-threatening arrhythmias including bradycardia (Fig. 37.3) and asystole [195, 197]. Other symptoms of toxicity may be more vague and include fatigue, dizziness, syncope, hyperkalemia, and gastrointestinal upset, which is the most common. A rather unusual reported symptom of toxicity is visual disturbances with yellow-green discoloration and halos. Digoxin toxicity can be acute, chronic, or acute-on-chronic, and specific symptoms may be more or less meaningful in each setting [50, 195]. For example, hyperkalemia in acute toxicity is a maker for a severe poisoning event

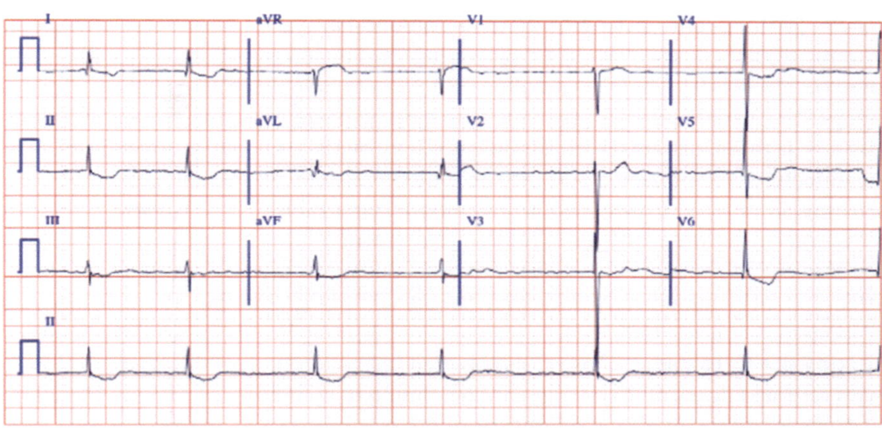

Fig. 37.3 Digitalis toxicity electrocardiogram [166]

but may have less meaning in the setting of chronic toxicity secondary to renal impairment [195]. In all cases, the causes should be sought and symptomology, not digoxin levels, should drive the treatment plan. Digoxin is predominately renally excreted and has a half-life of between 1.5 and 2 days leading to the opportunity for accumulation, particularly with renal impairment and advanced age, and is a major factor in the development of chronic toxicity [50, 195]. Despite the narrow therapeutic window, digoxin levels have proven an unreliable means of establishing toxicity [195]. Typically, the suggested therapeutic range is from 0.5 to 0.9 ng/mL in heart failure patients [198–200]. However, appropriate target serum levels in patients being treated for atrial fibrillation is much less clear with the recent ARISTOTLE trial demonstrated increased mortality with serum digoxin levels in excess of 1.2 ng/mL [201, 202]. Based on the targeted therapeutic range in heart failure and known increase in toxicity as digoxin levels exceed 2 ng/mL, most labs currently report the digoxin therapeutic range as 0.5–2 ng/mL [199]. Values above 2 ng/mL are associated with increased toxicity; however, patients may experience symptoms of toxicity below this level [195, 199].

Management of digoxin toxicity in the chronic, asymptomatic, and mildly symptomatic setting is largely reducing or stopping digoxin dosing [50]. It is important to ensure cardiology support is present as the decrease in circulating digoxin may result in a decline in the control of the treated condition. Additionally, hypokalemia can increase the severity of digoxin toxicity so monitoring and management of electrolytes should be a priority [203]. The backbone of treatment of life-threatening digoxin toxicity is the use of digoxin immune Fab [50, 197]. As with most severe intoxications, immediate management of life-threatening digoxin toxicity is key. Digoxin levels should be drawn and sent immediately however, in the presences of ECG demonstrating life-threatening toxicity treatment should not be delayed for lab results [50]. Specific dosing of digoxin immune Fab varies based on acute versus chronic toxicity, known versus unknown ingested quantities of digoxin, and current digoxin levels [49]. There is an online calculator to help determine appropriate dosing per the manufacturer for patients who have an acute ingestion of a known quantity or in those patients with chronic toxicity with a known digoxin level. The manufacturer recommends 800 mg for acute ingestions of unknown quantities and 240 mg in chronic toxicity with unknown levels (Table 37.4). However, there is variation in the dose utilized worldwide, a recent European consensus statement recommends for patients in cardiac arrest secondary to digoxin overdose to administer 200 mg immediately followed by an additional 200 mg if an inadequate response is achieved [50, 204]. In patients not currently in cardiac arrest but demonstrating life-threatening signs of intoxication, administration of 40–80 mg followed with repeated doses of 40–80 mg until resolution of symptoms of toxicity [50]. This consensus statement also supports use of digoxin immune Fab in patient with very high digoxin levels (>12 ng/mL) regardless of symptomology at a dose adequate to neutralize half of the circulating digoxin. Post treatment with digoxin immune Fab, digoxin levels circulating bound digoxin may still be present for days to weeks depending on the patient's renal function [49]. As a result, digoxin levels that include both bound and unbound digoxin are unlikely to provide any significant insight to the status of toxicity.

Digoxin is not dialyzable (Table 37.7), however, in conjunction with digoxin immune Fab as primary therapy bradyarrhythmias may benefit from atropine and ventricular arrhythmias from lidocaine or magnesium [50, 197]. Phenytoin may also be considered until digoxin immune Fab can be administered [197]. Additional treatment options include cardiac pacing but should be reserved to patients where digoxin immune Fab is not available [50, 197].

37.14 Beta-Blockers

Beta-blockers are currently, and have historically been, one of the most prescribed medications in the United States [205, 206]. This can be attributed, in part, to the long-standing position of beta-blockers as recommended therapy in various guidelines for multiple cardiovascular related conditions as well as a variety of other medical conditions [207–209]. With the ready availability of medications within this class, it is no surprise that it is a major source of both accidental and intentional overdose and related toxicity [210, 211]. Fortunately, although considered as having a high potential for fatal outcomes, with prompt and proper treatment, the vast majority of these events are not fatal. This doesn't diminish the importance of co-ingestion of other substances in the clinical course of a beta-blocker toxicity although studies have not shown co-ingestion to be associated with a significantly worse outcome [212].

Beta-receptors are present throughout the body and, when stimulated by catecholamines, are responsible for a wide variety of biological responses. The toxicology of a beta-blocker overdose is fairly simple as the large dose of beta-blocker will result in non-selective blockade of these receptors preventing normal physiologic response to circulating catecholamines [210]. In the case of the cardiovascular system, this results in bradycardia or heart block with accompanying hypotension as well as depressed cardiac contractility and output [209, 210, 213–215]. Gluconeogenesis and glycogenolysis are also dependent on stimulation of beta-receptors and result in hypoglycemia during acute intoxication. In patients with asthma or COPD, bronchospasm may occur. Based on the unique pharmacokinetic properties of the ingested beta-blocker, other symptoms can appear such as CNS depression and seizures in lipophilic beta-blockers [209, 210]. Timing is also variable based on the specific ingested beta-blocker as some beta-blockers come in extended-release forms or are associated with longer half-lives [209, 210, 213–215]. Kinetics may also be impacted by other co-ingested agents due to decreased gastrointestinal motility [210]. Typically, beta-blockers are rapidly absorbed with peak levels 1–4 h after ingestion and a relatively short half-life in most cases [209, 210, 213–215]. Some beta-blockers, such as sotalol, have additional mechanisms of action that result in the prolongation of the cardiac action potential [216]. This has the additional effect of extending the QTc interval and increasing the risk for cardiac arrhythmias with overdose. The increased QTc interval can persist for several days and necessitates extended observation and management, as does extended-release formulations and beta-blockers with long half-lives [209, 210, 213–216].

Many branches of treatment exist for beta-blocker overdose based on the specific agent and presenting symptoms. The majority of treatment modalities initially focus on the immediate need for supportive care. In those patients with severe CNS depression, intubation may be needed [210]. However, caution may be needed, particularly in smaller patients and children, as vagal stimulation may occur and result in bradycardia. Bronchospasm secondary to beta-blocker toxicity may be treated with inhaled bronchodilators. Seizures should be managed with benzodiazepines as first-line therapy. Some patients, depending on the beta-blocker ingested, may experience widening of the QRS complex and QTc prolongation. Sodium bicarbonate should be administered in the case of QRS complex widening and magnesium sulfate for prolongation of the QTc complex. Gastric lavage, activated charcoal, and whole bowel irrigation may be considered based on the specific product ingested and the timeline of presentation.

Likely the most widely identified beta-blocker overdose symptomology is bradycardia and hypotension, thus a variety of treatment options exist. Atropine may be given, but is likely to only be effective when the bradycardia becomes symptomatic due to increased vagal tone [217]. Fluid boluses should be used to try to mitigate hypotension where possible, but caution should be used when the patient has concomitant diseases associated with and exacerbated by fluid overload such as systolic or diastolic cardiac dysfunction or pulmonary edema. Vasopressor therapy, particularly epinephrine and norepinephrine, at high doses, may be able to support blood pressure and heart rate in those patients not already responsive to fluids. First-line treatment of symptomatic beta-blocker toxicity when fluid boluses and vasopressors are ineffective includes the use of glucagon (Table 37.4). Glucagon can induce nausea and vomiting and should not be used when the patient is unable to protect their airway, but loading doses followed by continuous IV infusion titrated to patient blood pressure and/or heart rate response may be effective in overcoming the cardiovascular depression associated with a beta-blocker overdose [51–53]. Patients on glucagon therapy may experience hyperglycemia and hypocalcemia which should be appropriately monitored and managed. Treatment with calcium may be beneficial to patients who have overdosed on beta-blockers. If a patient proves refractory to all previous therapies, the patient should be considered for high-dose insulin, euglycemic therapy (HIET). This is a therapy where the patient is given high-dose insulin therapy along with dextrose to maintain a euglycemic state which may augment cardiac contractility [54–56]. Numerous animal studies along with human case studies have found effective management using HIET safe and effective and a readily acceptable therapy (Table 37.4). The risk of hypoglycemia is ever present with the high doses of administered insulin so care must be taken to maintain glucose, within the generally accepted goal of 150–200 mg/dL, thus bolus doses of dextrose and continuous infusions of 10% dextrose accompany the insulin infusion (Table 37.4). Although this is a safe and effective therapy, close attention must be paid to volume status, blood glucose, and potassium as these can change quickly and may need further titration of insulin, dextrose, or supplemental potassium. You may also have to consider the concentration of the insulin drip to ensure volume status is not overloaded.

In some patients, alternative treatments such as extracorporeal membrane oxygenation (ECMO) and dialysis may be considered (Table 37.7), but initiation parameters for these extend beyond the scope of this chapter.

37.15 Calcium Channel Blockers

Much like beta-blockers, calcium channel blockers are a commonly prescribed and guideline driven medication in the treatment of various cardiovascular disease states universally [205, 206, 208, 218]. Similar to beta-blockers, over ingestion can be both intentional or accidental; however, both causes can result in significant toxic symptomology and may, in some cases, lead to death [219]. Co-ingestion of other substances are associated with worse outcomes although most cases can be successfully treated if caught and managed promptly [212].

L-type voltage-gated calcium channels are prevalent throughout the body and are the targets of all types of calcium channel blockers [220]. These channels are responsible for several steps in the cardiac electrical conduction pathway including the depolarization for the sinoatrial node and the propagation of the impulse through the atrioventricular node. Calcium release from the sarcoplasmic reticulum in the cardiac muscle is also responsible for triggering myocardial contraction. Higher intracellular calcium levels are associated with the strength of contraction as well. Vascular smooth muscle tone is also maintained via cytosolic calcium concentrations. Calcium channel blockers come in three different classes: phenylalkylamines (verapamil), benzothiazepines (diltiazem), and dihydropyridines (nifedipine, amlodipine, and a host of others) [221–224]. Each of these has slightly different affinities for specific tissues and thus common effects. Both verapamil and diltiazem have potent impacts on the cardiac electrical conduction pathway. Verapamil has greater impact on decreasing smooth muscle tone versus diltiazem which decreases the cardiac chronotropy to a greater extent [225]. Dihydropyridines have less impact on cardiac contractility and electrical conduction but are highly effective vasodilators. Thus it would stand that those patients experiencing toxicity from verapamil would more likely present with cases of symptomatic bradycardia and heart block and those presenting with toxicity from a dihydropyridine would more likely have symptomatic hypotension. However, at toxic doses, the selectivity of these drugs for their respective tissues is lost and both verapamil and diltiazem will present with hypotension, bradycardia, and myocardial conduction abnormalities [226]. Dihydropyridine agents are more likely to develop severe hypotension and a reflex tachycardia [220]. Because of different formulations, onset of symptoms can begin anywhere from 2 h post-ingestion to 16 h post-ingestion and may start with nonspecific symptoms such as fatigue and dizziness. These neurologic symptoms may progress to altered mental status, coma, and even death.

Treatment of calcium channel blocker overdose follows treatment of beta-blocker overdose closely. Initial focus should be on stabilization and resuscitation of the patient. Some patients may benefit from activated charcoal or whole bowel irrigation, but depends on the timing of ingestion versus presentation and the drug and formulation ingested. Initial support should include fluid bolus and repletion as needed based on patient response [227]. Calcium infusion is a key component of treatment of calcium channel blocker overdose as any unblocked channels may allow calcium influx with higher serum calcium concentrations (Table 37.4). However, depending on the severity of intoxication, the value of this treatment may vary [57]. Although more frequent dosing or IV infusion has been used, there are significant side effects possible with aggressive dosing and alternative therapies should be considered prior to providing more aggressive calcium dosing [228]. Vasopressors should be considered, particularly norepinephrine and epinephrine to support blood pressure, heart rate, and cardiac contractility. Dobutamine may be added if the patient is exhibiting cardiogenic shock. High-dose insulin, euglycemic therapy (HIET) has proven beneficial in both the calcium channel blocker overdose population and the beta-blocker overdose population and has the added benefit of the same dosing algorithm (Table 37.4) [55, 58]. This makes early initiation of therapy easier as there is a short delay between starting therapy and clinical response, and early presentation may make the differentiation between beta-blocker overdose and calcium channel blocker overdose challenging. Due to the highly lipophilic nature of verapamil and diltiazem, dialysis is not an option (Table 37.7). However, the use of lipid emulsion therapy may be an option in the most refractory patients based on the theoretical benefit of the lipid emulsion serving as a lipid "sink" for these highly lipophilic medications (Table 37.4) [229–231]. Further, it is proposed that the lipid emulsion can provide an additional fatty energy source to myocytes under duress from the toxicity of the overdose and metabolites. It is important to do all necessary blood work prior to the infusion as serum triglycerides should be monitored and high-dose lipid emulsion can interfere with the accuracy of some other labs including serum glucose.

Although historically some have recommended therapies like glucagon and methylene blue, these were not recommended in the 2017 Expert Consensus for the Management of Calcium Channel Blocker Poisoning in Adults due to the limited number of case reports for methylene blue and the presence of more clearly effective therapies versus glucagon [227].

Non-medicinal therapies may also be considered, such as ECMO and pacemaker placement in severe refractory cases; however, specific criteria for initiation remain outside the scope of this chapter.

37.16 Toxicology Screens

Toxicology screens, while useful in confirming or ruling out etiology for patient presentation, do have potential for false results. Understanding the different types of drug screens and cross-reactivity between agents can assist in determining likelihood for false results and when to rely on patient presentation and history over screening. Saliva, sweat, and hair screenings will not be covered as these are more frequently utilized in outpatient settings; meconium screenings utilized in neonates will also not be covered [232].

Urine drug screens are the gold standard for inpatient testing as they are noninvasive collections and produce rapid results. Most medications and agents of abuse are readily found in the urine due to excretion of metabolites; however, identification of specific agents is a two-part process: immunoassay and mass spectrometry. Screening typically involves a minimum of 30 mL of urine which undergoes an initial immunoassay test, at most testing facilities this includes what is known as the "Federal 5" drugs of abuse: amphetamines, cocaine, marijuana, opiates, phencyclidine (PCP), and their respective metabolites [232, 233]. Additional agents that can be added to the immunoassay tests include barbiturates, benzodiazepines, buprenorphine, codeine, fentanyl, lysergic acid diethylamide (LSD), methadone, morphine, oxycodone, propoxyphene, tramadol, and tricyclic antidepressants [232–235]. The immunoassay tests used include enzymatic immunoassay (EIA), enzyme-linked immunosorbent assay (ELISA), and fluorescence polarization immunoassay [236]. These tests, while rapid, lack sensitivity and specificity, thus leading to increased potential of false positive and negative results. Often this is attributed to biochemical structural similarities between agents such as phencyclidine (PCP) and venlafaxine which may lead to false positives; false negatives may result from testing for specific metabolites that other drugs within the same class do not produce such as lorazepam and alprazolam with diazepam (Table 37.15) [235, 247]. Concentration cut-offs may also lead to false negatives in immunoassay tests depending on the agent tested and the concentration cut-offs determined as detectable or positive by such tests at each facility. This may be seen in medications with therapeutic

Table 37.15 Common false positive and false negative urine immunoassay drug screens [233, 235–246]

	Amph/Meth	Barb	BZD	CBD	MTD	OPI	PCP	LSD
False +	Amantadine Aripiprazole Atomoxetine Bisoprolol Bupropion Chloroquine Chlorpromazine Doxepin Ephedrine Esmolol Labetalol Metformin Metoprolol Mexiletine Promethazine Pseudoephedrine Ranitidine Selegiline Sildenafil Tramadol Trazodone	Ibuprofen Naproxen	Efavirenz Sertraline	Dronabinol Efavirenz Ibuprofen Lumacaftor/ Ivacaftor Naproxen Promethazine Pantoprazole	Chlorpromazine Clomipramine Doxylamine Diphenhydramine Quetiapine Verapamil	Imipramine Levofloxacin Naloxone Naltrexone Rifampin	Desvenlafaxine Dextromethorphan Diphenhydramine Ibuprofen Ketamine Lamotrigine Tramadol Venlafaxine Zolpidem	Amitriptyline Bupropion Buspirone Diltiazem Doxepin Doxylamine Fentanyl Fluoxetine Haloperidol Imipramine Labetalol Methylphenidate Metoclopramide Prochlorperazine Risperidone Sertraline Trazodone Verapamil

(continued)

Table 37.15 (continued)

	Amph/Meth	Barb	BZD	CBD	MTD	OPI	PCP	LSD
False −	MDMA or ecstasy	Sodium thiopental	Alprazolam Chlordiazepoxide Clonazepam Lorazepam Midazolam	Synthetics (spice, K2)		Buprenorphine Fentanyl Hydrocodone Hydromorphone Meperidine Methadone Oxycodone Tramadol		

+ positive, − negative, *Amph* amphetamines, *Meth* methamphetamines, *Barb* barbiturates, *BZD* benzodiazepines, *CBD* cannabinoids, *MTD* methadone, *OPI* opiates, *PCP* phencyclidine, *LSD* lysergic acid diethylamide, *TCA* tricyclic antidepressants, *MDMA* methylenedioxymethamphetamine indications such as some opioids where the deemed positive concentration may be different than considered therapeutic concentrations and thus could result in false negatives [233, 234, 248]. Due to their rapid utilization, immunoassay screens are considered "presumed positive" results and require confirmation by mass spectrometry due to potential for false positive results [234, 235]. Gas chromatography-mass spectrometry (GC-MS) and liquid chromatography-mass spectrometry (LC-MS) are considered the gold standard for confirmatory screens due to their specificity as well as quantitative results [232, 235, 236]. The downside is turn-around time; mass spectrometry testing for smaller institutions may require sending to larger testing sites. When evaluating intoxicated patients, drug screening may be useful, but understanding drug concentration cut-offs, types of testing, and the limitations, these tests carry are essential and support evaluating patient history as well as presentation and potential toxidromes to guide initial treatment.

37.17 Conclusion

Patients experiencing medication overdoses and intoxications can have highly variable clinical presentation, from asymptomatic to life-threatening deterioration, and require quick intervention utilizing a multi-disciplinary approach. Pharmacists are uniquely trained to support identification of toxidromes, communicate with poison control centers, and assist with emergent bedside care. Knowledge of drug mechanisms of action, interactions, metabolism, pharmacodynamics, and pharmacokinetics allows the pharmacists to help plan for monitoring needs, complications and to educate the patient and other caregivers about the anticipated course of the intoxication. The experience with the use and acquisition of specific antidotes that may be niche therapies as well as their dosing can be key to the early and successful treatment of these patient populations. Pharmacists should be engaged early in the care of any potential overdose to assist in optimizing patient outcomes.

References

1. National Poison Control Call Statistics. 2021. https://www.poison.org/poison-statistics-national. Accessed 6 Nov 2023.
2. Centers for Disease Control and Prevention, National Center for Injury Prevention and Control. Understanding the opioid overdose epidemic. 2023. https://www.cdc.gov/opioids/basics/epidemic.html. Accessed 6 Nov 2023.
3. Thim T, Krarup NHV, Grove EL, et al. Initial assessment and treatment with the airway, breathing, circulation, disability, exposure (ABCDE) approach. Int J Gen Med. 2012;5:117–21. https://doi.org/10.2147/IJGM.S28478.
4. Brocato C, Paley RJ Toxidromes: common poisoning syndromes to know—JEMS: EMS, Emergency Medical Services—Training, Paramedic. EMT News. https://www.jems.com/patient-care/common-poisoning-syndromes-to-know/. Accessed 23 Oct 2023.

5. Holstege CP, Borek HA. Toxidromes. Crit Care Clin. 2012;28:479–98. https://doi. org/10.1016/j.ccc.2012.07.008.
6. Broderick ED, Metheny H, Crosby B. Anticholinergic toxicity. In: StatPearls. Treasure Island: StatPearls Publishing; 2023.
7. By the 2023 American Geriatrics Society Beers Criteria® Update Expert Panel. American Geriatrics Society 2023 updated AGS Beers Criteria® for potentially inappropriate medication use in older adults. J Am Geriatr Soc. 2023;71:2052–81. https://doi.org/10.1111/ jgs.18372.
8. Taylor JR, Streetman DS, Castle SS. Medication bezoars: a literature review and report of a case. Ann Pharmacother. 1998;32:940–6. https://doi.org/10.1345/aph.17420.
9. Lott EL, Jones EB. Cholinergic toxicity. In: StatPearls. Treasure Island: StatPearls Publishing; 2022.
10. Robb EL, Baker MB. Organophosphate toxicity. In: StatPearls. Treasure Island: StatPearls Publishing; 2023.
11. The National Institute for Occupational Safety and Health (NIOSH). Sarin: Nerve Agent | NIOSH | CDC. 2011. https://www.cdc.gov/niosh/ershdb/emergencyresponsecard_29750001. html. Accessed 23 Oct 2023.
12. Goldstein S, Richards JR. Sympathomimetic toxicity. In: StatPearls. Treasure Island: StatPearls Publishing; 2023.
13. Simone CG, Bobrin BD. Anxiolytics and sedative-hypnotics toxicity. In: StatPearls. Treasure Island: StatPearls Publishing; 2023.
14. Gardner EA, McGrath SA, Dowling D, Bai D. The opioid crisis: prevalence and markets of opioids. Forensic Sci Rev. 2022;34:43–70.
15. Oelhaf RC, Del Pozo E, Azadfard M. Opioid toxicity. In: StatPearls. Treasure Island: StatPearls Publishing; 2023.
16. Schiller EY, Goyal A, Mechanic OJ. Opioid overdose. In: StatPearls. Treasure Island: StatPearls Publishing; 2023.
17. Lexi-Drugs/Naloxone. UpToDate Inc. Accessed 19 Feb 2024.
18. Goldfrank L, Weisman RS, Errick JK, Lo MW. A dosing nomogram for continuous infusion intravenous naloxone. Ann Emerg Med. 1986;15:566–70. https://doi.org/10.1016/ s0196-0644(86)80994-5.
19. Boyer EW. Management of opioid analgesic overdose. N Engl J Med. 2012;367:146–55. https://doi.org/10.1056/NEJMra1202561.
20. Kelly A, Kerr D, Koutsogiannis Z, et al. Randomised trial of intranasal versus intramuscular naloxone in prehospital treatment for suspected opioid overdose. Med J Aust. 2005;182:24–7. https://doi.org/10.5694/j.1326-5377.2005.tb06550.x.
21. Robertson TM, Hendey GW, Stroh G, Shalit M. Intranasal naloxone is a viable alternative to intravenous naloxone for prehospital narcotic overdose. Prehosp Emerg Care. 2009;13:512–5. https://doi.org/10.1080/10903120903144866.
22. Wong A, Graudins A. Simplification of the standard three-bag intravenous acetylcysteine regimen for paracetamol poisoning results in a lower incidence of adverse drug reactions. Clin Toxicol (Phila). 2016;54:115–9. https://doi.org/10.3109/15563650.2015.1115055.
23. Wong A, Isbister G, McNulty R, et al. Efficacy of a two bag acetylcysteine regimen to treat paracetamol overdose (2NAC study). EClinicalMedicine. 2020;20:100288. https://doi. org/10.1016/j.eclinm.2020.100288.
24. O'Callaghan C, Graudins A, Wong A. A two-bag acetylcysteine regimen is associated with shorter delays and interruptions in the treatment of paracetamol overdose. Clin Toxicol (Phila). 2022;60:319–23. https://doi.org/10.1080/15563650.2021.1966027.
25. Howland MA. Physostigmine salicylate. In: Nelson LS, Howland MA, Lewin NA, et al., editors. Goldfrank's toxicologic emergencies. 11th ed. New York: McGraw-Hill Education; 2019.
26. Proudfoot AT, Krenzelok EP, Vale JA. Position paper on urine alkalinization. J Toxicol Clin Toxicol. 2004;42:1–26. https://doi.org/10.1081/clt-120028740.

27. American College of Medical Toxicology. Guidance document: management priorities in salicylate toxicity. J Med Toxicol. 2015;11:149–52. https://doi.org/10.1007/s13181-013-0362-3.
28. Ashurst JV, Nappe TM. Methanol toxicity. In: StatPearls. Treasure Island: StatPearls Publishing; 2023.
29. Fomepizole injection [package insert]. Shirley: American Regent, Inc; 2020.
30. Iqbal A, Glagola JJ, Nappe TM. Ethylene glycol toxicity. In: StatPearls. Treasure Island: StatPearls Publishing; 2022.
31. McMartin K. Are calcium oxalate crystals involved in the mechanism of acute renal failure in ethylene glycol poisoning? Clin Toxicol (Phila). 2009;47:859–69. https://doi.org/10.3109/15563650903344793.
32. Howland MA. Antidotes in depth—Atropine. In: Goldfrank's toxicologic emergencies. 11th ed. New York: McGraw Hill.
33. Henretig FM, Kirk MA, McKay CA. Hazardous chemical emergencies and poisonings. N Engl J Med. 2019;380:1638–55. https://doi.org/10.1056/NEJMra1504690.
34. King AM, Aaron CK. Organophosphate and carbamate poisoning. Emerg Med Clin North Am. 2015;33:133–51. https://doi.org/10.1016/j.emc.2014.09.010.
35. Koenig KL, Boatright CJ, Hancock JA, et al. Health care facility-based decontamination of victims exposed to chemical, biological, and radiological materials. Am J Emerg Med. 2008;26:71–80. https://doi.org/10.1016/j.ajem.2007.07.004.
36. Roberts DM, Aaron CK. Management of acute organophosphorus pesticide poisoning. BMJ. 2007;334:629–34. https://doi.org/10.1136/bmj.39134.566979.BE.
37. Boyer EW, Shannon M. The serotonin syndrome. N Engl J Med. 2005;352:1112–20. https://doi.org/10.1056/NEJMra041867.
38. Body R, Bartram T, Azam F, Mackway-Jones K. Guidelines in emergency medicine network (GEMNet): guideline for the management of tricyclic antidepressant overdose. Emerg Med J. 2011;28:347–68. https://doi.org/10.1136/emj.2010.091553.
39. Bruccoleri RE, Burns MM. A literature review of the use of sodium bicarbonate for the treatment of QRS widening. J Med Toxicol. 2016;12:121–9. https://doi.org/10.1007/s13181-015-0483-y.
40. Khalid MM, Waseem M. Tricyclic antidepressant toxicity. In: StatPearls. Treasure Island: StatPearls Publishing; 2023.
41. Dougherty PP, Klein-Schwartz W. Octreotide's role in the management of sulfonylurea-induced hypoglycemia. J Med Toxicol. 2010;6:199–206. https://doi.org/10.1007/s13181-010-0064-z.
42. Fasano CJ, O'Malley G, Dominici P, et al. Comparison of octreotide and standard therapy versus standard therapy alone for the treatment of sulfonylurea-induced hypoglycemia. Ann Emerg Med. 2008;51:400–6. https://doi.org/10.1016/j.annemergmed.2007.06.493.
43. Rowden AK, Fasano CJ. Emergency management of oral hypoglycemic drug toxicity. Emerg Med Clin North Am. 2007;25:347–56; abstract viii. https://doi.org/10.1016/j.emc.2007.02.010.
44. Spiller HA, Sawyer TS. Toxicology of oral antidiabetic medications. Am J Health Syst Pharm. 2006;63:929–38. https://doi.org/10.2146/ajhp050500.
45. Clifton J, Leikin JB. Methylene blue. Am J Ther. 2003;10:289–91. https://doi.org/10.1097/00045391-200307000-00009.
46. Skold A, Cosco DL, Klein R. Methemoglobinemia: pathogenesis, diagnosis, and management. South Med J. 2011;104:757–61. https://doi.org/10.1097/SMJ.0b013e318232139f.
47. Yuen H-W, Becker W. Iron toxicity. In: StatPearls. Treasure Island: StatPearls Publishing; 2023.
48. Deferoxime Mesylate [package insert]. Lake Forest: Hospira; 2023.
49. DIGIFab dosing information & calculator | DIGIFab. https://digifab.health/en-us/dosing-digifab/dosing.html. Accessed 22 Mar 2024.
50. Andrews P, Anseeuw K, Kotecha D, et al. Diagnosis and practical management of digoxin toxicity: a narrative review and consensus. Eur J Emerg Med. 2023;30:395–401. https://doi.org/10.1097/MEJ.0000000000001065.

51. Peterson CD, Leeder JS, Sterner S. Glucagon therapy for beta-blocker overdose. Drug Intell Clin Pharm. 1984;18:394–8. https://doi.org/10.1177/106002808401800507.

52. Love JN, Howell JM. Glucagon therapy in the treatment of symptomatic bradycardia. Ann Emerg Med. 1997;29:181–3. https://doi.org/10.1016/S0196-0644(97)70327-5.

53. Shepherd G. Treatment of poisoning caused by β-adrenergic and calcium-channel blockers. Am J Health Syst Pharm. 2006;63:1828–35. https://doi.org/10.2146/ajhp060041.

54. Cole JB, Arens AM, Laes JR, et al. High dose insulin for beta-blocker and calcium channel-blocker poisoning. Am J Emerg Med. 2018;36:1817–24. https://doi.org/10.1016/j.ajem.2018.02.004.

55. Engebretsen KM, Kaczmarek KM, Morgan J, Holger JS. High-dose insulin therapy in beta-blocker and calcium channel-blocker poisoning. Clin Toxicol. 2011;49:277–83. https://doi.org/10.3109/15563650.2011.582471.

56. Holger JS, Engebretsen KM, Fritzlar SJ, et al. Insulin versus vasopressin and epinephrine to treat β-blocker toxicity. Clin Toxicol. 2007;45:396–401. https://doi.org/10.1080/15563650701285412.

57. Hofer CA, Smith JK, Tenholder MF. Verapamil intoxication: a literature review of overdoses and discussion of therapeutic options. Am J Med. 1993;95:431–8. https://doi.org/10.1016/0002-9343(93)90314-F.

58. Bailey B. Glucagon in beta-blocker and calcium channel blocker overdoses: a systematic review. J Toxicol Clin Toxicol. 2003;41:595–602. https://doi.org/10.1081/clt-120023761.

59. Bunchorntavakul C, Reddy KR. Acetaminophen-related hepatotoxicity. Clin Liver Dis. 2013;17:587–607. https://doi.org/10.1016/j.cld.2013.07.005.

60. Chiew AL, Buckley NA. Acetaminophen poisoning. Crit Care Clin. 2021;37:543–61. https://doi.org/10.1016/j.ccc.2021.03.005.

61. Michienzi A, Tobarran N, Hieger MA. Extended release acetaminophen overdose with delayed peak concentrations. Am J Ther. 2022;29:e655–6. https://doi.org/10.1097/MJT.0000000000001329.

62. Hodgman MJ, Garrard AR. A review of acetaminophen poisoning. Crit Care Clin. 2012;28:499–516. https://doi.org/10.1016/j.ccc.2012.07.006.

63. Hendrickson RG. What is the most appropriate dose of N-acetylcysteine after massive acetaminophen overdose? Clin Toxicol (Phila). 2019;57:686–91. https://doi.org/10.1080/15563650.2019.1579914.

64. Dart RC, Mullins ME, Matoushek T, et al. Management of acetaminophen poisoning in the US and Canada: a consensus statement. JAMA Netw Open. 2023;6:e2327739. https://doi.org/10.1001/jamanetworkopen.2023.27739.

65. Yan M, Huo Y, Yin S, Hu H. Mechanisms of acetaminophen-induced liver injury and its implications for therapeutic interventions. Redox Biol. 2018;17:274–83. https://doi.org/10.1016/j.redox.2018.04.019.

66. Wolf SJ, Heard K, Sloan EP, et al. Clinical policy: critical issues in the management of patients presenting to the emergency department with acetaminophen overdose. Ann Emerg Med. 2007;50:292–313. https://doi.org/10.1016/j.annemergmed.2007.06.014.

67. Chomchai S, Mekavuthikul P, Phuditshinnapatra J, Chomchai C. Sensitivity of dose-estimations for acute acetaminophen overdose in predicting hepatotoxicity risk using the Rumack-Matthew nomogram. Pharmacol Res Perspect. 2022;10:e00920. https://doi.org/10.1002/prp2.920.

68. Dart RC, Rumack BH. Patient-tailored acetylcysteine administration. Ann Emerg Med. 2007;50:280–1. https://doi.org/10.1016/j.annemergmed.2007.01.015.

69. Pourbagher-Shahri AM, Schimmel J, Shirazi FM, et al. Use of fomepizole (4-methylpyrazole) for acetaminophen poisoning: a scoping review. Toxicol Lett. 2022;355:47–61. https://doi.org/10.1016/j.toxlet.2021.11.005.

70. Tylenol for healthcare professionals. Guidelines for the management of acetaminophen overdose. https://www.tylenolprofessional.com/sites/tylenol_hcp_us/files/acetaminphen_overdose_treatment_info.pdf. Accessed 1 July 2023.

71. Akakpo JY, Ramachandran A, Curry SC, et al. Comparing N-acetylcysteine and 4-methylpyrazole as antidotes for acetaminophen overdose. Arch Toxicol. 2022;96:453–65. https://doi.org/10.1007/s00204-021-03211-z.

72. Rampon G, Wartman H, Osmon S, Scalzo A. Use of fomepizole as an adjunct in the treatment of acetaminophen overdose: a case series. Toxicol Commun. 2020;4:1–4. https://doi.org/1 0.1080/24734306.2019.1705596.

73. Kiernan EA, Fritzges JA, Henry KA, Katz KD. A case report of massive acetaminophen poisoning treated with a novel "triple therapy": N-acetylcysteine, 4-Methylpyrazole, and hemodialysis. Case Rep Emerg Med. 2019;2019:9301432. https://doi.org/10.1155/2019/9301432.

74. Palmer BF, Clegg DJ. Salicylate toxicity. N Engl J Med. 2020;382:2544–55. https://doi. org/10.1056/NEJMra2010852.

75. Gummin DD, Mowry JB, Spyker DA, et al. 2018 annual report of the American Association of Poison Control Centers' National Poison Data System (NPDS): 36th annual report. Clin Toxicol (Phila). 2019;57:1220–413. https://doi.org/10.1080/15563650.2019.1677022.

76. Thongprayoon C, Petnak T, Kaewput W, et al. Hospitalizations for acute salicylate intoxication in the United States. J Clin Med. 2020;9:2638. https://doi.org/10.3390/jcm9082638.

77. O'Malley GF. Emergency department management of the salicylate-poisoned patient. Emerg Med Clin North Am. 2007;25:333–46; abstract viii. https://doi.org/10.1016/j. emc.2007.02.012.

78. Chyka PA, Erdman AR, Christianson G, et al. Salicylate poisoning: an evidence-based consensus guideline for out-of-hospital management. Clin Toxicol (Phila). 2007;45:95–131. https://doi.org/10.1080/15563650600907140.

79. Thongprayoon C, Lapumnuaypol K, Kaewput W, et al. Gastrointestinal bleeding among hospitalizations for salicylate poisoning in the United States. QJM. 2021;114:190–5. https://doi. org/10.1093/qjmed/hcab034.

80. Runde TJ, Nappe TM. Salicylates toxicity. In: StatPearls. Treasure Island: StatPearls Publishing; 2023.

81. Lexi-Tox/Acetaminophen. UpToDate. Accessed 28 Oct 2023.

82. King JD, Kern MH, Jaar BG. Extracorporeal removal of poisons and toxins. Clin J Am Soc Nephrol. 2019;14:1408–15. https://doi.org/10.2215/CJN.02560319.

83. Gosselin S. Juurlink DN, Kielstein JT, et al. Extracorporeal treatment for acetaminophen poisoning: recommendations from the EXTRIP workgroup. Clin Toxicol (Phila). 2014;52:856–67. https://doi.org/10.3109/15563650.2014.946994.

84. Lexi-Tox/Salicylates. UpToDate. Accessed 28 Oct 2023.

85. Juurlink DN, Gosselin S, Kielstein JT, et al. Extracorporeal treatment for salicylate poisoning: systematic review and recommendations from the EXTRIP workgroup. Ann Emerg Med. 2015;66:165–81. https://doi.org/10.1016/j.annemergmed.2015.03.031.

86. Ashurst JV, Nappe TM. Isopropanol toxicity. In: StatPearls. Treasure Island: StatPearls Publishing; 2023.

87. Ghannoum M, Gosselin S, Hoffman RS, et al. Extracorporeal treatment for ethylene glycol poisoning: systematic review and recommendations from the EXTRIP workgroup. Crit Care. 2023;27:56. https://doi.org/10.1186/s13054-022-04227-2.

88. Roberts DM, Yates C, Megarbane B, et al. Recommendations for the role of extracorporeal treatments in the management of acute methanol poisoning: a systematic review and consensus statement. Crit Care Med. 2015;43:461–72. https://doi.org/10.1097/ CCM.0000000000000708.

89. Lexi-Tox/Antidepressants, tricyclic. UpToDate. Accessed 28 Oct 2023.

90. Yates C, Galvao T, Sowinski KM, et al. Extracorporeal treatment for tricyclic antidepressant poisoning: recommendations from the EXTRIP workgroup. Semin Dial. 2014;27:381. https://doi.org/10.1111/sdi.12227.

91. Lexi-Tox/Antidepressants, selective serotonin reuptake inhibitor. UpToDate. Accessed 1 Aug 2023.

92. Lexi-Tox/Antidepressants, serotonin/norepinephrine reuptake inhibitor. UpToDate. Accessed 9 Nov 2023.
93. Lexi-Tox/Bupropion. UpToDate. Accessed 9 Nov 2023.
94. Lexi-Tox/Sulfonylureas. UpToDate. Accessed 28 Oct 2023.
95. Gumber MR, Kute VB, Shah PR, et al. Successful treatment of severe iron intoxication with gastrointestinal decontamination, deferoxamine, and hemodialysis. Ren Fail. 2013;35:729–31. https://doi.org/10.3109/0886022X.2013.790299.
96. Bouchard J, Shepherd G, Hoffman RS, et al. Extracorporeal treatment for poisoning to beta-adrenergic antagonists: systematic review and recommendations from the EXTRIP workgroup. Crit Care. 2021;25:201. https://doi.org/10.1186/s13054-021-03585-7.
97. Tieu A, Velenosi TJ, Kucey AS, et al. β-blocker dialyzability in maintenance hemodialysis patients. Clin J Am Soc Nephrol. 2018;13:604–11. https://doi.org/10.2215/CJN.07470717.
98. Yeh T-H, Tu K-C, Hung K-C, et al. Impact of type of dialyzable beta-blockers on subsequent risk of mortality in patients receiving dialysis: a systematic review and meta-analysis. PLoS One. 2022;17:e0279680. https://doi.org/10.1371/journal.pone.0279680.
99. Lexi-Tox/Beta-Blockers. UpToDate. Accessed 28 Oct 2023.
100. Lexi-Tox/Calcium Channel Blockers. UpToDate. Accessed 28 Oct 2023.
101. Wong A, Hoffman RS, Walsh SJ, et al. Extracorporeal treatment for calcium channel blocker poisoning: systematic review and recommendations from the EXTRIP workgroup. Clin Toxicol (Phila). 2021;59:361–75. https://doi.org/10.1080/15563650.2020.1870123.
102. Mactier R, Laliberté M, Mardini J, et al. Extracorporeal treatment for barbiturate poisoning: recommendations from the EXTRIP workgroup. Am J Kidney Dis. 2014;64:347–58. https://doi.org/10.1053/j.ajkd.2014.04.031.
103. Coluzzi F, Caputi FF, Billeci D, et al. Safe use of opioids in chronic kidney disease and hemodialysis patients: tips and tricks for non-pain specialists. Ther Clin Risk Manag. 2020;16:821–37. https://doi.org/10.2147/TCRM.S262843.
104. Hassan H, Bastani B, Gellens M. Successful treatment of normeperidine neurotoxicity by hemodialysis. Am J Kidney Dis. 2000;35:146–9. https://doi.org/10.1016/S0272-6386(00)70314-3.
105. Lexi-Tox/Opioids. UpToDate. Accessed 10 Nov 2023.
106. Dialysis for Acute Poisonings—DynaMedex. https://www.dynamedex.com/management/dialysis-for-acute-poisonings#GUID-ABA87282-EB2B-46AA-BD58-C2E269719FDB. Accessed 9 Nov 2023.
107. Ghannoum M, Berling I, Lavergne V, et al. Recommendations from the EXTRIP workgroup on extracorporeal treatment for baclofen poisoning. Kidney Int. 2021;100:720–36. https://doi.org/10.1016/j.kint.2021.07.014.
108. Lexi-Tox/Baclofen. UpToDate. Accessed 10 Nov 2023.
109. Al Khalili Y, Sekhon S, Jain S. Carbamazepine toxicity. In: StatPearls. Treasure Island: StatPearls Publishing; 2023.
110. Lexi-Tox/Carbamazepine. UpToDate. Accessed 28 Oct 2023.
111. Ghannoum M, Yates C, Galvao TF, et al. Extracorporeal treatment for carbamazepine poisoning: systematic review and recommendations from the EXTRIP workgroup. Clin Toxicol (Phila). 2014;52:993–1004. https://doi.org/10.3109/15563650.2014.973572.
112. Lexi-Tox/Digoxin. UpToDate. Accessed 25 May 2023.
113. Mowry JB, Burdmann EA, Anseeuw K, et al. Extracorporeal treatment for digoxin poisoning: systematic review and recommendations from the EXTRIP workgroup. Clin Toxicol (Phila). 2016;54:103–14. https://doi.org/10.3109/15563650.2015.1118488.
114. Lexi-Tox/Lithium. UpToDate. Accessed 28 Oct 2023.
115. Decker BS, Goldfarb DS, Dargan PI, et al. Extracorporeal treatment for lithium poisoning: systematic review and recommendations from the EXTRIP workgroup. Clin J Am Soc Nephrol. 2015;10:875–87. https://doi.org/10.2215/CJN.10021014.
116. Lexi-Tox/Biguanides. UpToDate. Accessed 28 Oct 2023.
117. Calello DP, Liu KD, Wiegand TJ, et al. Extracorporeal treatment for metformin poisoning: systematic review and recommendations from the extracorporeal treatments in poisoning workgroup. Crit Care Med. 2015;43:1716–30. https://doi.org/10.1097/CCM.0000000000001002.

118. Lexi-Tox/Phenytoin and derivatives. UpToDate. Accessed 28 Oct 2023.
119. Anseeuw K, Mowry JB, Burdmann EA, et al. Extracorporeal treatment in phenytoin poisoning: systematic review and recommendations from the EXTRIP (extracorporeal treatments in poisoning) workgroup. Am J Kidney Dis. 2016;67:187–97. https://doi.org/10.1053/j.ajkd.2015.08.031.
120. Lexi-Tox/Valproic acid and derivatives. UpToDate. Accessed 28 Oct 2023.
121. Ghannoum M, Laliberté M, Nolin TD, et al. Extracorporeal treatment for valproic acid poisoning: systematic review and recommendations from the EXTRIP workgroup. Clin Toxicol (Phila). 2015;53:454–65. https://doi.org/10.3109/15563650.2015.1035441.
122. Bennett IL, Cary FH, Mitchell GL, Cooper MN. Acute methyl alcohol poisoning: a review based on experiences in an outbreak of 323 cases. Medicine (Baltimore). 1953;32:431–63. https://doi.org/10.1097/00005792-195312000-00002.
123. Ghannoum M, Hoffman RS, Mowry JB, Lavergne V. Trends in toxic alcohol exposures in the United States from 2000 to 2013: a focus on the use of antidotes and extracorporeal treatments. Semin Dial. 2014;27:395–401. https://doi.org/10.1111/sdi.12237.
124. Slaughter RJ, Mason RW, Beasley DMG, et al. Isopropanol poisoning. Clin Toxicol (Phila). 2014;52:470–8. https://doi.org/10.3109/15563650.2014.914527.
125. Robinson CN, Latimer B, Abreo F, et al. In-vivo evidence of nephrotoxicity and altered hepatic function in rats following administration of diglycolic acid, a metabolite of diethylene glycol. Clin Toxicol (Phila). 2017;55:196–205. https://doi.org/10.1080/15563650.2016.1271128.
126. Jacobsen D, McMartin KE. Methanol and ethylene glycol poisonings. Mechanism of toxicity, clinical course, diagnosis and treatment. Med Toxicol. 1986;1:309–34. https://doi.org/10.1007/BF03259846.
127. Hovda KE, Hunderi OH, Tafjord A-B, et al. Methanol outbreak in Norway 2002-2004: epidemiology, clinical features and prognostic signs. J Intern Med. 2005;258:181–90. https://doi.org/10.1111/j.1365-2796.2005.01521.x.
128. Karayel F, Turan AA, Sav A, et al. Methanol intoxication: pathological changes of central nervous system (17 cases). Am J Forensic Med Pathol. 2010;31:34–6. https://doi.org/10.1097/PAF.0b013e3181c160d9.
129. Alhamad T, Blandon J, Meza AT, et al. Acute kidney injury with oxalate deposition in a patient with a high anion gap metabolic acidosis and a normal osmolal gap. J Nephropathol. 2013;2:139–43. https://doi.org/10.12860/JNP.2013.23.
130. Kang M, Galuska MA, Ghassemzadeh S. Benzodiazepine toxicity. In: StatPearls. Treasure Island: StatPearls Publishing; 2023.
131. Zar T, Graeber C, Perazella MA. Recognition, treatment, and prevention of propylene glycol toxicity. Semin Dial. 2007;20:217–9. https://doi.org/10.1111/j.1525-139X.2007.00280.x.
132. Barceloux DG, Bond GR, Krenzelok EP, et al. American Academy of Clinical Toxicology practice guidelines on the treatment of methanol poisoning. J Toxicol Clin Toxicol. 2002;40:415–46. https://doi.org/10.1081/clt-120006745.
133. Brent J. Fomepizole for ethylene glycol and methanol poisoning. N Engl J Med. 2009;360:2216–23. https://doi.org/10.1056/NEJMct0806112.
134. Pappas AA, Ackerman BH, Olsen KM, Taylor EH. Isopropanol ingestion: a report of six episodes with isopropanol and acetone serum concentration time data. J Toxicol Clin Toxicol. 1991;29:11–21. https://doi.org/10.3109/15563659109038593.
135. Jha VK, Padmaprakash KV. Extracorporeal treatment in the management of acute poisoning: what an intensivist should know? Indian J Crit Care Med. 2018;22:862–9. https://doi.org/10.4103/ijccm.IJCCM_425_18.
136. Borron SW, Baud FJ, Garnier R. Intravenous 4-methylpyrazole as an antidote for diethylene glycol and triethylene glycol poisoning: a case report. Vet Hum Toxicol. 1997;39:26–8.
137. Seltzer JA, Corbett B, Lasoff DR, Clark RF. Symptomatic diethylene glycol ingestion successfully treated with fomepizole monotherapy. J Emerg Med. 2022;63:58–61. https://doi.org/10.1016/j.jemermed.2022.04.021.

138. Brophy PD, Tenenbein M, Gardner J, et al. Childhood diethylene glycol poisoning treated with alcohol dehydrogenase inhibitor fomepizole and hemodialysis. Am J Kidney Dis. 2000;35:958–62. https://doi.org/10.1016/s0272-6386(00)70270-8.

139. Pillai U, Hothi JC, Bhat ZY. Severe propylene glycol toxicity secondary to use of anti-epileptics. Am J Ther. 2014;21:e106–9. https://doi.org/10.1097/MJT.0b013e31824c407d.

140. Miller MA, Forni A, Yogaratnam D. Propylene glycol-induced lactic acidosis in a patient receiving continuous infusion pentobarbital. Ann Pharmacother. 2008;42:1502–6. https://doi.org/10.1345/aph.1L186.

141. Chowdhary S, Bhattacharyya R, Banerjee D. Acute organophosphorus poisoning. Clin Chim Acta. 2014;431:66–76. https://doi.org/10.1016/j.cca.2014.01.024.

142. Aman S, Paul S, Chowdhury FR. Management of organophosphorus poisoning: standard treatment and beyond. Crit Care Clin. 2021;37:673–86. https://doi.org/10.1016/j.ccc.2021.03.011.

143. Sam C, Bordoni B. Physiology, acetylcholine. In: StatPearls. Treasure Island: StatPearls Publishing; 2023.

144. Richardson KJ, Schwinck JL, Robinson MV. Organophosphate poisoning. Nurse Pract. 2021;46:18–21. https://doi.org/10.1097/01.NPR.0000743328.87750.d7.

145. Wadia RS, Sadagopan C, Amin RB, Sardesai HV. Neurological manifestations of organophosphorous insecticide poisoning. J Neurol Neurosurg Psychiatry. 1974;37:841–7. https://doi.org/10.1136/jnnp.37.7.841.

146. Hulse EJ, Haslam JD, Emmett SR, Woolley T. Organophosphorus nerve agent poisoning: managing the poisoned patient. Br J Anaesth. 2019;123:457–63. https://doi.org/10.1016/j.bja.2019.04.061.

147. Selden BS, Curry SC. Prolonged succinylcholine-induced paralysis in organophosphate insecticide poisoning. Ann Emerg Med. 1987;16:215–7. https://doi.org/10.1016/s0196-0644(87)80018-5.

148. Lexi-Tox/Carbamates. UpToDate. Accessed 1 Aug 2023.

149. Substance Abuse and Mental Health Services Administration. Key substance use and mental health indicators in the United States: results from the 2021 National Survey on Drug Use and Health; 2023.

150. Sarko J. Antidepressants, old and new. A review of their adverse effects and toxicity in overdose. Emerg Med Clin North Am. 2000;18:637–54. https://doi.org/10.1016/s0733-8627(05)70151-6.

151. Reilly TH, Kirk MA. Atypical antipsychotics and newer antidepressants. Emerg Med Clin North Am. 2007;25:477–97; abstract x. https://doi.org/10.1016/j.emc.2007.02.003.

152. Starr P, Klein-Schwartz W, Spiller H, et al. Incidence and onset of delayed seizures after overdoses of extended-release bupropion. Am J Emerg Med. 2009;27:911–5. https://doi.org/10.1016/j.ajem.2008.07.004.

153. Jasiak NM, Bostwick JR. Risk of QT/QTc prolongation among newer non-SSRI antidepressants. Ann Pharmacother. 2014;48:1620–8. https://doi.org/10.1177/1060028014550645.

154. Woolf AD, Erdman AR, Nelson LS, et al. Tricyclic antidepressant poisoning: an evidence-based consensus guideline for out-of-hospital management. Clin Toxicol (Phila). 2007;45:203–33. https://doi.org/10.1080/15563650701226192.

155. Buckley NA, Faunce TA. "Atypical" antidepressants in overdose: clinical considerations with respect to safety. Drug Saf. 2003;26:539–51. https://doi.org/10.2165/00002018-200326080-00002.

156. Thanacoody R, Caravati EM, Troutman B, et al. Position paper update: whole bowel irrigation for gastrointestinal decontamination of overdose patients. Clin Toxicol (Phila). 2015;53:5–12. https://doi.org/10.3109/15563650.2014.989326.

157. Dunkley EJC, Isbister GK, Sibbritt D, et al. The hunter serotonin toxicity criteria: simple and accurate diagnostic decision rules for serotonin toxicity. QJM. 2003;96:635–42. https://doi.org/10.1093/qjmed/hcg109.

158. Mikkelsen N, Damkier P, Pedersen SA. Serotonin syndrome—A focused review. Basic Clin Pharmacol Toxicol. 2023;133:124–9. https://doi.org/10.1111/bcpt.13912.
159. Boddy R, Ali R, Dowsett R. Use of sublingual olanzapine in serotonin syndrome. 2004. https://www.researchgate.net/publication/285981887_Use_of_sublingual_olanzapine_in_ serotonin_syndrome. Accessed 24 Oct 2023.
160. Overberg A, Purpura A, Nanagas K. "Ghost tablet" husks excreted in feces in large bupropion XL overdose. Clin Toxicol (Phila). 2019;57:141–2. https://doi.org/10.1080/15563650.201 8.1494276.
161. Druteika D, Zed PJ. Cardiotoxicity following bupropion overdose. Ann Pharmacother. 2002;36:1791–5. https://doi.org/10.1345/aph.1C045.
162. Curry SC, Kashani JS, LoVecchio F, Holubek W. Intraventricular conduction delay after bupropion overdose. J Emerg Med. 2005;29:299–305. https://doi.org/10.1016/j. jemermed.2005.01.027.
163. Reichert C, Reichert P, Monnet-Tschudi F, et al. Seizures after single-agent overdose with pharmaceutical drugs: analysis of cases reported to a poison center. Clin Toxicol (Phila). 2014;52:629–34. https://doi.org/10.3109/15563650.2014.918627.
164. Shepherd G, Velez LI, Keyes DC. Intentional bupropion overdoses. J Emerg Med. 2004;27:147–51. https://doi.org/10.1016/j.jemermed.2004.02.017.
165. Brooks DE, Levine M, O'Connor AD, et al. Toxicology in the ICU: part 2: specific toxins. Chest. 2011;140:1072–85. https://doi.org/10.1378/chest.10-2726.
166. Nathanson LA, McClennen S, Safran C, Goldberger AL. ECG wave-maven: an internet-based electrocardiography self-assessment program for students and clinicians. Med Educ Online. 2003;8:4339. https://doi.org/10.3402/meo.v8i.4339.
167. Kerr GW, McGuffie AC, Wilkie S. Tricyclic antidepressant overdose: a review. Emerg Med J. 2001;18:236–41. https://doi.org/10.1136/emj.18.4.236.
168. Thanacoody HKR, Thomas SHL. Tricyclic antidepressant poisoning: cardiovascular toxicity. Toxicol Rev. 2005;24:205–14. https://doi.org/10.2165/00139709-200524030-00013.
169. Blackman K, Brown SG, Wilkes GJ. Plasma alkalinization for tricyclic antidepressant toxicity: a systematic review. Emerg Med (Fremantle). 2001;13:204–10. https://doi. org/10.1046/j.1442-2026.2001.00213.x.
170. Wrenn K, Smith BA, Slovis CM. Profound alkalemia during treatment of tricyclic antide-pressant overdose: a potential hazard of combined hyperventilation and intravenous bicar-bonate. Am J Emerg Med. 1992;10:553–5. https://doi.org/10.1016/0735-6757(92)90183-x.
171. Harrigan RA, Nathan MS, Beattie P. Oral agents for the treatment of type 2 diabetes mel-litus: pharmacology, toxicity, and treatment. Ann Emerg Med. 2001;38:68–78. https://doi. org/10.1067/mem.2001.114314.
172. Glatstein M, Scolnik D, Bentur Y. Octreotide for the treatment of sulfonylurea poisoning. Clin Toxicol (Phila). 2012;50:795–804. https://doi.org/10.3109/15563650.2012.734626.
173. Lheureux PE, Zahir S, Penaloza A, Gris M. Bench-to-bedside review: antidotal treatment of sulfonylurea-induced hypoglycaemia with octreotide. Crit Care. 2005;9:543–9. https://doi. org/10.1186/cc3807.
174. Carr R, Zed PJ. Octreotide for sulfonylurea-induced hypoglycemia following overdose. Ann Pharmacother. 2002;36:1727–32. https://doi.org/10.1345/aph.1C076.
175. Klein-Schwartz W, Stassinos GL, Isbister GK. Treatment of sulfonylurea and insulin over-dose. Br J Clin Pharmacol. 2016;81:496–504. https://doi.org/10.1111/bcp.12822.
176. Curry S. Methemoglobinemia. Ann Emerg Med. 1982;11:214–21. https://doi.org/10.1016/ s0196-0644(82)80502-7.
177. Wright RO, Lewander WJ, Woolf AD. Methemoglobinemia: etiology, pharmacology, and clinical management. Ann Emerg Med. 1999;34:646–56. https://doi.org/10.1016/ s0196-0644(99)70167-8.
178. McNulty R, Kuchi N, Xu E, Gunja N. Food-induced methemoglobinemia: a systematic review. J Food Sci. 2022;87:1423–48. https://doi.org/10.1111/1750-3841.16090.

179. Office of the Commissioner. Ingesting or inhaling nitrite "poppers" can cause severe injury or death. US Food and Drug Administration; 2023.
180. Tello DM, Doodnauth AV, Patel KH, et al. Poppers-induced methemoglobinemia: a curious case of the blues. Cureus. 2021;13:e15276. https://doi.org/10.7759/cureus.15276.
181. Lefevre T, Nuzzo A, Mégarbane B. Poppers-induced life-threatening methemoglobinemia. Am J Respir Crit Care Med. 2018;198:e137–8. https://doi.org/10.1164/rccm.201806-1044IM.
182. Sonck E, Bourmanne E, Bruteyn J, Dolip W. Methemoglobinemia due to use of poppers: a case report. J Med Case Rep. 2022;16:244. https://doi.org/10.1186/s13256-022-03475-8.
183. Iolascon A, Bianchi P, Andolfo I, et al. Recommendations for diagnosis and treatment of methemoglobinemia. Am J Hematol. 2021;96:1666–78. https://doi.org/10.1002/ajh.26340.
184. Office of Dietary Supplements—Iron. https://ods.od.nih.gov/factsheets/Iron-HealthProfessional/. Accessed 20 Oct 2023.
185. Pestaner JP, Ishak KG, Mullick FG, Centeno JA. Ferrous sulfate toxicity: a review of autopsy findings. Biol Trace Elem Res. 1999;69:191–8. https://doi.org/10.1007/BF02783871.
186. Morris CC. Pediatric iron poisonings in the United States. South Med J. 2000;93:352–8.
187. Mowry JB, Spyker DA, Cantilena LR, et al. 2013 annual report of the American Association of Poison Control Centers' National Poison Data System (NPDS): 31st annual report. Clin Toxicol (Phila). 2014;52:1032–283. https://doi.org/10.3109/15563650.2014.987397.
188. Gummin DD, Mowry JB, Spyker DA, et al. 2016 annual report of the American Association of Poison Control Centers' National Poison Data System (NPDS): 34th annual report. Clin Toxicol. 2017;55:1072–254. https://doi.org/10.1080/15563650.2017.1388087.
189. Fine JS. Iron poisoning. Curr Probl Pediatr. 2000;30:71–90. https://doi.org/10.1067/mps.2000.104055.
190. Chyka PA, Butler AY, Holley JE. Serum iron concentrations and symptoms of acute iron poisoning in children. Pharmacotherapy. 1996;16:1053–8.
191. Chyka P, Banner W Jr. Hematopoietic agents. In: Medical toxicology. 3rd ed. Philadelphia: Lippincott Williams & Wilkins; 2003. p. 605–15.
192. Peck MG, Rogers JF, Rivenbark JF. Use of high doses of deferoxamine (Desferal) in an adult patient with acute iron overdosage. J Toxicol Clin Toxicol. 1982;19:865–9. https://doi.org/10.3109/15563658208992521.
193. David MNV, Shetty M. Digoxin. In: StatPearls. Treasure Island: StatPearls Publishing; 2023.
194. Burchell HB. Digitalis poisoning: historical and forensic aspects. J Am Coll Cardiol. 1983;1:506–16. https://doi.org/10.1016/S0735-1097(83)80080-1.
195. Cummings ED, Swoboda HD. Digoxin toxicity. In: StatPearls. Treasure Island: StatPearls Publishing; 2023.
196. Haynes K, Heitjan D, Kanetsky P, Hennessy S. Declining public health burden of digoxin toxicity from 1991 to 2004. Clin Pharmacol Ther. 2008;84:90–4. https://doi.org/10.1038/sj.clpt.6100458.
197. Lavonas EJ, Akpunonu PD, Arens AM, et al. 2023 American Heart Association focused update on the management of patients with cardiac arrest or life-threatening toxicity due to poisoning: an update to the American Heart Association guidelines for cardiopulmonary resuscitation and emergency cardiovascular care. Circulation. 2023;148:e149–84. https://doi.org/10.1161/CIR.0000000000001161.
198. Yancy CW, Jessup M, Bozkurt B, et al. 2013 ACCF/AHA guideline for the management of heart failure: a report of the American College of Cardiology Foundation/American Heart Association task force on practice guidelines. J Am Coll Cardiol. 2013;62:e147–239. https://doi.org/10.1016/j.jacc.2013.05.019.
199. Drug Result Page—Quick Answers—Medication Safety—Monitoring. In: Digoxin. https://www.micromedexsolutions.com/micromedex2/librarian/CS/707E84/ND_PR/evidencexpert/ND_P/evidencexpert/DUPLICATIONSHIELDSYNC/E7CC7D/ND_PG/evidencexpert/ND_B/evidencexpert/ND_AppProduct/evidencexpert/ND_T/evidencexpert/PFActionId/evidencexpert.DoIntegratedSearch?SearchTerm=digoxin&UserSearchTerm=digoxin&SearchFilter=filterNone&navitem=searchALL#cite9_dp. Accessed 21 Mar 2024.

200. Ahmed A, Gambassi G, Weaver MT, et al. Effects of discontinuation of digoxin versus continuation at low serum digoxin concentrations in chronic heart failure. Am J Cardiol. 2007;100:280–4. https://doi.org/10.1016/j.amjcard.2007.02.099.
201. Lopes RD, Rordorf R, De Ferrari GM, et al. Digoxin and mortality in patients with atrial fibrillation. J Am Coll Cardiol. 2018;71:1063–74. https://doi.org/10.1016/j.jacc.2017.12.060.
202. Ferrari F, Santander IRMF, Stein R. Digoxin in atrial fibrillation: an old topic revisited. Curr Cardiol Rev. 2020;16:141–6. https://doi.org/10.2174/1573403X15666190618110941.
203. Hall RJ, Gelbart A, Billingham M, et al. Effect of chronic potassium depletion on digitalis-induced inotropy and arrhythmias. Cardiovasc Res. 1981;15:98–107. https://doi.org/10.1093/cvr/15.2.98.
204. Chan BSH, Buckley NA. Digoxin-specific antibody fragments in the treatment of digoxin toxicity. Clin Toxicol. 2014;52:824–36. https://doi.org/10.3109/15563650.2014.943907.
205. Kane SP. ClinCalc DrugStats 2021 update—The Most commonly prescribed drugs in the United States—ClinCalc.com. 2021. https://clincalc.com/blog/2021/09/clincalc-drugstats-2021-update-the-most-commonly-prescribed-drugs-in-the-united-states/. Accessed 29 Sep 2023.
206. Kane SP. The top 200 of 2020. https://clincalc.com/DrugStats/Top200Drugs.aspx. Accessed 29 Sept 2023.
207. Heidenreich PA, Bozkurt B, Aguilar D, et al. 2022 AHA/ACC/HFSA guideline for the management of heart failure: a report of the American College of Cardiology/American Heart Association joint committee on clinical practice guidelines. Circulation. 2022;145:e895–e1032. https://doi.org/10.1161/CIR.0000000000001063.
208. Unger T, Borghi C, Charchar F, et al. 2020 international society of hypertension global hypertension practice guidelines. Hypertension. 2020;75:1334–57. https://doi.org/10.1161/HYPERTENSIONAHA.120.15026.
209. Drug Result Page—Quick Answers—Dosing/Administration—Adult Dosing. In: Propranolol. https://www.micromedexsolutions.com/micromedex2/librarian/CS/0ECE9D/ND_PR/evidencexpert/ND_P/evidencexpert/DUPLICATIONSHIELDSYNC/1246C1/ND_PG/evidencexpert/ND_B/evidencexpert/ND_AppProduct/evidencexpert/ND_T/evidencexpert/PFActionId/evidencexpert.GoToDashboard?docId=488725&contentSetId=100&title=Propranolol+Hydrochloride&servicesTitle=Propranolol+Hydrochloride&brandName=Propranol&UserMdxSearchTerm=Propranol&=null#. Accessed 29 Sept 2023.
210. Khalid MM, Galuska MA, Hamilton RJ. Beta-blocker toxicity. In: StatPearls. Treasure Island: StatPearls Publishing; 2023.
211. Eizadi-Mood N, Adib M, Otroshi A, et al. A clinical-epidemiological study on beta-blocker poisonings based on the type of drug overdose. J Toxicol. 2023;2023:e1064955. https://doi.org/10.1155/2023/1064955.
212. Lauterbach M. Clinical toxicology of beta-blocker overdose in adults. Basic Clin Pharmacol Toxicol. 2019;125:178–86. https://doi.org/10.1111/bcpt.13231.
213. Drug Result Page—Quick Answers—Dosing/Administration—Adult Dosing. In: Metoprolol tartrate. https://www.micromedexsolutions.com/micromedex2/librarian/CS/9A7DA6/ND_PR/evidencexpert/ND_P/evidencexpert/DUPLICATIONSHIELDSYNC/3BBC9F/ND_PG/evidencexpert/ND_B/evidencexpert/ND_AppProduct/evidencexpert/ND_T/evidencexpert/PFActionId/evidencexpert.DoIntegratedSearch?SearchTerm=Metoprolol+Tartrate&fromInterSaltBase=true&UserMdxSearchTerm=%24userMdxSearchTerm&false=null&=null#. Accessed 29 Sept 2023.
214. Drug Result Page—Quick Answers—Dosing/Administration—Adult Dosing. In: Metoprolol succinate. https://www.micromedexsolutions.com/micromedex2/librarian/CS/9A7DA6/ND_PR/evidencexpert/ND_P/evidencexpert/DUPLICATIONSHIELDSYNC/3BBC9F/ND_PG/evidencexpert/ND_B/evidencexpert/ND_AppProduct/evidencexpert/ND_T/evidencexpert/PFActionId/evidencexpert.DoIntegratedSearch?SearchTerm=Metoprolol+Succinate&fromInterSaltBase=true&UserMdxSearchTerm=%24userMdxSearchTerm&false=null&=null#. Accessed 29 Sept 2023.

215. Drug Result Page—Quick Answers—Dosing/Administration—Adult Dosing. In: Atenolol. https://www.micromedexsolutions.com/micromedex2/librarian/CS/D6A9F9/ND_PR/evidencexpert/ND_P/evidencexpert/DUPLICATIONSHIELDSYNC/2839B1/ND_PG/evidencexpert/ND_B/evidencexpert/ND_AppProduct/evidencexpert/ND_T/evidencexpert/PFActionId/evidencexpert.DoIntegratedSearch?SearchTerm=atenolol&UserSearchTerm=atenolol&SearchFilter=filterNone&navitem=searchALL#. Accessed 29 Sept 2023.

216. Drug Result Page—Quick Answers—Dosing/Administration—Adult Dosing. In: Sotalol. https://www.micromedexsolutions.com/micromedex2/librarian/CS/D6A9F9/ND_PR/evidencexpert/ND_P/evidencexpert/DUPLICATIONSHIELDSYNC/2839B1/ND_PG/evidencexpert/ND_B/evidencexpert/ND_AppProduct/evidencexpert/ND_T/evidencexpert/PFActionId/evidencexpert.DoIntegratedSearch?SearchTerm=sotalol&UserSearchTerm=sotalol&SearchFilter=filterNone&navitem=searchALL#. Accessed 29 Sept 2023.

217. Mundan A Beta Adrenergic Blocker Toxicity—Emergency Management—DynaMedex. https://www.dynamedex.com/management/beta-adrenergic-blocker-toxicity-emergency-management. Accessed 15 Oct 2023.

218. Hindricks G, Potpara T, Dagres N, et al. 2020 ESC guidelines for the diagnosis and management of atrial fibrillation developed in collaboration with the European Association for Cardio-Thoracic Surgery (EACTS): the task force for the diagnosis and management of atrial fibrillation of the European Society of Cardiology (ESC) developed with the special contribution of the European Heart Rhythm Association (EHRA) of the ESC. Eur Heart J. 2021;42:373–498. https://doi.org/10.1093/eurheartj/ehaa612.

219. Salhanick SD, Shannon MW. Management of calcium channel antagonist overdose. Drug Saf. 2003;26:65–79. https://doi.org/10.2165/00002018-200326020-00001.

220. Chakraborty RK, Hamilton RJ. Calcium channel blocker toxicity. In: StatPearls. Treasure Island: StatPearls Publishing; 2023.

221. Drug Result Page—Quick Answers—Dosing/Administration—Adult Dosing. In: Verapamil. https://www.micromedexsolutions.com/micromedex2/librarian/CS/38F371/ND_PR/evidencexpert/ND_P/evidencexpert/DUPLICATIONSHIELDSYNC/A52138/ND_PG/evidencexpert/ND_B/evidencexpert/ND_AppProduct/evidencexpert/ND_T/evidencexpert/PFActionId/evidencexpert.DoIntegratedSearch?SearchTerm=Amlodipine&fromInterSaltBase=true&UserMdxSearchTerm=%24userMdxSearchTerm&false=null&=null#. Accessed 15 Oct 2023.

222. Drug Result Page—Quick Answers—Dosing/Administration—Adult Dosing. In: Diltiazem. https://www.micromedexsolutions.com/micromedex2/librarian/PFDefaultActionId/evidencexpert.DoIntegratedSearch?navitem=topHome&isToolPage=true#. Accessed 15 Oct 2023.

223. Drug Result Page—Quick Answers—Dosing/Administration—Adult Dosing. In: Nifedipine. https://www.micromedexsolutions.com/micromedex2/librarian/PFDefaultActionId/evidencexpert.DoIntegratedSearch?navitem=topHome&isToolPage=true#. Accessed 15 Oct 2023.

224. Drug Result Page—Quick Answers—Dosing/Administration—Adult Dosing. In: Amlodipine. https://www.micromedexsolutions.com/micromedex2/librarian/PFDefaultActionId/evidencexpert.DoIntegratedSearch?navitem=topHome&isToolPage=true#. Accessed 15 Oct 2023.

225. Ramoska EA, Spiller HA, Winter M, Borys D. A one-year evaluation of calcium channel blocker overdoses: toxicity and treatment. Ann Emerg Med. 1993;22:196–200. https://doi.org/10.1016/S0196-0644(05)80202-1.

226. Proano L, Chiang WK, Wang RY. Calcium channel blocker overdose. https://pubmed.ncbi.nlm.nih.gov/7605536/. Accessed 15 Oct 2023.

227. St-Onge M, Anseeuw K, Cantrell FL, et al. Experts consensus recommendations for the management of calcium channel blocker poisoning in adults. Crit Care Med. 2017;45:e306–15. https://doi.org/10.1097/CCM.0000000000002087.

228. Drug Result Page—In-Depth Answers—Medication Safety—Adverse effects. In: Calcium chloride. https://www.micromedexsolutions.com/micromedex2/librarian/CS/082335/ND_PR/evidencexpert/ND_P/evidencexpert/DUPLICATIONSHIELDSYNC/4FB1EC/ND_PG/evidencexpert/ND_B/evidencexpert/ND_AppProduct/evidencexpert/ND_T/evidencexpert/PFActionId/evidencexpert.DoIntegratedSearch?SearchTerm=calcium%20

chloride&UserSearchTerm=calcium%20chloride&SearchFilter=filterNone&navitem=searchALL#. Accessed 7 Nov 2023.

229. Montiel V, Gougnard T, Hantson P. Diltiazem poisoning treated with hyperinsulinemic euglycemia therapy and intravenous lipid emulsion. Eur J Emerg Med. 2011;18:121. https://doi.org/10.1097/MEJ.0b013e32834130ab.

230. Grunbaum AM, Gilfix BM, Gosselin S, Blank DW. Analytical interferences resulting from intravenous lipid emulsion. Clin Toxicol. 2012;50:812–7. https://doi.org/10.3109/15563650.2012.731509.

231. Sebe A, Dişel NR, Açıkalın Akpınar A, Karakoç E. Role of intravenous lipid emulsions in the management of calcium channel blocker and β-blocker overdose: 3 years experience of a university hospital. Postgrad Med. 2015;127:119–24. https://doi.org/10.1080/00325481.2015.1012480.

232. Tamama K. Advances in drugs of abuse testing. Clin Chim Acta. 2021;514:40–7. https://doi.org/10.1016/j.cca.2020.12.010.

233. Raouf M, Bettinger JJ, Fudin J. A practical guide to urine drug monitoring. Fed Pract. 2018;35:38–44.

234. Saitman A, Park H-D, Fitzgerald RL. False-positive interferences of common urine drug screen immunoassays: a review. J Anal Toxicol. 2014;38:387–96. https://doi.org/10.1093/jat/bku075.

235. Nelson ZJ, Stellpflug SJ, Engebretsen KM. What can a urine drug screening immunoassay really tell us? J Pharm Pract. 2016;29:516–26. https://doi.org/10.1177/0897190015579611.

236. Moeller KE, Kissack JC, Atayee RS, Lee KC. Clinical interpretation of urine drug tests: what clinicians need to know about urine drug screens. Mayo Clin Proc. 2017;92:774–96. https://doi.org/10.1016/j.mayocp.2016.12.007.

237. Brahm NC, Yeager LL, Fox MD, et al. Commonly prescribed medications and potential false-positive urine drug screens. Am J Health Syst Pharm. 2010;67:1344–50. https://doi.org/10.2146/ajhp090477.

238. Caricasole V, Spagnolo G, Di Bernardo I, et al. Aripiprazole causing false positive urine amphetamine drug screen in an adult patient with bipolar disorder. Compr Psychiatry. 2019;94:152126. https://doi.org/10.1016/j.comppsych.2019.152126.

239. Kissner D, LeFlore Y, Narayan SB, et al. False-positive cannabinoid screens in adult cystic fibrosis patients treated with lumacaftor/ivacaftor. J Cyst Fibros. 2018;17:e51–3. https://doi.org/10.1016/j.jcf.2018.08.006.

240. Farley TM, Anderson EN, Feller JN. False-positive phencyclidine (PCP) on urine drug screen attributed to desvenlafaxine (Pristiq) use. BMJ Case Rep. 2017;2017:bcr2017222106. https://doi.org/10.1136/bcr-2017-222106.

241. Syed H, Som S, Khan N, Faltas W. Doxylamine toxicity: seizure, rhabdomyolysis and false positive urine drug screen for methadone. BMJ Case Rep. 2009;2009:bcr09.2008.0879. https://doi.org/10.1136/bcr.09.2008.0879.

242. Bithi N, Merrigan SD, McMillin GA. Does labetalol trigger false positive drug testing results? J Addict Med. 2023;17:e209–10. https://doi.org/10.1097/ADM.0000000000001117.

243. Adashek JJ, Khadilkar A, Enciso J, et al A case of esmolol-induced false-positive amphetamine urine drug test. Cureus. 2021;13:e12429. https://doi.org/10.7759/cureus.12429.

244. Pope JD, Drummer OH, Schneider HG. False-positive amphetamines in urine drug screens: a 6-year review. J Anal Toxicol. 2023;47:263–70. https://doi.org/10.1093/jat/bkac089.

245. Cole J. Case report of a phencyclidine false positive due to lamotrigine use with confirmatory testing. Am J Emerg Med. 2022;61:234.e5–6. https://doi.org/10.1016/j.ajem.2022.08.010.

246. Tenore PL. Advanced urine toxicology testing. J Addict Dis. 2010;29:436–48. https://doi.org/10.1080/10550887.2010.509277.

247. Tamama K, Lynch MJ. Newly emerging drugs of abuse. Handb Exp Pharmacol. 2020;258:463–502. https://doi.org/10.1007/164_2019_260.

248. Abou El Hassan M, Colantonio D, Likhodii S, Nassar BA. The analytical performance of six urine drug screens on cobas 6000 and ARCHITECT i2000 compared to LC-MS/MS gold standard. Clin Biochem. 2021;93:99–103. https://doi.org/10.1016/j.clinbiochem.2021.04.003.

Chapter 38
The Management of Critical Illness in Obstetric Patients

Kayla Popova

Abbreviations

ACEi	Angiotensin converting enzyme inhibitor
ACLS	Advanced cardiac life support
AFE	Amniotic fluid embolism
AFLP	Acute fatty liver in pregnancy
ALT	Alanine transaminase
aPTT	Activated partial thromboplastin time
ARDS	Acute respiratory distress syndrome
AST	Aspartate aminotransferase
BP	Blood pressure
CPR	Cardiopulmonary resuscitation
COP	Colloid osmotic pressure
COP-PCOP	Colloid osmotic pressure-pulmonary capillary occlusion pressure
CT	Computed tomography
CVP	Central venous pressure
CYP	Cytochrome
DBP	Diastolic blood pressure
DIC	Disseminated intravascular coagulation
DVT	Deep vein thrombosis
ECMO	Extracorporeal membrane oxygenation
ER	Extended-release
ERV	Expiratory reserve volume
FAOD	Fatty acid oxidation defects
FFP	Fresh frozen plasma

K. Popova (✉)
University of Michigan Health—Michigan Medicine, Ann Arbor, MI, USA
e-mail: khardie@umich.edu

© The Author(s), under exclusive license to Springer Nature
Switzerland AG 2025

Y. Alzaidi, M. A. Gebily (eds.), *The Pharmacist's Expanded Role in Critical
Care Medicine*, https://doi.org/10.1007/978-3-031-77335-8_38

Fi$_{O2}$	Fraction of inspired oxygen
FRC	Functional residual volume
g	Grams
g/h	Grams per hour
GBS	Group B streptococcus
GFR	Glomerular filtration rate
HELLP	Hemolysis, elevated liver enzymes, low platelets
Hgb	Hemoglobin
HIT	Heparin-induced thromboembolism
H$_2$O	Water
ICU	Intensive care unit
INR	International normalized ratio
IR	Immediate release
IVC	Inferior vena cava
LCHAD	Long-chain 3-hydroxylacyl-CoA dehydrogenase
LDH	Lactate dehydrogenase
LFTs	Liver transaminases
LMWH	Low-molecular-weight-heparin
mcg/min	Microgram per minute
MEOWS	Modified early obstetric warning scoring
mg	Milligram
mg/dL	Milligrams per deciliter
mg/kg	Milligram per kilogram
microL	Microliter
mL	Milliliter
mmHg	Millimeter of mercury
MRSA	Methicillin-resistant *Staphylococcus aureus*
Pa$_{CO2}$	Partial pressure of carbon dioxide
Pa$_{O2}$	Partial pressure of oxygen
Pco$_2$	Partial pressure of carbon dioxide
PD	Pharmacodynamics
PE	Pulmonary embolism
PEEP	Positive end-expiratory pressure
PK	Pharmacokinetics
PPH	Postpartum hemorrhage
PT	Prothrombin time
PTT	Partial thromboplastin time
PVR	Pulmonary vascular resistance
OAT	Organic anion transporters
OCT	Organic cation transporters
RAAS	Renin-angiotensin-aldosterone system
RV	Residual volume
SBP	Systolic blood pressure
SOS	Sepsis in obstetrics

SVR	Systemic vascular resistance
TMP-SMX	Trimethoprim-sulfamethoxazole
TLC	Total lung capacity
UFH	Unfractionated heparin
UGT	Uridine 5′-diphosphate glucuronosyltransferase
UTI	Urinary tract infection
Vd	Volume of distribution
VQ	Ventilation-perfusion
VTE	Venous thromboembolism
VWF	von Willebrand factor
WBC	White blood cell

38.1 Introduction

Critical illness in pregnancy is complex given the need for the management of both mother and fetus and requires a multidisciplinary approach and an understanding of the physiology of pregnancy. Approximately 1–10 obstetric patients per 1000 deliveries will experience an intensive care unit (ICU) admission in the United States [1]. The physiologic changes of various organ systems can be challenging for medical management. Additionally, there are pharmacokinetic changes during pregnancy that can affect pharmacologic treatment and may guide changes to management, especially since the presentation of various disorders in pregnancy may be different. Also importantly to note is that a patient still falls within the obstetric classification not only during pregnancy but up to 6 weeks postpartum [2]. ICU admission rates in pregnancy are approximately 200–700 women per 100,000 deliveries so while it constitutes a small population of ICU patients, it remains an important one [2]. Major causes of ICU admissions in pregnancy are hypertensive disorders of pregnancy, such as preeclampsia and eclampsia, major hemorrhage, trauma, respiratory conditions, cardiovascular disorders, diabetic ketoacidosis, and sepsis [1, 3, 4]. This chapter will review the physiology of pregnancy and the pathophysiology and management of several disorders associated with critical illness in obstetric patients.

38.2 Physiology of Pregnancy

Several physiologic changes occur throughout pregnancy which affect many organ systems, including the cardiovascular system, hematological system, respiratory system, urinary system, and gastrointestinal system. The systems pertinent to critical care are cardiovascular, hematological, and respiratory which will be discussed in more detail below.

38.2.1 Cardiovascular System

As it pertains to the cardiovascular system, several hemodynamic and circulatory processes change throughout pregnancy, beginning in the first trimester and peaking at the end of the second trimester, to ensure and maximize adequate oxygen delivery to the fetus that then gradually return to prepregnancy levels during the postpartum period [2, 4–6]. The prominent pregnancy-induced changes for a healthy obstetric person include increased heart rate (by 10–15%), cardiac output (by 30–50%), blood volume (by 30–50%), and erythrocyte count (by 20–40%), and decreased blood pressure (BP) and systemic vascular resistance (SVR) [1–10]. Approximately 17% of the increased cardiac output is directed to the uterine arteries to increase the blood supply to the gravid uterus to a rate of 500 mL/min [9]. As will be noted later, such an increase in blood flow to the uterus leads to the profound blood loss that can occur with obstetric hemorrhage. Blood volume is thought to increase by 1200–1600 mL in a pregnant patient compared to a nonpregnant patient [9]. Since blood volume increases by a greater degree than erythrocyte count, a mild dilutional or relative anemia can occur [2, 4, 10]. This results in a decrease of hematocrit by about 12% [4]. In multifetal gestation, the increase in blood volume is even greater than singleton gestation so the dilutional anemia will be greater [4]. Increased extracellular blood volume, or plasma volume, is related to the renin-angiotensin-aldosterone system (RAAS) where there is increased sodium retention secondary to aldosterone production that leads to a decrease in serum albumin concentration and colloid osmotic pressure (COP) and mild peripheral edema [4, 9]. Additionally, increases in estrogen lead to hepatic production of renin which contributes to this sodium retention [9].

During the first trimester of pregnancy, BP will decrease by approximately 10% due to peripheral vasodilation from increases in estrogen and progesterone, and cardiac output will begin to increase as heart rate and stroke volume increase [1, 4–6, 10]. Heart rate will increase by 15–20 beats per minute above nonpregnant levels with some literature noting this increase can be up to 30 beats higher than prepregnancy baseline [1, 4, 10]. The stroke volume increase is mediated by an increased preload and decreased afterload [4]. Increased levels of relaxin result in additional vasodilatory effect on the vascular endothelium via nitric oxide resulting in decreased SVR and BP [5]. A decrease in SVR of 20–35% allows for a decreased afterload [4, 10]. As part of maternal hemodynamic compensation or adaptation for the reduced SVR and BP, increased sympathetic and baroreceptor sensitivity and activation of RAAS leads to an increased heart rate and cardiac output [5]. Pulse pressure will also increase, and there will be an improved myocardial function [8].

Pertinent to the critical care setting, other hemodynamic changes during pregnancy include decreased pulmonary vascular resistance (PVR), COP, and colloid osmotic pressure-pulmonary capillary occlusion pressure (COP-PCOP) while the pulmonary artery occlusion pressure and central venous pressure remain unchanged to the nonpregnant state [7, 11]. The decreased COP and COP-PCOP gradient may lead to an increased risk of fluid overload after rigorous fluid resuscitation due to third spacing in a pregnant person [1, 7]. Moreover, once a pregnant person reaches the third trimester, the blood volume increases to nearly 50% above the prepregnancy level, and this can be more significant in patients with multifetal gestations [7, 12]. This lends further to the risk of fluid overload. Additionally, heart rate and stroke volume are increased lending to an increased cardiac output [7]. However, the cardiac output of pregnant persons with heart disease like severe mitral stenosis may not experience an increase [7]. If invasive hemodynamic monitoring is required, SVR and PVR are decreased in pregnancy, particularly near term, which may confound determining whether a decrease in SVR is from endotoxin release associated with sepsis or the gravid state [7]. Cardiac output can be affected in pregnant patients, particularly during the third trimester, while in a supine position where cardiac output can decrease by up to 30% due to the gravid uterus compressing the vena cava and abdominal aorta [1, 4]. This compression is improved if patients layiin a left lateral decubitus position [4]. These cardiovascular changes must be taken into consideration in the critical care setting.

38.2.2   Hematological System

Hematologic changes that can occur in pregnancy include a relative leukocytosis, which may further increase during labor, decreased hemoglobin, increased production of factors VII, VIII, IX, X, XII, and von Willebrand factor (VWF), decreased protein S, and a reduction in fibrinolysis [7, 10]. The changes in the coagulation system place the pregnant person at a five-fold increased risk of venous thromboembolism (VTE) [7]. Additionally, the blood volume expansion of 40–60% that occurs during pregnancy coupled with a decrease in hematocrit results in a dilutional anemia [6]. The benefit of this increased blood volume and decreased blood viscosity is to prevent significant thromboembolic events given the hypercoagulable state of pregnancy [2]. This is another important consideration since critical illness is also a risk factor for VTE. The increased blood volume also allows for blood loss up to 1000 mL without significantly affecting hemoglobin levels [2].

38.2.3   Respiratory System

Several changes occur within the respiratory system as it relates to lung volume and capacity in pregnancy. During pregnancy, oxygen consumption increases by 20–35%, with some literature reporting up to a 60% increase, due to fetal and placental consumption and increased maternal need [1, 4, 9]. This increased use then leads to a 34–50% increase above baseline of carbon dioxide production [4]. Progesterone-mediated increases in respiratory rate may lead to a decreased buffering capacity which can play a role in critically ill pregnant patients [1]. Tidal volume is increased by 30–40% during pregnancy, which is driven by an increase in respiratory depth, but not rate, secondary to the increased progesterone levels [2, 7,

8, 10]. The increase in tidal volume leads to an increased minute volume that peaks in the third trimester at 20–40% above baseline that also lowers arterial Pco_2 to 30 mmHg leading to a primary respiratory alkalosis in pregnancy [2, 4, 7, 10]. This results in reduced serum bicarbonate to levels of 18–21 mEq/L because of renal compensation that ultimately leads to an alkalemic maternal pH of 7.40–7.45 [3, 4, 7]. The increased compensated respiratory alkalosis decreases buffering capacity and increases acidosis during CPR [1]. There is also a 5% increase in inspiratory capacity [8]. Finally during pregnancy, the residual volume (RV) and expiratory reserve volume (ERV) decrease affecting the functional residual capacity (FRC) and total lung capacity (TLC) [2, 6–8]. The FRC, ERV, and RV are all thought to be decreased by up to 20% in pregnancy due to a diaphragm elevation that may increase up to 4 cm because of the gravid uterus and chest wall changes from hormones while the TLC is decreased by 5% [2, 3, 6, 8, 9]. The FRC can decrease further when a pregnancy patient is in the supine position [9]. The combination of decreased FRC and increased oxygen consumption leads to a decreased oxygen reserve [4, 9]. Given these changes in the setting of hypoventilation, there is an increased risk of faster desaturation due to apnea and hypoxia for both the pregnant patient and fetus which is an important consideration during intubation [4, 9]. Respiratory parameters that are unchanged in pregnancy include vital capacity and inspiratory reserve volume [4, 6, 8]. Supine positional changes again play in role and can lead to positional hypoxemia due to an increased alveolar-to-arterial oxygen gradient [4]. It is recommended to obtain arterial blood gases in a seated position [4].

38.2.4 Renal System

In the first and second trimesters, renal blood flow increases by 60–80% above pre-pregnancy levels [4]. Since relaxin has a vasodilatoy effect on endothelium to cause a decreased SVR and BP, it also leads to a 50% increase in renal blood flow and glomerular filtration by the end of the first trimester [2, 4, 5, 10]. There are also changes to the renal system in pregnancy where plasma flow to the kidney increases and glomerular filtration (mL/min) increases throughout pregnancy, peaking in the third trimester [6, 8]. Such changes in renal physiology lead to serum creatinine levels of 0.5–0.7 mg/dL (or <0.8 mg/dL), and normal serum creatinine levels as seen in nonpregnant patients may be indicative of renal dysfunction in pregnant patients [2, 4]. Given these changes in renal function in pregnancy, renal insufficiency in pregnancy can be defined by a serum creatinine >1 mg/dL and requires renally adjusting medications appropriately [2]. Additionally, pregnant patients commonly experience glycosuria that may not be correlated with serum blood glucose levels [6].

Understanding the physiologic changes that occur in pregnancy can be helpful to optimize treatment management, and it is pathway for pharmacists to play an integral role in dosing medications for changes in renal function in critically ill pregnant patients.

38.3   Pharmacokinetic and Pharmacodynamic Changes During Pregnancy

Pharmacokinetic (PK) and pharmacodynamic (PD) changes occur throughout pregnancy because of changes in physiology that can influence drug concentration in the body. PK relates to how the body affects the drug and thus the time course of drug concentration in the body [13]. PK changes include those related to drug absorption, distribution, metabolism, and elimination. Not all changes in PK during pregnancy are clinically significant, particularly for medications with a wide therapeutic window relative to mediations with a narrow therapeutic window [14]. Having an understanding of the physiological changes and the subsequent effects on PK and PD are important considerations, and an area where a pharmacist can play a key role in determining changes in dose, frequency, and monitoring to optimize the safety and efficacy of medications.

Drug absorption is affected during pregnancy. For pregnant patients who experience nausea and vomiting, the amount of drug actually absorbed following oral administration can be altered [13]. This is particularly important during the first trimester when nausea and vomiting are more common, but some pregnant patients can experience nausea and vomiting for the duration of pregnancy. Progesterone also leads to a slowing of gastric emptying and gastrointestinal motility which then reduces drug absorption and bioavailability [12, 13]. Additionally, gastrointestinal transit time is slowed because of reduced intrinsic contractility and pressure from the gravid uterus [12]. There is also an increase in gastric acid pH in pregnancy due to decreased gastric acid production affecting the ionization of medications [13]. There can be increased ionization of medications that are weak acids leading to reduced absorption, and for medications that are weak bases, they will remain largely unionized and can be more easily absorbed [13]. Despite the changes potentially reducing drug absorption, it is important to note that increased cardiac output and intestinal perfusion may aid in medication absorption [13]. The clinical significance of all the potential changes of drug absorption in pregnancy still needs to be validated.

As discussed previously, intravascular volume is increased during pregnancy, beginning in the first trimester and peaking in the third trimester [12]. A pregnant patient's volume of distribution (Vd) can increase by up to 50%, and this increase is largely driven by estrogen activation of the RAAS and can lead to several alterations in drug PK [12, 14]. The distribution of medications occurs after entry of a medication into systemic circulation where Vd describes the extent of that distribution [13]. Medications with a high Vd are highly bound to tissues, medications with a Vd that approximates plasma volume largely remain in the intravascular space, and medications with a low Vd tend to be highly protein bound [13]. The increased Vd causes a dilutional effect to serum drug concentration where there is reduced drug concentration, particularly for polar and large molecular weight medications [12]. However, the dilutional effect also reduces circulating protein concentrations, which in turn, can lead to increased availability of unbound or active drug [12]. With the increased extracellular and total body water in pregnancy, Vd will increase for hydrophilic medications; yet, there is also an increase in fat during pregnancy which can increase the absorption of lipophilic medications and thus the Vd of those medications [13, 14]. Such changes in Vd can affect therapeutic effect and adverse effects [13]. Pharmacists can play an important role in helping to determine optimal dosing by taking into account the changes in Vd of medications.

The concentrations of albumin and alpha 1-acid glycoprotein are decreased during pregnancy which then affects the plasma protein binding of medications [13]. Acidic and neutral medications bind to albumin where basic medications bind to alpha 1-acid glycoprotein [14]. Albumin levels are thought to be reduced by up to 70–80% and alpha 1-acid glycoprotein levels by 52% in the third trimester [14]. A reduction in plasma protein binding leads to increased free drug [13]. Medications that are highly protein bound with a narrow therapeutic index require therapeutic drug monitoring (i.e., tacrolimus) and should be closely monitored during pregnancy given these PK changes.

Pregnancy also affects the activity of cytochrome P450 or CYP450 enzymes, which play a key role in drug metabolism. CYP3A4, CYP2A6, CYP2D6, and CYP2C9 are all increased in pregnancy while CYP1A1 and CYP2C19 are decreased during pregnancy [12–14]. Such effects on CYP enzymes can decrease or increase levels of drug in body. Additionally, uridine 5′-diphosphate glucuronosyltransferase (UGT) 1A4 is increased by up to 300% at the end of pregnancy [12, 13]. Despite the changes in CYP450 enzymes, another confounding factor when considering drug metabolism in pregnancy is a reduction in cardiac output perfusing the liver because while there is an increase in cardiac output during pregnancy, hepatic blood flow remains constant ultimately leading to a reduction in hepatic first-pass metabolism [12].

Given the increased cardiac output by 30–50% at term, there is an increase in renal plasma flow and creatinine clearance which can result in an increased clearance of renally excreted medications [12]. Glomerular filtration rate (GFR) is increased by 30–50% by the third trimester which can increase the renal clearance of medications and their metabolites, particularly those solely excreted by glomerular filtration [13, 14]. Again, consideration should still be given to medications that are highly protein bound but renally eliminated because the reduced protein binding in pregnancy can lead to more free drug available. This needs to be balanced against the increased renal elimination before increasing the dose or dosing frequency of medications [12]. Another consideration for the renal elimination of medications is the degree of renal tubular transport [13]. There is an upregulation of renal P-gp, certain organic cation transporters (OCT), and organic anion transporters (OAT) [14]. Despite the increased GFR in pregnancy, the magnitude of change of elimination of a medication may not align because of renal tubular transport [13]. For example, digoxin clearance is 20–30% higher in pregnancy despite 80% being renally eliminated [13].

Consideration of the pharmacologic properties of medications and how the alterations in the PK of pregnant persons may affect drug concentration within the body will be important for determining the optimal medication, dose, and frequency for a critically ill pregnant patient.

38.4 Hypertensive Disorders of Pregnancy

One of the leading causes for a pregnant person to need ICU admission is due to hypertensive disorders of pregnancy. Hypertension during pregnancy can be classified as gestational hypertension, chronic hypertension, chronic hypertension with superimposed preeclampsia, and preeclampsia/eclampsia/HELLP (hemolysis, elevated liver enzymes, and low platelets) [8]. Gestational hypertension is diagnosed after 20 weeks of gestation and is the new onset of elevated BP with a systolic blood pressure (SBP) $\geq$140 mmHg or a diastolic blood pressure (DBP) $\geq$90 mmHg on two or more occasions and at least 4 h apart with the absence of proteinuria [8, 15, 16]. Chronic hypertension is hypertension before pregnancy, whereas chronic hypertension with superimposed preeclampsia is chronic hypertension that is complicated by preeclampsia after 20 weeks of gestation [8, 15]. Preeclampsia is hypertension after 20 weeks of gestation that is associated with other signs and symptoms besides the elevated BP parameters above, such as new onset proteinuria, right upper quadrant or epigastric pain, new onset headache unresponsive to medication, thrombocytopenia, renal insufficiency, and increased liver transaminases (LFTs) [6, 15, 16]. Preeclampsia with severe features can be diagnosed in a patient with gestational hypertension presenting with a severe range BP which is defined by an SBP $\geq$ 160 mmHg or DBP $\geq$ 110 mmHg or any additional severe signs or symptoms defined in Table 38.1 [3, 15].

Preeclampsia occurs in 2–8% of pregnancies and is associated with endothelial dysfunction, hypertension, and proteinuria [4]. While the etiology of preeclampsia is not fully known, several mechanisms have been proposed. It is thought to be due to the abnormal development of blood vessels supplying the placenta leading to placental ischemia and oxidative stress [4, 15]. This then leads to angiogenic factors being released into maternal circulation resulting in downstream endothelial dysfunction, such as increased vascular permeability, increased sensitivity to endogenous/exogenous vasopressors, and activated coagulation cascade [4, 15]. Other etiologies are chronic uteroplacental ischemia, immune maladaptation, very low density lipoprotein toxicity, genetic imprinting, increased trophoblast apoptosis or necrosis, and maternal inflammatory response to the trophoblasts [15]. Primigravida, multifetal gestations, history of preeclampsia, family history of preeclampsia, chronic hypertension, chronic renal disease, diabetes mellitus, obesity, age $\geq$40 years, autoimmune disease, and antiphospholipid antibodies are all risk factors for developing preeclampsia [4]. Preeclampsia can be a significant cause of ICU admissions among pregnant and postpartum patients [4].

Several organ systems can be affected in preeclampsia, which includes the central nervous system, clotting cascade, heart, kidneys, liver, respiratory system, and systemic vasculature [4]. Intense vasospasm occurs in preeclampsia due to an interaction between endogenous vasodilators and vasoconstrictors, such as prostacyclin, thromboxane A_2, nitric oxide, and endothelins [15]. Progression of preeclampsia to eclampsia can occur rapidly resulting in convulsions [4, 15]. New onset tonic-clonic, focal, or multifocal seizures, not due to an alternative diagnosis, mark the evolution of preeclampsia to

Table 38.1 Preeclampsia and preeclampsia with severe features diagnostic criteria [15]

Preeclampsia		
Blood pressure (after 20 weeks of gestation)		
SBP ≥ 140 mmHg or DBP ≥ 90 mmHg on 2 or more occasions and at least 4 h apart		
SBP ≥ 160 mmHg or DBP ≥ 110 mmHg		
AND		
Proteinuria with ≥300 mg on 24 h urine collection	*OR*	Protein/creatinine ratio of ≥0.3 Or Dipstick reading of 2+
OR (if no proteinuria and new onset hypertension plus any of the criteria below)		
Elevated LFTs twice the ULN		
New onset headache refractory to medication and not alternative diagnoses for headache or visual symptoms		
Pulmonary edema		
Serum creatinine concentrations >1.1 mg/dL or doubling of serum creatinine in the absence of renal disease		
Platelet count <100 × 10^9/L		
Preeclampsia with severe features		
SBP ≥ 160 mmHg or DBP ≥ 110 mmHg on ≥2 occasions at least 4 h apart		
Elevated LFTs twice the ULN or severe persistent RUQ pain or epigastric pain unresponsive to medication		
New onset headache refractory to medication and not alternative diagnoses for headache		
Pulmonary edema		
Serum creatinine concentrations >1.1 mg/dL or doubling of serum creatinine in the absence of renal disease		
Platelet count <100 × 10^9/L		
Visual disturbances		

SBP systolic blood pressure, *DBP* diastolic blood pressure, *LFT* liver transaminase, *ULN* upper limit of normal, *RUQ* right upper quadrant
Adapted from Gestational Hypertension and Preeclampsia. Obstetrics & Gynecology. 2020;135(6):e237-e260. https://doi.org/10.1097/AOG.0000000000003891

eclampsia [15]. The convulsions or seizures are due to cerebral vasospasm, ischemia, edema, and/or hypertensive encephalopathy [4]. Eclamptic seizures can result in maternal aspiration pneumonia, trauma, or maternal hypoxia with up to one fourth of women who experience eclampsia developing white matter loss [15]. Hematologic changes during preeclampsia include thrombocytopenia from increased platelet activation, aggregation, and consumption [15]. Renal dysfunction can also result from ischemia, intravascular volume depletion, and/or glomeruloendotheliosis [4, 15]. Respiratory compromise may occur because of pulmonary edema from the increased capillary permeability associated with preeclampsia as well as increased left ventricular afterload, myocardial dysfunction, decreased COP associated with the proteinuria, and/or vigorous fluid resuscitation [4]. Eclampsia, if not promptly treated, can be lethal [4]. Patients are at risk for preeclampsia and eclampsia up to 1 month postpartum [4].

Another complication of preeclampsia that is associated with adverse maternal and fetal outcomes is HELLP syndrome which can occur in 10–20% of severe preeclampsia cases [4]. The acronym for HELLP syndrome stands for hemolysis (H), elevated liver enzymes (E-L), and low platelet count (L-P). There is more significant multi-organ dysfunction with HELLP compared to preeclampsia because of secondary fibrin deposition and hypoperfusion [4]. Periportal or focal parenchymal necrosis may occur and be associated with the significant elevated liver enzymes noted in HELLP, and microangiopathic hemolytic anemia and consumptive coagulopathy can also result in disseminated intravascular coagulation (DIC) [4].

Patients with preeclampsia or eclampsia do not experience the significant increase in fluid volume, or hypervolemia, as seen in healthy pregnant persons [7, 15]. This ultimately leads to a form of relative hemoconcentration; however, severe preeclampsia also results in vascular permeability leading to peripheral edema [7]. This is an important consideration in the setting of fluid resuscitation which could be ineffective and even lead to life-threatening elevated pulmonary capillary wedge pressure and pulmonary edema if not managed correctly [7, 15]. Additionally, given the intravascular hypovolemia associated with preeclampsia, these patients do not tolerate blood loss from obstetric hemorrhage as well, and it can result in more significant hemodynamic effects and instability coupled with the relative hemoconcentration increases the risk of thromboembolic events [2].

Hypertension in pregnancy is defined by a SBP >140 mmHg or DBP >90 mmHg where severe range hypertension is defined by a SBP $\geq$160 mmHg or DBP $\geq$110 mmHg [4, 16]. Diagnosing preeclampsia during pregnancy is sometimes difficult in certain patients who may present with mild hypertension and minimal or absent proteinuria [4]. Edema can be a nonspecific finding since many pregnant patients experience edema at some point during pregnancy given the increased Vd associated with pregnancy [4]. Preeclampsia is diagnosed by new onset hypertension with a SBP $\geq$140 mmHg or DBP $\geq$90 mmHg on two or more occasions plus $\geq$300 mg of protein in a 24-h urine collection [4, 6, 15, 16]. Typically this begins after 20 weeks of gestation, and the presentation can be subtle [4]. Preeclampsia with severe features is marked by an SBP $\geq$160 mmHg or DBP $\geq$110 mmHg, proteinuria $\geq$300 mg/dL in 24 h or protein/creatinine ratio $\geq$0.3 in a random urine specimen, early onset disease (<34–35 weeks of gestation), and the presence of oliguria, pulmonary edema, or an intractable headache that does not respond to treatment [3, 4]. Other signs and symptoms may be malaise, headache, visual changes, nausea, vomiting, and right upper quadrant pain [4]. Diagnosis of HELLP includes hemolysis on a peripheral blood smear, increased serum bilirubin, increased serum transaminases, and thrombocytopenia.

Management of a patient diagnosed with preeclampsia will include early diagnosis, close medical observation, including prolonged hospitalization during the antepartum period until the time of delivery, and a timed delivery that will optimize maternal and fetal well-being [3, 4]. From a laboratory standpoint, collecting a complete blood cell count, serum creatinine, lactate dehydrogenase (LDH), aspartate aminotransferase (AST), alanine transaminase (ALT), and testing for proteinuria will be important in the diagnosis of preeclampsia [6, 15]. Since the removal of the placenta is the only curative treatment, timing of delivery will be an important consideration in weighing both maternal and fetal health [4, 6, 16]. Delivery is recommended in patients with preeclampsia with severe features affecting organ function or an intractable headache unresponsive to treatment, HELLP syndrome, or fetal distress at 34 0/7 weeks of gestation [4]. The use of antihypertensives will be important to manage blood pressure to prevent end-organ damage; however, the disease will continue to progress despite blood pressure management [4]. Treatment includes the use of intravenous labetalol, oral nifedipine immediate release (IR), or intravenous hydralazine for patients who present with severe range blood pressures (SBP $\geq$160 mmHg or DBP $\geq$ 90 mmHg) [3, 15]. Medication should be given within 30–60 min of identification of a severe range BP, and although literature does not show one agent to be more effective than another, intravenous labetalol and hydralazine are typically considered to be first-line for the treatment of severe hypertension in pregnancy [15, 17]. Dosing for intravenous labetalol includes 10–20 mg over 2 min for one dose followed by 20–80 mg intravenously every 10–30 min to a maximum cumulative dose of 300 mg/24 h [3, 15, 18]. A typical dose titration would be labetalol 10–20 mg intravenously over 2 min, repeat BP in 10 min; if BP remains elevated at $\geq$160 mmHg or $\geq$110 mmHg, administer labetalol 20 mg intravenously over 2 min, repeat BP in 10 min; if BP is still elevated at $\geq$160 mmHg or $\geq$110 mmHg, administer labetalol 80 mg intravenously over 2 min [3, 18]. The onset of action is 1–2 min [15]. Labetalol should be avoided in patients with uncontrolled asthma, preexisting myocardial disease, decompensated heart failure, heart block, and bradycardia [15, 19]. Dosing for intravenous hydralazine begins at 5 mg for one dose followed by 5–10 mg intravenously every 20–40 min to a maximum cumulative dose of 20 mg/24 h [15]. A typical dose titration will be hydralazine 5–10 mg intravenously over 2 min, repeat BP in 20 min; if BP remains elevated at $\geq$160 mmHg or $\geq$110 mmHg, administer hydralazine 10 mg intravenously over 2 min, repeat BP in 20 min; if BP remains elevated at $\geq$160 mmHg or $\geq$110 mmHg, give labetalol 20 mg intravenously over 2 min [3, 20]. The onset of action is 10–20 min, and adverse effects include increased risk of maternal hypotensive with successive doses, headache, and changes in fetal heart rate [15]. Finally for nifedipine IR, initial dosing is 10–20 mg orally for one dose followed by 10–20 mg in 20 min if blood pressure remains within severe range [15, 21]. Thereafter dosing can be repeated every 2–6 h to a maximum dose of 180 mg/24 h [15]. A typical dose titration would be nifedipine IR 10 mg orally for one dose, repeat BP in 20 min; if BP remains elevated at $\geq$160 mmHg or $\geq$110 mmHg, give nifedipine IR 20 mg orally for one dose, repeat BP in 20 min; if BP remains elevated at $\geq$160 mmHg or $\geq$110 mmHg, give a second dose of nifedipine IR 20 mg orally for one dose [3, 21]. The onset of action is 5–10 min, and adverse effects include reflex tachycardia and headaches [15]. Patients in the ICU may require continuous infusions of labetalol, esmolol, nicardipine, or nitroglycerin to control BP. Nitroprusside should be avoided due to the risk of fetal cyanide poisoning [6].

Chronic management of severe range BP in patients with preeclampsia includes oral labetalol, oral nifedipine extended-release (ER), and oral hydralazine. The starting dose of labetalol is 200 mg orally every 12 h which may be increased up to a maximum of 2400 mg/day or 800 mg orally every 8 h [15]. Nifedipine ER starting dose is 30 mg orally once daily and can be increased up to a maximum dose of 60 mg orally twice daily. Once the maximum tolerated dose of one agent is used, the addition of a second agent can be considered. Diuretics like hydrochlorothiazide can be considered with caution to monitor intravascular volume depletion which can occur in preeclampsia. The use of nitroprusside and angiotensin-converting enzyme inhibitors (ACEi) is contraindicated during pregnancy [4].

Additionally, patients who present with preeclampsia with severe features should be started on a magnesium sulfate infusion to prevent eclamptic seizures and placental abruption [3, 4, 6]. Magnesium sulfate helps to reduce the risk of preeclampsia progressing to eclampsia by 50% in some literature and decreases the risk of maternal death [4, 15]. Patients should continue on a magnesium sulfate infusion through delivery and for 24 h after delivery [6]. While a goal magnesium serum concentration has not be adequately established in the literature, typical dose recommendations include a bolus dose of magnesium sulfate 4–6 g over 20–30 min followed by an infusion rate of 1–2 g/h to maintain appropriate serum magnesium levels that range from 4.8 to 8.4 mg/dL in order to increase the seizure threshold [3, 4, 6, 15]. This takes into consideration the larger volume of distribution in pregnant patients and higher BMI [15]. In the setting of difficult intravenous access, alternative dosing for magnesium sulfate is 10 g intramuscularly as a loading dose (5 g in each buttock) followed by 5 g intramuscularly every 4 h [15]. Adverse effects to monitor with the administration of high magnesium doses are deep tendon reflexes given the ultimate concern for respiratory depression and cardiac arrest [15]. Since magnesium is primarily excreted via the urine, patients who have acute or chronic renal sufficiency should have serum magnesium levels closely monitored every 4 h with consideration for lower magnesium sulfate infusion dosing, such as a 4–6 g loading dose followed by a continuous rate of 1 g/h [15]. In the event of respiratory depression requiring intubation, calcium gluconate 1 g intravenously over 3 min should be administered as a reversal agent [15].

38.5   Obstetric Hemorrhage

Both antepartum and postpartum hemorrhage (PPH) can be life threatening in pregnant patients and are a leading cause of maternal morbidity and mortality worldwide [4, 6]. Antepartum hemorrhage is often attributed to placental abruption, placenta previa, or uterine rupture where postpartum hemorrhage is most often associated with uterine atony, obstetric trauma, prolonged labor, or chorioamnionitis; however, uterine inversion and DIC may also be causes [4, 6]. It is critical to quickly identify the source of bleeding (cervical, perianal, periclitoral, perineal, periurethral, rectal, and vaginal) [22]. Careful monitoring of maternal heart rate and BP, in addition to the physical signs of hemorrhage, is important to promptly detect and treat a maternal hemorrhage.

PPH is defined as a cumulative blood loss greater than or equal to 1000 mL in the first 24 h of delivery or blood loss with signs and symptoms of hypovolemia, such as hypotension and tachycardia [3, 22]. The amount is not dependent on the type of delivery. If PPH is diagnosed based on signs and symptoms, it should be noted that these signs typically do not present until there has been significant blood loss, which is around 25% of a pregnant patient's blood volume or greater than or equal to 1500 mL [6, 22]. PPH can be primary or secondary where primary PPH occurs within the first 24 h of birth, and secondary occurs greater than 24 h after birth and up to 12 weeks postpartum [16, 22]. The rate of PPH has increased from 1994 to 2006 to 25% while the rate of maternal mortality from PPH has decreased to approximately 10% of maternal mortalities [22]. The most common cause of postpartum hemorrhage is uterine atony, which may be secondary to several factors, including cesarean section, oxytocin use, prolonged labor, uterine overdistension, placental abruption, or retained contents and accounts for 70–80% of PPH cases [3, 4, 6, 16, 22]. First-line treatment for uterine atony is the use of uterotonics [22]. Typically, the first-line uterotonic is considered to be intravenous oxytocin, but there is allowance for provider discretion since no one uterotonic has been shown to be more efficacious than another [4, 22]. Often more than one uterotonic will be used for PPH pending contraindications to certain agents where a second agent is used 3–25% of the time [22]. The use of a second uterotonic is needed in 3–25% of PPH cases, the most common of which are methylergonovine, 15-methyl prostaglandin $F_{2\alpha}$, or misoprostol [22]. Postpartum hemorrhage can lead to further consequences including adult respiratory distress syndrome (ARDS), shock, DIC, acute renal failure, loss of fertility, and pituitary necrosis (Sheehan syndrome) [22]. Assessment of a patient's coagulation status requires assessment of thrombin and may necessitate the need for administration of clotting factors and fibrinogen [22]. Retention of placental tissue or products of conception typically requires manual removal or uterine curettage [22].

Active management of PPH includes ensuring intravenous access, volume replacement, and emptying of the bladder along with oxytocin administration with a bolus dose of 10 units intravenously followed by an infusion not to exceed 40 units [3, 6, 16, 22]. For patients who do not have intravenous access, an alternative would be to administer oxytocin 10 units intramuscularly [22]. Administration of methylergonovine plus oxytocin or misoprostol plus oxytocin has not been shown to be more effective than oxytocin alone [22]. The typical suggested sequence of uterotonics, if no contraindications exist, is oxytocin, followed by methergine, then carboprost, and finally misoprostol [16]. Oxytocin receptors begin to be expressed in the uterus at approximately 13 weeks of gestation and increase in number until term [23, 24]. Oxytocin will bind to these oxytocin receptors to cause the release of intracellular calcium and production of prostaglandin, both of which will ultimately lead to uterine contraction to mitigate bleeding [23]. Saturation of oxytocin receptors can occur due to the number of oxytocin receptors present in the gravid uterus [24]. Additionally, repeated dosing of oxytocin can lead to desensitization [24]. Adverse effects associated with oxytocin include cardiac arrhythmias, QTc prolongation, tachycardia, nausea, vomiting, and hyponatremia [4, 23]. The optimal oxytocin dosing for postpartum hemorrhage has not been establish and is often institution-specific [25].

Another first-line uterotonic is methylergonovine (Methergine) which is an ergot derivative and acts directly on the smooth muscle of the uterus to cause sustained contractions by increasing tone, rate, and amplitude of contractions [4, 26]. Adverse effects associated with methylergonovine are angina pectoris, atrioventricular block, bradycardia, hypertension, coronary artery vasospasm, tachycardia, dizziness, headache, diaphoresis, nausea, vomiting, leg cramps, and dyspnea [26]. Since methylergonovine is associated with a hypertensive effect, it is contraindicated in patients with chronic hypertension or hypertensive disorders of pregnancy due to its potential to cause cerebral hemorrhagic from its blood pressure raising effects [4].

A third uterotonic for consideration is misoprostol which is a synthetic prostaglandin E1 analog that works by binding to smooth muscle cells lining the uterus to cause a uterotonic effect [27]. Adverse effects associated with misoprostol include abdominal pain, bronchospasm, headache, diarrhea, nausea, vomiting, shivering/chills, hypotension, tachycardia, urine rupture, and thrombosis [4, 27, 28]. Misoprostol should be avoided in patients with a history of cardiac or pulmonary disease [4].

For patients with blood loss of 1000 mL or greater, adjunctive treatment with tranexamic acid 1 g at 1 mL/min with consideration for a second 1 g dose 30 min later if bleeding is not controlled [3]. Tranexamic acid is an agent that inhibits fibrinolysis by forming a reversible complex that displaces plasminogen from fibrin [29]. Adjunctive treatment with tranexamic acid can be considered when other medical management with uterotonics fails and if administered within 3 h of delivery given the reduction in mortality from obstetric hemorrhage noted in the WOMAN trial [22, 30]. Adverse effects include abdominal pain, headache, back pain, musculoskeletal pain, and sinus symptoms [29]. Rare postmarketing side effects are thromboembolism and seizure, although the 1 g dosing used in the WOMAN trial did not show increased rates of VTE with tranexamic acid [22, 29].

See Table 38.2 for more information on agents used for the medical management of PPH. The use of prothrombin complex (PCC), fibrinogen concentrates, and recombinant factor VII are limited [22]. Use should be reserved for refractory cases after multiple rounds of uterotonics and massive transfusion protocol [22]. The use of uterotonics plays a pivotal role in managing uterine atony, along with uterine massage, bimanual compression, surgical techniques to control bleeding, or uterine artery embolization; however, cases of refractory or uncontrolled PPH may require a hysterectomy [3, 6, 16, 22].

DIC, while a less common cause of PPH, is a consumptive coagulopathy that can have quick onset before or after delivery and is associated with a high maternal and fetal mortality [4]. Pregnancy is known to be a hypercoagulable state with increased levels of fibrinogen, VWF, and clotting factors VII, VIII, and X; however, in DIC, hemorrhage occurs despite the hypercoagulable conditions of pregnancy due to procoagulant depletion [4, 32]. Certain conditions are associated with a higher risk of DIC, including amniotic fluid embolism, fetal death, HELLP, and placental abruption [4, 22]. The likely etiologies of coagulopathy in pregnancy are amniotic fluid

Table 38.2 Medications used to treat PPH [22, 23, 26, 28, 29, 31]

Medication	Mechanism of action	Dose/Route	Frequency	Adverse effects	Contraindications
Carboprost	Synthetic prostaglandin $F_{2\alpha}$ analog that induces uterine contractions	0.25 mg IM	Q15–90 min (up to max of 8 doses)	• Nausea • Vomiting • Fever • Headache • Chills • Shivering • Bronchospasm	• Asthma • Hypertension • Active hepatic disease • Active pulmonary disease • Active cardiac disease
Methylergonovine	Increases tone, rate, and amplitude of contractions	0.2 mg IM[a]	q2–4h	• Nausea • Vomiting • Severe hypertension	• Hypertension • Preeclampsia • Cardiovascular disease • Hypersenstivity to methylergonovine
Misoprostol	Synthetic prostaglandin E_1 analog that induces uterine contractions	600–1000 mcg PO, SL, rectal	One-time dose	• Nausea • Vomiting • Diarrhea • Shivering • Fever • Headache	• Hypersensitivity to misoprostol or other prostaglandins

Oxytocin	Binds to oxytocin receptors to cause the release of calcium and local prostaglandin production to induce contractions	10 units IM 10–40 units in 500–1000 mL as continuous infusion	IM: One-time dose IV: Continuous infusion	• Nausea • Vomiting • Hyponatremia (prolonged dosing) Hypotension (from IV push)	• Hypersensitivity oxytocin
Tranexamic acid	Inhibits fibrinolysis by displacing plasminogen from fibrin	1 g IV over 10–20 min	One-time dose, may repeat in 30 min if bleeding continues	• Abdominal pain • Headache • Musculoskeletal pain • Sinus symptoms • VTE • Seizure	• Active thrombus • Subarachnoid hemorrhage

IM intramuscular, *PO* oral, *SL* sublingual

Adapted from Practice Bulletin No. 183: Postpartum Hemorrhage. Obstetrics & Gynecology. 2017;130(4):e168-e186. https://doi.org/10.1097/AOG.0000000000002351

[a] Can consider IV in life-threatening situations. IV route is associated with severe hypertension

embolism and placental abruption [22]. For amniotic fluid embolism, profound coagulopathy or DIC should almost always be expected and treated promptly with volume replacement, and an interdisciplinary team should initiate an institution's massive transfusion protocol as soon as possible [22]. Further discussion of amniotic fluid embolism is included below. Placental abruption is typically manifested by vaginal bleeding, tachysystole, pain, and the need for implementation of a massive transfusion protocol for 17% of cases [22]. If a provider is concerned for pregnancy-related DIC, assessment of a peripheral blood smear, platelet count, prothrombin time (PT), partial thromboplastin time (PTT), or fibrinogen should occur [4].

In the setting of DIC (and PPH in general), management continues to include immediate volume replacement with crystalloids and supplemental oxygen [4, 6]. In the setting of hemorrhagic shock or a drop in hemoglobin (Hgb), administration of packed red blood cells should be given [4]. Dilutional coagulopathy and thrombocytopenia can occur with massive blood loss, and administration of fresh frozen plasma (FFP) may be indicated [4]. If a patient has low platelet levels <50,000, platelet transfusions should be given [4]. Similarly, if a patient has low fibrinogen levels, administration of fibrinogen and/or cryoprecipitate should be considered [4]. Intubation and mechanical ventilation may be required for hypoxia associated with hemorrhagic shock [4]. Further pharmacologic management of hemorrhage will depend on the etiology of the hemorrhage.

While the goal of PPH is to use nonsurgical methods or medical management initially, refractory uterine bleeding may require arterial embolization, uterine shunting, or uterine packing; however, uncontrolled postpartum hemorrhage can require a hysterectomy to be lifesaving [4, 16, 22]. Overall, critical care management of an obstetric hemorrhage aligns with other major hemorrhages where controlling of the bleed, correcting any coagulopathy, monitoring for continued or rebleeding and transfusion reactions, and stabilizing serum lactate, temperature, and volume status are vital [16].

38.6 Sepsis and Septic Shock

A cause of critical illness in pregnancy which is also a leading cause of maternal morbidity with a high mortality rate, up to 13%, is sepsis [4, 33]. There are three definitions or categories to be utilized per the Third International Consensus Definition for Sepsis and Septic Shock (Sepsis-3), and those are infection, sepsis, and septic shock where sepsis is an infection with organ dysfunction, and septic shock is sepsis requiring vasopressor support after adequate fluid resuscitation [1]. The Quick Sequential Organ Failure Assessment parameters have not been adjusted or externally validated in pregnancy [1, 10]. The modified early obstetric warning scoring (MEOWS) system and sepsis in obstetrics (SOS) score can be used to stratify sepsis in pregnancy, but they are not validated [10]. Further complications from sepsis include ARDS, cardiac dysfunction, fetal demise, multi-organ failure, neonatal neurological abnormalities, shock, and potentially irreversible multi-organ failure [4, 33]. It can be difficult to define maternal sepsis due to the physiologic changes of pregnancy [34]. Not only do these physiologic changes potentially mask a septic picture, they can make maternal response to sepsis difficult [33]. While the physiology of pregnant patients includes a decrease in vascular resistance and increase in heart rate that can serve to mask sepsis, rapid or drastic changes from a patient's baseline in blood pressure and/or heart rate can be concerning for sepsis [4, 16]. Additionally, while an increase in white blood cell (WBC) count is expected in late pregnancy, a significant elevation above maternal baseline could indicate infection [4]. The presence of delirium or altered mental status should also be concerning [16]. The National Partnership for Maternal Safety developed Maternal Early Warning Criteria to serve as parameters for vital signs necessitating evaluation [1, 35]. These criteria include SBP, DBP, heart rate, respiratory rate, oxygen saturation, oliguria, maternal agitation, confusion, or unresponsiveness. See Table 38.3 for further information.

Causes of sepsis in pregnancy can be obstetric, nonobstetric, and/or procedure-related, which may include abscess, antepartum pyelonephritis, chorioamnionitis, postpartum endometritis, septic abortion or pelvic thrombophlebitis, appendicitis, cholecystitis, pneumonia, amniocentesis, or surgical site infection [4, 6, 16]. In the setting of chorioamnionitis, endometritis, intra-abdominal or pelvic abscess, septic abortion, or surgical site infections, causative organisms tend to be those that colonize the skin or lower genital tract [4]. Obstetric-based infections are often polymicrobial, and consideration should be given to cover Gram positive, Gram negative, and anaerobic microorganisms [4]. The major causes of infection and sepsis in pregnancy that will be discussed below include pyelonephritis, endometritis, and chorioamnionitis for treatment management.

Management of septic pregnant patients should include prompt achievement of hemodynamic stability since blood flow during pregnancy plays a vital role in fetal

Table 38.3 Maternal early warning criteria [1, 35]

Criteria	Parameter
Systolic blood pressure (mmHg)	<90 or >160
Diastolic blood pressure (mmHg)	>100
Heart rate (beats per min)	<50 or >120
Respiratory rate (breaths per min)	<10 or >30
Oxygen saturation (%)	<95
Oliguria (mL/h for ≥2 h)	<35
Mental status	• Maternal agitation, confusion, or unresponsiveness • Non-remitting headache or shortness of breath in preeclampsia

Derived from ACOG Practice Bulletin No. 211: Critical Care in Pregnancy. Obstetrics & Gynecology. 2019;133(5):e303-e319. https://doi.org/10.1097/AOG.0000000000003241

oxygen delivery, and the need to initiate broad-spectrum antimicrobial therapy and fluid resuscitation within the first hour [1, 4, 16, 36]. Assessment of hypoperfusion during sepsis in pregnancy should include preload, afterload, and myocardial contractility [4]. Central venous pressure (CVP) is typically unchanged in pregnancy relative to prepregnancy so utilizing CVP to determine circulating volume helps determine the magnitude of volume resuscitation that is required [4]. However, CVP is less reliable for determining volume status in pregnant patients with valvular disease, heart failure, pericardial disease, and other conditions associated with obstruction [4]. The signs of septic shock in pregnancy can be difficult to decipher since increased heart rate and decreased BP are normal physiologic changes associated with pregnancy [9]. Assessing for trends and changes from baseline play a vital role in helping to determine the onset of sepsis versus a normal pregnancy state. In early pregnancy, pulse pressure can be used to determine a pregnant patient's response to fluid resuscitation; however, this is less reliable later in pregnancy because of the gravid uterus [4]. The use of echocardiography may be helpful in determining volume status and assessing the inferior vena cava (IVC) [4]. During the assessment of sepsis, a central venous oxygen saturation lower than 70% can be a normal finding later in pregnancy where otherwise that would be considered an indicator of sepsis in nonpregnant individuals [4]. Ensuring tissue perfusion for the pregnant patient will also ensure adequate placental blood flow which depends on uterine perfusion pressure, maternal BP, and maternal cardiac output [9]. Dobutamine can be used for pregnant patients with sepsis complicated by cardiac dysfunction based on elevated cardiac filling pressures, narrow pulse pressure, slow capillary return, and cool, clammy extremities [4].

Vasoactive agents can be utilized in pregnant patients with continued hypotension and hypoperfusion despite fluid resuscitation [4]. The selection of the optimal vasopressor would be one that has the least effect on decreasing uterine perfusion since no specific guidelines exist for preferred vasopressors [9, 10]. Uterine vessels at maximal dilation have only alpha-adrenergic receptors [37]. In animal studies with baboons and sheep, dopamine, which is a dopaminergic, alpha-1, and beta-1 agonist, has been shown to reduce uterine artery blood flow, but no studies have assessed fetal effects in humans [9]. Dobutamine, a beta-1 and beta-2 agonist, has been used for myocardial infarction and cardiopulmonary bypass in human pregnancies and has not increased the risk of congenital abnormalities in animal studies [9, 38]. The effect on uterine blood flow is not known [9]. Epinephrine, an alpha-1 and beta-1 agonist with some beta-2 agonism, has been shown to increase uterine activity and uterine vasoconstriction in studies with monkeys but may also lead to uterine relaxation given the lesser beta-2 activity [9]. The use of epinephrine at any time in pregnancy has been associated with inguinal hernia; however, this may have been related to maternal illness [39]. Norepinephrine, an alpha-1 and beta-1 agonist, was shown to decrease placental blood flow and result in decreas fetal oxygenation, fetal urine flow, and lung liquid flow when given in high doses (40 mcg/min) [40]. Since doses used for hemodynamic stability are lower, the clinical significance of these adverse effects is not clear [40]. Phenylephrine is an alpha-1 agonist commonly used for maternal hypotension after spinal and epidural anesthesia; however, given its pure alpha-1 agonism and uterine expression of alpha-adrenergic receptors, it can lead to constriction of uterine vessels and decrease uterine blood flow [37]. This can have adverse fetal outcomes including fetal hypoxia and bradycardia [37]. There is also an association between fetal malformations and phenylephrine use during the first trimester; nevertheless, a 2018 study showed similar maternal BP, and maternal, neonatal umbilical artery, and venous acid-base measurements in patients who received either phenylephrine or ephedrine for maternal hypotension from spinal anesthesia [39, 41]. The phenylephrine group did have lower umbilical vein partial pressure of oxygen [41]. Both phenylephrine and ephedrine are associated with reduced fetal pH with better Apgar scores and incidence of fetal acidosis with phenylephrine [42]. Finally for vasopressin, a direct vasoconstrictor that increases systemic vascular resistance and mean arterial pressure via stimulation of the arginine vasopressin (AVP) R1a receptors, can be considered in refractory cases of hypotension and hemodynamic compromise [9, 43]. There have been no reports of adverse fetal outcomes with the use of vasopressin during pregnancy; however, vasopressin may induce uterine activity which has been reported with intramuscular and intranasal formulations [44]. Notably during pregnancy, the levels of endogenous vasopressin undergo at threefold increase in the third trimester of pregnancy [45]. The 2016 Society of Critical Care Medicine Guidelines support the use of norepinephrine as a first-line vasopressor in septic pregnant patients [10, 46]. Phenylephrine and ephedrine may be considered as second-line agents given extrapolated use from studies with spinal anesthesia; however, they both exhibit tachyphylaxis [10, 47]. Given the least effect on placental and uterine perfusion, the use of phenylephrine would be a preferred vasoactive agent in the setting of continued hypotension despite fluid resuscitation. Caution should be noted for phenylephrine's ability to cause maternal reflex bradycardia and reduced cardiac output [10, 47].

The general workup for sepsis in pregnancy patients should include blood and urine cultures as well as cultures from other sites concerning for the source of infection [4]. Initiation of broad-spectrum antimicrobial therapy and working to achieve source control are critical [4, 16]. Antimicrobial coverage should include Gram positive, Gram negative, and anaerobic coverage, where anaerobic coverage is important if there is concern for an obstetric source [4]. Preferred antimicrobials in pregnancy include penicillins, cephalosporins, clindamycin, trimethoprim-sulfamethoxazole (TMP-SMX), and vancomycin [48]. If a pregnant patient is at risk for nosocomial or resistant bacteria, the antimicrobial regimen should be broadened to cover for those microbes [4]. For example, in the setting of skin and soft tissue infection in pregnant patients, utilizing antibiotics to cover methicillin-resistant *Staphylococcus aureus* (MRSA) is reasonable given levels of community-acquired MRSA [4].

Other measures including mechanical intubation, treatment of fevers with acetaminophen and cooling blankets, and glucose control are all important for maternal and fetal health. In refractory shock, the use of corticosteroids can be indicated, especially if concerned for adrenal insufficiency [4]. Additional parameters for optimization include nutritional supports, mitigating oversedation, VTE prevention, gastrointestinal prophylaxis, and prevention of secondary infections [4].

38.6.1 Pyelonephritis

Bacteriuria and asymptomatic bacteremia are common in pregnancy, and urinary tract infections (UTIs) account for 3.5% of antepartum admissions [48, 49]. Consequently, untreated UTIs can progress to pyelonephritis in a small portion of pregnant patients which is a leading cause of septic shock during pregnancy and occurs in up to 10% of patients [4, 48]. Of pregnant patients diagnosed with pyelonephritis, 15–20% will have bacteremia as well [50]. Pregnancy increases the risk of pyelonephritis due to ureteral stasis [4, 6, 48, 50, 51]. Urinary stasis is the result of several physiologic changes. Progesterone causes smooth muscle relaxation which leads to ureteral and renal calyces dilation [6, 10, 48, 50]. The gravid uterus also causes ureteral compression and a reduction in bladder capacity, and decreased detrusor tone can result in incomplete emptying of the bladder [10, 48, 50]. These changes all make pregnant patients prone to UTIs and subsequently pyelonephritis.

Causative microbes for pyelonephritis in pregnancy are mostly Gram-negative rods but also Gram-positive microorganisms can be seen [4]. *Escherichia coli* is the most common, causing up to 82.5–85% of pyelonephritis cases in pregnancy followed by *Klebsiella pneumoniae*, and *Staphylococcus*, *Streptococcus*, *Proteus*, and *Enterococcus* species [10, 48, 50, 52]. Endotoxin release from Gram-negative microorganisms leads to the release of cytokines, histamine, and bradykinins resulting in endothelial damage and decreased cardiac output and vascular resistance [10, 50]. Additionally, the endotoxin release can result in pulmonary edema and ARDS because of alveolar damage [48, 50]. This sequela results in the need for respiratory support with mechanical ventilation and ICU admission.

Management of pyelonephritis in pregnancy requires hospital admission given the potential for rapid progression to septic shock and ARDS [10, 48, 50]. Prompt initiation of intravenous antimicrobial therapy that cover the microorganisms of concern is necessary to prevent the progression of pyelonephritis to septic shock and ARDS in 1–8% of cases [10]. As noted above, penicillins and cephalosporins are preferred agents in pregnancy as well as clindamycin, TMP-SMX, vancomycin, and nitrofurantoin [48]. During the first and last trimester of pregnancy, TMP-SMX should be avoided. There is concern for an increased risk of congenital malformations, including neural tube defects, cardiovascular malformations, urinary tract defects, oral clefts, club foot with TMP-SMX use during the first trimester owing to TMP's effect on folic acid metabolism resulting in decreases folic acid levels [53]. During the last trimester of pregnancy, there is concern for TMP-SMX increasing the risk of hyperbilirubinemia and kernicterus, with extra consideration given to infants who are born prematurely [48]. The suggested initial empiric therapy for a pregnant patient who presents with pyelonephritis is ceftriaxone 2 g intravenous once daily and then tailored to sensitivities. If broad-spectrum antimicrobial therapy is needed in the setting of septic shock, consideration should be given for piperacillin-tazobactam 4.5 g intravenously every 6 h plus vancomycin 15 mg/kg intravenously every 8 h and renally dose adjusted in the setting of acute kidney injury or chronic kidney disease. In the setting of penicillin allergies, the use of intravenous cephalosporins, aztreonam, metronidazole, and aminoglycosides should be considered. Once antibiotic therapy is initiated, there may be a worsening of a patient's clinical status because of cell kill of the Gram-negative bacteria leading to further endotoxin release [48]. This is important to note so that it is not thought that the antimicrobial agents are not providing adequate coverage. A treatment duration of 14 days is recommended.

The recurrence of pyelonephritis in pregnancy is approximately 20% which lends to the recommendation to place pregnant patients on suppressive therapy with nitrofurantoin 100 mg orally at bedtime or cephalexin 500 mg orally once daily at bedtime after a treatment course [48, 50, 51]. By administering the suppressive antimicrobial agent at bedtime, this allows for the medication to concentrate in the urine overnight when patients are less likely to void.

38.6.2 Chorioamnionitis

Intraamniotic infection is commonly known as chorioamnionitis and affects approximately 4% of pregnant patients and 2 to 5% of deliveries [4, 54]. An intraamniotic infection is an infection marked by inflammation that can affect the amniotic fluid, placenta, fetus, fetal membranes, and/or decidua [6, 54]. This type of infection can rarely be caused by invasive procedures or hematogenous spread, for example, by *Listeria monocytogenes*, but more commonly occurs because of ascending bacterial translocation from the lower genital tract [54]. Risk factors for intraamniotic infection are internal uterine and fetal monitors, low parity, meconium-stained fluid, multiple digital exams, and certain genital tract pathogens, such as group B strep (GBS) and sexually transmitted diseases. It is important to treat chorioamnionitis early to prevent progression to sepsis and improve maternal and fetal outcomes [4, 54].

Neonatal morbidity from intraamniotic infection includes neonatal pneumonia, meningitis, sepsis, and even death with long-term complications including bronchopulmonary dysplasia and cerebral palsy [54]. Administration of antimicrobial therapy either as part of GBS prophylaxis during labor or for the treatment of chorioamnionitis has been shown to decrease GBS-specific neonatal sepsis ten-fold [54]. There is also maternal morbidity to consider including dysfunctional labor, postpartum hemorrhage from uterine atony, endometritis, peritonitis, sepsis, ARDS, and death [54]. For chorioamnionitis, patients will typically present with fever, maternal or fetal tachycardia, abdominal tenderness, and foul-smelling amniotic fluid. If a pregnant patient presents with sepsis or ARDS, chorioamnionitis should be on the differential [4]. The use of antimicrobial therapy alone for chorioamnionitis will not be adequate and source control will require the delivery of the fetus for both maternal and fetal well-being [4].

Diagnosis of an intraamniotic infection is most often via a clinical diagnosis but can also be done via amniotic fluid culture including Gram stain, and/or biochemical analysis leading to three different categories of infection [54]. The categories are isolated maternal fever, suspected intraamniotic infection, and confirmed intraamniotic infection [54]. A suspected intraamniotic infection is based on the clinical criteria that include a maternal intrapartum fever, defined as a single oral temperature of $\geq$39 °C or an oral temperature 38–38.9 °C that persists after 30 min, and one or more of the following criteria, fetal tachycardia, maternal leukocytosis, and/or purulent cervical drainage [54]. An amniotic fluid test that is positive either from Gram stain, glucose level, or culture results or placental pathology positive for placental infection or inflammation confirm a diagnosis of intraamniotic infection; however, this most often is not done until after delivery so suspected infection tends to largely be a clinical diagnosis [54].

Management of intraamniotic infection includes prompt initiation of antimicrobial therapy with the addition of antipyretics such as acetaminophen for the management of fever and augmentation of labor or need for cesarean delivery [54]. Recommended antimicrobial therapy includes ampicillin 2 g intravenously every 6 h plus gentamicin 2 mg/kg intravenously for one dose as a load followed by 1.5 mg/kg intravenously every 8 h or 5 mg/kg intravenously every 24 h [54]. Per ACOG, in the setting of allergies, the recommendation for antimicrobial therapy for mild penicillin allergy is cefazolin 2 g intravenously every 8 h plus gentamicin 2 mg/kg intravenously for one dose as a load followed by 1.5 mg/kg intravenously every 8 h or 5 mg/kg intravenously every 24 h and for severe penicillin allergy, the recommendation is for clindamycin 900 mg intravenously every 8 h plus gentamicin 2 mg/kg intravenously for one dose as a load followed by 1.5 mg/kg intravenously every 8 h or 5 mg/kg intravenously every 24 h OR vancomycin 1 g intravenously every 12 h plus gentamicin 2 mg/kg intravenously for one dose as a load followed by 1.5 mg/kg intravenously every 8 h or 5 mg/kg intravenously every 24 h [54]. Other regimens that can be considered consist of ampicillin-sulbactam, piperacillin-tazobactam, cefotetan, cefoxitin, or ertapenem [10]. For sepsis without subsequent bacteremia, treatment duration should be 7–14 days with step down to oral antibiotics upon clinical stability. For sepsis with bacteremia, treatment duration is 7–14 days from the first negative blood culture. See Table 38.4 for more information.

38.6.3 Endometritis

Endometritis occurs as a postpartum infection and in severe and rare instances, as sepsis [4]. Risk factors for postpartum endometritis include cesarean section and GBS colonization. Severe cases of endometritis are associated with toxin-producing strains of clostridium, staphylococcus, and streptococcus [4]. In general, the infection is polymicrobial with a majority being attributed to anaerobic microorganisms,

Table 38.4 Antimicrobial regimens for the treatment of intraamniotic infections [53]

Antibiotic and dose
Recommended antibiotics
Ampicillin 2 g IV q6h <u>Plus</u> Gentamicin 2 g IV × 1 dose followed by 1.5 mg/kg IV q8h or 5 mg/kg IV q24h[a] (two possible gentamicin dosing modalities)
Mild PCN allergy
Cefazolin 2 g IV q8h <u>Plus</u> Gentamicin 2 g IV × 1 dose followed by 1.5 mg/kg IV q8h or 5 mg/kg IV q24h[a]
Severe PCN allergy
Clindamycin 900 mg IV q8h <u>Plus</u> Gentamicin 2 g IV × 1 dose followed by 1.5 mg/kg IV q8h or 5 mg/kg IV q24h[a] **OR** Vancomycin 1 g IV q12h (for GBS vaginal/rectal culture that clindamycin resistant) <u>Plus</u> Gentamicin 2 g IV × 1 dose followed by 1.5 mg/kg IV q8h or 5 mg/kg IV q24h[a]
Alternative regimens
Ampicillin-sulbactam 3 g IV q6h OR Cefotetan 2 g IV q12h OR Cefoxitin 2 g IV q8h OR Ertapenem 1 g IV q24h OR Piperacillin-tazobactam 3.375 g IV q6h or 4.5 g IV q8h
Additional dosing post-delivery indicated for cesarean section only

IV intravenous, *PCN* penicillin, *GBS* Group B streptococcus
Adapted from Committee Opinion No. 712: Intrapartum Management of Intraamniotic Infection. Obstetrics & Gynecology. 2017;130(2):e95-e101. doi:10.1097/AOG.0000000000002236
[a] Two possible gentamicin dosing modalities

such as *Bacteriodes*, *Clostridium*, and *Peptostreptococcus* sp and to a lesser extent with aerobic microorganisms, such as GBS, *E. coli*, and enterococcus [10]. Toxic shock syndrome from *Streptococcus pyogenes* or *Staphylococcus aureus* often has the presence of a hematoma and can be fatal if not promptly identified and treated [4, 10]. Patients who underwent vaginal delivery are less likely to experience a complication with postpartum endometritis relative to cesarean deliveries [54]. Patients whose pregnancy or labor was complicated by chorioamnionitis and underwent a cesarean section should be given an additional dose of antibiotic therapy postpartum [54]. Patients with endometritis may present with a fever, uterine tenderness, abdominal tenderness, and/or purulent vaginal discharge or lochia [4, 10]. The use of cervical cultures can yield normal vaginal flora microbes leading to contamination of the culture itself since it is not representative of the infectious etiology [4]. Treatment should consist of intravenous antimicrobial therapy with cefazolin 2 g intravenously every 8 h plus metronidazole 500 mg orally or intravenously every 8 h as empiric therapy for uncomplicated endometritis. This should be continued until the patient is clinically improved and afebrile for 24–48 h. If concerned for sepsis, empiric therapy should be escalated to piperacillin-tazobactam

4.5 g intravenously every 6 h and vancomycin 15 mg/kg intravenously every 8 h with both antibiotics adjusted for renal function. Alternative regimens in the setting of penicillin allergies include cefepime 2 g intravenously every 8 h plus metronidazole 500 mg orally or intravenously every 8 h and vancomycin 15 mg/kg intravenously every 8 h with cefepime and vancomycin dose adjusted for renal function and finally aztreonam 2 g intravenously every 8 h plus metronidazole 500 mg orally or intravenously every 8 h plus vancomycin 15 mg/kg intravenously every 8 h with aztreonam and vancomycin dose adjusted for renal function. Antimicrobial therapy should be continued until clinical improvement and stability and afebrile for 24 h. Timely identification and management of intraamniotic infections are important to prevent maternal and neonatal morbidity and mortality.

38.7 Amniotic Fluid Embolism

Amniotic fluid embolism (AFE) is a rare and potentially lethal event that may occur during delivery or the immediate postpartum period leading to a significant cause of maternal mortality [3, 4, 8]. It is unpreventable with an occurrence of 1 in 40,000 pregnancies and associated with a 20–60% mortality [8]. Patients who survive an AFE, even with optimal management, can still suffer high rates of morbidity, such as central nervous system dysfunction [4, 55]. AFE is classified as the vascular transfer of amniotic fluid or other material, such as fetal squamous cells, from the fetal compartment into maternal circulation, eventually reaching pulmonary circulation that triggers an acute event [6, 8, 55]. This fluid can contain lanugo, vernix, meconium, and thromboplastic substances [8]. This transfer causes activation of proinflammatory mediator systems leading a response similar to systemic inflammatory response syndrome [55]. Despite this fluid entering maternal circulation, pulmonary obstruction from the contents of the fluid is considered a minor factor in the pathophysiology of AFE [4]. Another unproven etiology is AFE is a type of anaphylactoid reaction from fetal content circulating in the fluid [4]. With AFE, an acute increase in PVR leads to right heart failure; however, some patients only have minimal increases in PVR with profound left ventricular dysfunction instead leading to pulmonary edema, circulatory collapse, and ultimately cardiopulmonary arrest [3, 4, 6].

The presentation of AFE is a sudden onset of maternal distress marked by sudden hypoxia and hypotension as well as neurological symptoms in 33% of patients, which includes altered mental status, seizures, and coma [3, 8, 55]. Patients with an abrupt onset of respiratory failure demonstrate shortness of breath, pulmonary edema, ARDS, and cyanosis [4, 8]. Other effects include sudden cardiovascular collapse, significant hypotension, cardiac dysrhythmias, myocardial infarction, DIC (80–83% of patients), and hemorrhage [4, 8, 55]. A less common initial presentation for AFE is bleeding and shock only, but this remains a presentation to keep on the AFE differential, particularly if it is followed by cardiovascular collapse, cardiovascular arrest, seizures, and respiratory difficulty [4, 55]. The fetus may show signs of distress before the acute event with decelerations on the tocometer as well as a loss of variability and possibly terminal fetal bradycardia due to uterine hypoperfusion due to uterine hypertonus from catecholamine release [55]. The diagnosis of AFE is initially a clinical diagnosis [55].

There can be fetal, maternal, and obstetrical factors that predispose the occurrence of AFE, some of which include fetal distress, fetal macrosomia, placenta accreta or previa, placental abruption, polyhydramnios, premature rupture of membranes, advanced maternal age (>35 years old), diabetes, multiparity, cesarean section, eclampsia, induction of labor, oxytocin use, and uterine rupture [6, 8, 54]. The hypoxic injury associated with AFE can result in severe hypoxemia, tissue hypoxia, and left heart failure/dysfunction. Other pathophysiology includes pulmonary hypertension leading to decreased cardiac output and pulmonary edema [8].

Acute management includes intubation with mechanical ventilation/positive end-expiratory pressure (PEEP) support to ensure adequate oxygenation, volume support ± blood products to help control bleeding, and vasopressor support for profound hypotension to stabilize circulation [4, 6, 8]. With ventilatory support, PEEP will be titrated to achieve a Pa_{O2} >90 mmHg and fraction of inspired oxygen Fi_{O2} ≤0.6 [4]. Sedation should be used during intubation and paralytics can be considered to help allow complete rest of respiratory muscles [4]. In patients who experience cardiac arrest, immediate initiation of cardiopulmonary resuscitation is necessary [54]. In the advanced cardiac life support (ACLS) algorithm, the use of vasopressors, antiarrhythmic agents, and defibrillating doses can all be used [54]. In the setting of concern for heart failure, an urgent echocardiogram should be ordered to help determine the type and degree of heart failure [4]. If heart failure is present, milrinone can be considered, and bronchodilators like nitric oxide or inhaled epoprostenol for pulmonary hypertension [8]. For DIC or hemorrhage associated with AFE, rapid administration of blood product should be performed; platelet transfusion for a platelet count <50,000/microL, FFP to normalize international normalized ratio (INR), and FFP, fibrinogen, and cryoprecipitate for a fibrinogen <200 mL/dL should also be considered [6, 8]. Fluid resuscitation should also occur for volume repletion with consideration still given to the presence of heart failure [4]. The use of vasoactive medications should also be utilized for BP support, especially in cases where the BP is refractory to volume resuscitation and continued profound vasodilation [4]. Laboratory monitoring would include PT, PTT, D-dimer, fibrinogen, INR, complete blood cell count, arterial blood gas, and diagnostic studies should include chest X-ray, electrocardiogram, and echocardiogram [8].

38.8   Venous Thromboembolism

Pregnant patients are at a four- to five-fold higher risk of venous thromboembolism (VTE), manifested by deep vein thrombosis (DVT) and pulmonary embolism (PE) compared to nonpregnant patients due to the hypercoagulable state of pregnancy and venous stasis with the VTE risk extending up to 6 weeks postpartum [4, 11, 56]. Of thromboembolic events, approximately 80% are attributed to VTE, which contributes to 9.3% of maternal deaths in the United States [11]. DVT accounts for 75–80% of VTE cases, whereas 20–25% are due to PE [6, 11]. Given the prevalence of VTE in pregnancy and potentially significant consequences, having an understanding of the pathophysiology, risk factors, and management of critically ill obstetric patients who present with this complication is an important consideration.

Several factors contribute to the promotion of VTE in pregnancy, some of which include compression of the inferior vena cava and pelvic veins secondary to an enlarging uterus, decreased mobility, hypercoagulability, and increased venous stasis [3, 11]. The compression of the left iliac vein by the right iliac artery and compressed vena cava by the enlarging uterus leads to a DVT more commonly occurring in the left leg in pregnant patients compared to nonpregnant patients [11]. Coagulation factors are also altered in pregnancy where the procoagulant fibrinogen, Factor VII, Factor VIII, Factor X, VWF, and plasminogen activator inhibitor-1 and -2 are all increased [3, 11]. Additionally that natural anticoagulant protein S is decreased, and there is no change in protein C and antithrombin [11]. The risk of VTE in pregnancy is present throughout all trimesters with increased risk occurring in the second and third trimester [11]. The postpartum period is also a time of continuous increased thrombogenic risk with the first week postpartum comprising the greatest risk [11]. Individual risk factors can also play in role for VTE in pregnancy. The most significant is a person history of thrombosis which has a three-fold to four-fold risk of recurrent VTE (RR 3.5, CI 1.6–5.8) followed by presence of thrombophilia [11]. Other factors to consider for the increased risk of VTE are cesarean delivery, postpartum hemorrhage, obesity, hypertension, autoimmune disease, heart disease, sickle cell disease, multiple gestation, and preeclampsia [11, 56].

DVT usually presents as pain and swelling unilaterally within an extremity, and particularly for pregnancy, the DVT will often be iliofemoral (64%) and iliac thromboses (17%) rather than distal DVT [11]. Using Doppler ultrasonography with a deep vein ultrasound (DVU) to assess for VTE is an important initial assessment [11]. For PE, patients may present with symptoms, such as dyspnea, chest pain, tachycardia, and dizziness [56]. There are instances where empiric therapeutic anticoagulation can be considered for a clinicalt picture strongly concerning for VTE, and diagnostic testing cannot be obtained [11]. It is not recommended to obtain D-dimer levels in pregnant patients because of the progressive increase in D-dimer levels that occurs as pregnancy progresses [11]. If concerned for a PE, the use of a ventilation-perfusion (VQ) scan or computed tomographic (CT) scan is recommended [6, 11, 56]. While there may be concern for radiation exposure, the rate of this exposure for both a VQ scan and CT is low at approximately 0.32–0.64 mGY and up to 0.0513–0.1308 mGY in the third trimester, respectively [6, 11].

The treatment of VTE in obstetric patients includes low-molecular-weight heparin (LMWH), unfractionated heparin (UFH), and warfarin with the preferred agents being LMWH and heparin compounds since these agents do not cross the placenta [6, 11, 56]. It is important to remember the various PK changes in pregnancy that can affect LMWH and UFH. The increase in maternal blood volume by up to 50% is a consideration for hydrophilic medications and increase in maternal glomerular filtration for renally cleared medications, such as for LMWH [11]. There is also increased protein binding of heparin. These effects can result in a lower peak plasma concentration and shorter half-life potentially requiring increased doses of these medications [11]. LMWH has a more predictable PK and is easier to administer so it tends to be preferred over UFH in pregnancy. Other advantages of LMWH over UFH are fewer bleeding episodes, lower risk of heparin-induced thromboembolism (HIT), longer half-life, and lower risk of bone mineral density loss [11]. Monitoring of therapeutic anticoagulation can be done using institution-specific guidelines with either anti-Xa or activated partial thromboplastin time (aPTT). Therapeutic dosing of enoxaparin is 1 mg/kg subcutaneously every 12 h for a target peak anti-Xa of 0.5–1 units/mL (some literature recommends 0.6–1 units/mL) drawn 4 h after the third dose [6, 11]. Therapeutic dosing of UFH is 10,000 units or more subcutaneously every 12 h adjusted to aPTT of 1.5–2.5 times the control drawn 6 h after the last injection [11]. Moreover, for critically ill obstetric patients in the ICU, the use of UFH as an infusion per hospital protocol for VTE is appropriate and may be preferred, especially in cases where the decision for delivery could be rapid and if the pregnant patient is at risk of bleeding or has an acute kidney injury.

The use of warfarin during the first trimester is contraindicated due to teratogenic effects, thought to be dose dependent, including coumarin embryopathy which consists of nasal and limb hypoplasia [57]. CNS abnormalities may also occur such as ventral midline dysplasia and dorsal midline dysplasia [57]. However, given the high risk of thrombosis associated with a mechanical heart valve, consideration can be given to resuming warfarin in the second trimester of pregnancy [57]. In the setting of critical illness for an obstetric patient on warfarin requiring immediate delivery, cesarean section should be considered, and the neonate may require vitamin K administration and fresh frozen plasma since the risk for fetal hemorrhage with maternal warfarin use is the highest at the time of delivery [11].

The use of oral anti-Xa inhibitors, such as apixaban, edoxaban, rivaroxaban, and oral direct thrombin inhibitors is not recommended in pregnancy or lactation and should be immediately discontinued in patients who are pregnant, planning to become pregnant, or who are breastfeeding given insufficient safety data [11].

For pregnant patients with severe cutaneous allergies or HIT, fondaparinux may be a preferred alternative anticoagulant [11]. Despite literature demonstrating no adverse effects to the infant, anticoagulant activity has been detected in the cord blood after maternal use of fondaparinux [11]. Patients who require parenteral therapeutic anticoagulation with a direct thrombin inhibitor can consider argatroban dosed and monitored per institution protocol for the shortest duration needed [11].

For obstetric patients not admitted with VTE but who are critically ill in the ICU, the use of chemoprophylaxis will be important given the hypercoagulability of pregnancy or postpartum in addition to the risk factors of critical illness. Thromboprophylaxis should be tailored to the patient and their risk factors using clinical practice guidelines [11]. Dosing for VTE prophylaxis with enoxaparin can be 40 mg subcutaneously once daily or with an intermediate-dose of enoxaparin 40 mg subcutaneously every 12 h [11]. Prophylactic dosing for UFH is based on trimester, with UFH 5000–7500 units subcutaneously every 12 h recommended in the first trimester, UFH 7500–10,000 units subcutaneously every 12 h in the second trimester, and UFH 10,000 units subcutaneously every 12 h in the third trimester [11]. In the setting of prophylactic dosing, the importance of selecting LMWH versus UFH largely revolves around the need for neuraxial anesthesia since a LMWH like enoxaparin has a longer half-life and depending on the dose, may need to be held for a longer duration than UFH if a patient needs neuraxial anesthesia for delivery.

38.9 Acute Fatty Liver in Pregnancy

Acute fatty liver in pregnancy (AFLP) is a rare but potentially fatal obstetric emergency that typically begins in the third trimester, most commonly after 30 weeks of gestation, and has an incidence of 1 in 7000–15,000 pregnancies [3, 4, 6, 58–60]. In the 1980s, maternal mortality from AFLP was up to 70% with mortality rates now at 2%; however, infant mortality still ranges from 10% to 20% [60]. Risk factors identified for AFLP are multigravida, male sex of the fetus, another diagnosis of liver disease in pregnancy (i.e., HELLP, preeclampsia), and a prior episode of AFLP [58, 60]. While increases in liver function tests (LFTs) can be noted with HELLP syndrome and preeclampsia due to periportal or focal parenchymal necrosis and fibrin deposition, this disease can lead to intraparenchymal hemorrhage, hepatic rupture/infarction, or subcapsular hematoma [4]. Physiologic changes in pregnancy lead to increased maternal serum fatty acids due to the decreased oxidation of long- and medium-chain fatty acids [60]. Long-chain 3-hydroxylacyl-CoA dehydrogenase (LCHAD) deficiency has been associated as a susceptibility to AFLP [6, 58, 60]. In addition, fetal fatty acid oxidation defects (FAOD), which include enzymes involved in fatty acid mitochondrial metabolism, is thought to be a risk factor for AFLP [4, 58]. Maternal hormone-sensitive lipase activity is increased, and insulin resistance mediated by the placenta can increase triglyceride levels which are then broken down into free fatty acids [58]. There is an increased demand for fatty acids during pregnancy for fetal and placental growth where mitochondrial oxidation of those fatty acids can be altered [58]. If fatty acid oxidation fails in the fetus and placenta, products of metabolism accumulate leading to toxic metabolic intermediate accumulation in maternal hepatocytes which results in hepatic dysfunction from microvesicular fatty steatosis of the liver [58, 60]. Fatty acid infiltration also occurs in the kidney leading to renal impairment and dysfunction [60]. This accumulation of fatty acids and their metabolites in maternal blood can result in increased reactive oxygen species, inflammatory pathway activation, and cellular necrosis ensuing in hepatic failure in the pregnant patient [58]. Additionally, there can be increased fatty acids in the placenta resulting in placental dysfunction and impaired oxygen delivery to the fetus [60].

The prompt diagnosis of AFLP is difficult because other liver diseases associated with pregnancy share similar features; however, a marked difference between AFLP and other liver diseases associated with pregnancy is the presence of true liver dysfunction [58]. Signs and symptoms include malaise, nausea, vomiting, anorexia, encephalopathy, right upper quadrant pain, jaundice, polydipsia, and polyuria [3, 4, 6, 58, 60]. Rapid, escalating symptoms of AFLP are coagulopathy, hypoglycemia, and renal failure [3, 58]. To help distinguish AFLP from HELLP and preeclampsia, the presence of hypoglycemia, elevated INR, and other symptoms, including encephalopathy and DIC, are noted in AFLP [58]. Other laboratory findings include hyperbilirubinemia, elevated γ-glutamyl transpeptidase, elevated ammonia, hyperuricemia, elevated creatinine and blood urea nitrogen, thrombocytopenia, and elevated lipase [6, 60]. If a liver biopsy is obtained, histology of AFLP shows microvesicular infiltration of hepatocytes of the pericentral zone and not periportal zone [58]. The use of imaging in diagnosing AFLP is unclear since ultrasound can be nonspecific, but imaging with MRI may be more helpful [58]. A proposed diagnostic tool for AFLP is the Swansea criteria that have an 85% positive predictive value and 100% negative predictive value [58, 60, 61]. It can be used in the absence of another diagnosis for liver dysfunction in pregnancy [58, 60, 61]. However, it has been suggested that this criterion is more helpful once patients are already critically ill [58].

With concern for AFLP, and the presence of liver dysfunction and coagulopathy, acute management includes the need for urgent delivery [3, 6, 58]. Treatment thereafter is supportive; however in the setting of fulminant liver failure, the AFLP may be not reversible and requires liver transplantation [3, 58]. Postpartum acute management could include the complications of acute liver failure with encephalopathy, acute renal failure, DIC, and gastrointestinal bleeding [58]. There is also the possibility for hepatic rupture or hematoma with AFLP [58]. ICU care will involve correction of hypoglycemia, monitoring for coagulopathy, administration of blood products, plasmapheresis, dialysis, and/or mechanical ventilation for acute respiratory distress syndrome, monitoring for coagulopathy [6, 58]. Use of lactulose 20–30 g by mouth every 4–6 h can be considered to help with elevated ammonia levels and promote loss via feces [6]. While often AFLP is reversible within 1–3 weeks postpartum, in instances where recovery is not occurring and liver function worsens, liver transplantation may need to be considered [4, 58].

Recovery from AFLP depends on the comorbid complications. Typically decreasing LFTs occurs in 1–2 days post-delivery where it may take 3–4 days to see a decline in cholesterol and bilirubin [58]. If acute kidney injury was part of the clinical picture that will typically resolve in 7–10 days; however, histological changes may continue for up to 5 weeks [58]. It is vital that AFLP is diagnosed as early as possible to improve maternal and fetal outcomes.

38.10 Acute Respiratory Failure

Acute respiratory distress syndrome (ARDS) is the acute onset of diffuse inflammation and subsequent pulmonary edema from increased vascular permeability resulting in a Pa_{O2} to Fi_{O2} ratio <200 and has a maternal mortality that varies from 9% to 44% [1, 4, 56]. An increasing $PaCO_2$ indicates that work of breathing for a pregnant patient may be too high; however, extra consideration of the compensated respiratory alkalosis state in pregnancy is needed because a normal Pa_{CO_2} in nonpregnant patients may be very concerning in pregnant patients [1, 6, 62]. Pregnant patients are at an increased risk of developing ARDS, and when they present with pulmonary symptoms, progression to ARDS can be rapid [1]. While this pulmonary edema is noncardiogenic, it is commonly caused by sepsis due to pyelonephritis or influenza and is associated with maternal and fetal mortality, perinatal asphyxia, and premature delivery [1, 4]. Preeclampsia and AFE are obstetrical causes that can lead to ARDS [1, 4, 56]. Additionally, if a pregnant patient is using tocolytic therapy with a beta-2 agonist in the setting of preterm labor, steroids for fetal lung maturation, magnesium sulfate, and intravenous hydration can all also contribute to an iatrogenic pulmonary edema [56].

Acute treatment should include airway management with low tidal volume mechanical ventilation and evaluation for infection with prompt initiation of broad-spectrum antimicrobial agents [1, 4, 9, 63]. If a pregnant patient presents with unstable hemodynamics and worsening hypoxemia, intubation and mechanical ventilation should be strongly considered [4]. The use of early mechanical intubation can increase the prompt stabilization of the pregnant patient and fetus [4]. However, in pregnant patients, there are challenges with airway management owing to the pregnancy anatomy and physiology [1]. Hypoxemia can occur rapidly due to increased minute ventilation and decreased functional residual capacity [1]. The risk of tracheal intubation failure is eight times more likely relative to the general surgical population due to the changes in physiology described above, including increased airway edema and breast size, and other disease states in pregnancy, such as obesity and preeclampsia [1, 9, 56]. If a pregnant patient is receiving magnesium sulfate due to a hypertensive disorder of pregnancy or for neuroprotection in the setting of prematurity, the minimum effective dose and duration should be used [56]. If diuresis is needed due to fluid overload, diuretics can be considered, again selecting for the lowest dose to achieve adequate urine output and close attention paid to maintain adequate uterine perfusion [56].

Ventilator management for ARDS in pregnancy includes the general principles of a low tidal volume of 6 mL/kg to prevent overdistention of alveoli and plateau pressures <30 cm H_2O to decrease barotrauma risk [4]. Additional considerations are the presence of pharyngeal, laryngeal, and vocal cord enema in pregnancy that can make intubation more difficult [4]. Delayed gastric emptying occurs in pregnancy which can increase the risk of aspiration during endotracheal intubation, as well as during seizures and altered mental status [1, 2]. Avoiding significant acidemia will be important from a fetal standpoint since acidemia will impair fetal carbon dioxide transfer and oxygen extraction [4]. While a mild increase in maternal Pa_{CO_2} can be tolerated, significant hypercapnia and resulting respiratory acidosis should be avoided [4]. If acidosis results, caution should be employed with the use of intravenous sodium bicarbonate because exogenous sodium bicarbonate will increase serum carbon dioxide which can rapidly cross the placenta and cause an acidosis in the fetus [4]. Significant alkalosis should also be avoided to prevent decreased placental blood flow and subsequent impairment of fetal Pa_{O_2} [4]. Hypoxemia should be corrected to $Fi_{O_2} < 0.6$, and a goal $Pa_{O_2} > 90$ mmHg should be achieved to prevent fetal distress [4]. To help decrease oxygen consumption and avoid intrathoracic pressure effects with mechanical ventilation, the use of neuromuscular blockers or paralytics can be considered [4]. Cisatracurium, pancuronium, vecuronium, and atracurium, all nondepolarizing neuromuscular blockers, can be used in pregnancy and show no significant adverse fetal effects [4]. Cisatracurium does not depend on hepatic or renal function so it may be a preferred neuromuscular blocker in pregnancy [4]. From a sedation standpoint during mechanical intubation, morphine and fentanyl are acceptable agents to use in pregnancy [4]. The use of benzodiazepines during pregnancy should be avoided during the first trimester due to the theoretical risk of cleft palate and other birth defects; however, in later trimesters, use can be considered at the lowest dose and shortest duration [4]. Fetal monitoring should occur for all pregnant patients who are critically ill on mechanical ventilation. Extracorporeal membrane oxygenation (ECMO) can be considered during pregnancy for life-threatening refractory hypoxemia [4].

38.11   Conclusion

Medication management of critically ill obstetric patients requires a multidisciplinary approach with the intensivist, maternal-fetal medicine obstetrician, and pharmacist. Medications should not be withheld if they are needed for maternal hemodynamic stability or are maternal life-saving measures [1]. The same applies for the use of diagnostic imaging [1]. However, when selecting treatment or a medication, care should be given to the least teratogenic medication, especially if a pregnant patient is in the first trimester of pregnancy, and attempt to select for medications that do not significantly affect placental blood flow [1]. Fetal heart rate monitoring with a tocometer is necessary given critical maternal status and high likelihood of the administration of medications that may affect fetal cardiac function. Additionally, having an understanding of the physiological changes in pregnancy and how those changes can affect the presentation of a critically ill obstetric patient as well as the pharmacokinetic and pharmacodynamic properties of medications will be important to optimize maternal and fetal outcomes.

References

1. ACOG practice bulletin no. 211: critical care in pregnancy. Obstet Gynecol. 2019;133(5):e303–e319. https://doi.org/10.1097/AOG.0000000000003241.
2. Guntupalli KK, Hall N, Karnad DR, Bandi V, Belfort M. Critical illness in pregnancy. Chest. 2015;148(4):1093–104. https://doi.org/10.1378/chest.14-1998.
3. Griffin KM, Oxford-Horrey C, Bourjeily G. Obstetric disorders and critical illness. Clin Chest Med. 2022;43(3):471–88. https://doi.org/10.1016/j.ccm.2022.04.008.
4. Patterson K, O'Connor M, Hall J, Strek M. Chapter 127: critical illness in pregnancy. 4th ed. McGraw-Hill; 2014.

5. Khedagi AM, Bello NA. Hypertensive disorders of pregnancy. Cardiol Clin. 2021;39(1):77–90. https://doi.org/10.1016/j.ccl.2020.09.005.

6. Dulu A, Ragsdale E, Dena G. Critical care issues in pregnancy. In: Critical Care. McGraw-Hill Education.

7. Yeomans ER, Gilstrap LC. Physiologic changes in pregnancy and their impact on critical care. Crit Care Med. 2005;33(Supplement):S256–8. https://doi.org/10.1097/01. CCM.0000183540.69405.90.

8. Varon J. Critical care of the pregnant patient. In: Handbook of critical and intensive care medicine. Springer International Publishing; 2021. pp. 429–460. https://doi. org/10.1007/978-3-030-68270-5_12.

9. Zouein E, Bourjeily G. Management principles of the critically ill obstetric patient. In: Medical management of the pregnant patient. New York: Springer; 2015. p. 21–31. https://doi. org/10.1007/978-1-4614-1244-1_2.

10. Bridwell R, Carius B, Long B, Oliver J, Schmitz G. Sepsis in pregnancy: recognition and resuscitation. West J Emerg Med. 2019;20(5):822–32. https://doi.org/10.5811/westjem.2019.6.43369.

11. ACOG practice bulletin no. 196: thromboembolism in pregnancy. Obstet Gynecol. 2018;132(1):e1-e17. https://doi.org/10.1097/AOG.0000000000002706.

12. Ward RM, Varner MW. Principles of pharmacokinetics in the pregnant woman and fetus. Clin Perinatol. 2019;46(2):383–98. https://doi.org/10.1016/j.clp.2019.02.014.

13. Feghali M, Venkataramanan R, Caritis S. Pharmacokinetics of drugs in pregnancy. Semin Perinatol. 2015;39(7):512–9. https://doi.org/10.1053/j.semperi.2015.08.003.

14. Pinheiro EA, Stika CS. Drugs in pregnancy: pharmacologic and physiologic changes that affect clinical care. Semin Perinatol. 2020;44(3):151221. https://doi.org/10.1016/j. semperi.2020.151221.

15. Gestational hypertension and preeclampsia. Obstet Gynecol. 2020;135(6):e237–e260. https:// doi.org/10.1097/AOG.0000000000003891.

16. Banerjee A, Cantellow S. Maternal critical care: part II. BJA Educ. 2021;21(5):164–71. https:// doi.org/10.1016/j.bjae.2020.12.004.

17. Emergent therapy for acute-onset, severe hypertension during pregnancy and the postpartum period. Obstet Gynecol. 2017;129(4):e90–e95. https://doi.org/10.1097/ AOG.0000000000002019.

18. American College of Obstetricians and Gynecologists (ACOG). Severe hypertension in pregnancy bundle. Algorithm: labetalol. https://www.acog.org/-/media/project/acog/acogorg/files/ forms/districts/smi-hypertension-bundle-labetalol-algorithm.pdf.

19. Labetalol injection [prescribing information]. Berkeley Heights: Hikma Pharmaceuticals USA Inc; 2023.

20. American College of Obstetricians and Gynecologists (ACOG). Severe hypertension in pregnancy bundle. Algorithm: hydralazine. 2020. https://www.acog.org/-/media/project/acog/aco-gorg/files/forms/districts/smi-hypertension-bundle-hydralazine-algorithm.pdf.

21. American College of Obstetricians and Gynecologists (ACOG). Severe hypertension in pregnancy bundle. Algorithm: nifedipine. 2020. https://www.acog.org/-/media/project/acog/aco-gorg/files/forms/districts/smi-hypertension-bundle-oral-nifedipine-algorithm.pdf.

22. Practice bulletin no. 183: postpartum hemorrhage. Obstet Gynecol. 2017;130(4):e168–e186. https://doi.org/10.1097/AOG.0000000000002351.

23. Pitocin (oxytocin) [prescribing information]. Chestnut Ridge: Par Pharmaceutical; 2021.

24. Vallera C, Choi LO, Cha CM, Hong RW. Uterotonic medications. Anesthesiol Clin. 2017;35(2):207–19. https://doi.org/10.1016/j.anclin.2017.01.007.

25. Guidelines for active management of the third stage of labor using oxytocin: AWHONN practice brief number 12. J Obstet Gynecol Neonatal Nurs. 2021;50(4):499–502. https://doi. org/10.1016/j.jogn.2021.04.006.

26. Methylergonovine maleate [prescribing information]. Berlin: Breckenridge Pharmaceutical; 2019.

27. Krugh M, Maani CV. Misoprostol. StatPearls [Internet]. Treasure Island: StatPearls Publishing; 2023.

28. Cytotec (misoprostol) [prescribing information]. New York: Pfizer; 2021.
29. Tranexamic acid in sodium chloride injection [prescribing information]. Exela Pharma Sciences LLC; 2020.
30. Shakur H, Roberts I, Fawole B, et al. Effect of early tranexamic acid administration on mortality, hysterectomy, and other morbidities in women with post-partum haemorrhage (WOMAN): an international, randomised, double-blind, placebo-controlled trial. Lancet. 2017;389(10084):2105–16. https://doi.org/10.1016/S0140-6736(17)30638-4.
31. Hemabate (carboprost tromethamine injection) [prescribing information]. New York: Pfizer; 2022.
32. Kujovich JL. Hormones and pregnancy: thromboembolic risks for women. Br J Haematol. 2004;126(4):443–54. https://doi.org/10.1111/j.1365-2141.2004.05041.x.
33. Greer O, Shah NM, Johnson MR. Maternal sepsis update: current management and controversies. Obstet Gynaecol. 2020;22(1):45–55. https://doi.org/10.1111/tog.12623.
34. Vaught AJ. Maternal sepsis. Semin Perinatol. 2018;42(1):9–12. https://doi.org/10.1053/j.semperi.2017.11.003.
35. Mhyre JM, D'Oria R, Hameed AB, et al. The maternal early warning criteria. Obstet Gynecol. 2014;124(4):782–6. https://doi.org/10.1097/AOG.0000000000000480.
36. Rhodes A, Evans LE, Alhazzani W, et al. Surviving sepsis campaign: international guidelines for management of sepsis and septic shock: 2016. Intensive Care Med. 2017;43(3):304–77. https://doi.org/10.1007/s00134-017-4683-6.
37. Smith NT, Corbascio AN. The use and misuse of pressor agents. Anesthesiology. 1970;33(1):58–101. https://doi.org/10.1097/00000542-197007000-00019.
38. Dobutamine injection [prescribing information]. Hospira Inc; 2020.
39. Heinonen O, Slone D, Shapiro S. Birth defects and drugs in pregnancy. Publishing Sciences Group; 1977.
40. Stevens AD, Lumbers ER. Effects of intravenous infusions of noradrenaline into the pregnant ewe on uterine blood flow, fetal renal function, and lung liquid flow. Can J Physiol Pharmacol. 1995;73(2):202–8. https://doi.org/10.1139/y95-029.
41. Dyer RA, Emmanuel A, Adams SC, et al. A randomised comparison of bolus phenylephrine and ephedrine for the management of spinal hypotension in patients with severe preeclampsia and fetal compromise. Int J Obstet Anesth. 2018;33:23–31. https://doi.org/10.1016/j.ijoa.2017.08.001.
42. Lee A, Ngan Kee WD, Gin T. A quantitative, systematic review of randomized controlled trials of ephedrine versus phenylephrine for the management of hypotension during spinal anesthesia for cesarean delivery. Anesth Analg. 2002;94(4):920–6. https://doi.org/10.1097/00000539-200204000-00028.
43. Vasostrict (vasopressin) [prescribing information]. Chestnut Ridge: Par Pharmaceutical; 2022.
44. Oravec D, Lichardus B. Management of diabetes insipidus in pregnancy. BMJ. 1972;4(5832):114–5. https://doi.org/10.1136/bmj.4.5832.114-c.
45. Robinson KW, Hawker RW, Robertson PA. Antidiuretic hormone (ADH) in the human female. J Clin Endocrinol Metab. 1957;17(2):320–2. https://doi.org/10.1210/jcem-17-2-320.
46. Morgan J, Roberts S. Maternal sepsis. Obstet Gynecol Clin North Am. 2013;40(1):69–87. https://doi.org/10.1016/j.ogc.2012.11.007.
47. Nag DS. Vasopressors in obstetric anesthesia: a current perspective. World J Clin Cases. 2015;3(1):58. https://doi.org/10.12998/wjcc.v3.i1.58.
48. Habak PJ, Griggs JRP. Urinary tract infection in pregnancy. StatPearls [Internet]. 2022. https://www.ncbi.nlm.nih.gov/books/NBK537047/. Accessed 3 Apr 2023.
49. Gazmararian J. Hospitalizations during pregnancy among managed care enrollees. Obstet Gynecol. 2002;100(1):94–100. https://doi.org/10.1016/S0029-7844(02)02024-0.
50. Jolley JA, Wing DA. Pyelonephritis in pregnancy. Drugs. 2010;70(13):1643–55. https://doi.org/10.2165/11538050-000000000-00000.

51. Grette K, Cassity S, Holliday N, Rimawi BH. Acute pyelonephritis during pregnancy: a systematic review of the aetiology, timing, and reported adverse perinatal risks during pregnancy. J Obstet Gynaecol. 2020;40(6):739–48. https://doi.org/10.1080/01443615.2019.1647524.

52. Wing DA, Fassett MJ, Getahun D. Acute pyelonephritis in pregnancy: an 18-year retrospective analysis. Am J Obstet Gynecol. 2014;210(3):219.e1–6. https://doi.org/10.1016/j.ajog.2013.10.006.

53. Matok I, Gorodischer R, Koren G, Landau D, Wiznitzer A, Levy A. Exposure to folic acid antagonists during the first trimester of pregnancy and the risk of major malformations. Br J Clin Pharmacol. 2009;68(6):956–62. https://doi.org/10.1111/j.1365-2125.2009.03544.x.

54. Committee opinion no. 712: intrapartum management of intraamniotic infection. Obstet Gynecol. 2017;130(2):e95-e101. https://doi.org/10.1097/AOG.0000000000002236.

55. Pacheco LD, Saade G, Hankins GDV, Clark SL. Amniotic fluid embolism: diagnosis and management. Am J Obstet Gynecol. 2016;215(2):B16–24. https://doi.org/10.1016/j.ajog.2016.03.012.

56. Mighty HE. Acute respiratory failure in pregnancy. Clin Obstet Gynecol. 2010;53(2):360–8. https://doi.org/10.1097/GRF.0b013e3181deb3f1.

57. Otto CM, Nishimura RA, Bonow RO, et al. 2020 ACC/AHA guideline for the management of patients with valvular heart disease: a report of the American College of Cardiology/American Heart Association joint committee on clinical practice guidelines. Circulation. 2021;143(5):e35–71. https://doi.org/10.1161/CIR.0000000000000923.

58. Liu J, Ghaziani TT, Wolf JL. Acute fatty liver disease of pregnancy: updates in pathogenesis, diagnosis, and management. Am J Gastroenterol. 2017;112(6):838–46. https://doi.org/10.1038/ajg.2017.54.

59. Nelson DB, Yost NP, Cunningham FG. Acute fatty liver of pregnancy: clinical outcomes and expected duration of recovery. Am J Obstet Gynecol. 2013;209(5):456.e1–7. https://doi.org/10.1016/j.ajog.2013.07.006.

60. Naoum EE, Leffert LR, Chitilian HV, Gray KJ, Bateman BT. Acute fatty liver of pregnancy. Anesthesiology. 2019;130(3):446–61. https://doi.org/10.1097/ALN.0000000000002597.

61. Ch'ng CL. Prospective study of liver dysfunction in pregnancy in Southwest Wales. Gut. 2002;51(6):876–80. https://doi.org/10.1136/gut.51.6.876.

62. Hegewald MJ, Crapo RO. Respiratory physiology in pregnancy. Clin Chest Med. 2011;32(1):1–13. https://doi.org/10.1016/j.ccm.2010.11.001.

63. Ventilation with lower tidal volumes as compared with traditional tidal volumes for acute lung injury and the acute respiratory distress syndrome. N Engl J Med. 2000;342(18):1301–1308. https://doi.org/10.1056/NEJM200005043421801.

Chapter 39
Critical Care of the Burn Patient

Zachary Drabick

39.1 Introduction

According to the American Burn Association (ABA), over 30,000 burn injuries are treated annually at a burn center in the United States (USA) [1]. An estimated 1 in 10,000 people in the USA required hospitalization for burn injuries in the five-year period of 2018–2022. Most burn injuries occur in people between the ages of 20 and 69 years old, and the majority occur in males (66%). Forty percent of all incidents were caused by flame or flash burns, with over 90% of them being accidental. Just below 10,000 cases in the year 2022 required intensive care unit (ICU) admission. The majority (~56%) of burns in 2022 affected less than 10% of the Total Body Surface Area (TBSA) with large burns (≥20% TBSA) accounting for roughly 6% of burn injuries that year. The overall mortality rate for all burns was 3.3%, which increased to ~25% if inhalation injury was involved.

39.2 Classification of Burns

Burns are classified into categories according to their depth and the underlying structures that are affected (Table 39.1), though many burn wounds are a mixture of different depths [2]. First-degree burns affect only the epidermal skin and are not counted toward a patient's TBSA burns as they will heal on their own with no or minimal outpatient treatment. Partial and deep burns are counted as a patient's TBSA and usually require assessment and treatment by a clinician. Quick estimation of burn sizes can be accomplished by the palmar method or the rule of nines,

Z. Drabick (✉)
Department of Pharmacy, University of Florida Health, Jacksonville, FL, USA
e-mail: zdra0001@shands.ufl.edu

© The Author(s), under exclusive license to Springer Nature Switzerland AG 2025

Y. Alzaidi, M. A. Gebily (eds.), *The Pharmacist's Expanded Role in Critical Care Medicine*, https://doi.org/10.1007/978-3-031-77335-8_39

Table 39.1 Depths and descriptions of burns

	Superficial (First degree)	Partial thickness (Second degree)		Deep/full thickness		
		Superficial	Deep	Third degree	Fourth degree[a]	Fifth degree[a]
Affects	Epidermis (not counted as part of TBSA)	Top layers of dermis	Middle/bottom layers of dermis	All of dermis into subcutaneous fat	Involves fascia and/or muscle	Deep tissue destruction
Appearance	Bright red	Red or pink	Pale	White/gray/yellow, leathery	Complete skin loss	Complete skin loss
Sensation	Painful	Painful	Dull	Insensate	Insensate	Insensate
Medical care	Usually heals on its own or with dressing	Usually heals with dressing and topical antimicrobials	Likely to need STSG	STSG	STSG, flap	Amputation

STSG Split Thickness Skin Graft

[a] Fourth- and fifth-degree burns are grouped with third degree in some classification systems, and are classified separately in others

but detailed calculation of TBSA is usually performed using a Lund and Browder Chart. Burns are also categorized by their mechanism: flash/flame, scald, contact, chemical, and electrical. Knowing the mechanism of how the burn occurred provides valuable context for evaluation and treatment.

39.3 Surgical Treatment

Many partial thickness and most, if not all, deep burns will require inpatient medical treatment [3]. Figure 39.1 outlines a simplified operative course for these patients whose wounds require grafting. Patients with large burns (≥20% TBSA) will usually spend multiple weeks in the hospital, while those with the largest TBSAs (≥40%) will usually spend months or even a year in the inpatient setting with a significant amount of that time as ICU level of care [2]. These patients will also make multiple trips to the operating room for staged grafting, which involves grafting different areas of the body at different times. It's usually not practical to graft all burned areas at one time, especially if both the anterior and posterior sides of the body are affected. If the burn wound does not appear to have the granulation potential to support an autograft, a temporary covering is applied to the wound to provide physical protection and to stimulate regeneration of dermal elements [4, 5]. Allograft is one common temporary covering that is taken from deceased human donors [6]. There are a number of synthetic dressings available on the market that can be used as well depending on the quality and depth of the burn. Most synthetic dressings are

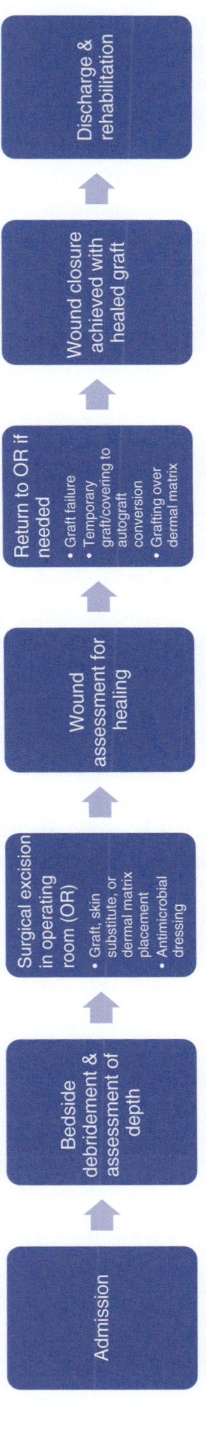

Fig. 39.1 Simplified admission course for burns

impregnated with silver ions that provide antimicrobial activity. As deep third-degree burns destroy the entire dermal layer, some surgeons may opt to place a dermal substitute product on the wound prior to, or even in-lieu of, autografting to provide a substrate for dermal regeneration [4, 5]. If the wounds appear to have the granulation potential for healing, then healthy, unburned skin from the patient's body is harvested, creating a donor site, placed on top of the wound, and covered with a dressing. The dressings are taken down in the post-operative period, usually day 3 or 4, and assessed for engraftment. If successful, then those wounds are considered closed. However, complications such as infection, comorbidities that affect wound healing (especially diabetes), can result in graft failure. Those patients will likely need more rounds of excision, coverings, and dressings before they can fully heal.

39.4 Burn Wound Infection and Topical Antibiotics/ Antiseptics

Burn wounds are initially colonized with gram-positive organisms such as staphylococci in the first 3–5 days after the injury occurs [7, 8]. Gram-negative organisms will become the predominant colonizers around days 5–7 of admission and are the major causes of burn wound infections [7, 8]. Fungal burn wound infections can occur after the first 1–2 weeks of admission and are associated with high mortality rates if invasive [9, 10]. Open burn wounds will require topical antimicrobials or antiseptics to prevent progression of colonization to infection. Intravenous antimicrobials are not required unless the patient displays signs of cellulitis, or of systemic infection, or the infecting pathogen has become invasive. Table 39.2 lists some common topical medications used to prevent or treat burn wound infections [11–24].

Table 39.2 Common topical antiseptics and antimicrobials

	Formulations	Spectrum	Notes
Hypochlorous acid	0.024–0.025%, ≤0.033%	Bactericidal Gram-positive and Gram-negative bacteria, yeasts, molds	Not cytotoxic in commercially available formulations Unclear duration of effects
Sodium hypochlorite	0.5%, 0.25%, 0.125%, 0.0125%	Gram-positive, Gram-negative, yeasts, molds	Concentration-dependent cytotoxicity Short duration of effects (~10 min) requires frequent reapplication
Chlorhexidine	0.05%	Bactericidal Gram-positive and Gram-negative bacteria, yeasts, some viruses	Cytotoxicity limits use on healing wounds
Iodine	Many	Bactericidal Gram-positive and Gram-negative bacteria, fungicidal, tuberculocidal, virucidal, and sporicidal	Irritating, stains, slows healing process
Acetic acid	0.25–5%	Bactericidal Gram-positive and Gram-negative bacteria, yeasts, molds	Concentration-dependent cytotoxicity and irritation
Bacitracin	Cream, ointment	Bacteriostatic Gram-positive and Gram-negative bacteria	Less activity against multidrug-resistant organisms (MDROs)
Mupirocin	Ointment	Bactericidal Primarily staphylococcal species, including MRSA	No cytotoxicity
Mafenide	11.1% cream Powder for 5% solution (discontinued)	Bacteriostatic Gram-positive and Gram-negative bacteria	Powder form discontinued in 2023, cream remains available Effective against some MDROs
Medical honey	Sterile, medical grade forms, food-grade are not sterile	Bactericidal Gram-positive and Gram-negative bacteria	May promote wound healing
Silver nitrate	0.5% solution	Gram-positive and Gram-negative bacteria, some candida species	Silver may slow healing process Stains
Silver sulfadiazine	1% cream	Bactericidal Gram-positive and Gram-negative bacteria, some candida species, herpes viruses	Silver may slow healing process Effective against some MDROs Best for prevention, not treatment of infection

39.5 Resuscitation

Large burns (≥20% TBSA) are at risk of developing shock, multiorgan dysfunction, and increased mortality [25]. One of the most important interventions for patients with large burns is to provide adequate fluid resuscitation. Most, if not all, burn centers will have a protocol for resuscitation, with some being primarily provider-driven, others nurse-directed, and others guided with software programs. Many different formulas have been developed to estimate the amount of fluids a patient with large burns may require in the first 24 h after injury. Two of the most widely used are the Parkland formula (4 mL × weight (kg) × TBSA) and the Modified Brooke Formula (2 mL × weight (kg) × TBSA). The 2023 ABA Guidelines on Burn Shock Resuscitation recommend that clinicians consider using the Modified Brooke Formula to calculate initial fluid infusion rates as it may lead to comparable clinical outcomes and less overall fluid than the Parkland formula [26]. These formulas are primarily used to calculate an initial fluid infusion rate and should not be thought of as fluid goals that are meant to be achieved in the first 24 h of burn injury. This initial fluid rate will usually be titrated hourly to maintain adequate urine output (UO) or hemodynamic stability. Adequate urine output of 0.5 mL/kg/h still remains the most widely used standard to guide resuscitation and titrate fluids, though others such as mean atrial pressure (MAP), trends in hemoglobin (HGB) or lactate, cardiac output (CO), stroke volume variation (SVV), or transpulmonary thermodilution (TPTD) may be used depending on the center [27]. Lactated Ringer's (LR) remains the fluid of choice for resuscitation due to its lower sodium and chloride content than 0.9% sodium chloride solution, as well as the addition of a buffering agent (lactate).

Compartment syndrome remains the most feared complication of burn resuscitation, as abdominal compartment syndrome is associated with high mortality rates. A cumulative fluid volume exceeding 250 mL/kg in the first 24 h of resuscitation has been identified as a major risk factor for developing compartment syndrome and has been termed the Ivy Index [28]. Patients nearing that cumulative volume should have bladder pressure monitoring initiated, and intraabdominal hypertension (>20 mmHg) should prompt interventions to limit further fluid administration. Albumin [29–33], ascorbic acid infusions [34–50], and continuous renal replacement therapy (CRRT) [51–56] have been proposed and used as adjuncts to crystalloid resuscitation to try and decrease the total amount of fluid and reduce the risk of compartment syndrome (Fig. 39.2). The implementation of these adjuncts is highly center- and clinician-specific and will require assistance from the pharmacist clinician to implement well. A randomized-controlled trial is currently enrolling patients to compare the impact of an LR-based resuscitation to an LR + albumin-based resuscitation on total fluid administered (NCT04356859). Using fresh frozen plasma in place of albumin has also been advocated by some clinicians, as it may help regenerate the endothelial glycocalyx [57].

Albumin	Ascorbic Acid IV	CRRT
• Rate based: Convert 1/3 of infusing LR and titrate both to maintain urine output 0.5-1 mL/kg/hr • TBSA based: • 30-49%: 50 mL/hr • 50-69%: 100 mL/hr • ≥70%: 150 mL/hr	• High dose: 66 mg/kg/hr continuous infusion for 24-36 hrs • Low dose: 3.5 g/day	• High volume femofiltration (HVHF): 65-70 mL/kg/hr for first 48-72 hrs after burn injury • Standard volume hemofiltration: 20-35 mL/kg/hr

Fig. 39.2 Selected adjuncts to crystalloid resuscitation

39.6 Inhalation Injury

Another major contributor to burn injury morbidity and mortality is the presence of inhalation injury. True inhalation injury occurs when a patient is exposed to smoke for an extended amount of time in an enclosed space. Inhalation of soot particles and chemicals produced from burning furniture, plastic, wood, and other materials moves past the glottis and into the lower airway to cause direct injury to lung tissue [58]. Thermal injury from heat will affect the area above the glottis and can result in upper airway edema and swelling leading to obstruction. Facial burns, singed nasal hairs, soot in the upper airway, and voice hoarseness are signs that subglottic inhalation injury may be present. Early intubation is indicated if inhalation injury is suspected so that an endotracheal tube can be passed through the airway before swelling occurs. Diagnosis of inhalation injury can be made on the patient's clinical signs and symptoms; however, a fiberoptic bronchoscopy is the preferred method used to visualize the lower airway for signs that subglottic injury has occurred. Subglottic injury is primarily chemical in nature and can result in mucosal hyperemia, bronchospasm, cast and fibrin clot formation, mucosal sloughing and epithelial necrosis, loss of surfactant, free radical damage, and decreased mucociliary clearance [59].

Standard treatment of inhalation injury is largely supportive. Intubation with mechanical ventilation is indicated for clinically significant injury. Bronchial lavages may help by physically removing obstructive material like mucous plugs, clots/casts, and soot from the airways. However, supporting the patient's lungs with mechanical ventilation and giving them time to heal are still needed. Adjunctive treatments have been studied but are not universally accepted (Table 39.3) [60–75]. Nebulized heparin, N-acetylcysteine, and albuterol are the most commonly given adjuncts and are administered sequentially or mixed together to exert a synergistic

Table 39.3 Adjunctive treatments for inhalation injury

Intervention	Regimen	Effects
Nebulized unfractionated heparin (undiluted IV formulation)	5000–10,000 units every 4 h for 5–7 days	Inhibition of airway clot formation, decreased inflammation
Nebulized N-acetylcysteine (20% nebulizer solution)	4 mL every 4 h for 5–7 days	Mucolysis, free radical scavenger
Nebulized albuterol sulfate (0.5% nebulizer solution)	3 mL every 4 h for 5–7 days	Bronchodilation, prevention of bronchospasm from other nebulized agents
Nebulized sodium bicarbonate (IV formulation diluted to 2–5%, or used undiluted at 4.2–8.4%)	3–4 mL every 4 h for 5–7 days	Alternative to N-acetylcysteine, may counteract chlorine gas inhalation
Nebulized racemic epinephrine (2.25% nebulizer solution)	0.5 mL every 4 h for 5–7 days	Reduction of airway blood flow and mucous secretion, increased ventilation

effect. This "inhalation cocktail" may reduce the duration of mechanical ventilation and mortality, though high-quality trials are lacking. Racemic epinephrine has also been studied but is not routinely employed. Other interventions such as surfactant and steroids have not shown a consistent benefit.

Systemic toxicities from significant cyanide and carbon monoxide (CO) exposure can also follow inhalation injury. Both these substances are produced from combustion of materials commonly found in homes, furniture, buildings, and automobiles [58, 59]. Cyanide interrupts mitochondrial oxidative phosphorylation and shifts aerobic respiration to anaerobic metabolism, producing lactate [76]. Carbon monoxide binds iron-bound hemoglobin, producing carboxyhemoglobin and reducing its binding capacity of oxygen (O_2). Lack of O_2 then requires tissues to produce energy via anaerobic metabolism, leading to increased lactate production [76]. Blood carboxyhemoglobin concentrations of >10% are usually required to produce clinically significant toxicity [59, 76].

Unfortunately, detection of cyanide and/or CO toxicity is challenging due to lack of widely and quickly available detection methods and nonspecific clinical symptoms. The blood carboxyhemoglobin concentration can be rapidly obtained via a CO-oximetry device or on an arterial blood gas. Detecting cyanide toxicity is harder. It has been proposed that a very high lactate of >8–10 mg/dL, along with respiratory failure, shock, and/or altered mental status are reasonable clinical criteria [77]. If the blood carboxyhemoglobin concentration exceeds 10%, then it may also be reasonable to suspect significant cyanide exposure and absorption as well [78]. Treatment of CO toxicity consists of administering 100% O_2 until blood carboxyhemoglobin concentrations decrease to <10% or until toxicity symptoms subside. Cyanide toxicity is treated with hydroxocobalamin 5 g IV over 15 min, which may be repeated for continued signs of toxicity like persistently elevated lactate. Hydroxocobalamin is usually well tolerated, producing only red or pink colored urine, though concerns about increased acute kidney injury have been introduced recently [78]. Older treatments such as sodium nitrite, sodium thiosulfate, and methylene blue are now relegated to alternatives in case of unavailability of hydroxocobalamin.

39.7 Infections and Antimicrobial Dosing

Infections are the main cause of mortality amongst burn patients who survive their initial injury and resuscitation. Burn wounds are a major cause of sepsis, with pneumonia, central catheters, and urinary tract infections being significant sources. Patients with large burn injuries ($\geq$20 TBSA) are usually hospitalized for long lengths of time and are therefore exposed to many different hospital-acquired organisms. Consequently, infections with Gram-negative organisms such as *Pseudomonas spp*, *Enterobacter cloacae*, *Acinetobacter spp*, *Stenotrophomonas maltophilia* and *Klebsiella spp* are common. As these patients are exposed to multiple courses of different antimicrobials, resistance tends to develop and multidrug resistant (MDR) and extensively drug resistant (XDR) organisms can proliferate, requiring newer, broader antimicrobials to be used or more aggressive dosing of conventional antimicrobials to account for the elevated minimum inhibitory concentrations (MICs). Invasive fungal and mold infections also put burn patients at high risk of mortality and often require extensive excision or even amputation in addition to antifungal therapy. *Candida*, *Aspergillus*, *Mucorales*, *Fusarium*, and *Trichosporon* species are some examples of fungal organisms that can colonize burn wounds and then invade the surrounding healthy tissue and blood vessels, which can result in systemic exposure and seeding of secondary foci leading to deep-seeded infections like endocarditis and meningitis.

Burn patients also present a unique challenge to the pharmacist clinician given their altered pharmacokinetic profiles. These patients will often have increased total body fluid from resuscitation and high maintenance needs, fluid shifts and third spacing, increased glomerular filtration and hepatic extraction from increased cardiac output, altered plasma protein concentrations, and increased exudate losses from open burn wounds. These often result in many medications having an increased volume of distribution, increased total and renal clearances (augmented renal clearance), changes in the unbound fraction, and shorter half-lives than would be found in comparable patients without burns. Beta-lactam antimicrobials remain the first line and most widely studied treatments for infections in patients with burns. Table 39.4 displays commonly used beta-lactam antimicrobials and their recommended dosing regimens for patients with large burns. Pharmacist clinicians can also utilize therapeutic drug monitoring (TDM) for some of these antimicrobials to optimize the pharmacodynamic parameters associated with clinical efficacy and possibly reduction of resistance [79–83].

Burn-unit specific antibiograms can be useful in identifying first-line empiric antibiotics and trends in resistance but have limitations. CLSI guidelines recommend that only the first isolate be used, and only species with $\geq$30 isolates should be included in a routine antibiogram [84]. However, large burn patients are

Table 39.4 Beta-lactam dosing in patients with large burn injury

	Suggested regimens for augmented renal clearance (ARC)	High MIC regimens
Ceftazidime	2 g every 6–8 h 1 g every 4 h	2 g every 4 h 2 g loading dose followed by 6 g/24 h continuous infusion
Cefepime	2 g every 8 h extended infusion over 3–4 h 1 g every 4 h	2 g loading dose followed by 6–8 g/24 h continuous infusion
Piperacillin-tazobactam	4.5 g every 6–8 h extended infusion over 3 h	4.5 g loading dose followed by 18-24 g/24 h continuous infusion
Imipenem-cilastatin	500 mg every 6 h	1000 mg every 6 h
Meropenem	2 g every 8 h extended infusion over 3–4 h	2 g loading dose followed by 6–9 g/24 h continuous infusion
Aztreonam	2 g every 8 h	2 g every 6 h 2 g loading dose followed by 6–8 g/24 h continuous infusion
Ceftolozane-tazobactam	3 g every 8 h extended infusion over 3 h	Unknown, can consider 3 g loading dose followed by 9 g/24 h continuous infusion
Ceftazidime-avibactam	2.5 g every 8 h extended infusion over 2 h	Unknown, can consider 2.5 g loading dose followed by 7.5 g/24 h continuous infusion
Meropenem-vaborbactam	4 g every 8 h extended infusion over 3 h	Unknown, can consider 4 g loading dose followed by 12 g/24 h continuous infusion
Imipenem-cilastatin-relebactam	1.25 g every 6 h	Unknown, continuous infusion may not be practicable due to short stability at room temperature (2 h)
Cefiderocol	2 g every 6 h extended infusion over 3 h	Unknown, can consider 2 g loading dose followed by 8 g/24 h continuous infusion

frequently admitted for multiple months, are exposed to multiple courses of antimicrobials, and are frequently colonized and/or develop infections with organisms harboring resistance. Additionally, many burn units are small, limiting the number of isolates that are collected in a year's timeframe. It may be advantageous for the pharmacist clinician to develop multiple antibiograms at different time points, e.g., at monthly intervals, at 1, 3, and/or 6 month intervals, or after the first and/or second courses of antimicrobials to capture resistance patterns later in the patients' stay [85]. Combining antibiograms from two or more years may also be required so that an adequate number of isolates can be analyzed and reported. Another unique idea that has been proposed would be to develop a topical antibiogram that would display susceptibilities for the common topical medications that are used against isolates cultured from burn wound areas [86]. Clinicians could then choose the topical medication with highest activity against colonizing or infecting organism.

39.8   Hypermetabolism

Another major component of caring for patients with large burns is mitigating the hypermetabolism that develops soon after injury. Hypermetabolism is a complex process and is characterized in part by increased basal body temperature, CO_2 production, O_2 consumption, glucose consumption and resistance, proteolysis, and lipolysis [87]. These processes are mediated through hormonal changes and increased catecholamine release during the stressed state. The result is loss of lean body/muscle mass, decreased bone mineral density, and poor wound healing leading to poor outcomes [88]. The hypermetabolic response has been documented to persist for 1–2 years postburn injury [89] and its magnitude increases with burn size [90].

Management of hypermetabolism can be grouped into non-pharmacological and pharmacological modalities [88]. Non-pharmacological treatments include environmental management, early wound excision and closure, and early nutrition. Environmental strategies include raising the ambient room temperature in both the patient's room and the operating room and using occlusive dressings to prevent bodily heat loss [91]. Early wound excision and closure can decrease muscle protein catabolism and remove devitalized tissue that provides a substrate for microbial infection, thus decreasing risk of early sepsis [91, 92]. Providing early, high carbohydrate and high protein nutrition, particularly through the enteral route, contributes to increased preservation of muscle mass [91]. Overall calories can be estimated by applying a stress factor to the Harris-Benedict eq. (1.4–1.6 × basal energy expenditure (BEE)), or via another equation such as the Toronto formula. Ideally, indirect calorimetry would be used to measure the resting energy expenditure (REE) instead of estimating it via an equation; however, this is often not available. Delivering protein doses of 1.5–2 g/kg/day in adults and up to 3 g/kg/day in children has been suggested. Protein intakes above 2–2.5 g/kg/day may increase urea production without a corresponding increase in muscle protein synthesis. Limiting calories from fat to no more than 15% of overall calories may be helpful as carbohydrates are the preferred energy source in large burns and excess free fatty acids can accumulate in the liver [93].

Two of the more extensively studied pharmacological treatments for hypermetabolism include beta-antagonists and anabolic steroids. Since catecholamines are a major driver of burn hypermetabolism, beta-antagonists, propranolol in particular, have been studied in mitigating this response. Propranolol has been studied in both children and adults and has been shown to decrease resting heart rate, lipolysis, and muscle protein catabolism [94–99]. Propranolol was chosen due to its non-specificity and ability to inhibit β_2-related metabolic processes; however, it is currently unknown if a β_1-specific antagonist would produce the same reduction in metabolic rate or proteolysis [100]. Anabolic steroids are another class of medications widely studied and used to counteract the loss of lean body mass after a large burn injury. Prior to its removal from the market in 2023, oxandrolone was the medication of choice for burn patients as it showed more specificity for anabolic receptors and less activity at androgenic receptors than testosterone [101–110]. However, it was removed by the Food and Drug Administration (FDA) due to concerns of hepatoxicity, which was rarely identified in burn patients [111–113]. While testosterone and its oral analogue, methyltestosterone remain available in the USA, most of the other Schedule III anabolic steroids have been removed from the market. Evidence using testosterone in patients with large burn injury is extremely limited [110, 114].

Other medications that have been studied to combat hypermetabolism, but are less widely used include metformin, insulin infusions, and recombinant human growth hormone (rhGH). Metformin is a biguanide that increases muscle uptake of glucose and decreases hepatic glucose production and glucose absorption from the GI tract. It has been studied in adult burn patients as an anti-catabolic and anti-inflammatory agent with beneficial effects seen in small trials [115–122]. Insulin acts as an anabolic agent, especially when titrated to a tight blood glucose range or given as high dose infusions, as, similar to metformin, it provides glucose to muscle cells, thereby enabling increased protein synthesis [123–133]. Lastly, rhGH has been studied in pediatric patients with large burns with increased weight, height, lean body mass, and bone density [114, 134]. The dosing and monitoring for these agents are summarized in Table 39.5.

Table 39.5 Commonly used anti-catabolic medications

Agent	Dosing	Monitoring parameters
Propranolol	0.2 mg/kg/dose PO q6–8h titrated up daily to reduce baseline HR by ~20%	Heart rate, blood pressure
Oxandrolone	10 mg PO twice daily	Weekly transaminases and bilirubin
Testosterone	Ideal dosing unknown, 200 mcg IM every week used in one small trial	Weekly transaminases and bilirubin, hirsutism
Metformin	500 mg PO every 8 h for patients receiving enteral feeding, increase to 850 mg PO every 8 h if tolerating 500 mg PO twice daily with meals for patients on a regular diet, increase to 1000 mg PO twice daily with meals if tolerating	GI discomfort, nausea, diarrhea, lactic acidosis, renal function (eGFR < 30 mL/min)
Insulin infusion	Intensive: insulin infusion titrated to blood glucose (BG) 80–110 mg/dL or 90–120 mg/dL or 100–140 mg/dL Conventional: insulin infusion titrated to BG: 120–180 mg/dL or 140–180 mg/dL High dose insulin infusion: 7.5 mUnits/kg/min to target plasma insulin concentration of ~900 mcgU/mL Submaximal insulin infusion: 2.6 mU/kg/min	Hypoglycemia
Recombinant human growth hormone (rhGH)	Pediatrics only 0.1–0.2 mg/kg SC/IM daily	Hyperglycemia (insulin resistance), injection site reactions

39.9 Pain and Analgesics

Pain from burn injury is considered to be one of the most intense among all injuries. Treatment of burn injury in the form of operations, creation of donor sites, dressing changes, debridements, and physical and occupational therapy also contribute to pain beyond that of the initial burn wound [135, 136]. Burn pain is multifactorial and complex, with nociceptive, neuropathic, and psychogenic aspects. Burn pain is also different depending on what phase of care the patient is in; though most patients will have background, breakthrough, procedural, and anticipatory pain. Opioids remain the most widely used and most effective medications for treating burn pain. Adjunctive medications and methods such as dexmedetomidine [137], ketamine [137–141], gabapentin [142–147], pregabalin [145, 148–151], acetaminophen, non-steroidal anti-inflammatory drugs (NSAIDs) [152–157], duloxetine [158], lidocaine [159–162], regional anesthesia, hypnosis, distraction/virtual reality, music, relaxation, and massage have also been studied and are used clinically Table 39.6 includes common dosing for adjuncts when used to treat burn pain.

Table 39.6 Analgesia adjuncts for burn pain

Agent	Dosing	Monitoring parameters
Acetaminophen	650–1000 mg PO every 4–6 h	Transaminases
Ketorolac	15–30 mg IV every 6 h for a maximum of 5 days	Renal function, bleeding
Ibuprofen	400–800 mg PO/IV every 6–8 h	Renal function, bleeding
Gabapentin	100–300 mg PO three times daily, titrated daily up to 1200 mg PO three times daily or 900 mg PO four times daily for neuropathic/adjunct pain relief	Renal function, over sedation
Pregabalin	50–75 mg PO twice daily, titrated up to 300 mg PO every 8–12 h for neuropathic/adjunct pain relief	Renal function, sedation
Duloxetine	60 mg PO daily	Nausea, insomnia, serotonin syndrome
Ketamine	Procedures: 0.5 mg/kg IV push or 0.3–0.9 mg/kg/h continuous infusion Post-operative: 0.1–0.5 mg/kg/h continuous infusion	Over sedation, blood pressure, heart rate, secretions, hallucinations, dysphoria
Dexmedetomidine	Post-operative or procedures: 0.2–1.5 mcg/kg/min IV continuous infusion	Bradycardia, hypotension
Lidocaine	Post-operative: 4 mg/min IV infusion for 4 h, then 3 mg/min IV continuous infusion	Renal function, numbness, tingling, tinnitus, metallic taste, muscle twitching, seizures, arrhythmias

39.10 Micronutrients

Not only is nutrition important for burn patients to support optimal healing, but also repletion of vitamins and trace elements may also produce benefits such as reduction of skin protein catabolism, reduction in pneumonia, improvement in wound healing, and a shorter hospital stay [163–171]. Zinc, selenium, and copper have been the most studied of the trace elements, as each is involved in vital cellular processes involved in immunity, healing, and recovery. Copper contributes to collagen synthesis, dopamine synthesis, and immunity. Zinc is a cofactor for multiple enzymes involved in metabolic pathways, protein synthesis, gene replication, and antioxidant defenses. Selenium is essential for the antioxidant activity of glutathione peroxidases and NFkB expression. Large burn injury has been found to result in losses of these and other micronutrients through open burn wound exudative losses and increased losses in urine [172–178]. Unfortunately, most common laboratory methods of assessing for deficiency (usually via serum concentrations) may not actually reflect overall deficiency as their serum concentrations are altered in the presence of inflammation [179, 180]. Thus it may be prudent to replicate the doses used in small trials, as they seem to be well tolerated. Figure 39.3 displays the micronutrients and doses studied in large burn injury.

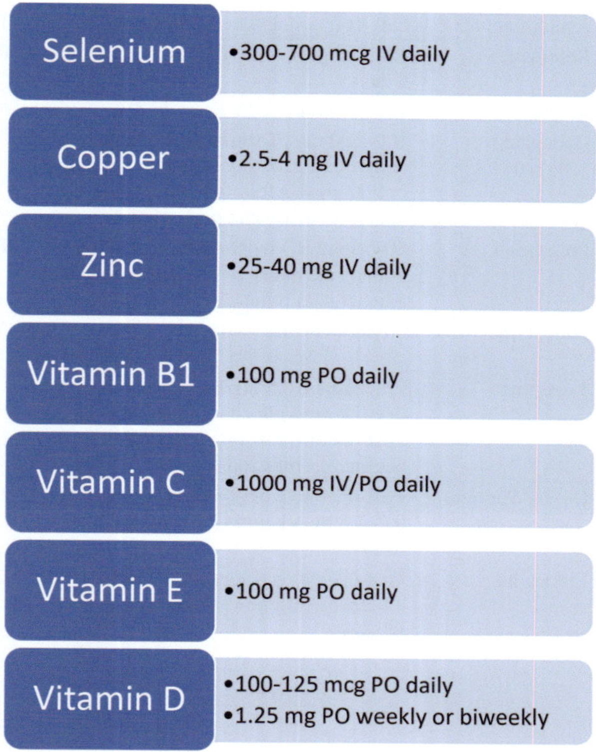

Fig. 39.3 Vitamin and trace element dosing in large burn injury

39.11 Venous Thromboembolism Prophylaxis

Finally, another area where the pharmacist clinician can contribute is in the area of VTE prophylaxis [181–188]. While some burn centers use heparin for prophylaxis, many have shifted to using a low molecular weight heparin, mainly enoxaparin, as many in the trauma community have done [189]. It has been recognized in both the trauma and burn populations that standard enoxaparin doses of 40 mg SC daily or 30 mg SC twice daily are likely not enough to achieve prophylactic concentrations [190]. Hypermetabolism, augmented renal clearance, altered skin blood flow, and obesity are likely contributing factors. Even changing practice to 40 mg SC twice daily may not achieve prophylactic concentrations in some patients [191–195]. Some centers have implemented peak Anti-Xa monitoring with dose adjustments to target a prophylactic range of 0.1–0.3 units/mL or 0.2–0.4 units/mL, depending on their lab's calibration [196, 197]. One center did a regression analysis and developed a formula used to predict empiric doses of enoxaparin that would be required based on a patient's TBSA and total body weight. After implementing a dosing protocol based on that equation, doses up to 80 mg SC twice daily were required to achieve prophylactic concentrations [198]. It is still currently unknown if adjusting enoxaparin to achieve prophylactic peak anti-Xa concentrations results in reductions in VTE rates, and although there is some suggestion from the trauma patient population that this may be the case, there are conflicting results and more studies are needed [195, 199–205].

References

1. American Burn Association. 2023 annual burn injury summary report [Internet]. 2023 [cited 2023 Dec 15]. https://ameriburn.org/wp-content/uploads/2023/11/2023-aba-bisr-overview-v2023113-pdf-standard.pdf.
2. Kagan RJ, Peck MD, Ahrenholz DH, et al. Surgical management of the burn wound and use of skin substitutes. J Burn Care Res. 2013;34(2):e60–79.
3. Sheridan RL, Chang P. Acute burn procedures. Surg Clin North Am. 2014;94(4):755–64.
4. Nyame TT, Chiang HA, Orgill DP. Clinical applications of skin substitutes. Surg Clin North Am. 2014;94(4):839–50.
5. Hill DM, Hickerson WL, Carter JE. A risk-benefit review of currently used dermal substitutes for burn wounds. J Burn Care Res. 2023;44(1):S26–32.
6. Tognetti L, Pianigiani E, Ierardi F, et al. Current insights into skin banking: storage, preservation and clinical importance of skin allografts. J Biorepository Sci Appl Med. 2017;5:41–56.
7. Church D, Elsayed S, Reid O, Winston B, Lindsay R. Burn wound infections. Clin Microbiol Rev. 2006;19(2):403–34.
8. Weinstein RA, Mayhall CG. The epidemiology of burn wound infections: then and now. Clin Infect Dis. 2003;37(4):543–50.
9. Struck MF, Gille J. Fungal infections in burns: a comprehensive review. Ann Burns Fire Disasters. 2013;26(3):147–53.
10. Pruskowski KA, Mitchell TA, Kiley JL, Wellington T, Britton GW, Cancio LC. Diagnosis and management of invasive fungal wound infections in burn patients. Eur Burn J. 2021;2(4):168–83.

11. Neely AN, Gardner J, Durkee P, et al. Are topical antimicrobials effective against bacteria that are highly resistant to systemic antibiotics? J Burn Care Res. 2009;30(1):19–29.
12. Glasser JS, Guymon CH, Mende K, Wolf SE, Hospenthal DR, Murray CK. Activity of topical antimicrobial agents against multidrug-resistant bacteria recovered from burn patients. Burns. 2010;36(8):1172–84.
13. McDonnell G, Russell AD. Antiseptics and disinfectants: activity, action, and resistance. Clin Microbiol Rev. 1999;12(1):147–79.
14. Harriott MM, Bhindi N, Kassis S, et al. Comparative antimicrobial activity of commercial wound care solutions on bacterial and fungal biofilms. Ann Plast Surg. 2019;83(4):404–10.
15. Georgiadis J, Nascimento VB, Donat C, Okereke I, Shoja MM. Dakin's solution: "one of the most important and far-reaching contributions to the armamentarium of the surgeons". Burns. 2019;45(7):1509–17.
16. Barsoumian A, Sanchez CJ, Mende K, et al. In vitro toxicity and activity of Dakin's solution, mafenide acetate, and amphotericin B on filamentous fungi and human cells. J Orthop Trauma. 2013;27(8):428–36.
17. Wang L, Bassiri M, Najafi R, et al. Hypochlorous acid as a potential wound care agent: part I. Stabilized hypochlorous acid: a component of the inorganic armamentarium of innate immunity. J Burns Wounds. 2007;6:e5.
18. Heggers JP, Sazy JA, Stenberg BD, et al. Bactericidal and wound-healing properties of sodium hypochlorite solutions: the 1991 Lindberg award. J Burn Care Rehabil. 1991;12(5):420–4.
19. Sakarya S, Gunay N, Karakulak M, Ozturk B, Ertugrul B. Hypochlorous acid: an ideal wound care agent with powerful microbicidal, antibiofilm, and wound healing potency. Wounds. 2014;26(12):342–50.
20. Boecker D, Zhang Z, Breves R, Herth F, Kramer A, Bulitta C. Antimicrobial efficacy, mode of action and in vivo use of hypochlorous acid (HOCl) for prevention or therapeutic support of infections. GMS Hyg Infect Control. 2023;18:Doc07.
21. Boyce ST, Warden GD, Holder IA. Cytotoxicity testing of topical antimicrobial agents on human keratinocytes and fibroblasts for cultured skin grafts. J Burn Care Rehabil. 1995;16(2):97–103.
22. Agrawal KS, Sarda AV, Shrotriya R, Bachhav M, Puri V, Nataraj G. Acetic acid dressings: finding the holy grail for infected wound management. Indian J Plast Surg. 2017;50(3):273–80.
23. Halstead FD, Rauf M, Moiemen NS, et al. The antibacterial activity of acetic acid against biofilm-producing pathogens of relevance to burns patients. PLoS One. 2015;10(9):e0136190.
24. Hajská M, Dragúňová J, Koller J. Cytotoxicity testing of burn wound dressings: first results. Cell Tissue Bank. 2017;18(2):143–51.
25. Rae L, Fidler P, Gibran N. The physiologic basis of burn shock and the need for aggressive fluid resuscitation. Crit Care Clin. 2016;32(4):491–505.
26. Cartotto R, Johnson LS, Savetamal A, et al. American Burn Association clinical practice guidelines on burn shock resuscitation. J Burn Care Res. 2024;45:565–89.
27. Cancio LC, Bohanon FJ, Kramer GC. Burn resuscitation. In: Herndon DN, editor. Total burn care. Elsevier Inc.; 2018. p. 77–86.
28. Ivy ME, Atweh NA, Palmer J, Possenti PP, Pineau M, D'Aiuto M. Intra-abdominal hypertension and abdominal compartment syndrome in burn patients. J Trauma. 2000;49(3):387–91.
29. Cartotto R, Greenhalgh D. Colloids in acute burn resuscitation. Crit Care Clin. 2016;32(4):507–23.
30. Cartotto R, Callum J. A review of the use of human albumin in burn patients. J Burn Care Res. 2012;33(6):702–17.
31. O'Mara MS, Slater H, Goldfarb IW, Caushaj PF. A prospective, randomized evaluation of intra-abdominal pressures with crystalloid and colloid resuscitation in burn patients. J Trauma. 2005;58(5):1011–8.
32. Navickis RJ, Greenhalgh DG, Wilkes MM. Albumin in burn shock resuscitation: a meta-analysis of controlled clinical studies. J Burn Care Res. 2016;37(3):e268–78.

33. Park SH, Hemmila MR, Wahl WL. Early albumin use improves mortality in difficult to resuscitate burn patients. J Trauma Acute Care Surg. 2012;73(5):1294–7.
34. Buehner M, Pamplin J, Studer L, et al. Oxalate nephropathy after continuous infusion of high-dose vitamin C as an adjunct to burn resuscitation. J Burn Care Res. 2016;37(4):e374–9.
35. Nagel SS, Radu CA, Kremer T, et al. Safety, pharmacodynamics, and efficacy of high- versus low-dose ascorbic acid in severely burned adults. J Burn Care Res. 2020;41(4):871–7.
36. Flores E, Sánchez-Sánchez M, Gutierrez C, et al. High dose ascorbic acid during acute resuscitation in critically burn patients. J Burn Care Res. 2022;43(1):149–55.
37. Kahn SA, Lentz CW. Fictitious hyperglycemia: point-of-care glucose measurement is inaccurate during high-dose vitamin C infusion for burn shock resuscitation. J Burn Care Res. 2015;36(2):e67–71.
38. Kremer T, Harenberg P, Hernekamp F, et al. High-dose vitamin C treatment reduces capillary leakage after burn plasma transfer in rats. J Burn Care Res. 2010;31(3):470–9.
39. Kahn SA, Beers RJ, Lentz CW. Resuscitation after severe burn injury using high-dose ascorbic acid: a retrospective review. J Burn Care Res. 2011;32(1):110–7.
40. Lin J, Falwell S, Greenhalgh D, Palmieri T, Sen S. High-dose ascorbic acid for burn shock resuscitation may not improve outcomes. J Burn Care Res. 2018;39(5):708–12.
41. Tanaka H, Matsuda T, Miyagantani Y, Yukioka T, Matsuda H, Shimazaki S. Reduction of resuscitation fluid volumes in severely burned patients using ascorbic acid administration: a randomized, prospective study. Arch Surg. 2000;135(3):326–31.
42. Nakajima M, Kojiro M, Aso S, et al. Effect of high-dose vitamin C therapy on severe burn patients: a nationwide cohort study. Crit Care. 2019;23(1):407.
43. Tanaka H, Lund T, Wiig H, et al. High dose vitamin C counteracts the negative interstitial fluid hydrostatic pressure and early edema generation in thermally injured rats. Burns. 1999;25(7):569–74.
44. Tanaka H, Matsuda H, Shimazaki S, Hanumadass M, Matsuda T. Reduced resuscitation fluid volume for second-degree burns with delayed initiation of ascorbic acid therapy. Arch Surg. 1997;132(2):158–61.
45. Dubick MA, Williams C, Elgjo GI, Kramer GC. High-dose vitamin C infusion reduces fluid requirements in the resuscitation of burn-injured sheep. Shock. 2005;24(2):139–44.
46. Hollinshead MB, Spillert CR, Lazaro EJ. The beneficial effects of ascorbic acid on murine burns. J Burn Care Rehabil. 1985;6(1):50–4.
47. Matsuda T, Tanaka H, Williams S, Hanumadass M, Abcarian H, Reyes H. Reduced fluid volume requirement for resuscitation of third-degree burns with high-dose vitamin C. J Burn Care Rehabil. 1991;12(6):525–32.
48. Tanaka H, Hanumadass M, Matsuda H, Shimazaki S, Walter RJ, Matsuda T. Hemodynamic effects of delayed initiation of antioxidant therapy (beginning two hours after burn) in extensive third-degree burns. J Burn Care Rehabil. 1995;16(6):610–5.
49. Rizzo JA, Rowan MP, Driscoll IR, Chung KK, Friedman BC. Vitamin C in burn resuscitation. Crit Care Clin. 2016;32(4):539–46.
50. May JM. How does ascorbic acid prevent endothelial dysfunction? Free Radic Biol Med. 2000;28(9):1421–9.
51. Chung KK, Juncos LA, Wolf SE, et al. Continuous renal replacement therapy improves survival in severely burned military casualties with acute kidney injury. J Trauma. 2008;64(2 Suppl):S179–85; discussion S185–7.
52. Chung KK, Coates EC, Hickerson WL, et al. Renal replacement therapy in severe burns: a multicenter observational study. J Burn Care Res. 2018;39(6):1017–21.
53. You B, Zhang YL, Luo GX, et al. Early application of continuous high-volume haemofiltration can reduce sepsis and improve the prognosis of patients with severe burns. Crit Care. 2018;22(1):173.
54. Chung KK, Coates EC, Smith DJ, et al. High-volume hemofiltration in adult burn patients with septic shock and acute kidney injury: a multicenter randomized controlled trial. Crit Care. 2017;21(1):289.

55. Hill DM, Rizzo JA, Aden JK, Hickerson WL, Chung KK. Continuous venovenous hemofiltration is associated with improved survival in burn patients with shock: a subset analysis of a multicenter observational study. Blood Purif. 2021;50(4–5):473–80.

56. Chung KK, Lundy JB, Matson JJ, et al. Continuous venovenous hemofiltration in severely burned patients with acute kidney injury: a cohort study. Crit Care. 2009;13(3):R62.

57. Milford EM, Reade MC. Resuscitation fluid choices to preserve the endothelial glycocalyx. Crit Care. 2019;23(1):77.

58. Sheridan RL. Fire-related inhalation injury. N Engl J Med. 2016;375(5):464–9.

59. Foncerrada G, Culnan DM, Capek KD, et al. Inhalation injury in the burned patient. Ann Plast Surg. 2018;80(3 Suppl 2):S98–105.

60. Miller AC, Elamin EM, Suffredini AF. Inhaled anticoagulation regimens for the treatment of smoke inhalation-associated acute lung injury: a systematic review. Crit Care Med. 2014;42(2):413–9.

61. Ashraf U, Bajantri B, Roa-Gomez G, Venkatram S, Cantin A, Diaz-Fuentes G. Nebulized heparin and N-acetylcysteine for smoke inhalational injury: a case report. Medicine (Baltimore). 2018;97(19):2–5.

62. Kashefi NS, Nathan JI, Dissanaike S. Does a nebulized heparin/N-acetylcysteine protocol improve outcomes in adult smoke inhalation? Plast Reconstr Surg. 2014;134(1):1–6.

63. Foster KN, Holmes JH. Inhalation injury: state of the science 2016. J Burn Care Res. 2017;38(3):137–41.

64. Bartley AC, Edgar DW, Wood FM. Pharmaco-management of inhalation injuries for burn survivors. Drug Des Devel Ther. 2008;2:9.

65. Desai MH, Mlcak R, Richardson J, Nichols R, Herndon DN. Reduction in mortality in pediatric patients with inhalation injury with aerosolized heparin/acetylcystine therapy. J Burn Care Rehabil. 1998;19(3):210–2.

66. Miller AC, Rivero A, Ziad S, Smith DJ, Elamin EM. Influence of nebulized unfractionated heparin and N-acetylcysteine in acute lung injury after smoke inhalation injury. J Burn Care Res [Internet]. 2009;30(2):249–256. http://www.ncbi.nlm.nih.gov/pubmed/19165116.

67. Lange M, Hamahata A, Traber DL, et al. Preclinical evaluation of epinephrine nebulization to reduce airway hyperemia and improve oxygenation after smoke inhalation injury. Crit Care Med. 2011;39(4):718–24.

68. McGinn KA, Weigartz K, Lintner A, Scalese MJ, Kahn SA. Nebulized heparin with N-acetylcysteine and albuterol reduces duration of mechanical ventilation in patients with inhalation injury. J Pharm Pract. 2019;32(2):163–6.

69. Lopez E, Fujiwara O, Lima-Lopez F, et al. Nebulized epinephrine limits pulmonary vascular hyperpermeability to water and protein in ovine with burn and smoke inhalation injury. Crit Care Med. 2016;44(2):e89–96.

70. Foncerrada G, Lima F, Clayton RP, et al. Safety of nebulized epinephrine in smoke inhalation injury. J Burn Care Res. 2017;38(6):396–402.

71. Fukuda S, Lopez E, Ihara K, et al. Superior effects of nebulized epinephrine to nebulized albuterol and phenylephrine in burn and smoke inhalation-induced acute lung injury. Shock. 2020;54(6):774–82.

72. Vajner JE, Lung D. Case files of the University of California San Francisco Medical Toxicology fellowship: acute chlorine gas inhalation and the utility of nebulized sodium bicarbonate. J Med Toxicol. 2013;9(3):259–65.

73. Cox CL, McIntire AM, Bolton KJ, et al. A multicenter evaluation of outcomes following the use of nebulized heparin for inhalation injury (HIHI2 study). J Burn Care Res. 2020;41:1004–8.

74. Miller AC, Rivero A, Ziad S, Smith DJ, Elamin EM. Influence of nebulized unfractionated heparin and N-acetylcysteine in acute lung injury after smoke inhalation injury. J Burn Care Res. 2009;30(2):249–56.

75. McIntire AM, Harris SA, Whitten JA, et al. Outcomes following the use of nebulized heparin for inhalation injury (HIHI study). J Burn Care Res. 2017;38(1):45–52.

76. Dries DJ, Endorf FW. Inhalation injury: epidemiology, pathology, treatment strategies. 2013.
77. Baud FJ, Borron SW, Mégarbane B, et al. Value of lactic acidosis in the assessment of the severity of acute cyanide poisoning. Crit Care Med. 2002;30(9):2044–50.
78. Sheckter CC, Mandell S. Say no to cyanokit. Pause at the 10, 10 threshold. Burns. 2022;48(6):1516–8.
79. Fournier A, Eggimann P, Pagani JL, et al. Impact of the introduction of real-time therapeutic drug monitoring on empirical doses of carbapenems in critically ill burn patients. Burns. 2015;41(5):956–68.
80. Alshaer M, Mazirka P, Burch G, Peloquin C, Drabick Z, Carson J. Experience with implementing a beta-lactam therapeutic drug monitoring service in a Burn Intensive Care Unit: a retrospective chart review. J Burn Care Res. 2023;44(1):121–8.
81. Magréault S, Jauréguy F, Carbonnelle E, Zahar JR. When and how to use MIC in clinical practice? Antibiotics (Basel). 2022;11(12):1748.
82. Machado AS, Oliveira MS, Sanches C, et al. Clinical outcome and antimicrobial therapeutic drug monitoring for the treatment of infections in acute burn patients. Clin Ther. 2017;39(8):1649–1657.e3.
83. Patel BM, Paratz J, See NC, et al. Therapeutic drug monitoring of beta-lactam antibiotics in burns patients—a one-year prospective study. Ther Drug Monit. 2012;34(2):160–4.
84. Simner PJ, Hindler JA, Bhowmick T, et al. What's new in antibiograms? Updating CLSI M39 guidance with current trends. J Clin Microbiol. 2022;60(10):e0221021.
85. Hill DM, Arif F, Sultan-Ali I, Velamuri SR. 515 deficiencies of rule-based technology generated antibiograms and application in patients with prolonged lengths of stay. J Burn Care Res. 2022;43(Supplement_1):S92–3.
86. Robinson AD, Walroth TA, Spera LJ, et al. 52 developing a topical antibiogram in the burn unit. J Burn Care Res. 2020;41(Supplement_1):S34–5.
87. Jeschke MG, Chinkes DL, Finnerty CC, et al. Pathophysiologic response to severe burn injury. Transactions of the Meeting of the American Surgical Association. 2008;126(3):37–51.
88. Porter C, Tompkins RG, Finnerty CC, Sidossis LS, Suman OE, Herndon DN. The metabolic stress response to burn trauma: current understanding and therapies. Lancet. 2016;388(10052):1417–26.
89. Jeschke MG, Gauglitz GG, Kulp GA, et al. Long-term persistance of the pathophysiologic response to severe burn injury. PLoS One. 2011;6(7):e21245.
90. Jeschke MG, Mlcak RP, Finnerty CC, et al. Burn size determines the inflammatory and hypermetabolic response. Crit Care. 2007;11(4):1–11.
91. Herndon DN, Tompkins RG. Support of the metabolic response to burn injury. Lancet. 2004;363(9424):1895–902.
92. Hart DW, Wolf SE, Chinkes DL, et al. Effects of early excision and aggressive enteral feeding on hypermetabolism, catabolism, and sepsis after severe burn. J Trauma. 2003;54(4):755–64.
93. Clark A, Imran J, Madni T, Wolf SE. Nutrition and metabolism in burn patients. Burns Trauma. 2017;5(1):11.
94. Ali A, Herndon DN, Mamachen A, et al. Propranolol attenuates hemorrhage and accelerates wound healing in severely burned adults. Crit Care. 2015;19(1):1–9.
95. Jeschke MG, Norbury WB, Finnerty CC, Branski LK, Herndon DN. Propranolol does not increase inflammation, sepsis, or infectious episodes in severely burned children. J Trauma. 2007;62(3):676–81.
96. Herndon D, Carson J, Fagan SP, et al. 288 propranolol use in adult burn patients: results from a multi-center safety and efficacy trial. J Burn Care Res. 2023;44(Supplement_2):S184.
97. Herndon DN, Hart DW, Wolf SE, Chinkes DL, Wolfe RR. Reversal of catabolism by beta-blockade after severe burns. N Engl J Med. 2001;345(17):1223–9.
98. Flores O, Stockton K, Roberts JA, Muller MJ, Paratz JD. The efficacy and safety of adrenergic blockade after burn injury: a systematic review and meta-analysis. J Trauma Acute Care Surg. 2016;80(1):146–55.

99. Núñez-Villaveirán T, Sánchez M, Millán P, García-de-Lorenzo A. Systematic review of the effect of propanolol on hypermetabolism in burn injuries. Med Intensiva. 2015;39(2):101–13.
100. Herndon DN, Nguyen TT, Wolfe RR, et al. Lipolysis in burned patients is stimulated by the β2-receptor for catecholamines. Arch Surg. 1994;129(12):1301–4; discussion 1304–5.
101. Ahmad A, Herndon DN, Szabo C. Oxandrolone protects against the development of multiorgan failure, modulates the systemic inflammatory response and promotes wound healing during burn injury. Burns. 2019;45(3):671–81.
102. Li H, Guo Y, Yang Z, Roy M, Guo Q. The efficacy and safety of oxandrolone treatment for patients with severe burns: a systematic review and meta-analysis. Burns. 2016;42(4):717–27.
103. Wolf SE, Edelman LS, Kemalyan N, et al. Effects of oxandrolone on outcome measures in the severely burned: a multicenter prospective randomized double-blind trial. J Burn Care Res. 2006;27(2):131–9.
104. Reeves PT, Herndon DN, Tanksley JD, et al. Five-year outcomes after long-term oxandrolone administration in severely burned children: a randomized clinical trial. Shock. 2016;45(4):367–74.
105. Jeschke MG, Finnerty CC, Suman OE, Kulp G, Mlcak RP, Herndon DN. The effect of oxandrolone on the endocrinologic, inflammatory, and hypermetabolic responses during the acute phase postburn. Ann Surg. 2007;246(3):351–60.
106. Pham TN, Klein MB, Gibran NS, et al. Impact of oxandrolone treatment on acute outcomes after severe burn injury. J Burn Care Res. 2008;29(6):902–6.
107. Demling RH, DeSanti L. The rate of restoration of body weight after burn injury, using the anabolic agent oxandrolone, is not age dependent. Burns. 2001;27(1):46–51.
108. Miller JT, Btaiche IF. Oxandrolone treatment in adults with severe thermal injury. Pharmacotherapy. 2009;29(2):213–26.
109. Hart DW, Wolf SE, Ramzy PI, et al. Anabolic effects of oxandrolone after severe burn. Ann Surg. 2001;233(4):556–64.
110. Ferrando AA, Sheffield-Moore M, Wolf SE, Herndon DN, Wolfe RR. Testosterone administration in severe burns ameliorates muscle catabolism. Crit Care Med. 2001;29(10):1936–42.
111. McCullough MC, Namias N, Schulman C, et al. Incidence of hepatic dysfunction is equivalent in burn patients receiving oxandrolone and controls. J Burn Care Res. 2007;28(3):412–20.
112. Kiracofe B, Coffey R, Jones LM, et al. Incidence of oxandrolone induced hepatic transaminitis in patients with burn injury. Burns. 2019;45(4):891–7.
113. Kiracofe B, Zavala S, Gayed RM, et al. Risk factors associated with the development of transaminitis in oxandrolone-treated adult burn patients. J Burn Care Res. 2019;40(4):406–11.
114. Demling RH. Comparison of the anabolic effects and complications of human growth hormone and the testosterone analog, oxandrolone, after severe burn injury. Burns. 1999;25(3):215–21.
115. Riesenman PJ, Braithwaite SS, Cairns BA. Metformin-associated lactic acidosis in a burn patient. J Burn Care Res. 2007;28(2):342–7.
116. Gore DC, Wolf SE, Herndon DN, Wolfe RR. Metformin blunts stress-induced hyperglycemia after thermal injury. J Trauma. 2003;54(3):555–61.
117. Jeschke MG, Abdullahi A, Burnett M, Rehou S, Stanojcic M. Glucose control in severely burned patients using metformin: an interim safety and efficacy analysis of a phase II randomized controlled trial. Ann Surg. 2016;264(3):518–27.
118. Shi L, Jiang Z, Li J, et al. Metformin improves burn wound healing by modulating microenvironmental fibroblasts and macrophages. Cells. 2022;11(24):1–24.
119. Gore DC, Wolf SE, Sanford A, Herndon DN, Wolfe RR. Influence of metformin on glucose intolerance and muscle catabolism following severe burn injury. Ann Surg. 2005;241(2):334–42.
120. Hiyama Y, Marshall AH, Kraft R, et al. Effects of metformin on burn-induced hepatic endoplasmic reticulum stress in male rats. Mol Med. 2013;19(1):1–6.
121. Yousuf Y, Datu A, Barnes B, Amini-Nik S, Jeschke MG. Metformin alleviates muscle wasting post-thermal injury by increasing Pax7-positive muscle progenitor cells. Stem Cell Res Ther. 2020;11(1):1–14.

122. Rivas E, Herndon DN, Porter C, Meyer W, Suman OE. Short-term metformin and exercise training effects on strength, aerobic capacity, glycemic control, and mitochondrial function in children with burn injury. Am J Physiol Endocrinol Metab. 2018;314(3):E232–40.
123. Cree MG, Zwetsloot JJ, Herndon DN, et al. Insulin sensitivity is related to fat oxidation and protein kinase C activity in children with acute burn injury. J Burn Care Res. 2008;29(4):585–94.
124. Gibson BR, Galiatsatos P, Rabiee A, et al. Intensive insulin therapy confers a similar survival benefit in the burn intensive care unit to the surgical intensive care unit. Surgery. 2009;146(5):922–30.
125. Fram RY, Cree MG, Wolfe RR, et al. Intensive insulin therapy improves insulin sensitivity and mitochondrial function in severely burned children. Crit Care Med. 2010;38(6):1475–83.
126. Hemmila MR, Taddonio MA, Arbabi S, Maggio PM, Wahl WL. Intensive insulin therapy is associated with reduced infectious complications in burn patients. Surgery. 2008;144(4):629–37.
127. Jeschke MG, Kulp GA, Kraft R, et al. Intensive insulin therapy in severely burned pediatric patients: a prospective randomized trial. Am J Respir Crit Care Med. 2010;182(3):351–9.
128. Jeschke MG, Boehning DF, Finnerty CC, Herndon DN. Effect of insulin on the inflammatory and acute phase response after burn injury. Crit Care Med. 2007;35(9 Suppl):S519–23.
129. Ballian N, Rabiee A, Andersen DK, Elahi D, Gibson BR. Glucose metabolism in burn patients: the role of insulin and other endocrine hormones. Burns. 2010;36(5):599–605.
130. Gore DC, Herndon DN, Wolfe RR, Cioffi WG, Pruitt B. Comparison of peripheral metabolic effects of insulin and metformin following severe burn injury. J Trauma. 2005;59(2):316–23.
131. Sakurai Y, Aarsland A, Herndon DN, et al. Stimulation of muscle protein synthesis by long-term insulin infusion in severely burned patients. Ann Surg. 1995;222(3):283–97.
132. Ferrando AA, Chinkes DL, Wolf SE, Matin S, Herndon DN, Wolfe RR. A submaximal dose of insulin promotes net skeletal muscle protein synthesis in patients with severe burns. Ann Surg. 1999;229(1):11–8.
133. Mojtahedzadeh M, Jafarieh A, Najafi A, Khajavi MR, Khalili N. Comparison of metformin and insulin in the control of hyperglycaemia in non-diabetic critically ill patients. Endokrynol Pol. 2012;63(3):206–11.
134. Gauglitz GG, Williams FN, Herndon DN, Jeschke MG. Burns: where are we standing with propranolol, oxandrolone, recombinant human growth hormone, and the new incretin analogs? Curr Opin Clin Nutr Metab Care. 2011;14(2):176–81.
135. Romanowski KS, Carson J, Pape K, et al. American Burn Association guidelines on the management of acute pain in the adult burn patient: a review of the literature, a compilation of expert opinion, and next steps. J Burn Care Res. 2020;41(6):1129–51.
136. Moffatt C, Franks PJ, Hollinworth H, et al. Pain at wound dressing changes. Eur Wound Manag Assoc. 2002:1–17.
137. Kundra P, Velayudhan S, Krishnamachari S, Gupta SL. Oral ketamine and dexmedetomidine in adults' burns wound dressing—A randomized double blind cross over study. Burns. 2013;39(6):1150–6.
138. Zor F, Ozturk S, Bilgin F, Isik S, Cosar A. Pain relief during dressing changes of major adult burns: ideal analgesic combination with ketamine. Burns. 2010;36(4):501–5.
139. Lintner AC, Brennan P, Miles MVP, Leonard C, Alexander KM, Kahn SA. Oral administration of injectable ketamine during burn wound dressing changes. J Pharm Pract. 2021;34(3):423–7.
140. Mcguinness SK, Wasiak J, Cleland H, et al. A systematic review of ketamine as an analgesic agent in adult burn injuries. Pain Med. 2011;12(10):1551–8.
141. Brennan PG, Landry JK, Miles MVP, Lintner AC, McGinn KA, Kahn SA. Intravenous ketamine as an adjunct to procedural sedation during burn wound care and dressing changes. J Burn Care Res. 2019;40(2):246–50.
142. Wibbenmeyer L, Eid A, Liao J, et al. Gabapentin is ineffective as an analgesic adjunct in the immediate postburn period. J Burn Care Res. 2014;35(2):136–42.

143. Gray P, Williams B, Cramond T. Successful use of gabapentin in acute pain management following burn injury: a case series. Pain Med. 2008;9(3):371–6.
144. Ahuja RB, Gupta R, Gupta G, Shrivastava P. A comparative analysis of cetirizine, gabapentin and their combination in the relief of post-burn pruritus. Burns. 2011;37(2):203–7.
145. Kaul I, Amin A, Rosenberg M, Rosenberg L, Meyer WJ. Use of gabapentin and pregabalin for pruritus and neuropathic pain associated with major burn injury: a retrospective chart review. Burns. 2018;44(2):414–22.
146. Kneib CJ, Sibbett SH, Carrougher GJ, Muffley LA, Gibran NS, Mandell SP. The effects of early neuropathic pain control with gabapentin on long-term chronic pain and itch in burn patients. J Burn Care Res. 2019;40(4):457–63.
147. Ahnood E, Bradley B, Kesey J, Larumbe E, Griswold J. 61 the use of methadone plus gabapentin as a multimodal pain regimen compared with traditional pain management protocols in burn patients: a retrospective study. J Burn Care Res. 2019;40(Supplement_1):S43.
148. Matsuda KM, Sharma D, Schonfeld AR, Kwatra SG. Gabapentin and pregabalin for the treatment of chronic pruritus. J Am Acad Dermatol. 2016;75(3):619–625.e6.
149. Gray P, Kirby J, Smith MT, et al. Pregabalin in severe burn injury pain: a double-blind, randomised placebo-controlled trial. Pain. 2011;152(6):1279–88.
150. Ahuja RB, Gupta GK. A four arm, double blind, randomized and placebo controlled study of pregabalin in the management of post-burn pruritus. Burns. 2013;39(1):24–9.
151. Jones LM, Uribe AA, Coffey R, et al. Pregabalin in the reduction of pain and opioid consumption after burn injuries: a preliminary, randomized, double-blind, placebo-controlled study. Medicine (Baltimore). 2019;98(18):e15343.
152. Barrow RE, Ramirez RJ, Zhang XJ. Ibuprofen modulates tissue perfusion in partial-thickness burns. Burns. 2000;26(4):341–6.
153. Waymack JP. The effect of ibuprofen on postburn metabolic and immunologic function. J Surg Res. 1989;46(2):172–6.
154. Dong YL, Declan Fleming RY, Yan TZ, Herndon DN, Waymack JP. Effect of ibuprofen on the inflammatory response to surgical wounds. J Trauma. 1993;35(3):340–3.
155. Waymack JP, Jenkins M, Gottschlich M, Alexander JW, Warden GD. Effect of ibuprofen on the postburn hypermetabolic response: a case report. J Burn Care Rehabil. 1990;11(4):340–2.
156. Wallace BH, Caldwell FT, Cone JB. Ibuprofen lowers body temperature and metabolic rate of humans with burn injury. J Trauma. 1992;32(2):154–7.
157. Promes JT, Safcsak K, Pavliv L, Voss B, Rock A. A prospective, multicenter, randomized, double-blind trial of IV ibuprofen for treatment of fever and pain in burn patients. J Burn Care Res. 2011;32(1):79–90.
158. Najafi A, Zeinali Nejad H, Nikvarz N. Evaluation of the analgesic effects of duloxetine in burn patients: an open-label randomized controlled trial. Burns. 2019;45(3):598–609.
159. Wasiak J, Mahar PD, Mcguinness SK, et al. Intravenous lidocaine for the treatment of background or procedural burn pain. Cochrane Database Syst Rev. 2014;2014(10):CD005622.
160. Mattsson U, Cassuto J, Tarnow P, Jönsson A, Jontell M. Intravenous lidocaine infusion in the treatment of experimental human skin burns—Digital colour image analysis of erythema development. Burns. 2000;26(8):710–5.
161. Wasiak J, Spinks A, Costello V, et al. Adjuvant use of intravenous lidocaine for procedural burn pain relief: a randomized double-blind, placebo-controlled, cross-over trial. Burns. 2011;37(6):951–7.
162. Abdelrahman I, Steinvall I, Elmasry M, Sjoberg F. Lidocaine infusion has a 25% opioid-sparing effect on background pain after burns: a prospective, randomised, double-blind, controlled trial. Burns. 2020;46(2):465–71.
163. Berger MM. Antioxidant micronutrients in major trauma and burns: evidence and practice. Nutr Clin Pract. 2006;21(5):438–49.
164. Kurmis R, Greenwood J, Aromataris E. Trace element supplementation following severe burn injury: a systematic review and meta-analysis. J Burn Care Res. 2016;37(3):143–59.

165. Pantet O, Stoecklin P, Charrière M, Voirol P, Vernay A, Berger MM. Trace element repletion following severe burn injury: a dose-finding cohort study. Clin Nutr. 2019;38(1):246–51.
166. Berger MM, Baines M, Raffoul W, et al. Trace element supplementation after major burns modulates antioxidant status and clinical course by way of increased tissue trace element concentrations. Am J Clin Nutr. 2007;85(5):1293–300.
167. Berger MM, Spertini F, Shenkin A, et al. Trace element supplementation modulates pulmonary infection rates after major burns: a double-blind, placebo-controlled trial. Am J Clin Nutr. 1998;68(2):365–71.
168. Berger MM, Binnert C, Chiolero RL, et al. Trace element supplementation after major burns increases burned skin trace element concentrations and modulates local protein metabolism but not whole-body substrate metabolism. Am J Clin Nutr. 2007;85(5):1301–6.
169. Rehou S, Shahrokhi S, Natanson R, Stanojcic M, Jeschke MG. Antioxidant and trace element supplementation reduce the inflammatory response in critically ill burn patients. J Burn Care Res. 2018;39(1):1–9.
170. Sahib AS, Al-Jawad FH, Alkaisy AA. Effect of antioxidants on the incidence of wound infection in burn patients. Ann Burns Fire Disasters. 2010;23(4):199–205.
171. Berger MM, Eggimann P, Heyland DK, et al. Reduction of nosocomial pneumonia after major burns by trace element supplementation: aggregation of two randomised trials. Crit Care. 2006;10(6):R153.
172. Sampson B, Constantinescu MA, Chandarana I, Cussons PD. Severe hypocupraemia in a patient with extensive burn injuries. Ann Clin Biochem. 1996;33(5):462–4.
173. Berger MM, Shenkin A. Trace element requirements in critically ill burned patients. J Trace Elem Med Biol. 2007;21(Suppl. 1):44–8.
174. Stucki P, Perez MH, Cotting J, Shenkin A, Berger MM. Substitution of exudative trace element losses in burned children. Crit Care. 2010;14(1):439.
175. Cunningham JJ, Lydon MK, Emerson R, Harmatz PR. Low ceruloplasmin levels during recovery from major burn injury: influence of open wound size and copper supplementation. Nutrition. 1996;12(2):83–8.
176. Berger MM, Cavadini C, Bart A, et al. Cutaneous copper and zinc losses in burns. Burns. 1992;18(5):373–80.
177. Berger MM, Rothen C, Cavadini C, Chiolero RL. Exudative mineral losses after serious burns: a clue to the alterations of magnesium and phosphate metabolism. Am J Clin Nutr. 1997;65(5):1473–81.
178. Shewmake KB, Talbert GE, Bowser-Wallace BH, Caldwell FT, Cone JB. Alterations in plasma copper, zinc, and ceruloplasmin levels in patients with thermal trauma. J Burn Care Rehabil. 1988;9(1):13–7.
179. Berger MM, Talwar D, Shenkin A. Pitfalls in the interpretation of blood tests used to assess and monitor micronutrient nutrition status. Nutr Clin Pract. 2023;38(1):56–69.
180. Oakes EJC, Lyon TDB, Duncan A, Gray A, Talwar D, O'Reilly DSJ. Acute inflammatory response does not affect erythrocyte concentrations of copper, zinc and selenium. Clin Nutr. 2008;27(1):115–20.
181. Rue LW, Cioffi WG, Rush R, McManus WF, Pruitt BA. Thromboembolic complications in thermally injured patients. World J Surg. 1992;16(6):1151–4.
182. Li Q, Ba T, Wang LF, Chen Q, Li F, Xue Y. Stratification of venous thromboembolism risk in burn patients by Caprini score. Burns. 2019;45(1):140–5.
183. Ahuja RB, Bansal P, Pradhan GS, Subberwal M. An analysis of deep vein thrombosis in burn patients (part 1): comparison of D-dimer and Doppler ultrasound as screening tools. Burns. 2016;42(8):1686–92.
184. Pannucci CJ, Osborne NH, Wahl WL. Acquired inpatient risk factors for venous thromboembolism after thermal injury: reply. J Burn Care Res. 2013;34(4):e273.
185. Van Haren RM, Thorson CM, Valle EJ, et al. Hypercoagulability after burn injury. J Trauma Acute Care Surg. 2013;75(1):37–43.

186. Meizoso J, Ray J, Allen C, et al. Hypercoagulability and venous thromboembolism in burn patients. Semin Thromb Hemost. 2015;41(1):43–8.
187. Harrington DT, Mozingo DW, Cancio L, Bird P, Jordan B, Goodwin CW. Thermally injured patients are at significant risk for thromboembolic complications. J Trauma. 2001;50(3):495–9.
188. Pannucci CJ, Osborne NH, Park HS, Wahl WL. Acquired inpatient risk factors for venous thromboembolism after thermal injury. J Burn Care Res. 2012;33(1):84–8.
189. Bushwitz J, Leclaire A, He J, Mozingo D. Clinically significant venous thromboembolic complications in burn patients receiving unfractionated heparin or enoxaparin as prophylaxis. J Burn Care Res. 2011;32(6):578–82.
190. Cronin BJ, Godat LN, Berndtson AE, et al. Anti-Xa guided enoxaparin dose adjustment improves pharmacologic deep venous thrombosis prophylaxis in burn patients. Burns. 2019;45(4):818–24.
191. Lu P, Harms K-A, Paul E, Bortz H, Lo C, Cleland H. Venous thromboembolism in burns patients: are we underestimating the risk and underdosing our prophylaxis? J Plast Reconstr Aesthet Surg. 2021;74(8):1814–23.
192. Liu A, Minasian RA, Maniago E, Justin Gillenwater T, Garner WL, Yenikomshian HA. Venous thromboembolism chemoprophylaxis in burn patients: a literature review and single-institution experience. J Burn Care Res. 2021;42(1):18–22.
193. Blake M, Roadley-Battin R, Torlinski T. Prophylactic anti-coagulation after severe burn injury in critical care settings. Acta Med Litu. 2019;26(1):38–45.
194. Godat LN, Cronin BJ, Pham A, et al. 30 above and beyond: enoxaparin dose adjustment is required for adequate VTE prophylaxis in burn patients. J Burn Care Res. 2018;39(suppl_1):S20.
195. Malinoski D, Jafari F, Ewing T, et al. Standard prophylactic enoxaparin dosing leads to inadequate anti-Xa levels and increased deep venous thrombosis rates in critically ill trauma and surgical patients. J Trauma. 2010;68(4):874–80.
196. Lin H, Faraklas I, Cochran A, Saffle J. Enoxaparin and antifactor Xa levels in acute burn patients. J Burn Care Res. 2011;32(1):1–5.
197. Lin H, Faraklas I, Saffle J, Cochran A. Enoxaparin dose adjustment is associated with low incidence of venous thromboembolic events in acute burn patients. J Trauma. 2011;71(6):1557–61.
198. Faraklas I, Ghanem M, Brown A, Cochran A. Evaluation of an enoxaparin dosing calculator using burn size and weight. J Burn Care Res. 2013;34(6):621–7.
199. Karcutskie CA, Dharmaraja A, Patel J, et al. Relation of antifactor-Xa peak levels and venous thromboembolism after trauma. J Trauma Acute Care Surg. 2017;83(6):1102–7.
200. Costantini TW, Min E, Box K, et al. Dose adjusting enoxaparin is necessary to achieve adequate venous thromboembolism prophylaxis in trauma patients. J Trauma Acute Care Surg. 2013;74(1):128–35.
201. Karcutskie CA, Dharmaraja A, Patel J, et al. Association of anti–factor Xa–guided dosing of enoxaparin with venous thromboembolism after trauma. JAMA Surg. 2018;153(2):144.
202. Singer GA, Riggi G, Karcutskie CA, et al. Anti-Xa–guided enoxaparin thromboprophylaxis reduces rate of deep venous thromboembolism in high-risk trauma patients. J Trauma Acute Care Surg. 2016;81(6):1101–8.
203. Ko A, Harada MY, Barmparas G, et al. Association between enoxaparin dosage adjusted by anti–factor Xa trough level and clinically evident venous thromboembolism after trauma. JAMA Surg. 2016;151(11):1006.
204. Rostas JW, Brevard SB, Ahmed N, et al. Standard dosing of enoxaparin for venous thromboembolism prophylaxis is not sufficient for most patients within a trauma intensive care unit. Am Surg. 2015;81(9):889–92.
205. Rodier SG, Bukur M, Moore S, et al. Weight-based enoxaparin with anti-factor Xa assay-based dose adjustment for venous thromboembolic event prophylaxis in adult trauma patients results in improved prophylactic range targeting. Eur J Trauma Emerg Surg. 2021;47(1):145–51.

Chapter 40
Management of the Solid Organ Transplant Recipients in the Intensive Care Unit

Sarah Bova, Chelsey Song, and Heather Johnson

40.1 Introduction to Solid Organ Transplant

Transplantation is life-saving for patients with liver, heart, and pulmonary failure and provides increased quantity and quality of life for those living with end-stage kidney disease. In 2023, over 46,000 transplants were performed and there were over 6900 living donors in the United States [1]. Transplant patients are medically complex. Beyond transplantation, these patients often have multiple pre-existing comorbidities with related polypharmacy and are likely to benefit from the critical care pharmacist for both transplant-related and non-transplant-related health care needs. The ICU and emergency medicine pharmacists are likely to encounter transplant patients in all phases of care, from pre-transplant evaluation to post-operative management as well as acute management of patients with a remote history of transplant [2].

Pharmacist involvement is essential when caring for transplant recipients. While transplant evaluations are the bylaws of the Organ Procurement and Transplantation Network published in 2023 indicate that "Each transplant program should identify at least one Clinical Transplant Pharmacist on staff who will provide pharmaceutical expertise to transplant recipients..," the CMS established guidance still does not explicitly specify that a pharmacist be a member of the transplant team, instead indicating that the team include "individuals with appropriate qualifications, training and experience in the relevant areas of medicine, nursing, nutrition, social

S. Bova (✉) · C. Song
University of Maryland Medical Center, Baltimore, MD, USA
e-mail: Sarah.Bova@umm.edu

H. Johnson
University of Pittsburgh Medical Center, Pittsburgh, PA, USA

University of Pittsburgh, Pittsburgh, PA, USA

© The Author(s), under exclusive license to Springer Nature Switzerland AG 2025
Y. Alzaidi, M. A. Gebily (eds.), *The Pharmacist's Expanded Role in Critical Care Medicine*, https://doi.org/10.1007/978-3-031-77335-8_40

services, transplant coordination, and pharmacology" [3, 4]. While most transplant centers will have a transplant pharmacist working closely with the team, critical care pharmacists may also serve this role.

The role of the pharmacist includes transplant evaluation, perioperative care along with the post-transplant phase and ambulatory setting, for both living donors and transplant recipients. While transplant evaluations are often completed in the outpatient setting, in cases of acute organ failure it is conceivable that evaluation for heart, liver, or lung and even small bowel transplant could occur in the ICU. Pharmacist evaluation of transplant candidates includes a thorough medication history and an assessment of a candidate's pharmacologic and nonpharmacologic risks related to transplantation. Targeted assessment should include allergies along with reactions, anticoagulation, drug interactions, hormonal contraception and replacement therapy, vaccination history, as well as chronic pain management and existing immunosuppressive or immune-modulating agents. Nonpharmacologic assessment includes assessment of adherence and medication access as well as health literacy. Documentation of the evaluation will be dependent on center-specific policy developed to meet the CMS Conditions of Participation and UNOS policy. Pharmacists are uniquely qualified to provide systematic assessment and mitigation plans. In the setting of acute illness in the ICU, the pharmacist may need to engage caregivers and family members where appropriate to obtain complete information [5].

In the peri-transplant phase, pharmacists should be able to provide evidence (i.e., documentation) of collaboration as is related to medication-related care plans. The ICU pharmacist is often in a position to collaborate with the transplant pharmacist in this regard and in some instances may even be responsible for documentation per hospital policy. Transplant pharmacists also provide a significant amount of patient and caregiver education prior to discharge. While not generally the norm for most transplant patients, there may be instances in which the ICU pharmacist is in a position to provide and document discharge education. Most importantly, given the need for ICU care for most perioperative transplant patients, critical care pharmacists collaborate with transplant pharmacists to facilitate transitions of care.

40.2 Immunosuppression

Following solid organ transplantation, appropriate immunosuppression is essential to prevent allograft rejection. As the medication expert, critical care pharmacists in any setting should be familiar with the implications of pharmacologic immunosuppression as well as their specific adverse effects. Moreover, close monitoring of these medications is essential in the critically ill patient and the ICU pharmacist is uniquely positioned to do this. Without immunosuppression, the recipient's immune system will recognize antigens on the donor cells as non-self which can lead to immune activation and tissue damage. Although immunologic risk is optimized pre-transplant through ABO matching, reducing the number of mismatched human leukocyte antigens, and testing for pre-existing antibodies, immunosuppression is still needed to prevent rejection. Immunosuppression prevents allograft rejection by inhibiting T-cell activation. The three signals or steps to T-cell activation include recognition of donor antigen, costimulation, and proliferation of T-cells [6]. Recipient T-cells recognize major histocompatibility complex molecules on donor antigen presenting cells. When this recognition is followed by the binding of costimulatory molecules, interleukin-2 and other cytokines are produced and trigger nucleotide synthesis and T-cell proliferation. These T-cells then cause tissue damage to the transplanted organ.

Immunosuppression can be divided into three phases: induction, maintenance, and treatment of rejection. Induction immunosuppression can be used to prevent rejection and to facilitate minimization of maintenance immunosuppression. Induction immunosuppression agents are further divided into lymphocyte depleting agents and non-lymphocyte depleting agents. Rabbit anti-thymocyte globulin is a polyclonal antibody which targets numerous T-cell receptors leading to lysis and cell death and is the most common lymphocyte depleting agent used in solid organ transplant. Dosing varies by center and organ type with most patients receiving 1.5–2 mg/kg on the day of transplant followed by three to five additional doses. Leukopenia and thrombocytopenia are common, and subsequent doses are adjusted based on white blood cell and platelet counts. There is also a risk of infusion reaction and patients should receive corticosteroids, diphenhydramine, and acetaminophen 1 h prior to infusion, and infusion should be given over 4–6 h through a 0.22 μm filter. Alemtuzumab is a lymphocyte depleting monoclonal antibody that targets the CD52 receptor and causes lysis and cell death of both T and B cells. Alemtuzumab is typically given as a single dose of 30 mg intravenous on the day of transplant. Of note, alemtuzumab (Campath) is no longer commercially available and is provided only to transplant centers enrolled in the manufacturer's distribution program. Basiliximab is a non-lymphocyte depleting monoclonal antibody that binds the interleukin-2 receptor preventing T-cell activation. Basiliximab is well tolerated and is given as two 20 mg doses intravenously over 30 min on day of transplant and post-operative day four.

The decision to give induction immunosuppression and choice of induction agent depends largely on the organ being transplanted and the transplant center protocol. In 2021, 91.3% of kidney recipients, 31.1% of liver recipients, 49% of heart recipients, and 82.2% of lung recipients received induction immunosuppression according to the Scientific Registry of Transplant Recipients [7]. It is common for kidney recipients to receive either rabbit anti-thymocyte globulin or alemtuzumab. Basiliximab is typically reserved for kidney recipients at low risk of rejection including elderly patients and those with non-kidney allografts already on maintenance immunosuppression. Data on use of induction for liver, heart, and lung transplant recipients is limited leading to variability in practice. Cost is also an important factor to consider as both rabbit anti-thymocyte globulin and basiliximab are high cost medications.

Maintenance immunosuppression is used to prevent rejection lifelong. Calcineurin inhibitors, including cyclosporine and tacrolimus, are the backbone of maintenance immunosuppression for most transplant recipients. Cyclosporine is available as non-modified cyclosporine (Sandimmune) and modified cyclosporine (Neoral or Gengraf) (Table 40.1). These formulations are not interchangeable, and use of modified cyclosporine is preferred over non-modified due to improved absorption and pharmacokinetics. Tacrolimus is the most common calcineurin inhibitor used today. Tacrolimus is available as immediate release (Prograf) and

Table 40.1 Maintenance immunosuppressants

Drug	Formulations available	Adverse effects	Pearls
Tacrolimus (Prograf)	0.5 mg, 1 mg, and 5 mg capsules Oral suspension Intravenous solution	Nephrotoxicity Neurotoxicity Hyperkalemia Hypomagnesemia Hyperglycemia Hypertension QT prolongation Alopecia	– Intravenous administration avoided due to risk of nephrotoxicity – Oral suspension may be given through enteral feeding tubes
Tacrolimus ER (Envarsus XR)	0.75 mg, 1 mg, and 4 mg tablets		– Do not crush or break tablets
Tacrolimus XL (Astagraf)	0.5 mg, 1 mg, and 5 mg capsules		– Tacrolimus XL ≈ total daily dose of tacrolimus IR – Tacrolimus XR ≈ 0.8 (total daily dose of tacrolimus IR)
Cyclosporine modified (Neoral, Gengraf)	25 mg, 50 mg, and 100 mg capsules Oral solution Intravenous solution	Nephrotoxicity Neurotoxicity Hyperkalemia Hypomagnesemia Hyperglycemia Hypertension Gingival hyperplasia Hirsutism	– Intravenous administration avoided due to risk of nephrotoxicity – Oral solution may be given through enteral feeding tubes
Mycophenolate mofetil (Cellcept)	250 mg capsules 500 mg tablets Oral suspension Intravenous solution	Nausea Vomiting Diarrhea Leukopenia	– REMS program due to teratogenicity – Do not crush or break tablets – 250 mg mycophenolate mofetil = 180 mg mycophenolate sodium
Mycophenolate sodium (Myfortic)	180 mg and 360 mg tablets		
Azathioprine (Imuran)	50 mg, 75 mg, and 100 mg tablets	Leukopenia Thrombocytopenia Hepatotoxicity	– Check thiopurine methyltransferase (TPMT) before initiating
Sirolimus (Rapamune)	0.5 mg, 1 mg, and 2 mg tablets Oral solution	Peripheral edema Hypercholesterolemia Hypertriglyceridemia Impaired wound healing Proteinuria	– Administered every 24 h – Typically HELD around surgical procedures due to impaired wound healing
Everolimus (Zortress)	0.25 mg, 0.5 mg, 0.75 mg, and 1 mg tablets		– Administered every 12 h – Typically HELD around surgical procedures due to impaired wound healing

extended release (Astagraf XL and Envarsus XR). Like cyclosporine, these formulations are not interchangeable. Tacrolimus immediate release is administered every 12 h while both extended release products are administered every 24 h. For patients unable to receive enteral tacrolimus, it is possible to administer the powder from tacrolimus immediate release capsules sublingually. It is important to note that when administering tacrolimus sublingually, it bypasses first-pass metabolism and significant dose reductions are needed when converting from enteral tacrolimus. When switching patients between enteral and sublingual as well as switching between tacrolimus immediate release and extended release formulations, it is recommended to contact the transplant pharmacist for dosing recommendations.

Calcineurin inhibitors have a narrow therapeutic index as well as significant inter- and intra- patient variability requiring therapeutic drug monitoring to ensure safety and efficacy. The goal trough level will vary depending on center protocol, organ transplanted, time since transplant, and individual risk of rejection. Levels for cyclosporine and for tacrolimus immediate release should be drawn 12 h after a dose where levels for tacrolimus extended release should be drawn 24 h after a dose. Pharmacists should pay particular attention to admission levels, which are often uninterpretable as they do not reflect 12- or 24-h troughs. Factors that can increase tacrolimus exposure include diarrhea, hepatic dysfunction, marijuana use, and grapefruit consumption. Factors that can decrease tacrolimus exposure include administration with food and history of gastric bypass. Tacrolimus is metabolized by the liver and excreted in bile with minimal renal excretion, and tacrolimus exposure is not affected by renal dysfunction. Tacrolimus is metabolized by CYP3A4 and has several significant drug–drug interactions. Strong CYP3A4 inhibitors and inducers require tacrolimus dose adjustments when starting or stopping. Strong CYP3A4 inhibitors include erythromycin, azole antifungals, protease inhibitors, and non-dihydropyridine calcium channel blockers. Strong CYP3A4 inducers include rifampin, rifabutin, carbamazepine, phenytoin, and phenobarbital. Non-steroidal anti-inflammatory drugs, angiotensin converting enzyme inhibitors, and angiotensin receptor blockers can decrease renal perfusion when used with calcineurin inhibitors, and this combination is generally avoided especially in the early post-transplant period.

Antimetabolites, including mycophenolate and azathioprine, are often used in combination with calcineurin inhibitors for maintenance immunosuppression. Mycophenolate is available in two formulations: mycophenolate mofetil (Cellcept) and mycophenolate sodium (Myfortic) (Table 40.1). Dose reductions of mycophenolate due to infection, leukopenia, and diarrhea are common. Mycophenolate has been documented to cause significant birth defects and has a REMS program. Women of child bearing potential should be counseled to use two forms of birth control while taking mycophenolate. Azathioprine is safe to use in patients who are pregnant.

Steroids may also be used as part of induction and maintenance immunosuppression depending on center protocol. Patients typically receive methylprednisolone doses of 500–1000 mg on the day of transplant followed by a taper. For steroid withdrawal protocols, patients will typically be tapered off steroids by 1 month post-transplant. Prednisone may be restarted if a patient is unable to tolerate other maintenance immunosuppressants or if there are concerns for rejection. Steroids are also a first line agent for the treatment of acute cellular rejection.

Use of mTOR inhibitors, including sirolimus and everolimus, is generally avoided in the immediate post-transplant period due to impaired wound healing and risk of graft thrombosis. Patients may be transitioned to an mTOR inhibitor later on due to infection, malignancy, or inability to tolerate calcineurin inhibitors or anti-metabolites. Heart transplant recipients may also have mTOR inhibitors added to their maintenance immunosuppression regimens to prevent cardiac allograft vasculopathy. Use of mTOR inhibitors is often limited by adverse effects. Like calcineurin inhibitors, mTOR inhibitors also have a narrow therapeutic index and require therapeutic drug monitoring.

40.3 Pharmacokinetic and Pharmacodynamic Considerations with Transplanted Organs

Critical illness results in changes that can significantly impact drug disposition. Clinicians should be prepared for fluctuations in drug exposure and dosing in the immediate post-transplant settings. In kidney transplant recipients, for example, the presence of delayed graft function presents many challenges in fluid management and prediction of medication clearance, especially in patients who may require intermittent dialysis. A comprehensive evaluation of kidney function (i.e., trend of total urine output, electrolyte clearance, and creatinine clearance evaluations) should be considered in dosing of medications that are renally eliminated. Often times, when possible one-time doses are preferred to assess the true clearance of medications in the setting of renally toxic medications (i.e., vancomycin). Due to the hepatic metabolism of tacrolimus, liver transplant recipients with severe cholestasis may have decreased tacrolimus drug clearance and ultimately supra-therapeutic or toxic trough levels, acute kidney injury, and electrolyte abnormalities.

Site of delivery may also impact absorption of immunosuppressive agents. Changing of delivery site from gastric to duodenal or jejunal may impact absorption as CYP3A expression tends to decrease more distally. Oral bioavailability is also influenced by intestinal motility, with diarrhea increasing tacrolimus exposure as upwards of 50% of intestinal P-glycoprotein is oftentimes sloughed off during diarrhea, causing increased bioavailability and potential toxicity of tacrolimus [8]. Inflammatory cytokines such as TNF-alpha and IL-6 may down-regulate cytochrome P450 enzymes as well as higher-IL-18 and IFN-gamma levels, often seen in liver transplant patients, will exhibit lower dose normalized tacrolimus levels [9].

Fluid management is often challenging post-transplant and may be managed differently depending on the organ transplanted. Kidney transplant recipients often require aggressive fluid repletion in the setting of profound urine output to avoid dehydration, hypotension, and subsequent graft ischemia. The type of fluid replacement is controversial and oftentimes patient or center specific. Colloid repletion such as albumin is attractive for the theoretical increase in intravascular oncotic pressure and volume, improvement in protein administration, as well as various antioxidant and anti-inflammatory properties. However, crystalloid repletion has shown comparative outcomes in terms of overall clinical efficacy among kidney transplant recipients.

Fluid resuscitation among liver transplant is even more challenging. While the same benefits of increase in oncotic pressure and potential decrease in oxidative stress still hold true, the real benefit of albumin repletion is in the management of acute kidney injury in hepato-renal syndrome, spontaneous bacterial peritonitis, and large volume paracentesis. This includes Jackson-Pratt (JP) drain management for the large amount of ascitic fluid that may be lost during the first couple post-operative days.

40.4 Transplant Complications

40.4.1 Graft Rejection

Graft or immune tolerance between the recipient and the donor is the ultimate goal within the field of transplantation. However, until that goal can be medically achieved, allograft rejection can occur at any time post-transplant with the highest incidence early post-operatively around 3–6 months. There are multiple risk factors that may lead to rejection including under immunosuppression, high degree of donor to recipient HLA mismatches, degree of recipient humoral sensitization, delayed graft function, recipient race, systemic infection, cause of organ failure, as well as medication non-adherence [10]. Rejection is often described as T-cell mediated rejection (TCMR) and antibody-mediated rejection (AMR). While each organ has their own respective criteria for severity of rejection as well as treatment management, the overall concepts are similar across all organ types.

T-cell mediated rejection (TCMR), typically a result of under immunosuppression, is secondary to allorecognition either by donor or recipient antigen-presenting cell and leads to tissue inflammation and damage. TCMR is largely steroid responsive with T-cell quiescence occurring rapidly with two to three large pulses of systemic steroids (i.e., methylprednisolone 500–1000 mg/dose) followed by steroid taper to maintenance goal. If the allograft is not responsive after steroid therapy, T-cell depleting agents such as rabbit anti-thymocyte globulin (rATG) can be added on to further salvage the allograft. When T-cell depleting therapies are used, it is prudent to add on opportunistic infection prophylaxis, such as *pneumocystis jirovecii pneumonia* (PJP) and/or cytomegalovirus (CMV) per institutional guidelines.

Antibody-mediated rejection (AMR) is typically a result of human leukocyte antigens (HLA) antibodies produced by the recipient against the donor allograft that can either cause direct cytotoxic endothelial damage or trigger complement activation. The overall treatment approach is to remove the circulating donor specific antibodies (DSA) via procedures such as plasmapheresis and infusion of intravenous immunoglobulin (IVIG) to bind and neutralize the existing DSAs before tissue damage results. Depending on the severity of AMR, patients typically undergo 5–6 sessions of plasmapheresis with a goal IVIG infusion of 1.5–2 g/kg during a treatment course. Unlike TCMR, AMR is more B-cell dependent and treatment success is often variable [11]. It is worth noting that procedures such as plasmapheresis will remove not only large antibody molecules (i.e., IgG and IgM) but also clotting factors and proteins as well. Patients undergoing plasmapheresis should have their anticoagulation plan as well as other high protein, low volume of distribution medications evaluated by a pharmacist to ensure proper medication management. For refractory AMR that is unresponsive to PLEX and IVIG, anti-CD20 monoclonal antibodies such as rituximab and proteasome inhibitors such as bortezomib can be added to prevent additional antibody production [12].

Overall, for the treatment of allograft rejection, either TCMR or AMR, the patient's maintenance immunosuppression such as calcineurin inhibitor and anti-metabolite should also be optimized as the duration of effect of rejection treatments is limited.

Reliable clinical markers for monitoring graft health are critical for the outcome and management of transplanted organs. While having certain laboratory markers such as serum creatinine as an indicator for kidney function, and markers of liver injury are helpful in the acute and long-term evaluation of organ function, they're not perfect. Oftentimes, especially in the concern for organ rejection, clinical markers lag behind actual tissue damage and by the time that clinical markers are increased the tissue damage has already occurred. The gold standard for diagnosing tissue rejection is still tissue biopsy, and some centers will do surveillance biopsies at pre-specified time points post-transplant while other centers will only biopsy the transplanted organ if there is a concern for rejection. However due to limitations of time and risks associated with the procedure, biopsy is not always attainable or feasible. The development of non-invasive biomarker assays such as donor derived cell free DNA (dd-cfDNAa) and gene expression profiling (GEP) are groundbreaking developments in the management of solid organ transplant recipients. When tissue necrosis or damage occurs, either intentional (i.e., procedure) or unintentional (i.e., organ rejection), small amounts of donor DNA are released in the recipient blood stream and are quantifiable utilizing a variety of commercially available assays (Table 40.2). The utility of the dd-cfDNA assays is currently institutionally specific. These assays have a higher negative predictor value for ruling out rejection in kidney, heart, and liver patients with greater sensitivity than positive predictor for ruling in rejection in lieu of biopsy data. Alternatively, GEP is the analysis of molecular expression of specific genes which are associated with heightened immune response in cases such organ rejection or infection. It provides more granular data in allograft function, however often times used in combination with dd-cfDNA to provide the clearest depiction of graft function.

Table 40.2 Non-invasive monitoring for graft rejection [13–16]

	Allosure	Prospera	TruGraf	Vitagraf
Test type	cfDNA	cfDNA	57 gene GEP microarray	cdDNA
NPV	84%	83%	78%	98%
PPV	75%	61%	71%	74%
Sensitivity	59% in indication for biopsy	74% in indication for biopsy	48% in surveillance biopsy	73% in surveillance biopsy

40.4.2   Infectious Complications

Given immunosuppression required to prevent rejection, infections are common after solid organ transplant. A patient's risk of infection is based on epidemiologic exposures and the net state of immunosuppression [17]. Type of infection is often dependent on time post-transplant, with surgical and donor-derived infections being most common in the first month and opportunistic infections emerging later in the first year. Transplant recipients may not present with typical symptoms of infection and may become infected with a wider spectrum of pathogens than immunocompetent patients. For more on infectious complications after solid organ transplant, please refer to the "Infections in Solid Organ Transplant Recipients in the ICU" chapter.

40.4.3   Neurologic Complications

Neurologic complications are common in transplant recipients and often highest in liver and lung transplant recipients. Encephalopathy (altered mental status) may occur in as many as 30–40% of liver, lung, and small bowel recipients. Graft failure may also precipitate encephalopathy whether related to hypoxia with lung transplant, hypotension or prolonged need for bypass after heart transplantation, and both hepatic and uremic encephalopathy. Delayed clearance of anesthetics and neuromuscular blocking agents may occur more frequently with hepatic or renal dysfunction. Pre-operative risks may also impact the risk such as history of hepatic encephalopathy or alcohol or drug use. Post-operative metabolic changes such as hyponatremia, uremia, and hypercalcemia also play a role [18]. Risk factors for the development of delirium in transplant recipients include CNI use, cardiopulmonary bypass, and reduced intraoperative cerebral perfusion [19]. Additionally high doses of corticosteroids used intra-operatively and post-operatively may contribute to delirium and agitation. Lung transplant recipients may develop severe hyperammonemia possibly due to infection with mycoplasma or ureaplasma species. This can lead to development of severe encephalopathy and may be fatal.

Neurotoxicity after transplantation impacts about 5% of patients and has variable presentation including tremors and headache as well as neuropathy, seizures, catatonic stupor, and cortical blindness. It has been proposed that alterations in the blood–brain barrier may impact CNS exposure of CNIs and this may in part explain the presence of neurologic changes even at low CNI systemic concentrations or delay in resolution of neurologic symptoms after the cessation or reduction of CNI exposure [20]. Pharmacists should recognize medications that dramatically increase CNI exposure such as azole antifungals, macrolides, and protease inhibitors and implement preemptive CNI dose reduction to avoid toxicities. Akinetic mutism may also be the result of CNIs and should reverse upon cessation of these agents [18].

Seizures are estimated to occur in 5–10% of transplant recipients, and current prevalence is probably lower than historical estimates due to more judicious dosing of CNIs. Seizures associated with CNI can be either focal or generalized. While the management of seizures in the transplant patient does not differ from the non-transplant patient, there are some important caveats in solid organ transplant. Antiepileptic drugs (AED) such as phenytoin, phenobarbital, and carbamazepine are cytochrome P450 inducers that not only increase the metabolism of CNIs and mTORs, but may also increase the elimination of azole antifungals. Additionally, fluctuating organ function may significantly impact drug disposition and dosing. Moreover, rapid administration of phenytoin may lead to arrhythmias and hypotension. Free phenytoin levels may be elevated in patients with malnutrition and hypo-albuminemia. Of note, phenytoin has been employed to dramatically decrease CNI levels in the setting of CNI toxicity [21]. Due to significant drug interactions with phenytoin and CNIs, levetiracetam and lacosamide are preferred agents. Transplant patients will not generally require prolonged anticonvulsant therapy after initial treatment if the inciting cause is removed.

Posterior reversible encephalopathy syndrome (PRES) may present as a combination of altered mental status, seizure activity, headache, visual abnormalities, as well as nausea/vomiting. In solid organ transplant recipients, calcineurin inhibitors have been most often implicated in the cause of PRES, but mTOR inhibitors and mycophenolate mofetil have also been implicated [22–24]. Other risk factors for the development of PRES include hypomagnesemia, hypocholesterolemia, hypertension, and renal failure. MRI findings for PRES include hyper intense signals on T1- and T2-weighted images, likely related to vasogenic edema. PRES can occur at any time after transplant with a median onset of 17 days post-transplant and can occur even with therapeutic concentrations of CNIs. Treatment includes cessation or minimization of offending agents and blood pressure control as well as supportive care. Resolution of neurologic signs is variable and often lags behind reduction in CNI concentrations. PRES is rare, with an estimated incidence of 0.5–5% of transplant patients, and along with the presence of neurologic symptoms, risk factors, and imaging consistent with PRES, other alternative diagnoses should be excluded before a diagnosis of PRES can be made. Primary CNS insults such as infection, stroke, and osmotic demyelination should be considered as well. Post-transplant lymphoproliferative disorder (PTLD) may also present with seizure or neurologic changes if there is CNS involvement.

40.4.4   Thromboembolic Complications

Transplant recipients have a significantly increased incidence of VTE with the highest incidence in heart and lung recipients [25]. The majority of VTE events occur in the first year after transplant, likely related to thrombophilic states, hospitalizations, surgeries, central catheters, and immunosuppressive medications. In a large study, transplant recipients treated for VTE had an increased risk of non-major, major, and fatal bleeding over non-transplant patients, largely driven by bleeding in liver transplant recipients [25]. Other risk factors for bleeding included older age, anemia, thrombocytopenia, use of corticosteroids, and creatinine clearance <60 mL/min. In this cohort transplant, recipients were less likely to receive DOACs and more likely to receive maintenance low-molecular weight heparins, albeit with lower per kg doses compared to non-transplant patients. Transplant recipients with bleeding complications were more likely to have creatinine clearance <60 mL/min.

Risk factors leading to VTE in kidney transplant recipients include hypercoagulability acquired prior to transplant, manipulation of iliac vein, immunosuppressive medications, immobility, smoking, older age, peritoneal dialysis, delayed graft function, and use of mTOR inhibitors. One study reported a VTE incidence of 0.9% in the first 30 days after kidney transplant, in a setting without routine thromboprophylaxis [26]. The decision to use pharmacologic anticoagulation following transplant is limited by potential for post-operative bleeding, anemia requiring blood transfusions, and the potential need for invasive procedures such as biopsy. Graft thrombosis occurs in 2–3% of kidney transplant recipients, with most resulting in graft loss. It has been suggested that low-dose aspirin could reduce the rate of allograft thrombosis; however, more research is needed to evaluate risk versus benefit [27]. About 40–70% of kidney transplant recipients will require blood transfusions in the post-operative period. This anemia may be related to surgical blood losses, delayed production of erythropoietin, and adverse effects of immunosuppressive medications.

In contrast to patients with kidney disease who have an increased risk of VTE, the risk of VTE in liver transplant recipients is comparable to other major abdominal surgery [28]. Common risk factors for VTE include frailty, immobility, and prior VTE. While coagulopathy as measured by INR resolves quickly in the setting of successful liver transplant, thrombocytopenia generally takes weeks to resolve. In the absence of active bleeding, correction of elevated INR or reduced platelet count is not indicated as these should correct post-transplant. All liver transplant recipients should be screened for aberrations in liver blood flow with ultrasound within the first 24 h after transplant and any significant increase in liver transaminases. The decision to administer routine pharmacologic thromboprophylaxis post-liver transplant is provider specific, but should be strongly considered in patients with limited mobility and otherwise normal routine coagulation parameters. The decision to administer blood products in the setting of recent liver transplant should be made in collaboration with the transplant surgeon as administration of blood products can increase the risk of early thromboembolic events, hepatic artery thrombosis (HAT), in particular. The risk of HAT and PVT post-transplant is highly impacted by surgical technique and anastomotic issues of the donor and recipient. Therapeutic anticoagulation is indicated within 24 h post-transplant in patients with multiple risk factors for portal or hepatic vein thrombosis (pre-transplant PVT, slow portal flow, partial thrombectomy, nonphysiologic portal vein reconstruction, and thrombophilic disorder). It should be noted that early administration of the mTOR inhibitor sirolimus was associated with an increased risk of HAT, resulting in a black box warning and recommendations to delay use until at least 30 days post-transplant [29].

Lung and heart transplant recipients have significantly higher risk of VTE including stroke than other SOT recipients, with incidence of VTE for lung recipients of 17–30% at 1 month and up to 64% by 4 years. Risk factors for VTE in the lung transplant recipient include hypercoagulable state, older age, diabetes, hypercholesterolemia, ECMO , cardiopulmonary bypass, pneumonia, immobility, and sirolimus. Causes for stroke in these patients may be air embolism as well as pulmonary vein thrombosis at the left atrial anastomosis. Lung transplant recipients are also at increased risk of atrial fibrillation both pre- and post-transplant [19]. Despite this well-recognized risk, no standard approach to anticoagulation post-lung transplant exists [30]. Kainuma et al. evaluated heart transplant recipients who received peri-transplant UFH and compression stockings, reporting VTE in 42% of patients at 60 days post-transplant (28.2% in the first 30 days), with a median of 11 days [31]. Risk factors included history of DVT/PE, intubation for more than 3 days, and longer cardiac bypass time. ISHLT 2022 guidelines for the care of heart transplant recipients indicate that DOACs are reasonable alternatives to vitamin K antagonists for stroke prophylaxis as well as for the treatment of VTE [32]. However, in patients receiving cyclosporin (a strong p-gp inhibitor), there is a greater potential for increased DOAC exposure and thus bleeding if also combined with a strong CYP3A4 inhibitor. Moreover, decreased renal function may also require dose personalization in some situations and DOACs should be held at least 48 h prior to endomyocardial biopsy [32].

40.4.5 Acute Kidney Injury and Renal Failure

Kidney injury, acute and chronic, is a frequent complication in transplant recipients, owing in part to the complications of antecedent disease such as hypertension and diabetes as well as perioperative complications and calcineurin inhibitor toxicity (Table 40.3). CKD affects 10–20% of non-kidney transplant recipients resulting in approximately 5% of the kidney transplant waiting list being non-kidney transplant recipients (Table 40.4) [37]. AKI has been reported in up to 50% of liver transplant recipients, with some estimates of end-stage kidney failure and CKD at 4% and 25%, respectively, 10 years post-transplant [38]. For the transplant patient with CKD, efforts to preserve renal function often include CNI minimization or avoidance, balancing the potential improvement in renal function with increased risk of biopsy proven rejection.

Table 40.3 Risk factors for renal dysfunction in transplant recipients [20, 33–36]

Heart	Lung	Liver	Kidney
• Elevated pre-operative right heart pressures • Decreased pulmonary artery pulsatility index • Pre-existing CKD • Post-transplant hypotension • Volume depletion • High CNI concentrations	• ECMO • Post-operative complications • High CNI concentration	• Intraoperative hypotension and vasopressor use • Post-perfusion syndrome • Pre-existing CKD or AKI-HRS • High pre-transplant MELD • Donor age > 60, Donor BMI > 30, DCD donor • Type 2 diabetes • Hypertension • Female sex • Obesity • Alcohol-related liver disease • Viral hepatitis • Hepatocellular carcinoma • CNI	• Deceased donor kidney • Thrombosis • Rejection • Urinary obstruction • High CNI concentrations

Table 40.4 Reported incidence of renal dysfunction in non-renal transplant recipients [20, 33–36]

	Acute kidney injury	Chronic kidney disease	Dialysis
Liver	50%	25%	4%, 10 years
Heart	70%	10–40%, 3–7 years	5–10%, 9–10 years
Lung	52%	23%, 5 years 52%, 10 years	
Intestine		21.3%, 3 years	

The assessment of renal function in transplant recipients is also challenging. In patients with protein calorie malnutrition, creatinine production may be reduced due to sarcopenia. Equations containing creatinine perform poorly in lung transplant patients with low mid-arm muscle area, low body mass index as well as patients with cystic fibrosis, probably due to the decreased production of creatinine in these patients [39]. In such patients equations containing cystatin c performed better. Likewise, in patients with liver disease and liver transplant, serum creatinine as a marker of renal function may lead to over estimation of glomerular filtration rate. Low or normal serum creatinine may be the result of low muscle mass related to malnutrition, decreased hepatic production of creatinine as well as enlarged volume of distribution. The incorporation of urine output into the systematic evaluation of liver transplant recipients increases the number of patients identified with AKI [40]

40.4.6 *Cardiovascular Complications*

Cardiovascular complications including coronary artery disease, myocardial infarction, congestive heart failure, and arrhythmias significantly contribute to patient and graft survival following solid organ transplant. Cardiovascular complications are the leading cause of death in renal transplant recipients with up to 40% of renal recipients experiencing a cardiovascular event within the first 36 months post-transplant [41]. In liver transplant, cardiovascular disease is the third most common cause of death long term accounting for 12–16% of patients [42]. Many of the risk factors for cardiovascular disease post-transplant mirror those risk factors in the general non-transplant population. These risk factors include diabetes, hypertension, hyperlipidemia, increased age, obesity, and smoking [43]. In addition, transplant recipients may be at increased risk due to the immunosuppression medications used and to the development of chronic kidney disease post-transplant.

Pharmacists, including pharmacists in the intensive care units, can help to optimize medication regimens to decrease the risk of cardiovascular disease. The KDIGO guidelines for management of kidney transplant recipients recommend use of aspirin 65–100 mg/day for primary prevention of cardiovascular disease in patients with diabetes and for secondary prevention in patients with atherosclerotic cardiovascular disease [44]. In regard to statin therapy, the KDIGO guidelines recommend adults over age 50 with eGFR <60 mL/min and those with CKD and eGFR over 60 mL/min receive statin therapy [45]. These guidelines also recommend all adult kidney recipients receive treatment with a statin.

References

1. 2022 Annual Report of the U.S. Organ Procurement and Transplantation Network and the Scientific Registry of Transplant Recipients: Transplant Data 2012–2021.
2. Lichvar AB, Moss Chandran M, Cohen EA, et al. The expanded role of the transplant pharmacist: a 10-year follow-up. Am J Transplant. 2023;9:135–1387.
3. Organ Procurement and Transplantation Network (OPTN) Bylaws. OPTN; 2023. https://optn.transplant.hrsa.gov/. Accessed 15 August 2023.
4. 42 CFR Parts 405, 482, 488, and 498 Medicare Program; Hospital Conditions of Participation: Requirements for Approval and Re-Approval of Transplant Centers To Perform Organ Transplants; Final Rule (2007) Department of Health and Human Services Center for Medicare and Medicaid Services. www.cms.gov. Accessed 15 August 2023.
5. Maldonado AQ, Hall RC, Pilch NA, et al. ASHP guidelines on pharmacy services in solid organ transplantation. Am J Health-Syst Pharm. 2020;77:222–32.
6. Halloran PF. Immunosuppressive drugs for kidney transplantation. N Engl J Med. 2004;351:2715–29.
7. Organ Procurement and Transplantation Network (OPTN) and Scientific Registry of Transplant Recipients (SRTR). OPTN/SRTR 2021 Annual Data Report. Published 2023. Accessed [9/1/2023].
8. Lemahieu W, Maes B, Verbeke K, et al. Cytochrome P450 3A4 and P-glycoprotein activity and assimilation of tacrolimus in transplant patients with persistent diarrhea. Am J Transplant. 2005;5(6):1383–91.

9. Knops N, Levtchenko E, van den Heuvel B, Kuypers D. From gut to kidney: transporting and metabolizing calcineurin-inhibitors in solid organ transplantation. Int J Pharmaceut. 2013;452:14–35.

10. Nankivell BJ, Alexander SI. Rejection of the kidney allograft. N Engl J Med. 2010;363(15):1451–62.

11. Garces JC, Giusti S, Staffeld-Coit C, et al. Antibody-mediated rejection: a review. Ochsner J. 2017;17(1):46–55.

12. Schinstock CA, Mannon RB, Budde K, et al. Recommended treatment for antibody-mediated rejection after kidney transplantation: the 2019 Expert Consensus From the Transplantation Society Working Group. Transplantation. 2020;104(5):911–22.

13. Jordan SC, Bunnapradist S, Bromberg JS, et al. Donor-derived cell-free DNA identifies antibody-mediated rejection in donor specific antibody positive kidney transplant recipients. Transplant Direct. 2018;4:e379.

14. Peabody J, Billings P, Valdenor C, et al. Randomized clinical trial of a novel donor-derived cfDNA test to detect rejection in CPV-simulated renal transplant patients. Int Urol Nephrol. 2020;52(8):1593–601.

15. Friedewald JJ, Kurian SM, Heilman RL, et al. Clinical Trials in Organ Transplantation 08 (CTOT-08). Development and clinical validity of a novel blood-based molecular biomarker for subclinical acute rejection following kidney transplant. Am J Transplant. 2019;19(1):98–109.

16. Oellerich M, Shipkova M, Asendorf T, et al. Absolute quantification of donor-derived cell-free DNA as a marker of rejection and graft injury in kidney transplantation: results from a prospective observational study. Am J Transplant. 2019;19(11):3087.

17. Fishman JA. Infection in organ transplantation. Am J Transplant. 2017;17:856–79.

18. Dhar R. Neurologic complications of transplantation. Neurocrit Care. 2018;28:4–11.

19. Kanade R, Kler A, Banga A. Non-pulmonary complications after lung transplantation: part 1. Indian J Thorac Cardiovasc Surg. 2022;38:S280–9.

20. Van den Hoogen MWF, Seghers L, Manintveld OC, et al. Care for the organ transplant recipient in the intensive care unit. J Crit Care. 2021;64:37–44.

21. Meaney CJ, O'Connor M, McGowan M, et al. Treatment of prolonged tacrolimus toxicity using phenytoin in a haemodialysis patient. J Clin Pharm Ther. 2019;44:640643.

22. Chen S, Hu J, Xuu L, et al. Posterior reversible encephalopathy syndrome after transplantation: a review. Mol Neurobiol. 2016;53:6897–909.

23. Gersch K, Spencer TR. New-onset seizure activity in a transplant patient on immunosuppressive therapy. J Am AssocNurse Pract. 2020;32:824–8.

24. Song T, Rao Z, Tan Q, et al. Calcineurin inhibitors associated posterior reversible encephalopathy syndrome in solid organ transplantation. Medicine. 2016;95:1–8.

25. Garcia-Ortega A, Lopez-Reyes R, Anguera G, et al. Venous thromboembolism in solid-organ transplant recipients: findings from the RIETE registry. Thrombosis Res. 2021;201:131–8.

26. Massicotte-Azarniouch D, Sood MM, Fergusson DA, et al. The association of venous thromboembolism with blood transfusion in kidney transplant patients. Transfusion. 2022;62:2480–9.

27. Pegler AH, Hegerty K, Gately RP, et al. Incidence of thromboembolic complications following kidney transplantation with short and extended aspirin prophylaxis: a retrospective single-center study. Ann Transplant. 2023;28:e93914.

28. Sakowitz S, Bakhtiya SS, Verma A, et al. Risk and factors associated with venous thromboembolism following abdominal transplantation. Surg Open Sci. 2023;13:18–23.

29. Montalvá E, Rodríguez-Perálvarez M, Blasi A, et al. Consensus statement on hemostatic management, anticoagulation, and antiplatelet therapy in liver transplantation. Transplantation. 2022;106:1123–31.

30. Shepherd HM, Rr H, Witt CA, et al. Bleeding and thrombotic complications associated with anticoagulation prior to lung transplantation: a case series. J Thorac Dis. 2022;14:2917–26.

31. Kainuma A, Ning Y, Kurlansky PA, et al. Deep vein thrombosis and pulmonary embolism after heart transplantation. Clin Transplant. 2022;36:e14705.

32. Velleca A, Shullo MA, Dhital K, et al. The international society for heart and lung transplantation (ISHLT) guidelines for the care of heart transplant recipients. J Heart Lung Transplant. 2023;42(5):e1–e141.
33. Milson C, Considine A, Cramp ME, et al. Adult liver transplantation: UK clinical guideline—part 2: surgery and post-operation. Frontline Gastroenterol. 2020;11:385–96.
34. Dong V, Nadim MK, Karvella CJ. Post-liver transplant acute kidney injury. Liver Transplant. 2021;27:1653–64.
35. Janus N, Launay-Vacher V, Sebbag L, et al. Renal insufficiency, mortality, and drug management in heart transplant. Results of the CARIN study. Transplant Int. 2014;27:931–8.
36. Grootjans H, Verschuuren EAM, van Gemert JP, et al. Chronic kidney disease after lung transplantation in a changing era. Transplant Rev. 2022;36:100727.
37. Wiseman AC. CKD in recipients of non-kidney solid organ transplants: a review. Am J Kidney Dis. 2022;80:108–18.
38. Solà E, Ginès P. Chronic kidney disease: a major concern in liver transplantation in the XXI century. J Hepatol. 2014;61:196–7.
39. Degen DA, Janardan J, Barraclough KA. Predictive performance of different kidney function equations in lung transplant patients. Clin Biochem. 2017;50:385–93.
40. DellaVolpe J, Al-Khafaji A. Acute kidney injury before and after liver transplant. J Intensive Care Med. 2019;34:6867–695.
41. Shirali AC, Bia MJ. Management of cardiovascular disease in renal transplant recipients. Clin J Am Soc Nephrol. 2008;3(2):491–504.
42. Watt KDS, Pedersen KDS, Kremers WK, et al. Evolution of causes and risk factors for mortality post-liver transplant: results of the NIDDK long-term follow-up study. Am J Transplant. 2010;10(6):1420–7.
43. Devine PA, Courtney AE, Maxwell AP. Cardiovascular risk in renal transplant recipients. J Nephrol. 2019;32:389–99.
44. Kidney Disease: Improving Global Outcomes (KDIGO) Transplant Work Group. KDIGO clinical practice guideline for the care of kidney transplant recipients. Am J Transplant. 2009;9(Suppl. 3):S1–S157.
45. Kidney Disease: Improving Global Outcomes (KDIGO) Lipid Work Group. KDIGO clinical practice guideline for lipid management in chronic kidney disease. Kidney Int. 2013;3(3):259–305.

Chapter 41
Pharmacotherapy of Trauma and the Role of the Pharmacist

Ruben Santiago, Brian Gilbert, Lance Ray, and Erin Reichert

41.1 Introduction

Unintentional injuries and violence are the leading cause of death for Americans ≤ 44 years of age [1]. In 2022, unintentional injuries were the third leading cause of death, behind heart disease and cancer [2]. Prior to 1980, trauma care in the United States was described as inconsistent due to a lack of a standardized approach [3]. The "first hour" of trauma care was changed in the United States and in much of the rest of the world due to a tragedy that occurred in February 1976 [4, 5]. Piloting his plane in rural Nebraska, Dr. James Styner, an orthopedic surgeon, crashed his plane in a cornfield. The crash left him and three of his children with serious or critical injuries and resulted in the instant death of his wife. The initial hospital care that the family received was inadequate and upon recognizing this Styner stated, "When I can provide better care in the field with limited resources than what my children and I received at the primary care facility, there is something wrong with the system, and the system has to be changed" [5]. This tragedy was the inception for the Advanced Trauma Life Support (ATLS) course as we know it today. ATLS provides a systematic approach to the evaluation and management of patients with significant or life-threatening injuries [3, 6]. When properly implemented, the skills and knowledge provided through ATLS can lower early mortality in trauma patients by at least 15% [4].

R. Santiago (✉)
Department of Pharmacy, Jackson Memorial Hospital, Miami, FL, USA

B. Gilbert
Department of Pharmacy, Wesley Medical Center, Wichita, KS, USA

L. Ray
Department of Pharmacy, Denver Health Medical Center, Denver, CO, USA

E. Reichert
Department of Pharmacy, The Ohio State University Wexner Medical Center, Columbus, OH, USA

© The Author(s), under exclusive license to Springer Nature Switzerland AG 2025
Y. Alzaidi, M. A. Gebily (eds.), *The Pharmacist's Expanded Role in Critical Care Medicine*, https://doi.org/10.1007/978-3-031-77335-8_41

Initial management of the trauma patient includes the primary survey, which is composed of the following: Airway maintenance with restriction of cervical spine motion, Breathing and ventilation, Circulation with hemorrhage control, Disability (assessment of neurologic status), and Exposure/Environmental control or colloquial known as the ABCDE of trauma [3]. This mnemonic is meant to identify the most time sensitive interventions that should occur in the initial assessment of the trauma patient. For example, the loss of an airway is the most immediate threat to life, followed by an inability to breathe, then the reduction of circulating blood volume, and lastly an expanding intracranial mass lesion (hematoma or hemorrhage). This method prioritizes the identification and management of life-threatening conditions [3, 6]. Newer literature has pointed to a CAB approach to the management of the exsanguinating patient in hemorrhagic shock. When intubation occurs in this patient population, it may lead to vasodilation, worsening hypotension and subsequent organ perfusion. Further studies are needed to establish this shift in focus in trauma care [7, 8].

If a patient's airway is compromised (i.e., obstructed with foreign bodies, vomitus, and/or blood), has a traumatic insult such as facial or mandibular fractures, severe tracheal/laryngeal injuries, or is at risk secondary to head trauma, a definitive airway must be established via endotracheal intubation. Patients who are able to communicate verbally are not in immediate jeopardy; however, repeated assessment of the airway must be completed to ensure patency. Severely head-injured patients with altered mental status or a Glasgow Coma Scale (GCS) of 8 or lower may also require a definitive airway. Other indications for definitive airway placement include, but are not limited to, impending airway compromise due to injury or the inability to maintain adequate oxygenation [3, 6].

41.2   Rapid Sequence Intubation

Rapid sequence intubation (RSI) is a common strategy in emergency airway management and is defined as the administration of a sedative-hypnotic (induction) agent followed by a neuromuscular blocking agent (NMBA) in rapid succession with immediate placement of an endotracheal tube prior to assisted ventilation [9, 10]. RSI is the preferred method for securing the patient's airway in the emergency department (ED) as it reduces the risk of aspiration of gastric contents, attenuates the physiologic response to intubation, and optimizes intubation conditions [11]. Emergency medicine pharmacists are critical members of the emergency care team and must be familiar with medications used during RSI. This includes dosing, onset, duration of action, contraindications, and monitoring considerations. Table 41.1 provides information on the most common medications used during RSI.

Table 41.1 Characteristics of medications used during RSI

Medication	Dose	Onset	Duration	Considerations
Induction agents				
Etomidate	0.3 mg/kg	5–30 s	3–15 min	Minimal hemodynamic effects, inhibits cortisol synthesis, transient myoclonic movements
Ketamine	1–2 mg/kg	30–90 s	5–15 min	May increase BP, HR May use in hypotension; caution in catecholamine depleted patients May use in patients with reactive airway disease
Propofol	1–2.5 mg/kg	10–60 s	3–10 min	Consider alternatives in patients that are hemodynamically unstable
Methohexital	1–1.5 mg/kg	<30 s	5–10 min	Avoid in patients with hypotension and reactive airway disease Can cause laryngospasm
Midazolam	0.1–0.3 mg/kg	60–180 s	10–80 min[a]	Avoid in patients with hemodynamic instability, heart failure, elderly, hepatic disease Clearance prolonged in renal failure and obesity May consider use in patients with seizures
Paralytics				
Succinylcholine	1.5 mg/kg	30–60 s	5–15 min	Avoid in patients with history of malignant hyperthermia, hyperkalemia, or at risk of hyperkalemia Use actual body weight for dosing
Rocuronium	0.6–1.2 mg/kg	60–120 s	40–120 min	Higher dosing strategies lead to intubating conditions similar to succinylcholine Use ideal bodyweight in obese patients

[a]May be prolonged in patients with severe hepatic impairment

41.2.1 Pre-treatment

Medications used for pre-treatment are intended to decrease the negative physiologic response associated with intubation and are administered prior to induction and paralytic agents. Negative physiologic responses include hypertension, bradycardia, and abrupt increases in intracranial pressure (ICP). In trauma scenarios, these medications are not normally administered as they should be given 2–3 min prior to induction to achieve their desired effect. For a more in-depth review of pre-treatment medications, please refer to the chapter on Rapid Sequence Intubation [11–14].

41.2.2 Induction Agents

Induction agents produce a general state of anesthesia by rapidly producing unconsciousness, allowing the administration of paralytics, leading to ideal conditions for intubation. There are a variety of medications that may be used for induction for RSI and include etomidate, ketamine, propofol, barbiturates such as methohexital, and benzodiazepines such as midazolam. The pharmacist involved in RSI must be familiar with these agents as patient-specific characteristics and clinical picture will dictate which agent is the most appropriate [10, 12–14].

41.2.3 Etomidate

Etomidate, an imidazole-derived sedative hypnotic, exerts its effect by enhancing the effect of gamma-aminobutyric acid (GABA), inhibiting excitatory stimuli producing unconsciousness. It has a quick onset of action and short duration of action and also has a favorable hemodynamic profile, making it a useful agent in patients who are hypotensive and those with multisystem trauma. Etomidate causes a moderate reduction in intracranial pressure by decreasing cerebral blood flow and also causes a moderate reduction in intraocular pressure [12–14]. An adverse effect associated with the use of etomidate is its inhibition of the synthesis of cortisol. Etomidate inhibits 11-beta-hydroxylase, along with several other enzymes, leading to adrenal suppression. Clinical studies have shown that the extent and duration of adrenal suppression produced by one dose of etomidate for RSI are not associated with worse clinical outcomes, higher rates of nosocomial infections, or increased mortality [10, 11]. Myoclonus is also associated with the use of etomidate with rates ranging from 22% to 90%; however, this is not normally seen as it is quickly followed by a paralytic [10, 14]. Pre-treatment with short acting opioids, particularly fentanyl, has been shown as a safe and effective approach to prevent etomidate-induced myoclonus. While not necessary during RSI, this strategy may be best suited for procedural sedation with etomidate [15]. The dose range is 0.2–0.6 mg/kg with the most common dose for RSI being 0.3 mg/kg [14].

41.2.4 Ketamine

Ketamine, an n-methyl-d-aspartate (NMDA) receptor antagonist, is a phencyclidine derivative that is also used as an induction agent for RSI. Ketamine has a similar onset and duration of action when compared to etomidate. Ketamine is the only induction agent that has sedative as well as analgesic properties and produces a cataleptic-like state in the patient [13].

Ketamine produces a dose-related rise in heart rate and blood pressure in patients who are not catecholamine depleted [13]. This occurs as ketamine stimulates CNS outflow and lessens the reuptake of catecholamines [10, 14]. As a result of these sympathomimetic effects, ketamine may be an ideal induction agent for patients with hypotension; however, it can worsen hypotension and exacerbate myocardial depression in patients that are catecholamine depleted. Ketamine has direct negative cardiac inotropic effects; however, these effects are normally overridden by ketamine's sympathetic stimulation. Due to these negative effects, caution should be used in patients with severe heart failure [14]. A maximum dose of 1.5 mg/kg is recommended in patients who are catecholamine depleted [10, 13, 14].

Ketamine may also be the preferred induction agent in patients with reactive airway disease as it relieves bronchospasm by dilating the bronchial smooth muscle and stimulates the pulmonary beta receptors [14]. It also potentiates the bronchodilatory effects of epinephrine [13]. Historically, it has been recommended to avoid the use of ketamine in patients with increased ICP; however, recent studies have indicated that the use of ketamine in sedated and mechanically ventilated patients did not result in increased ICP [11, 14]. Ketamine may be a reasonable induction agent in patients with blunt head trauma and hypotension as ketamine maintains mean arterial pressure and is associated with a decrease in vasopressor requirements in this scenario. Additionally, in intubated, head-injured patients, cerebral perfusion pressure (CPP) remains stable when compared to benzodiazepine and opioid combinations for sedation and analgesia [10].

Adverse effects of ketamine can include an increase in oral secretions and in rare instances laryngospasm. Its use may also lead to emergence phenomenon; however, this is not often seen due to post-intubation sedation and analgesia management [11]. Due to ketamine's sympathomimetic effects, it may lead to an increase in myocardial oxygen demand, making it a suboptimal agent in patients with a history of heart failure or ischemic heart disease [10, 13, 14]. The recommended dose of ketamine for RSI is 1–2 mg/kg.

41.2.5 Propofol

Propofol is a GABA agonist that is highly lipophilic and crosses the blood–brain barrier, resulting in a quick onset of action [11, 14]. Similar to ketamine, it possesses some NMDA receptor antagonist activity [11]. Propofol has ideal attributes for an induction agent for RSI as it has a rapid onset of action and short duration of action [14]. Decreasing cerebral oxygen consumption and ICP, propofol remains an option in the hemodynamically stable patient with increased ICP [12–14]. Propofol also has mild bronchodilating properties, making it another choice for patients with reactive airway disease; however, its cardiovascular adverse effect profile described below precludes it from being used more frequently as an induction agent in RSI [13, 14].

Propofol has negative cardiovascular effects as it has been shown to decrease blood pressure by reducing preload and afterload and decreasing cardiac contractility [13]. It has calcium channel as well as beta-adrenergic antagonist properties. Therefore, it should be used with caution in patients who are hypovolemic, hypotensive, and/or have a reduced ejection fraction [14]. The trauma patient population is at higher risk of hypotension due to hypovolemia and blood loss sustained from their injuries [16]. The dose range for propofol is 1–2.5 mg/kg, but due to the risk of hemodynamic instability associated with large doses, it is suggested to start at the lower range of 1–1.5 mg/kg for induction [11]. Historically, propofol was contraindicated in patients with a hypersensitivity to soy, peanut, and egg proteins; however, newer evidence has determined that avoidance in patients with these allergies is no longer necessary [10].

41.2.6 Methohexital

Methohexital, an ultra-short acting barbiturate, is an alternative induction agent that works via agonism of GABA receptors. Due to other induction agents with favorable hemodynamic profiles and barbiturate shortages, the use of methohexital has fallen dramatically. Side effects associated with methohexital include respiratory depression, venodilation, and myocardial depression. This medication may decrease ICP and cerebral blood flow by decreasing cerebral oxygen demand; however, caution should be used in patients with TBI due to its propensity to cause hypotension [14].

A retrospective study conducted in a medical ICU compared the safety and efficacy of methohexital and etomidate for endotracheal intubation. Outcomes were similar between groups in regard to blood pressure change, rate of successful intubation, time from drug administration to intubation, and number of intubation attempts [17]. Another retrospective study compared the safety and effectiveness of methohexital or ketamine with etomidate for patients in the ED undergoing RSI. First success intubation rates were similar between etomidate and methohexital as the ketamine group was too small to draw any conclusions [18]. Methohexital preparation is not ideal for RSI as it requires reconstitution prior to administration which may delay the procedure. The dose for induction of methohexital is 1–1.5 mg/kg [14, 18].

41.2.7 Midazolam

Midazolam is a short-acting benzodiazepine that exerts its pharmacologic effect through direct binding of GABA receptors [11, 13]. It has a slow onset of action when compared to other induction agents, has a prolonged duration of action, and if not adequately dosed, may insufficiently sedate the patient for RSI. Dose-dependent hypotension may be observed due to decreased vascular tone and systemic vascular resistance [11, 14]. The induction dose of midazolam is 0.1–0.3 mg/kg. Therefore, like propofol, the dose often necessary for induction obviates its use as a preferred agent in RSI since patients could easily receive a dose of 20–30 mg. Due to its slow onset of action and deleterious hemodynamic effects, midazolam is a suboptimal agent for use as an induction agent during RSI. Midazolam for induction should be reserved for when other agents are not readily available [11].

41.2.8 Comparison of Induction Agents in Trauma

A prospective, randomized study compared etomidate to ketamine in an adult critically ill patient population (including trauma patients) requiring endotracheal intubation. Patients were randomly assigned to etomidate 0.3 mg/kg or ketamine 2 mg/kg followed by succinylcholine. There was no significant difference between maximum sequential organ failure assessment (SOFA) score, difficulty in intubation, early complications after intubation, and 28-day mortality between the groups [19]. A retrospective study in adult trauma patients compared etomidate 0.3 mg/kg to ketamine 1–2 mg/kg, followed by succinylcholine. Mortality was similar between groups along with peri-intubation outcomes (first-pass intubation success, need for rescue surgical airway, and peri-intubation cardiac arrest) [20]. A prehospital study conducted in the Netherlands evaluated etomidate versus S(+)-ketamine in traumatic brain injury. They found no difference in mortality at 30 days between groups [21].

A retrospective study of trauma patients intubated in the ED evaluated the rates of hypotension between propofol, etomidate, and midazolam. The use of propofol was associated with an increased risk of post-intubation hypotension (OR 3.64, p = 0.04) [16]. A multicenter retrospective study evaluated the hemodynamic effects of etomidate, propofol, and ketamine in adult trauma patients requiring RSI in the ED. This study found no significant difference between the induction agent used and hemodynamic effects [22]. It is worth noting that studying the hemodynamic effects of induction agents in trauma is challenging because of the confounding hypotension of hemorrhagic shock in trauma patients, as well as the fact that any neuroleptic medication inherently decreases sympathetic tone, thereby altering hemodynamics. Nevertheless, pharmacists on the trauma team and those involved in RSI must know the specific medication characteristics as well as patient-specific parameters when choosing an optimal induction agent.

41.2.9 Neuromuscular Blockers

Neuromuscular blocking agents (NMBAs) are administered after the induction agent and paralyze skeletal muscles, creating optimal intubation conditions while minimizing the risk of aspiration. NMBAs work at the level of the neuromuscular junction, antagonizing the action of acetylcholine on nicotinic receptors. They do not possess any sedative, amnestic, or analgesic properties. The two types of NMBAs are depolarizing and nondepolarizing neuromuscular blockers. Succinylcholine is a depolarizing NMBA and rocuronium is a common nondepolarizing NMBA used in RSI [11, 13].

41.2.10 Succinylcholine

Succinylcholine is an ideal paralytic for RSI as it has a rapid onset of action and short duration of action. A dimer of acetylcholine molecules, succinylcholine mimics the action of acetylcholine at the neuromuscular junction, resulting in transient muscle fasciculations when it initially binds (depolarization), followed by full paralysis as it blocks the action of acetylcholine by occupying the acetylcholine receptor [11–13]. Succinylcholine should be avoided in patients where hyperkalemia would be a concern, such as those with renal dysfunction or burn patients, given the transient increase in serum potassium values that occurs after administration [11, 13]. Succinylcholine may be used in patients up to 48 h after an acute burn injury; however, if patient presentation is delayed, an alternative agent should be used [23]. The slight rise in potassium possesses little threat as most patients can tolerate this shift; however, patients with a predisposition to hyperkalemia may suffer a serious dysrhythmia or cardiac arrest. Succinylcholine is also contraindicated in patients with a personal or family history of malignant hyperthermia [11–13]. The dose of succinylcholine for RSI is 1.5 mg/kg based on actual body weight [10].

41.2.11 Rocuronium

Rocuronium is a nondepolarizing neuromuscular blocker. It exerts its pharmacological effect by competing and blocking the effects of acetylcholine at the postjunctional cholinergic nicotinic receptors in the neuromuscular junction, resulting in paralysis without fasciculations [11, 13, 14]. The dose of rocuronium for RSI ranges from 0.6 to 1.2 mg/kg with the higher range (1–1.2 mg/kg) achieving an onset of action comparable to that of succinylcholine [11]. The dose is based on ideal body weight in obese patients [10]. Caution should be used, and the dose reduced in patients with a history of neuromuscular weakness such as those with myasthenia gravis [24].

41.2.12 Succinylcholine vs. Rocuronium

A 2015 Cochrane review composed 50 studies totaling 4151 patients compared succinylcholine to rocuronium for RSI. Their conclusion was that succinylcholine creates better intubation conditions than rocuronium for both excellent and clinically acceptable intubation conditions during RSI. This review included various dose ranges for rocuronium. When comparing rocuronium at a lower dosage range of 0.6 mg/kg to 0.7 mg/kg, succinylcholine created significantly more excellent intubation conditions; however, when reviewing studies that had a higher dosing strategy for rocuronium (0.9–1.2 mg/kg), there was no statistical difference between rocuronium and succinylcholine. Rocuronium remains a suitable alternative to succinylcholine and should be used when contraindications to succinylcholine exist. The dose used for rocuronium for RSI should be at least 1 mg/kg [25].

Patanwala et. al. evaluated the difference in mortality between succinylcholine and rocuronium in patients presenting with a TBI that received RSI in the ED. There were 233 patients included in the study with 149 patients in the succinylcholine group and 84 patients in the rocuronium group. There was an association with increased mortality in severe TBI patients that received succinylcholine [26]. The authors state that the increase in mortality may be due to a transient increase in ICP in the succinylcholine group, leading to greater intracranial injury. Patients in the succinylcholine group were also more likely to have hypotension, a predictor of mortality in patients suffering from a TBI.

Differences between succinylcholine and rocuronium include their mechanism of action and duration of action. Rocuronium lasts longer than succinylcholine; 40–120 min versus 5–15 min, respectively [11]. As a result, sedation and analgesia are paramount in patients who receive rocuronium as they may be paralyzed without being properly sedated. Lack of proper sedation can lead to awareness with paralysis which is discussed more in depth later in this chapter. There is no clear superior choice of paralytic for RSI. The decision to use succinylcholine or rocuronium is patient specific and depends on the clinical scenario.

41.2.13 Reversal of Rocuronium

The long duration of rocuronium may be undesirable in certain patient populations (i.e., patients necessitating a neurologic exam). A novel modified cyclodextrin, sugammadex, may be used to reverse the paralytic effects of rocuronium and vecuronium. This medication works by forming a complex with rocuronium or vecuronium, reducing the amount of the paralytic agent available to bind to nicotinic cholinergic receptors in the neuromuscular junction, resulting in reversal of neuromuscular blockade. Doses as high as 16 mg/kg are recommended when immediate reversal (within 3 min) is needed for rocuronium that was dosed at 1.2 mg/kg. Doses as low as 2–4 mg/kg are appropriate for most patients. Sugammadex is not recommended in the setting of severe renal disease because the NMBA-sugammadex complex is renally excreted, and the half-life of this complex is increased 17-fold [27]. The theoretical concern with this is potential dissociation of the NMBA from sugammadex over time followed by a return of some paralytic effect, although this has not been shown in case reports or other data. An adverse effect of sugammadex is marked bradycardia. Therefore, monitoring of hemodynamic changes after this medication is administered is required [10, 11, 27].

41.2.14 Role of the Pharmacist in RSI

Pharmacists are a vital member of the team when a patient requires RSI. Pharmacists can ensure that the most appropriate induction agent is selected based off patient's vital signs and their past medical history. Also, pharmacists assist in choosing the best paralytic agent by reviewing pertinent labs such as the patient's potassium level prior to intubation. If there is no laboratory information available, the pharmacist must communicate with the team to ensure the patient is not at risk of hyperkalemia prior to administering succinylcholine. Pharmacists can also help optimize the dose of medications that patients receive based off their weight. Bhat et al. evaluated the appropriate dosing of etomidate and succinylcholine in obese and nonobese patients and found that obese patients were more likely to be under dosed during RSI, whereas nonobese patients were more likely to be overdosed [28]. Pharmacists responding to RSI must know where supplies such as labels, syringes, and alcohol swabs are located in order to prepare medications. The emergency medicine and critical care pharmacists are perfectly positioned to assist with dosing and preparation, ensuring that post-intubation sedation and analgesia are administered in a timely manner. For a more in-depth review of RSI, please refer to the chapter on RSI.

41.3 Post-intubation Sedation and Analgesia

Providing adequate sedation and analgesia post-RSI in trauma patients cannot be understated, especially when long-acting paralytics, such as rocuronium, are utilized in the intubation process. Studies show that 10.8–53% of mechanically ventilated patients were not provided any post-intubation sedation or analgesia in the ED [29, 30]. In addition to paralytic choice, inherent differences in ED vs intensive care unit (ICU) workflow likely contribute. Such ED aspects include high patient-load, ED crowding, and lack of protocols for critically ill patients. EDs often lack protocols for sedation management and up to one-third of ED patients on mechanical ventilation do not receive an assessment of sedation depth [31]. Hospital crowding results in longer ED length-of-stay prior to ICU transfer, which also certainly contributes to slower optimal care and may even negatively affect overall mortality [32].

Literature indicates that ED patients treated with long-acting paralytics, such as rocuronium, experience lower doses and greater delays in post-intubation sedation initiation compared to those given succinylcholine [33, 34]. The ED-AWARENESS Study provided a much-needed light cast on the issue of undertreating pain and sedation in ED ventilated patients, particularly from the aspect of awareness with paralysis (AWP) after RSI. The primary outcome of AWP was assessed by investigators by interviewing patients after extubation and prior to hospital discharge. Individual clinical scenarios such as type and dose of paralytic were considered to help determine the potential or occurrence of AWP. Possible or definite AWP events were determined to be 2.6% of patients in this study. Administration of rocuronium in the ED was significantly associated with AWP (OR 5.1; 95% CI, 1.30–20.1). While there were several limitations to this study, the prevalence of AWP was 2.6% in this cohort, notably higher than previous operating room (OR) studies exploring AWP where prevalence is shown to be from 0.1% to 0.2% [35]. The OR has several advantages to help curb incidence of AWP including the presence of anesthesiologists, the use of inhaled anesthesia adjuncts to IV medication(s), and the typical elective-nature (non-critically ill) in a controlled setting. While the ED-AWARENESS rate of AWP (2.6%) may seem relatively low, this number is far from trivial. This rate of AWP translates to a large number of patients each year when considering the number of mechanically intubated patients in EDs annually. AWP may contribute to several long-term psychological effects such as major depression, anxiety, complex phobias, and post-traumatic stress disorder [36–38].

Pharmacists involved in RSI play a pivotal role in providing adequate sedation and analgesia during trauma. Rocuronium is an important risk factor to AWP [31]. Amini et al. found that the presence of a pharmacist led to a decreased time to sedation and analgesia in trauma patients undergoing RSI with rocuronium as the paralytic [39]. Several other studies have evaluated the role of the pharmacist on post-intubation sedation analgesia and have found that the presence of a pharmacist decreases time to sedation and analgesia [40, 41]. Thoughtful selection of the paralytic along with adequate sedation should be considered if a long-acting paralytic is used.

Clinical practice guidelines for pain, agitation/sedation, delirium, immobility, and sleep disruption in adult ICU patients (PADIS) were published in 2018 and focus on a variety of strategies that improve care and reduce delirium in critically ill adults [42]. Recommendations are applicable to trauma patients and stress the importance of protocolized, stepwise approach for pain and sedation while providing options to reduce opiates and provide light sedation when possible. Emergency department staff are often focused on other priorities including procedures, imaging, and further patient stabilization, which may preclude the strict adherence to pain and sedation protocols. For such reasons, pain and sedation medications are often given liberally when possible. Nonetheless, EDs should strive to have standard protocol-driven assessments and management of analgesia and sedation. Light sedation should be aimed for using short-acting agents and avoiding benzodiazepines when possible [42].

A common scoring tool used for sedation in ventilated patients is the Richmond Agitation-Sedation Scale (RASS). No strict definition of light sedation exists, but a RASS score of −2 to +1 (or equivalent using other scales) was used to evaluate light sedation literature in the PADIS guidelines. The SED-ED trial published in 2020 found that deep sedation was administered to the majority of ED patients across 15 study centers, a practice which carried over to the ICU setting in most cases [30]. Patients receiving deep sedation in the ED had more hospital-free days (OR 2.3;

95% CI: 0.26–4.32). Many other important outcomes, while not statistically significant, were numerically in favor of lighter sedation, such as ventilator-free days, ICU-free days, and mortality. These results show that ED sedation practice is often centered on deep sedation, and this practice carries over to the ICU setting, where it has been shown to result in poor patient outcomes including higher mortality [43–46].

In conclusion, sedation and analgesia are important aspects of patient care. While deep sedation should be avoided, light sedation can be challenging in the ED setting with various competing priorities. On the other hand, inadvertent inadequate sedation and analgesia can also be a concern in the ED, especially when long-acting paralytics are used [29]. Widespread provider and nursing education on medication traits such as duration of action, development of protocols, and order sets, along with bedside vigilance are key to optimal treatment of trauma patients.

41.4 Initial Analgesia Management and Local Anesthetics

Various intravenous agents can be administered for sedation and analgesia in acute trauma patients. Depending on intubation status, blood pressure, and level of pain, different medications and treatment modalities can be considered.

Fentanyl is a desirable first-line analgesic agent in the setting of trauma because of its quick onset, short duration, and relatively favorable adverse effect profile. Fentanyl is a synthetic opioid agonist and causes very little histamine release ([47]). Hypotension is therefore considered to occur to a lesser extent than with other opioids. Fentanyl's onset is rapid, and the duration of analgesic effect is 30–60 min after a single IV dose. Morphine and hydromorphone are also frequently used opioids in the acute trauma setting and typically utilized for their longer duration of action.

Nonsteroidal anti-inflammatory drugs (NSAIDS) are frequently used in traumatic injuries for analgesia. Since NSAIDs inhibit prostaglandin-mediated platelet aggregation, the primary concern of using NSAIDs in trauma patients is increased risk of bleeding. NSAIDs may portend an increased risk of bleeding but is seen after multiple doses in steady-state concentrations and found to be less than with antiplatelet and anticoagulant agents [48]. Ketorolac is a common NSAID used to treat acute pain. A randomized controlled trial performed in an ED setting found that ketorolac had equal analgesic effect when patients were given a 10 mg, 15 mg, or 30 mg single-dose [49].

It may be favorable to avoid NSAIDS in older adults or those with acute kidney injury due to risk of further renal injury. If opioids have been optimized in this case, an alternative choice may be acetaminophen. Intravenous acetaminophen was approved by the FDA in 2010 for the treatment of acute pain. IV acetaminophen use has been controversial and often has limited status on inpatient formularies due to studies showing no difference in pain reduction versus oral acetaminophen [50].

Nevertheless, IV acetaminophen remains an option for those unable to tolerate oral analgesia or have contraindications to other IV agents.

Ketamine in sub-dissociative doses has also been evaluated for the treatment of analgesia. Studies have shown that ketamine is as effective as morphine in relieving pain at 15 and 30 min [51]. The dose for this indication is 0.1–0.6 mg/kg, with the most studied dose being 0.3 mg/kg [51, 52]. It is recommended to administer ketamine as a slow infusion over 15 min to avoid adverse effects such as feelings of unreality and sedation [53]. This modality may be considered when initial medications are unable to control the patient's pain. Relative contraindications to sub-dissociative dose ketamine include poorly controlled cardiovascular disease, pregnancy, psychosis, hepatic disease, and elevated intracranial and intraocular pressure [54].

41.5 Local Anesthesia

Localized anesthesia is often desirable and necessary in various scenarios involving trauma. Trauma may involve lacerations or wounds that need suturing, debridement, or cleaning. Decompression of a pneumothorax with insertion of a chest tube may be warranted. In less urgent chest tube placements, local anesthesia can minimize discomfort in a conscious patient. However, such procedures may require procedural systemic analgesia and sedation if large and complex.

Local anesthesia is achieved by infiltrating soft tissue surrounding a nerve with a sodium channel blocker, inhibiting the propagation of action potential through the neurons. A variety of local anesthetics and formulations exist to maximize effect, minimize bleeding, and avoid toxicity. Lidocaine and bupivacaine are frequently used for laceration repair and wound debridement in the acute setting. Most local anesthetics are available with various concentrations of epinephrine. Adding a vasopressor to peripheral nerve blockade serves two purposes. First, vasopressors reduce absorption of the medication, thereby increasing the duration of nerve blockade while reducing the risk of systemic toxicity. Second, the addition of a vasoconstrictor can reduce bleeding if problematic. Medication profiles are shown in Table 41.2.

Table 41.2 Local anesthetic pharmacological profiles [55–59]

Local anesthetic	Maximum dose (24 h)	Half-life[a] (h)	Duration (h) after infiltration[a]	Lipid solubility
Lidocaine	4.5 mg/kg (max 300 mg) (7 mg/kg with epinephrine, max 500 mg)	1.6	1–2	+
Bupivacaine	2 mg/kg (max 175 mg) (2.5 mg/kg with epinephrine, max 225 mg)	2.7	3–4	+++
Ropivacaine	3 mg/kg (max 200 mg) (4 mg/kg with epinephrine, max 250 mg)	1.8	2–6	+

[a]Epinephrine will extend the tissue half-life and duration

Regional analgesia can be achieved with a neuraxial block such as an epidural, which is not typically performed in acute trauma, or a peripheral nerve block. Peripheral nerve blocks are increasingly being taught and performed in the ED setting for large lacerations, and joint and fracture reductions [60]. Utilization of regional nerve blocks compared to procedural sedation is endorsed by multiple professional physician societies and has been shown to decrease resource utilization, length of stay, and opioid use and improve patient recovery [61–63]. Ultrasound sonography is utilized for peripheral nerve blocks in order to locate and ensure specific nerve anatomy, and surrounding tissue is appropriately anesthetized with local anesthetics. The same sodium channel blocking local anesthetics may be used for peripheral nerve blocks, but there is a higher risk of inadvertent intravenous or intra-arterial injection with these procedures. Accordingly, regional nerve blocks require more vigilance with regard to maximum dose in order to avoid local anesthetic systemic toxicity (LAST).

Local anesthetic systemic toxicity is a rare but serious adverse event most commonly reported with regional nerve blocks. Mild symptoms include mild subjective symptoms such as sedation and confusion, but these can be prodromal to more severe adverse effects. Seizure, dysrhythmia, and cardiac arrest are signs of LAST that require prompt attention [64]. Seizures should be treated with benzodiazepines. When dysrhythmia, hypotension, or cardiac arrest occur, intravenous lipid emulsion (ILE) therapy should be administered. Unfortunately, most evidence supporting the use of lipid emulsion therapy is from animal studies, and only case reports exist for humans. Nevertheless, the recommended dose of ILE is 1.5 mL/kg of 20% lipid emulsion (max 100 mL) administered as a bolus dose over 2–3 min. If the patient continues to be unstable with no response, an additional bolus can be considered. A maximum dose of 10–12 mL/kg of 20% ILE has been suggested, and a continuous infusion may be considered but this approach is controversial [64, 65]. Toxicology or poison center consultation is recommended in all cases involving severe local anesthetic systemic toxicity.

41.6 Trauma-Induced Coagulopathy

Patients experiencing severe trauma face risks of hypercoagulable (excessive clotting), hypocoagulable (insufficient clotting), or mixed states. This variability can lead to significant bleeding, clot formation, or a combination of both, depending on the time elapsed since the injury [66] (Fig. 41.1).

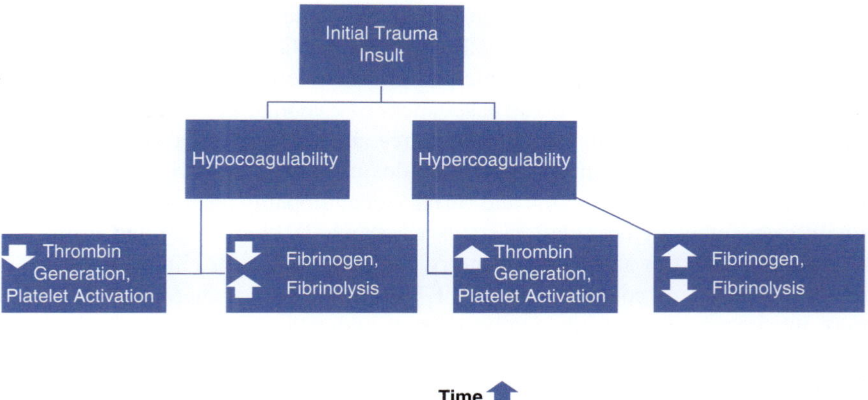

Fig. 41.1 Hyper- and hypocoagulability in trauma [66]

41.6.1 Coagulopathy

Trauma-induced coagulopathy (TIC) is a complex and multifactorial condition that occurs in patients suffering from severe trauma. The phenotypic expression of TIC is composed of disturbances in clotting factor activity, platelet aggregation, dysfibrinogenemia, and fibrinolysis. Other factors like hypocalcemia, hypothermia, and metabolic acidosis from impaired oxygen delivery also contribute to TIC directly and indirectly. As clinician understanding of pathological disturbances has evolved, more emphasis has been placed on the cellular components found in whole blood rather than just plasma derived factor issues [67]. This cell- based model emphasizes the role platelets have at primary hemostasis and is theorized to more closely mimic what is happening in vivo than the traditional model of coagulation.

One of the most challenging aspects of TIC is that no formal definition exists; therefore, consensus management and prognostic assessment become extremely difficult for clinical practice, as well as research. Effective management of TIC includes appropriate damage control as well as resuscitation with blood products, calcium, and mitigating coagulopathy induced from medications with reversal or prothrombotic agents [68, 69]. Additionally, timely diagnosis is vital to begin early definitive resuscitation measures [70]. Traditional laboratory tests such as prothrombin time/international normalized ratio (PT/INR), activated partial thromboplastin time (aPTT), fibrinogen levels, and platelet count, have been historically used in assessing coagulopathy in critically ill patients [71]. However, these tests have limitations in the context of acute trauma, with the most important being that they only provide quantitative data without functional assessment. Viscoelastic testing methods (VET), such as thromboelastography (TEG®) and rotational thromboelastometry (ROTEM®), have re-emerged as valuable prognostic and therapeutic tools offering real-time, functional assessment of coagulation dynamics in one single test. The differences in testing procedures and variables measured are outside the scope of this chapter but have been well documented. Patients experiencing TIC often present with hyperdynamic and variable coagulopathy phenotypes. Therefore, timely assessment of coagulation status using whole blood tests that mimic the hemostatic properties at the site of injury can be valuable for clinicians [72]. The cell-based model of coagulation and VET are interrelated where both provide a more integrated and physiologically relevant understanding of hemostasis. Some advantages and disadvantages of both traditional and VET methods are listed in Table 41.3.

The use of VET is unique in that they have been applied diagnostically, prognostically, and therapeutically in the management of trauma patients [73, 74]. Parameters of interest in the management of TIC include clotting factor dysfunction, dysfibrinogenemia, alterations in platelet aggregation, medication-induced coagulopathies contributing to TIC, and disturbances in physiological fibrinolysis. While no validated treatment algorithm exists, most literature will utilize prothrombin complex concentrates or fresh frozen plasma with retardation in clotting factor activity, fibrinogen concentrates or cryoprecipitate if dysfibrinogenemia is noted, desmopressin or platelet transfusion with reduced platelet aggregation noted, and antifibrinolytics such as tranexamic acid if hyperfibrinolysis is present [75]. Currently, the use of VET for guided resuscitation of medication-induced coagulopathy remains a promising area of ongoing research with slow adoption into clinical practice given market availability, paucity of associated literature, and lack of validated algorithms associated with their use in this cohort [76–78].

A recent systematic review evaluated the utility of VET in guiding hemostatic resuscitation for trauma patients [79]. The review incorporated ten studies—two randomized controlled trials (RCTs) and eight observational studies. These studies

Table 41.3 Strengths and limitations of tests utilized in assessing trauma-induced coagulopathy [71, 72]

Aspect	Traditional coagulation tests	Viscoelastic testing
Standardization	Well standardized with most formal training for clinicians based on these tests	Less standardized, variability across devices, not interchangeable
Turnaround time	Relative but most produce results within $\leq$45 min	Rapid results; can be monitored in real time
Evaluation of clot formation and lysis	Can provide quantitative assessment of factors II, VII, IX, and X; serial fibrinogen or D-dimer levels may be utilized but has limited sensitivity in trauma	Provides functional assessment of both clot initiation, speed, and fibrinolysis status in a single test; provides functional assessment of platelets at receptor sites
Cost	Lower initial costs and maintenance	May provide net benefit in overall healthcare costs

were assessed for their impact on various outcomes, including mortality, blood transfusion requirements, hospital length of stay (LOS), intensive care unit (ICU) LOS, incidence of massive transfusions, and serious adverse events (ADEs). In this cohort however, it's likely that mortality, blood product transfusion, and serious ADEs are the most relevant.

The review reported mixed outcomes regarding mortality. Two studies demonstrated a reduction in mortality with VET-guided strategies. Specifically, Cochrane et al. found significantly lower 24-h and 30-day mortalities in the post-TEG group [80]. Gonzalez et al. observed significantly lower 6-h and 28-day mortality rates in the TEG group compared to the conventional coagulation test (CCT) group [81]. However, eight other studies, including the only multicenter trial, ITACTIC, did not find significant differences in mortality between VET-guided and control groups [82]. Notably, the ITACTIC study did report reduced 28-day mortality in trauma patients with severe traumatic brain injury (TBI) when guided by VET. Interestingly, only a small number of patients in both cohorts required massive transfusion, and a large portion of patients in both groups did not receive any blood products. This may help explain why there was no significant difference observed between the treatment groups. Another study highlighted a significant reduction in total mortality among trauma patients under 30 years of age after implementing a TEG strategy, though no difference was observed in the overall trauma patient population [83].

The impact of VET-guided strategies on blood product usage was variable. Some studies noted that VHA implementation reduced blood product usage, while others did not find significant differences. For instance, one study reported that patients in the TEG group received less plasma and platelets in the first 2 h of resuscitation, though this difference was not significant over 24 h [84]. In the ITACTIC study, VET-guided patients received more fibrinogen equivalent and similar plasma between baseline and hemostasis, but less plasma at 24 h post-injury compared to the CCT group [82]. Additionally, patients were more likely to receive platelet transfusion, highlighting the overall emphasis that non-plasma-based coagulation disturbances are identified with VET use. Observational studies also varied, with some reporting reductions in blood product usage and others noting increases or no significant differences.

Serious adverse event incidence, including thromboembolic events, sepsis, and acute kidney injury, was similar between VET-guided and control groups according to the two RCTs included in the review [79]. Observational studies provided mixed results regarding the cost-effectiveness of VET-guided strategies, with some indicating higher costs for blood products in the post-VET group, while others reported lower or equal costs compared to pre-VET protocols.

TIC represents a major challenge in the management of severely injured patients. While conventional coagulation tests have been the cornerstone of diagnostic and treatment approaches, the use of VET has re-emerged as a possible adjunct or primary tool in the management of these patients. The use of VET methods offers significant advantages by delivering real-time, whole blood assessments of hemostasis, guiding targeted therapeutic interventions, and improving clinical outcomes. Evidence currently demonstrates a moderate benefit of their use over traditional testing. As more personnel are trained in their use, operational functions become more efficient, and our understanding of pathophysiology evolves, their use may eventually outgrow traditional assessments. It is likely that the integration of VET into trauma care protocols is likely to become more widespread, enhancing the management and prognosis of patients with TIC.

41.7 Shock Management for the Pharmacist

Shock, which is defined as inadequate perfusion and oxygenation leading to cellular and tissue hypoxia (Table 41.4), in trauma patients is a critical condition that requires prompt and effective management to prevent irreversible organ damage and death [85]. Management consists of a multifaceted and dynamic process that requires a thorough understanding of various interventions, including blood therapy resuscitation, the sparing use of vasopressors, and calcium supplementation. The etiology of shock when trauma patients initially present is considered to be hemorrhagic, until ruled out, as hemorrhage is the common cause of shock in this patient population. The concept of damage control is stratified into three parts: surgical control to obtain hemostasis, physiological restoration, and definitive surgical repair [86]. Since up to 40% of all trauma mortality is associated with blood loss, it is imperative pharmacists understand appropriate resuscitation strategies [85].

41.7.1 Integrative Approach to Shock Management

Effective shock management in trauma requires an integrative approach that combines the principles of damage control resuscitation (DCR) with appropriate use of vasopressors and calcium supplementation. Early recognition and treatment are crucial given that delayed care is associated with increased

Table 41.4 Hemorrhagic shock classification [85]

Class I hemorrhage	Class II hemorrhage	Class III hemorrhage	Class IV hemorrhage
• 15% blood loss • Tachycardia may or may not be present • Transfusion not required • Restoration of blood volume $\leq$24 h	• 15–30% blood volume loss • Clinical symptoms present • Requires fluid replacement with positive clinical findings	• 30–40% blood volume loss • Classic signs of inadequate perfusion • Require emergent transfusion and/or operation	• >40% blood volume loss • Life-threatening injury requiring massive blood transfusion and immediate surgical intervention

mortality [70]. Initial treatment should consist of early blood product resuscitation with limited crystalloid therapy. Continuous hemodynamic monitoring, along with frequent assessment of laboratory parameters, allows for real-time adjustments in resuscitation strategies. This ensures that the patient's physiological needs are met promptly, minimizing the risk of under-resuscitation or over-resuscitation. Management of shock in trauma patients requires a coordinated effort from a multidisciplinary team, including trauma surgeons, emergency physicians, anesthesiologists, pharmacists, nurses, respiratory therapist, spiritual support personnel, and other critical care specialists. Effective communication and collaboration among team members are essential for optimizing patient outcomes especially in a high stress resuscitative effort.

41.7.2 Transfusion Therapy

One of the largest parts of physiological restoration is by the use of DCR. Most cases of shock secondary to hemorrhage require passage through the emergency department or trauma bay. It is during this time frame that expedited identification of potential bleeding sites with physical exam and imaging are needed. Initial resuscitation begins with transfusion therapy pre- and intraoperatively during this time. Both hemostatic and hemodynamic resuscitation must be accounted for to ensure adequate blood flow to vital organs, while mitigating ongoing hemorrhage with permissive hypotension in the absence of any neurological injury. One aspect of resuscitation of trauma patients as opposed to other critically ill patients is the sparing use of crystalloid therapies [87]. The mitigation of acid–base disturbances, which can contribute to ongoing coagulopathy, and prevention of a dilutional effect on hemostasis are proposed rationales for avoiding their use.

Balanced transfusion, often referred to as a 1:1:1 ratio, involves the transfusion of packed red blood cells (PRBCs), fresh frozen plasma (FFP), and platelets. This approach aims to mimic whole blood, providing oxygen-carrying capacity, clotting factors, and platelets simultaneously, which is crucial for maintaining hemostasis in bleeding patients. Studies have shown that such balanced transfusion strategies improve survival rates in trauma patients with severe hemorrhage [88]. Recently, there has been a resurgence in the use of whole blood transfusion, particularly in military settings and civilian trauma centers with massive transfusion protocols. Whole blood provides all necessary components in one product, simplifying logistics and potentially improving outcomes, including 24-h mortality rates, by reducing the dilutional coagulopathy seen with the use of FFP, PRBCs, and platelet transfusions [89]. Adopting a goal-directed approach, where the decision to transfuse is based on physiological parameters and laboratory values (such as hemoglobin levels, lactate, and base deficit), helps in optimizing the balance between adequate resuscitation and the risk of transfusion-related complications [90]. Often, patients require large volume resuscitation of blood, triggering massive transfusion protocols (MTP). Determining when to initiate MTP is critical. Common triggers include hemodynamic instability, signs of shock, and significant ongoing hemorrhage [91]. MTPs are designed to provide rapid and structured delivery of blood products to patients with life-threatening hemorrhage, ensuring that transfusions are both timely and balanced. The early activation of MTPs has been shown to improve survival rates by maintaining hemodynamic stability and ensuring adequate tissue perfusion. Initiation, prediction, and monitoring of MTPs have been previously discussed with VET vs. traditional methods.

Blood transfusion is a critical component in the management of trauma patients. While it is necessary to replace lost blood volume and improve oxygen delivery to tissues, it carries significant risks. Complications such as transfusion-related acute lung injury (TRALI), characterized by acute respiratory distress, and transfusion-associated circulatory overload (TACO), resulting from volume overload, require immediate cessation of transfusion and initiation supportive care [92]. Caused by donor antibodies reacting with recipient leukocytes, TRALI is a serious condition, typically occurring within 6 h of transfusion. Symptoms include dyspnea, hypoxemia, fever, and bilateral pulmonary infiltrates. The incidence rate of TRALI in trauma patients is estimated to be around 0.08% to 15% [93]. Early recognition and supportive respiratory care are crucial for management. TACO results from the inability of the recipient's circulatory system to manage the volume of transfused blood, leading to pulmonary edema [94]. Symptoms include dyspnea, hypertension, tachycardia, and jugular venous distension. The incidence rate of TACO can range from 1% to 8% in surgical patients, with higher rates observed in those receiving massive transfusions. Management includes the utilization of diuretics, oxygen supplementation, and adjusting transfusion rates to mitigate fluid overload. In addition to TACO and TRALI, lesser prevalent transfusion-related reactions have been described associated with hemolytic and infectious processes. Electrolyte imbalances such as hypocalcemia and hyperkalemia from massive transfusions further complicate care [95].

41.7.3 Hypocalcemia in Trauma Patients

Hypocalcemia is a significant concern in trauma patients due to various mechanisms associated with trauma that can lead to this imbalance (Table 41.5). In fact, hypocalcemia has been recognized as such an important factor in the resuscitation of trauma patients that the classic "triad of death" in trauma patients (coagulopathy, hypothermia, acidosis) has been updated to include hypocalcemia, forming what is commonly referred to as the "death diamond." The incidence rate varies given that the definition and method used to identify are inconsistent in the literature, but some estimates of over 50% of patients with hemorrhagic shock in trauma will experience hypocalcemia [68]. The two biggest risk factors include massive blood transfusion, where citrate in stored blood products binds calcium, reducing ionized calcium levels, and hemorrhagic shock, which leads to hypocalcemia through dilutional effects of whole blood loss, dilution with resuscitation, and again citrate binding. Severe

Table 41.5 Common causes of hypocalcemia in trauma patients [96, 97]

Hypocalcemia cause	Description
Hemorrhagic shock	Loss of blood and components including calcium
Intracellular influx	Intracellular shift of calcium secondary to ischemia and hypoperfusion
Impaired homeostasis	Impaired calcium regulation post-traumatic insult
Increased sympathetic activity	Increased sympathetic activation can lead to hypocalcemia
Citrated blood transfusion	Citrated products that are not metabolized can chelate calcium
Hepatic dysfunction	Reduced citrate metabolism increases serum citrate levels and hypocalcemia

tissue injury can release intracellular components, disrupting calcium homeostasis, while renal dysfunction, common in trauma patients, impairs calcium regulation [98]. Hyperventilation-induced respiratory alkalosis increases calcium binding to albumin, lowering ionized calcium levels, and sepsis can further exacerbate hypocalcemia through increased capillary permeability and altered hormone levels (although is not often seen in the early stages of acute trauma).

Hypocalcemia is associated with increased mortality in trauma patients, with studies showing that low ionized calcium levels upon admission correlate with higher mortality, especially in patients with higher Injury Severity Scores (ISS) and persistent hypocalcemia during hospitalization, as well as an early predictor of the necessity for blood transfusion [99]. Management of hypocalcemia in trauma patients involves regular monitoring of ionized calcium levels, particularly in patients receiving massive transfusions, and timely administration of intravenous calcium (calcium gluconate or calcium chloride) to maintain normal levels, which improves hemodynamics and reduces transfusion requirements [100]. Balanced resuscitation strategies, including careful fluid management and the use of blood products and crystalloids, help maintain electrolyte balance, including calcium levels. Implementing trauma resuscitation protocols with guidelines for calcium management and involving a multidisciplinary team ensures comprehensive management of hypocalcemia and other metabolic disturbances, reducing complications and improving survival rates in trauma patients. In conclusion, prompt recognition and management of hypocalcemia through evidence-based strategies and a multidisciplinary approach are essential for reducing mortality and improving prognosis in trauma patients.

41.7.4   Vasopressor Support in Patients with Traumatic Injuries

The use of vasopressors in trauma patients, particularly those with hemorrhagic shock, presents both benefits and risks [101]. Beyond just pure volume loss, patients with trauma often exhibit reduced sympathetic tone leading to hypotension. Vasopressors can reduce the need for large volumes of resuscitation fluids, potentially preventing complications associated with fluid overload [102]. However, early administration and higher doses are linked to increased mortality, as often times they prevent rapid administration of blood products and increase organ ischemia. There are inconsistencies among trauma centers nationally and internationally on the appropriate use of vasopressors in traumatic shock with some advocating for early vasopressor use while others to omit entirely [103]. Additionally, in non-neurotrauma cohort's, permissive hypotension is often permitted to promote vasoconstriction and reduce newly formed clots from rupturing, but this is based on inconsistent data sets [104]. The optimal timing, agent, and dosing remain unknown. Lastly, it remains unknown if there is a selection bias toward increased mortality in patients with traumatic shock receiving vasopressors secondary to having more refractory cases than those that do not require them.

Norepinephrine is generally recommended as the first-line vasopressor in managing hypotensive shock in trauma patients due to its efficacy in increasing mean arterial pressure (MAP). Vasopressin, while also used, is often considered a second-line agent. However, the AVERT-Shock trial indicated that low-dose vasopressin (≤ 0.04 units/min) could decrease blood product requirements in hemorrhagic shock without increasing complications, although more research is needed to determine its optimal timing and dosage [105]. For spinal cord injuries, vasopressors such as norepinephrine and dopamine are crucial in managing neurogenic shock in maintaining a MAP of 85–90 mmHg for the first 7 days post-injury, as recommended by the Consortium for Spinal Cord Medicine guidelines, to optimize spinal cord perfusion and improve neurological outcomes [106]. Striving for an increased MAP is suspected to increase perfusion and reduce ischemia and secondary injuries. Currently, minimal data exists on the optimal agent in patients with spinal cord injuries. Similar to other cohorts, norepinephrine is generally utilized as first-line vasopressor with vasopressin, midodrine, phenylephrine, and pseudoephedrine all having been evaluated in this cohort. The use of corticosteroids remains polarizing in this population with proponents of the therapy advocating for their neuroprotective effects in reducing inflammation and secondary injury attenuation while improving sensory and motor functions [107, 108]. Opponents of their use discuss the paucity of evidence demonstrating benefit with increases in infection, gastrointestinal bleeding, hyperglycemia, and delayed wound healing.

The management of traumatic shock caused by tension pneumothorax and cardiac tamponade requires immediate recognition and prompt intervention due to their life-threatening nature. Tension pneumothorax occurs when air accumulates in the pleural space, leading to increased intrathoracic pressure, lung collapse, and compromised venous return, resulting in shock [109]. Immediate decompression is crucial, typically achieved by needle thoracostomy followed by chest tube placement to re-expand the lung and restore hemodynamic stability. Cardiac tamponade is caused by the accumulation of blood or fluid in the pericardial sac, compressing the heart and impeding its ability to pump effectively, leading to shock [110]. Rapid diagnosis via clinical signs and ultrasound is essential. Management involves pericardiocentesis to aspirate the accumulated fluid and relieve pressure around the heart. Both conditions require supportive care, including fluid resuscitation and oxygenation, alongside definitive surgical interventions to address the underlying injuries and prevent recurrence. Early recognition and intervention are critical to improving outcomes in patients with traumatic shock due to tension pneumothorax and cardiac tamponade.

Effective shock management in trauma patients hinges on a comprehensive approach that integrates blood therapy resuscitation, vasopressor utilization when indicated, and calcium supplementation. Each component plays a distinct but interrelated role in stabilizing the patient, preventing secondary complications, and improving survival rates. By adhering to evidence-based protocols and maintaining vigilant monitoring, healthcare providers can navigate the complexities of trauma-induced shock and deliver optimal care to this critically ill population.

41.8   Tranexamic Acid

During fibrinolysis, plasminogen binds to fibrin through its lysine binding site. The complex is cleaved by tissue plasminogen activator by converting plasminogen to plasmin. Tranexamic acid (TXA) is a synthetic lysine analog that inhibits the conversion of plasminogen to plasmin, preventing hemorrhage by stabilizing the fibrin clot [111]. Typical dosing of TXA in trauma is 1 g followed by an infusion of 1 g over 8 h [112]. Newer studies have utilized 2 g as a single bolus for ease of administration in the prehospital setting [113, 114]. Evidence supporting the use of TXA in trauma is mixed due to heterogeneity between mechanism of injury, timing of medication administration, and injury severity score. There does not appear to be increased risk of thromboembolic complications except in use of military patient population [115].

Clinical randomization of an antifibrinolytic in significant hemorrhage (CRASH-2) was the first study to show a decrease in all-cause mortality and death due to bleeding when TXA was given within 3 h of injury in trauma patients; however, the study also has limitations, including no injury severity score reported, majority of patients were from low to moderate income developing countries, only half of the patients included received a transfusion, and approximately 5% of patients had bleeding as cause of death [112]. The use of TXA is recommended for the bleeding patient or at risk for bleeding in the European guidelines for trauma coagulopathy [116]. Other studies have not shown a benefit in the prehospital setting [117, 118].

When looking at TXA in specific patient populations such as patients with mild to moderate traumatic brain injury, TXA decreased mortality when given within 3 h [119]. The CRASH-3 trial did not demonstrate mortality benefits in severe head injury patients. In military trauma, TXA decreased mortality with a benefit also seen in patients with massive transfusion [115]. The use of TXA in the bleeding combat patient is supported by the Joint Trauma System Tactical Combat Casualty Care (TCCC) Guidelines [120]. Other observational civilian trauma studies have shown mixed mortality benefits when used as an adjunct during massive transfusion [121–123]. Further studies are needed to elucidate the trauma patients that may benefit the most from TXA and the optimal dosing strategy.

41.9 Anticoagulation Reversal

The prehospital use of anticoagulants in injured trauma patients can lead to bleeding complications resulting in increased transfusions and mortality. Prompt identification of anticoagulant use can prevent worsening bleeding, especially in the elderly as anticoagulant use is common. The decision to reverse should be based upon the severity and location of bleeding, while also considering the anticoagulant pharmacokinetics (Table 41.6) and indication [124–128]. Obtaining information regarding the type of anticoagulant the patient uses, their last dose, and indication for use is not always available and may rely on collateral information and/or laboratory monitoring.

Apixaban, rivaroxaban, and edoxaban are factor Xa inhibitors or direct oral anticoagulants (DOACs). DOACs are the most common anticoagulant agents, especially in elderly patients. Unfortunately, there are limited blood tests to detect aberrations in coagulation due to these agents. Detection on thromboelastography has limited data and is variable, and the use of prothrombin time (PT) and activated partial thromboplastin time (PTT) is also variable depending on severity of coagulopathy [76, 78, 129].

Andexanet alfa is a recombinant human factor Xa protein used for life-threatening or uncontrolled bleeding for patients on factor Xa inhibitors taken within the last 24 hours. Andexanet alfa has two dosing regimens based upon last dose of factor Xa inhibitors and dose. The low-dose regimen is a 400 mg bolus followed by 4 mg/min for 120 min while the high dose is an 800 mg bolus followed by an 8 mg/min for infusion 120 min. Most of the data for Andexanet is for patients with an intracranial hemorrhage on a factor Xa inhibitor with a GCS of 13–15 [130, 131]. Prior to Andexanet's approval, 4-factor prothrombin complex concentrate (4F-PCC) was considered the standard of care for patients with life-threatening bleeding or requiring an operative procedure on a DOAC. 4F-PCC dosing strategies can be either a weight-based dose of 25–50 units/kg or a fixed dose strategy of 2000 units can be considered [132]. Guidelines currently recommend andexanet alfa with 4F-PCC as an alternative if andexanet alfa is not available for factor Xa reversal [133].

Table 41.6 Pharmacokinetics of oral anticoagulants

	Time to peak (h)	Half-life (h)	Hepatic metabolism	Renal elimination (%)
Apixaban	1–4	12	Yes	25
Rivaroxaban	2–4	5–9	Yes	33
Edoxaban	1–2	10–14	Yes	50
Warfarin	72–96	20–60	Yes	–
Dabigatran	1–2	11–13	Minimal	80

Table 41.7 Warfarin reversal strategy

	INR 2–<4	INR 4–6	INR > 6	Fixed dose non-intracranial bleed	Fixed dose ICH
4F-PCC dose	25 unit/kg (max 2500 unit)	35 units/kg (max 3500 unit)	50 units/kg (max 5000 unit)	1000 units	1500 units

Dabigatran is a direct thrombin inhibitor that's use has diminished since the approval of factor Xa inhibitors. Thrombin time (TT) is the most sensitive for detecting dabigatran in the plasma. A normal TT can rule out the presence of a significant amount of dabigatran. Activated partial thromboplastin time (aPTT) is likely to be often prolonged at the peak of dabigatran levels, but at trough, aPTT is likely to be prolonged only if that particular aPTT reagent is sensitive to dabigatran. Due to variability with aPTT and reagents, a normal aPTT cannot rule out the presence of dabigatran in the plasma. Idarucizumab is a humanized monoclonal antibody fragment that binds to free and bound dabigatran and is indicated for reversal of patients with severe bleeding. The recommended dose of idarucizumab is 5 g.

Warfarin inhibits vitamin k dependent clotting factors II, VII, IX, and X, in addition to protein C and S. For immediate reversal of major bleeding, prothrombin complex concentrate (PCC) is preferred due to faster time to reversal when compared to fresh frozen plasma. Dosing of 4F-PCC is weight based and dependent on INR (Table 41.7). A fixed dosing strategy of 1500 units for intracranial hemorrhage (ICH) or 1000 units for all other bleeds can also be utilized [132]. Due to the long half-life of warfarin and the potential for rebound INR, vitamin K 5–10 mg via an IV infusion over 30 minutes is also recommended in conjunction with PCC.

41.10 Traumatic Brain Injury

Traumatic brain injury (TBI) is a major cause of disability, morbidity, and mortality. Previous data estimate approximately 2.8 million TBI-related ED visits, 282,000 hospitalizations, and 5600 annual deaths in the United States. The highest rates of TBIs occurred in persons aged ≥ 75 years or <4 years due to falls or blunt force injury. Motor vehicle crashes account for the second most common mechanism in for those aged 15–44 years [134].

TBI pathophysiology is a complex process with many factors influencing presentation and response including primary injury, blunt or penetrating trauma, and secondary processes such as seizures, hematoma expansion, and neuroplasticity. Secondary injuries can happen minutes to days from the primary injury with a cascade of molecular, chemical, and inflammatory changes resulting in disruption in the blood–brain barrier and further cerebral damage.

During the primary survey, a brief neurologic exam assesses motor, verbal, and eye opening using the 15-poing Glasgow Coma Scale (GCS). Mild TBI is defined

Table 41.8 Glasgow Coma Scale

Score	Eye opening (*E*)	Verbal response (*V*)	Best motor response (*M*)
1	None	None	None
2	To pressure	Sounds	Extension
3	To sound	Words	Abnormal flexion
4	Spontaneous	Confused	Normal flexion
5	N/A	Oriented	Localizing
6	N/A	N/A	Obeys commands

[a]GCS score = *E* + *V* + *M* = Best possible score 15; worst possible score 3

Table 41.9 GCS classification and severity of brain injury

Score	Severity of injury
13–15	Mild
9–12	Moderate
3–8	Severe

as GCS $\geq$ 13, moderate TBI as GCS 9–12, and severe TBI as CGS $\leq$ 8 [135, 136]. Refer to Tables 41.8 and 41.9 above for calculation of GCS score and classification of severity of brain injury. A more in-depth neurologic evaluation of pupils and motor strength and sensation is completed during the secondary exam. Assessment of the intubated patient is difficult and relies on pupil reactivity, symmetry, and cough/gag reflexes. The intoxicated patient with alcohol, recreational drugs, and medications taken prior to arrival have the potential to impact the GCS exam and further imaging is needed. The prehospital use of anticoagulants is associated with a two to six times greater mortality rate, and rapid correction of coagulopathy must also be prioritized. The goal of treatment is to prevent secondary brain injury from hypoxia, cerebral hypoperfusion, and elevated intracranial pressure. This is achieved by establishment of an airway, adequate oxygenation, and ventilation, hemodynamic stability to maintain cerebral perfusion pressure, and reduction in ICP. Systolic blood pressure (SBP) should be maintained at $\geq$100 mmHg for patients 50–69 years of age or 110 mmHg for patient <50 years or >70 years of age as studies have shown better outcomes associated with mortality [137, 138]. In patients that are intubated, adequate sedation should be prioritized to slow down the overall metabolic process and consideration should be given to continuous infusion agents such as propofol, which can also reduce ICP. When administering fluid, either isotonic or hypertonic fluids are recommended.

41.11　Hyperosmolar Therapy

The initiation of hyperosmolar therapy may be based upon the patient's signs and symptoms of herniation such as Cushing's phenomenon. This phenomenon consists of bradycardia, irregular respirations, and hypertension or widened pulse pressure, imaging, or a combination. Hyperosmolar therapy, such as mannitol or hypertonic saline (HTS) may be a useful temporizing measure for lowering intracranial pressure and cerebral edema until more definitive treatment is established. The primary mechanism of action of mannitol in the reduction of ICP is by increasing the osmotic gradient across the blood–brain barrier, thereby creating an osmosis of water from the brain parenchyma to extracellular space. Dosing is variable from 0.5 to 1.5 g/kg. Retrospective studies showed that ICP lowering was not dependent on mannitol dose but potentially higher initial ICP [139]. The higher the ICP, the more disturbed the blood–brain barrier, resulting in a greater fluid shift across the blood–brain barrier. Since mannitol is an osmotic diuretic, mannitol can precipitate hypotension and caution is advised in patients with labile blood pressure and it should be avoided in patients with a systolic blood pressure (SBP) < 90 mmHg.

Hypertonic saline's predominant mechanism of action is an osmotic shift of fluid across the blood–brain barrier. Concentrations of HTS vary widely, from 2% to 23.4%, with little evidence to support a superior concentration, but may rely more on the osmolar load delivered to the patient. Ideally, a premade solution of HTS such as 3% or 5% should be utilized and stored in trauma areas to avoid delays. When utilizing 3% sodium chloride, 250 mL or 4 mL/kg can be administered as a bolus. During intracranial emergencies, there is sufficient evidence to support the peripheral administration of HTS. Both mannitol and HTS lower ICP but no evidence has shown either agent to improve neurologic outcome or mortality. A recent meta-analysis comparing hypertonic saline to mannitol showed lower ICP (after 90 min) and better cerebral perfusion pressure (CPP) with hypertonic saline [140].

41.12 Seizure Prophylaxis

Early post-traumatic seizures (PTS) are seizures that occur within 7 days of injury. Post-traumatic seizures are a significant concern in severe TBI patients and are associated with greater morbidity and mortality. Risk factors for early post-traumatic seizure include lower GCS, younger age, depressed skull fracture, and penetrating head trauma [138]. Prophylactic antiseizure medications have shown to decrease the incidence of early PTS [141]. However, in severe TBI, no agent is superior. Studies do not support the use of antiseizure medications for late PTS. The use of levetiracetam has become more common due to the favorable side effect profile and wider therapeutic index compared to other agents such as phenytoin. With lack heterogeneity in studies, dose ranges from 500 mg to 1000 mg every 12 h. For mild to moderate TBI, observational studies showed a small reduction in the incidence of early PTS with seizure prophylaxis, but the overall incidence of early PTS was low [142]. Further studies are needed to elucidate optimal patient population, antiseizure medication, and dose. For further information regarding TBI management, please refer to the TBI chapter.

41.13 Antibiotics in Trauma

Antibiotics play an adjunctive role as part of the complete care of the initial management of the trauma patient. Antibiotics are indicated in patients who present with open fractures. The type of open fracture, where it is located on the body (extremity vs. facial vs. skull), and the environment in which it occurred (land-based vs. aquatic) assists in determining the initial antibiotic regimen. Administering antibiotics as soon as possible, ideally within 1-h post insult, is necessary in trauma patients as a delay in antibiotics is associated with an increased risk of infection [3, 143]. The Eastern Association for the Surgery of Trauma (EAST) guidelines provide recommendations for initial antibiotic management in open fractures.

The EAST guidelines define an open fracture as a fracture that communicates with the environment through a break in the skin. They recommend that systemic antibiotic coverage targeting gram-positive organisms be initiated as soon as possible after injury. The Gustilo classification is a grading system used to classify open fractures (Table 41.10) [144]. This classification helps to determine prognosis, likelihood of infection, and antibiotic coverage needed.

Type I and type II open fractures require gram-positive coverage with additional gram-negative coverage needed for type III open fractures. A first-generation cephalosporin (i.e., cefazolin) is used for type I and type II open fractures with the guidelines recommending the addition of an aminoglycoside when there is a type III open fracture present. These guidelines recommend adding high-dose penicillin with open fractures that have the potential to be contaminated with fecal or clostridial organisms, such as in farm-related injuries [144].

Evaluating an evidence-based open fracture antibiotic prophylaxis protocol, Rodriguez et al. compared ceftriaxone for type III open fractures versus cefazolin and gentamicin from the pre-protocol group. This study found a significant decrease in the use of gentamicin without an increase in skin and soft tissue infection rates. [145] Depending on local institutional protocols and local susceptibility patterns, initial antibiotic choice may differ for open fractures.

In open extremity fractures, antibiotic therapy is targeted toward gram-positive organisms present on skin flora such as *Staphylococcus aureus* and *Streptococcus*

Table 41.10 Gustilo classification [144]

Type I	Open fracture with a skin wound <1 cm in length and clean
Type II	Open fracture with a laceration >1 cm without extensive soft tissue damage, flaps, or avulsions
Type III	Open segmental fracture with >10 cm wound with extensive soft tissue injury or a traumatic amputation (special categories in Type III include gunshot fractures and open fractures caused by farm injuries)
III_A	Adequate soft tissue coverage
III_B	Significant soft tissue loss with exposed bone that requires soft tissue transfer to achieve coverage
III_C	Associated vascular injury that requires repair for limb preservation

species [146]. If the injury occurred in the maxillofacial region, antibiotic coverage should be directed toward organisms present in the oral cavity and mucous membranes of the sinus and nasal passages and include gram-positive organisms (*S. aureus, Streptococcus* species, *Micrococcus* species, *Corynebacterium* species, and *Propionibacterium* species) and gram-negative anaerobic organisms (*Bacteroides* species, *Porphyromonas* species, *Prevotella* species, and *Fusobacterium* species) [146]. In penetrating abdominal trauma, aerobic and anaerobic coverage is needed [147, 148]. If the injury occurred in an aquatic environment, antibiotics should be tailored to the type of body of water where the trauma occurred (salt vs. fresh vs. brackish). In saltwater environments, antibiotics targeting *Vibrio* species are needed, whereas freshwater environments require coverage of *Aeromonas hydrophila* and *Pseudomonas spp.* Injuries exposed to brackish water require coverage of both *Vibrio* species and *Aeromonas hydrophila* [146, 149–151]. Table 41.11 provides an example of which antibiotic(s) to use based off the area where the trauma occurred and provides recommendations for traumas occurring in the aquatic environment.

The dose of cefazolin is weight dependent. For patients weighing >120 kg, it is recommended to administer cefazolin 3 g IV as a loading dose. Patients who present with a penicillin allergy may also reliably receive cephalosporins as cross reactivity is 1–2.55% and dependent on the molecular side chains of the medications involved [155].

A retrospective study compared initial antibiotic selection and timing in trauma patients presenting with open fractures between a trauma resuscitation team with a pharmacist and those without a pharmacist. Eighty-one percent of patients in the pharmacist group received guideline concordant antibiotics versus 47% in the group without a pharmacist present ($p < 0.01$). The median (IQR) time to antibiotics was 14 (11–20) min in the pharmacist group versus 20 min (12–27) without a pharmacist present [156]. As an integral member of the trauma resuscitation team, the pharmacist should provide recommendations for antibiotics based on the type of trauma that presents, the environment where the trauma occurred, and patient-specific characteristics. The responding pharmacist should also obtain and prepare antibiotics at the bedside when necessary to ensure that antibiotics are delivered in a timely manner.

41.13.1 Wound Management—Tetanus Prophylaxis

Tetanus is a potentially fatal, vaccine preventable noncommunicable disease caused by the neurotoxin (tetanospasmin) produced from *Clostridium tetani*. *Clostridium tetani* is a spore-forming, obligate, anaerobic gram-positive bacillus that is ubiquitous and found in high concentrations in soil and animal excrement [157]. Tetanospasmin prevents the release of GABA at the junction of inhibitory nerve synapses, producing excitatory nerve impulses that give rise to the typical clinical symptoms. Symptoms include sustained muscular contractions which may be

Table 41.11 Recommendations for antibiotics in trauma [146, 151–154]

Traumatic injury	Antibiotic regimen	Alternative agent for patients with severe penicillin/cephalosporin allergy	Recommended duration of therapy
Central nervous system			
Skull fracture	Cefazolin 2 g IV every 8 h	Fluoroquinolone[b] + Clindamycin 600–900 mg IV every 8 h	Varies on patient condition (approximately 5 days)
Penetrating brain injury	Ceftriaxone 2 g IV every 12 h + metronidazole 500 mg IV 6–8h	Fluoroquinolone[b] ± metronidazole 500 mg IV + vancomycin[d]	Varies on patient condition (approximately 5 days)
Maxillofacial	Ampicillin/sulbactam 3 g IV[a]	Clindamycin 600–900 mg IV every 8 h	Time of injury to 24 h after surgery
Open extremity fractures			
Type I	Cefazolin 2–3 g IV[a] Every 24 h to every 8 h	Clindamycin 600–900 mg IV every 8 h	24 h after wound closure
Type II	Cefazolin 2–3 g IV[a] Every 24 h to every 8 h	Clindamycin 600–900 mg IV every 8 h	24 h after wound closure
Type III	Ceftriaxone 2 g IV every 24 h Or Cefazolin 2–3 g IV[a] plus gentamicin[c]	Clindamycin 600–900 mg IV every 8 h + gentamicin IV[c]	Up to 72 h, not more than 24 h after wound closure
Penetrating abdominal injury	Cefoxitin 2 g IV[a] Or Ceftriaxone 1–2 g + metronidazole 500 mg	Clindamycin 600–900 mg every 8 h + gentamicin IV[c]	Do not continue for more than 24 h in the presence of hollow viscous injury; no further antibiotics needed in the absence of hollow viscous injury
Aquatic traumas			
Freshwater	Cefepime 1–2 g IV[a]	Levofloxacin 750 mg IV every 24 h	Varies on patient condition
Saltwater	Ceftazidime 2 g IV[a] or ceftriaxone 2 g every 24 h IV + Doxycycline 100 mg IV every 12 h	Levofloxacin 750 mg IV every 24 h ± doxycycline 100 mg IV	Varies on patient condition
Human and animal bites	Ampicillin sulbactam 3 g IV[a]	Doxycycline 100 mg IV every 12 h	3–5 days

[a]Frequency determined by renal function
[b]Ciprofloxacin, levofloxacin, moxifloxacin (if using moxifloxacin, no need for additional anaerobic coverage)
[c]Once daily extended interval dosing
[d]Dose based off institutional policy

Table 41.12 Tetanus prophylaxis in routine wound management [3, 157]

Number of doses of adsorbed tetanus toxoid containing vaccine	Clean and minor wound		All other wounds[a]	
	DTap, Tdap, or, Td	TIG	DTap, Tdap, or, Td	TIG
Unknown or <3	Yes	No	Yes	Yes
≥3	No	No	No	No

DTap diphtheria and tetanus toxoids and acellular pertussis vaccine, *Tdap* tetanus toxoid, reduced diphtheria toxoid, and acellular pertussis, *Td* tetanus and diphtheria toxoids, *TIG* tetanus immune globulin

[a]Wounds that are contaminated with dirt, feces, soil and saliva, puncture wounds, avulsions, missile wounds, crush wounds, bites, frost bite, and burns

DTaP is recommended for children aged < 7 years

Patients who have not completed their vaccine series and are ≥7 years should receive Tdap as part of their wound management

Patients with HIV or severe immunodeficiency who have contaminated wounds should also receive TIG, regardless of their vaccine history

generalized or localized. The most common direct cause of death from tetanus is respiratory failure. [3, 6, 157, 158]

Spores require a break in the skin to access the body and grow under low oxygen conditions. Puncture wounds and wounds with significant tissue destruction are more prone to the development of tetanus as spores are more likely to break through the skin in these traumas; however, minor and major wounds alike can cause tetanus. As spores gain access to the body through an open wound, the incubation period is 1–2 days and takes as long as 7–21 days from injury to symptom onset with extremes of 1 day to several months [157]. Treatment is supportive with prevention being the mainstay of management. All wounds should be cleaned and debrided if necessary [3, 157, 158].

Immunization is key in preventing tetanus. A tetanus toxoid containing vaccine as well as tetanus immunoglobulin (TIG), when needed, is a standard part of wound management. For patients who present with a clean, minor wound and have had completed a tetanus diphtheria series within the last 10 years, the vaccine is not indicated. If they have not completed the series or their status is unknown, Tdap is the preferred tetanus toxoid containing vaccine in patients ≥11 years of age. For patients with all other wounds, if it has been more than 5 years since their last tetanus dose, then a tetanus toxoid containing vaccine is indicated. Table 41.12 provides an overview on tetanus prophylaxis recommendations [3, 157].

41.14 Initial Management of the Burn Patient

Burns are a major source of unintentional injury and fatalities in the US and globally [159]. Many types of burns may present to the ED including chemical, electrical, and thermal. Burn severity is determined by a combination of factors including patient age, burn type, size, and thickness. Severe burns warrant transfer to a burn center for specialized management [160]. Other conditions such as frostbite and

Stevens-Johnson syndrome/toxic epidermal necrolysis may require burn center transfer and management. This section will focus on thermal burns as they are the most commonly encountered [161].

41.14.1 Fluid Management

In the first 24 h after burn injury, inflammatory and vasoactive mediators are released resulting in capillary leak and large extravascular fluid shifts. Catecholamine release causes increase in systemic vascular resistance (SVR) and potentiates hypovolemia and hypoperfusion. Therefore, acute fluid resuscitation is a pivotal intervention for severe burn patients. In general, burns covering > 20% total body surface area (TBSA) should receive acute fluid resuscitation, which is based on body size and surface area burned [160, 162]. The goal of fluid resuscitation is to prevent end-organ failure from hypovolemia while avoiding the "fluid creep" phenomenon, characterized as a progressive respiratory failure and intra-abdominal compartment syndrome due to fluid overload [163].

Total body surface area can be determined by multiple methods. A common easy method recommended by the American Burn Association (ABA) is the "Palmar method" where the patient's entire palmar surface (including fingers and thumb) represents approximately 1% of TBSA [164]. Burn centers often use the Lund-Browder Chart for the most accurate TBSA estimation [165]. It is important to note that any estimation tool can overestimate burn size, not because of the inaccuracy of such methods, but rather inherent biases in the human application of these measurement strategies. This overestimation may result in both inappropriate transfers to burn centers and over-fluid resuscitation [166].

Severe burns should be treated promptly with iso-osmotic crystalloids [167]. Hypertonic fluids and colloids have not shown benefit over iso-osmotic crystalloids. Physiologic or balanced salt solutions (e.g., lactated Ringers, Hartmann's solution, Plasma-Lyte A) are considered the preferred iso-osmotic crystalloids due to concern for hyperchloremic acidosis with large volumes of 0.9% sodium chloride [168]. The American Burn Association (ABA) recommends initial resuscitation with lactated ringers (LR) due to its availability and because its composition closely approximates physiologic electrolytes [165].

The Parkland and the Brooke formula were introduced in the mid-twentieth century to guide adequate fluid resuscitation in burn patients [169, 170]. The Parkland formula was considered a standard approach for many until the modified Brooke formula was championed and theorized to result in less fluid overload [171]. However, both protocols have come under scrutiny for fluid over-resuscitation [172]. The ABA currently recommends 2 mL/kg/%TBSA as an initial fluid resuscitation strategy, with further titration-based individualized, patient-centered care with close monitoring of hemodynamics and urine output [162, 173]. For example, higher fluid requirements can be anticipated in larger area full-thickness burns.

Table 41.13 Burn fluid resuscitation formulas

Formula	Amount	Fluid	Rate
Parkland	4 mL per kg per TBSA%	Lactated Ringer's (or other balanced crystalloid)	Administer ½ over 8 h, followed by ½ over 16 h
Modified Brooke	2 mL per kg per TBSA%		

Urine output should be strictly monitored hourly with a goal of 0.5–1 mL/kg/h in adults and 1.0–1.5 mL/kg/h in children (Table 41.13) [174].

As a more simplified option for empiric fluid resuscitation in burns, the ABA recommends LR at a rate of 500 mL/h for severe burns in ages 14 and over in the prehospital setting and initial ED management phase prior to transfer to a burn center [165].

41.14.1.1 Inhalation Injury

Smoke inhalation is a major cause of death at the scene of a closed-space fire. Carbon monoxide (CO) and cyanide (CN) are the most concerning toxicities in inhalation injury.

Carbon monoxide is an odorless nonirritating gas resulting from incomplete combustion of organic compounds which results in the formation of carboxyhemoglobin. Due to CO binding to hemoglobin with 200 times greater affinity than oxygen, tissue hypoxia rapidly affects the brain and heart. Serum carboxyhemoglobin (COHb) levels are readily available in most facilities and as a reliable marker for CO toxicity, especially because pulse oximetry is unreliable. While oxygen is still absorbed by the lungs, normal levels of dissolved oxygen will be present in the blood (PaO$_2$), and COHb does not negatively affect the color or wavelength absorption of blood so SaO$_2$ readings may be normal. While serum COHb levels of 5–10% are abnormal, chronic smokers may have such levels, which are rarely associated with symptoms. As COHb levels reach 10–20% headaches and peripheral vasodilation occur. More severe symptoms are seen above 30% and coma, seizures, and cardiac arrest occur at levels above 50–60%. Oxygen supplementation and potential intubation are first-line therapy for CO poisoning [165]. There are no pharmacotherapeutic options for CO toxicity. Hyperbaric oxygen therapy is controversial because of limited evidence and benefit when initiated early (<24 h) [175]. Additionally, few centers offer hyperbaric therapy and prioritizing this can delay other definitive care including transfer to a burn center.

Cyanide is an extremely toxic by-product of incomplete combustion and typically forms when synthetic substances such as rubber, acrylic, and plastic materials are burned which includes household items such as furniture, drapes, and upholstery. Cyanide readily passes to intracellular spaces and interferes with mitochondrial aerobic metabolism and ATP production which results in a shift to anaerobic respiration [165, 176]. Serum cyanide levels are not typically available for logistical reasons, but elevated lactate levels that are otherwise unexplained can be used as a surrogate. Plasma lactate levels exceeding 10 mmol/L were identified as a reliable marker for CN toxicity and found to estimate CN levels of greater than 1.0 mg/L, considered the lower toxic threshold [177].

Several medications have been studied and utilized for CN toxicity including sodium thiosulphate and sodium or amyl nitrite. However, due to desirable pharmacokinetics and efficacy, hydroxocobalamin is considered the first-line agent [165, 178]. Hydroxocobalamin (Cyanokit) is an intravenous medication available in a 5g vial as powderized drug that requires reconstitution prior to use and is infused over 15 min. Since hydroxocobalamin's mechanism of action involves substituting its hydroxyl group for CN, it is immediately transformed to cyanocobalamin, a water soluble vitamin (vitamin B-12). Hydroxocobalamin's adverse effects include transient hypertension, acute tubular necrosis, and skin and urine discoloration. Due to its dark-red hue, various laboratory interference is expected with colorimetric assays. Such interference varies by test and manufacturer; a full list of potential laboratory errors can be found in hydroxocobalamin's package insert [179].

Hydroxocobalamin may be given empirically including in the prehospital phase if CN toxicity is suspected, and even if severe CO poisoning is suspected (understanding that this agent will not improve CO poisoning). However, experts and guidelines recommend reserving empiric therapy for patients who are obtunded or undergoing CPR after suspected smoke inhalation [165, 180]. Regardless, a favorable risk-benefit profile of this antidote and the need for rapid treatment may warrant prudency and early empiric treatment.

41.14.1.2 Other Considerations

Burn patients require rapid assessment and prompt treatment. As with any severely injured patient, circulation, airway, and breathing are paramount to consider and support. Fluid resuscitation and treatment of inhalation injury are roles that can be enhanced with ED pharmacist support. However, other considerations warrant mention in providing optimal burn care in the ED.

41.14.1.3 Paralytics

Patients who require endotracheal intubation after severe burns are considered safe to receive succinylcholine for paralysis up to 48 h after injury [23]. It is after this time point where both electrolyte derangements and acetylcholine receptor upregulation create issues. After 48 h, and up to 1 year after severe burns, receptor upregulation results in hypersensitivity to succinylcholine and resistance to nondepolarizing neuromuscular blockers. This results in exaggerated effects (i.e., hyperkalemia) for depolarizing agents where use should generally be avoided. Conversely, increased dose requirements for nondepolarizing agents such as rocuronium are seen, particularly from 3 to 7 days after burn injury [23].

41.14.1.4 Pain

Opiates and benzodiazepines are recommended for pain and anxiety as it is often difficult to differentiate between the two. Frequent administration of IV opiates is recommended in burn patients, and required doses may exceed typical weight-based maximum dose recommendations. Intramuscular dosing of pain medications is not recommended in large area burns [165].

41.14.1.5 Vasopressors

Vasopressors should be avoided in the early treatment of severe burns especially when fluid resuscitation has yet to be optimized. Burn patients are at risk for extremity hyperperfusion, and vasopressors can exacerbate this and lead to worse outcomes. There is currently no confirmed specific role for vasopressors in burn patients [181]. If vasopressors are deemed necessary, there is no evidence to support the decision to use norepinephrine over vasopressin and both are considered acceptable [162].

41.15 Antibiotic Prophylaxis

There is no role for systemic antibiotic prophylaxis in the early treatment of burn patients. Patients with severe burns and long hospital stays are at high risk for long-term bacterial and fungal infections with resistant organisms, and prophylactic antibiotics can promote such scenarios. Prophylactic antibiotics have been postulated to improve all-cause mortality but evidence to support this is weak [182, 183]. Broad consensus over time has advised against the use of prophylactic systemic antibiotics because of the lack of supporting data and increased prevalence of antibiotic resistance. However, individual consideration may be warranted in specific cases of severe burns in patients who are mechanically ventilated or have multiple early skin grafting. Topical antibiotic ointments or ophthalmic drops may be considered for minor skin burns and corneal burns. Burn center consultation is recommended for specific antibiotic selection [165].

41.16   Trauma in Burn Patients

Trauma is often associated with burns such as blast injuries and trauma encountered while escaping fire. A core principle is that trauma workup and care should always precede burn treatment which improves survival [165].

41.17   Obstetrical Trauma

Trauma affects 7% of all pregnancies and requires admission in 4 out 1000 pregnancies [184]. It accounts for nearly half of all deaths of pregnant women [185]. The most common causes of trauma in pregnancy include assault, motor vehicle crashes, and falls. Pregnancy can introduce complexities with additional team members such as obstetrician and/or the neonatology team. Pregnancy is associated with physiological changes such as a decrease in systemic vascular resistance (SVR) from baseline by 35–40%, beginning in the first trimester, until the middle of the second trimester where the SVR remains decreased until after delivery. Blood volume, cardiac output, and the size of the heart are all increased during pregnancy. Supine pregnant patients around 20 weeks can cause compression of the inferior vena cava (IVC) leading to decreased cardiac output and hypotension. The patient should be placed on their left lateral if possible to avoid the uterus compressing the IVC and aorta.

Standard ATLS is followed for the pregnant patient and takes priority. Fetal monitoring is coordinated with the trauma team and obstetric team after stabilization of the pregnant patient. The normal range for fetal heart rate is 120–160 beats per minute. The fetus is considered viable at a gestational age of ≥23 weeks [184]. If fetal distress is detected or maternal arrest occurs, an emergent cesarean section, also known as resuscitative hysterotomy, can be performed. Due to aortocaval compression by the uterus, cardiopulmonary resuscitation with chest compressions is thought to be less effective in pregnant patients. The sooner this procedure occurs at the onset of cardiac arrest, the better the outcomes [185]. The pharmacists must also be prepared for neonatal resuscitation. It is important to have protocols in place and dedicated teams for the pregnant patient and fetus while also ensuring access to medications for post-partum hemorrhage (PPH) such as oxytocin, methylergonovine, carboprost, misoprostol, and TXA. TXA may be considered when initial medical therapy fails [186]. A 2018 Cochrane review demonstrated that the use of TXA within 3 h reduced mortality due to bleeding in patients with primary PPH [187]. Considerations for medications in the management of PPH are shown in Table 41.14.

Sedatives and analgesics will cross the placenta but are considered safe to administer as the fetus is fully developed. If an emergency cesarean section is performed, the newborn might have a lower APGAR score which is a rapid assessment of the newborn reported at 1 min and 5 min after birth. The score includes five components

Table 41.14 Common medications for PPH [186]

	Oxytocin (Pitocin®)	Methylergonovine (Methergine®)	Hemabate (Carboprost®) Prostaglandin F2 alpha analogue	Misoprostol (Cytotec®) (Prostaglandin E$_1$ analog)
Dose/route	10–40 units/L NS or LR continuous infusion Can also give 10 units IM	0.2 mg IM or IMM every 2–4 h IV for urgent use	250 mcg IM or IMM every 15–90 min Not to exceed 8 doses	800–1000 mcg Rectally
Adverse effects	• Nausea and vomiting • Undiluted rapid IV can cause hypotension	• Nausea and vomiting • Hypertension • Diarrhea • Diaphoresis • Cramping • Headache • Dizziness • Bradycardia or tachycardia	• Nausea and vomiting • Diarrhea • Shivering • Fever and chills	• Nausea and vomiting • Shivering • Diarrhea • Fever
Contraindications	Allergy to oxytocin	• Hypertension • Toxemia	• Avoid in asthma • Relative contraindications: cardiac, pulmonary, hepatic, or renal disease	Allergy to PG
Disadvantage /Cautions	IV administration: associated with hypertension, intracerebral hemorrhage, myocardial infarction	Refrigeration required, light sensitive	Expensive Refrigeration required	Only available in 100 & 200 mcg tablets
Storage	Room temperature	Refrigeration Light sensitive	Refrigeration	Room temperature

color, heart rate, reflexes, muscle tone, and respirations, and each component is given a score of 0, 1, or 2.

Traumatic placental injury can also result in fetomaternal hemorrhage (FMH). In Rh-negative mothers, FMH may stimulate an immune reaction in the mother leading to the formation of antibodies or alloimmunization. The transplacental passage of these antibodies may lead to hemolytic disease in the fetus and if untreated or undiagnosed, can lead to significant fetal morbidity and mortality [188].

O-negative blood should be transfused when needed until type and screen are available to avoid rhesus D (Rh) alloimmunization in Rh-negative mothers. Anti-D immunoglobulin should be given to all rhesus D-negative pregnant trauma patients within 72 h. A single dose of 300 mcg, administered within 72 h of injury, provides protection against sensitization for up to 30 mL of fetal blood in the maternal circulation [189, 190].

Pregnant patients can receive X-rays, computed tomography (CT) scan, and magnetic resonance imaging (MRI) [191]. Mandatory shielding of the fetus for all but pelvic and lumbar spine films should be performed. Tests should be ordered judiciously, and redundancy should be eliminated. Low osmolality iodinated contrast and gadolinium contrast can cross the placenta. Human and animal studies do not indicate harm to the fetus with iodinated contrast, while human and animal studies with gadolinium contrast are sparse and the risk vs benefit should be considered when considering use [3, 192].

41.18 Cardiac Arrest in Trauma

Cardiac arrest in the setting of trauma is associated with a low survival rate and high neurological disability in survivors. Survival rates vary greatly depending on the mechanism of trauma, prehospital transport time, and capability of trauma receiving centers. Traumatic cardiac arrest survival rates have seen improvement in developed countries, with recent data suggesting overall survival rate of around 7% and as high as 9.2% with the caveat that arrest happens after EMS arrival [193–195]. To put this into context, prehospital traumatic arrest survival is comparable to those of out-of-hospital cardiac arrest stemming from any cause, which typically ranges from 8.2% to 10.4% [196]. In contrast to medical arrest, trauma patients most often have a healthy heart. Therefore, priority is focused on repairing the underlying injury and addressing hemorrhagic shock.

Important time points after traumatic arrest inform resuscitation in the trauma bay. Resuscitative efforts are considered futile if the patient has received prehospital CPR for greater than 15 min after any mechanism [197]. The Western Trauma Association further delineates this to 10 min after blunt trauma (e.g., vehicle impact or fall) or 15 min after penetrating trauma (e.g., stab or gunshot wound) [198]. For pulseless trauma patients who arrive within these time windows, a resuscitative thoracotomy is indicated. The purpose of this procedure is to explore and repair cardiac or great vessel injuries and/or cross-clamp the aorta to prevent further exsanguination while preserving perfusion to the brain and coronary arteries. Similar to the concept of aortic cross-clamp, Resuscitative Endovascular Balloon Occlusion of the Aorta (REBOA) is a progressive device providing a less invasive alternative to thoracotomy. Similar to the concept of aortic cross-clamp, REBOA is intended to tamponade the aorta and thereby control bleeding from injuries below the diaphragm. While endorsed by EM physicians and surgeons in the US, evidence is currently conflicting on its survival benefit and specific trauma application [199–202].

Traumatic arrest creates a different set of priorities than conventional medical arrest. Procedures such as thoracotomy and central large-bore vein or artery access often trump conventional ACLS interventions [203]. Once in the ED, chest compressions are unlikely helpful and may result in harm as different priorities compete. Intravenous epinephrine (i.e., 1 mg every 3–5 min) has shown no survival benefit and is generally not endorsed in the setting of traumatic arrest [204, 205]. Rather, focus should be on administration of blood and emergent surgical procedures aimed at reversing hemorrhagic shock.

Administration of intracardiac epinephrine during emergent thoracotomy is controversial [206]. Scant evidence is provided from case reports dating back 100 years, yet no studies have formally evaluated this practice [207, 208]. If intracardiac epinephrine is employed, 1 mg is the accepted dose and either common concentration of epinephrine is acceptable (1 mg/mL or 1 mg/10 mL) depending on availability. In fact, our contemporary dose of epinephrine in ACLS (1 mg) was extrapolated from surgeons historical experience with intracardiac epinephrine [209]. For intracardiac epinephrine, we recommend a longer (>1.5″) and smaller gauge (>22G) needle in order to ensure administration into the left ventricular chamber and avoid myocardial wall tissue injury. Intramural epinephrine can result in profound myocardial ischemia and malignant arrhythmias.

While traumatic arrest is largely aimed at procedures to repair the injury and provide resuscitative blood products, pharmacist involvement is crucial in advising on medication selection, administration methods, and overall medical management strategies. Many of the same general post-arrest care principles apply in traumatic arrest including timely administration of sedation and analgesia where the pharmacist can provide valuable care [210, 211].

41.19 Venous Thromboembolism Prophylaxis in the Trauma Patient

41.19.1 Epidemiology and Pathophysiology

Venous thromboembolism (VTE) is a significant cause of morbidity and mortality in trauma patients, necessitating effective thromboprophylaxis strategies [212]. Previous data has estimated the incidence of deep venous thrombosis (DVT) in trauma patients to be as high as 18% with a pulmonary embolism (PE) rate of 11% compared to 0.2% total VTE rate in non-traumatic cohorts. Mortality-associated PEs in the trauma cohort account for upwards of 5% of preventable deaths [213]. Trauma patients are inherently at high risk for VTE due to multiple factors, including the severity of injury, prolonged immobilization, surgical interventions, comorbidities, and systemic inflammatory responses (Table 41.15) [214–216].

Virchow's Triad, which has historically described VTE development, remains consistent in trauma patients. First, patients often remain immobile secondary to injury and post-surgical procedures leading to venous stasis. Prolonged immobilization, common in orthopedic fractures and traumatic spinal injuries, are well-known risk factors within this cohort. For this subset of trauma patients, the incidence of VTE development has been estimated to be as high as 80% [215]. Second, after the initial trauma insult, patients have a massive systemic procoagulant sequelae that promotes clot formation, resulting in a hypercoagulable state. Higher injury severity scores correlate with an increased risk of VTE, as severe injuries are often associated with increased hypercoagulability. Lastly, trauma itself may cause direct endothelial or vessel wall damage which can lead to VTE. Like other critically ill medical cohorts, trauma patients also may be at increased

Table 41.15 Examples of modifiable and non-modifiable risk factors for venous thromboembolism in trauma patients [214]

Category	Risk factor	Explanation
Non-modifiable	Age	Weakened vascular integrity associated with advanced age increase VTE risk
	Gender	Male gender is associated with increased VTE risk
	Severity of injury	An increased injury severity score increases risk of VTE given higher inflammatory response and tissue/vasculature damage
Modifiable	Immobilization	Prolonged immobilization secondary to injury or surgery increases risk for VTE given pronounced venous stasis
	Surgical interventions	Vessel injuries and postoperative recovery from surgery increase VTE risk
	Blood transfusions	Increased activation of procoagulant mediators and increased blood viscosity from transfusions have all been implicated in increased VTE rates with trauma patients
	Inadequate VTE prophylaxis	Failure to implement timely and appropriate intensity of prophylaxis have been implemented with higher VTE rates

risk for VTE development secondary to comorbidities like cancer, obesity, and genetic polymorphisms such as factor V Leiden disease [217].

41.19.2 Venous Thromboembolism Prophylaxis

Chemical prophylaxis in trauma patients is a cornerstone in preventing VTE and involves anticoagulants that inhibit clot formation. Low molecular weight heparins (LMWH), particularly enoxaparin, is frequently used due to its predictable pharmacokinetics and ease of administration, with a historical dosing regimen of 30 mg subcutaneously every 12 h; however, as the body habitus of the public has increased, there has been more data to suggest that weight-based dosing regimens reach target anti-Xa activity more often. However, a recent meta-analysis demonstrated that this has not correlated with reduced VTE incidence [218]. Unfractionated Heparin (UFH) remains an option for those with renal dysfunction or other contraindications, but LMWH should be utilized as it has demonstrated superiority for efficacy at reducing VTE, DVT, and PE incidence in comparison [219]. Standard UFH dosing is considered 5000 units every 8 h; however, higher dosing regimens, up to 7500 units every 8 h, have been explored with uncertainty with respect to efficacy and safety in non-trauma cohorts. The use of factor Xa inhibitors, such as apixaban and rivaroxaban, is not routinely utilized in the trauma cohort due to uncertainty of safety and efficacy, but a recent pilot study by Hamidi et al. demonstrated that there may be a cohort of patients where these agents could be utilized safely [220]. Ultimately, the initial agent and dose selection must be personalized to the patient, with much consideration given to the risk of bleeding, comorbidities, and risk factors for thrombosis.

Mechanical prophylaxis serves as an adjunct or a lesser alternative, especially when chemical prophylaxis is contraindicated due to bleeding risks. Intermittent pneumatic compression (IPC) devices, which cyclically inflate and deflate around the legs to promote venous return and induce possible antithrombotic effects, are commonly utilized [221]. The estimated effect on the use of IPCs, chemical prophylaxis, both strategies alone, or in some combination remains relatively unknown given the minimal randomized-controlled data available. However, data available from a recent Cochrane analysis would suggest the addition of IPCs to a chemical prophylactic regimen appears to reduce the incidence of DVT, PE, and VTE without compromising safety [222]. One issue associated with IPCs is that compliance remains relatively low despite documented benefits. In one study it was found that <30% of patients were compliant in a non-trauma cohort with discomfort, itching, or non-reapplication after bathing or ambulating being the most common reason for non-utilization [223]. In cases where anticoagulation is contraindicated or in patients with recurrent VTE despite adequate anticoagulation, inferior vena cava (IVC) filters may be placed to prevent emboli from reaching the lungs. While IVCs may prevent PEs, they have not demonstrated mortality benefit in the trauma cohort, indicating careful patient selection must occur when considering this strategy [224].

Dose optimization of VTE prophylaxis has been of interest in recent years as our understanding of pharmacokinetic variances seen in trauma patients has evolved. Trauma patients often display a hyperdynamic response known as augmented renal clearance (ARC) in approximately 50% of patients, placing them at risk for under dosing of certain medication classes such as LMWH for VTE prophylaxis [225]. Additionally, when patients have extremes in body habitus, the volume of distribution may not follow population kinetics in trauma patients making dosing challenging [226]. Monitoring anti-factor Xa levels can guide dosing in patients with extremes of body weight or ARC to ensure therapeutic levels are achieved without increasing bleeding risk [227]. In a recent meta-analysis, higher anti-Xa levels were associated with reduced VTE risk and anti-Xa guided chemoprophylaxis improves anti-Xa target achievement, but dose adjustment protocols may not significantly reduce VTE incidence. Currently, the role of monitoring and dose adjustment protocols as opposed to earlier weight-based regimens, and their role in VTE prevention remains unknown.

The outcomes of VTE prophylaxis in trauma patients highlight the delicate balance between preventing VTE and managing bleeding risks. Effective prophylaxis significantly lowers the incidence of DVT and PE, major contributors to morbidity and mortality in this population. The use of VTE prophylaxis is associated with reduced mortality, as PE is a leading cause of death in trauma patients. Optimal initial dosing, regimen changes, and appropriate monitoring still require higher quality data to elucidate appropriate strategies for VTE prevention.

41.20 Role of the Pharmacist

As a critical member of the trauma response team, the pharmacist plays an integral role in patient care. By preparing, obtaining, and ultimately expediting medications needed for the patient, the pharmacist helps to reduce medication errors, provides safe and appropriate medications in a timely manner, advocates for the patient, and ensures guideline concordant medications are delivered. By being involved in the secondary survey, pharmacists may also assess potential medication allergies, retrieving/review the patient's medication history, and review the patient's immunization status. An "AMPLE" history is performed on all patients during the secondary survey and consists of Allergies, Medication history, Past medical history, Last meal, and Events/Environment surrounding the trauma [3, 6]

A dedicated pharmacist as a part of the trauma team helps to decrease time to medication administration for antibiotics, analgesics, sedatives, paralytics, and medications for RSI. Studies also show that there are fewer medication errors when the pharmacist is part of the trauma team [228]. In a survey conducted in a US medical academic medical/trauma center, 97% of physicians and 83% of nurses agreed or strongly agreed that the "presence of the emergency pharmacist during trauma and medical resuscitations" enhanced their ability to deliver safe, quality care to patients [229]. One study described the interventions and activities of the pharmacist on the trauma response team at a level 1 trauma center and documented 304 interventions in 264 patients. These consisted of dosage recommendations (60%), drug information (27%), alternative therapy recommendations (6%), drug discontinuation recommendations (3%), drug recommendations (2%), and drug wastage avoidance (2%). The top medications involved were analgesics (26%), sedatives (17%), antimicrobials (17%), vaccines (12%), and fluids (7%). Facilitating the administration of medications comprised 83% of interventions [230]. Another study looked at the pharmacist's impact on acute pain management during trauma resuscitation and found that pharmacists reduced time to first analgesia (17 min versus 21 min without a pharmacist, $p = 0.03$) [231].

A follow-up survey conducted in trauma centers identified through the American College of Surgeons showed that there was an increase in pharmacist participation on the trauma team from 23% in 2007 to 70% in 2017 ($p < 0.001$). Ninety-seven percent of centers who had a pharmacist on the trauma team described their involvement as "valuable" or "extremely valuable." Pharmacist services provided during trauma resuscitations included provision of drug information, dosage calculations, and medication procurement and preparation [232]. A 2024 randomized trial compared the presence of an emergency medicine pharmacist on trauma resuscitation to no pharmacist and evaluated time to analgesia within 30 min. The cohort with a pharmacist present were more likely to provide analgesia within 30 min of arrival compared to no pharmacist, 83.7% versus 64.1% ($p = 0.042$), respectively. Other medications provided by the pharmacist during this trial included anticoagulation reversal, sedation and analgesia post-RSI, local anesthetics, antimicrobials, and tetanus prophylaxis [233].

41.21   Conclusion

The 2021 American Society of Health-Systems Pharmacists statement on emergency medicine pharmacist services states that pharmacists should be involved in all critical and acute resuscitative efforts, including trauma resuscitation as studies have shown improved safety and expedited time to medication administration [211]. Pharmacists serve many roles on the trauma team, from preparing medications at the bedside to ensuring the safe use of medications in the acutely ill trauma patient. The role of the pharmacist is essential as they are the medication experts, providing vital drug information in time sensitive cases.

References

1. Centers for Disease Control and Prevention, National Center for Injury Prevention and Control. Injury Prevention and Control. Injuries and violence are leading causes of death. Last reviewed May 13, 2024. Accessed July 10, 2024. https://www.cdc.gov/injury/wisqars/animated-leading-causes.html.

2. Kochanek KD, Murphy SL, Xu JQ, Arias E. Mortality in the United States, 2022. NCHS Data Brief, no 492. Hyattsville, MD: National Center for Health Statistics; 2024. https://doi.org/10.15620/cdc:135850.

3. American College of Surgeons. Advanced Trauma Life Support, 10th Edition; 2017. Copyright 2018. American College of Surgeons 633 N. Saint Clair Street Chicago, IL 60611-3211. Advanced Trauma Life Support Student Course Manual. Library of Congress Control Number: 2017907997 ISBN 78-0-9968262-3-5.

4. Pasha SM. How one plane crash changed the way we work. Neth J Med. 2017;75(3):98.

5. Bridgewater F. Forty years on from an event that changed the management of trauma around the world: what actually happened that night forty years ago? Mil Med. 2016;181(10):1176–81. https://doi.org/10.7205/MILMED-D-15-00554.

6. Scarponcini T, Edwards C, Rudis M, Jasiak K, Hays D. The role of the emergency pharmacist in trauma resuscitation. J Pharm Pract. 2011;24(2):146–59. https://doi.org/10.1177/0897190011400550.

7. Ferrada P. Shifting priorities from intubation to circulation first in hypotensive trauma patients. Am Surg. 2018;84(2):e75–6.

8. Ferrada P, Ferrada R, Jacobs L, et al. Prioritizing circulation to improve outcomes for patients with exsanguinating injury: a literature review and techniques to help clinicians achieve bleeding control. J Am Coll Surg. 2024;238(1):129–36.

9. Acquisto NM, Mosier J, Bittner E, Patanwala A, Hirsch K, Hargwood P, et. al. Society of critical care medicine clinical practice guidelines for rapid sequence intubation in the critically ill adult patient. Crit Care Med 2023; 51(10):1411-1430. doi: https://doi.org/10.1097/CCM.0000000000006000

10. Hampton J, Hommer K, Musselman M, Bilhimer M. Rapid sequence intubation and the role of the emergency medicine pharmacist: 2022 update. Am J Health Syst Pharm. 2023;80(4):182–95. https://doi.org/10.1093/ajhp/zxac326.

11. Engstrom K, Brown C, Mattson A, Lyons N, Rech M. Pharmacotherapy optimization for rapid sequence intubation in the emergency department. Am J Emerg Med. 2023;70:19–29. https://doi.org/10.1016/j.ajem.2023.05.004.

12. Reynolds S, Heffner J. Airway management of the critically ill patient: rapid-sequence intubation. Chest. 2005;127(4):1397–412. https://doi.org/10.1378/chest.127.4.1397.

13. Hampton J. Rapid-sequence intubation and the role of the emergency department pharmacist. Am J Health Syst Pharm. 2011;68(14):1320–30. https://doi.org/10.2146/ajhp100437.

14. Stollings J, Diedrich D, Oyen L, Brown D. Rapid-sequence intubation: a review of the process and considerations when choosing medications. Ann Pharmacother. 2014;48(1):62–76. https://doi.org/10.1177/1060028013510488.

15. Wang J, Li QB, Wu YY, Wang BN, Kang JL, Xu XW. Efficacy and safety of opioids for the prevention of etomidate-induced myoclonus: a meta-analysis. Am J Ther. 2018;25(5):e517–23. https://doi.org/10.1097/MJT.0000000000000404.

16. Dietrich S, Mixon M, Rogoszewski R, Delgado S, Knapp V, Floren M, Dunn J. Hemodynamic effects of propofol for induction of rapid sequence intubation in traumatically injured patients. Am Surg. 2018;84(9):1504–8.

17. Diaz-Guzman E, Mireles-Cabodevila E, Heresi G, Bauer S, Arroliga A. A comparison of methohexital versus etomidate for endotracheal intubation of critically ill patients. Am J Crit Care. 2010;19(1):48–54. https://doi.org/10.4037/ajcc2010562.

18. Farrell N, Killius K, Kue R, Langlois B, Nelson K, Golenia P. A comparison of etomidate, ketamine, and methohexital in emergency department rapid sequence intubation. J Emerg Med. 2020;59(4):508–14. https://doi.org/10.1016/j.jemermed.2020.06.054.

19. Jabre P, Combes X, Lapostolle F, Dhaouadi M, Ricard-Hibon A, Vivien B, et al. Etomidate versus ketamine for rapid sequence intubation in acutely ill patients: a multicentre randomised controlled trial. Lancet. 2009;374(9686):293–300. https://doi.org/10.1016/S0140-6736(09)60949-1.

20. Upchurch C, Grijalva C, Russ S, Collins S, Semler M, Rice T, et al. Comparison of etomidate and ketamine for induction during rapid sequence intubation of adult trauma patients. Ann Emerg Med. 2017;69(1):24–33.e2. https://doi.org/10.1016/j.annemergmed.2016.08.009.
21. Mansvelder F, Bossers S, Loer S, Bloemers F, Lieshout E, Hartog D, et al. Etomidate versus ketamine as prehospital induction agent in patients with suspected severe traumatic brain injury. Anesthesiology. 2024;140(4):742–51. https://doi.org/10.1097/ALN.0000000000004894.
22. Leede E, Kempema J, Wilson C, et. al. A multicenter investigation of the hemodynamic effects of induction agents for trauma rapid sequence intubation. J Trauma Acute Care Surg 2021; 90(6):1009-1013. doi: https://doi.org/10.1097/TA.0000000000003132.
23. Bittner EA, Shank E, Woodson L, Martyn JAJ. Acute and perioperative care of the burn-injured patient. Anesthesiology. 2015;122(2):448–64. https://doi.org/10.1097/ALN.0000000000000559.
24. Roper J, Fleming E, Long B, Koyfman A. Myasthenia gravis and crisis: evaluation and management in the emergency department. J Emerg Med. 2017;53(6):843–53.
25. Tran D, Newton E, Mount V, Lee J, Wells G, Perry J. Rocuronium versus succinylcholine for rapid sequence induction intubation. Cochrane Database Syst Rev. 2015;2015(10):CD002788. https://doi.org/10.1002/14651858.CD002788.pub3.
26. Patanwala A, Erstad B, Roe D, Sakles J. Succinylcholine is associated with increased mortality when used for rapid sequence intubation of severely brain injured patients in the emergency department. Pharmacotherapy. 2016;36(1):57–63. https://doi.org/10.1002/phar.1683.
27. Bridion (sugammadex) [package insert]. Greenville, NC. Patheon Manufacturing Services LLC; 2015.
28. Bhat R, Mazer-Amirshahi M, Sun C, et al. Accuracy of rapid sequence intubation medication dosing in obese patients intubated in the ED. Am J Emerg Med. 2016;34(12):2423–5. https://doi.org/10.1016/j.ajem.2016.09.056.
29. Bonomo JB, Butler AS, Lindsell CJ, Venkat A. Inadequate provision of postintubation anxiolysis and analgesia in the ED. Am J Emerg Med. 2008;26(4):469–72. https://doi.org/10.1016/j.ajem.2007.05.024.
30. Fuller BM, Roberts BW, Mohr NM, et al. The ed-sed study: a multicenter, prospective cohort study of practice patterns and clinical outcomes associated with emergency department sedation for mechanically ventilated patients. Crit Care Med. 2019;47(11):1539–48. https://doi.org/10.1097/CCM.0000000000003928.
31. Pappal R, Roberts B, Mohr N, et al. The ED-AWARENESS study: a prospective, observational cohort study of awareness with paralysis in mechanically ventilated patients admitted from the emergency department. Ann Emerg Med. 2021;77(5):532–44. https://doi.org/10.1016/j.annemergmed.2020.10.012. Epub 2021 Jan 21
32. Angotti LB, Richards JB, Fisher DF, et al. Duration of mechanical ventilation in the emergency department. West J Emerg Med. 2017;18(5):972–9. https://doi.org/10.5811/westjem.2017.5.34099.
33. Korinek JD, Thomas RM, Goddard LA, St John AE, Sakles JC, Patanwala AE. Comparison of rocuronium and succinylcholine on postintubation sedative and analgesic dosing in the emergency department. Eur J Emerg Med. 2014;21(3):206–11. https://doi.org/10.1097/MEJ.0b013e3283606b89.
34. Watt JM, Amini A, Traylor BR, Amini R, Sakles JC, Patanwala AE. Effect of paralytic type on time to post-intubation sedative use in the emergency department. Emerg Med J. 2013;30(11):893–5. https://doi.org/10.1136/emermed-2012-201812.
35. Sebel PS, Bowdle TA, Ghoneim MM, et al. The incidence of awareness during anesthesia: a multicenter United States study. Anesth Analg. 2004;99(3):833–9. https://doi.org/10.1213/01.ANE.0000130261.90896.6C.
36. Cook TM, Andrade J, Bogod DG, et al. 5th National Audit Project (Nap5) on accidental awareness during general anaesthesia: patient experiences, human factors, sedation, consent, and medicolegal issues. Br J Anaesth. 2014;113(4):560–74. https://doi.org/10.1093/bja/aeu314.

37. Pandit JJ, Andrade J, Bogod DG, et al. 5th National Audit Project (Nap5) on accidental awareness during general anaesthesia: summary of main findings and risk factors. Br J Anaesth. 2014;113(4):549–59. https://doi.org/10.1093/bja/aeu313.

38. Leslie K, Chan MTV, Myles PS, Forbes A, McCulloch TJ. Posttraumatic stress disorder in aware patients from the B-aware trial. Anesth Analg. 2010;110(3):823–8. https://doi.org/10.1213/ANE.0b013e3181b8b6ca.

39. Amini A, Faucett E, Watt J, et al. Effect of a pharmacist on timing of postintubation sedative and analgesic use in trauma resuscitations. Am J Health Syst Pharm. 2013;70(17):1513–7. https://doi.org/10.2146/ajhp120673.

40. Johnson E, Meier A, Shirakbari A, Weant K, Justice S. Impact of rocuronium and succinylcholine on sedation initiation after rapid sequence intubation. J Emerg Med. 2015;49(1):43–9. https://doi.org/10.1016/j.jemermed.2014.12.028.

41. Robey-Gavin E, Abuakar L. Impact of clinical pharmacists on initiation of postintubation analgesia in the emergency department. J Emerg Med. 2016;50(2):308–14. https://doi.org/10.1016/j.jemermed.2015.07.029.

42. Devlin JW, Skrobik Y, Gélinas C, et al. Executive summary: clinical practice guidelines for the prevention and management of pain, agitation/sedation, delirium, immobility, and sleep disruption in adult patients in the ICU. Crit Care Med. 2018;46(9):1532–48. https://doi.org/10.1097/CCM.0000000000003259.

43. Stephens RJ, Ablordeppey E, Drewry AM, et al. Analgosedation practices and the impact of sedation depth on clinical outcomes among patients requiring mechanical ventilation in the ed: a cohort study. Chest. 2017;152(5):963–71. https://doi.org/10.1016/j.chest.2017.05.041.

44. Stephens RJ, Dettmer MR, Roberts BW, et al. Practice patterns and outcomes associated with early sedation depth in mechanically ventilated patients: a systematic review and meta-analysis. Crit Care Med. 2018;46(3):471–9. https://doi.org/10.1097/CCM.0000000000002885.

45. Shehabi Y, Bellomo R, Reade MC, et al. Early intensive care sedation predicts long-term mortality in ventilated critically ill patients. Am J Respir Crit Care Med. 2012;186(8):724–31. https://doi.org/10.1164/rccm.201203-0522OC.

46. Shehabi Y, Bellomo R, Kadiman S, et al. Sedation intensity in the first 48 hours of mechanical ventilation and 180-day mortality: a multinational prospective longitudinal cohort study. Crit Care Med. 2018;46(6):850–9. https://doi.org/10.1097/CCM.0000000000003071.

47. Fentanyl [package insert]. Lake Forest, IL. Pfizer; Hospira; 2023.

48. Greer IA. Effects of ketorolac tromethamine on hemostasis. Pharmacotherapy. 1990;(10, 6 Pt 2):71S–6S.

49. Motov S, Yasavolian M, Likourezos A, et al. Comparison of intravenous ketorolac at three single-dose regimens for treating acute pain in the emergency department: a randomized controlled trial. Ann Emerg Med. 2017a;70(2):177–84. https://doi.org/10.1016/j.annemergmed.2016.10.014.

50. Antill AC, Frye SW, McMillen JC, et al. Treatment with oral versus intravenous acetaminophen in elderly trauma patients with rib fractures: a prospective randomized trial. Am Surg. 2020;86(8):926–32. https://doi.org/10.1177/0003134820940268.

51. Motov S, Rockoff B, Cohen V, et al. Intravenous subdissociative-dose ketamine versus morphine for analgesia in the emergency department: a randomized controlled trial. Ann Emerg Med. 2015;66(3):222–9.

52. Lovett S, Reed T, Riggs R, et al. A randomized, noninferiority, controlled trial of two doses of intravenous subdissociative ketamine for analgesia in the emergency department. Acad Emerg Med. 2021;28(6):647–54.

53. Motov S, Mai M, Pushkar I, et al. A prospective randomized, double-dummy trial comparing IV push low dose ketamine to short infusion of low dose ketamine for treatment of pain in the ED. Am J Emerg Med. 2017b;35(8):1095–100.

54. Schwenk E, Viscusi E, Buvanendran A, et al. Consensus guidelines on the use of intravenous ketamine infusions for acute pain management from the American Society of Regional

Anesthesia and Pain Medicine, the American Academy of Pain Medicine, and the American Society of Anesthesiologists. Reg Anesth Pain Med. 2018;43(5):456–66. https://doi.org/10.1097/AAP.0000000000000806.

55. Heavner JE. Local anesthetics. Curr Opin Anaesthesiol. 2007;20(4):336–42. https://doi.org/10.1097/ACO.0b013e3281c10a08.

56. Lidocaine injection [Package Insert]. Lake Forest, Il: Hospira; 2021.

57. Ropivacaine [Package Insert]. Lake Forest, Il: Hospira; 2023.

58. Hyland SJ, Wolfe RC, Patel G, Johnson EG. Perioperative medical emergencies: the role of clinical pharmacists and a review of pharmacotherapy considerations. J Am Coll Clin Pharm. 2023;6(9):1053–70. https://doi.org/10.1002/jac5.1762.

59. Marcaine® (Bupivacaine) [Package Insert]. Lake Forest, Il: Hospira; 2023.

60. ACEP Policy Statement—ultrasound-guided nerve blocks; 2024. https://www.acep.org/patient-care/policy-statements/ultrasound-guided-nerve-blocks. Accessed July 12, 2024.

61. Blaivas M, Adhikari S, Lander L. A prospective comparison of procedural sedation and ultrasound-guided interscalene nerve block for shoulder reduction in the emergency department. Acad Emerg Med. 2011;18(9):922–7. https://doi.org/10.1111/j.1553-2712.2011.01140.x.

62. Tezel O, Kaldirim U, Bilgic S, et al. A comparison of suprascapular nerve block and procedural sedation analgesia in shoulder dislocation reduction. Am J Emerg Med. 2014;32(6):549–52. https://doi.org/10.1016/j.ajem.2014.02.014.

63. Bhoi S, Chandra A, Galwankar S. Ultrasound-guided nerve blocks in the emergency department. J Emerg Trauma Shock. 2010;3(1):82–8. https://doi.org/10.4103/0974-2700.58655.

64. Neal JM, Barrington MJ, Fettiplace MR, et al. The third American society of regional anesthesia and pain medicine practice advisory on local anesthetic systemic toxicity: executive summary 2017. Reg Anesth Pain Med. 2018;43(2):113–23. https://doi.org/10.1097/AAP.0000000000000720.

65. American College of Medical Toxicology. ACMT position statement: guidance for the use of intravenous lipid emulsion. J Med Toxicol. 2017;13(1):124–5. https://doi.org/10.1007/s13181-016-0550-z.

66. Moore EE, Moore HB, Kornblith LZ, Neal MD, Hoffman M, Mutch NJ, Schöchl H, Hunt BJ, Sauaia A. Trauma-induced coagulopathy. Nat Rev Dis Primers. 2021;7(1):30.

67. Ho KM, Pavey W. Applying the cell-based coagulation model in the management of critical bleeding. Anaesth Intensive Care. 2017;45(2):166–76.

68. Wray JP, Bridwell RE, Schauer SG, Shackelford SA, Bebarta VS, Wright FL, Bynum J, Long B. The diamond of death: hypocalcemia in trauma and resuscitation. Am J Emerg Med. 2021;41:104–9.

69. Gonzalez E, Moore EE, Moore HB. Management of trauma-induced coagulopathy with thrombelastography. Crit Care Clin. 2017;33(1):119–34.

70. Hsieh SL, Hsiao CH, Chiang WC, Shin SD, Jamaluddin SF, Son DN, Hong KJ, Jen-Tang S, Tsai W, Chien DK, Chang WH, Chen TH. PATOS Clinical Research Network. Association between the time to definitive care and trauma patient outcomes: every minute in the golden hour matters. Eur J Trauma Emerg Surg. 2022;48(4):2709–16.

71. Gilbert BW, Bissell BD, Santiago RD, Rech MA. Tracing the lines: a review of viscoelastography for emergency medicine clinicians. J Emerg Med. 2020;59(2):201–15.

72. Rech MA, Gilbert BW, Nei S, Garg R, Brown CS. The clot thickens: how to use viscoelastic testing in critical illness. J Am Coll Clin Pharm. 2023;6(8):954–63. https://doi.org/10.1002/jac5.1829.

73. Hartmann J, Walsh M, Grisoli A, Thomas AV, Shariff F, McCauley R, Vande Lune S, Zackariya N, Patel S, Farrell MS, Sixta S, March R, Evans E, Tracy R, Campello E, Scărlătescu E, Agostini V, Dias J, Greve S, Thomas S. Diagnosis and Treatment of Trauma-Induced Coagulopathy by Viscoelastography. Semin Thromb Hemost. 2020;46(2):134–46.

74. Laursen TH, Meyer MAS, Meyer ASP, Gaarder T, Naess PA, Stensballe J, Ostrowski SR, Johansson PI. Thrombelastography early amplitudes in bleeding and coagulopathic trauma patients: results from a multicenter study. J Trauma Acute Care Surg. 2018;84(2):334–41.

75. Baksaas-Aasen K, Gall L, Eaglestone S, Rourke C, Juffermans NP, Goslings JC, Naess PA, van Dieren S, Ostrowski SR, Stensballe J, Maegele M, Stanworth SJ, Gaarder C, Brohi K, Johansson PI. iTACTIC—implementing treatment algorithms for the correction of trauma-induced coagulopathy: study protocol for a multicentre, randomised controlled trial. Trials. 2017;18(1):486.

76. Dias JD, Lopez-Espina CG, Ippolito J, Hsiao LH, Zaman F, Muresan AA, Thomas SG, Walsh M, Jones AJ, Grisoli A, Thurston BC, Artang R, Bilden KP, Hartmann J, Achneck HE. Rapid point-of-care detection and classification of direct-acting oral anticoagulants with the TEG 6s: implications for trauma and acute care surgery. J Trauma Acute Care Surg. 2019a;87(2):364–70.

77. Connelly CR, Yonge JD, McCully SP, Hart KD, Hilliard TC, Lape DE, Watson JJ, Rick B, Houser B, Deloughery TG, Schreiber MA, Kiraly LN. Assessment of three point-of-care platelet function assays in adult trauma patients. J Surg Res. 2017;212:260–9.

78. Dias JD, Lopez-Espina CG, Ippolito J, et al. Rapid point of care detection and classification of direct-acting oral anticoagulants with the TEG 6s: implication for trauma and acute care surgery. J Trauma Acute Care Surg. 2019b;97:364–70.

79. Zhu Z, Yu Y, Hong K, Luo M, Ke Y. Utility of viscoelastic hemostatic assay to guide hemostatic resuscitation in trauma patients: a systematic review. World J Emerg Surg. 2022;17(1):48.

80. Cochrane C, Chinna S, Um JY, Dias JD, Hartmann J, Bradley J, Brooks A. Site-of-care visco-elastic assay in major trauma improves outcomes and is cost neutral compared with standard coagulation tests. Diagnostics (Basel). 2020;10(7):486.

81. Gonzalez E, Moore EE, Moore HB, Chapman MP, Chin TL, Ghasabyan A, Wohlauer MV, Barnett CC, Bensard DD, Biffl WL, Burlew CC, Johnson JL, Pieracci FM, Jurkovich GJ, Banerjee A, Silliman CC, Sauaia A. Goal-directed hemostatic resuscitation of trauma-induced coagulopathy: a pragmatic randomized clinical trial comparing a viscoelastic assay to conventional coagulation assays. Ann Surg. 2016;263(6):1051–9.

82. Baksaas-Aasen K, Gall LS, Stensballe J, Juffermans NP, Curry N, Maegele M, Brooks A, Rourke C, Gillespie S, Murphy J, Maroni R, Vulliamy P, Henriksen HH, Pedersen KH, Kolstadbraaten KM, Wirtz MR, Kleinveld DJB, Schäfer N, Chinna S, Davenport RA, Naess PA, Goslings JC, Eaglestone S, Stanworth S, Johansson PI, Gaarder C, Brohi K. Viscoelastic haemostatic assay augmented protocols for major trauma haemorrhage (ITACTIC): a randomized, controlled trial. Intensive Care Med. 2021;47(1):49–59.

83. Mohamed M, Majeske K, Sachwani GR, Kennedy K, Salib M, McCann M. The impact of early thromboelastography directed therapy in trauma resuscitation. Scand J Trauma Resusc Emerg Med. 2017;25(1):99.

84. Tapia NM, Chang A, Norman M, Welsh F, Scott B, Wall MJ Jr, Mattox KL, Suliburk J. TEG-guided resuscitation is superior to standardized MTP resuscitation in massively transfused penetrating trauma patients. J Trauma Acute Care Surg. 2013;74(2):378–85.

85. Cannon JW. Hemorrhagic shock. N Engl J Med. 2018;378(4):370–9.

86. Malgras B, Prunet B, Lesaffre X, Boddaert G, Travers S, Cungi PJ, Hornez E, Barbier O, Lefort H, Beaume S, Bignand M, Cotte J, Esnault P, Daban JL, Bordes J, Meaudre E, Tourtier JP, Gaujoux S, Bonnet S. Damage control: concept and implementation. J Visc Surg. 2017;154(Suppl. 1):S19–29.

87. Ertmer C, Kampmeier T, Rehberg S, Lange M. Fluid resuscitation in multiple trauma patients. Curr Opin Anaesthesiol. 2011;24(2):202–8.

88. Holcomb JB, Tilley BC, Baraniuk S, Fox EE, Wade CE, Podbielski JM, del Junco DJ, Brasel KJ, Bulger EM, Callcut RA, Cohen MJ, Cotton BA, Fabian TC, Inaba K, Kerby JD, Muskat P, O'Keeffe T, Rizoli S, Robinson BR, Scalea TM, Schreiber MA, Stein DM, Weinberg JA, Callum JL, Hess JR, Matijevic N, Miller CN, Pittet JF, Hoyt DB, Pearson GD, Leroux B, van Belle G, PROPPR Study Group. Transfusion of plasma, platelets, and red blood cells in a

1:1:1 vs a 1:1:2 ratio and mortality in patients with severe trauma: the PROPPR randomized clinical trial. JAMA. 2015;313(5):471–82.

89. van der Horst RA, Rijnhout TWH, Noorman F, Borger van der Burg BLS, van Waes OJF, Verhofstad MHJ, Hoencamp R. Whole blood transfusion in the treatment of acute hemorrhage, a systematic review and meta-analysis. J Trauma Acute Care Surg. 2023;95(2):256–66.

90. Cable CA, Razavi SA, Roback JD, Murphy DJ. RBC transfusion strategies in the ICU: a concise review. Crit Care Med. 2019;47(11):1637–44.

91. Maier CL, Brohi K, Curry N, Juffermans NP, Mora Miquel L, Neal MD, Shaz BH, Vlaar APJ, Helms J. Contemporary management of major haemorrhage in critical care. Intensive Care Med. 2024;50(3):319–31.

92. Roubinian N. TACO and TRALI: biology, risk factors, and prevention strategies. Hematol Am Soc Hematol Educ Program. 2018;2018(1):585–94.

93. Hu L, Wang B, Jiang Y, Zhu B, Wang C, Yu Q, Hou W, Xia Z, Wu G, Sun Y. Risk factors for transfusion-related acute lung injury. Respir Care. 2021;66(6):1029–38.

94. Li G, Kojicic M, Reriani MK, Fernández Pérez ER, Thakur L, Kashyap R, Van Buskirk CM, Gajic O. Long-term survival and quality of life after transfusion-associated pulmonary edema in critically ill medical patients. Chest. 2010;137(4):783–9.

95. Sharma S, Sharma P, Tyler LN. Transfusion of blood and blood products: indications and complications. Am Fam Physician. 2011;83(6):719–24.

96. Vasudeva M, Mathew JK, Groombridge C, Tee JW, Johnny CS, Maini A, Fitzgerald MC. Hypocalcemia in trauma patients: a systematic review. J Trauma Acute Care Surg. 2021;90(2):396–402.

97. Moore HB, Tessmer MT, Moore EE, et al. Forgot calcium? Admission ionized-calcium in two civilian randomized controlled trials of pre-hospital plasma for traumatic hemorrhagic shock. J Trauma Acute Care Surg. 2020;88:588–96.

98. DeBot M, Sauaia A, Schaid T, Moore EE. Trauma-induced hypocalcemia. Transfusion. 2022;62(Suppl. 1):S274–80.

99. Kronstedt S, Roberts N, Ditzel R, Elder J, Steen A, Thompson K, Anderson J, Siegler J. Hypocalcemia as a predictor of mortality and transfusion. A scoping review of hypocalcemia in trauma and hemostatic resuscitation. Transfusion. 2022;62(Suppl. 1):S158–66.

100. Shandaliy Y, Busey K, Scaturo N. Impact of a calcium replacement protocol during massive transfusion in trauma patients at a level 2 trauma center. Am J Health Syst Pharm. 2024:zxae099. https://doi.org/10.1093/ajhp/zxae099.

101. Richards JE, Harris T, Dünser MW, Bouzat P, Gauss T. Vasopressors in trauma: a never event? Anesth Analg. 2021;133(1):68–79.

102. Sims CA, Guan Y, Bergey M, Jaffe R, Holmes-Maguire L, Martin N, Reilly P. Arginine vasopressin, copeptin, and the development of relative AVP deficiency in hemorrhagic shock. Am J Surg. 2017;214(4):589–95.

103. Gauss T, Richards JE, Tortù C, Ageron FX, Hamada S, Josse J, Husson F, Harrois A, Scalea TM, Vivant V, Meaudre E, Morrison JJ, Galvagno S, Bouzat P, French Trauma Research Initiative. Association of early norepinephrine administration with 24-hour mortality among patients with blunt trauma and hemorrhagic shock. JAMA Netw Open. 2022;5(10):e2234258.

104. Tran A, Yates J, Lau A, Lampron J, Matar M. Permissive hypotension versus conventional resuscitation strategies in adult trauma patients with hemorrhagic shock: a systematic review and meta-analysis of randomized controlled trials. J Trauma Acute Care Surg. 2018;84(5):802–8.

105. Sims CA, Holena D, Kim P, Pascual J, Smith B, Martin N, Seamon M, Shiroff A, Raza S, Kaplan L, Grill E, Zimmerman N, Mason C, Abella B, Reilly P. Effect of low-dose supplementation of arginine vasopressin on need for blood product transfusions in patients with trauma and hemorrhagic shock: a randomized clinical trial. JAMA Surg. 2019;154(11):994–1003.

106. Yue JK, Tsolinas RE, Burke JF, Deng H, Upadhyayula PS, Robinson CK, Lee YM, Chan AK, Winkler EA, Dhall SS. Vasopressor support in managing acute spinal cord injury: current knowledge. J Neurosurg Sci. 2019;63(3):308–17.

107. Ahuja CS, Wilson JR, Nori S, Kotter MRN, Druschel C, Curt A, Fehlings MG. Traumatic spinal cord injury. Nat Rev Dis Primers. 2017;3:17018.
108. Bracken MB. Steroids for acute spinal cord injury. Cochrane Database Syst Rev. 2012;1(1):CD001046.
109. Leech C, Turner J. Shock in trauma. Emerg Med Clin North Am. 2023;41(1):1–17.
110. Pendleton AC, Leichtle SW. Cardiac tamponade from blunt trauma. Am Surg. 2022;88(6):1319–21.
111. Wang K, Santiago R. Tranexamic acid—a narrative review for the emergency medicine clinician. Am J Emerg Med. 2022;56:33–44. https://doi.org/10.1016/j.ajem.2022.03.027. Epub 2022 Mar 22
112. CRASH-2 Trial Collaborators, Shakur H, Roberts I, Bautista R, et al. Effects of tranexamic acid on death, vascular occlusive events, and blood transfusion in trauma patients with significant hemorrhage: a randomized placebo-controlled trial. Lancet. 2010;376(9734):23–32.
113. Androski CP, Bianchi W, Robinson DL, et al. Case series on 2g tranexamic acid flush from the 75th ranger regiment casualty database. J Spec Oper Med. 2020;20(4):85–91. https://doi.org/10.55460/CG6S-N11M.
114. Drew B, Auten JD, Cap AP, et al. The use of tranexamic acid in tactical combat casualty care: TCCC proposed change 20-02. J Spec Oper Med. 2020;20(3):36–43. https://doi.org/10.55460/ZWV3-5CBW.
115. Morrison JJ, Dubose JJ, Rasmussen TE, Midwinter MJ. Military application of tranexamic acid in trauma emergency resuscitation (MATTERs) study. Arch Surg. 2012;147(2):113–9.
116. Rossaint R, Afshari A, Bouillon B, et al. The European guideline on management of major bleeding and coagulopathy following trauma (6th edition). Crit Care. 2023;27(1):80.
117. PATCH-Trauma Investigators and the ANZICS Clinical Trials Group. Prehospital tranexamic acid for severe trauma. N Engl J Med. 2023;389:127–36.
118. Guyette FX, Brown JB, Zenati MS, et al. Tranexamic acid during prehospital transport at risk for hemorrhage after injury. JAMA Surg. 2021;1156:11–20.
119. CRASH-3 Trial Collaborators. Effects of tranexamic acid on death, disability, vascular occlusive events and other morbidities in patients with acute traumatic brain injury (CRASH-3): a randomised, placebo-controlled trial. Lancet. 2019;394(10210):1713–23.
120. Deaton T, Drew B, Montgomery H, et al. Joint trauma system tactical combat casualty care guidelines. 2024 January 25. https://learning-media.allogy.com/api/v1/pdf/f4cf1d4e-3191-443a-befc-415838fb04f2/contents.
121. Neeki MM, Fanglong D, Toy J, et al. Tranexamic acid in civilian trauma care in the California prehospital antifibrinolytic therapy study. West J Emerg Med. 2018;19:977–86.
122. Rivas L, Estroff J, Sparks A, et al. The incidence of venous thromboembolic events in trauma patients after tranexamic administration: an EAST multicenter study. Blood Coag Fibrinol. 2021;32:27–43.
123. Duchesne J, Taghavi S, Ninokawa S, et al. After 800 mtp events, mortality due to hemorrhagic shock remains high and unchanged despite several in-hospital hemorrhage control advancements. Shock. 2021;56:70–8.
124. Eliquis (apixaban). Package insert. Princeton, NJ: Bristol-Myers Squibb; September 2021.
125. Xarelto (rivaroxaban). Package insert. Titusville, NJ: Janssen Pharmaceuticals; February 2023.
126. Savaysa (edoxaban). Package insert. Tokyo: Daiichi Sankyo Co; January 2015.
127. Pradaxa (dabigatran). Package insert. Ridgefield, CT: Boehringer Ingelheim Pharmaceuticals; November 2011
128. Coumadin (warfarin). Package insert. Princeton, NJ: Bristol-Myers Squibb; October 2011
129. Kobayashi LM, Britio A, Barmparas G, et al. Laboratory measures of coagulation among trauma patients on NOAs: result of the AAST-MIT. Trauma Surg Acute Care Open. 2018;3:e000231.
130. ANNEXA-4 Investigators. Full study report of Andexanet alfa for bleeding associated with factor xa inhibitors. N Engl J Med 2019;380:1326-1335.

131. ANNEXA-I Investigators. Andexanet for factor xa inhibitor-associated acute intracerebral hemorrhage. N Engl J Med 2024:390:1745-1755.
132. Tomaselli GE, Mahaffey KW, Cuker A, et al. 2020 ACC expert consensus decision pathway on management of bleeding in patients on oral anticoagulants: a report of the American College of Cardiology Solution Set Oversight Committee. J Am Coll Cardiology. 2020;76(5):594–622.
133. Greenberg S, Ziai W, Cordonnier C, et al. 2022 Guideline for the Management of Patients With Spontaneous Intracerebral Hemorrhage: A Guideline From the American Heart Association/American Stroke Association. Stroke. 2022;53(7):e282–361. https://doi.org/10.1161/STR.0000000000000407. Epub 2022 May 17
134. Taylor CA, Bell JM, Breiding MJ, Xu L. Traumatic brain injury–related emergency department visits, hospitalizations, and deaths—United States, 2007 and 2013. MMWR Surveill Summ. 2017;66(SS-9):1–16.
135. Kay T, Harrington D, Adams R, et al. Definition of mild traumatic brain injury. J Head Trauma Rehabil. 1993;8:86–7.
136. Foulkes M, Eisenberg H, Jane J, et al. The traumatic coma data bank: design, methods, and baseline characteristics. J Neurosurg. 1991;75:S8–13.
137. Berry C, Ley EJ, Bukur M, et al. Redefining hypotension in traumatic brain injury. Injury. 2012;43(11):1833–7.
138. Carney N, Totten AM, O'Reilly C, et al. Guidelines for the management of severe traumatic brain injury, 4th edition. Neurosurgery. 2017;80(1):6–15.
139. Sorani MD, Morabito D, Rosenthal G, et al. Characterizing the dose-response relationship between mannitol and intracranial pressure in traumatic brain injury patients using a high-frequency physiological data collection system. J Neurotrauma. 2008;25:291–8.
140. Schwimmbeck F, Voellger B, Chappell D, et al. Hypertonic saline vs mannitol for traumatic brain injury: a systematic review and meta-analysis with trial sequential analysis. J Neurosurg Anesthes. 2021;33(1):10–20.
141. Temkin NR, Dikmen SS, Wilensky AJ, et al. N Engl J Med. 1990;323:497–502.
142. Pease M, Mittal A, Merkaj S, et al. Early seizure prophylaxis in mild and moderate traumatic brain injury a systematic review and meta-analysis. JAMA Neurol. 2024;81(5):507–14.
143. ACS TQIP Best Practices in the Management of Orthopaedic Trauma. American College of Surgeons. Orthopaedic Trauma Association. 2015. https://www.facs.org/media/mkbnhqtw/ortho_guidelines.pdf.
144. Hoff W, Bonadies J, Cachecho R, Dorlac W. East Practice Management Guidelines Work Group: update to practice management guidelines for prophylactic antibiotic use in open fractures. J Trauma. 2011;70(3):751–4. https://doi.org/10.1097/TA.0b013e31820930e5.
145. Rodriguez L, Jung HS, Goulet J, Cicalo A, Machado-Aranda D, Napolitano L. Evidence-based protocol for prophylactic antibiotics in open fractures: improved antibiotic stewardship with no increase in infection rates. J Trauma Acute Care Surg. 2014;77(3):400–7.; discussion 407-8; quiz 524. https://doi.org/10.1097/TA.0000000000000398.
146. Hopkins T, Daley M, Rose D, Jaso T, Brown C. Presumptive antibiotic therapy for civilian trauma injuries. J Trauma Acute Care Surg. 2016;81(4):765–74. https://doi.org/10.1097/TA.0000000000001164.
147. Coccolini F, Sartelli M, Sawyer R, et al. Antibiotic prophylaxis in trauma: global alliance for infection in surgery, surgical infection society Europe, World Surgical Infection Society, American Association for the Surgery of Trauma, and World Society of Emergency Surgery guidelines. J Trauma Acute Care Surg. 2024;96(4):674–82. https://doi.org/10.1097/TA.0000000000004233.
148. Goldberg S, Anand R, Como J, et al. Prophylactic antibiotic use in penetrating abdominal trauma: an Eastern Association for the Surgery of Trauma practice management guideline. J Trauma Acute Care Surg. 2012;73(5 Suppl. 4):S321–5. https://doi.org/10.1097/TA.0b013e3182701902.

149. Snyckers CH, Visser A, Hoosien E, et al. Management of open tibia fracture following fresh water contamination. SA Orthop J. 2010:41–6.
150. Diaz J, Lopez F. Skin, soft tissue and systemic bacterial infections following aquatic injuries and exposures. Am J Med Sci. 2015;349(3):269–75. https://doi.org/10.1097/MAJ.0000000000000366.
151. Appelbaum R, Farrell M, Gelbard R, et al. Antibiotic prophylaxis in injury: an American Association for the Surgery of Trauma Critical Care Committee clinical consensus document. Trauma Surg Acute Care Open. 2024;9(1):e001304. https://doi.org/10.1136/tsaco-2023-001304.
152. Hospenthal D, Murray C, Andersen R, et al. Guidelines for the prevention of infections associated with combat-related injuries: 2011 update: endorsed by the Infectious Diseases Society of America and the Surgical Infection Society. J Trauma. 2011;71(2 Suppl 2):S210–34. https://doi.org/10.1097/TA.0b013e318227ac4b.
153. Stevens D, Bisno A, Chambers H, et al. Practice guidelines for the diagnosis and management of skin and soft tissue infections: 2014 update by the Infectious Diseases Society of America. Clin Infect Dis. 2014;59(2):e10–52. https://doi.org/10.1093/cid/ciu444.
154. Ganga A, Leary O, Sastry R, et al. Antibiotic prophylaxis in penetrating traumatic brain injury: analysis of a single-center series and systematic review of the literature. Acta Neurochir (Wien). 2023;165(2):303–13. https://doi.org/10.1007/s00701-022-05432-2.
155. Campagna J, Bond M, Schabelman E, Hayes B. The use of cephalosporins in penicillin-allergic patients: a literature review. J Emerg Med. 2012;42(5):612–20. https://doi.org/10.1016/j.jemermed.2011.05.035.
156. Impact of an emergency medicine pharmacist on initial antibiotic prophylaxis for open fractures in trauma patients The American Journal of Emergency Medicine 2018;36(2):290–293. https://doi.org/10.1016/j.ajem.2017.10.039.
157. Liang J, Tiwari T, Moro P, et al. Prevention of pertussis, tetanus, and diphtheria with vaccines in the United States: Recommendations of the Advisory Committee on Immunization Practices (ACIP). MMWR Recomm Rep. 2018;67(2):1–44. https://doi.org/10.15585/mmwr.rr6702a1.
158. Rhee P, Nunley M, Demetriades D, Velmahos G, Doucet J. Tetanus and trauma: a review and recommendations. J Trauma. 2005;58(5):1082–8. https://doi.org/10.1097/01.ta.0000162148.03280.02.
159. Brigham PA, McLoughlin E. Burn incidence and medical care use in the United States: estimates, trends, and data sources. J Burn Care Rehabil. 1996;17(2):95–107. https://doi.org/10.1097/00004630-199603000-00003.
160. Bettencourt AP, Romanowski KS, Joe V, et al. Updating the burn center referral criteria: results from the 2018 edelphi consensus study. J Burn Care Res. 2020;41(5):1052–62. https://doi.org/10.1093/jbcr/iraa038.
161. Burns. https://www.who.int/news-room/fact-sheets/detail/burns. Accessed July 24, 2024.
162. Cartotto R, Johnson LS, Savetamal A, et al. American burn association clinical practice guidelines on burn shock resuscitation. J Burn Care Res. 2024;45(3):565–89. https://doi.org/10.1093/jbcr/irad125.
163. Pruitt BA. Protection from excessive resuscitation: "pushing the pendulum back". J Trauma. 2000;49(3):567–8. https://doi.org/10.1097/00005373-200009000-00030.
164. Guidelines for Burn Patient Referral—American Burn Association. https://ameriburn.org/resources/burnreferral/. Accessed July 24, 2024.
165. American Burn Association. 2018 Advanced Burn Life Support Course Provider Manual; 2018. https://ameriburn.org/wp-content/uploads/2019/08/2018-abls-providermanual.pdf (Accessed July 24, 2024).
166. Pham C, Collier Z, Gillenwater J. Changing the way we think about burn size estimation. J Burn Care Res. 2019;40(1):1–11. https://doi.org/10.1093/jbcr/iry050.

167. Perel P, Roberts I, Ker K. Colloids versus crystalloids for fluid resuscitation in critically ill patients. Cochrane Database Syst Rev. 2013;(2):CD000567. https://doi.org/10.1002/14651858.CD000567.pub6.
168. Young JB, Utter GH, Schermer CR, et al. Saline versus plasma-Lyte A in initial resuscitation of trauma patients: a randomized trial. Ann Surg. 2014;259(2):255–62. https://doi.org/10.1097/SLA.0b013e318295feba.
169. Baxter CR, Shires T. Physiological response to crystalloid resuscitation of severe burns. Ann N Y Acad Sci. 1968;150(3):874–94. https://doi.org/10.1111/j.1749-6632.1968.tb14738.x.
170. Reiss E, Stirmann JA, Artz CP, Davis JH, Amspacher WH. Fluid and electrolyte balance in burns. J Am Med Assoc. 1953;152(14):1309–13. https://doi.org/10.1001/jama.1953.03690140017004.
171. Pruitt BA. Fluid and electrolyte replacement in the burned patient. Surg Clin North Am. 1978;58(6):1291–312. https://doi.org/10.1016/s0039-6109(16)41692-0.
172. Dahl R, Galet C, Lilienthal M, Dwars B, Wibbenmeyer L. Regional burn review: neither Parkland nor Brooke formulas reach 85% accuracy mark for burn resuscitation. J Burn Care Res. 2023;44(6):1452–9. https://doi.org/10.1093/jbcr/irad047.
173. Blumetti J, Hunt JL, Arnoldo BD, Parks JK, Purdue GF. The Parkland formula under fire: is the criticism justified? J Burn Care Res. 2008;29(1):180–6. https://doi.org/10.1097/BCR.0b013e31815f5a62.
174. Pham TN, Cancio LC, Gibran NS, American Burn Association. American Burn Association practice guidelines burn shock resuscitation. J Burn Care Res. 2008;29(1):257–66. https://doi.org/10.1097/BCR.0b013e31815f3876.
175. Huang CC, Ho CH, Chen YC, et al. Hyperbaric oxygen therapy is associated with lower short- and long-term mortality in patients with carbon monoxide poisoning. Chest. 2017;152(5):943–53. https://doi.org/10.1016/j.chest.2017.03.049.
176. MacLennan L, Moiemen N. Management of cyanide toxicity in patients with burns. Burns. 2015;41(1):18–24. https://doi.org/10.1016/j.burns.2014.06.001.
177. Baud FJ, Barriot P, Toffis V, et al. Elevated blood cyanide concentrations in victims of smoke inhalation. N Engl J Med. 1991;325(25):1761–6. https://doi.org/10.1056/NEJM199112193252502.
178. Shepherd G, Velez LI. Role of hydroxocobalamin in acute cyanide poisoning. Ann Pharmacother. 2008;42(5):661–9. https://doi.org/10.1345/aph.1K559.
179. CYANOKIT® (hydroxocobalamin) [package insert]. West Conshohocken, PA. BTG International Ltd.; 2021.
180. Mintegi S, Clerigue N, Tipo V, et al. Pediatric cyanide poisoning by fire smoke inhalation: a European expert consensus. Toxicology surveillance system of the intoxications working group of the Spanish society of paediatric emergencies. Pediatr Emerg Care. 2013;29(11):1234–40. https://doi.org/10.1097/PEC.0b013e3182aa4ee1.
181. Knappskog K, Andersen NG, Guttormsen AB, Onarheim H, Almeland SK, Beitland S. Vasoactive and/or inotropic drugs in initial resuscitation of burn injuries: a systematic review. Acta Anaesthesiol Scand. 2022;66(7):795–802. https://doi.org/10.1111/aas.14095.
182. Meulenbroek LFP, de Jong FICRS. Voice quality in relation to voice complaints and vocal fold condition during the screening of female student teachers. J Voice. 2011;25(4):462–6. https://doi.org/10.1016/j.jvoice.2010.01.003.
183. Ramos G, Cornistein W, Cerino GT, Nacif G. Systemic antimicrobial prophylaxis in burn patients: systematic review. J Hosp Infect. 2017;97(2):105–14. https://doi.org/10.1016/j.jhin.2017.06.015.
184. Barraco RD, Chiu WC, Clancy TV, et al. Practice management guidelines for the diagnosis and management of injury in the pregnant patient: the EAST practice management guidelines work group. J Trauma. 2010;69:211–4.
185. April M, Long B. Trauma in pregnancy: a narrative review of the current literature. Am J Emerg Med. 2024;81:53–61. https://doi.org/10.1016/j.ajem.2024.04.029.

186. Shields L, Goffman D, Caughey A. Practice Bulletin No. 183: postpartum hemorrhage. Obstet Gynecol. 2017;130(4):e168–86. https://doi.org/10.1097/AOG.0000000000002351.
187. Shakur H, Beaumont D, Pavord S, et. al. Antifibrinolytic drugs for treating primary postpartum haemorrhage. Cochrane Database Syst Rev 2018;2(2):CD012964. doi: https://doi.org/10.1002/14651858.CD012964.
188. Guidelines for diagnostic imaging during pregnancy and lactation. ACOG Committee Opinion No. 723. American College of Obstetricians and Gynecologists. Obstet Gynecol 2017;130(4):210-16.
189. Jain V, Chari R, Maslovitz S, et al. Guidelines for the management of a pregnant trauma patient. J Obstet Gynacecol Can. 2015;37(6):553–71.
190. Prevention of Rh D Alloimmunization. Practice Bulletin No. 181. American College of Obstetricians and Gynecologists. Obstet Gynecol. 2017;130:e57–70.
191. ACR-SPR Practice parameter for imaging pregnant or potentially pregnant patients with ionizing radiation. American College of Radiology. 2023a. https://www.acr.org/-/media/acr/files/practice-parameters/pregnant-pts.pdf.
192. ACR manual on contrast media. American College of Radiology. 2023b. https://www.acr.org/-/media/ACR/Files/Clinical-Resources/Contrast_Media.pdf.
193. Alremeithi R, Tran Q, Quintana M, et al. Approach to traumatic cardiac arrest in the emergency department: a narrative literature review for emergency providers. World J Emerg Med. 2024;15(1):3–9. https://doi.org/10.5847/wjem.j.1920-8642.2023.085.
194. Deasy C, Bray J, Smith K, et al. Traumatic out-of-hospital cardiac arrests in Melbourne, Australia. Resuscitation. 2012;83(4):465–70. https://doi.org/10.1016/j.resuscitation.2011.09.025. Epub 2011 Oct 10
195. Shi D, McLaren C, Evans C. Neurological outcomes after traumatic cardiopulmonary arrest: a systematic review. Trauma Surg Acute Care Open. 2021;6(1):e000817. https://doi.org/10.1136/tsaco-2021-000817. eCollection 2021
196. Daya MR, Schmicker RH, Zive DM, et al. Out-of-hospital cardiac arrest survival improving over time: results from the Resuscitation Outcomes Consortium (Roc). Resuscitation. 2015;91:108–15. https://doi.org/10.1016/j.resuscitation.2015.02.003.
197. Seamon MJ, Haut ER, Van Arendonk K, et al. An evidence-based approach to patient selection for emergency department thoracotomy: a practice management guideline from the Eastern Association for the Surgery of Trauma. J Trauma Acute Care Surg. 2015;79(1):159–73. https://doi.org/10.1097/TA.0000000000000648.
198. Burlew CC, Moore EE, Moore FA, et al. Western Trauma Association critical decisions in trauma: resuscitative thoracotomy. J Trauma Acute Care Surg. 2012;73(6):1359–63. https://doi.org/10.1097/TA.0b013e318270d2df.
199. Brenner M, Bulger EM, Perina DG, et al. Joint statement from the American college of surgeons committee on trauma (Acs cot) and the American college of emergency physicians (ACEP) regarding the clinical use of resuscitative endovascular balloon occlusion of the aorta(REBOA). Trauma Surg Acute Care Open. 2018;3(1):e000154. https://doi.org/10.1136/tsaco-2017-000154.
200. Morrison JJ, Galgon RE, Jansen JO, Cannon JW, Rasmussen TE, Eliason JL. A systematic review of the use of resuscitative endovascular balloon occlusion of the aorta in the management of hemorrhagic shock. J Trauma Acute Care Surg. 2016;80(2):324–34. https://doi.org/10.1097/TA.0000000000000913.
201. Castellini G, Gianola S, Biffi A, et al. Resuscitative endovascular balloon occlusion of the aorta (Reboa) in patients with major trauma and uncontrolled haemorrhagic shock: a systematic review with meta-analysis. World J Emerg Surg. 2021;16(1):41. https://doi.org/10.1186/s13017-021-00386-9.
202. Jansen JO, Hudson J, Cochran C, et al. Emergency department resuscitative endovascular balloon occlusion of the aorta in trauma patients with exsanguinating hemorrhage: the UK-REBOA randomized clinical trial. JAMA. 2023;330(19):1862–71. https://doi.org/10.1001/jama.2023.20850.

203. Monsieurs KG, Nolan JP, Bossaert LL, et al. European resuscitation council guidelines for resuscitation 2015: section 1. Executive summary. Resuscitation. 2015;95:1–80. https://doi.org/10.1016/j.resuscitation.2015.07.038.
204. ECC Committee, Subcommittees and Task Forces of the American Heart Association. 2005 American Heart Association Guidelines for cardiopulmonary resuscitation and emergency cardiovascular care. Circulation. 2005;112(Suppl. 24):IV1–203. https://doi.org/10.1161/CIRCULATIONAHA.105.166550.
205. Wongtanasarasin W, Thepchinda T, Kasirawat C, Saetiao S, Leungvorawat J, Kittivorakanchai N. Treatment outcomes of epinephrine for traumatic out-of-hospital cardiac arrest: a systematic review and meta-analysis. J Emerg Trauma Shock. 2021;14(4):195–200. https://doi.org/10.4103/JETS.JETS_35_21.
206. Lamberg JJ, Malhotra AK. Intracardiac epinephrine injection during open thoracotomy and circulatory arrest. J Anesth Clin Res. 2013;04(07) https://doi.org/10.4172/2155-6148.1000341.
207. Gottesman J. Resuscitation by the intracardiac injection of epinephrin. JAMA. 1922;79(16):1334. https://doi.org/10.1001/jama.1922.02640160054018.
208. Bodon C, Rath K. The intracardiac injection of adrenalin. Lancet. 1923;201(5195):586–90. https://doi.org/10.1016/S0140-6736(00)71763-6.
209. European Resuscitation Council. Part 6: advanced cardiovascular life support. Section 6: pharmacology II: agents to optimize cardiac output and blood pressure. European Resuscitation Council. Resuscitation. 2000;46(1–3):155–62. https://doi.org/10.1016/s0300-9572(00)00279-3.
210. Farmer BM, Hayes BD, Rao R, Farrell N, Nelson L. The role of clinical pharmacists in the emergency department. J Med Toxicol. 2018;14(1):114–6. https://doi.org/10.1007/s13181-017-0634-4.
211. Ortmann MJ, Johnson EG, Jarrell DH, et al. ASHP guidelines on emergency medicine pharmacist services. Am J Health Syst Pharm. 2021;78(3):261–75. https://doi.org/10.1093/ajhp/zxaa378.
212. Ruskin KJ. Deep vein thrombosis and venous thromboembolism in trauma. Curr Opin Anaesthesiol. 2018;31(2):215–8.
213. Ho KM, Burrell M, Rao S, Baker R. Incidence and risk factors for fatal pulmonary embolism after major trauma: a nested cohort study. Br J Anaesth. 2010;105(05):596–602.
214. Pastori D, Cormaci VM, Marucci S, Franchino G, Del Sole F, Capozza A, Fallarino A, Corso C, Valeriani E, Menichelli D, Pignatelli P. A comprehensive review of risk factors for venous thromboembolism: from epidemiology to pathophysiology. Int J Mol Sci. 2023;24(4):3169.
215. Geerts WH, Code KI, Jay RM, Chen E, Szalai JP. A prospective study of venous thromboembolism after major trauma. N Engl J Med. 1994;331(24):1601–6.
216. Beckman MG, Hooper WC, Critchley SE, Ortel TL. Venous thromboembolism: a public health concern. Am J Prev Med. 2010;38(Suppl. 4):S495–501.
217. Gao X, Zeng L, Wang H, Zeng S, Tian J, Chen L, Peng T. Prevalence of venous thromboembolism in intensive care units: a meta-analysis. J Clin Med. 2022;11(22):6691.
218. Ebeid A, Cole E, Stallwood-Hall C. The efficacy of weight-based enoxaparin dosing for venous thromboembolism prophylaxis in trauma patients: a systematic review and meta-analysis. J Trauma Acute Care Surg. 2022;93(2):e71–9.
219. Tran A, Fernando SM, Carrier M, Siegal DM, Inaba K, Vogt K, Engels PT, English SW, Kanji S, Kyeremanteng K, Lampron J, Kim D, Rochwerg B. Efficacy and safety of low molecular weight heparin versus unfractionated heparin for prevention of venous thromboembolism in trauma patients: a systematic review and meta-analysis. Ann Surg. 2022;275(1):19–28.
220. Hamidi M, Zeeshan M, Kulvatunyou N, Mitra HS, Hanna K, Tang A, Northcutt A, O'Keeffe T, Joseph B. Operative spinal trauma: thromboprophylaxis with low molecular weight heparin or a direct oral anticoagulant. J Thromb Haemost. 2019;17(6):925–33.
221. Chouhan VD, Comerota AJ, Sun L, Harada R, Gaughan JP, Rao AK. Inhibition of tissue factor pathway during intermittent pneumatic compression: a possible mechanism for anti-thrombotic effect. Arterioscler Thromb Vasc Biol. 1999;19(11):2812–7.

222. Kakkos S, Kirkilesis G, Caprini JA, Geroulakos G, Nicolaides A, Stansby G, Reddy DJ. Combined intermittent pneumatic leg compression and pharmacological prophylaxis for prevention of venous thromboembolism. Cochrane Database Syst Rev. 2022;1(1):CD005258.

223. Brady D, Raingruber B, Peterson J, Varnau W, Denman J, Resuello R, De Contreaus R, Mahnke J. The use of knee-length versus thigh-length compression stockings and sequential compression devices. Crit Care Nurs Q. 2007;30(3):255–62.

224. Kelkar AH, Rajasekhar A. Do prophylactic inferior vena cava filters in trauma patients reduce the risk of mortality or pulmonary embolism? Hematol Am Soc Hematol Educ Program. 2020;2020(1):629–33.

225. Mulder MB, Eidelson SA, Sussman MS, Schulman CI, Lineen EB, Iyenger RS, Namias N, Proctor KG. Risk factors and clinical outcomes associated with augmented renal clearance in trauma patients. J Surg Res. 2019;244:477–83.

226. Farrar JE, Droege ME, Philpott CD, Mueller EW, Ernst NE, Makley AT, Deichstetter KM, Droege CA. Impact of weight on anti-Xa attainment in high-risk trauma patients on enoxaparin chemoprophylaxis. J Surg Res. 2021;264:425–34.

227. Verhoeff K, Raffael K, Connell M, Kung JY, Strickland M, Parker A, Anantha RV. Relationship between anti-Xa level achieved with prophylactic low-molecular weight heparin and venous thromboembolism in trauma patients: a systematic review and meta-analysis. J Trauma Acute Care Surg. 2022;93(2):e61–70.

228. Rudis M, Attwood R. Emergency medicine pharmacy practice. J Pharm Pract. 2011;24(2):135–45. https://doi.org/10.1177/0897190011400549.

229. Fairbanks R, Hildebrand J, Kolstee K, Schneider S, Shah M. Medical and nursing staff highly value clinical pharmacists in the emergency department. Emerg Med J. 2007;24(10):716–8. https://doi.org/10.1136/emj.2006.044313.

230. Patanwala A, Hays D. Pharmacist's activities on a trauma response team in the emergency department. Am J Health Syst Pharm. 2010;67(18):1536–8. https://doi.org/10.2146/ajhp090311.

231. Montgomery K, Hall B, Keriazes G. Pharmacist's impact on acute pain management during trauma resuscitation. J Trauma Nurs. 2015;22(2):87–90. https://doi.org/10.1097/JTN.0000000000000112.

232. Porter B, Zaeem M, Hewes P, et al. Pharmacist involvement in trauma resuscitation across the United States: a 10-year follow-up survey. Am J Health Syst Pharm. 2019;76(16):1226–30. https://doi.org/10.1093/ajhp/zxz124.

233. Roman C, Dooley M, Fitzgerald M, et al. Pharmacists in trauma: a randomised controlled trial of emergency medicine pharmacists in trauma response teams. Emerg Med J. 2024;41(7):397–403. https://doi.org/10.1136/emermed-2022-212934.

Part X
Special Considerations in Critical Care

Chapter 42
Prescription for Prevention: A Focus on Preventing Complications in the ICU

Katherine Spezzano

42.1 Introduction

The foundation of critical care medicine is high-quality supportive care and frequent assessments to support a patient through their illness—all while preventing hospital-acquired complications. Prevention of the many hospital-acquired complications is key to reduce ICU length of stay and improve outcomes. Mnemonics such as FAST HUG and FAST HUGS BID have been specifically created to improve the quality of care for critically ill patients and ensure all aspects of general care are met [1, 2]. These mnemonics were created by intensivists, and FASTHUG-MAIDENS was created by pharmacists specifically to target medication-related problems [3]. Implementation of FASTHUG-MAIDENS by pharmacy residents has been shown to increase the identification of medication-related problems and increases the contribution a pharmacist can make during rounds [4]. This chapter will focus on various aspects of these mnemonics and hospital-acquired complications that prophylaxis is implemented for routinely during the care of a critically ill patient.

42.2 Venous Thromboembolism Prophylaxis

Venous thromboembolism (VTE) is a relatively common diagnosis; however, VTE as a result of hospitalization or critical illness is preventable. Despite this, about 50% of VTE events occur due to a current or recent hospital stay [5]. This could be due to patient's individual risk factors, inability to receive prophylaxis against VTE, suboptimal agent selection, or inappropriate dosing. The critical care pharmacist, in

K. Spezzano (✉)
University of Kentucky HealthCare, Lexington, KY, USA
e-mail: kat.spezzano@uky.edu

© The Author(s), under exclusive license to Springer Nature
Switzerland AG 2025
Y. Alzaidi, M. A. Gebily (eds.), *The Pharmacist's Expanded Role in Critical Care Medicine*, https://doi.org/10.1007/978-3-031-77335-8_42

conjunction with the medical team, is able to ensure appropriateness of VTE prophylaxis for a given patient while optimizing agent choice and dosing.

The American Society of Hematology recommends using pharmacologic VTE prophylaxis compared to no prophylaxis in critically ill patients [5]. However, in clinical practice this decision isn't always as black and white. Patients can have a compilation of factors that may make them a higher bleeding risk but concomitantly have a high risk to develop a VTE. An abbreviated list of risk factors for VTE and factors that increase bleeding risk can be found in Table 42.1. Risk stratification scores have been created to assist clinicians in assessing a patient's risk for VTE, especially when a patient has one or more factors associated with increased bleed risk. The Caprini score can be utilized for surgical patients and has been validated in many different types of surgical patients; the Padua Prediction Score is thought to be the best model for medical patients [6, 7].

There are several options for pharmacologic prevention of VTE including low-molecular weight heparins (LMWH), unfractionated heparin (UFH), and fondaparinux. These medications are indirect anticoagulants that bind to antithrombin III and form a covalent bond with coagulation enzymes to inhibit their procoagulant activity [8]. The difference between them are the length of the chains after the pentasaccharide responsible for binding antithrombin III, with heparin having the longest, variable chains, and fondaparinux being synthesized only to be the pentasaccharide sequence [8]. The general dosing strategies can be found in Table 42.2. Generally, LMWH, such as enoxaparin and dalteparin, is preferred over UFH due to increased efficacy in preventing deep venous thrombosis [9]. There are certain instances where you would preferentially utilize UFH; patients with a creatinine clearance under 30 mL/min or increased bleeding risk often receive UFH. UFH has a comparatively shorter half-life (1.5 h compared to 7 h), is not renally metabolized, and can be more completely reversed by protamine if necessary, though prophylactic doses often do not require reversal [8]. Alternatively, the dose of enoxaparin can be decreased in patients with a creatinine clearance of <30 mL/min, but switching to UFH is generally deemed the safer option [8]. Fondaparinux is reserved for patients with a history of heparin-induced thrombocytopenia (HIT) since it will not provoke the same immunologic reaction as our other pharmacologic agents. This agent is also renally metabolized and contraindicated with a creatinine clearance

Table 42.1 Risk factors for VTE and increased bleeding risk [5]

Increased VTE risk	Increased bleeding risk
• Reduced mobility	• GFR < 60 mL/min/m^2
• Active cancer	• Age > 40
• Previous VTE	• Active cancer
• Known thrombophilic condition	• Intensive Care Unit stay
• Trauma or surgery within 1 month	• INR > 1.5
• Age > 70	• Bleeding within 3 months
• Ongoing hormonal treatment	
• Body mass index >30	
• Active infection	
• Pregnancy	

GFR glomerular filtration rate, *INR* international normalized ratio

Table 42.2 Dosing of pharmacologic agents for VTE prophylaxis [8, 10]

Pharmacologic options	Dosing strategy	Body weight considerations
Unfractionated Heparin	5000 units SQ every 8 h	BMI $\geq$ 40 mg/m^2: 7500 units SQ every 8 h
Enoxaparin	40 mg SQ every 24 h	40 $\leq$ BMI < 50 mg/m^2: 40 mg SQ every 12 h BMI $\geq$ 50 mg/m^2: 60 mg SQ every 12 h
Dalteparin	5000 mg SQ every 24 h	BMI $\geq$ 40 mg/m^2: 7500 units SQ every 24 h
Fondaparinux	2.5 mg SQ every 24 h	Contraindicated if body weight < 50 kg

SQ subcutaneous, *BMI* body mass index

<30 mL/min [8]. It also uniquely is contraindicated in patients with low body weight, limiting its potential utilization further. There is little additional monitoring than renal function, signs of bleeding, and platelets, as mentioned above. Anti-Xa monitoring is utilized for therapeutic dosing of LMWH, however very infrequent for prophylactic dosing. Acceptable ranges for anti-Xa levels are not widely agreed upon for this indication, however 0.2–0.59 units/mL can be considered.

Besides increased bleeding risk, HIT is the largest adverse effect that we must monitor for when utilizing either LMWH or UFH for VTE prophylaxis. This can affect up to 5% of patients who receive UFH and 1% who receive LMWH; however, it is more prevalent in the cardiothoracic surgery patient population due to their increased exposure to heparin products [11, 12]. This effect is an immunologic response of IgG antibodies binding to heparin-PF4 complexes. PF4 is a molecule released upon platelet activation and is attracted to heparin due to their opposite charges. Once IgG attaches to this complex, it can further activate platelets, releasing more PF4, creating a cyclic process and induce a severely hypercoagulable state also associated with a high bleeding risk due to consumption of platelets [11]. The hallmark sign of HIT is this reduction in platelets, typically seen 5–10 days from the onset of heparin exposure, or within 1 day if the patient has had prior exposure. What makes identification challenging is that there are many confounding factors that can lead to thrombocytopenia in a critically ill patient. Continuous venovenous hemodialysis, medication side effects, mechanical support devices, and sepsis are common confounders in the diagnosis of HIT. The 4 T score is a predictive tool that can assess a patient's likelihood for experiencing HIT based on the level of thrombocytopenia, timing of platelet fall, presence of thrombosis, and presence of any other confounding causes [13]. The negative predictive value of this tool is 99.8%, so if a patient's score is <3 a HIT diagnosis is unlikely [13]. A higher score with this tool may warrant laboratory testing, holding additional heparin products, and considering anticoagulation with direct thrombin inhibitors while the results are pending.

Patients should not also receive VTE prophylaxis if they are thrombocytopenic from other causes. Generally, VTE prophylaxis is withheld if a patient's platelets fall below 50,000/mm^3. This is based off surgical data regarding risk of hemorrhage during surgery with this level of thrombocytopenia [14]. If the risk of developing a VTE in a patient is deemed to be extremely high, the evidence suggests that platelets <10,000 /mm^3 is when there is a risk for spontaneous intracranial hemorrhage and prophylaxis should definitely be withheld [15]. In practice, we generally stick to the 50,000/mm³ cutoff. Patients experiencing active bleeding or have experienced recent severe hemorrhage should also not receive VTE prophylaxis. The timing of re-initiating therapy depends on numerous factors such as severity of the bleed, site of the bleed, and the patient's assessed risk for developing a VTE. More critical locations of bleeding, such as intracranial hemorrhage, may require holding prophylaxis (and anticoagulation) for a month, while gastro-intestinal (GI) bleeding only requires withholding VTE prophylaxis if managed aggressively only until the condition has been managed, and conservatively up to 14 days [16]. These recommendations come from resumption of full anticoagulation, so pending a patient's risk for development of a VTE, prophylaxis may be considered sooner. While patients cannot receive pharmacologic prophylaxis, there are several non-pharmacologic prophylactic options that can be utilized. Options include intermittent pneumatic compression devices and graduated compression stockings. These therapies are often utilized in combination with pharmacologic prophylaxis though the literature does not support a benefit to this practice [9]. Inferior vena cava filters are another option, however requires an invasive procedure and typically limited to patients who have an indication for therapeutic anticoagulation but cannot tolerate it.

Other considerations when deciding on selecting and dosing VTE prophylaxis is patient body mass index (BMI), patient population, and medical history. Patients with elevated BMI require increased dosing of both LMWH and UFH [17, 18]. Refer to Table 42.2 for this dosing information. Patients who also present as a trauma or undergo orthopedic surgery require increased dosing of LMWH. Enoxaparin 30 mg subcutaneously every 12 h was shown to be more effective at reducing the incidence of deep venous thrombosis than UFH in patients who have experienced major trauma, so this dosing has been adopted for the trauma patient population [19]. Finally, patients with a history or new diagnosis of liver disease may have an elevated INR. While in a typical patient, increases in INR are typically associated with an anticoagulant effect, this does not have the same meaning in this population. Both anticoagulant and procoagulant factors are decreased in liver disease, meaning their risk for both bleeding and thromboembolism is increased. These patients still require VTE prophylaxis, despite an elevated INR.

42.3   Stress Ulcer Prophylaxis

Critically ill patients can develop stress ulcers while hospitalized, which can progress to gastrointestinal (GI) hemorrhage. These ulcers are thought to occur due to reduced gastric blood flow, mucosal ischemia, and reperfusion injury [20]. Patients at higher risk for developing stress ulcers are candidates for stress ulcer prophylaxis (SUP). Risk factors are commonly divided into major and minor factors; one major risk factor or two minor risk factors are indications for SUP [21–25]. A summary of risk factors can be found in Table 42.3.

Table 42.3 Risk factors for SUP [21–25]

Major risk factors	Minor risk factors
• Mechanical ventilation > 48 h • Platelet count < 50,000/mm³ • INR > 1.5 or PTT 2× control • Burns >30% TBSA • Spinal cord injury/head trauma	• Renal failure • Septic shock • Hydrocortisone > 250 mg/day[a] • GI bleed or perforation within 1 year

TBSA total body surface area, *INR* international normalized ratio, *PTT* partial thromboplastin time
[a]or equivalent doses of other corticosteroids

Table 42.4 Dosing of pharmacologic options for SUP

Pharmacologic agent	Dosing
Proton pump inhibitors	
Omeprazole	20 mg PO daily
Pantoprazole	40 mg PO/NG/IV daily
Esomeprazole	40 mg PO/NG daily
Lansoprazole	30 mg PO/NG daily
Rabeprazole	20 mg PO/NG daily
Histamine type-2 receptor antagonists	
Famotidine	20 mg PO/NG/IV twice daily
Cimetidine	300 mg PO four times daily

PO by mouth, *NG* per nasogastric tube, *IV* intravenous

Pharmacologic agents to prevent stress ulcers focus on increasing the intragastric pH; a pH of <4 has been correlated with the degree of esophageal injury [26]. Proton pump inhibitors (PPIs) or histamine Type-2 receptor antagonists (H2RAs) have been shown to increase the intragastric pH > 4 [26, 27]; Other acid-lowering pharmacologic therapies, such as antacids and sucralfate, have been shown to be inferior to these therapies [23, 28]. PPIs irreversibly inhibit the stomach's H^+/K^+ ATPase proton pump, thereby inhibiting the secretion of gastric acid. Typical dosing for stress ulcer prevention is only once daily, which can lead to 70% of enzymes being inhibited [27]. Reaching steady state takes 2–3 days with acid inhibition of an enzyme lasting up to 48 h due to the irreversible binding to the H^+/K^+ ATPase proton pump [27]. A summary of dosing for the different PPIs can be found in Table 42.4. H2RAs lower the secretion of gastric acid by reversibly inhibiting histamine H2 receptors on gastric parietal cells. These cells are responsible for secreting gastric acid. The onset of action for these medications is approximately 60 minutes and have a much longer half-life than PPIs (4–10 h versus 90 min) making them ideal for on-demand treatment and quick onset [10, 27]. However, due to their reversible binding, at least twice daily dosing is required. A summary of standard H2RA dosing schemes can be found in Table 42.4. H2RAs are renally metabolized, so will require a dose adjustment for patients who have renal impairment.

There has been much debate over which pharmacologic agent is the best choice for pharmacologic prevention of stress ulcers and resulting GI hemorrhage. The

PEPTIC trial in 2020 examined if there was any difference in 90-day mortality in utilizing either PPIs or H2RAs for SUP. This trial found no difference in mortality (18.3% vs 17.5%; 95% CI 1.00–1.10); however, a high rate of cross-over from the H2RA cohort muddies these results [29]. Due to a wide acceptance that these two pharmacologic classes are equal, the agent with lower side effects seems to be the logical choice. While the long-term side effect of bone density loss associated with PPIs is not relevant to its use for this indication, there are still risks of acute interstitial nephritis, Clostridium difficile infections, and pneumonia [30] with these agents. Recent studies also indicate an increased risk for developing extended-spectrum β-lactamase- or carbapenemase-producing Enterobacterales with PPI therapy [31]. H2RAs are generally well tolerated with the most common side effects including headache, drowsiness, abdominal pain, constipation, and diarrhea [10]. Delirium and/or confusion can be seen with H2RAs in elderly patients or those with renal or liver impairment; however, this can be mitigated with proper renal dose adjustments and avoidance of cimetidine [32]. However, PPIs can be considered over H2RAs for patients who are on PPI therapy at home, have symptoms of GI reflux despite H2RA therapy, or cannot tolerate H2RAs.

Pharmacotherapy for SUP may not be required. Recent literature suggests that enteral nutrition may be enough to provide prophylaxis from developing stress ulcers. The mechanism for this protective effect has not been elucidated, but it is postulated to be due to dilutional alkalization or stimulating gastric blood flow [33, 34]. A systematic review of pharmacologic SUP to either placebo or no prophylaxis in critically ill patients who were receiving enteral nutrition found that there was no difference between GI bleeding (RR 0.80; 95% CI 0.49–1.31) [35]. Due to low risk of starting enteral nutrition and the elevated risk with pharmacologic SUP, especially PPIs, utilizing enteral nutrition as SUP may be reasonable. However, current practice has been hesitant to adopt this practice and pharmacologic SUP is often utilized despite a patient's nutrition status. There are still many unknowns about enteral nutrition as SUP, such as rate of feeds, location of feeding, and additional patient selection, prior to this being adopted into practice.

42.4 Prevention of Infection

Critically ill patients often require invasive lines, drains, and mechanical ventilation through an endotracheal tube. All these foreign objects are a source of acquired infection, and the risk increases the longer they are present [36]. The assessment of any indwelling lines or catheters is even a part of the FAST HUGS BID mnemonic in order to draw attention to their presence and hopefully encourage their early removal [2]. Without their removal, patients are at risk for developing central line-associated bloodstream infections (CLABSIs) or catheter-associated urinary tract infections (CAUTIs). Intensive care units are often assessed on how frequent these infections happen, and there is a large institutional push to reduce the rate of them as much as possible.

The most common indications for indwelling lines can be found in Table 42.5. Hemodynamic monitoring is indicated when patients are either on continuous vasoactive or antihypertensive medications and typically done through an arterial line. This allows the medical team to get more accurate measurements of blood pressure so that these medications can be titrated appropriately. In practice, if a patient is on low-dose hemodynamic support and is thought that they will only need support for 24–48 hours, the team may defer placing an arterial line as long as the cuff blood pressure is thought to be accurate. This is one way in practice to prevent placement of central access and reduce a patient's infectious risk. Placement of a central line is also needed for medications considered vesicants or irritants to reduce the likelihood of extravasation or infiltrations [37, 38]. Extravasation is leakage of a vesicant into surrounding tissues which can cause soft tissue damage from blistering and tissue necrosis while infiltrations are caused by irritants leaking into the surrounding tissues [38]. Cytotoxic chemotherapy medications are common vesicants but noncytotoxic medications are less described. Table 42.6 provides a summary of some common vesicants utilized in the critically ill patient. Of note, vasopressors are classified as a vesicant, but more literature is being published about the safety of peripheral vasopressor administration, at least for short duration. The recent CLOVERS trial assessing fluid management strategies in septic shock allowed for the use of peripheral vasopressors and 63% of patients were started via this route [39]. Of the patients utilizing peripheral access to receive vasopressors, only three patients (0.006%) experienced extravasation, showcasing the overall safety of this practice [39].

Despite practices to limit the utilization of central lines, often they are still required during the course of a critically ill patient. There are still several options to reduce the rate of CLABSIs and CAUTIs rather than removing the access. The first is the adherence to central line insertion bundle. The proposed bundle is separated into things to do prior to, during, and after insertion of a central venous catheter. Before insertion, it is recommended to have an evidence-based list of indications for central access, require education for those involved in the insertion, and give patients admitted to the ICU chlorhexidine baths daily [42]. During insertion providers should adhere to infection prevention practices such as the aseptic technique and maximal barrier precautions, perform hand hygiene, utilize an all-inclusive catheter

Table 42.5 Common indications for indwelling lines [37, 40]

Central venous lines	Urinary catheters
• Hemodynamic monitoring	• Assessment of urinary output
• Administration of vesicants or irritants	• Urinary retention
• Frequent lab draws	• Bladder outlet obstruction
• Poor venous access, limited peripheral lines	• Assist healing of open sacral or perineal wounds
• Acute renal failure requiring HD or CRRT	
• Plasmapheresis	
• Bradycardia requiring transvenous pacing	

HD hemodialysis, *CRRT* continuous renal replacement therapy

Table 42.6 Common vesicants in the critically ill [38, 41]

Vesicants
• Acyclovir
• Albumin
• Amiodarone
• Amphotericin
• Ampicillin
• Calcium salts
• Contrast
• Dextrose solutions $\geq 10\%$
• Dobutamine
• Immunoglobulin
• Lorazepam
• Mannitol
• Parenteral nutrition, lipids
• Phenytoin
• Potassium chloride
• Propofol
• Sodium bicarbonate
• Valproic acid
• Vancomycin
• Vasopressors

kit, and bathe the patient's skin around the insertion site in chlorhexidine [42]. If internal jugular access is required, it is recommended to do this guided by an ultrasound machine [42]. Additionally, while not addressed for all patients in the guidelines, the femoral access site for central lines has been found to have an increased rate of CLABSIs compared to intrajugular access (58.3% vs 41.7%; $p = 0.0008$) [43]. The internal jugular site has also been shown to be more prone to CLABSIs compared to the subclavian location [44]. After insertion, ensure optimal nursing ratios, disinfect catheter hubs, needleless connectors, and injection ports before accessing the central line, appropriately care for each line type and change dressings as recommended, remove central lines as soon as able, and perform surveillance for CLABSIs [42]. Pharmacists can help with the timely removal of central lines or urinary catheters by incorporating it into their daily review. We can note when medications requiring central access are discontinued, provide recommendations on appropriate alternatives to vesicants, and if no diuretics or large volume input is expected, ask the team if the urinary catheter is necessary.

Another common hospital-acquired infection that requires routine prevention and surveillance is ventilator-associated pneumonia (VAP). VAP occurs in approximately 10% of critically ill patients who require mechanical ventilation and requires longer duration of mechanical ventilation and hospital length of stay [45–47]. The Society for Healthcare Epidemiology, Infectious Diseases Society of America, American Hospital Association, Association for Professionals in Infection Control and Epidemiology, and The Joint Commission have recommendations for preventing this acquired infection [48]. Their recommendations are summarized in Table 42.7. Notably, minimizing sedation and implementing sedation awakening trials and

Table 42.7 VAP prevention strategies [48]

Essential practices	Considerations	Not recommended
• Avoid intubation and reintubation • Minimize sedation • Elevate the head-of-bed to 30–45° • Provide oral care with a toothbrush • Provide early nutrition – Enteral nutrition is preferred	• If there is a low prevalence of antibiotic resistant organisms, consider selective decontamination • Early tracheostomy • Postpyloric feeding	• Oral care with chlorhexidine • Chlorhexidine bathing • Probiotics • Monitoring residual gastric volumes

spontaneous breathing trials have shown to increase the amount of days free from the ventilator (14.7 days vs 11.6 days; $p = 0.02$) [49]. Additionally, in stark difference to the CLABSI recommendations in favor of chlorhexidine bathing, the VAP prevention guidelines recommend against this practice [48]. This is due to meta-analyses not showing improvements in rate of VAP when only double-blind studies were analyzed (RR, 0.88 [95% CI, 0.66–1.16]) and with potential for increased rate of mortality (OR 1.25, 1.05–1.50) [50, 51]. Due to these conflicting recommendations and unclear correlation with mortality, many institutions still utilize chlorhexidine oral care and bathing for the prevention of hospital-acquired infections.

Many institutions still implement selective decolonization to methicillin-resistant staphylococcus aureus (MRSA), a common organism implicated in VAP. Two pharmacologic agents exist for this indication, mupirocin ointment and iodophor. The most common iodophor in practice is povidone-iodine. Two decolonization strategies exist: universal decolonization to all patients admitted to the ICU and selective decontamination to patients who tested positive for MRSA in their nares via nasal swabbing. Huang and colleagues found that the universal decolonization strategy with mupirocin was more effective in reducing MRSA clinical isolates [52]. However, it was unclear which option was more efficacious. In combination with chlorhexidine bathing, povidone-iodine was not found to be noninferior to mupirocin in reducing the incidence of *staphylococcus aureus* and MRSA clinical cultures [53]. If an institution deems that it would like to utilize universal decolonization based on their prevalence of antibiotic resistance, mupirocin plus chlorhexidine bathing seems to be a reasonable strategy.

An additional therapy that has been used to prevent VAP is the empiric use of antibiotics. Various regimens have been studied including administration of intravenous (IV) ampicillin-sulbactam, IV ceftriaxone, nebulized aminoglycosides, nebulized ceftazidime, and nebulized colistin [54–59]. In a meta-analysis of comparative trials regarding this indication, it was found that the use of prophylactic antibiotics resulted in lower VAP rates compared with control groups (RR = 0.62) [60]. This practice has still not been widely adopted due to concerns regarding selection bias in many of the studies investigating prophylactic antibiotics.

## 42.5	Prevention of Hypoglycemia

Spontaneous episodes of severe hypoglycemia happen in <1.5% of critically ill patients but can have profound effects on morbidity and mortality, if untreated [61, 62]. Hypoglycemia is more common in patients with fulminant hepatic failure, overt adrenal failure during septic shock, malnutrition, chronic liver cirrhosis, and chronic renal failure [63]. Hypoglycemia is commonly defined as a blood glucose level <70 mg/dL; however, symptoms may not be present at this threshold [64]. Severe hypoglycemia is considered as a blood glucose level <40 mg/dL, and patients will almost always be symptomatic at this level [65]. Hypoglycemia may have such an impact on morbidity and mortality since glucose is the brain's primary source of energy [66]. A reduction in this supply can cause impairment in neuronal function [66]. Additionally, the catecholamine release in response to hypoglycemia can cause myocardial ischemia, hypokalemia, and prolongation of the QTc interval causing arrhythmias [67]. Historically, it was thought that strict blood glucose control to levels of 80–110 mg/dL was optimal; however, the NICE_SUGAR trial actually showed this practice increased mortality compared to the target of 140–180 mg/dL [62, 65]. This could be related to the higher incidence of severe hypoglycemia in the intensive glucose control cohort (6.8% vs 0.5%; $p < 0.001$) [62]. Therefore, in practice the glucose target range of 140–180 mg/dL has been adopted.

As mentioned above, patients with impaired liver or renal function are at a higher risk for hypoglycemia. Insulin is metabolized and cleared through both the liver and the kidney. Endogenous insulin secreted by the pancreas is 80% cleared through first pass metabolism as it is transported to the liver prior to systematic circulation via the portal vein [68]. Then any systemic insulin is filtered by the glomeruli and reabsorbed in the proximal tubule [69]. The liver is also pivotal in glucose homeostasis, regulating glucose production and storage through gluconeogenesis and glycogenolysis [70]. If there are no glycogen stores due to impaired glycogenesis, hypoglycemia can occur if means of nutrition and glucose source is stopped. For these patients, increased monitoring while NPO and a reduced threshold for starting a dextrose infusion during that time is warranted. With renal impairment, impaired clearance of insulin can lead to dose-stacking. Due to this, 5 units of regular insulin is now recommended for treatment of hyperkalemia in patients with renal dysfunction, compared to 10 units, due to reduced rates of hypoglycemia (15.6% versus 6.1%; $p = 0.004$) with the same level of potassium reduction [71].

Selecting the appropriate insulin regimen for critically ill patients also is an important factor in preventing hypoglycemia. Patients with Type 2 diabetes mellitus (DM) may have prior to admission oral antihyperglycemic medications. On admission to the ICU, these agents are stopped due to potential adverse effects from their continuance. The two main examples of this are development of lactic acidosis with continuation of metformin if acute kidney injury develops and hypoglycemia if sulfonylureas are continued [72, 73]. Patients with Type 2 DM may also be on home subcutaneous insulin therapy. The nutrition provided to critically ill patients is variable, so a 20% reduction in the home basal insulin dose is widely adopted and the basal dose should be around 50% of the insulin regimen [74]. The 20% correction factor is due to the variable nutrition and often unknown compliance however there may be an increased requirement due to critical illness, so clinical judgment is needed. For patients with Type 1 DM, there is no endogenous insulin production so their home regimens typically consist only of subcutaneous insulin and could be delivered via an insulin pump. There should be no interruption of basal insulin for patients with Type 1 DM due to the potential development of diabetic ketoacidosis (DKA) [75]. The same correction factor as patients with Type 2 DM can be considered, but likely a more conservative adjustment should be applied given the risk for development of DKA. If a patient is managed with an insulin pump at home, most institutions require patients to be able to manage this independently to continue this while admitted. Many critically ill patients lack this capacity, so the pump should be stopped and this can be converted to a basal dose of insulin depending on the pump's settings.

Patient's insulin requirements may initially be increased comparatively from home due to stress hyperglycemia related to their critical illness. The basal insulin discussed above should be given either as insulin glargine or regular insulin. Insulin glargine is typically dosed every 24 hours, either in the morning or evening, due to its long half-life, however twice daily dosing can be considered based on a patient's home regimen or total insulin requirements [10]. This long half-life is what also makes this option less frequently utilized in practice in the ICU. Patients may go NPO spontaneously, and despite that fact that the glargine should be dosed solely on a patient's basal requirement, it may lead to hypoglycemia if nutrition is stopped and the glargine is still on board due to impaired clearance mechanisms reviewed above. This is why utilizing a basal-bolus regimen for insulin management is so important. Only proven basal requirements should be covered with insulin glargine for a critically ill patient. Another option for basal insulin administration is regular insulin, dosed every 6 hours based on its half-life of 1.5 h [10]. This option has less of risk of hypoglycemia if tube feeds are stopped since the half-life is shorter. In addition to any basal requirements a patient may have, patients may require additional boluses of insulin depending on a patient's diet or critical illness. A good indicator of how much to increase a patient's insulin regimen is by how much of their sliding scale they are requiring. Sliding scales can either be "regular" or increased to "resistant." Resistant insulin sliding scale may be appropriate if a patient is on over 40 units of insulin a day prior to admission or if it is noted that the blood glucose readings are not decreasing after an appropriate dose of the regular insulin sliding scale [76]. If a patient is receiving full tube feeding, increasing the dose of regular insulin by an average of the sliding scale amount is appropriate. If utilizing insulin glargine, the dose should only be increased if the fasting blood glucose reading is above 180 mg/dL and all checks throughout the day have been elevated. Of note, for patients experiencing hyperglycemia, sliding scale insulin alone is not sufficient. The basal-bolus regimen has been shown to have improved blood glucose control without an increase in hypoglycemia compared to utilizing sliding scale alone [77]. Patients should be switched over to receiving insulin lispro when/if they tolerate oral feeds since it closer replicates normal insulin secretion due to its rapid onset and short half-life [10, 78]. Due to the constant changes in caring for critically ill patients, an activatable hypoglycemia protocol should be ordered on all patients receiving insulin [79].

Despite the American Diabetes Association recommending that all critically ill patients be treated with intravenous insulin, this is not as common in practice [80]. The rationale behind this recommendation is to achieve rapid control over hyperglycemia due to the mortality benefits [65]. There are some disease states, such as DKA, hyperosmolar hyperglycemia syndrome, or hypertriglyceridemia-induced pancreatitis, that require utilization of this therapy. However, these protocols are outside the scope of this chapter since they are not solely targeting therapy to a blood glucose level of 140–180 mg/dL. Insulin drips are typically nursing-protocol driven, require more frequent monitoring than subcutaneous administration, and are considered a high-risk medication. Due to this, subcutaneous administration is often chosen as an initial strategy, in the face of recommendations that critically ill patients be managed with intravenous insulin. The Critical Care Medicine guidelines expand upon this further stating that patients who are not appropriate for subcutaneous insulin are patients with Type 1 DM, hemodynamically unstable, hypothermia, edema, or frequent interruption of dextrose intake [81]. Once patients have stabilized, they suggest that it is then they can be switched to a subcutaneous regimen [81]. However, if patients are persistently above goal with subcutaneous therapy and it is thought that they will not reach the goal with adjustments in this regimen, or if there is concerns about impaired subcutaneous absorption, which can be seen with elevated doses of vasopressors or fluid overload, patients may be switched to an intravenous infusion.

42.6 Prevention of Delirium

Delirium occurs in up to 80% of critically ill patients and can increase six month mortality [82, 83]. The incidence is lower in patients who are in the ICU but not requiring mechanical ventilation, however can still reach up to 50% [82]. In addition to increased mortality, patients with delirium have an increased time on mechanical ventilation, increased ICU length of stay, hospital length of stay, and cost [84, 85]. Unfortunately, there is no guideline recommended treatment for delirium, only recommendations for prevention [86]. Both the MIND-USA trial and the AID-ICU trial assessed treating delirium with antipsychotics, and found they did not change mortality or days without delirium compared to placebo [87, 88]. Prevention is paramount to address delirium prior to it escalating in severity to being addressed with sedating medications for patient and/or staff safety or increasing barriers to extubation or liberation from the ICU.

Several components make up the guideline recommended prevention strategies. As a bundled approach, these components have been shown to decrease the development of delirium and reduce the amount of time spent with delirium, if diagnosed [89]. One component of these bundles is re-orientation done by either family members or staff. Re-orientation done by a family member is often more successful due to patient's familiarity with them and also due to limitations on staff's time and nursing ratios [90]. Upon admittance to the ICU, ensuring patients have access to any vision or hearing aids they may require and as are appropriate, also helps in preventing delirium [91]. Sleep hygiene is frequently implicated in the development of delirium, so optimizing this has also shown to be helpful [86]. Having the blinds up in a patient's room during the day, minimizing light and sounds at night, and ensuring television use only during waking hours are all steps to encourage maintenance of the sleep-wake cycle. Finally, stewardship of medications linked to delirium should be considered. Medications linked to delirium are summarized in Table 42.8, frequently due to requiring renal adjustments. While some of these medications may be necessary in a patient's disease course; risk versus benefit discussions are warranted when there are appropriate alternatives in a patient at risk or diagnosed with delirium.

Scoring tools have been validated in the critically ill population to diagnose delirium. These tools are the Confusion Assessment Method for the ICU, or CAM-ICU, score and the Intensive Care Delirium Screening Checklist, or ICDSC [86]. These assessments are done at a minimum once every 12 hours since the hallmark of delirium is a waxing and waning state. As mentioned previously, there is no recommended treatment for delirium if it develops. Routine practice is to enforce any preventative measures and assess if any medications linked to delirium can be discontinued. Antipsychotic or sedative medications should only be considered if a patient is a harm to themselves or others. Delirium typically lasts for three days, however can last up to several weeks, and supportive therapy is continued until improvement [94].

Table 42.8 Medications associated with delirium [92, 93]

Medications
• Corticosteroids
• Sedatives
– Especially benzodiazepines
• Opioids
• Anticholinergic medication
– Antihistamines
– Scopolamine
• Non-steroidal anti-inflammatory drugs
• Skeletal muscle relaxants
• Digoxin
• Tricyclic antidepressants
• Fluoroquinolones
• Anticonvulsants
• Dihydropyridines

42.7   Prevention of Acute Kidney Injury

Acute kidney injury (AKI) occurs in up to 50% of critically ill patients and has been associated with increased time on mechanical ventilation, incidence of chronic kidney disease, hospital length of stay, and mortality [95–97]. The risk factors associated with the development of AKI in critically ill patients are listed in Table 42.9. Pharmacists can play a key role in modifying the nephrotoxic drug administration risk factor. When a pharmacist is involved in the recommendations of drug selection, routes, dose adjustment, drug–drug interactions, drug side effect management, and more, the incidence of AKI decreases [98]

Pharmacist are uniquely poised to assist with nephrotoxin stewardship since the literature assessing different nephrotoxins is continually updated. For example, the concomitant administration of vancomycin and piperacillin-tazobactam was believed to cause an increased incidence of AKI, compared to administration with other beta-lactams [100]. However, more recent evidence suggests that this is a pseudotoxicity [101]. While serum creatinine appears to increase with this combination therapy, no other markers of nephrotoxicity, including cystatin C, requirement of dialysis, or mortality, were increased compared to other combination beta-lactam therapy [101]. While practice had swung to avoid this combination for several years, now pharmacists can educate the medical team about this new data and open up therapy options for patients without question of risk.

The reason that the combination of vancomycin and piperacillin-tazobactam was associated with development of AKI was due to the criteria for diagnosing AKI. In literature examining this complication, an increase in serum creatinine was often utilized [100]. However, creatinine is not the perfect measurement of renal function since it is not only filtered through the glomerulus but secreted into the tubules, as well [102]. Both vancomycin and piperacillin-tazobactam bind to renal transporters that mediate the secretion of creatinine, potentially leading to this increase in secretion and an elevation in creatinine. If creatinine was the only measurement monitored, an increase in serum creatinine would seem to correlate to a decrease in glomerular filtration, instead of an

Table 42.9 Risk factors associated with the development of AKI [99]

Risk factors
• Diabetes
• Emergency surgery
• Heart failure
• High-risk surgery
• Higher baseline creatinine
• Higher severity of disease scores
• Hypertension
• Longer time in cardiopulmonary bypass pump
• Older age
• Sepsis
• Use of intra-aortic balloon pump
• Use of nephrotoxic drugs
• Use of vasopressors/inotropes

increase in tubular secretion. Markers of kidney function, such as cystatin C, may be a more accurate depiction of changes in glomerular filtration since it is produced by all nucleated cells and freely filtered by the glomerulus and not returned to circulation [103]. Cystatin C has been shown to be a better marker for early detection of AKI and is not affected by gender, age, race, protein intake, and muscle mass, like serum creatinine [104]. Despite most medications relying on creatinine clearance cutoffs, a systematic review of multiple medications showed that utilizing cystatin C to estimate glomerular filtration rate predicted drug clearance as well, or better, than serum creatinine [105]. Pharmacists can consider utilizing cystatin C to inform them of a patient's dynamic renal function and utilize this information in conjunction with other clinical references to decide on renal dose adjustments of medications.

42.8   Prevention of Torsade de Pointe

Torsade de Pointe is one of the most feared medication-induced side effects due to its ability to precipitate to ventricular fibrillation and cardiac arrest. It is a polymorphic ventricular arrhythmia associated with a prolonged QT interval, meaning the time from ventricular depolarization to repolarization is prolonged. QT prolongation can be congenital or acquired; medications are not the only etiology of acquired-QT prolongation, electrolyte disturbances and cardiac ischemia can cause a prolongation, as well [106, 107].

Part of the medication approval process now assesses a medication's proarrhythmic potential [108]. A list of common QT-prolonging medications can be found in Table 42.10. QT-prolonging medications have also been shown to have an additive effect [106]. In practice, the corrected QT interval, or QTc, is calculated to account for heart rate in the assessment of the QT interval. A prolonged QTc for males is >450 ms and > 460 ms for females. However, it is not until the QTc reaches 500 ms that the clinical team will typically adjust medications. A QTc of >500 ms is what has been shown to increase mortality as compared to lower values [109]. Even this

Table 42.10 Common QT-prolonging medications in the ICU [106, 108, 111–113]

Medications
• Procainamide
• Azithromycin
• Haloperidol
• Droperidol
• Tricyclic antidepressants
• Fluoroquinolones
• Methadone
• Ondansetron
• Propofol
• Azole antifungals
• Erythromycin
• Loop diuretics

cutoff doesn't go without scrutiny; if the QRS complex is prolonged in addition to the QTc more calculations can be done to assess a patient's true risk for arrhythmia. The JTc interval is defined as the end of the QRS complex (the J point) to the start of the T wave and characterizes repolarization and can be easily calculated by subtracting the duration of the QRS from the QTc. The JTc interval has been shown to be a better predictor of cardiac events than QTc if the QRS is >120 ms [110]. A prolonged JTc is defined as >430 ms.

Electrolyte management plays just as large a role for prevention of Torsade de Pointes as medication management. Electrolytes are often checked daily in critically ill patients and pharmacists should ensure they are appropriately repleted. Hypokalemia and hypocalcemia were the strongest independent risk factors for QTc prolongation in a study assessing risk factors for Torsade de Pointes [106]. Nursing-driven electrolyte replacement protocols can be implemented to assist with replacement of these electrolytes. They have been shown to reduce the time to electrolyte repletion and number of necessary repletions missed, without increasing high post-replacement measurements [114]. Even if institutions implement these protocols, pharmacists can still be helpful in recommending additional potassium monitoring or supplementation for patients receiving loop diuretics or patients at risk for refeeding syndrome.

If on a routine electrocardiogram, a patient has a prolonged QTc >500 ms, the first step is to evaluate the QRS. If this is prolonged more than 120 ms, consider calculating the JTc to assess if the prolonged QRS is elevating the QTc, or the patient still may be at risk for arrhythmia. If this is still prolonged or the patient's QRS was not prolonged, assess a patient's electrolytes and replete them, as necessary. After repletion, check another electrocardiogram to see if this resolved the prolonged QTc. Once electrolyte derangements are ruled out as the cause of a prolonged QTc, assess the medication list for any agents associated with a prolonged QTc. Withdraw these medications as able and substitute with alternatives than do not prolong the QTc. Examples of this is substitution of doxycycline for azithromycin for atypical coverage of community acquired pneumonia of prochlorperazine for ondansetron for the treatment of postoperative nausea and vomiting. Additionally, since QTc prolongation is additive, if a patient's QTc interval is borderline elevated and another QTc prolonging medication is added to their regimen, consider obtaining another electrocardiogram after initiation to ensure therapy is safe.

References

1. Vincent JL. Give your patient a fast hug (at least) once a day. Crit Care Med. 2005;33(6):1225–9.
2. Vincent WR 3rd. and K.W. Hatton, Critically ill patients need "FAST HUGS BID" (an updated mnemonic). Crit Care Med. 2009;37(7):2326–7. author reply 2327
3. Mabasa VH, et al. A standardized, structured approach to identifying drug-related problems in the intensive care unit: FASTHUG-MAIDENS. Can J Hosp Pharm. 2011;64(5):366–9.
4. Masson SC, et al. Validity evidence for FASTHUG-MAIDENS, a mnemonic for identifying drug-related problems in the intensive care unit. Can J Hosp Pharm. 2013;66(3):157–62.

5. Schünemann HJ, et al. American Society of Hematology 2018 guidelines for management of venous thromboembolism: prophylaxis for hospitalized and nonhospitalized medical patients. Blood Adv. 2018;2(22):3198–225.

6. Gould MK, et al. Prevention of VTE in nonorthopedic surgical patients: Antithrombotic Therapy and Prevention of Thrombosis, 9th ed: American College of Chest Physicians Evidence-Based Clinical Practice Guidelines. Chest. 2012;141(2 Suppl):e227S.

7. Kahn SR, et al. Prevention of VTE in nonsurgical patients: Antithrombotic Therapy and Prevention of Thrombosis, 9th ed: American College of Chest Physicians Evidence-Based Clinical Practice Guidelines. Chest. 2012;141(Suppl. 2):e195S–226S.

8. Hirsh J, et al. Parenteral anticoagulants: American College of Chest Physicians Evidence-Based Clinical Practice Guidelines (8th edition). Chest. 2008;133(Suppl. 6):141s–59s.

9. Fernando SM, et al. VTE Prophylaxis in critically Ill adults: a systematic review and network meta-analysis. Chest. 2022;161(2):418–28.

10. Lexicomp Online, Lexi-Drugs. UpToDate, Inc.

11. Lee GM, Arepally GM. Heparin-induced thrombocytopenia. Hematology Am Soc Hematol Educ Program. 2013;2013:668–74.

12. Solanki J, et al. Heparin-induced thrombocytopenia and cardiac surgery. Semin Thorac Cardiovasc Surg. 2019;31(3):335–44.

13. Lo GK, et al. Evaluation of pretest clinical score (4 T's) for the diagnosis of heparin-induced thrombocytopenia in two clinical settings. J Thromb Haemost. 2006;4(4):759–65.

14. Easaw JC, et al. Canadian consensus recommendations on the management of venous thromboembolism in patients with cancer. Part 2: treatment. Curr Oncol. 2015;22(2):144–55.

15. Guidelines for the use of platelet transfusions. Br J Haematol. 2003;122(1):10–23.

16. Witt DM. What to do after the bleed: resuming anticoagulation after major bleeding. Hematology Am Soc Hematol Educ Program. 2016;2016(1):620–4.

17. Freeman AL, Pendleton RC, Rondina MT. Prevention of venous thromboembolism in obesity. Expert Rev Cardiovasc Ther. 2010;8(12):1711–21.

18. Joy M, et al. Safety and efficacy of high-dose unfractionated heparin for prevention of venous thromboembolism in overweight and obese patients. Pharmacotherapy. 2016;36(7):740–8.

19. Geerts WH, et al. A comparison of low-dose heparin with low-molecular-weight heparin as prophylaxis against venous thromboembolism after major trauma. N Engl J Med. 1996;335(10):701–7.

20. Plummer MP, Blaser AR, Deane AM. Stress ulceration: prevalence, pathology and association with adverse outcomes. Crit Care. 2014;18(2):213.

21. Cook DJ, et al. Risk factors for gastrointestinal bleeding in critically ill patients. Canadian Critical Care Trials Group. N Engl J Med. 1994;330(6):377–81.

22. Simons RK, et al. A risk analysis of stress ulceration after trauma. J Trauma. 1995;39(2):289–93. discussion 293–4

23. Cook D, et al. Risk factors for clinically important upper gastrointestinal bleeding in patients requiring mechanical ventilation. Canadian Critical Care Trials Group. Crit Care Med. 1999;27(12):2812–7.

24. Rhodes A, et al. Surviving sepsis campaign: international guidelines for management of sepsis and septic shock: *2016*. Crit Care Med. 2017;45(3):486–552.

25. ASHP Therapeutic Guidelines on Stress Ulcer Prophylaxis. ASHP Commission on Therapeutics and approved by the ASHP Board of Directors on November 14, 1998. Am J Health Syst Pharm. 1999;56(4):347–79.

26. Hunt RH. Importance of pH control in the management of GERD. Arch Intern Med. 1999;159(7):649–57.

27. Shin JM, Sachs G. Pharmacology of proton pump inhibitors. Curr Gastroenterol Rep. 2008;10(6):528–34.

28. Cook D, et al. A comparison of sucralfate and ranitidine for the prevention of upper gastrointestinal bleeding in patients requiring mechanical ventilation. Canadian Critical Care Trials Group. N Engl J Med. 1998;338(12):791–7.

29. Young PJ, et al. Effect of stress ulcer prophylaxis with proton pump inhibitors vs histamine-2 receptor blockers on in-hospital mortality among ICU patients receiving invasive mechanical ventilation: the PEPTIC Randomized Clinical Trial. JAMA. 2020;323(7):616–26.

30. Yibirin M, et al. Adverse effects associated with proton pump inhibitor use. Cureus. 2021;13(1):e12759.

31. Willems RPJ, et al. Association of proton pump inhibitor use with risk of acquiring drug-resistant enterobacterales. JAMA Netw Open. 2023;6(2):e230470.

32. Werbel T, Cohen PR. Ranitidine-associated sleep disturbance: case report and review of H2 antihistamine-related central nervous system adverse effects. Cureus. 2018;10(4):e2414.

33. Pingleton SK, Hadzima SK. Enteral alimentation and gastrointestinal bleeding in mechanically ventilated patients. Crit Care Med. 1983;11(1):13–6.

34. Ephgrave KS, Kleiman-Wexler RL, Adair CG. Enteral nutrients prevent stress ulceration and increase intragastric volume. Crit Care Med. 1990;18(6):621–4.

35. Huang HB, et al. Stress ulcer prophylaxis in intensive care unit patients receiving enteral nutrition: a systematic review and meta-analysis. Crit Care. 2018;22(1):20.

36. Miller A, Vujcich E, Brown J. Effect of central line duration and other risk factors on central line-associated bloodstream infection in severe adult burns patients at a large tertiary referral burns centre: a 5-year retrospective study. Eur Burn J. 2022;3(1):18–26.

37. Chopra V, et al. The Michigan Appropriateness Guide for Intravenous Catheters (MAGIC): results from a multispecialty panel using the RAND/UCLA appropriateness method. Ann Intern Med. 2015;163(Suppl. 6):S1–40.

38. Le A, Patel S. Extravasation of noncytotoxic drugs: a review of the literature. Ann Pharmacother. 2014;48(7):870–86.

39. Shapiro NI, et al. Early restrictive or liberal fluid management for sepsis-induced hypotension. N Engl J Med. 2023;388(6):499–510.

40. Wong ES. Guideline for prevention of catheter-associated urinary tract infections. Am J Infect Control. 1983;11(1):28–36.

41. Hadaway L. Infiltration and extravasation. Am J Nurs. 2007;107(8):64–72.

42. Marschall J, et al. Strategies to prevent central line-associated bloodstream infections in acute care hospitals: 2014 update. Infect Control Hosp Epidemiol. 2014;35(7):753–71.

43. Hafeez SB, et al. Catheter-related bloodstream infection with femoral central access versus internal jugular access in patients admitting to medical intensive care unit. Cureus. 2022;14(9):e29416.

44. Charalambous C, et al. Risk factors and clinical impact of central line infections in the surgical intensive care unit. Arch Surg. 1998;133(11):1241–6.

45. Wang Y, et al. National trends in patient safety for four common conditions, 2005–2011. N Engl J Med. 2014;370(4):341–51.

46. Muscedere JG, Day A, Heyland DK. Mortality, attributable mortality, and clinical events as end points for clinical trials of ventilator-associated pneumonia and hospital-acquired pneumonia. Clin Infect Dis. 2010;51(Suppl. 1):S120–5.

47. Kollef MH, Hamilton CW, Ernst FR. Economic impact of ventilator-associated pneumonia in a large matched cohort. Infect Control Hosp Epidemiol. 2012;33(3):250–6.

48. Klompas M, et al. Strategies to prevent ventilator-associated pneumonia, ventilator-associated events, and nonventilator hospital-acquired pneumonia in acute-care hospitals: 2022 Update. Infect Control Hosp Epidemiol. 2022;43(6):687–713.

49. Girard TD, et al. Efficacy and safety of a paired sedation and ventilator weaning protocol for mechanically ventilated patients in intensive care (Awakening and Breathing Controlled trial): a randomised controlled trial. Lancet. 2008;371(9607):126–34.

50. Klompas M, et al. Reappraisal of routine oral care with chlorhexidine gluconate for patients receiving mechanical ventilation: systematic review and meta-analysis. JAMA Intern Med. 2014;174(5):751–61.

51. Price R, MacLennan G, Glen J. Selective digestive or oropharyngeal decontamination and topical oropharyngeal chlorhexidine for prevention of death in general intensive care: systematic review and network meta-analysis. BMJ. 2014;348:g2197.
52. Huang SS, et al. Targeted versus universal decolonization to prevent ICU infection. N Engl J Med. 2013;368(24):2255–65.
53. Huang SS, et al. Nasal iodophor antiseptic vs nasal mupirocin antibiotic in the setting of chlorhexidine bathing to prevent infections in adult ICUs: a randomized clinical trial. JAMA. 2023;330(14):1337–47.
54. Karvouniaris M, et al. Nebulised colistin for ventilator-associated pneumonia prevention. Eur Respir J. 2015;46(6):1732–9.
55. Claridge JA, et al. Aerosolized ceftazidime prophylaxis against ventilator-associated pneumonia in high-risk trauma patients: results of a double-blind randomized study. Surg Infect. 2007;8(1):83–90.
56. Acquarolo A, et al. Antibiotic prophylaxis of early onset pneumonia in critically ill comatose patients. A randomized study Intensive Care Med. 2005;31(4):510–6.
57. Vallés J, et al. Efficacy of single-dose antibiotic against early-onset pneumonia in comatose patients who are ventilated. Chest. 2013;143(5):1219–25.
58. Lode H, et al. Systemic and endotracheal antibiotic prophylaxis of nosocomial pneumonia in ICU. Intensive Care Med. 1992;18(Suppl. 1):S24–7.
59. Rathgeber J, et al. Prevention of pneumonia by endotracheal micronebulization of tobramycin. Anasthesiol Intensivmed Notfallmed Schmerzther. 1993;28(1):23–9.
60. Zha S, et al. Prophylactic antibiotics for preventing ventilator-associated pneumonia: a pairwise and Bayesian network meta-analysis. Eur J Med Res. 2023;28(1):348.
61. Bagshaw SM, et al. The impact of early hypoglycemia and blood glucose variability on outcome in critical illness. Crit Care. 2009;13(3):R91.
62. Finfer S, et al. Intensive versus conventional glucose control in critically ill patients. N Engl J Med. 2009;360(13):1283–97.
63. Lacherade JC, Jacqueminet S, Preiser JC. An overview of hypoglycemia in the critically ill. J Diabetes Sci Technol. 2009;3(6):1242–9.
64. Cryer PE, Davis SN, Shamoon H. Hypoglycemia in diabetes. Diabetes Care. 2003;26(6):1902–12.
65. van den Berghe G, et al. Intensive insulin therapy in critically ill patients. N Engl J Med. 2001;345(19):1359–67.
66. Mergenthaler P, et al. Sugar for the brain: the role of glucose in physiological and pathological brain function. Trends Neurosci. 2013;36(10):587–97.
67. Laitinen T, et al. Electrocardiographic alterations during hyperinsulinemic hypoglycemia in healthy subjects. Ann Noninvasive Electrocardiol. 2008;13(2):97–105.
68. Najjar SM, Perdomo G. Hepatic insulin clearance: mechanism and physiology. Physiology (Bethesda). 2019;34(3):198–215.
69. Rabkin R, Ryan MP, Duckworth WC. The renal metabolism of insulin. Diabetologia. 1984;27(3):351–7.
70. Nordlie RC, Foster JD, Lange AJ. Regulation of glucose production by the liver. Annu Rev Nutr. 1999;19:379–406.
71. Keeney KP, et al. Assessment of intravenous insulin dosing strategies for the treatment of acute hyperkalemia in the emergency department. Am J Emerg Med. 2020;38(6):1082–5.
72. Rajasurya V, Anjum H, Surani S. Metformin use and metformin-associated lactic acidosis in intensive care unit patients with diabetes. Cureus. 2019;11(5):e4739.
73. Deusenberry CM, et al. Hypoglycemia in hospitalized patients treated with sulfonylureas. Pharmacotherapy. 2012;32(7):613–7.
74. Maynard G, et al. Improved inpatient use of basal insulin, reduced hypoglycemia, and improved glycemic control: effect of structured subcutaneous insulin orders and an insulin management algorithm. J Hosp Med. 2009;4(1):3–15.

75. Mendez CE, Umpierrez G. Management of the hospitalized patient with type 1 diabetes mellitus. Hosp Pract (1995). 2013;41(3):89–100.
76. Magaji V, Johnston JM. Inpatient management of hyperglycemia and diabetes. Clin Diabet. 2011;29(1):3–9.
77. Umpierrez GE, et al. Randomized study of basal-bolus insulin therapy in the inpatient management of patients with type 2 diabetes (RABBIT 2 trial). Diabetes Care. 2007;30(9):2181–6.
78. Griffen SC, et al. Administration of Lispro insulin with meals improves glycemic control, increases circulating leptin, and suppresses ghrelin, compared with regular/NPH insulin in female patients with type 1 diabetes. J Clin Endocrinol Metab. 2006;91(2):485–91.
79. American Diabetes Association. 13. Diabetes care in the hospital. Diabetes Care. 2016;39(Suppl. 1):S99–104.
80. Committee ADAPP. 16. Diabetes care in the hospital: standards of medical care in diabetes—2022. Diabetes Care. 2021;45(Suppl. 1):S244–53.
81. Jacobi J, et al. Guidelines for the use of an insulin infusion for the management of hyperglycemia in critically ill patients. Critical Care Med. 2012;40(12):3251–76.
82. Sadaf F, et al. Prevalence and risk factors of delirium in patients admitted to intensive care units: a multicentric cross-sectional study. Cureus. 2023;15(9):e44827.
83. Ely EW, et al. Delirium as a predictor of mortality in mechanically ventilated patients in the intensive care unit. JAMA. 2004;291(14):1753–62.
84. Salluh JI, et al. Outcome of delirium in critically ill patients: systematic review and meta-analysis. BMJ. 2015;350:h2538.
85. Zhang Z, Pan L, Ni H. Impact of delirium on clinical outcome in critically ill patients: a meta-analysis. Gen Hosp Psychiatry. 2013;35(2):105–11.
86. Devlin JW, et al. Clinical practice guidelines for the prevention and management of pain, agitation/sedation, delirium, immobility, and sleep disruption in adult patients in the ICU. Crit Care Med. 2018;46(9):e825–73.
87. Girard TD, et al. Haloperidol and ziprasidone for treatment of delirium in critical illness. N Engl J Med. 2018;379(26):2506–16.
88. Andersen-Ranberg NC, et al. Haloperidol for the treatment of delirium in ICU patients. N Engl J Med. 2022;387(26):2425–35.
89. Rivosecchi RM, et al. The implementation of a nonpharmacologic protocol to prevent intensive care delirium. J Crit Care. 2016;31(1):206–11.
90. Munro CL, et al. Delirium prevention in critically ill adults through an automated reorientation intervention—a pilot randomized controlled trial. Heart Lung. 2017;46(4):234–8.
91. Morandi A, et al. Visual and hearing impairment are associated with delirium in hospitalized patients: results of a multisite prevalence study. J Am Med Dir Assoc. 2021;22(6):1162–7.
92. Alagiakrishnan K, Wiens CA. An approach to drug induced delirium in the elderly. Postgrad Med J. 2004;80(945):388–93.
93. Clegg A, Young JB. Which medications to avoid in people at risk of delirium: a systematic review. Age Ageing. 2011;40(1):23–9.
94. Slooter AJ, Van De Leur RR, Zaal IJ. Delirium in critically ill patients. Handb Clin Neurol. 2017;141:449–66.
95. Vieira JM Jr, et al. Effect of acute kidney injury on weaning from mechanical ventilation in critically ill patients. Crit Care Med. 2007;35(1):184–91.
96. Melo FAF, et al. A systematic review and meta-analysis of acute kidney injury in the intensive care units of developed and developing countries. PLoS One. 2020;15(1):e0226325.
97. Coca SG, Singanamala S, Parikh CR. Chronic kidney disease after acute kidney injury: a systematic review and meta-analysis. Kidney Int. 2012;81(5):442–8.
98. Polat EC, Koc A, Demirkan K. The role of the clinical pharmacist in the prevention of drug-induced acute kidney injury in the intensive care unit. J Clin Pharm Ther. 2022;47(12):2287–94.
99. Cartin-Ceba R, et al. Risk factors for development of acute kidney injury in critically ill patients: a systematic review and meta-analysis of observational studies. Crit Care Res Pract. 2012;2012:691013.

100. Hammond DA, et al. Systematic review and meta-analysis of acute kidney injury associated with concomitant vancomycin and piperacillin/tazobactam. Clin Infect Dis. 2017;64(5):666–74.
101. Miano TA, et al. Association of vancomycin plus piperacillin-tazobactam with early changes in creatinine versus cystatin C in critically ill adults: a prospective cohort study. Intensive Care Med. 2022;48(9):1144–55.
102. Rahn KH, Heidenreich S, Brückner D. How to assess glomerular function and damage in humans. J Hypertens. 1999;17(3):309–17.
103. Kumaresan R, Giri P. A comparison of serum cystatin C and creatinine with glomerular filtration rate in Indian patients with chronic kidney disease. Oman Med J. 2011;26(6):421–5.
104. Murty MS, et al. Serum cystatin C as a marker of renal function in detection of early acute kidney injury. Indian J Nephrol. 2013;23(3):180–3.
105. Barreto EF, Rule AD, Murad MH, Kashani KB, Lieske JC, Erwin PJ, Steckelberg JM, Gajic O, Reid JM, Kane-Gill SL. Prediction of the Renal Elimination of Drugs With Cystatin C vs. Creatinine: A Systematic Review. Mayo Clin Proc. 2019;94:500–14.
106. Heemskerk CPM, et al. Risk factors for QTc interval prolongation. Eur J Clin Pharmacol. 2018;74(2):183–91.
107. Kenigsberg DN, et al. Prolongation of the QTc interval is seen uniformly during early transmural ischemia. J Am Coll Cardiol. 2007;49(12):1299–305.
108. Turner JR, et al. Drug-induced Proarrhythmia and Torsade de Pointes: a primer for students and practitioners of medicine and pharmacy. J Clin Pharmacol. 2018;58(8):997–1012.
109. Haugaa KH, et al. Institution-wide QT alert system identifies patients with a high risk of mortality. Mayo Clin Proc. 2013;88(4):315–25.
110. Crow RS, Hannan PJ, Folsom AR. Prognostic significance of corrected QT and corrected JT interval for incident coronary heart disease in a general population sample stratified by presence or absence of wide QRS complex: the ARIC Study with 13 years of follow-up. Circulation. 2003;108(16):1985–9.
111. Thomas SH, Behr ER. Pharmacological treatment of acquired QT prolongation and torsades de pointes. Br J Clin Pharmacol. 2016;81(3):420–7.
112. Drew BJ, et al. Prevention of torsade de pointes in hospital settings: a scientific statement from the American Heart Association and the American College of Cardiology Foundation. Circulation. 2010;121(8):1047–60.
113. Al-Khatib SM, et al. 2017 AHA/ACC/HRS Guideline for management of patients with ventricular arrhythmias and the prevention of sudden cardiac death: executive summary: a report of the American College of Cardiology/American Heart Association Task Force on Clinical Practice Guidelines and the Heart Rhythm Society. Circulation. 2018;138(13):e210–71.
114. Hijazi M, Al-Ansari M. Protocol-driven vs. physician-driven electrolyte replacement in adult critically ill patients. Ann Saudi Med. 2005;25(2):105–10.

Chapter 43
Comprehensive Fluid Therapy in Critical Care: Guidelines and Best Practices for Fluid Stewardship

Manu L. N. G. Malbrain

43.1 Introduction

Intravenous (IV) fluid therapy is an essential component of patient management in critical care settings like the emergency department, intensive care unit, and the operating room, but also outside the acute care environment on regular medical and surgical wards [1, 2]. However, inappropriate administration can lead to significant morbidity, like acid–base and electrolyte disturbances, fluid accumulation syndrome (FAS) with increased intra-abdominal pressure (IAP), pulmonary edema, venous congestion, and mortality [3]. Fluid stewardship involves a coordinated approach to ensure judicious use of IV fluids, optimizing clinical outcomes while minimizing risks [1, 4, 5]. This chapter provides a detailed overview on various aspects of fluid therapy, focusing on evidence-based practices and guidelines. The following sections will cover definitions, 10 Ds and principles of fluid therapy, methods for resuscitation and maintenance, considerations for special populations, and strategies for effective fluid stewardship.

M. L. N. G. Malbrain (✉)
First Department of Anaesthesiology and Intensive Therapy, Medical University Lublin, Lublin, Poland

Medical Data Management, Medaman, Geel, Belgium

International Fluid Academy, Lovenjoel, Belgium
e-mail: manu.malbrain@umlub.pl

© The Author(s), under exclusive license to Springer Nature Switzerland AG 2025
Y. Alzaidi, M. A. Gebily (eds.), *The Pharmacist's Expanded Role in Critical Care Medicine*, https://doi.org/10.1007/978-3-031-77335-8_43

43.2 The 10 Ds of Fluid Therapy

For more information on this topic, we refer to a recently published book on rational use of IV fluids [6].

1. **Definitions**: Establishing clear and universal definitions for various types of fluids and their use is crucial. This includes differentiating between maintenance fluids (to cover daily needs), resuscitation fluids (to restore shock and save lives), replacement fluids (to cover the ongoing losses), and nutrition fluids (to cover daily caloric needs). This also includes definitions for volume status and fluid responsiveness.
2. **Diagnosis**: Accurate diagnosis of the patient's fluid volume status and fluid needs based on their clinical condition is essential. This involves identifying underlying pathologies, co-morbidities and assessing the extent of fluid deficits as well as assessment of fluid responsiveness and unresponsiveness.
3. **Distribution**: Understanding the distribution of fluids within different compartments of the body helps in tailoring fluid therapy. This includes knowledge of intravascular, extravascular, interstitial, intracellular, and extracellular fluid spaces. The concepts of osmolality and tonicity (or effective osmolality) are equally important. One must be aware that all fluids are lost to the interstitial space at some point. The volume expanding effect of 1 L of crystalloid after 1 h is 25%, for hypotonic solutions like 5% glucose or dextrose, this is 8% and for colloids, this is 100%. However, the half-life is context sensitive and in situations of severe shock or hypotension (e.g., during surgery or after anesthesia induction), the volume expansion effect of crystalloids and colloids may be similar as long as they are infused and shock persists [1, 2].
4. **Drug**: Fluids are drugs and should only be given when needed and with caution. The best fluid may be the one that was not administered unnecessarily (withholding). In analogy to the very well-known concept of antibiotic stewardship, we should now also consider and think fluid stewardship. Selecting the appropriate type of fluid (crystalloid or colloid, isotonic or hypotonic or hypertonic, balanced or unbalanced) should be based on the patient's condition and treatment goals.
5. **Dose**: Determining the correct volume and rate of fluid administration in relation to the indication to achieve the desired therapeutic effect without causing harm.
6. **Duration**: Specifying the appropriate length and duration of fluid therapy based on the patient's ongoing needs and response to treatment.
7. **De-escalation**: Reducing or stopping fluid therapy (withdrawing) when it is no longer needed (e.g., when the patient can take oral fluids or when shock has resolved) to avoid fluid overload, FAS and related complications.
8. **Documentation**: Ensuring thorough documentation of all aspects of fluid therapy, including type, volume, rate, and patient response. It is all about giving the right fluid, in the right dose, at the right rate, to the right patient at the right time.
9. **Diligence (Stewardship)**: Implementing diligent oversight and management of fluid therapy practices to optimize patient outcomes and minimize risks implies

a plan do check act cycle following up on key performance indicators. This will be discussed further.

10. **Discussion**: Engaging in multidisciplinary discussions and reviews of fluid therapy practices (including adverse effects and IV fluid-related complications) to ensure continuous improvement and adherence to best practices. This implies change management and transformation and needs authentic leadership to tackle human factors and resistance to change.

43.3 Resuscitation Fluid Therapy

Fluid resuscitation is a critical intervention in restoring hemodynamic stability in critically ill patients in order to save lives. Resuscitation fluids refer to the fluids administered in the early initial phase of shock to restore adequate organ perfusion [1]. They should only be given in case of low preload and presence of fluid responsiveness, and they should always be given as a fluid challenge, i.e., assessing fluid status and fluid responsiveness before and after [7]. The choice of fluid, volume, and rate of administration should be guided by the patient's clinical condition and response to therapy. Commonly used resuscitation fluids include crystalloids (e.g., normal saline NaCl 0.9%, lactated Ringer's (LR) or Hartmann's solution, acetated Ringer's solution, or PlasmaLyte, among others) and colloids (e.g., albumin, starches, or gelatins). It must be noted that LR is slightly hypotonic and thus not ideal as a resuscitation fluid. The goal of resuscitation is to restore effective circulating volume, improve the microcirculation and tissue perfusion-related mismatch between oxygen delivery and consumption, and stabilize macrohemodynamic parameters (heart rate, blood pressure, stroke volume) in shocked patients. A recent study showed that from all the fluids administered only 6% are for resuscitation [8].

1. **Initial assessment**: Evaluate the patient's volume status, hemodynamic parameters, and underlying condition [6]. This may involve clinical examination (body weight, fluid balance, capillary refill time, central to peripheral temperature difference, saturation and pleth variability index, urine output,…), hemodynamic monitoring (blood pressure, heart rate, cardiac output), laboratory tests (hemoconcentration, inflammation, capillary leak index, kidney function and electrolytes, acid-base status, and lactate), radiology imaging and POCUS or point of care ultrasound (inferior vena cava collapsibility, left ventricular outflow tract velocity time integral) or advanced hemodynamic monitoring (transpulmonary thermodilution with assessment of global end-diastolic volume, lung water, functional hemodynamics with pulse pressure and stroke volume variation, bioelectrical impedance analysis, Swan-Ganz).

2. **Choice of fluid**: Balanced isotonic crystalloids are typically the first choice for resuscitation due to their effectiveness in expanding intravascular volume, lower cost, and greater safety. A recent meta-analysis showed that balanced solutions (mainly PlasmaLyte) have a 90% probability for reducing mortality with about

1% (ranging from a 1% increase to a 9% decrease), and thus should be used preferably (also in diabetic keto-acidosis, sepsis, burns, and acute kidney injury) except for patients with neurologic problems like traumatic brain injury or intra-cranial hypertension where normal saline NaCl 0.9% remains the best option as well as in patients with gastrointestinal losses (and metabolic alkalosis) [9]. In fact, there is nothing normal about saline as human plasma does not contain 154 mmol/L of Na nor 154 mmol/L of Cl and therefore we should just refer to saline or NaCl 0.9%, likewise we also do not talk about "normal" albumin but just albumin. The strong ion difference (SID) of the ideal fluid should be around 24–26 mmol/L, while the SID of saline is 0 mmol/L [10]. Albumin 20% may be considered at a later stage (de-resuscitation), or in specific situations, such as severe hypoalbuminemia or large-volume fluid losses (after paracentesis).

3. **Volume and rate**: Most often they are given as a bolus of 4 ml/kg over 10–15 min, and fluid status and responsiveness should be reassessed. The initial dose of crystalloid fluid in septic shock is usually 30 ml/kg according to the surviving sepsis campaign guidelines, administered over 1–2 h [11]; however, one size does not fit all and fluids should always be personalized, individualized, and tailored the patient's actual needs [12]. This can be adjusted based on the patient's response and ongoing losses. For colloids (e.g., albumin 20%), a smaller volume may be sufficient due to their higher oncotic pressure.

4. **Monitoring response**: Fluids should always be given as a "challenge" and their effect should be monitored. Continuous monitoring of hemodynamic parameters, urine output, and laboratory tests (lactate, urine analysis) are essential to assess the response to fluid resuscitation. Recent studies point towards the fact that abdominal (APP) or renal perfusion pressure (RPP) [13, 14] may be a better resuscitation endpoint or target than mean arterial pressure (MAP). APP can be calculated as MAP minus intra-abdominal pressure (IAP) and RPP as MAP minus IAP minus central venous pressure (CVP). Signs of adequate resuscitation include improved stroke volume, blood pressure, heart rate, urine output, lactate, and mental status.

5. **Adjustments**: Based on the patient's response, additional fluid boluses/challenges may be administered, or the infusion rate adjusted (e.g., in burns). If the patient shows signs of fluid overload or accumulation, consider reducing the fluid rate or initiating de-resuscitation as will be discussed further.

43.4 Maintenance Fluid Therapy

Maintenance fluids are a source of water, electrolytes, and also potentially glucose. Maintenance therapy aims to meet the patient's daily fluid, glucose, and electrolyte requirements when oral intake is inadequate or if the patients' need is not met through other sources (i.e., nutrition). This involves calculating daily needs for water, glucose, and electrolytes, and choosing appropriate fluids to maintain homeostasis. The aim of maintenance fluid is to prevent dehydration, starvation ketosis, and electrolyte disorders.

43.4.1   Daily Fluid Requirements

1. **Water**: Approximately 25–30 ml/kg/day or 1 ml/kg/h, adjusted based on patient's age, weight, and clinical condition.
2. **Electrolytes**: Sodium (1–2 mmol/kg/day), potassium (1 mmol/kg/day), and chloride (1 mmol/kg/day).
3. **Glucose**: 1–1.5 g/kg/day to prevent starvation ketosis.

43.4.2   Choosing Maintenance Fluids

1. **Isotonic crystalloids**: Balanced crystalloids (e.g., lactated Ringer's, PlasmaLyte) are often administered for maintenance therapy due to their more physiological electrolyte composition; however, these are isotonic solutions that do not contain glucose and therefore should only be given for resuscitation.
2. **Hypotonic solutions**: In most situations, hypotonic balanced maintenance solutions are the best first choice (e.g., Glucion 5%, Maintelyte 5%, GNaK). Recent studies showed that the sodium content and sodium balance may even be more important than the fluid balance in relation to FAS and outcomes [15–17]. In children there is still controversy, and the consensus is that hypotonic solutions should be administered with caution to avoid hyponatremia [18].
3. **Monitoring**: Regular monitoring of fluid balance, body weight, electrolytes, and glucose levels is essential to avoid complications such as electrolyte imbalances and fluid overload or FAS. De-escalation of maintenance solutions should be initiated if the patient receives fluids from other sources to avoid fluid creep, a term that refers to the unintentional and unmeasured fluid volumes administered in the process of delivering other medication (antibiotics, sedatives, painkillers, etc.) and/or nutrition through enteral and parenteral routes [8, 17]. Usually, ICU patients receive enough fluids from other sources (e.g., drug dilution) to cover the daily needs so that maintenance fluids are rarely indicated.

43.5   Fluid Therapy in Special Populations

Certain populations, such as patients with renal or cardiac dysfunction, require tailored fluid management strategies to avoid exacerbating their conditions. Volume-restricted patients, in particular, need careful monitoring and precise adjustments to fluid therapy.

43.5.1 Renal Dysfunction

Fluid management in critically ill patients requires careful fluid choice, volume control, and continuous monitoring. Isotonic crystalloids should be used cautiously, avoiding fluids high in potassium or phosphate. However, it's a misconception that balanced crystalloids (containing potassium) are more harmful than saline (not containing potassium) and patients with acute kidney injury (AKI) and increased potassium levels; studies indicate that saline NaCl 0.9% can increase potassium levels due to hyperchloremic metabolic acidosis.

Recent research indicates that hydroxyethyl starch (HES) solutions increase the risk of AKI, RRT use, and mortality compared to crystalloids [19]. Gelatin solutions also show nephrotoxic effects, though evidence is less robust [19]. The benefits and harms of different crystalloid solutions have been studied, and a recent meta-analysis showed that balanced solutions are more favorable compared to saline NaCl 0.9% with respect to the development of major adverse kidney events on day 30 (MAKE30) [9, 20]. Research continues on the efficacy of fluid boluses for oliguria and the negative impacts of higher fluid volumes. Ensuring the right fluid is given to the right patient at the right time aims to improve care and outcomes for critically ill patients with kidney injury.

Monitoring daily and cumulative fluid balance and body weight is crucial to avoid overload and FAS, and diuretics (or a combination of diuretics) and/or renal replacement therapy with net ultrafiltration may be necessary. Additionally, regular assessment of renal function, acid-base status, and electrolytes (serum and urine) is essential. Optimal fluid management is vital for critically ill patients at risk of or with acute kidney injury (AKI), as incorrect fluid choice, timing, rate, and volume can lead to venous congestion harming these patients. New technologies like POCUS with VExUS score, or bioelectrical impedance (vector) analysis (BI(V)A) show promise in assessing blood volume and hydration status [21, 22].

43.5.2 Cardiac Dysfunction

Fluid management strategies required for patients with cardiogenic shock should use distinct approaches for right heart failure (RHF) and left heart failure (LHF). Cardiogenic shock, a condition marked by inadequate cardiac output leading to tissue hypoperfusion, requires precise management tailored to the specific type of heart failure involved [6].

In RHF, the right ventricle struggles to pump blood effectively to the lungs, resulting in systemic congestion and fluid overload. Managing fluid in RHF is particularly challenging because the heart is highly sensitive to fluid overload, which can exacerbate congestion. Preload optimization is crucial and is often guided by dynamic assessments, such as echocardiography, central venous pressure (CVP) monitoring, or passive leg raising. However, fluid administration must be approached with caution, as the right ventricle may already be operating at its maximum capacity. Advanced monitoring tools like the PICCO system, which measures global end-diastolic volume (GEDV), can be particularly misleading in RHF due to factors like the presence of chronic dilation, atrial enlargement or valvular disease, potentially leading to inaccurate readings that underestimate or overestimate true fluid volume. Furthermore, caution is advised in RHF, particularly when interpreting preload versus afterload variations, which can be tricky in mechanically ventilated patients. All monitoring tools should be used carefully and context-specific, in conjunction with other clinical data, to avoid inappropriate fluid management.

Conversely, LHF is characterized by the left ventricle's inability to pump blood effectively into the systemic circulation, often leading to pulmonary congestion and reduced systemic perfusion. Fluid resuscitation in LHF presents a different set of challenges, as the left ventricle is often intolerant to volume overload. Fluid boluses in these patients must be carefully titrated to achieve specific end points, such as improved tissue oxygen delivery and end-organ perfusion. Echocardiography and dynamic measures of fluid responsiveness are essential in guiding this therapy. While the pulmonary artery (PA) catheter remains the gold standard for assessing hemodynamics in LHF, less invasive methods are increasingly recognized for their potential to provide similar insights. However, tools like PICCO may present challenges in LHF due to their susceptibility to influences from conditions like valvular disease or chronic heart failure.

There is significant debate about the fluid tolerance of patients with cardiogenic shock who present with congestion ("cold and wet"). These patients often have poor fluid tolerance, raising questions about the common practice of administering fluids in such cases. When indicated, isotonic crystalloids should be used and rapid fluid administration or excessive sodium intake should be avoided to prevent exacerbation of heart failure and pulmonary edema. Monitoring in patients with HF should focus on signs of fluid overload, such as pulmonary edema (check for B-lines on lung ultrasound or extravascular lung water with transpulmonary thermodilution) or elevated IAP or CVP. When available, continuous monitoring of hemodynamic parameters, IAP, APP, and cardiac function should be performed.

43.5.3 Volume-Restricted Patients

In volume-restricted patients, the use of IV fluids requires a meticulous approach to ensure optimal outcomes while avoiding complications from fluid overload. A thorough assessment of the patient's fluid status, including daily monitoring of body weight and fluid balance, is essential for guiding fluid administration. Careful planning is critical to determine the appropriate type and amount of fluid. Balanced crystalloids are generally preferred, but their use should be approached with caution, ensuring that unnecessary fluid administration is minimized. This includes avoiding maintenance fluids that are not absolutely necessary and preventing "fluid creep," which refers to the inadvertent administration of fluids through various routes. Frequent monitoring of the patient's fluid balance, electrolytes, and overall clinical status is crucial to adjust fluid therapy as needed and to promptly identify any signs of fluid overload or imbalance. This careful and tailored approach helps manage the delicate balance required in volume-restricted patients.

43.6 Volume Status Assessment

Accurate assessment of volume status is critical in guiding fluid therapy. Techniques include clinical examination, laboratory, radiologic imaging and POCUS, hemodynamic monitoring, and the use of dynamic indices such as functional hemodynamics passive leg raising test and other fluid responsiveness tests [7]. These are summarized in Figs. 43.1 and 43.2.

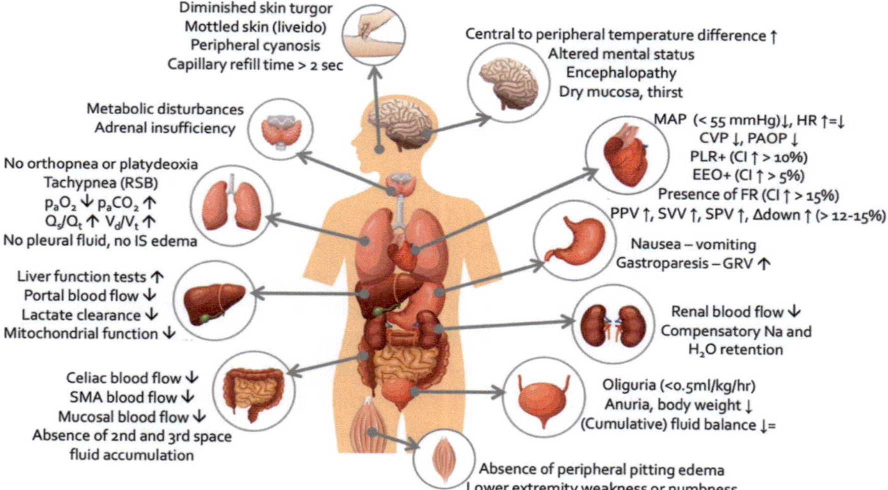

Fig. 43.1 Clinical signs and symptoms related to hypovolemia and hypoperfusion. Adapted with permission from Malbrain et al. according to the Open Access CC BY License 4.0 [6]*CVP* central venous pressure, *EEO* end-expiratory occlusion, *FR* fluid responsiveness, *GRV* gastric residual volume, *HR* heart rate, *MAP* mean arterial blood pressure, *Na* sodium, *PAOP* pulmonary artery occlusion pressure, *PLR* passive leg raising, *PPV* pulse pressure variation, *Qs/Qt* shunt fraction, *RSB* rapid shallow breathing, *SMA* superior mesenteric artery, *SPV* systolic pressure variation, *SVV* stroke volume variation, *Vt/Vd* dead space ventilation

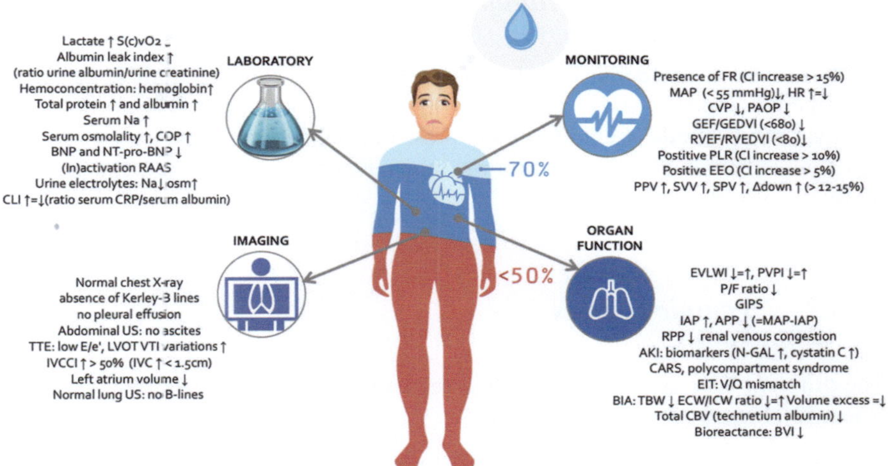

Fig. 43.2 Laboratory, imaging, hemodynamic, and organ function signs and symptoms related to hypovolemia and hypoperfusion. Total body water accounts for 70% of body weight. Overt signs and symptoms of hypovolemia occur when circulating blood volume is reduced with more than 50%. Adapted with permission from Malbrain et al. according to the Open Access CC BY Licence 4.0 [6]*AKI* acute kidney injury, *APP* abdominal perfusion pressure, *BIA* bioelectrical impedance analysis, *BNP* brain natriuretic peptide, *BVI* blood volume index, *CARS* cardio-abdominal-renal syndrome, *CBV* circulating blood volume, *CI* cardiac index, *CLI* capillary leak index, *COP* colloid oncotic pressure, *CRP* C-reactive protein, *CVP* central venous pressure, *ECW* extracellular water, *EIT* electrical impedance tomography, *EEO* end-expiratory occlusion, *EVWLI* extravascular lung water index, *FR* fluid responsiveness, *GEDVI* global end-diastolic volume index, *GEF* global ejection fraction, *GIPS* global increased permeability syndrome, *HR* heart rate, *IAP* intra-abdominal pressure, *ICW* intracellular water, *IVC* inferior vena cava, *IVCCI* inferior vena cava collapsibility index, *LVOT* left ventricular outflow tract, *MAP* mean arterial blood pressure, *Na* sodium, *P/F ratio* pO$_2$ over FiO$_2$ ratio, *PAOP* pulmonary artery occlusion pressure, *PLR* passive leg raising, *PPV* pulse pressure variation, *PVPI* pulmonary vascular permeability index, *RAAS* renin angiotensin aldosterone system, *RPP* renal perfusion pressure, *RVEDVI* right ventricular end-diastolic volume index, *RVEF* right ventricular ejection fraction, *ScvO2* mixed central venous oxygen saturation, *SPV* systolic pressure variation, *SVV* stroke volume variation, *TBW* total body water, *TTE* transthoracic echocardiography, *US* ultrasound, *V/Q* ventilation/perfusion, *VTI* velocity time integral

43.6.1   *Clinical Examination*

1. **Signs of hypovolemia**: Tachycardia, hypotension (mean arterial pressure < 65 mmHg or abdominal perfusion pressure < 55 mmHg), dry mucous membranes, decreased skin turgor, oliguria (<1 ml/kg/h), increased capillary refill time (>2–3 s).
2. **Signs of hypervolemia**: Edema (pitting, anasarca), elevated jugular venous pressure, pulmonary crackles, weight gain, positive (cumulative) fluid balance.

43.6.2 Hemodynamic Monitoring

1. **Non-invasive methods**: Blood pressure, heart rate, capillary refill time, pleth variability index.
2. **Invasive methods**: Central venous pressure, pulmonary artery pressure, (un) calibrated cardiac output monitoring, transpulmonary thermodilution (volumetric monitoring).

43.6.3 Dynamic Indices

The different tests are summarized in a recent review paper and briefly discussed below [7]. Figure 43.3 gives an overview.

1. **Fluid responsiveness**: Is defined as a 15% increase in stroke volume or cardiac output after a fluid challenge (4 ml/kg over 5–10 min or 500 ml/15 min).
2. **Functional hemodynamics**: Pulse pressure (PPV) and stroke volume variation (SVV) above 15% indicate fluid responsiveness. In situations of increased intra-thoracic pressure (PEEP, intra-abdominal hypertension), thresholds need to be revised to 20–25%.
3. **Passive leg raising test**: Transient increase in venous return (from the legs and splanchnic mesenteric venous capacitance pool) simulates a fluid challenge

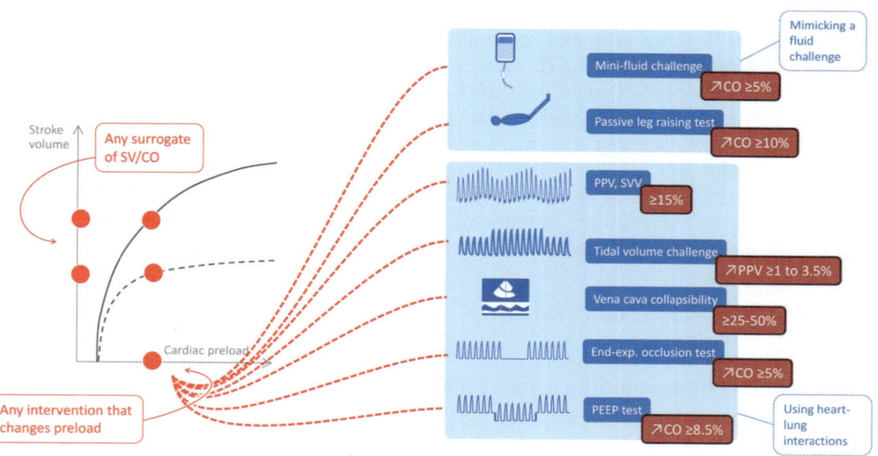

Fig. 43.3 Tests and indices of preload responsiveness. The principle of the dynamic assessment of preload responsiveness is to observe spontaneous or induced changes in cardiac preload, and the resulting change in cardiac output, stroke volume, or their surrogates. Some tests or indices use heart–lung interactions in mechanically ventilated patients, while some others mimic a classical fluid challenge. Diagnostic threshold and year of description are indicated. Adapted with permission from Malbrain et al. according to the Open Access CC BY License 4.0 [6] *CO* cardiac output, *PPV* pulse pressure variation

without one single drop of fluid (250–300 ml). Monitoring hemodynamic response (with a 10% increase in stroke volume or cardiac output) allows to predict fluid responsiveness or unresponsiveness.

4. **Other fluid responsiveness tests**:

   (a) Mini fluid challenge test: Administration of a small fluid bolus (1 ml/kg over 1–5 min) and monitoring of changes in stroke volume or cardiac output (threshold 5%).

   (b) End-expiratory occlusion test: Performing an end-expiratory hold for 15 s and monitoring of changes in stroke volume or cardiac output (threshold 5%).

   (c) Tidal volume variation test: Stepwise increase tidal volume (with 2 ml/kg) from 4 to 8 ml/kg and monitoring functional hemodynamics (threshold PPV increase $\geq$1 to 3.5%).

43.7 De-resuscitation

De-resuscitation involves the careful removal of excess fluids to prevent fluid overload and its associated complications. Strategies include the medical (diuretics) or mechanical (RRT and UF) interventions and adjustments based on dynamic assessments of fluid status and fluid (un)responsiveness [3, 23]. Figure 43.4 gives a schematic overview of FAS.

The prevention and management of FAS are shown in Table 43.1 and can be summarized as follows [3].

1. **Assessment**: Evaluate the patient's daily and cumulative fluid balance, body weight, hemodynamic status, and signs of fluid overload or FAS (e.g., edema, respiratory distress). This may involve clinical examination, ultrasound, bioelectrical impedance, and laboratory tests.

2. **Fluid restriction**: In some cases, fluid restriction (withholding) or fluid de-escalation (withdrawing and de-resuscitation) may be necessary to prevent further fluid accumulation. This involves limiting oral and IV fluid intake based on the patient's fluid balance and clinical condition.

3. **Diuretics**: Loop diuretics (e.g., furosemide) are commonly used to promote diuresis and remove excess fluids. The dose and frequency should be tailored to the patient's needs and response and sometimes a combination of diuretics can be necessary (Table 43.1).

4. **Mechanical fluid removal**: In case of limited response to diuretics, renal replacement therapy with net ultrafiltration can be considered.

5. **Monitoring**: Continuous monitoring of hemodynamic parameters, body weight, fluid balance, urine output, and (serum and urine) electrolyte levels is essential during de-resuscitation. Adjustments to the diuretic dose or fluid restriction may be needed based on the patient's response.

6. **Transition**: Once the patient's fluid status is stabilized, transitioning from IV to oral fluids and gradual reduction of diuretic therapy can be attempted, ensuring appropriate follow-up.

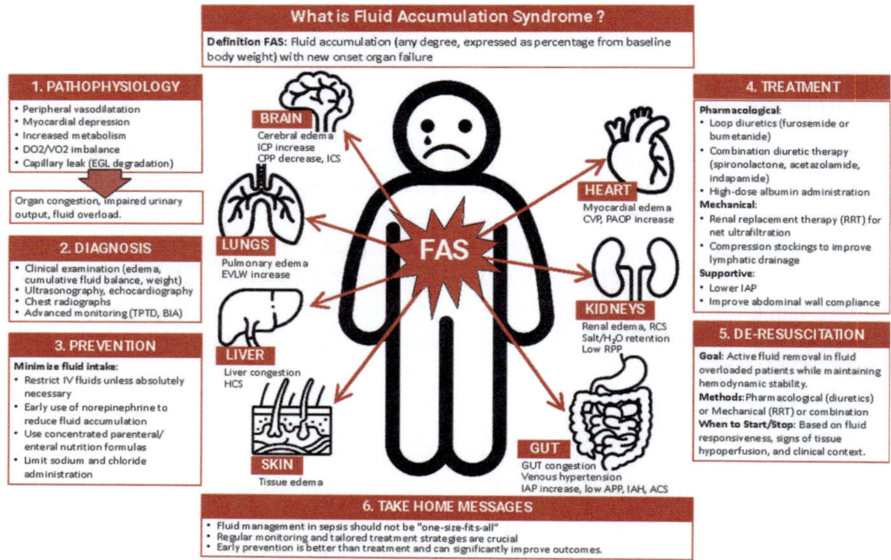

Fig. 43.4 Fluid accumulation syndrome. Adapted with permission from Pfortmueller et al. according to the Open Access CC BY License 4.0 [3]*ACS* abdominal compartment syndrome, *BIA* bioelectrical impedance analysis, *CVP* central venous pressure, *EGL* endothelial glycocalyx layer, *EVLW* extravascular lung water, *HCS* hepatic compartment syndrome, *IAH* intra-abdominal hypertension, *IAP* intra-abdominal pressure, *ICH* intracranial hypertension, *ICP* intracranial pressure, *RCS* renal compartment syndrome, *RPP* renal perfusion pressure, *TPTD* transpulmonary thermodilution

This table presents some suggestions for prevention and treatment of fluid accumulation based on personal experience of the author. It does not aim to provide an exhaustive, graded, and concise overview of the literature as current evidence is mostly limited to observational, retrospective, or small clinical studies, and more randomized trials are needed to better establish a personalized approach to fluid management. For more information, we refer the reader to some recent review papers on this topic [1, 24]. Adapted from Pfortmueller et al. with permission, according to the Open Access CC BY License 4.0 [3].

EN: enteral nutrition EVLWI: extravascular lung water index, FA: fluid accumulation, APP: abdominal perfusion pressure (MAP minus IAP), IAP: intra-abdominal pressure, PEEP: positive end-expiratory pressure, PF: P_aO_2 over F_iO_2 ratio, PPV: pulse pressure variation.

The four phases of fluid therapy according to the ROSE model with resuscitation, optimization, stabilization, and evacuation phases are illustrated in Fig. 43.5 as well as some triggers to start and stop IV fluids and to start and stop FAS treatment.

Table 43.1 Prevention and management of FAS

Treatment options	Description
Prevention	*Monitoring* – Basic monitoring (i.e., arterial and central venous line) – In case of unresolved shock, consider echocardiography and advanced hemodynamic monitoring – Obtain baseline body weight (scale, estimate, retrieve from medical records) – Monitor for risk for fluid accumulation, i.e., daily body weight, daily and cumulative fluid balance, edema formation, sonography – Assess for impaired end-organ function: IAP, APP, PF ratio, success of EN, EVLWI, PVPI, BIA – Assess fluid responsiveness with functional hemodynamics (i.e., PPV or SVV, passive leg raising test, end-expiratory occlusion test) – Assess for signs of tissue hypoperfusion (DO_2/VO_2 mismatch, i.e., elevated lactate, increased mottling score, increased capillary refill time) **Note**: Fluids should only be administrated when the patient is hypovolemic, fluid responsiveness, fluid tolerant, AND without risk for fluid accumulation AND signs of impaired tissue perfusion present **(A) Fluids are required**: – Use a restrictive fluid management regime – Frequently re-assess fluid responsiveness/tissue perfusion – Stop fluid administration once fluid responsiveness and/or tissue perfusion are absent **(B) Fluids are not required: de-escalation** – Limit fluid intake (withholding and withdrawing) – Limit sodium and chloride intake – Limit/avoid maintenance solutions – Limit/avoid fluid creep – Improve lymphatic drainage (i.e., use leg compression bandages) – Use high density or concentrated enteral formula's (i.e., 2 Kcal/ml)

(continued)

Table 43.1 (continued)

Treatment options	Description
De-resuscitation	**Note**: Fluids should only be removed when there is fluid UNresponsiveness AND absence of signs of impaired tissue perfusion (normal lactate) AND presence of FAS (Fluid accumulation (any percentage) AND impaired end-organ function AND presence of GIPS (global increased permeability syndrome) AND venous congestion (VExUS) AND low dose of vasopressors (<0.3) **(A) Pharmacological measures** – Perform furosemide stress test: patient passes test if UO > 200 ml over the next 2 h after furosemide bolus of 1 mg/kg (naive) or 1.5 mg/kg (previous use) – Apply loop diuretic (i.e., furosemide): high dose and continuous furosemide (1 mg/kg bolus and 10 mg/h) If de-resuscitation is insufficient, a combination therapy of diuretics may be applied: – Carbonic anhydrase inhibitors (Acetazolamide, 250–500 mg IV bolus): inhibition of Na reabsorption in proximal tubule in case of metabolic alkalosis – Thiazide (Indapamide, 2.5–5 mg PO): inhibition of Na reabsorption in distal tubule in case of hypernatremia – Potassium sparing (Spironolactone, 25–50 mg PO): aldosterone receptor antagonist, reduction of Na reabsorption at the collector duct (ENaC channel)

	Na^+	K^+	pH	Ca^{2+}	Mg^{2+}
Loop diuretic	↑↓	↓	↑	↓	↓
Carbonic anhydrase inhibitors	–	↓	↓	–	–
Thiazide	↓	↓	↑	↑	↓
Potassium sparing	–	↑	↓	–	↑

(B) Mechanical measures
– Start RRT (continuous or intermittent) with net ultrafiltration

(C) Supportive measures
– Lower IAP and increase abdominal perfusion pressure
    Improve abdominal wall compliance (sedation, neuromuscular blockers, body positioning)
    Reduce intraluminal volume (ileus)
    Reduce intra-abdominal volume (ascites)
– Increase/support cardiac function
    Inotropes (i.e., dobutamine, milrinone)
    Low dose vasopressors to maintain APP
– Use vasodilators (i.e., calcium antagonists)
    Increase renal blood flow
– Lung protective ventilation with application of PEEP (to counteract IAP) and limiting driving pressures below 14 cmH_2O
– Administer albumin 20% (only if serum albumin levels below 30 g/L)

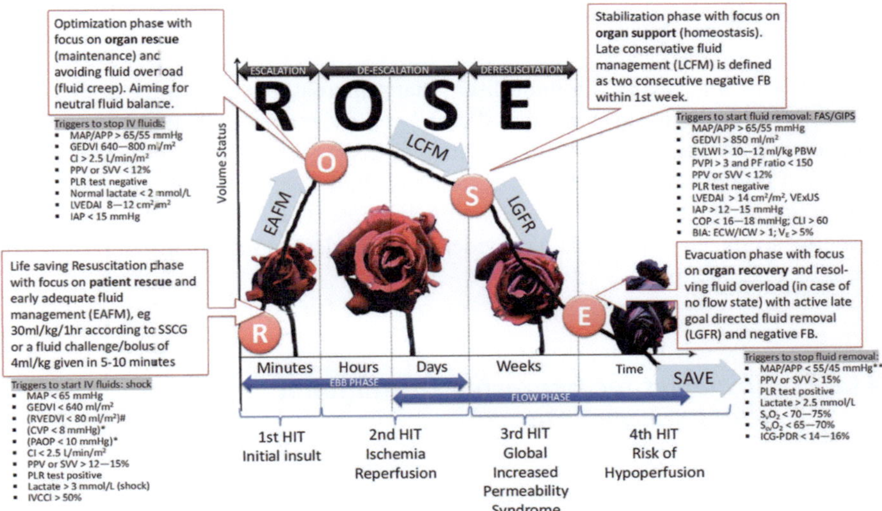

Fig. 43.5 The four phases conceptual model and deleterious effects of fluid accumulation syndrome. Graph showing the four-hit model of shock with evolution of patients' cumulative fluid volume status over time during the five distinct phases of resuscitation: Resuscitation (R), Optimization (O), Stabilization (S), and Evacuation (E) (ROSE), followed by a possible risk of hypoperfusion in case of too aggressive de-resuscitation. On admission, patients are often hypovolemic, followed by normovolemia after fluid resuscitation (escalation or EAFM, early adequate fluid management), and possible fluid overload, again followed by a phase returning to normovolemia with de-escalation via achieving zero fluid balance or late conservative fluid management (LCFM) and followed by late goal-directed fluid removal (LGFR) or de-resuscitation. In case of hypovolemia, O_2 cannot get into the tissue because of convective problems, in case of hypervolemia O_2 cannot get into the tissue because of diffusion problems related to interstitial and pulmonary edema and gut edema (ileus and abdominal hypertension). Adapted from Malbrain et al. with permission, according to the Open Access CC BY Licence 4.0 [6]

*Volumetric preload indicators such as GEDVI, LVEDAI, or RVEDVI are preferred over barometric ones such as CVP or PAOP

**Vasopressor can be started or increased to maintain MAP/APP above 55/45 during de-resuscitation phase

#Can only be measured via Swan-Ganz pulmonary artery catheter (PAC) and became obsolete

APP abdominal perfusion pressure (APP = MAP-IAP), *BIA* bioelectrical impedance analysis, *CI* cardiac index, *CLI* capillary leak index (serum CRP divided by serum albumin), *COP* colloid oncotic pressure, *CVP* central venous pressure, *EAFM* early adequate fluid management, *ECW/ICW* extracellular/intracellular water, *EVLWI* extravascular lung water index, *FAS* fluid accumulation syndrome, *GEDVI* global end-diastolic volume index, *GIPS* global increased permeability syndrome, *IAP* intra-abdominal pressure, *ICG-PDR* indocyanine green plasma disappearance rate, *IVCCI* inferior vena cava collapsibility index, *LCFM* late conservative fluid management, *LGFR* late goal-directed fluid removal, *LVEDAI* left ventricular end-diastolic area index, *MAP* mean arterial pressure, *PAOP* pulmonary artery occlusion pressure, *PF* P_aO_2 over F_iO_2 ratio, *PLR* passive leg raising, *PPV* pulse pressure variation, *PVPI* pulmonary vascular permeability index, *RVEDVI* right ventricular end-diastolic volume index, $S_{cv}O_2$ central venous oxygen saturation, *SSCG* surviving sepsis campaign guidelines, S_vO_2 mixed venous oxygen saturation, *SVV* stroke volume variation, V_E volume excess (from baseline body weight), *VExUS* venous congestion by ultrasound

43.8 Fluid Stewardship

Fluid stewardship involves a multidisciplinary approach to ensure the appropriate use of IV fluids. Fluid stewardship is defined as a series of coordinated interventions for judicious IV fluid administration, with a primary goal of limiting the deleterious effects of inappropriate fluid prescription and fluid overload or accumulation and optimizing the clinical outcomes and reducing costs [6]. This includes developing guidelines, educating healthcare providers, and implementing quality improvement initiatives [1, 25, 26].

43.8.1 Strategies for Improving Institutional Fluid Stewardship

A recent multidisciplinary report concluded that significant gaps currently exist in consistent education and training on fluid management, and innovative solutions are needed to drive change and transformation [25]. Healthcare institutions should therefore implement programs on fluid stewardship to achieve their quality improvement and patient safety goals.

The fundamental concept of IV fluid therapy is to "restore and maintain tissue oxygen, fluid and electrolyte homeostasis, and central euvolemia." This should be combined with an understanding of proper fluid management goals in resuscitation, replacement, nutrition, dilution (for other medications), and maintenance settings (Fig. 43.6). A recent study showed that on average from all fluids administered 3%

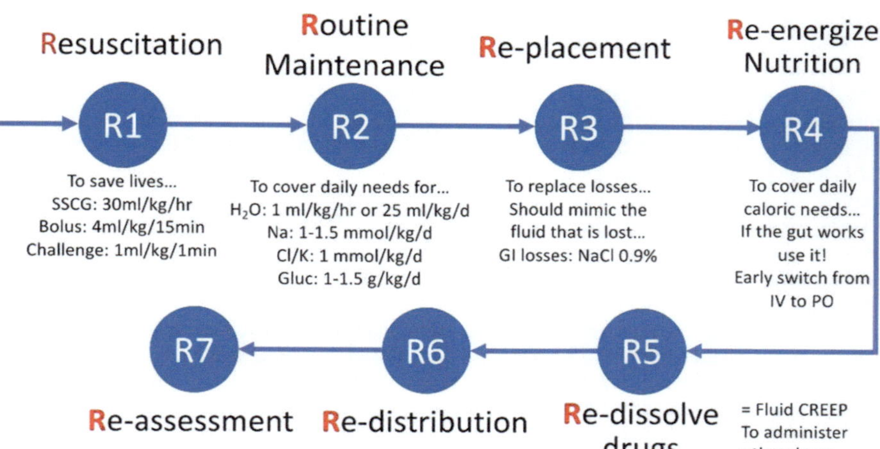

Fig. 43.6 The 7 Rs framework with the five indications for fluid administration (resuscitation, routine maintenance, replacement, dilution, or nutrition)

are blood products, 6% are resuscitation, 25% maintenance and replacement, 33% nutrition, and the other 33% are creep fluids [8].

The National Institute for Health and Care Excellence fluid guidelines provide a good starting point for fluid stewardship interventions, and these should include [27, 28]:

- An understanding of the physiology of water and electrolyte homeostasis.
- Knowledge of the risks, benefits, and harms of IV fluids.
- Assessment of fluid and electrolyte needs.
- Assessment of fluid and volume status and fluid (un)responsiveness.
- Prescribing IV fluids properly to each patient.
- Evaluating and documenting changes.
- Monitoring the response to IV fluids.
- Taking further action as required.
- Reporting complications of fluid management or administration as incidents that require investigation, to provide a basis for learning and improvement.

43.8.2   Improving Education and Training for Fluid Management

The foundation of effective fluid stewardship hinges on establishing an educational framework that caters to healthcare providers at various career levels. Analysis from previous surveys targeting fluid management clinicians—from novices to experts—revealed deficient knowledge levels [29]. Furthermore, a significant number of these professionals reported witnessing severe, yet unreported, fluid-related complications.

It is imperative for educators to adopt fresh perspectives that deviate from outdated, compartmentalized thinking, embracing a systems-oriented educational approach that enhances patient outcomes. This approach promotes collaborative practices across various specialties, fostering transparent communication and breaking down barriers within fluid management teams.

To embody this holistic educational strategy, training programs should incorporate diverse, cutting-edge learning tools, engaging personnel across all specialties involved in fluid management. Such comprehensive training is crucial for fostering a shift in the attitudes and practices of both new and seasoned clinicians. Identifying leaders within the institution, such as fluid stewards and advocates for change, who can secure administrative support is also vital.

Consideration should be given to modern virtual learning environments that offer flexibility for staff schedules, ensuring that all team members responsible for fluid decisions receive targeted training.

43.8.3 Guidelines, KPIs, and Data

Regular training should lead to the establishment of consistent guidelines to manage fluid therapy effectively. Proposed guidelines should cover the spectrum of assessment, prescription, monitoring, and ongoing clinical reviews. Local analyses of fluid usage metrics, such as total fluids per patient and bed occupancy days, should support the development of fluid stewardship programs.

While poor fluid management may not directly cause mortality, it significantly impacts outcomes like acid–base and electrolyte imbalances, fluid overload, FAS, and renal issues, potentially increasing morbidity and mortality rates. Approximately 20% of patients experience adverse effects from improper fluid management, stemming from both excessive and insufficient fluid administration.

Institutions should perform cost-benefit analyses of effective fluid management strategies, utilizing extensive data sources beyond local snapshots, including prescription and laboratory data, imaging, and patient records.

43.8.4 Best Practices for Fluid Stewardship

All institutions should consider a commitment to effective fluid stewardship at the local level. Institutions that have yet to implement standardized fluid stewardship can follow some key steps for success, as seen in Fig. 43.7. For the attending clinician, the process of fluid prescription can be condensed to four questions:

1. Does my patient need fluid, and is there a potential benefit of fluid administration?
2. If so, why? This question considers whether it is for maintenance, replacement of losses, or resuscitation, or if the patient requires fluid restriction.
3. Which fluid should be used in these differing scenarios?
4. How much should I give to the patient, when and for how long? This question considers the dosing, rate, speed, timing, duration, and route of administration.

After starting an IV fluid, the next four questions that should be addressed are as follows:

1. When to stop IV fluids? When shock has been resolved.
2. When to start fluid de-escalation? E.g., when to stop maintenance fluids or when to start hypercaloric enteral feeding to reduce fluid intake and the risk of fluid accumulation.
3. When to start active fluid removal or de-resuscitation? When the presence of fluid accumulation or global increased permeability syndrome negatively impacts end-organ function.
4. When to stop fluid removal? This question addresses the risks of fluid removal (e.g., causing hypoperfusion).

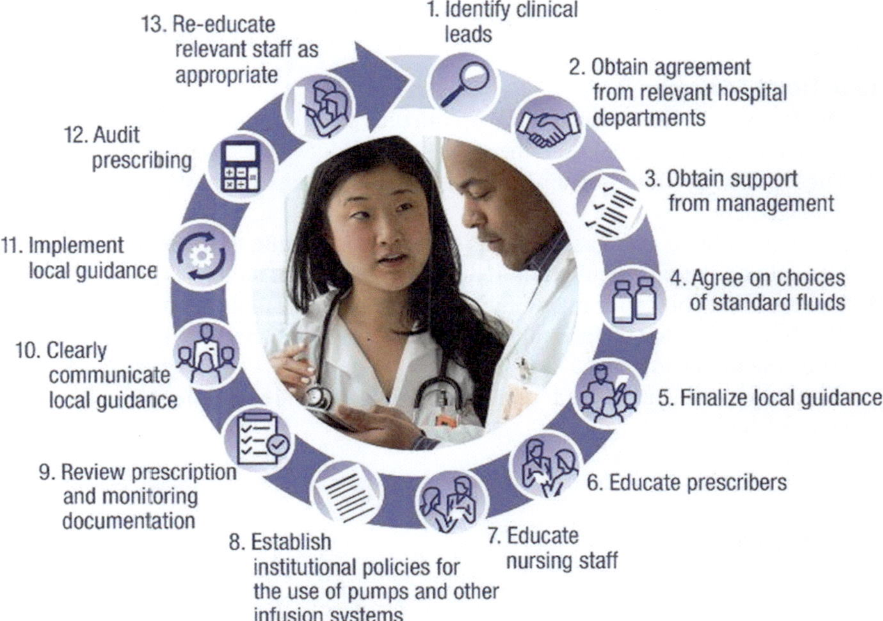

Fig. 43.7 Strategies to achieve institutional best practices in fluid stewardship. Adapted with permission from Malbrain MLNG et al. according to the Open Access CC BY license 4.0 [25]

All staff responsible for fluid management should regularly monitor patients for the appropriateness of fluid prescriptions, including initial patient assessment, decisions on fluid indication, fluid prescription, and regular fluid management.

43.9 Conclusion

In conclusion, comprehensive fluid therapy in critical care should focus on meticulous fluid stewardship to optimize clinical outcomes and minimize risks. The 10 D framework provides a structured approach to fluid management, encompassing definitions, diagnosis, distribution, drug selection, dosing, duration, de-escalation, documentation, diligence, and discussion. This systematic method ensures precise fluid resuscitation, maintenance, and de-resuscitation, tailored to individual patient needs and specific clinical scenarios. Special populations, such as those with renal or cardiac dysfunction, require careful and customized fluid strategies to prevent exacerbation of their conditions. Effective fluid stewardship involves a multidisciplinary effort, integrating evidence-based guidelines, continuous education, and robust monitoring systems to ensure the judicious use of IV fluids. By fostering collaboration and maintaining vigilance in fluid management practices, healthcare providers can significantly enhance patient safety and treatment efficacy in critical care settings.

Take Home Messages

1. Fluid stewardship is essential for optimizing patient outcomes and minimizing risks associated with IV fluid therapy.
2. The 10 Ds of fluid therapy provide a comprehensive framework for fluid management.
3. Accurate volume status assessment is crucial for guiding fluid therapy decisions.
4. Special populations require tailored fluid management strategies.
5. The best first choice for resuscitation is a balanced isotonic crystalloid solution.
6. The best option for maintenance (if needed at all) is a balanced hypotonic glucose containing solution.
7. Continuous education and quality improvement are key to effective fluid stewardship.

References

1. Malbrain M, Van Regenmortel N, Saugel B, De Tavernier B, Van Gaal PJ, Joannes-Boyau O, et al. Principles of fluid management and stewardship in septic shock: it is time to consider the four D's and the four phases of fluid therapy. Ann Intensive Care. 2018;8(1):66.
2. Malbrain M, Langer T, Annane D, Gattinoni L, Elbers P, Hahn RG, et al. Intravenous fluid therapy in the perioperative and critical care setting: executive summary of the International Fluid Academy (IFA). Ann Intensive Care. 2020;10(1):64.
3. Pfortmueller CA, Dabrowski W, Wise R, van Regenmortel N, Malbrain M. Fluid accumulation syndrome in sepsis and septic shock: pathophysiology, relevance and treatment—a comprehensive review. Ann Intensive Care. 2024;14(1):115.
4. Jacobs R, Jonckheer J, Malbrain M. Fluid overload FADEs away! Time for fluid stewardship. J Crit Care. 2018;48:458–61.
5. Malbrain MLNG, Rice TW, Mythen M, Wuyts S. It is time for improved fluid stewardship. ICU Manage Pract. 2018;18(3):158–62.
6. Malbrain MLNG, Wong A, Nasa P, Ghosh S. In: Malbrain MLNG, editor. Rational use of intravenous fluids in critically ill patients. Berlin: Springer Cham; 2023. p. 595.
7. Monnet X, Malbrain M, Pinsky MR. The prediction of fluid responsiveness. Intensive Care Med. 2023;49(1):83–6.
8. Van Regenmortel N, Verbrugghe W, Roelant E, Van den Wyngaert T, Jorens PG. Maintenance fluid therapy and fluid creep impose more significant fluid, sodium, and chloride burdens than resuscitation fluids in critically ill patients: a retrospective study in a tertiary mixed ICU population. Intensive Care Med. 2018;44(4):409–17.
9. Hammond NE, Zampieri FG, Tanna GLD, Garside T, Adigbli D, Cavalcanti AB, et al. Balanced crystalloids versus saline in critically Ill adults—a systematic review with meta-analysis. NEJM Evid. 2022;1(2):EVIDoa2100010.
10. Langer T, Santini A, Scotti E, Van Regenmortel N, Malbrain ML, Caironi P. Intravenous balanced solutions: from physiology to clinical evidence. Anaesthesiol Intensive Ther. 2015;47(1):78–88.
11. Evans L, Rhodes A, Alhazzani W, Antonelli M, Coopersmith CM, French C, et al. Executive summary: surviving sepsis campaign: international guidelines for the management of sepsis and septic shock 2021. Crit Care Med. 2021;49(11):1974–82.

12. Vandervelden S, Malbrain ML. Initial resuscitation from severe sepsis: one size does not fit all. Anaesthesiol Intensive Ther. 2015;47(1):44–55.

13. Moll V, Khanna AK, Kurz A, Huang J, Smit M, Swaminathan M, et al. Optimization of kidney function in cardiac surgery patients with intra-abdominal hypertension: expert opinion. Perioper Med. 2024;13(1):72.

14. Malbrain MLNG, De Keulenaer BL, Khanna AK. Continuous intra-abdominal pressure: is it ready for prime time? Intensive Care Med. 2022;48(10):1501–4.

15. Van Regenmortel N, Hendrickx S, Roelant E, Baar I, Dams K, Van Vlimmeren K, et al. 154 compared to 54 mmol per liter of sodium in intravenous maintenance fluid therapy for adult patients undergoing major thoracic surgery (TOPMAST): a single-center randomized controlled double-blind trial. Intensive Care Med. 2019;45(10):1422–32.

16. Van Regenmortel N, Langer T, De Weerdt T, Roelant E, Malbrain M, Van den Wyngaert T, et al. Effect of sodium administration on fluid balance and sodium balance in health and the perioperative setting. Extended summary with additional insights from the MIHMoSA and TOPMAST studies. J Crit Care. 2022;67:157–65.

17. Van Regenmortel N, Moers L, Langer T, Roelant E, De Weerdt T, Caironi P, et al. Fluid-induced harm in the hospital: look beyond volume and start considering sodium. From physiology towards recommendations for daily practice in hospitalized adults. Ann Intensive Care. 2021;11(1):79.

18. Brossier DW, Tume LN, Briant AR, Jotterand Chaparro C, Moullet C, Rooze S, et al. ESPNIC clinical practice guidelines: intravenous maintenance fluid therapy in acute and critically ill children—a systematic review and meta-analysis. Intensive Care Med. 2022;48(12):1691–708.

19. Perner A, Prowle J, Joannidis M, Young P, Hjortrup PB, Pettila V. Fluid management in acute kidney injury. Intensive Care Med. 2017;43(6):807–15.

20. Zampieri FG, Cavalcanti AB, Di Tanna GL, Damiani LP, Hammond NE, Machado FR, et al. Balanced crystalloids versus saline for critically ill patients (BEST-Living): a systematic review and individual patient data meta-analysis. Lancet Respir Med. 2024;12(3):237–46.

21. Samoni S, Vigo V, Resendiz LI, Villa G, De Rosa S, Nalesso F, et al. Impact of hyperhydration on the mortality risk in critically ill patients admitted in intensive care units: comparison between bioelectrical impedance vector analysis and cumulative fluid balance recording. Crit Care (London, England). 2016;20:95.

22. Cleymaet R, D'Hondt M, Scheinok T, Malbrain L, De Laet I, Schoonheydt K, et al. Comparison of bioelectrical impedance analysis (BIA)-derived parameters in healthy volunteers and critically ill patients. Life (Basel). 2023;14(1):27.

23. Malbrain M, Martin G, Ostermann M. Everything you need to know about deresuscitation. Intensive Care Med. 2022;48(12):1781–6.

24. Wiedermann CJ. Phases of fluid management and the roles of human albumin solution in perioperative and critically ill patients. Curr Med Res Opin. 2020;36(12):1961–73.

25. Malbrain M, Caironi P, Hahn RG, Llau JV, McDougall M, Patrao L, et al. Multidisciplinary expert panel report on fluid stewardship: perspectives and practice. Ann Intensive Care. 2023;13(1):89.

26. Malbrain ML, Mythen M, Rice TW, Wuyts S. It is time for improved fluid stewardship. ICU Manage Pract. 2018;18(3):158–62.

27. Padhi S, Bullock I, Li L, Stroud M, National Institute for H, Care Excellence Guideline Development G. Intravenous fluid therapy for adults in hospital: summary of NICE guidance. BMJ. 2013;347:f7073.

28. McDougall M, Guthrie B, Doyle A, Timmins A, Bateson M, Ridley E, et al. Introducing NICE guidelines for intravenous fluid therapy into a district general hospital. BMJ Open Qual. 2022;11(1):e001636.

29. Nasa P, Wise R, Elbers PWG, Wong A, Dabrowski W, Regenmortel NV, et al. Intravenous fluid therapy in perioperative and critical care setting-knowledge test and practice: an international cross-sectional survey. J Crit Care. 2022;71:154122.

Chapter 44
Approach to Thrombocytopenia in the ICU

Nidhi Kataria and Justin Kreuter

44.1 Thrombocytopenia

Platelets are small anucleate blood cells that are fragmented from megakaryocytes. They are most recognized as a critical component of primary hemostasis (i.e., formation of the platelet plug), but also play a role in immune function [1]. Once a platelet is released from a megakaryocyte, it will circulate in the blood for approximately 7–10 days. The typical normal range for platelet counts in healthy individuals ranges from 150×10^9/L to 400×10^9/L. The normal platelet count is maintained by thrombopoietin, which is made in the liver and absorbed by circulating platelets. Circulating thrombopoietin is a signal for megakaryocytes to increase platelet production. Therefore, when circulating platelets are few, less thrombopoietin is scavenged, and more thrombopoietin signal is received by megakaryocytes. The opposite is true when circulating platelets are many.

Thrombocytopenia is defined as a platelet count below the lower limit of the reference range, commonly <150,000/µL ($<150 \times 10^9$/L). However, thrombocytopenia is often further subdivided into mild ($100–149 \times 10^9$/L), moderate ($50–99 \times 10^9$/L), and severe ($<50 \times 10^9$/L). In mild thrombocytopenia, the number may be flagged as below the reference range, but clinical symptoms are absent. In moderate thrombocytopenia, there may be detectable deficits in laboratory assessment of hemostasis, but clinical symptoms remain absent. In severe thrombocytopenia, there may be impaired ability to form a thrombus as the number of circulating platelets decrease.

Thrombocytopenia is a common issue in patients admitted to the ICU. According to one systematic review, the prevalence of thrombocytopenia on admission to the ICU ranged from 8.3% to 67.6% and the incidence of thrombocytopenia acquired

N. Kataria · J. Kreuter (✉)
Department of Laboratory Medicine and Pathology, Mayo Clinic, Rochester, MN, USA
e-mail: Kreuter.Justin@mayo.edu

© The Author(s), under exclusive license to Springer Nature Switzerland AG 2025
Y. Alzaidi, M. A. Gebily (eds.), *The Pharmacist's Expanded Role in Critical Care Medicine*, https://doi.org/10.1007/978-3-031-77335-8_44

during the ICU stay ranged from 13.0% to 44.1% [2]. Although common, it remains clinically challenging because there are a variety of causes, which may require different treatment strategies. This is why, despite a patient with multiple issues, thrombocytopenia remains an important issue to get sorted out. A methodological approach is the cornerstone of evaluating a complex thrombocytopenic patient well.

44.2   Evaluation of Thrombocytopenia

The clinical history should begin with a review of prior platelet counts, both recent and older, if available in the clinical record. Pay attention to how platelet counts relate to key clinical events, such as hemostatic challenges and the starting/restarting of medications. Episodes of excessive bleeding should be explored for the type of bleeding (i.e., the site of bleeding and timing relative to a hemostatic challenge). And finally, the patient's background should be explored for medications, dietary habits, menstrual history, and comorbidities (e.g., malignancy, recent infection, autoimmune conditions, extracorporeal circuits) may help understand the patient's thrombocytopenia. While the clinical record should always be used to initially gather this information, speaking with the patient, their family, or their previous care team often are helpful perspectives to add to the evaluation. Similarly, a complete physical exam is important for understanding the patient's current clinical state. Examination of the skin and joints is important to recognize findings such as petechiae and hemarthroses, which tend to be related to platelet and coagulation factor deficiencies, respectively. An enlarged or nodular liver may suggest poor synthetic function of thrombopoietin. Splenomegaly may suggest sequestration of circulating platelets. Fever may suggest activation of the immune system and an increased rate of platelet consumption. An additional tool for awareness is the International Society on Thrombosis and Haemostasis (ISTH) Bleeding Assessment Tool (BAT) [3] provides an objective way of assessing platelet-related bleeding [4].

44.3   Laboratory Diagnosis

Platelet count is just the first step in the laboratory diagnosis of thrombocytopenia. Before diving into the nuances of how laboratory testing may contribute to sorting out an apparent thrombocytopenia, remember that laboratory medicine is a branch of medicine and that engagement with local experts from the laboratory will likely be helpful, as local practices may promote a particular way of efficiently evaluating the differential diagnosis of thrombocytopenia.

Automated cell counters are typically used to determine the circulating platelet count and may sometimes give a falsely low platelet count. Samples are usually collected into an ethylenediaminetetraacetic acid (EDTA) tube (i.e., purple top test tube) and EDTA is known to cause platelet clumping. These aggregates of platelets are not recognized by the analyzer as platelets. When this occurs, either reviewing the peripheral blood smear or repeating the platelet count in a sample that is collected in sodium citrate (i.e., light blue top test tube) will reveal the pseudothrombocytopenia [5]. Review of the peripheral smear may also reveal if the patient has giant platelets or cold agglutinin-induced platelet agglutination, which may similarly fail to be recognized by modern platelet analyzers. The additional benefit of the peripheral smear is that it may detect additional etiologic clues, such as the presence of schistocytes in microangiopathic conditions, blasts/immature white blood cells in leukemia, toxic granulation in sepsis. Failing to consider the full differential diagnosis may result in unnecessary platelet transfusions, additional costs of testing, and delayed procedures.

Mean Platelet Volume (MPV), an often-ignored parameter available on many analyzers, may provide important insights into the causes of a low platelet count. The normal reference range is between 7 and 10 fL. Increased MPV could be an indicator of the hereditary macrothrombocytopenias, accelerated platelet clearance as in ITP or gestational thrombocytopenia whereas decreased MPV may be seen in cases of Wiskott-Aldrich syndrome and in some cases of bone marrow failure.

And finally, situational awareness can keep a differential diagnosis grounded. The ICU setting is a place where infusion of fluids, transfusion of blood products, and bleeding may impact the circulating platelet count.

44.4 Clinical Meaning of Thrombocytopenia

Even though thrombocytopenia is defined by a number, the goal should be to treat the patient and not the number. The platelet transfusion guidelines for adults from the Association for the Advancement of Blood and Biotherapies (AABB) clarify how distinct levels of thrombocytopenia are significant in clinical practice [6]. The rate of intracranial bleeding has been noted to increase when the platelet count is below 5×10^9/L [7]; hence, most hospitals will try to keep patients above 10×10^9/L [8]. If a patient has a reason for increased platelet consumption (e.g., sepsis) or will be having an elective central line placement, then a platelet count below 20×10^9/L may indicate a need for platelet transfusion. If a patient is actively bleeding or will be going for a lumbar puncture, then a platelet count below 50×10^9/L may indicate a need for platelet transfusion. If a patient is going for an invasive procedure involving a closed anatomic space (e.g., central nervous system or eye), then a platelet count below 100×10^9/L may indicate a need for platelet transfusion.

44.5 Platelet Function Testing

In addition to numerical assessment, there are tests that evaluate platelet function. Some tests are commonly seen in ICU practice, such as Platelet Function Analyzer (PFA-100), VerifyNow, and Viscoelastic testing. Other tests are less commonly seen because they require subspecialized laboratory expertise, such as flow cytometry and platelet aggregometry.

The PFA-100 works by a relatively straightforward principle. Whole blood is aspirated through an aperture that is coated with either collagen/epinephrine or collagen/adenosine diphosphate (ADP). In this test, either epinephrine or ADP is the platelet activator and collagen is the substrate that the activated platelet can bind. Notice that the PFA-100 is creating an in vitro mimic of a bleeding vessel. The time it takes for a clot to occlude the aperture, closure time, is prolonged if platelet function is impaired.

The VerifyNow test is a modified aggregometry test that uses fibrinogen-coated beads to agglutinate platelets in whole blood. There is a VerifyNow Aspirin Test, which is used to assess a patient's platelet function when that patient has been taking aspirin. A second test available on the platform, VerifyNow PRUTest, is used to assess platelet function in patients taking P2Y12 inhibitors.

There are currently three viscoelastic testing platforms: Thromboelastography (TEG), Rotational Thromboelastometry (ROTEM), and Quantra. These tests are intended to provide an overview of several aspects of coagulation. Rather than measuring a single endpoint such as a clotting time, they create a tracing that illustrates clot formation over time. The variables most relevant to platelet function in each of the viscoelastic platforms are maximal amplitude (MA) in TEG, maximum clot firmness (MCF) in ROTEM, and platelet contribution to clot stiffness (PCS) in Quantra.

Flow cytometry can analyze many aspects of platelet function due to the development of different antibody targets. Because of the advantage of flow cytometry's ability to unique ability to examine many rare events in a sample, it is one of the few techniques that is not adversely affected by thrombocytopenia.

Platelet aggregometry is typically considered the gold standard of platelet function testing. It works by assessing platelet aggregation in response to different agonists (ristocetin, adenosine diphosphate, collagen, epinephrine, arachidonic acid) is detected by light transmission through the cuvette. Interpretation depends on the pattern of response to specific agonists.

44.6 Clinical Evaluation

Thrombocytopenia can happen due to a variety of reasons which can be broadly divided into four categories: increased platelet consumption, increased platelet destruction, platelet sequestration, and decreased platelet production. In the ICU setting, thrombocytopenia is often multifactorial due to the complexity of the ICU patient. However, it remains important to identify contributing factors for an effective treatment strategy. After the cause of thrombocytopenia is effectively addressed, assuming a normal bone marrow, the platelet count should return to normal within 5 days.

The most straightforward cause of thrombocytopenia in ICU patients is increased platelet consumption, which may occur due to bleeding, extracorporeal circuits (e.g., cardiopulmonary bypass, dialysis), and disseminated intravascular coagulation (DIC). Extracorporeal circuits are particularly challenging due to the balance between anticoagulation necessary to prevent clotting in the circuit and microvascular bleeding from systemic anticoagulation. The requirement for anticoagulation when a circuit is involved is a reminder that blood will clot when exposed to anything other than a normal blood vessel.

DIC occurs when localized control of coagulation is lost. In pathophysiologic terms, this occurs when thrombin and plasmin are freely circulating. Thrombin is the main procoagulant enzyme and plasmin is the main fibrinolytic enzyme. Regulatory control of these important enzymes is the definition of a normal coagulation system. When aberrant coagulation occurs, platelets and fibrinogen are consumed, and d-dimers are generated. Important causes of DIC include sepsis, malignancy, trauma, surgery, obstetric complications, snake bites, burns, etc. Treatment of the underlying cause along with symptomatic support is the cornerstone therapeutic approach [9].

Thrombotic microangiopathies (TMAs) are a spectrum of disorders with common features of vascular thrombosis, microangiopathic hemolytic anemia, and thrombocytopenia. TMAs group include thrombotic thrombocytopenic purpura (TTP), hemolytic uremic syndrome (HUS), as well as an atypical HUS (aHUS). Platelet consumption occurs within thrombi in thrombotic microangiopathies [10].

Heparin-induced thrombocytopenia (HIT) is a potential life-threatening complication associated with the use of unfractionated or low molecular weight heparin resulting in critical thrombocytopenia and thrombosis. It is an immune-mediated phenomenon with platelet-activating antibodies directed against PF4 complexed with heparin. Given that heparin is a widely used anticoagulant, the incidence of HIT has been reported to be higher in an ICU setting as compared to non-ICU setting (8.5% vs. 4.5%) [11]. It usually manifests between 5 and 10 days after exposure to heparin. The 4 T score (thrombocytopenia, timing of onset after heparin exposure, thrombosis, and other causes of thrombocytopenia) serves as an important pretest probability marker for the working diagnosis of HIT. Laboratory testing includes testing for anti-PF4-heparin antibodies by screening immunoassays confirmed by functional assays. Timely diagnosis and management involving stopping the heparin containing anticoagulants and switching to a non-heparin anticoagulant is essential to prevent adverse sequelae associated with this entity [12].

Immune Thrombocytopenia (ITP) is an immune-mediated thrombocytopenia mostly with autoantibodies directed against the platelet membrane glycoproteins leading to accelerated destruction and inhibition of platelet production. ITP is a diagnosis of exclusion and is categorized as primary or secondary type with underlying causes such as infections, malignancy, and autoimmune diseases. The management should be patient centric with a goal to treat or prevent significant bleeding and not focused on the platelet count. The treatment modalities include corticosteroids, IVIG, and anti-RhD. Platelet transfusions are used to prevent and treat life-threatening hemorrhage. In non-responding patient, therapies to increase platelet production including TPO mimetics can be used. The newer modalities like fosta-matinib splenic tyrosine kinase (SYK) inhibitor able to reduce the anti-platelet activity of phagocytes can be used in refractory cases [13].

Post-Transfusion Purpura (PTP) is a transfusion reaction characterized by severe thrombocytopenia (<10,000 platelets/µL) usually occurring 5–10 days after transfusion of platelet-containing blood products. More commonly seen in patients with history of pregnancy and blood transfusions (i.e., opportunities for alloimmunization) and is an antibody response against HPA. The unusual thing about the antibodies in PTP is that the antibody binds to both transfused platelets and the patient's own platelets, causing rapid destruction by macrophages. The patient's own platelets should be negative for the antigen, but in this clinical situation the antibody is said to have a "bystander" effect. The most common antigen implicated is human platelet antigen (HPA)-1a. It is self-limited with IVIG as first line of treatment. Therapeutic plasma exchange (TPE) could be considered, but this is not a first- or second-line treatment for PTP [14].

Given the polypharmacy during the management of critically ill patients paying a close attention to the patient's medication list becomes important as drugs can lead to both decreased production and increased destruction of platelets [15]. Drug-induced immune thrombocytopenia (DITP) involves antibody-mediated platelet destruction caused by exposure to a drug that leads to severe isolated thrombocytopenia and mucocutaneous bleeding. The clinical criteria for DITP are that thrombocytopenia occurs sometime after receiving the drug, discontinuation of the drug permits recovery of the platelet count, all other causes of thrombocytopenia have been excluded, and if the medication is readministered it will result in recurrence of thrombocytopenia [16]. Various drugs implicated in this category include quinine, quinidine, penicillin, vancomycin, digoxin, tirofiban, eptifibatide, abciximab, gold, herbal supplement, food, beverage, etc. It is a difficult diagnosis given the lack of an easily accessible diagnostic test, multiple comorbidities which can also lead to thrombocytopenia, polypharmacy during the management of critically ill patients and the challenge of finding alternative treatment. Clinical suspicion plays a significant role in getting the ball rolling followed by confirmation with detection of drug-dependent platelet antibodies in vitro.

Platelet refractoriness is a state where the patient fails to increment with platelet transfusion. Although not a cause of primary thrombocytopenia, this entity may be seen in thrombocytopenic patients. It is most often practically defined as the failure of an adult to increment by at least $10 \times 10^9/L$, when assessed by a 1-h post-transfusion platelet count. Unfortunately, in 80% of cases the blood bank is unable to identify compatible platelets for patients. Presumably, this is when the cause is non-immune. In the remaining 20% of cases, patient antibodies recognize human leukocyte antigens (HLA) or HPAs. When there is an immune cause, the ability for the blood bank to identify compatible platelets depends on the degree of patient alloimmunization [17]. Patients become alloimmunized from transfusions, transplantation, and pregnancy; therefore, being particularly judicious about when to transfuse is important to limit further alloimmunization.

Platelet sequestration, as it is recognized clinically, is an exaggeration of a normal process that occurs when the spleen is enlarged. In a normally sized spleen, one-third of the patient's platelet mass is found in the spleen. This is in a dynamic equilibrium with the circulating platelet pool. With increasing splenomegaly, an increasing fraction of the total platelet mass is sequestered in the spleen, resulting in mild to moderate thrombocytopenia [18]. The most important clinical aspect is to understand that platelet transfusion in this context will not result in a platelet increment. When transfused, most platelets will sequester in the spleen. Importantly, sequestered platelets are not destroyed and are released from the spleen into circulation during periods of stress. Therefore, thrombocytopenia due to splenic sequestration is a rare cause of bleeding.

Uremic platelet syndrome is not a cause of primary thrombocytopenia, rather it causes impaired platelet function. As a result, bleeding is a frequent concern among patients with uremia. The exact etiology remains controversial but is mostly centered around defective interaction of vWF with platelets. The management strategy involves dialysis, use of desmopressin (DDAVP) which helps in releasing vWF from endothelial cells, elevation of hematocrit using red blood cell transfusion or recombinant erythropoietin (associated with risk of thrombosis), cryoprecipitate infusion, conjugated estrogens, and limited role of platelet transfusions.

44.7 Clinical Management

Platelet transfusions are used therapeutically and prophylactically to treat or prevent bleeding, respectively. There are two main sources of platelets. A bag may be comprised of platelets from several whole blood donations. Alternatively, a unit may be collected via apheresis by a single donor. A typical apheresis platelet (3×10^{11}) is equivalent of 6 or more units of whole blood derived platelet (5×10^{10} platelets) [19]. Platelets are a critical resource that is in constant short supply. Although a platelet unit will have a shelf-life of 5–7 days, depending on the method to minimize bacterial contamination, most hospitals have less than a 2-day supply. Given the demand-supply imbalance and limited shelf-life judicial use of platelets is essential. Although a bleeding patient with severe thrombocytopenia will benefit from platelet transfusions, prophylactic platelet transfusions tend to lack supporting data.

Analogous to erythropoietin (red blood cells growth factor), the platelet growth factor is called Thrombopoietin (TPO). It is a protein produced primarily in liver parenchymal cells that acts through the TPO receptor, c-Mpl. It inhibits the apoptosis of megakaryocytes and enhances the production and maturation of megakaryocytes and platelets [20]. The first-generation thrombopoietic agents include recombinant human TPO (rhTPO) and pegylated recombinant human megakaryocyte growth and development factor (PEG-rHuMGDF or MGDF). The PEG-rHuMGDF has been associated with paradoxical thrombocytopenia because of antibodies to both the recombinant and endogenous TPO. The second-generation thrombopoietic agents also referred to as thrombopoietin receptor agonists bind to and activate TPO-R but have a different peptide sequence from endogenous TPO [21]. The second-generation TPO medications are particularly useful in oncology, autoimmune, and drug-induced causes of thrombocytopenia [22].

Intravenous immunoglobulin (IVIG) is a concentrate of the pooled immunoglobulins obtained via collection and pooling of human plasma from hundreds to thousands of donors which increases the lifespan of platelets in vivo by reducing the splenic clearance of platelets (136), via Fc-dependent mechanism. IVIg is recommended for ITP patients who are not responding to corticosteroids or cannot tolerate corticosteroids, as an emergency rescue procedure and under critical bleeding condition. Either IVIg or anti-D be used as a first-line treatment if corticosteroids are contraindicated. If IVIg is used, the dose should initially be 1 g/kg as a one-time dose. This dosage may be repeated if necessary. Pregnant patients with ITP can be treated with either corticosteroids or IVIg [23].

Anti-RhD is concentrated antibody preparations prepared from the plasma of immunized Rh-negative human donors and is Food and Drug Administration (FDA) approved for the treatment of immune thrombocytopenia in nonsplenectomized Rh-positive patients. Initial dosing recommendations range from 50 to 75 mcg/kg intravenously. Infusion of anti-RhD in Rh-positive individuals leads to antibody coating of circulating erythrocytes that are cleared primarily by the spleen. This immune-mediated clearance of sensitized erythrocytes occupies the reticuloendothelial system and allows survival of antibody-coated platelets [24]. The side effects include hemolysis, headache, fever, chills, and vomiting and rarely disseminated intravascular coagulation (DIC) and renal failure [25].

Fibrinolysis is an endogenous process for breaking-down clots. Excessive fibrinolysis may occur following trauma or childbirth and can lead to excessive bleeding. Hemostatic agents like antifibrinolytic agents and DDAVP are increasingly being used to control bleeding and prevent unnecessary blood transfusions. The antifibrinolytic agents approved for use in the United States are synthetic lysine analogs: tranexamic acid and epsilon aminocaproic acid and natural serine protease inhibitor aprotinin. They act by competitively and reversibly inhibiting the activation and binding of plasminogen to fibrin, thus stabilizing the clot. The CRASH 2 randomized controlled trial conducted in United Kingdom in 2013 showed that early administration of TXA (given within 1 h) reduced the risk of death in bleeding trauma patients with no increased incidence of side effects [26–29].

Desmopressin, DDAVP (1-deamino-8-D-arginine vasopressin), is a synthetic analog of the vasopressin that acts through V2 receptors inducing the release of von Willebrand factor from Weibel Palade bodies of the endothelial cells [30]. It has provided hemostatic benefit and thus reduced blood usage in the management of von Willebrand disease, hemophilia A, and platelet function defects. Routes of administration include intravenous, subcutaneous, sublingual, and intranasal routes. The dose for both intravenous and subcutaneous routes is 0.3 μg/kg. The side effect profile includes tachycardia, flushing, and headache being the common ones; hyponatremia and seizures and thrombotic events, such as stroke or acute myocardial infarction being rare ones.

In conclusion, thrombocytopenia is a frequent problem encountered in ICU with varying severity and clinical significance. The clinical situation, differential diagnosis, and laboratory testing should be kept in mind while working up a patient with thrombocytopenia.

References

1. Ali RA, Wuescher LM, Worth RG. Platelets: essential components of the immune system. Curr Trends Immunol. 2015;16:65–78.
2. Hui P, Cook DJ, Lim W, Fraser GA, Arnold DM. The frequency and clinical significance of thrombocytopenia complicating critical illness: a systematic review. Chest. 2011;139(2):271–8.
3. Rodeghiero F, Tosetto A, Abshire T, Arnold DM, Coller B, James P, ISTH/SSC Joint VWF and Perinatal/Pediatric Hemostasis Subcommittees Working Group, et al. STH/SSC bleeding assessment tool: a standardized questionnaire and a proposal for a new bleeding score for inherited bleeding disorders. J Thromb Haemost. 2010;8(9):2063–5.
4. Shahbazi M, Ahmadinejad M, Teimourpour A. Utility of the international society on thrombosis and hemostasis-bleeding assessment tool in the diagnosis of patients who suspected of platelet function disorders. Blood Coagul Fibrinolysis. 2024;35(1):8–13.
5. Nagalla S, Bray P. Platelet disorders (inherited and acquired). In: Reference module in biomedical sciences; 2014. https://doi.org/10.1016/B978-0-12-801238-3.00063-5.
6. Kaufman RM, Djulbegovic B, Gernsheimer T, Kleinman S, Tinmouth AT, Capocelli KE, et al. Platelet transfusion: a clinical practice guideline from the AABB. Ann Intern Med. 2015;162(3):205–13.
7. Slichter SJ, Kaufman RM, Assmann SF, McCullough J, Triulzi DJ, Strauss RG, et al. Dose of prophylactic platelet transfusions and prevention of hemorrhage. N Engl J Med. 2010;362(7):600–13.
8. Gaydos LA, Freireich EJ, Mantel N. The quantitative relation between platelet count and hemorrhage in patients with acute leukemia. N Engl J Med. 1962;266:905–9.
9. Papageorgiou C, Jourdi G, Adjambri E, Walborn A, Patel P, Fareed J, et al. Disseminated intravascular coagulation: an update on pathogenesis, diagnosis, and therapeutic strategies. Clin Appl Thromb Hemost. 2018;24(Suppl. 9):8S–28S.
10. Abou-Ismail MY, Kapoor S, Citla Sridhar D, Nayak L, Ahuja S. Thrombotic microangiopathies: an illustrated review. Res Pract Thromb Haemost. 2022;6(3):e12708.
11. Mushtaq AH, Rasheed AW, Jamil MG, Maghrabi K, Khoja O, Sajid MR, et al. A retrospective analysis of the frequency of heparin-induced thrombocytopenia in the intensive care unit at a tertiary care center in Riyadh, Saudi Arabia. Am J Blood Res. 2023;13(6):198–06.
12. Nicolas D, Nicolas S, Hodgens A, Reed M. Heparin-induced thrombocytopenia. Treasure Island (FL): StatPearls; 2024.
13. Provan D, Arnold DM, Bussel JB, Chong BH, Cooper N, Gernsheimer T, et al. Updated international consensus report on the investigation and management of primary immune thrombocytopenia. Blood Adv. 2019;3(22):3780–17.
14. Hawkins J, Aster RH, Curtis BR. Post-transfusion purpura: current perspectives. J Blood Med. 2019;10:405–15.
15. Vayne C, Guery EA, Rollin J, Baglo T, Petermann R, Gruel Y. Pathophysiology and diagnosis of drug-induced immune thrombocytopenia. J Clin Med. 2020;9(7):2212. https://doi.org/10.3390/jcm9072212.
16. Arnold DM, Kukaswadia S, Nazi I, Esmail A, Dewar L, Smith JW, et al. A systematic evaluation of laboratory testing for drug-induced immune thrombocytopenia. J Thromb Haemost. 2013;11(1):169–76.

17. Juskewitch JE, Norgan AP, De Goey SR, Duellman PM, Wakefield LL, Gandhi MJ, et al. How do I … Manage the platelet transfusion-refractory patient? Transfusion. 2017;57(12):2828–35.
18. Aster RH. Pooling of platelets in the spleen: role in the pathogenesis of "hypersplenic" thrombocytopenia. J Clin Invest. 1966;45(5):645–57.
19. Yuan S, Otrock ZK. Platelet transfusion: an update on indications and guidelines. Clin Lab Med. 2021;41(4):621–34.
20. Kuter DJ, Begley CG. Recombinant human thrombopoietin: basic biology and evaluation of clinical studies. Blood. 2002;100(10):3457–69.
21. Soff GA, Ray-Coquard I, Rivera LJM, Fryzek J, Mullins M, Bylsma LC, et al. Systematic literature review and meta-analysis on use of thrombopoietic agents for chemotherapy-induced thrombocytopenia. PLoS One. 2022;17(6):e0257673.
22. Gilreath J, Lo M, Bubalo J. Thrombopoietin receptor agonists (TPO-RAs): drug class considerations for pharmacists. Drugs. 2021;81(11):1285–305.
23. Neunert C, Terrell DR, Arnold DM, Buchanan G, Cines DB, Cooper N, et al. American Society of Hematology 2019 guidelines for immune thrombocytopenia. Blood Adv. 2019;3(23):3829–66.
24. Ware RE, Zimmerman SA. Anti-D: mechanisms of action. Semin Hematol. 1998;35(1 Suppl. 1):14–22.
25. Khan AM, Mydra H, Nevarez A. Clinical practice updates in the management of immune thrombocytopenia. Pharmacy Therapeut. 2017;42(12):756–63.
26. Roberts I, Shakur H, Coats T, Hunt B, Balogun E, Barnetson L, et al. The CRASH-2 trial: a randomised controlled trial and economic evaluation of the effects of tranexamic acid on death, vascular occlusive events and transfusion requirement in bleeding trauma patients. Health Technol Assess. 2013;17(10):1–79.
27. Levy JH, Koster A, Quinones QJ, Milling TJ, Key NS. Antifibrinolytic therapy and perioperative considerations. Anesthesiology. 2018;128(3):657–70.
28. Slaughter TF, Greenberg CS. Antifibrinolytic drugs and perioperative hemostasis. Am J Hematol. 1997;56(1):32–6.
29. Mannucci PM. Hemostatic drugs. N Engl J Med. 1998;339(4):245–53.
30. Ozgonenel B, Rajpurkar M, Lusher JM. How do you treat bleeding disorders with desmopressin? Postgrad Med J. 2007;83(977):159–63.

Chapter 45
Sustainable Pharmacy Practice in the ICU

Nicole G. M. Hunfeld and Amy L. Dzierba

45.1 Introduction

The healthcare sector is responsible for almost 5% of global (GHG) emissions [1] and has a carbon footprint equivalent to 514 coal-fired power plants [2]. A carbon footprint (or greenhouse gas footprint) is described as the impact of an activity, product, or service on the environment [3]. Burning of fossil fuels produces greenhouse gas (GHG) emissions, carbon dioxide being the most abundant, resulting in pollution and global warming. Hospitals and other healthcare facilities use significant amounts of energy, food, materials, and medicines, generating substantial waste and carbon emissions, thereby contributing to environmental pollution and health-related consequences. If the sector were a country, it would be the fifth largest polluter on Earth [4]. Under a "business as usual" scenario, emissions from healthcare could triple by 2050 (Fig. 45.1).

Health systems contribute to climate change primarily through GHG emissions falling under three scopes (Fig. 45.2): (1) scope 1 includes emissions under direct control of the healthcare facility such as fleet vehicles; (2) scope 2 encompasses indirect activities such as heating and electricity p; and (3) scope 3 includes all other indirect emissions, such as those from supply chains [2]. Emissions from supply chains include the production, transport, and disposal of medications, food, medical devices, and hospital equipment. The majority of GHG emissions results from

N. G. M. Hunfeld (✉)
Department of Intensive Care Adults and Department of Hospital Pharmacy,
Erasmus University Medical Center, Rotterdam, The Netherlands
e-mail: n.hunfeld@erasmusmc.nl

A. L. Dzierba
Department of Medicine, New York University Langone Health, New York, NY, USA
e-mail: Amy.Dzierba@nylangone.org

© The Author(s), under exclusive license to Springer Nature Switzerland AG 2025

Y. Alzaidi, M. A. Gebily (eds.), *The Pharmacist's Expanded Role in Critical Care Medicine*, https://doi.org/10.1007/978-3-031-77335-8_45

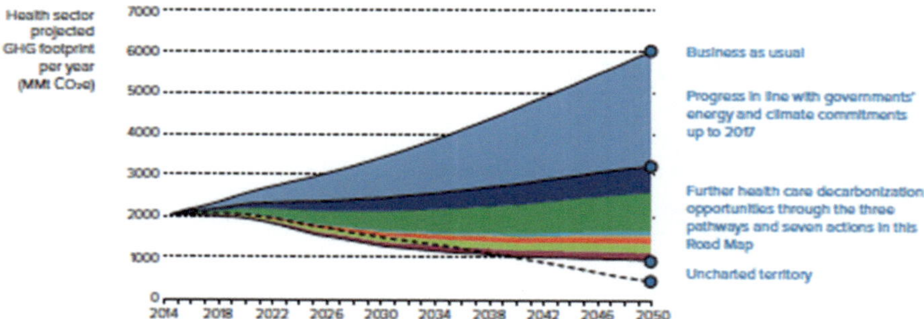

Fig. 45.1 Illustration of GHG emissions from 2014 to 2050. Figure originated from Healthcare without harm [4]

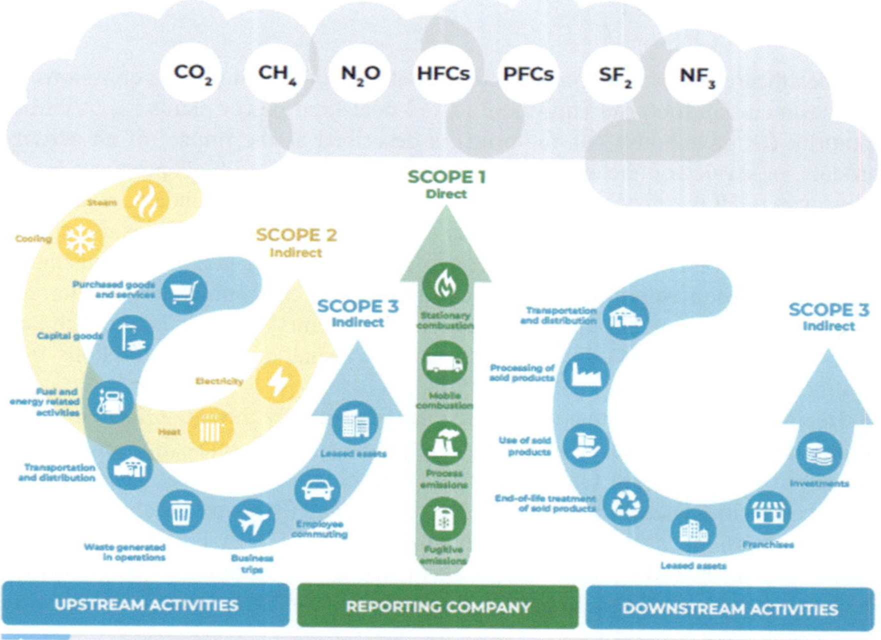

Fig. 45.2 Scope 1, 2, and 3 sources of emissions. Derived from [5]

indirect emissions under scope 3. Up to 60% of scope 3 emissions were identified in a large academic hospital in the Netherlands [6].

As the burden of disease increases, more pressure will be placed on health systems worldwide to provide an increasing number of hospital stays and medical appointments. Increasing demand and inefficiencies (such as overprescribing, preventable medical errors, and delivery of low-value care) will further increase emissions from health systems [2, 7] (Fig. 45.3). Environmental sustainability is germane

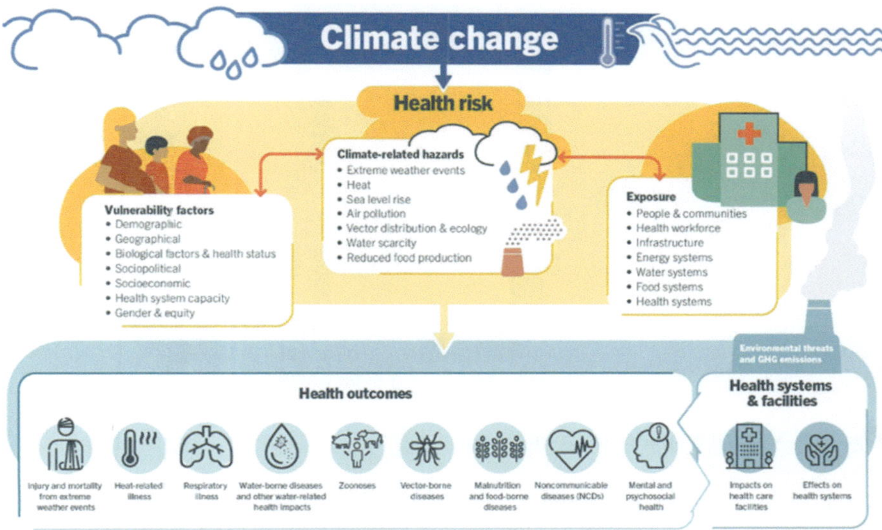

Fig. 45.3 The effect of climate change on health outcomes (from [7])

to the intensive care unit (ICU), a high resource area, generating 1.3 times more waste and 3.1 times more GHG as compared to acute inpatient units [8]

45.2 How to Measure Impact of Healthcare on the Environment?

Measuring the environmental impact of healthcare is a relatively new area of research. Different approaches exist to measure the environmental impact. The most common methods include a material flow analysis, a life cycle assessment, and a waste audit.

Material flow analysis (MFA) is an analytical method to quantify flows and stocks of material, substance, or product flows across different industrial sectors or within a specific system (Fig. 45.4). MFA is an important tool to study the biophysical aspects of human activity on different spatial and temporal scales. This method can also be applied to a single industrial installation, for example, tracking nutrient flows through a wastewater treatment plant. It is considered a core method of industrial ecology or anthropogenic, urban, social, and industrial metabolism. A MFA from Erasmus MC's ICU in Rotterdam, The Netherlands, observed a material mass inflow of 247,000 kg in 2019. The outflow showed that 50,000 kg was incinerated as (hazardous) hospital waste [10, 11]. The environmental impact per ICU patient was calculated based on the MFA data and resulted in 17 kg of mass, 12 kg CO_2 eq, 300 L of water usage, and 4 m^2 of agricultural land occupation per

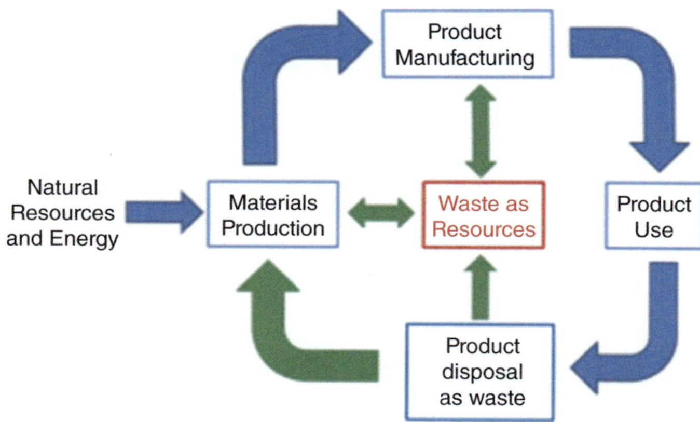

Fig. 45.4 Material flow analysis (from Balanay [9])

day. Five hotspots were identified: non-sterile gloves, isolation gowns, bed liners, surgical masks, and syringes. Continuous infusion fluids and continuous renal replacement therapy (CRRT) fluids were included in this analysis, as well as syringes, intravenous bags, infusion lines, and their packaging. The environmental impact of medications has not been analyzed to date.

Life cycle assessment (LCA), also known as life cycle analysis, is a methodology for assessing environmental impacts associated with all the stages of the life cycle of a commercial product, process, or service (Fig. 45.5). For instance, in the case of a manufactured product, environmental impacts are assessed from raw material extraction and processing (cradle), through the product's manufacture, distribution, and use, to the recycling or final disposal of the materials composing it (grave) [12, 13].

An LCA study involves a thorough inventory of the energy and materials that are required across the supply chain and value chain of a product, process, or service, and calculates the corresponding emissions to the environment, thus assessing cumulative potential environmental impacts. The aim is to document and improve the overall environmental profile of the product by serving as a holistic baseline upon which carbon footprints can be accurately compared.

Widely recognized procedures for conducting LCAs are included in the 14,000 series of environmental management standards of the International Organization for Standardization (ISO) ([14], https://www.iso.org/standards/popular/iso-14000-family). The general categories of environmental impacts needing consideration include resource use, human health, and ecological consequences.

General and specific cases (e.g., in the consistency of the methodology, the difficulty in performing, the cost in performing, revealing of intellectual property, and the understanding of system boundaries) limitations exist with the LCA approach. When LCA methodology wanes, it may be completed based on a practitioner's views or the economic and political incentives of the sponsoring entity (an issue plaguing all known data-gathering practices). As such, an LCA completed by 10

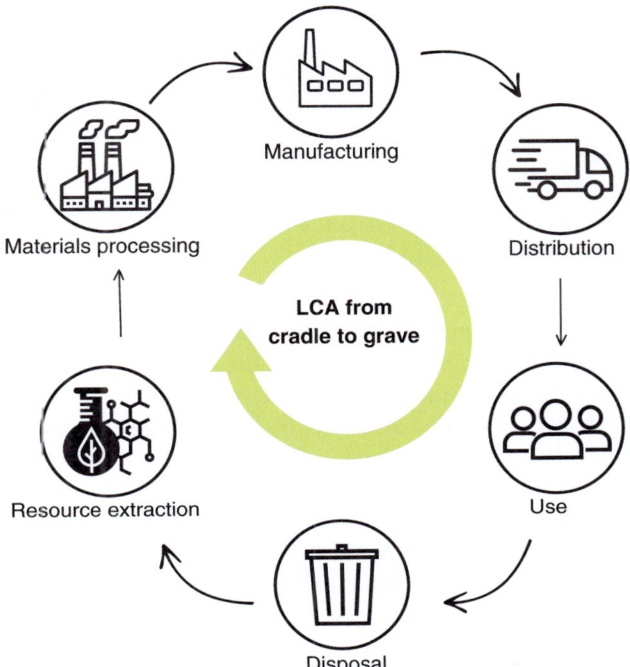

Fig. 45.5 Life cycle assessment (from: https://en.wikipedia.org/wiki/Life-cycle_assessment)

different parties could yield 10 different results. The ISO LCA Standard aims to normalize this; however, the guidelines are not overly restrictive and 10 different answers may still be generated [15]

Waste audit (WA) is a study of how much and what type of waste the business is producing. The idea is to break down how much waste is being recycled, composted, or sent to landfills or for incineration. It also helps to evaluate the contamination in each stream, what could have been recyclable, or what should not have been in the recycling. The results from a WA will help improve recommendations, signage, and education for healthcare professionals.

A hospital or ICU can do its own periodical WA by simply collecting trash, for a given period of time, sorting it into categories and weighing each one. During this process, one may note how clean and sorted recycling products are. It is important to equip employees so they can work safely (e.g., providing rubber gloves and face masks). A deeper dive will involve a waste composition study. This goes beyond a typical WA, breaking down waste even further by department or operational area. For example, recyclable waste could be broken down into subcategories like bottles, cans, plastic, and metal.

Examples of WA in healthcare are summarized in a systematic description of best practices by Slutzman and colleagues [16]. The authors identified 156 studies involving direct measurement of waste in medical facilities from 37 countries and concluded that there were significant differences in methods and results between high-and low-income countries. Furthermore, the quality of the studies was variable with general methodologic inconsistency. This publication provides a guideline for WA in healthcare.

45.3   The Environmental Impact of Medications Administered in the ICU

Data from the United Kingdom (UK) and the Netherlands demonstrated that 20–40% of the GHG emissions are caused by drugs and chemicals [6, 17, 18]. To date, no specific data exist of the environmental burden of drugs used in ICUs. Data from the MFA of an ICU showed that water (from CRRT and intravenous bags) was the main ingredient, accounting for 61% of the mass of the inflow [10, 11]. Data from general waste audits from the ICU in Erasmus MC showed that waste from medication accounts for 24% of the waste stream [19] (Fig. 45.6). Paper boxes, leaflets, and cardboard boxes were excluded from these audits, since the paper stream is a separate recycling stream within the hospital.

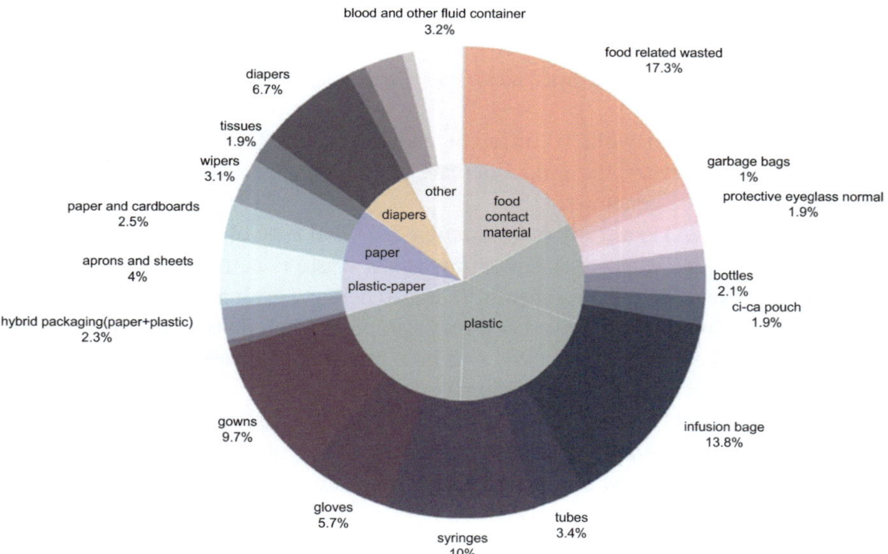

Fig. 45.6 Data from a waste audit from an intensive care unit https://repository.tudelft.nl/island-ora/object/uuid%3A58bb3d8c-cca3-4786-9e60-ff0f6f2edb3a?collection=education

45.4   The Cycle of the Drug: From Industry to Waste Water

45.4.1   Morphine: Life Cycle Analysis

In determining the environmental impact of a drug, a cradle-to-grave approach is needed. McAlister and colleagues performed an analysis for intravenous morphine. The authors examined the environmental life cycle (e.g., CO_2 equivalent ("CO_2 e") emissions and water use) from poppy farming through to production of 100 mg in 100 mL of intravenous morphine (standard infusion bag) in Australia [20]. All aspects of morphine production from poppy farming, pelletizing, bulk morphine manufacture to final formulation were measured (Fig. 45.7). Industry and inventory-sourced databases were used for most inputs. Their results showed that morphine sulfate had a climate change effect of 204 g CO_2 e (95% CI 189 to 280 g CO_2 e), approximating the CO_2 e emissions of driving an average car 1 km. Water use was 7.8 L (95% CI 6.7–9.0 L), primarily stemming from farming (6.7 L). All other environmental effects were minor and several orders of magnitude <CO_2 e emissions and water use. Almost 90% of CO_2 e emissions occurred during the final stages of 100 mg of morphine sulfate manufacture. Packaging of morphine sulfate contributed 95 g CO_2 e, which accounted for 46% of the total CO_2 e (95% CI 82–155 g CO_2 e). Mixing, filling, and sterilization of 100 mg morphine sulfate bags added a further 86 g CO_2 e, which accounted for 42% (95% CI 80–92 g CO_2 e). Poppy farming (6 g CO_2 e, 3%), pelletizing, and manufacturing (18 g CO_2 e, 9%) made smaller contributions to CO2 emissions. Overall, the environmental effects of growing opium poppies and manufacturing bulk morphine sulfate were small. The final stages of morphine production, particularly sterilization and packaging, contributed to almost 90% of morphine sulfate's carbon footprint. Focused measures to improve the energy efficiency and sources for drug sterilization and packaging could be explored as these are relevant to all drugs. The authors were unable to compare the environmental footprint of morphine in 10 mg glass vials (another common preparation) as no companies were willing to make their data available. More data on the impact of

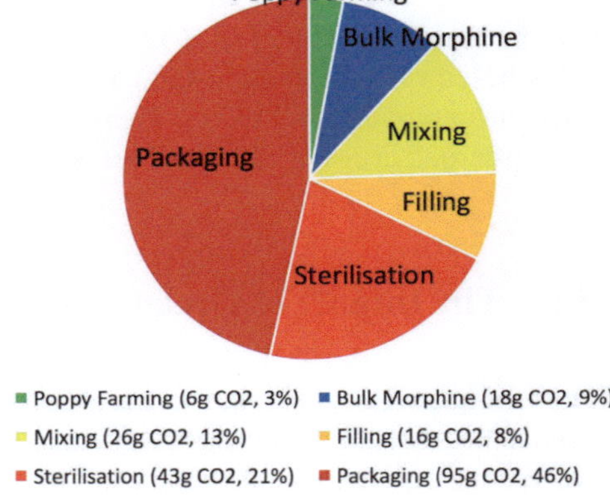

Fig. 45.7 Greenhouse gas impacts (g CO_2 and %) by stage of morphine's life cycle (205 g CO_2 total). The individual listing of the final steps in the process of morphine production (mixing, filling, sterilizing, and packaging) indicates that they are the most important contributors to morphine CO_2 emissions (from: [20])

the production of other drugs and comparisons between oral and intravenous preparations on the environment are needed. In the future, LCAs will rely on industry data for inputs beyond what was obtained directly.

45.4.2 Paracetamol and Its Environmental Impact

Estimated GHG emissions (expressed as carbon dioxide equivalents CO_2e) associated with intravenous and oral formulations of paracetamol (including one acetaminophen formulation in the USA) used in the perioperative period were assessed in 26 hospitals in the USA, UK, and Australia. [21]. For those surgical patients for whom oral formulations were indicated, CO_2e and costs of actual prescribing practices for intravenous or oral doses were compared with optimal oral prescribing. The carbon footprint for a 1 g dose was 38 g CO_2e (oral tablet), 151 g CO_2e (oral liquid), and 310–628 g CO_2e (intravenous, depending on type of packaging used and administration supplies used). Substituting oral tablets for intravenous paracetamol (used in 66–80% of patients) for elective surgical patients in 2019, ~5.7 kt CO_2e could have been avoided and would save 98.3% of financial costs. The authors concluded that intravenous paracetamol has a 12-fold greater life-cycle carbon emissions than the oral tablet. Additionally, glass vials have higher GHG emissions than plastic vials. As such, intravenous administration of paracetamol should be reserved for patients in which oral formulations are not feasible.

Another study compared different formulations of paracetamol in pediatric patients [22]. They estimated the embodied carbon of different formulations of paracetamol, its packaging, and the consumables used in administration. The cost was estimated from average contract pricing and converted to kilograms of carbon dioxide equivalent ($KgCO_2e$) using the emission factors. The results demonstrated a 6 g/CO_2e for one 750 mg tablet (administered in a paper medication cup) and 674 g/CO_2e for intravenous (administered in a 100 mL bag of 0.9% sodium chloride and a flush to clear the intravenous line). The authors observed a 100-fold higher emission with intravenous compared to tablets. The data of Davies et al. [21], found a 12-fold higher emission with intravenous compared to tablets. The large differences between these two LCAs may be a result of differences in cost calculations (spend based versus company data). Ecological toxicity was not studied in either the morphine or paracetamol LCAs. There is the potential that ecological toxicity exists from discarded drugs or excreta from patients entering our waste water [23].

45.5 The Impact of Green Teams

The consequences of the impact of healthcare on our climate, together with environmental data, plea for the individual ICUs to create "green teams," as one of the ways to tackle the environmental problems [24]. The "Guide for creating effective green teams in healthcare" ([25], practicegreenhealth.org) can be helpful in starting a green team in the ICU. Green teams can start the change toward a circular economy with the ICU hotspots as low hanging fruit [10, 11]. Furthermore, the publication "Create intensive care green teams, there is no time to waste" provides a list of practical tips from ICU environmental champions in New Zealand, Australia, Canada, and Belgium [26]. These themes emerged which align with advice for effective green teams in general (practicegreenhealth.org):

- Identify multidisciplinary green champions who are passionate about sustainability. Nurses often lead ICU green teams and are key to success at the bedside.
- Do not wait to be asked. Grassroots drive is a necessary condition for success strengthened by the top-down support of leadership. Leadership can strengthen groups by giving them autonomy to problem-solve, positive acknowledgment to the wider unit and appropriate financial resourcing of initiatives. A green team mission statement that aligns with the health care organization's values will demonstrate fitting as part of the quality framework.
- Map existing initiatives, plan next steps in conjunction with leadership teams, and set specific, measurable, achievable, realistic, and timely (SMART) goals. Meet regularly and set deadlines for actions.
- Sustainability should not be separate, it should be firmly embedded in quality frameworks. Make daily ICU processes and procedures more efficient, starting with process mapping your day.
- Communicate initiatives widely with regular reminders and updates at ward meetings, on posters, notice boards, in ICU newsletters and social media. Collaborate/share/copy ideas from others and get support to achieve targets from roles like hospital sustainability officers.
- Celebrate your success. Promote it. Keep it fun, be creative and show appreciation of all ideas, bring people along with you with encouragement, feedback, and education. If there are financial or health co-benefits, highlight these, and demonstrate how they can be invested back into patient care. Reframe the inevitable barriers encountered into opportunities.

Based on the experience of Erasmus MC and other ICUs in Europe, four other points can be added:

- Pharmacists need to be part of the ICU green team. Pharmacists can play an important role, given the high impact of medication on the environment and their knowledge of and engagement in the total medication process.
- Furthermore, the ICU cannot be considered as an isolated entity. Others, from outside the hospital are needed to help with a green transition, such as societies, faculties, industry, and healthcare policymakers [27].
- The 10R principle (see below) can be used as a tool in educating people about the environmental impact of a green intervention and it can help in showing the value of a green intervention.
- A green wall in an ICU can be an inspiration for all people that work or visit the ICU. The green wall can show green initiatives that have been implemented. It

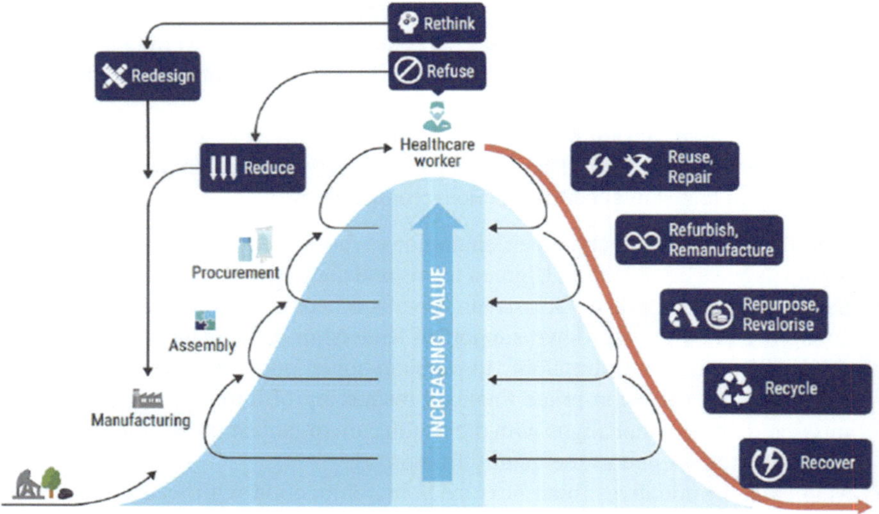

Fig. 45.8 Value hill with 10R strategy

can also invite others (family or relatives) to add new ideas about green interventions.

45.5.1   10R Approach

Based on the environmental issues and hotspots, the 10R strategies can be used as a starting point for circular interventions by healthcare staff [28] (Fig. 45.8). The 10Rs represent Refuse, Rethink, Reduce, Reuse, Repair, Refurbish, Remanufacture, Repurpose, Recycle, and Recover. Refuse (meaning not buying/using the product in the first place) is the strategy with the highest impact in the hierarchy of circular interventions, while Recover (generating energy from incineration of waste) represents the strategy with the lowest impact. In the transition from a linear to a circular system, knowledge about the environmental impact of products and actions is needed in order to determine environmental hotspots and to use the 10R strategies.

45.6   Examples of Green Team Activities for Pharmacists and Pharmacy Team

Table 45.1 shows a selection of green team activities led by the ICU pharmacist, based on the different steps in the medication process.

Table 45.1 Examples of green ICU pharmacy practices

Intervention	Information	R strategy
Prescribing		
Dose reduction	Acceptance of 10% deviation of prescribed dose, so one vial can be used instead of two	Reduce
Automated stop of medication order	Implements a 48-h automatic stop time for certain drugs. Metoclopramide and erythromycin either have an effect within 48 h or not	Reduce
Challenge	A national paracetamol challenge (by social media) was started to engage hospitals (and ICUs in particular) to decrease the amount of iv paracetamol with 25%. At ward level, we used posters and education to inspire intensivists to make this switch	Reduce
Dispensing		
Use of PFSS syringes (PreFilled sterilized syringes) for continuous administration	Use of national produced 50 mL PFSS. These syringes are sterilized after filling and can be administered over 7 days (instead of 24 h)	Reduce
Use of ready to administer (RTA) syringes	RTA syringes are being prescribed and dispensed as much as possible. This is, for example, protocolized together with ED and OR for intubation sets and cardiac arrest sets	Reduce
Redispensing of unused medication	Within the hospital unused drugs that are ordered for a specific patient are being transferred to the central stock room of the pharmacy for redispensing purpose	Reuse
Administration		
Decreased flow rate	Flow of infusion as flush (NaCl) is decreased from 3 mL/h to 2 mL/h. this saves 1500 iv bags and 5000 syringes per year	Reduce
Lowest volume of iv bag	Use of lowest volume of bag (50 mL is standard) (see also: Fluid stewardship)	Reduce
Use of RTA syringes instead of iv drip	Use of ready to administer syringes instead of iv bags: this saves 30.000 iv bags per year	Reduce
Therapeutic drug monitoring		
TDM with strict protocol	TDM is performed based on a protocol with pharmacist involvement (to minimize useless sampling)	Reduce
Vancomycin validated in arterial blood gas samples	Vancomycin is stable in ABG samples. We validated the method and left over ABG can be used to measure the vancomycin concentration [29]	Refuse
Waste reduction interventions		
Recycling of CRRT bags (packaging and bag itself)	Recycling of CRRT bags and packaging. The connectors are being cut off before disposing in separate bag	Recycle
Collection of zip lock bags from compounded syringes	Reuse of zip lock bags by pharmacy. Bags are being collected in dedicated box in ICU pharmacy room	Reuse

All the interventions should be part of the annual plan of the ICU green team and discussed during regular green teams meetings. Ideally, each intervention should be implemented by 2–3 green team members. Implementation occurs by communicating the green intervention in the ICU (e.g., weekly newsletters, advertisement on computer screens, and during rounds).

Two other interventions that directly correlate to the environment (refuse and reduce) and in which ICU pharmacists are often involved are antimicrobial and fluid stewardship.

45.7 Antimicrobial Stewardship

The benefits of antimicrobials in critically ill patients are well documented; however, there are significant environmental consequences with indiscriminate use [30]. The production, packaging, and transportation of antimicrobials contribute to GHG emissions. Furthermore, the use of extended or continuous infusions along with expanded therapeutic drug monitoring to optimize the pharmacokinetics and pharmacodynamics of antimicrobials increases resource use. Another environmental consequence of antimicrobial use is the release of active drug or metabolites into the environment whether from human feces and/or urine, or improper disposal leading to the development of antibiotic-resistant genes and bacteria [31]. Antimicrobial resistance is a global health concern resulting in prolonged hospitalization and increased mortality [32].

Antimicrobial parent compounds and active metabolites persist in the environment largely due to their resistance to degradation exerting toxic effects on the ecosystem. Various physicochemical methods and bioremediation have been used to mitigate the toxic effects of antimicrobials to the environment, particularly through wastewater [33]. However, cost, ease of accessibility, and effectiveness must be considered when adopting these technologies. Antimicrobial stewardship (AS) programs aim to minimize the negative effects of antimicrobial use and improve patient outcomes. Additionally, AS may have a positive impact on the environment although many knowledge gaps persist. The benefits of pharmacist involvement on critically ill patients with infections have been documented [34]. One large study reported lower mortality, shorter ICU length of stay, and lower hospital charges with ICUs with ICU pharmacists as compared to those that did not. The greatest benefit was in patients with nosocomial infections where mortality was 23.6% higher in the absence of clinical pharmacy services.

The ecological effects of antibiotics require a different approach [30]. The impacts come from various factors. Besides, the impact related to the production, packaging, and transportation, the production of pharmaceuticals is often a complex process requiring a lot of energy and raw materials, and resulting in considerable emissions into the soil, water, and air. While the impact of antimicrobial use on the hospital's microbial ecosystem and resistance patterns is reasonably well understood, antimicrobials have additional impacts on the wider ecosystem outside of hospitals. Antimicrobials are often not metabolized in the body and are excreted unchanged, mainly in the urine. These antimicrobials are then released directly into the effluent of the hospital, resulting in concentrations in hospital wastewater that are much higher when compared to wastewater from cities. One systematic review found that 57 antibiotics were reported to be present at least once in water or sediment of lakes around the world. In France, fluoroquinolones and trimethoprim concentrations in the environment were at increased, risking the selection of resistant bacteria. Pathogens may also be present in the wastewater from hospitals, including antimicrobial-resistant bacteria (ARB), as well as their resistance genes (ARG). Even when the bacteria are not viable, the genes may be transmitted to other bacteria in a cell-free manner further propagating antimicrobial resistance (AMR) in the environment. Wastewater treatment plants (WWTP) are able to remove significant proportions of these antimicrobials, ARBs and ARGs. However, removal efficacy is variable, resulting in the release of these drugs, pathogens, and genes into the wider environment. In many hospitals, antimicrobial stewardship programs (ASP) aim to improve the use of antimicrobials. The main goal of these ASPs is to reduce antimicrobial exposure and thus limit the development of AMR, and ICU pharmacists have a key role in these programs. While preventing the development and spread of AMR within the hospital environment remains the primary aim, ASPs also have a role to play in limiting AMR development and dissemination in the wider ecosystem. Optimizing the use of antimicrobials in hospitals will also have an impact beyond the hospital walls (Fig. 45.9).

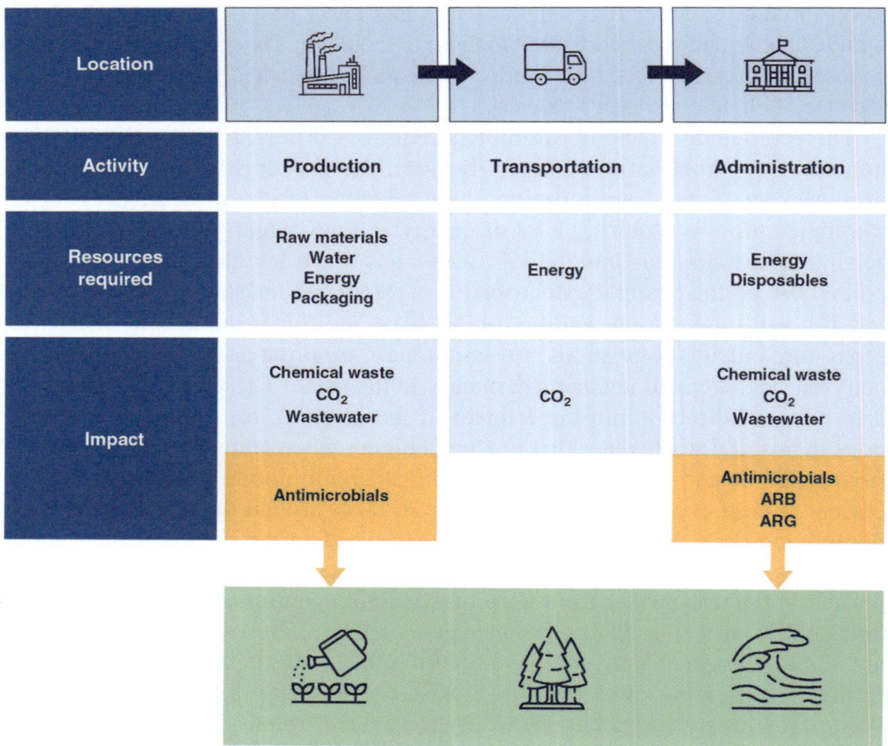

Fig. 45.9 Schematic overview of the impact of production, transport, administration, and disposal of antimicrobials, and the impact on the environment at the different stages. *ARB* antimicrobial-resistant bacteria, *ARG* antimicrobial resistance genes. Copied from Intensive Care Medicine with permission

45.8 Fluid Stewardship

Administration of intravenous fluids is ubiquitous in the intensive care unit for resuscitation and hemodynamic stabilization, replacement, flushes, and diluents for intravenous drugs. For example, more than 200 million liters of saline are consumed annually in the USA [35]. Compared to resuscitation fluids, maintenance and replacement fluids (volume for electrolyte replacement, fluids to keep veins patent, and for medication administration) account for more total daily fluid volume [36]. In a single-center study, 63% of the total IV volume resulted from medication diluents for patients admitted to a medical ICU [37].

Sequelae of fluid overload, defined as an increase in body weight over 10%, includes increased mortality, prolonged intensive care unit stay, and organ dysfunction mainly acute kidney and lung injury [38–40]. Mitigation strategies for fluid overload and associated adverse effects have been described using the "4 D's of fluid therapy" and the "4 rights" of fluid stewardship [41, 42]. Providing fluid

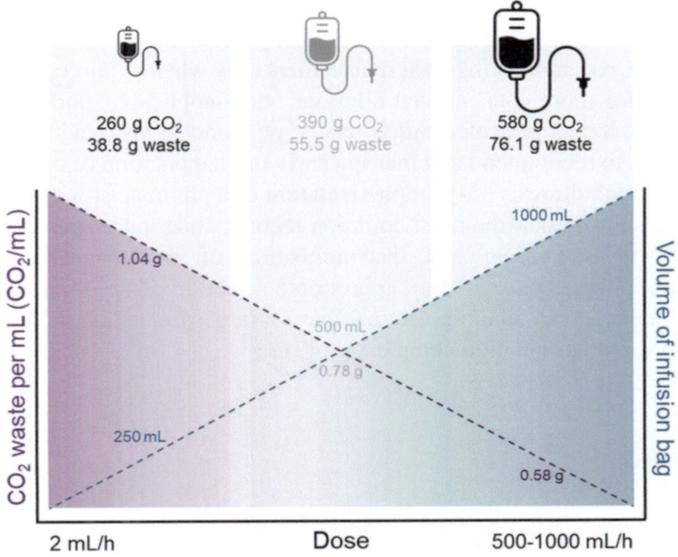

Fig. 45.10 Carbon dioxide (CO₂) emissions and waste production of different sizes of intravenous (IV) bags (Copied from Intensive Care Medicine with permission)

stewardship practices is not only essential to optimize care and prevent adverse events associated with fluid overload, but also an important consideration in reducing the environmental burden.

The MFA conducted at Erasmus University Medical Center identified 61% of the total mass of materials used in 1 year for all patients in the ICU came from sterile water, predominantly infusions and dialysis fluids [10, 11]. Hunfeld et al. underscored the environmental significance of fluid resuscitation in Dutch ICUs, revealing an annual IV bag waste generation of 3600 kg [43]. The production, transport, and disposal of intravenous bags generate a substantial carbon footprint, which contributes to climate change. The impact of the fluid itself (e.g., NaCl or ringer) is negligible (<1% of the total impact), while the CO_2 emissions for different bag sizes (50, 100, 250, and 1000 mL) vary greatly. A life cycle assessment of the different infusion bags results in the following CO_2 emissions per bag: 50 mL–130 g CO_2, 100 mL–150 g CO_2, 250 mL–260 g CO_2, 500 mL–390 g CO_2, and 1000 mL–580 g CO_2 (data on file Radboudumc, Nijmegen, The Netherlands) (Fig. 45.10). Thus, smaller bags have a lower absolute emission, while larger bags have a lower emission per mL fluid. By selecting the appropriate intravenous bag size for each patient at any time, we can reduce both the carbon footprint and the amount of medical waste generated.

To date no analysis on material flow, life cycle analysis or waste audit has been conducted for intravenous fluids such as albumin or crystalloids administered to patients in the ICU. Although the direct impact of ICU fluid stewardship on the environmental impact is still largely unknown, pharmacists can play a role in fluid stewardship potentially reducing daily materials used in fluid management. Critical care pharmacists help mitigate fluid overload by assessing the indication for fluid administration, recommending fluid replacement only when required, advising dilution changes for more concentrated dilutions when applicable, and discontinuing fluids when no longer indicated. Additionally, pharmacists work with the multidisciplinary team to recommend and manage early implementation of de-resuscitation strategies through diuresis [44]. Implementation of a pharmacist-led fluid stewardship service showed that the most common recommendations were conversion of intravenous to oral route and discontinuation of maintenance fluids [45]. Furthermore, pharmacists can help appropriate selection of fluid based on indication [46]. Reduction in albumin use may have a larger impact on the environment given its increased production complexity [47].

References

1. Watts N, Amann M, Arnell N, Ayeb-Karlsson S, Beagley J, Belesova K, et al. The 2020 report of The Lancet Countdown on health and climate change: responding to converging crises. Lancet. 2021;397(10269):129–70. https://doi.org/10.1016/S0140-6736(20)32290-X.
2. Healthcare without harm and ARUP 2019: How the Health Sector Contributes to the Global Climate Crisis and Opportunities for Action; 2019. Report: https://noharm-global.org/documents/health-care-climate-footprint-report (accessed May 11th, 2024).
3. Gaetani M, Uleryk E, Halgren C, Maratta C. The carbon footprint of critical care: a systematic review. Intensive Care Med. 2024;50(5):731–45. https://doi.org/10.1007/s00134-023-07307-1.
4. Healthcare without harm 2021: Global road map for health care decarbonization; 2021. https://healthcareclimateaction.org/roadmap (accessed May 11th, 2024).
5. Erasmus MC, Carbon footprint of Erasmus MC; 2021. https://www.erasmusmc.nl/-/media/erasmusmc/pdf/2-themaoverstijgend/duurzaam-erasmus-mc/erasmus_erasmus_sbt_landscapereport_def_msg.pdf (accessed May 29th, 2024).
6. Lau I, Burdorf A, Hesseling S, Wijk L, Tauber M, Hunfeld N. The carbon footprint of a Dutch academic hospital—using a hybrid assessment method to identify driving activities and departments. Front Public Health. 2024;12:1380400.
7. World Health Organization. Operational framework for building climate resilient and low carbon health systems. Geneva: World Health Organization; 2023.
8. Prasad PA, Joshi D, Lighter J, et al. Environmental footprint of regular and intensive inpatient care in a large US hospital. Int J Life Cycle Assess. 2022;27:38–49. https://doi.org/10.1007/s11367-021-01998-8.
9. Balanay R, Halog A. Tools for circular economy: review and some potential applications for the Philippine textile industry. In: Muthu SS, editor. The textile institute book series, circular economy in textiles and apparel. Woodhead Publishing; 2019. p. 49–75. ISBN 9780081026304.
10. Hunfeld N, Diehl JC, Timmermann M, van Exter P, Bouwens J, Browne-Wilkinson S, de Planque N, Gommers D. Circular material flow in the intensive care unit-environmental effects and identification of hotspots. Intensive Care Med. 2023a;49(1):65–74. https://doi.org/10.1007/s00134-022-06940-6.
11. Hunfeld N, Diehl JC, Gommers D, van der Zee S, van Raaij E. The Green Intensive care: from environmental hotspot to action. ICU Manage Pract. 2023b;23(3)
12. Ilgin MA, Gupta SM. Environmentally conscious manufacturing and product recovery (ECMPRO): a review of the state of the art. J Environ Manage. 2010;91(3):563–91. https://doi.org/10.1016/j.jenvman.2009.09.037.

13. United States Environmental Protection Agency, Life Cycle Assessment; 2024. http://www.epa.gov/nrmrl/std/lca/lca.html. Accessed May 14th 2024.

14. International Standardization Organisation; 2024. https://www.iso.org/standards/popular/iso-14000family. Accessed May 14th 2024.

15. Matthews HS, Hendrickson CT, Matthews DH. Life cycle assessment: quantitative approaches for decisions that matter. In: Open access textbook; 2014. p. 83–95.

16. Slutzman JE, Bockius H, Gordon IO, Greene HC, Hsu S, Huang Y, Lam MH, Roberts T, Thiel CL. Waste audits in healthcare: a systematic review and description of best practices. Waste Manag Res. 2023;41(1):3–17. https://doi.org/10.1177/0734242X221101531.

17. NHS Delivering a 'Net Zero' National Health Service 2022. https://www.england.nhs.uk/greenernhs/wp-content/uploads/sites/51/2022/07/B1728-delivering-a-net-zero-nhs-july-2022.pdf. Accessed May 14th 2024.

18. Steenmeijer MA, Rodrigues JFD, Zijp MC, Waaijers-van der Loop SL. The environmental impact of the Dutch healthcare sector beyond climate change: an input–output analysis. Lancet Planet Health. 2022;6(12):e949–57.

19. Julia Pongratz. Report master thesis; 2023. http://resolver.tudelft.nl/uuid:58bb3d8c-cca3-4786-9e60-ff0f6f2edb3a.

20. McAlister S, Ou Y, Neff E, Hapgood K, Story D, Mealey P, McGain F. The Environmental footprint of morphine: a life cycle assessment from opium poppy farming to the packaged drug. BMJ Open. 2016;6(10):e013302. https://doi.org/10.1136/bmjopen-2016-013302.

21. Davies JF, McAlister S, Eckelman MJ, McGain F, Seglenieks R, Gutman EN, Groome J, Palipane N, Latoff K, Nielsen D, Sherman JD, TRA2SH, GASP, and WAAREN collaborators. Environmental and financial impacts of perioperative paracetamol use: a multicentre international life-cycle analysis. Br J Anaesth. 2024.:S0007-0912(23)00725-0; https://doi.org/10.1016/j.bja.2023.11.053.

22. Wilson N, Dalton C. The embodied carbon of paracetamol and the consumables associated with different routes of administration in pediatrics. J Clim Change Health. 2024;16:100298. https://doi.org/10.1016/j.joclim.2024.100298.

23. Boxall AB. The environmental side effects of medication. EMBO Rep. 2004;5(12):1110–6. https://doi.org/10.1038/sj.embor.7400307.

24. McDermott-Levy R. The nurse's role on green teams: an environmental health opportunity. Pennsylvania Nurse. 2011;66(1):17–21.

25. PRACTICE Green Health. www.practicegreenhealth.org; 2024. Accessed May 14th 2024.

26. Trent L, Law J, Grimaldi D. Create intensive care green teams, there is no time to waste. Intensive Care Med. 2023;49(4):440–3. https://doi.org/10.1007/s00134-023-07015-w.

27. Hinrichs-Krapels S, Diehl JC, Hunfeld N, van Raaij E. Towards sustainability for medical devices and consumables: the radical and incremental challenges in the technology ecosystem. J Health Serv Res Policy. 2022;27(4):253–4. https://doi.org/10.1177/13558196221110416.

28. Reike D, Vermeulen W, Witjes S. The circular economy: new or refurbished as CE 3.0? Exploring controversies in the conceptualization of the circular economy through a focus on history and resource value retention options. Resour Conserv Recycl. 2018;135:246–64.

29. Smeets TJL, van de Velde D, Koch BCP, Endeman H, Hunfeld NGM. Using residual blood from the arterial blood gas test to perform therapeutic drug monitoring of vancomycin: an example of good clinical practice moving towards a sustainable intensive care unit. Crit Care Res Pract. 2022;27(2022):9107591. https://doi.org/10.1155/2022/9107591.

30. De Waele JJ, Leroux-Roels I, Conway-Morris A. Environmental sustainability and antimicrobials: an underestimated problem with far-reaching consequences. Intensive Care Med. 2024;50(3):453–6. https://doi.org/10.1007/s00134-024-07319-5.

31. Singer AC, Shaw H, Rhodes V, Hart A. Review of antimicrobial resistance in the environment and its relevance to environmental regulators. Front Microbiol. 2016;7:1728.

32. Nelson RE, Slayton RB, Stevens VW, et al. Attributable mortality of healthcare-associated infections due to multidrug-resistant gram-negative bacteria and methicillin-resistant *Staphylococcus aureus*. Infect Control Hosp Epidemiol. 2017;38:848–56.

33. Hunfeld N, Salinas Gabiña I, Weinbren M. Five sustainable tips about water in the ICU: reduction of water use and decrease of the amount of antibiotics in wastewater. Intensive Care Med. 2024;50(3):446–8. https://doi.org/10.1007/s00134-023-07317-z.
34. MacLaren R, Bond CA, Martin SJ, Fike D. Clinical and economic outcomes of involving pharmacists in the direct care of critically ill patients with infections. Crit Care Med. 2008;36:3184–9.
35. Myburgh JA, Mythen MG. Resuscitation fluids. N Engl J Med. 2013;369:1243–51.
36. Van Regenmortel N, Verbrugghe W, Roelant E, Van den Wyngaert T, Jorens PG. Maintenance fluid therapy and fluid creep impose more significant fluid, sodium, and chloride burdens than resuscitation fluids in critically ill patients: a retrospective study in a tertiary mixed ICU population. Intensive Care Med. 2018;44:409–17.
37. Magee CA, Bastin MLT, Laine ME, et al. Insidious harm of medication diluents as a contributor to cumulative volume and hyperchloremia: a prospective, open-label, sequential period pilot study. Crit Care Med. 2018;46:1217–23.
38. Bouchard J, Soroko SB, Chertow GM, Himmelfarb J, Ikizler TA, Paganini EP, et al. Fluid accumulation, survival and recovery of kidney function in critically ill patients with acute kidney injury. Kidney Int. 2009;76:422–7.
39. Boyd JH, Forbes J, Nakada TA, Walley KR, Russell JA. Fluid resuscitation in septic shock: a positive fluid balance and elevated central venous pressure are associated with increased mortality. Crit Care Med. 2011;39:259–65.
40. Murphy CV, Schramm GE, Doherty JA, Reichley RM, Gajic O, Afessa B, et al. The importance of fluid management in acute lung injury secondary to septic shock. Chest. 2009;136:102–9.
41. Hawkins WA, Smith SE, Newsome AS, et al. Fluid stewardship during critical illness: a call to action. J Pharm Pract. 2020;33:863–73.
42. Malbrain M, Van Regenmortel N, Saugel B, et al. Principles of fluid management and stewardship in septic shock: it is time to consider the four D's and the four phases of fluid therapy. Ann Intensive Care. 2018;8:66.
43. Touw H, Stobernack T, NGM H, Pickkers P. Size does matter. Sustainable choice of intravenous bags. Intensive Care Med. 2023;49(12):1529–30. https://doi.org/10.1007/s00134-023-07240-3.
44. Bissell BD, Laine ME, Bastin ML, et al. Impact of protocolized diuresis for de-resuscitation in the intensive care unit. Crit Care. 2020;24(1):70.
45. Hawkins WA, Smith SE, Newsome AS, Carr JR, Bland CM, Branan TN. Fluid Stewardship During Critical Illness: A Call to Action. J Pharm Pract. 2020;33(6):863–873. https://doi.org/10.1177/0897190019853979. Epub 2019 Jun 30. PMID: 31256705; PMCID: PMC7675763.
46. Callum J, Skubas NJ, Bathla A, Keshavarz H, Clark EG, Rochwerg B, Fergusson D, Arbous S, Bauer SR, China L, Fung M. Use of intravenous albumin: a guideline from the international collaboration for transfusion medicine guidelines. Chest. 2024;4. S0012-3692(24)00285-X
47. Matejtschuk P, Dash CH, Gascoigne. Production of human albumin solution: a continually developing colloid. Br J Anaesth. 2000;85:887–95.

Part XI
Supportive Care in Critical Illness

Chapter 46
Pain and Sedation: Assessment, Prevention, and Treatment in the Intensive Care Unit

Joanna L. Stollings and Sybil E. Watkins

46.1 Introduction

The Society of Critical Care Medicine (SCCM) published updated guidelines for the management of Pain Agitation/Sedation, Delirium, Immobility, and Sleep Disruption (PADIS) in adult ICU patients in 2018 [1]. These guidelines, together with recently published research, help guide ICU clinicians in the challenging task of optimizing patient comfort and outcomes while avoiding the complications of under- or oversedation. Rigorous research has developed our understanding of the complexities and importance of the assessment, prevention, and treatment of pain and agitation.

46.2 Analgesia

Severe pain is reported by more than 50% of patients following an ICU stay as their most traumatic memory. Uncontrolled pain in the ICU results in both short and long-term sequelae. Although pain is more overt in surgical, trauma, or burn patients, pain may occur in any type of ICU patient. Management of pain requires an individualized approach for optimization [2].

J. L. Stollings (✉)
Department of Pharmaceutical Services, Vanderbilt University Medical Center, Nashville, TN, USA

Critical Illness, Brain Dysfunction, and Survivorship (CIBS) Center, Vanderbilt University Medical Center, Nashville, TN, USA
e-mail: joanna.stollings@vumc.org

S. E. Watkins
Department of Internal Medicine, Vanderbilt University Medical Center, Nashville, TN, USA

© The Author(s), under exclusive license to Springer Nature Switzerland AG 2025

Y. Alzaidi, M. A. Gebily (eds.), *The Pharmacist's Expanded Role in Critical Care Medicine*, https://doi.org/10.1007/978-3-031-77335-8_46

A comprehensive review of nursing care that may cause discomfort, procedural-based pain and other causes of acute and chronic pain should be conducted by the interprofessional team. There are many causes of pain in the ICU including acute trauma, burns, postoperative pain, exacerbation of chronic pain, heart disease, ischemia, cancer pain, pancreatitis, or other abdominal pathology. Routine nursing care such as endotracheal tube suctioning, wound care, insertion of Foley catheters, chest tube management, bed positioning, bathing, and physical and occupational therapy can induce pain. Additionally, the following procedures performed in the ICU can also cause pain: intravenous line placement, endoscopy and bronchoscopy, chest tube placement or removal, paracentesis, lumbar puncture, biopsies, and fracture reductions [3].

Uncontrolled pain in the ICU results in both short- and long-term sequelae. A hypercatabolic state, decreased tissue perfusion, and impaired wound healing can all result from acute pain. Uncontrolled pain can result in a decreased immune response to infection by suppressing natural killer cell activity and neutrophil function. Severe pain is reported by more than 50% of patients following an ICU stay as their most traumatic memory [3]. Long-term studies, particularly those including trauma victims, show impaired physiologic and psychological function in patients who recall significant pain during their hospitalization. Additionally, health-related quality of life is reduced in up to 20% of patients. Chronic pain is reported in up to 40% of patients, while posttraumatic stress disorder is reported in 5–20% of patients [4].

The SCCM PADIS Guidelines recommend self-reporting of pain using a numeric rating scale (NRS) as the gold standard for assessment in patients that can verbalize [1]. An NRS of 4 or greater is indicative of pain. Non-verbal pain assessments can be utilized in patients that cannot adequately communicate their degree of pain but retain motor activity [5]. The PADIS Guidelines recommend using one of two validated behavioral pain scales in non-verbal patients: the Behavioral Pain Scale (BPS) (Table 46.1) and the Critical Care Pain Observation Tool (CPOT) [1] (Table 46.2). A BPS >5 or a CPOT score of 3 or greater is indicative of pain. Assessment of pain using validated scales should be conducted two to three times per nursing shift. Trends in pain scores should be used to help formulate daily titrations in pain medications. The use of vital signs alone such as tachycardia and hypertension is not recommended for assessing pain in the ICU patient [3]. However, they can be used as an indicator to perform a validated assessment tool for pain [6, 7].

Timing of pain medication administration is key. Patients should be treated within 30 min of a "significant pain" score. It is also imperative to reassess the degree of pain within about 30 min to 1 h after administering an "as-needed" pain medication to determine the efficacy of the drug and dose [8].

Intravenous opioids are recommended to treat pain in the ICU per the PADIS Guidelines [1]. Opiates bind to mu-opioid receptors in the central nervous system (CNS). The most commonly used intravenous opioids in the ICU are fentanyl, morphine, hydromorphone, remifentanil, and methadone. Properties of different opioids vary necessitating opioid choice according to patient comorbidities and needs (Table 46.3). Patients can develop tolerance to opiates quickly resulting in need for dose increase. Equianalgesic dosing should be used when switching from one opioid to another [2].

Table 46.1 Behavioral Pain Scale (BPS)

Item	Description	Score
Facial expression	Relaxed	1
	Partly tightened (e.g., brow lowering	2
	Fully tightened (e.g., eyelid closing)	3
	Grimacing	4
Upper limbs	No movement	1
	Partly bent	2
	Fully bent with finger flexion	3
	Permanently retracted	4
Compliance with ventilation	Tolerating movement	1
	Coughing but tolerating ventilation most of the time	2
	Fighting ventilator	3
	Unable to control ventilation	4

Table 46.2 Critical Care Pain Observation Tool (CPOT)

Indicator	Description	Score	
Facial expression	No muscular tension observed	Relaxed, neutral	0
	Presence of frowning, brow lowering, orbit tightening, and levator contraction	Tense	1
	All of the above facial movements plus eyelids tightly close	Grimacing	2
Body movements	Does not move at all (does not necessarily mean absence of pain)	Absence of movement	0
	Slow, cautious movements; touching or rubbing the pain site: seeking attention through movements	Protection	1
	Pulling tube, trying to sit up, moving limbs/thrashing, not following commands, striking at staff, trying to climb out of bed	Restlessness	2
Muscle extension (evaluated by passive flexion and extension of upper extremities)	No resistance to passive movements	Relaxed	0
	Resistance to passive movements	Tense, rigid	1
	Strong resistance to passive movements, inability to complete them	Very tense or rigid	2
Compliance with the ventilator (intubated patients)	Alarms not activated, easy ventilation	Tolerating ventilator or movement	0
	Alarms stop spontaneously	Coughing but tolerating	1
	Asynchrony: Blocking ventilation, alarms, often activated	Fighting ventilator	2
OR Vocalization (extubated patients)	Talking in normal tone or no sound	Talking in normal tone or no sound	0
	Sighing, moaning	Sighing, moaning	1
	Crying out, sobbing	Crying out, sobbing	2
Total, range			0–8

Table 46.3 Properties of opiates commonly used in the intensive care unit

Drug	Metabolic/drug interactions	Starting dose of continuous infusion	Drug-specific adverse effects	Drug accumulation
Fentanyl	3A4 major substrate	12.5–25 mcg/h; 0.35–0.5 mcg/kg loading dose followed by 12.5–25 mcg/h	Muscle rigidity	Hepatic failure; high volume of distribution; high lipophilicity; unpredictable clearance (long context-sensitive half-time) with prolonged infusion
Morphine	Glucuronidation	1–2 mg/h	Hypotension, bradycardia from histamine release	Hepatic failure; active metabolite (3- and 6-morphine glucuronide) accumulates in renal failure
Hydromorphone	Glucuronidation	0.25–0.5 mg/h	N/A	Hepatic failure
Methadone	3A4 and 2B6 major substrates	N/A	QTc prolongation, serotonin syndrome	Long half-life; hepatic and renal failure delay clearance
Remifentanil	Blood and tissue esterases	Loading dose: 1.5 mcg/kg Infusion: 0.5–15 mcg/kg/h	Chest wall rigidity; rebound pain upon discontinuation	N/A

h hour, *Mcg* micrograms, *mg* milligram, *N/A* not available

The most common adverse effects associated with opioids include: depressed respiratory drive, decreased blood pressure and heart rate, constipation, gastrointestinal (GI) intolerance, and altered sensorium [2, 9]. A bowel regimen should be initiated on day 1 unless contraindicated, with assessment for efficacy every 24–48 h as patients never get tolerance to constipation secondary to opioids. Constipation may also contribute to agitation or delirium [10, 11]. Opiates may induce a sedative effect as well as an altered sensorium in some patients [12].

Fentanyl is the most commonly used intravenous opioid in American adult ICUs. Fentanyl undergoes hepatic metabolism via cytochrome P450 (CYP) 3A4 substrate. Fentanyl has a quick onset of action, a short duration of action, and lacks a pharmacologically active metabolite [12]. Fentanyl comes in many dosage forms: Injectable (intravenous, intramuscular, intrathecal, epidural), transdermal, transmucosal, and nasal spray. The fentanyl patch is not generally appropriate for use in the ICU due to its latent onset (about 12 h) and potential for erratic absorption in febrile patients. A unique side effect associated with fentanyl is the risk of serotonin syndrome when used with other serotonergic agents [2, 9].

Morphine undergoes hepatic metabolism via glucuronidation to two major active metabolites, morphine-3-glucuronide (45–55%) and morphine-6-glucuronide

(10–15%). The glucuronide metabolites of morphine are both renally eliminated and can accumulate in patients with renal dysfunction. Continuous morphine infusions are rarely used for analgesia in the ICU setting due to many critically ill patients having impaired renal function. Morphine can be administered many ways intravenous, subcutaneous, intrathecal, epidural, and oral. Morphine can cause histamine release which can result in significant hypotension [2, 9].

Hydromorphone undergoes hepatic metabolism by glucuronidation to an inactive metabolite. Hydromorphone can be administered via multiple routes: intravenous, subcutaneous and oral [2, 9].

Remifentanil is metabolized by blood and tissue esterase function independent of renal and liver function. Remifentanil's onset and short duration of action result in little to no accumulation. Remifentanil can cause rebound pain and withdrawal symptoms due to its quick onset and short duration of action [9, 13].

Methadone undergoes phase I hepatic metabolism to inactive metabolites. It is a major substrate of CYP 2B6 and 3A4, moderate inhibitor of CYP2D6, and weak inhibitor of CYP3A4 resulting in a high potential for drug interactions. Methadone has a relatively long duration of action (12–48 h). It may accumulate in patients with hepatic failure or renal failure. The d-isomer of methadone works as both a partial mu-agonist and an N-methyl-D-aspartate receptor antagonist while the l-isomer is a full mu-agonist. The D-isomer properties are thought to decrease the tolerance effect to other opioids. Steady state and peak analgesic effect of oral methadone may not be reached for 3–5 days upon starting. Oversedation and respiratory depression may occur if titrated too quickly. Methadone is available in multiple dosage forms: Injectable (intravenous, intramuscular, subcutaneous) and oral. Methadone has been associated with dose-dependent QTc prolongation and risk of serotonin syndrome when used with other serotonergic agents [1, 2].

To reduce opioid requirements, non-opioid pain medications should serve as adjuncts. The PADIS guidelines suggest using acetaminophen as an adjunct to opioids to decrease pain intensity and opioid consumption [1]. Total daily acetaminophen doses should be added from all acetaminophen containing products, with a maximum dose of 4 g per day. In patients with significant liver disease, decreased total daily dosing should be considered. Dosage adjustment is necessary in patients receiving continuous renal replacement therapy or those with renal impairment. As compared to oral or rectal formulations, intravenous acetaminophen is significantly more expensive. Hypotension is also associated with intravenous acetaminophen [1].

The PADIS guidelines suggest not routinely using a COX-1 selective Nonsteroidal Anti-inflammatory Drugs (NSAID) as an adjunct to opioid therapy for pain management in critically ill adult patients [1]. NSAIDs may increase the risk of bleeding or acute renal failure in critically ill adult patients. The PADIS guidelines do not recommend the use of lidocaine in critically ill patients [1].

The PADIS guidelines suggest using low-dose ketamine (1–2 mcg/kg/h) as an adjunct to opioid therapy when seeking to reduce opioid consumption in postsurgical adults admitted to the ICU [1]. Ketamine may decrease dosing requirements of concurrently administered opioids. Ketamine has significant adverse effects including the following: mild to severe emergence reactions (e.g., confusion, excitement, irrational behavior, hallucinations, delirium), enhanced skeletal muscle tone, tachycardia, hypertension, and hypotension [2].

The PADIS guidelines suggest using a neuropathic pain medication such as gabapentin, carbamazepine, or pregabalin with opioids for neuropathic pain management in critically ill patients [1]. The PADIS guidelines also recommend using opioids with neuropathic pain medications for management of pain in adult ICU adults following cardiovascular surgery [1].

Gabapentin is initiated at 300–600 mg per day in two to daily doses. Gabapentin requires dosage adjustment in patients with impaired renal function. The target dose of gabapentin is 900–3600 mg per day in divided doses. It has been associated with depression, delirium, paresthesias, and asthenias [3, 13].

Carbamazepine's starting dose for neuropathic pain is 50–100 mg twice daily with a target dose of 100–200 mg every 4–6 h. The maximum dose is 1200 mg/day. Carbamazepine requires dosage in patients with renal dysfunction and should be used with caution in patients with liver dysfunction. Carbamazepine is an inducer of many CYP enzymes and a substrate of CYP3A4 resulting in a high potential for drug interactions. Carbamazepine is associated with somnolence, severe skin reactions (e.g., Stevens-Johnson syndrome, toxic epidermal necrolysis), pancytopenia, and syndrome of inappropriate antidiuretic hormone [1–3].

Pregabalin is initiated at 50 mg three times daily for neuropathic pain. It may be increased in 1 week to a maximum dose of 100 mg three times daily. Pregabalin requires dosage adjustment in patients with renal dysfunction. Pregabalin is associated with peripheral edema, dizziness, drowsiness, headache, fatigue, weight gain, xerostomia, visual field loss, and blurred vision [1, 2].

The PADIS guidelines suggest not offering cybertherapy or hypnosis for pain management in critically ill adults [1]. The PADIS guidelines suggest offering massage for pain management in critically ill adults [1]. The PADIS guidelines suggest offering music therapy to relieve both nonprocedural and procedural pain in critically ill adults [1].

Analgosedation advocates the use of opiate medications before prescribing an anxiolytic/hypnotic medication to provide patient comfort in the ICU [14, 15]. The PADIS guidelines recommend analgosedation (analgesia is used before a sedative to reach the sedative goal) or analgesia-based sedation (an opioid is used instead of a sedative to reach the sedative goal) [1]. Agitation and use of anxiolytics may be negated by providing pain relief early in the ICU stay.

Preprocedural pain management should be considered in all ICU patients. As many as 60% of patients do not receive preprocedural systemic pain medications for common procedures and wound care in the ICU [16]. A 2014 study by Puntillo et al. found the procedures most likely to double the patient's pain intensity score (from baseline to during-procedure) were chest tube removal, wound drain removal, and arterial line insertion. This study also found that higher-intensity pain and pain distress pre-procedure were associated with a high risk of increased pain during the procedure [17].

The PADIS guidelines suggest using the lowest effective dose of an opioid for procedural pain management in critically ill patients undergoing a procedure [1]. The PADIS guidelines recommend not using inhaled volatile anesthetics for procedural pain management. The PADIS guidelines also suggest using an NSAID administered intravenously, orally, or rectally as an opioid alternative for pain management during procedures in critically ill adults. Use of an NSAID topical gel for procedural pain management in critically ill adults is not recommended. In addition to nonpharmacologic relation techniques, preemptive analgesia for chest tube removal is recommended. Local analgesia and nitrous oxide are not recommended by the PADIS Guidelines for pain management during chest tube removal [1]. Postoperative thoracic epidural anesthesia/analgesia is recommended for patients following treatment of an abdominal aortic aneurysm. For traumatic rib fractures in the ICU, thoracic epidural anesthesia is suggested. Cold therapy and relation techniques are recommended by the PADIS guidelines for procedural pain management in critically ill adults [1]. Music therapy is suggested for both nonprocedural and procedural pain [1].

46.3 Agitation

Agitation is common in critically ill adult patients. Common causes of agitation in the ICU include pain, delirium, hypoxia, hypoglycemia, dehydration, and drug or alcohol withdrawal. Consequences of either under- or overtreating agitation in the ICU include Post Traumatic Stress Disorder, delirium, dementia, and anxiety. Medications used for agitation include propofol, dexmedetomidine, and benzodiazepines [1].

The PADIS Guidelines recommend 1 of 2 validated sedation scales: the Richmond Agitation Scale (RASS) (Table 46.4) and the Riker Sedation-Agitation Scale (SAS) (Table 46.5) [1]. The PADIS Guidelines recommend titration to a "light" versus "deep" level of sedation, unless clinically contraindicated and a daily spontaneous awakening trial (SAT) [1].

SATs are turning off the sedation and analgesia daily in mechanically ventilated patients. Spontaneous Breathing Trials (SBTs) are putting the patient on 5 of PEEP and 5 of pressure support with FiO_2 <50% once daily. SAT safety screen (If any are present, discontinue the protocol and repeat in 24 h or according to hospital protocol): Current RASS >2, goal for deeper sedation (e.g., RASS −3 to −5), Active seizures requiring a continuous infusion of a sedative to control, active alcohol withdrawal requiring a continuous infusion of a sedative to control, FiO_2 of 70% or greater, neuromuscular blockade, myocardial ischemia in previous 24 h or ongoing myocardial ischemia, intracranial pressure (ICP) >20 mmHg or need for control of intracranial pressure (ICP) [18].

If the patient passes the SAT safety screen, the SAT is conducted. Bolus opioids are recommended for breakthrough pain during the SAT. In the presence of active pain that does not respond three or more boluses, continuous opioid infusions are

Table 46.4 Richmond agitation sedation scale

Score	Term	Description
+4	Combative	Overtly combative or violent; immediate danger to staff
+3	Very agitated	Pulls on or removes tube(s) or has aggressive behavior toward staff
+2	Agitated	Frequently nonpurposeful movement or patient-ventilator dyssynchrony
+1	Restless	Anxious or apprehensive, but movements not aggressive or vigorous
0	Alert and calm	
−1	Drowsy	Not fully alert but has sustained (>10 s) awakening, with eye contact, to voice
−2	Light sedation	Briefly (<10 s) awakens with eye contact to voice
−3	Moderate sedation	Any movement (but no eye contact) to voice
−4	Deep sedation	No response to voice, but any movement to physical stimulation
−5	Unarousable	No response to voice or physical stimulation

Table 46.5 Sedation-agitation scale

7	Dangerous agitation	Pulling at ETT, trying to remove catheters, climbing over bedrail, striking at staff, thrashing side to side
6	Very agitated	Does not calm despite frequent verbal reminding of limits, requires physical restraints, biting ETT
5	Agitated	Anxious or mildly agitated, trying to sit up, calms down to verbal instructions
4	Calm and cooperative	Calm and cooperative, awakens easily, follows commands
3	Sedated	Difficult to arouse, awakens to verbal stimuli or gentle shaking but drifts off again, follows simple commands
2	Very sedated	Arouses to physical stimuli but does not communicate or follow commands, may move spontaneously
1	Unarousable	Minimal or no response to noxious stimuli, does not communicate or follow commands

ETT endotracheal tube

allowed to continue. If the patient "passes" the SAT, continue to the SBT safety screen. However, if agitation is precluding extubation, sometimes dexmedetomidine will be left during the SBT. SAT failure if any of the following happen: Anxiety/agitation/pain present (e.g., RASS >+1 for 5 min or more), respiratory rate >35 breaths/min for 5 min or more, oxygen saturation <88% for 5 min or more, ICP >20 mmHg, acute cardiac ischemia or arrhythmia, or respiratory or cardiac distress (e.g., heart rate increase of 20 beats/min or greater, heart rate, <55 beats/min, use of accessory muscles, abdominal paradox, diaphoresis, or dyspnea). If the patient fails the SAT, reinitiate the sedative infusion at half the previous dose and titrate to goal. The SAT should be repeated again the following AM [18].

The patient fails the SBT safety screen with any of the following: Agitation, oxygen saturation <88%, FiO_2 >50%, PEEP (positive end-expiratory pressure) of 7 cm H_2O or greater, myocardial ischemia in previous 24 h, increasing vasopressor requirements, or lack of inspiratory efforts. If a patient tolerates the SBT for 30–120 min, the patient is evaluated for extubation. The following indicate SBT failure: Respiratory rate >35 breaths/min (for more than 5 min) or <8 breaths/min, oxygen saturation <88% for more than 5 min, intracranial pressure >20 mmHg, mental status change, acute cardiac ischemia or arrhythmia, respiratory distress (use of accessory muscles, abdominal paradox, diaphoresis, and dyspnea). If the patient fails the SBT, the patient is placed on prior ventilator settings and retired again the following day [18].

Studies comparing a standard sedation protocol with daily pairing of a SAT with SBT have shown decreased days on mechanical ventilation, days in the ICU, and mortality when the SAT is paired with the SBT. The Awakening and Breathing Coordination (ABC) trial [18] included 336 mechanically ventilated patients from four hospitals. Patients were randomized to patient-targeted sedation protocol plus the SBT (control group), or a daily SAT paired with the SBT (intervention group). Both groups were deeply sedated on enrolment (RASS-4) and had been admitted for 2.2 days before enrollment. The mean ventilator-free days was 11.6 days in the usual care control group versus 14.7 days in the SAT plus SBT group ($p = 0.02$). The time to discharge was 12.9 days in the control group versus 9.1 days in the intervention group ($p = 0.01$). Self-extubations were higher in the intervention group, but there was no difference in self-extubations requiring reintubation between groups [18].

A nested cohort study of the ABC trial [19], evaluated 140 patients in which hourly doses of benzodiazepines and propofol during the daytime (7 a.m.–11 a.m.) and nighttime (11 p.m.–7 a.m.) for 5 days were measured. Greater daytime benzodiazepine doses were independently associated with failed SBT, extubation, and subsequent delirium in adjusted models ($p < 0.02$ for all). Nighttime increases in benzodiazepine doses were associated with failed SBT ($p < 0.01$) and delirium ($p = 0.05$).

The SLEAP study [20] evaluated the outcomes of patients receiving a daily sedation protocol alone versus patients utilizing a sedation protocol plus a daily sedation interruption. This study included 430 patients were enrolled from 16 tertiary care medical and surgical ICUs. Only opiate and benzodiazepine infusions were allowed in the study. In the sedation-alone protocol, the RASS goal was −3 to 0, and the Sedation-Agitation Scale (SAS) goal was 3 or 4. Nurses assessed sedation levels on an hourly basis and titrated medications every 15–30 min to achieve goal sedation. If patients were oversedated in either group, infusions were discontinued. According to the sedation protocol with daily sedation interruption, nurses performed daily SATs assessed hourly for wakefulness.

There was no difference in the primary outcome of time to successful extubation between the two groups. There was a significant difference in time to extubation in the prespecified surgical/trauma group between sedation protocol with daily sedation interruption and sedation protocol alone (6 vs. 13 days; hazard ratio [HR] 2.55; 95% CI, 1.40–5.44). No difference in time to extubation was detected between groups among medical ICU patients (9 vs. 8 days; HR 0.92; 95% CI, 0.72–1.18). Significantly lower daily doses of both benzodiazepines and opiates boluses and continuous infusions were used in the sedation protocol–alone group than in the sedation protocol plus interruption group [20].

Titration of medications using a sedation protocol to a goal level of sedation decrease time on mechanical ventilation, decrease ICU length of stay, and decrease rates of tracheostomy. The goal level of sedation should be reassessed daily, documented, and communicated clearly to the nursing and medical staff. Level of sedation should be assessed every 2–4 h throughout the day and every 4 h at night to minimize sleep disruption [1].

Shehabi et al. evaluated 251 medical/surgical patients who were ventilated and sedated for 24 h or more in a multicenter, prospective, longitudinal study in Australia and New Zealand. Deep sedation occurred in 191 patients (76.1%) and in 171 patients (68%) at 48 h within 4 h of initiating ventilation. Early deep sedation was an independent predictor of time to extubation (HR 0.90; 95% CI, 0.87–0.94; $p < 0.001$), hospital death (HR 1.11, 95% CI, 1.02–1.20; $p = 0.01$), and 180-day mortality (HR 1.08, 95% CI, 1.01–1.16; $p = 0.026$) [21].

The PADIS Guidelines recommend the following with regard to managing agitation in the ICU: We suggest using either propofol or dexmedetomidine over benzodiazepines [midazolam or lorazepam] for sedation in critically ill, mechanically ventilated adults and those after cardiac surgery. Benzodiazepines increase the risk of delirium in critically ill adults [1]. The properties of these different sedative agents must also be considered in drug selection (Table 46.6).

The MENDS study [22] compared the sedative effects of lorazepam and dexmedetomidine in medical and surgical adult ICU patients ($n = 103$). Dexmedetomidine had more delirium and coma-free days when compared to lorazepam (7 vs. 3 days, $p = 0.01$). The prevalence of "delirium or coma" was lower in the dexmedetomidine group (87% vs. 98%, $p = 0.03$). More patients were within 1 point of their RASS goal with dexmedetomidine (67%) than with lorazepam (55%), $p = 0.008$. There was no difference in mechanical ventilator-free days, ICU length of stay, or 28-day mortality. This study has been criticized because both groups received continuous infusions of sedatives without the option to bolus first. Also, patients were not required to have a spontaneous awakening trial (SAT).

The SEDCOM study [23] compared the sedative effects of midazolam with those of dexmedetomidine in medical and surgical adult ICU patients ($n = 366$). The prevalence of delirium was lower in the dexmedetomidine group (54%) than in the midazolam group (76.6%), $p < 0.001$. Median time to extubation was shorter in the dexmedetomidine group (3.7 days) than in the midazolam group (5.6 days), $p < 0.01$; however, the times in target sedation range, ICU length of stay, and mortality were no different between the two groups. This study did allow bolus dosing of study drugs, and patients were required to have an SAT if safety criteria were met.

A meta-analysis, "Benzodiazepine versus Nonbenzodiazepine-Based Sedation for Mechanically Ventilated Critically Ill Adults," [24] included trials from 1996 to 2013. Studies were included that met the following criteria: (1) randomized controlled parallel-group design; (2) medical and surgical adult ICU patients on mechanical ventilation receiving intravenous sedation; (3) patients receiving a

Table 46.6 Sedatives properties

Drug	Onset and duration	Precautions for use	CYP substrate (major)	Usual dose	Significant adverse effects
Propofol	Onset: 1 min Duration: short term: 0.5–1 h; long term >7 days: variable; 25–50 h has been observed (depends on depth and time on sedation)	Hypotension, bradycardia, hepatic/renal failure, pancreatitis	2B6	5–50 mcg/kg/min; 0.3–3 mg/kg/h	Hypotension, respiratory depression, bradycardia, PRIS
Dexmedetomidine	Onset: 5–10 min (with LD) 1–2 h (without LD) Duration: 1–2 h	Hepatic failure; symptomatic bradycardia	2A6	LD: 0.5–1 mcg/kg (optional) MD: 0.2–0.7 mcg/kg/h	Hypo/hypertension, bradycardia, pyrexia
Lorazepam	Onset: 5–20 min Duration: 4–8 h; prolonged with continuous infusion	Delirium, renal failure	N/A	Intermittent: 1–4 mg IV every 4–6 h	Oversedation, propylene glycol toxicity
Midazolam	Onset: 3–5 min Duration: 2–6 h, prolonged with continuous infusion	Hepatic failure, end-stage renal failure or dialysis, delirium	3A4	0.02–0.1 mg/kg/h	Oversedation

CI continuous infusion, *IV* intravenously, *LD* loading dose, *MD* maintenance dose, *N/A* not applicable; *PRIS* propofol-related infusion syndrome

non-benzodiazepine (propofol 1% or dexmedetomidine) compared with a benzodiazepine (lorazepam or midazolam); and (4) patients having predefined outcomes. Patients following cardiac surgery and obstetric patients were excluded. ICU length of stay was longer in a benzodiazepine strategy than in a non-benzodiazepine-based strategy (mean difference 1.6 days; 95% confidence interval [CI], 0.72–2.5; $p = 0.0005$). Longer duration of mechanical ventilation was found in the benzodiazepine-based strategy than in a non-benzodiazepine-based strategy (mean difference 1.9 days; 95% CI, 1.7–2.09; $p = 0.00001$). No difference in delirium prevalence was found between a benzodiazepine and a non-benzodiazepine-based strategy (relative risk [RR] 0.98; 95% CI, 0.76–1.27; $p = 0.94$). No difference in short-term mortality was found between a benzodiazepine and a non-benzodiazepine-based strategy (RR 0.98; 95% CI, 0.76–1.27, $p = 0.94$).

Propofol is one of the most commonly used sedatives in the ICU. Propofol works by potentiation of the GABAA receptor and may inhibit N-methyl-D-aspartate receptor activity at high doses. Propofol results in direct cardiac depressive effects by decreasing cardiac β-adrenergic responsiveness and attenuates β-adrenergic signal transduction in cardiac myocytes. Propofol undergoes hepatic conjugation. Propofol has extensive tissue distribution due to its high lipophilicity and large volume of distribution. Propofol is a substrate of CYP 2B6, 2C9, 2C19, and 3A4. Propofol is a 1% (10 mg/mL) lipid emulsion containing 1.1 kcal/mL (0.1 g of fat per 1 mL of propofol). This must be accounted for when considering patients' nutritional requirements. The usual starting dose of propofol is 5–10 mcg/kg/min, titrated every 5–10 min to goal sedative effect [2, 9].

NONSEDA [25] is a randomized, clinical parallel-group, multinational superiority study comparing no sedation (bolus doses of morphine) and light sedation (propofol for 48 h then midazolam titrated to a RASS of −2 to −3). No difference was found in 90-day mortality between groups (no sedation 148 [42.4%] vs. light sedation 130 [37%]; 95% CI −2.2–12.2; $p = 0.65$). Twenty seven percent of the no-sedation group crossed over to receive sedation within the first 24 h after randomization.

PRODEX [26] compared propofol with dexmedetomidine for sedation in mechanical ventilated patients. Patients in both groups were treated with daily sedation interruption trials and spontaneous breathing trials (SBTs). Pain was treated with fentanyl boluses. Proportion of time in target RASS (0, −3) without rescue therapy was the same in the propofol group (65%) and in the dexmedetomidine group (65%). There was no difference in median time on mechanical ventilation in the propofol (5 days) and dexmedetomidine (4 days) groups, $p = 0.24$. Patients were better able to communicate discomfort in the dexmedetomidine group. The prevalence of hypotension and bradycardia were similar between the two groups. Critical illness polyneuropathy occurred more often in the propofol group ($n = 11$) than in the dexmedetomidine group ($n = 2$), $p < 0.02$. The composite outcome of agitation, anxiety, and delirium occurred in 295 of the propofol group as compared to 18% of the dexmedetomidine group ($p = 0.008$).

The most common adverse effects associated with propofol include the following: bradycardia, hypotension, respiratory depression, hypertriglyceridemia pancreatitis with or without hypertriglyceridemia, and Propofol-Related Infusion Syndrome (PRIS) [9].

PRIS is a rare, life-threatening complication of propofol most often occurring at doses >50 mcg/kg/min for 48 h or more. PRIS occurs secondary to alterations in hepatic metabolism leading to an accumulation of ketone bodies and lactate and/or disruptions in the mitochondrial respiratory chain and inhibition of oxidative phosphorylation. Patients with urea cycle disorders are at high risk for PRIS. PRIS is associated with a high mortality rate. Prevention is key. Discontinuation of propofol should occur if any of the following signs or symptoms thought to be associated with PRIS develop: Metabolic acidosis, acute renal failure, cardiovascular collapse, cardiac arrhythmias including Brugada-like syndrome, rhabdomyolysis, myoglobinemia, myoglobinuria, hyperkalemia, hypertriglyceridemia, elevated creatine kinase concentrations. Risk factors for PRIS include the following: neurologic injury, sepsis, use of vasoactive medications, high-dose propofol, and acute liver failure [9, 27].

The PADIS Guidelines suggest that in adult ICU patients with delirium unrelated to alcohol or benzodiazepine withdrawal, dexmedetomidine infusions rather than benzodiazepine infusions should be administered for sedation to reduce the duration of delirium [1]. Dexmedetomidine is an α2-adrenoceptor agonist. Dexmedetomidine provides a sedative effect through inhibition of norepinephrine release from the locus coeruleus. It also produces a weak antinociceptive effect through inhibition of neuronal transmission through presynaptic C-fibers, release of substance P, and hyperpolarization of postsynaptic α receptors in the dorsal horn of the spinal column. Dexmedetomidine does not cause respiratory suppression. Thus, intubation is not required to use it. Dexmedetomidine does not have amnestic effects, and it is not appropriate to use in a chemically paralyzed patient [1, 9].

Dexmedetomidine is metabolized hepatically by glucuronidation. Dexmedetomidine has an onset of action of 20 min. Dexmedetomidine is highly protein bound. The loading dose of dexmedetomidine is not usually administered due to bradycardia. Dexmedetomidine's infusion rate is 0.2–0.7 mcg/kg/h. Randomized trials have administered rates up to 1.5 mcg/kg/h up to 5–7 days [9].

The Dexmedetomidine to Lessen ICU Agitation (DahLIA) [28] study was a multicenter, double-blind placebo controlled, parallel-group randomized clinical trial of 39 patients were randomized to dexmedetomidine and 32 patients to placebo. Dexmedetomidine increased ventilator-free hours compared with placebo (median, 144.8 h vs. 127.5 h, 95% CI 4–33.2 h, $p = 0.01$) at 7 days. The dexmedetomidine group had decreased time to extubation compared with placebo (median 21.9 h vs. 44.3 h, 95% CI 5.3–3.1 h, $p < 0.001$). Delirium resolved faster in the dexmedetomidine group compared with placebo (median, 23 h vs. 40 h, 95% CI, 3–28 h, $p = 0.01$). However, propofol use was common in both groups (72% in the dexmedetomidine group vs. 88% in the placebo group) (median cumulative dose 980 mg (IQR 280–3050) vs. 5390 mg (IQR 1880–10,803), $p < 0.001$).

The DESIRE [29] trial was an open-label, multicenter randomized clinical trial conducted in Japan in which 100 patients with sepsis were randomized to dexmedetomidine and 101 patients were randomized to placebo. Mortality at 28 days did not differ between the two groups (23% in the dexmedetomidine group vs. 31% in the placebo group; HR 0.69; 95% CI, 0.38–1.22; $p = 0.20$). Ventilator-free days did not differ between groups (median 20 days (IQR 5–24) in the dexmedetomidine group vs. 18 days (IQR 0.5–23) in the control group ($p = 0.20$).

SPICE III [30] is an open-label, randomized controlled trial comparing dexmedetomidine with usual care (propofol, midazolam, or other sedation) in patients receiving <12 h of mechanical ventilation who are expected to be on the ventilator for at least one additional day. The goal target RASS was −2 to +1. Death at 90 days occurred in 569 of 1956 (29.1%) of the usual care group and 566 of 1948 (29.1%) of the dexmedetomidine group (adjusted risk difference 0.0 percentage points; 95% CI, −2.9 to 2.8). In the dexmedetomidine group, 64% of patients additionally received propofol, 3% received midazolam, and 7% received both during the first

2 days after randomization. Sixty percent of patients received propofol, 12% received midazolam, and 20% received both in the usual care group. Application of the results of this study is very difficult given the many sedatives administered in both groups. Bradycardia and hypotension occurred in 5.1% and 2.7% of patients in the dexmedetomidine group. A post hoc analysis of SPICE III of 703 mechanically ventilated patients was conducted. Over the first 5 ICU days, more patients in the dexmedetomidine group had a temperature of 38.3 °C or greater (43.3% vs. 32.7%, $p = 0.004$) and 39.0 °C or greater (19.4% vs. 12.5%, $p = 0.013$).

MENDS 2 [31] is multicenter, double-blind trial comparing dexmedetomidine to propofol. No difference was found between either drug in the number of days alive and without delirium of coma (adjusted median 10.7 vs. 10.8 days; odds ratio, 0.96; 95% CI 0.74–1.26), ventilator-free days (adjusted median, 23.07 vs. 24 days, odds ratio 0.98; 95% CI, 0.63–1.51), or death at 90 days 38% vs 39%; hazard ratio, 1.06; 95% CI0.74–1.52).

A total of 77 randomized trials evaluating dexmedetomidine with other sedation in critically ill mechanically ventilated adults were evaluated. Compared with other sedatives, dexmedetomidine reduced the risk of delirium (RR 0.67; 95% CI, 0.55–0.81; moderate certainty), duration of mechanical ventilation (mean difference [MD] −1.8 h; 95% CI, −2.89 to −0.71; low certainty), and ICU length of stay (MD −0.32 days; 95% CI, −0.42 to −0.22; low certainty). Bradycardia (RR 2.39; 95% CI, 1.82–3.13; moderate certainty) and hypotension (RR 1.32; 95% CI, 1.07–1.63; low certainty) were increased with dexmedetomidine [32].

A rapid practice guideline was published looking at use of dexmedetomidine for sedation in mechanically ventilated adult patients in the ICU. The rapid practice guideline suggested use of dexmedetomidine over other sedative agents if the reduction in delirium was more highly valued than the potential for hypotension and bradycardia [33].

Tachycardia, pyrexia bradycardia, hypertension, fever, hypotension, and dry mouth are adverse effects associated with dexmedetomidine. Dexmedetomidine should be avoided in patients with acute decompensated heart failure or advanced heart block [9, 34].

Lorazepam is a benzodiazepine that binds to the postsynaptic GABAA receptor, undergoes hepatic clearance by conjugation to inactive compounds, moderate to high volume of distribution, and high protein binding. Lorazepam has an intermediate onset of action of 15–30 min. Its duration of action when dosed intermittently is 4–8 h. Lorazepam has amnestic effects. Lorazepam is intermittently dosed at 1–4 mg every 4–6 h. Lorazepam can also be administered as a continuous infusion [35].

A study was conducted to evaluate the number of days on mechanical ventilation in medical ICU patients receiving intermittent lorazepam ($n = 64$) compared with continuous infusion propofol ($n = 68$). Both groups underwent daily interruption of sedation if the fraction of inspired oxygen (FiO_2) was <80%. Median time on mechanical ventilation was 9 days in the lorazepam group as compared to 4.4 days in the propofol group, $p = 0.006$. ICU length of stay was 12.7 days in the lorazepam group as compared to 8.6 days in the propofol group ($p = 0.05$). No difference was found between groups in hospital mortality [36].

Injectable lorazepam is diluted in propylene glycol. Propylene glycol toxicity can occur with lorazepam infusions for more than 48 h, particularly at doses of 6–8 mg/h or greater. Symptoms of propylene glycol toxicity include: new-onset renal failure, respiratory failure, metabolic acidosis, and altered mental status. An elevated osmolar gap (>10 mOsm/kg) and elevated anion gap with new metabolic acidosis are recommended for assessment. If these metabolic abnormalities are present while a patient is receiving a lorazepam infusion, it should be discontinued. Lorazepam can also cause delirium, paradoxical agitation, confusion, prolonged duration of sedative action, respiratory depression, hypotension, and bradycardia [9, 37, 38].

Midazolam is a benzodiazepine that binds to the postsynaptic GABAA receptor. It undergoes phase I hepatic metabolism to an active glucuronidated metabolite, α1-hydroxymidazolam, which undergoes renal excretion. Midazolam is a short-acting benzodiazepine. It is a CYP3A4 substrate and interacts with numerous medications. Midazolam is highly lipophilic, has a large volume of distribution, and is highly protein bound. Clearance of midazolam or its metabolite is significantly impaired in patients with hepatic or renal dysfunction. Continuous renal replacement therapy partly clears the active metabolite but does not effectively clear the parent compound [39]. Midazolam has amnestic properties. Intermittent dosing of midazolam is 1–4 mg every 2–4 h intermittently. Midazolam may also be administered as a continuous infusion. Common adverse effects of midazolam include: delirium, paradoxical agitation prolonged duration of sedative action, respiratory depression, hypotension, and bradycardia [40, 41].

The MIDEX study [26] compared midazolam ($n = 251$) with dexmedetomidine ($n = 249$) for sedation in prolonged mechanical ventilation. Patients in both groups were treated with daily sedation interruption trials and SBTs. Pain was treated with fentanyl boluses. Target RASS goal was 0 to −3. There was no difference in the proportion of time at target RASS without rescue therapy in the midazolam group (56%) versus the dexmedetomidine group (60%). Median time on mechanical ventilation was lower in the dexmedetomidine group (5 days) than in the midazolam group (6.8 days), $p = 0.03$. Patients in the dexmedetomidine group were more arousable, more cooperative, and better able to communicate discomfort or pain to than the patients in the midazolam group. Hypotension occurred more often in the dexmedetomidine group (20.6%) than in the midazolam group (11.6%; $p = 0.007$. Bradycardia was more common in the dexmedetomidine group (14.2%) than in the midazolam group (5.2%; $p < 0.001$). Agitation, anxiety, and delirium did not differ between the two groups at 48 h.

Certain situations arise in the ICU setting in which sedation with propofol and appropriate concomitant analgesia are not sufficient to achieve patient comfort on the ventilator, often leading to ventilator desynchrony and complications secondary to this [42]. While propofol is the preferred agent for ICU sedation, if deeper sedation is required, benzodiazepines are occasionally used for improved ventilator synchrony and patient comfort. Benzodiazepines are also the preferred agent in the setting of PRIS [43].

Even with appropriate levels of sedation and analgesia, situations arise in which neuromuscular blockade is required to achieve ventilator synchrony and avoid adverse effects in ventilated patients. Neuromuscular blockers (NMBs) are divided into two groups, depolarizing and non-depolarizing agents. NMBs have various uses in the critical care setting, including muscle relaxation prior to rapid sequence intubation, therapeutic hypothermia following cardiac arrest, acute respiratory distress syndrome, status asthmaticus, and notably for patient-ventilator asynchrony [44]. Depolarizing NMBs (i.e., succinylcholine) function at the motor endplate of the neuromuscular junction (NMJ), and result in depolarization of the membrane. This leaves the motor endplate refractory to the effects of acetylcholine and therefore results in inability of muscle contraction. Non-depolarizing NMBs (i.e., vecuronium) block the binding of acetylcholine to the motor endplate via binding of the alpha subunit of the nicotinic receptor, inhibiting muscle contraction.

NMBs have been recommended for patients with severe ARDS defined by a P:F ratio of <100 mmHg. To test whether NMB results in improved ventilator synchrony, a one-time dose of vecuronium is trialed. If there is improvement in ventilator synchrony, continuous NMB with cisatracurium is initiated. Two major trials have looked at the adverse events related to continuous NMB. The ACURASYS trial (2010) suggested that paralysis with cisatracurium for 48 h in patients with early severe ARDS improved 90-day survival, increased ventilator-free days, reduced levels of inflammation, and reduced barotrauma [45]. The ROSE trial (2019) countered the aforementioned results and suggested that early NMB does not reduce mortality when using light sedation protocols and was associated with an increase in ICU-acquired weakness and serious cardiovascular events [46]. The Intensive Care Medicine Rapid Practice Guideline (ICM-RPG) group published a rapid practice guideline in October of 2020 regarding the use of NMBs. The ICM-RPG panel issued one recommendation and two suggestions regarding the use of NMBs in adults with ARDS. Current evidence does not support the early routine use of an NMBA infusion in adults with ARDS of any severity. It favors avoiding a continuous infusion of NMBA for patients who are ventilated using a lighter sedation strategy. However, for patients who require deep sedation to facilitate lung protective ventilation or prone positioning, and require neuromuscular blockade, an infusion of an NMB for 48 h is a reasonable option [47].

46.4 The ABCDEF Bundle

Incorporating multiple concomitant patient care interventions like management of pain and agitation into one consolidated bundle is an effective strategy that has been shown to be an effective strategy to improve clinical outcomes in critically ill patients. SCCM recommends implementing the ICU Liberation or "ABCDEF" bundle to align and coordinate care using an interprofessional approach. A: Assess, prevent, and manage pain, B: Both SATs and SBTs, C: Choice of analgesia and sedation, D: Delirium: Assess, prevent, and manage, E: Early mobility and exercise, F: Family engagement and empowerment [48].

In a prospective, multicenter, cohort study from 68 academic, community, and federal ICUs during a 20-month collection period, performance of the complete ABCDEF bundle was associated with a lower likelihood of death within 7 days (HR 0.32; CI, 0.17–0.62), next-day mechanical ventilation (OR 0.28; CI, 0.22–0.36), coma (OR 0.35; CI, 0.22–0.56), delirium (OR 0.60; CI, 0.49–0.72), physical restraint use (OR 0.37; CI, 0.30–0.46), ICU readmission (OR 0.54; CI, 0.37–0.79), and discharge to a facility other than home (OR 0.64; CI, 0.51–0.80). There was a dose response in between higher proportional bundle performance and improvement in each clinical outcome ($p < 0.002$). Pain was more commonly reported as bundle performance increased ($p = 0.0001$), probably because more patients were awake [48]. These results have been replicated in multiple studies [49–51]. Additionally, utilization of the ABCDEF Bundle has been shown to decrease cost [52, 53].

46.5   Conclusion

Identification of pain and agitation is key in the management of critically ill adults. Choosing the right agents or agents is imperative in both the prevention and treatment of pain and agitation.

Financial Support   None.

Conflicts of Interest   None.

Sources of Funding   None.

References

1. Devlin JW, Skrobik Y, Gelinas C, et al. Clinical practice guidelines for the prevention and management of pain, agitation/sedation, delirium, immobility, and sleep disruption in adult patients in the ICU. Crit Care Med. 2018;46(9):e825–e73.
2. Erstad BL, Puntillo K, Gilbert HC, et al. Pain management principles in the critically ill. Chest. 2009;135(4):1075–86.
3. Barr J, Fraser GL, Puntillo K, et al. Clinical practice guidelines for the management of pain, agitation, and delirium in adult patients in the intensive care unit. Crit Care Med. 2013;41(1):263–306.
4. Rotondi AJ, Chelluri L, Sirio C, et al. Patients' recollections of stressful experiences while receiving prolonged mechanical ventilation in an intensive care unit. Crit Care Med. 2002;30(4):746–52.
5. Puntillo K, Pasero C, Li D, et al. Evaluation of pain in ICU patients. Chest. 2009;135(4):1069–74.

6. Gelinas C, Fillion L, Puntillo KA, Viens C, Fortier M. Validation of the critical-care pain observation tool in adult patients. Am J Crit Care. 2006;15(4):420–7.

7. Payen JF, Bru O, Bosson JL, et al. Assessing pain in critically ill sedated patients by using a behavioral pain scale. Crit Care Med. 2001;29(12):2258–63.

8. Puntillo K, Ley SJ. Appropriately timed analgesics control pain due to chest tube removal. Am J Crit Care. 2004;13(4):292–301. discussion 302; quiz 303–294

9. Devlin JW, Mallow-Corbett S, Riker RR. Adverse drug events associated with the use of analgesics, sedatives, and antipsychotics in the intensive care unit. Crit Care Med. 2010;38(Suppl. 6):S231–43.

10. Mostafa SM, Bhandari S, Ritchie G, Gratton N, Wenstone R. Constipation and its implications in the critically ill patient. Br J Anaesth. 2003;91(6):815–9.

11. Nguyen T, Frenette AJ, Johanson C, et al. Impaired gastrointestinal transit and its associated morbidity in the intensive care unit. J Crit Care. 2013;28(4):537.

12. Mather LE. Clinical pharmacokinetics of fentanyl and its newer derivatives. Clin Pharmacokinet. 1983;8(5):422–46.

13. Park CM, Inouye SK, Marcantonio ER, et al. Perioperative gabapentin use and in-hospital adverse clinical events among older adults after major surgery. JAMA Intern Med. 2022;182(11):1117–27.

14. Breen D, Karabinis A, Malbrain M, et al. Decreased duration of mechanical ventilation when comparing analgesia-based sedation using remifentanil with standard hypnotic-based sedation for up to 10 days in intensive care unit patients: a randomised trial [ISRCTN47583497]. Crit Care. 2005;9(3):R200–10.

15. Strom T, Martinussen T, Toft P. A protocol of no sedation for critically ill patients receiving mechanical ventilation: a randomised trial. Lancet. 2010;375(9713):475–80.

16. Czarnecki ML, Turner HN, Collins PM, Doellman D, Wrona S, Reynolds J. Procedural pain management: a position statement with clinical practice recommendations. Pain Manag Nurs. 2011;12(2):95–111.

17. Puntillo KA, Max A, Timsit JF, et al. Determinants of procedural pain intensity in the intensive care unit. The Europain(R) study. Am J Respir Crit Care Med. 2014;189(1):39–47.

18. Girard TD, Kress JP, Fuchs BD, et al. Efficacy and safety of a paired sedation and ventilator weaning protocol for mechanically ventilated patients in intensive care (Awakening and Breathing Controlled trial): a randomised controlled trial. Lancet. 2008;371(9607):126–34.

19. Seymour CW, Pandharipande PP, Koestner T, et al. Diurnal sedative changes during intensive care: impact on liberation from mechanical ventilation and delirium. Crit Care Med. 2012;40(10):2788–96.

20. Mehta S, Burry L, Cook D, et al. Daily sedation interruption in mechanically ventilated critically ill patients cared for with a sedation protocol: a randomized controlled trial. JAMA. 2012;308(19):1985–92.

21. Shehabi Y, Bellomo R, Reade MC, et al. Early intensive care sedation predicts long-term mortality in ventilated critically ill patients. Am J Respir Crit Care Med. 2012;186(8):724–31.

22. Pandharipande PP, Pun BT, Herr DL, et al. Effect of sedation with dexmedetomidine vs lorazepam on acute brain dysfunction in mechanically ventilated patients: the MENDS randomized controlled trial. JAMA. 2007;298(22):2644–53.

23. Riker RR, Shehabi Y, Bokesch PM, et al. Dexmedetomidine vs midazolam for sedation of critically ill patients: a randomized trial. JAMA. 2009;301(5):489–99.

24. Fraser GL, Devlin JW, Worby CP, et al. Benzodiazepine versus nonbenzodiazepine-based sedation for mechanically ventilated, critically ill adults: a systematic review and meta-analysis of randomized trials. Crit Care Med. 2013;41(9 Suppl. 1):S30–8.

25. Olsen HT, Nedergaard HK, Toft P. Nonsedation or light sedation in critically ill, mechanically ventilated patients. N Engl J Med. 2020;382(26):e107.

26. Jakob SM, Ruokonen E, Grounds RM, et al. Dexmedetomidine vs midazolam or propofol for sedation during prolonged mechanical ventilation: two randomized controlled trials. JAMA. 2012;307(11):1151–60.

27. Fodale V, La Monaca E. Propofol infusion syndrome: an overview of a perplexing disease. Drug Saf. 2008;31(4):293–303.
28. Reade MC, Eastwood GM, Bellomo R, et al. Effect of dexmedetomidine added to standard care on ventilator-free time in patients with agitated delirium: a randomized clinical trial. JAMA. 2016;315(14):1460–8.
29. Kawazoe Y, Miyamoto K, Morimoto T, et al. Effect of dexmedetomidine on mortality and ventilator-free days in patients requiring mechanical ventilation with sepsis: a randomized clinical trial. JAMA. 2017;317(13):1321–8.
30. Shehabi Y, Howe BD, Bellomo R, et al. Early sedation with dexmedetomidine in critically ill patients. N Engl J Med. 2019;380(26):2506–17.
31. Hughes CG, Mailloux PT, Devlin JW, et al. Dexmedetomidine or propofol for sedation in mechanically ventilated adults with sepsis. N Engl J Med. 2021;
32. Lewis K, Alshamsi F, Carayannopoulos KL, et al. Dexmedetomidine vs other sedatives in critically ill mechanically ventilated adults: a systematic review and meta-analysis of randomized trials. Intensive Care Med. 2022;48(7):811–40.
33. Moller MH, Alhazzani W, Lewis K, et al. Use of dexmedetomidine for sedation in mechanically ventilated adult ICU patients: a rapid practice guideline. Intensive Care Med. 2022;48(7):801–10.
34. Grayson KE, Bailey M, Balachandran M, et al. The effect of early sedation with dexmedetomidine on body temperature in critically ill patients. Crit Care Med. 2021;49(7):1118–28.
35. Swart EL, de Jongh J, Zuideveld KP, Danhof M, Thijs LG, Strack van Schijndel RJ. Population pharmacokinetics of lorazepam and midazolam and their metabolites in intensive care patients on continuous venovenous hemofiltration. Am J Kidney Dis. 2005;45(2):360–71.
36. Carson SS, Kress JP, Rodgers JE, et al. A randomized trial of intermittent lorazepam versus propofol with daily interruption in mechanically ventilated patients. Crit Care Med. 2006;34(5):1326–32.
37. Barnes BJ, Gerst C, Smith JR, Terrell AR, Mullins ME. Osmol gap as a surrogate marker for serum propylene glycol concentrations in patients receiving lorazepam for sedation. Pharmacotherapy. 2006;26(1):23–33.
38. Pandharipande P, Shintani A, Peterson J, et al. Lorazepam is an independent risk factor for transitioning to delirium in intensive care unit patients. Anesthesiology. 2006;104(1):21–6.
39. Beigmohammadi MT, Hanifeh M, Rouini MR, Sheikholeslami B, Mojtahedzadeh M. Pharmacokinetics alterations of midazolam infusion versus bolus administration in mechanically ventilated critically ill patients. Iran J Pharm Res. 2013;12(2):483–8.
40. Honiden S, Siegel MD. Analytic reviews: managing the agitated patient in the ICU: sedation, analgesia, and neuromuscular blockade. J Intensive Care Med. 2010;25(4):187–204.
41. Shafer A. Complications of sedation with midazolam in the intensive care unit and a comparison with other sedative regimens. Crit Care Med. 1998;26(5):947–56.
42. Blanch L, Villagra A, Sales B, et al. Asynchronies during mechanical ventilation are associated with mortality. Intensive Care Med. 2015;41(4):633–41.
43. Pearson SD, Patel BK. Evolving targets for sedation during mechanical ventilation. Curr Opin Crit Care. 2020;26(1):47–52.
44. Adeyinka A, Layer DA. Neuromuscular blocking agents. In: StatPearls. Treasure Island (FL) ineligible companies. Disclosure: David Layer declares no relevant financial relationships with ineligible companies.2024.
45. Papazian L, Forel JM, Gacouin A, et al. Neuromuscular blockers in early acute respiratory distress syndrome. N Engl J Med. 2010;363(12):1107–16.
46. National Heart L, Blood Institute PCTN, Moss M, et al. Early neuromuscular blockade in the acute respiratory distress syndrome. N Engl J Med. 2019;380(21):1997–2008.
47. Alhazzani W, Belley-Cote E, Moller MH, et al. Neuromuscular blockade in patients with ARDS: a rapid practice guideline. Intensive Care Med. 2020;46(11):1977–86.
48. Pun BT, Balas MC, Barnes-Daly MA, et al. Caring for critically ill patients with the ABCDEF bundle: results of the ICU liberation collaborative in over 15,000 adults. Crit Care Med. 2019;47(1):3–14.

49. Balas MC, Vasilevskis EE, Olsen KM, et al. Effectiveness and safety of the awakening and breathing coordination, delirium monitoring/management, and early exercise/mobility bundle. Crit Care Med. 2014;42(5):1024–36.
50. Barnes-Daly MA, Phillips G, Ely EW. Improving hospital survival and reducing brain dysfunction at seven california community hospitals: implementing PAD guidelines via the ABCDEF bundle in 6064 patients. Crit Care Med. 2017;45(2):171–8.
51. Barr J, Downs B, Ferrell K, et al. Improving outcomes in mechanically ventilated adult ICU patients following implementation of the ICU liberation (ABCDEF) bundle across a large healthcare system. Crit Care Explor. 2024;6(1):e1001.
52. Hsieh SJ, Otusanya O, Gershengorn HB, et al. Staged implementation of awakening and breathing, coordination, delirium monitoring and management, and early mobilization bundle improves patient outcomes and reduces hospital costs. Crit Care Med. 2019;47(7):885–93.
53. Collinsworth AW, Priest EL, Masica AL. Evaluating the cost-effectiveness of the ABCDE bundle: impact of bundle adherence on inpatient and 1-year mortality and costs of care. Crit Care Med. 2020;48(12):1752–9.

Chapter 47
Neuromuscular Blockade in Critically Ill Adults

Omar Elnaggar, Michael Chen, and Hassan Farhan

47.1 The Neuromuscular Junction

The neuromuscular junction (NMJ) is the functional unit of all skeletal muscle activity. Each NMJ consists of one motor neuron axon terminal and one skeletal muscle fiber. Consisting of specialized intracellular and extracellular structures, the NMJ and its neurotransmitter acetylcholine are responsible for initiation of the action potential required for skeletal muscle movement. It is helpful to consider the NMJ in three separate regions:

47.1.1 Axon Terminal

Motor neuron axons from the spinal column deliver signals to multiple muscle fibers via branching axon terminals. Each axon terminal forms an NMJ with one muscle fiber. Within this unit exist all necessary structures in synthesis, release, and reuptake of acetylcholine. More specifically, mitochondria, endoplasmic reticulum, synaptic vesicles, SNARE protein complexes, and voltage-gated calcium channels [1, 2].

Acetylcholine is synthesized by the combination of choline and acetyl-coenzyme A (acetyl-CoA). This reaction takes place in the axon terminal and is facilitated by choline acetyltransferase [3]. A large portion of choline molecules are produced by the degradation of acetylcholine in the synaptic cleft and transferred into the axon

O. Elnaggar · M. Chen · H. Farhan (✉)
Anesthesiology, Perioperative and Pain Medicine, Stanford Hospital, Stanford, CA, USA
e-mail: hfarhan@stanford.edu

© The Author(s), under exclusive license to Springer Nature Switzerland AG 2025

Y. Alzaidi, M. A. Gebily (eds.), *The Pharmacist's Expanded Role in Critical Care Medicine*, https://doi.org/10.1007/978-3-031-77335-8_47

terminal by active transport proteins. Acetyl-CoA is produced in the mitochondria. Acetylcholine is actively transported into synaptic vesicles located near membrane-bound voltage-gated calcium channels [4].

Once a depolarizing action potential reaches the axon terminal, voltage-gated calcium channels are activated to allow influx of calcium ions, prompting acetylcholine vesicles to be released. To facilitate acetylcholine exocytosis into the synaptic cleft, synaptic vesicles must fuse with the axon terminal membrane. This is done by a process involving SNARE (soluble N-ethylmaleimide-sensitive fusion protein attachment protein receptors) proteins. SNAREs are high-affinity membrane-bound proteins existing on both the synaptic vesicle membrane (v-SNARE, such as synaptobrevin) and the axon plasma membrane (t-SNARE, such as syntaxin and SNAP) [5]. Calcium-mediated binding of vesicle and plasma membrane SNAREs forms a SNARE complex, allowing synaptic vesicle and plasma membrane fusion and release of vesicle contents into the synaptic cleft [4].

Lastly, the axon terminal is home to pre-junctional acetylcholine receptors. These receptors act as a positive feedback loop that signals additional production of acetylcholine in the axon terminal [6].

47.1.2 Synaptic Cleft

Between the axon terminal and motor endplate exists a 20–50 nm space termed the synaptic cleft. This arrangement is unique from synapses in the central nervous system, in that the neuron and muscle do not make direct contact [7].

Acetylcholine is released from the axon terminal to the synaptic cleft before binding to their receptors on the motor endplate. The synaptic cleft also contains acetylcholinesterase which is responsible for the hydrolysis of acetylcholine to choline and acetate. This reaction takes place rapidly, allowing large amounts of acetylcholine molecules to be hydrolyzed each second [7]. Recycled choline molecules are then transported into the axon terminal to be used for acetylcholine synthesis [3].

47.1.3 Motor Endplate

The motor endplate is composed of a highly specialized cell membrane termed the sarcolemma. The sarcolemma is unique in that its extracellular matrix allows tight connections with surrounding muscle cells creating a cohesive unit that can contract together. The motor endplate is highly concentrated with nicotinic acetylcholine receptors [8]. Acetylcholine receptors are formed of five polypeptide subunits. Mature receptors have two alpha subunits and one beta, delta, and epsilon subunit. Two acetylcholine bind to the alpha subunits producing a conformational change which permits influx of cations into the muscle fiber [9]. While all cations can pass through the channel, sodium influx predominates [8]. Increased membrane potential from sodium influx opens additional voltage-gated sodium channels, further increasing the membrane potential and triggering a muscle action potential.

Immature acetylcholine receptors are formed by the presence of a gamma subunit in place of the epsilon subunit. These are also referred to as fetal acetylcholine receptors due to their presence throughout fetal muscle tissue [9]. As discussed later in this chapter, administration of depolarizing neuromuscular blocking agents to patients with increased immature acetylcholine receptor expression can lead to life-threatening hyperkalemia [10].

A distinction should be made between nicotinic and muscarinic acetylcholine receptors. While nicotinic receptors are found in skeletal muscle, muscarinic receptors are primarily mediated by G protein-coupled acetylcholine receptors involved in parasympathetic nervous system activity and found in nearly all organ systems [11].

47.2 Neuromuscular Blocking Agents

Neuromuscular blocking agents, or neuromuscular blocking drugs (NMBD), have multiple indications in the critical care setting. This includes but is not limited to intubation, facilitating mechanical ventilation, and providing immobility for procedures. NMBDs are classified into two categories: depolarizing and nondepolarizing agents. Depolarizing agents bind to the acetylcholine receptor causing depolarization and contraction of the muscle fiber with subsequent relaxation. Nondepolarizing agents competitively antagonize the acetylcholine receptor and prevent depolarization.

47.2.1 General Pharmacological Considerations

Dosage of NMBDs is discussed in the context of ED95 (effective dose 95%). ED95 is the dose at which 50% of adults will have 95% suppression of a single twitch response to nerve stimulation. Commonly listed doses are those required to facilitate endotracheal intubation. Most intubating doses are two to three times the ED95. Clinical duration of action is the time from dose administration to recovery of 25% of T1 height [12].

Potency is inversely related to the onset of action. Less potent medications require a higher dosage [13]. This higher dosage creates a concentration gradient that quickly displaces the medication into the NMJ, facilitating fast blockade. Duration of action is influenced by multiple factors including dose, alterations in elimination and metabolism due to organ dysfunction, and volume of distribution. Most NMBDs undergo hepatic or renal elimination. In patients with liver and kidney dysfunction, duration of action can be prolonged [14]. Furthermore, physiological changes with age can significantly impact dosing, onset, and duration. Elderly patients are prone to renal and hepatic dysfunction as well as increased volume of distribution for most medications. While this may prolong half-life, its effect on clinically prolonged neuromuscular blockade is unpredictable [14–17].

Careful consideration of the appropriate weight-based dosing of NMBDs is important given the increased incidence of obesity in the critical care population. Obesity alters pharmacokinetic properties by changes in volume of distribution, cardiac output, and total blood volume. Obesity commonly presents with hepatic steatosis and renal dysfunction from other comorbidities such as diabetes and hypertension, potentially influencing hepatic and renal elimination [18]. Medications can be dosed by total, lean, and ideal body weight. Inappropriate administration of total body weight-based dosing can unnecessarily prolong blockade and increase the risk of adverse effects. Conversely, underdosing can lead to ventilator dyssynchrony and poor intubating conditions [19]. In normal weight individuals, total, lean, and ideal body weight are similar. Thus, dosing all medications by total body weight (TBW) in normal weight patients may be inconsequential. Fat mass makes up a disproportionate amount of total body weight in obese patients. The increased cardiac output seen in obese patients is directed toward vessel-rich groups. Therefore, administering total body weight dosing to obese patients can result in overdose [19]. With regard to NMBDs, all medications should be dosed by ideal body weight (IBW), with the exception of succinylcholine. Total body weight dosing of nondepolarizing medications unnecessarily prolongs blockade [20]. In obesity, patients have greater levels of pseudocholinesterase, responsible for the metabolism of succinylcholine. IBW dosing of succinylcholine produces poorer intubating conditions compared with TBW dosing [21]. This is particularly concerning in obese patients who are more likely to be difficult to intubate and ventilate compared with normal weight adults [22].

47.2.2 Depolarizing Agents (Succinylcholine)

While numerous depolarizing agents have been developed, succinylcholine remains the only one used today [10]. Due to its potency (ED95 0.3 mg/kg) and quick onset of action (60 s), succinylcholine has historically been the agent of choice to facilitate muscle relaxation for rapid sequence endotracheal intubation [23–25].

Succinylcholine is structurally similar to two acetylcholine molecules. Thus, only one succinylcholine molecule is required to activate the acetylcholine receptor. As with acetylcholine, binding of succinylcholine promotes an influx of sodium ions and depolarization of the muscle fiber. Unlike acetylcholine which quickly dissociates from the receptor, succinylcholine is more stably bound to the receptor causing a prolonged depolarization. This results in the commonly seen muscle fasciculations after administration [26]. Repolarization is delayed, preventing additional sodium influx and muscle contractions. Metabolism of succinylcholine is by hydrolysis via plasma pseudocholinesterase which exists outside of the neuromuscular junction [27]. Thus, the limiting factor in its duration of action is the diffusion out of the neuromuscular junction and into the extracellular fluid, of which takes place in less than 10 min assuming proper function and quantity of the plasma pseudocholinesterase enzyme [27, 28].

Despite its rapid and reliable muscle relaxation, succinylcholine has special considerations and contraindications making its clinical utility controversial. This is especially true with the growing use of nondepolarizing agents and the development of fast acting, hemodynamically stable reversal agents [23, 29]. The most feared complication from succinylcholine is life-threatening hyperkalemia. With its contraction-inducing mechanism of action, healthy individuals may experience mild, transient elevations of serum potassium as high as 0.5–1.0 mEq/L. [10] However, succinylcholine activation of immature acetylcholine receptors causes a profound release of potassium from skeletal muscle. Patients at risk for increased immature receptor expression and severe hyperkalemia are listed below [10, 26, 30, 31].

- Thermal injuries >48 h
- Upper and lower motor neuron injuries, including spinal cord injury and cerebral vascular injury
- Major trauma, crush injury, or rhabdomyolysis
- Prolonged immobility, paraplegia, quadriplegia
- Myopathies and neuromuscular disorders such as Duchenne Muscular Dystrophy, Guillain-Barre Syndrome, and Amyotrophic Lateral Sclerosis

Another feared and potentially fatal complication from succinylcholine is malignant hyperthermia (MH). This is an inherited hyper-metabolic disorder involving skeletal muscle. When exposed to a trigger agent, patients may develop hyperthermia, widespread muscular contraction, rhabdomyolysis, metabolic and respiratory acidosis, tachycardia, hypertension, and multiorgan failure [32, 33]. Management requires prompt diagnosis and timely administration of dantrolene to prevent ongoing calcium release in the skeletal muscle sarcoplasmic reticulum [34]. Furthermore, aggressive hemodynamic support and resuscitation may be required in an ICU setting.

Patients with atypical or deficient pseudocholinesterase should avoid succinylcholine administration given concern for significantly prolonged duration of action [27]. This may require ICU admission and continued mechanical ventilation until the medication is metabolized and the patient regains strength required for adequate ventilation. Assessment for the presence of atypical pseudocholinesterase is done by measuring the ability of dibucaine, an amide local anesthetic, to inhibit benzoylcholine hydrolysis by pseudocholinesterase [28]. In normal individuals, dibucaine should inhibit the action of pseudocholinesterase by greater than 70%. Atypical pseudocholinesterase is inherited in an autosomal recessive manner due to mutations in the butyrylcholinesterase gene. Patients with heterozygous inheritance may have increased duration of action of succinylcholine of up to 30%. Those with homozygous inheritance may be severely affected and experience paralysis for up to 4 h. Acquired pseudocholinesterase deficiency can occur in specific disease states or with the use of certain medications. This includes hepatic and renal dysfunction, pregnancy, thermal injury, infection, and the use of MAO inhibitors and anticholinesterase agents.

Other clinically significant adverse effects are listed below [26, 35]:

- Bradycardia, hypotension, and increased secretions due to binding to muscarinic acetylcholine receptors.
- Myalgias (50–90%).
- Increased intraocular pressures. The clinical significance of this is controversial. That said, it is reasonable to withhold administration in the setting of open globe injuries.
- Flushing, hypotension, tachycardia from histamine release.

47.2.3 Nondepolarizing Agents (Rocuronium, Vecuronium, Pancuronium, Cisatracurium, Atracurium, Mivacurium)

Nondepolarizing neuromuscular blocking agents block acetylcholine binding to alpha subunits on nicotinic receptors in the motor endplate. This prevents depolarization and leads to widespread paralysis [36]. Unlike succinylcholine, nondepolarizing agents are commonly used in settings requiring ongoing paralysis, such as therapeutic hypothermia and promoting ventilator synchrony. Larger doses of nondepolarizing agents can produce intubation conditions at speeds that rival that of succinylcholine [23]. Nondepolarizers vary greatly in onset, duration of action, metabolism, elimination, and side effect profile [24, 29]. There are two classes of nondepolarizing blocking agents: aminosteroid ("steroidal") and benzylisoquinolinium ("nonsteroidal"). These classes also differ in their ability to be reversed by sugammadex, which will be discussed in more detail in further sections [37].

Aminosteroid agents derive their name from the bulky steroid center in their chemical structure. These medications include rocuronium, vecuronium, and pancuronium.

Rocuronium and Vecuronium are two of the most widely used nondepolarizing agents in the ICU and operating room [38]. Vecuronium is a derivative of pancuronium and the first intermediate-acting nondepolarizing agent produced. Rocuronium and vecuronium are the paralytic of choice at many institutions given their potential for quick onset and intermediate duration of action [23, 39]. Vecuronium is much more potent than rocuronium (ED95, 0.05 mg/kg vs. 0.3 mg/kg, respectively), leading to slower onset of action at typical intubating doses (3.5–4 min vs. 1.5–2 min, respectively) [12, 40]. However, with doses five to six times ED95, Vecuronium can produce more rapid intubating conditions [12]. While both agents have a duration of action of approximately 40 min they have a clinically significant difference in their elimination profile [41]. Rocuronium undergoes elimination almost entirely unchanged, with 80% through the hepatobiliary system and

20% renally. Thus, in patients with hepatic and renal dysfunction, rocuronium duration of action can be prolonged due to increases in volume of distribution and half-life [42–44]. Vecuronium is primarily eliminated unchanged in the biliary and renal system, 40% and 30%, respectively. The rest is metabolized in the liver, forming 3-desacetyl vecuronium, a renally excreted metabolite with neuromuscular blocking properties. Significant increases in Vecuronium's duration of action in renal dysfunction are attributed to the accumulation of this active metabolite, especially when administered as a prolonged infusion [12, 45]. Thus, in the ICU setting, infusion dosing should be decreased with significant renal impairment [46]. Hepatic impairment can also affect vecuronium pharmacokinetics although this is more predictable because it is primarily eliminated through the biliary system.

Despite being the first steroid agent produced and introduced to the market in the 1960s, pancuronium has fallen out of favor. With an ED95 of 0.07 mg/kg, its onset on action of upwards of 5 min and duration of action nearing 90 min has little clinical utility today [47, 48]. Furthermore, pancuronium is known for its high degree of renal excretion, making up about 80% of its elimination profile. The presence of an active metabolite, 3-desacetylpancuronium, is problematic in the critical care setting where kidney injury is a common occurrence [29]. Pancuronium is also unique in that it blocks muscarinic receptors in the myocardium, leading to tachycardia and increased cardiac output [49].

The benzylisoquinolinium class includes cisatracurium, atracurium, and mivacurium. Aside from chemical structure, these agents differ from the nonsteroidal class mostly in their metabolism, elimination, and propensity for histamine release.

Atracurium and its 1R cis-1'R cis isomer cisatracurium are intermediate acting agents with a duration of action of approximately 45r min [12]. However, with an ED95 of 0.05 mg/kg, cisatracurium has a potency three times that of atracurium. Thus, cisatracurium has a slower onset of action of 5–6 min compared to approximately 2 min with atracurium [12, 50–52].

Cisatracurium is unique in that its elimination occurs almost exclusively by a temperature and pH-dependent and organ-independent process called Hoffman elimination. Hoffman elimination degrades an amine to an alkene and is slowed by acidosis and hypothermia, prolonging blockade. Small amounts of renal elimination occur, but to clinically insignificant degrees as shown by its use in patients with renal dysfunction [17]. Atracurium also undergoes Hoffman elimination but to a lesser degree (40% vs. 80% with cisatracurium). The remainder of its elimination is by hydrolysis via nonspecific plasma esterase. Both Hoffman elimination and degradation by nonspecific esterases are unsaturable processes, thus pharmacokinetics will not experience major changes with bolus dosing versus continuous infusion (elimination half-life approximately 20 min). This makes these agents a popular choice for sustained neuromuscular blockade in the ICU [53]. Cisatracurium infusions can be dosed as a fixed dose or titratable infusion. Fixed dosing of 37.5 mg/h has been used in multiple major trials [54, 55]. Dosing for TOF-titratable protocols range from 1 to 3 mcg/kg/min and have shown evidence of reduced total dosage and cost [56–58]. One primary metabolite of cisatracurium and atracurium is laudanosine, which is renally and hepatically cleared. While not an active neuromuscular blocker, it is associated with hypotension and central nervous system excitation. Prolonged infusions may cause accumulation of laudanosine, with animal studies showing excitatory EEG tracings and sustained seizures at high levels. In contrast, this has not been reported in adults [59, 60].

Mivacurium is unique to all nondepolarizing agents. Aside from its mechanism of action, Mivacurium shares multiple similarities with its depolarizing counterpart succinylcholine. The ED95 is 0.08 mg/kg, with an onset of action of 60–90 s at 2.5 times ED95 dose and duration of action of approximately 20 min [61]. This makes mivacurium the fastest onset and shortest duration of all nondepolarizing agents. Larger doses and rapid administration can lead to hemodynamic instability due to histamine release. Mivacurium also shares the same mechanism of clearance as succinylcholine via plasma pseudocholinesterase, further explaining its short duration of action [62]. For this reason, it is relatively contraindicated in patients with atypical or deficient pseudocholinesterase [28]. While it may seem that mivacurium offers all the benefits of succinylcholine without the adverse effects of a depolarizing agent, it unfortunately was discontinued from circulation in the United States in 2006 but has recently been reintroduced [63].

47.3 Neuromuscular Monitoring

To determine proper depth of neuromuscular blockade and subsequent blockade reversal, objective monitoring with nerve stimulation is paramount. Assessment with physical exam alone can significantly underestimate the degree of muscle relaxation and should not be a replacement for neuromonitoring [64]. Given concern for the adverse effects associated with deep neuromuscular blockade and the risk of residual blockade, international organizations have recommended quantitative monitoring for patients receiving neuromuscular blocking agents and reversal agents [64–66].

47.3.1 Nerve Stimulation

Quantitative monitoring requires stimulation of a peripheral nerve and measuring the associated muscular response. The peripheral nerve should be close to the skin, have a motor component and be able to elicit a muscle response that can be qualitatively or quantitatively monitored [67]. Nerve stimulation is done by transcutaneous transmission of an electrical signal via an electrode. Given that one motor neuron can communicate with many muscle fibers, the electrical signal must be of adequate strength and duration to stimulate all muscle fibers. Consideration should be given to the resistance in the skin as well. Skin temperature, oils and fluids, electrode application, and certain disease states can affect signal transmission [67]. Furthermore, stimulators are dual polar. The negative electrode is placed on the most superficial aspect of the nerve and the positive electrode placed elsewhere along the path of the nerve, avoiding direct stimulation of the muscle. Nerve stimulation can be delivered in a variety of ways depending on the strength, duration, and number of stimuli.

The most basic application of neurostimulation is via the single twitch measurement. A single electrical stimulus is applied for 0.1–0.3 ms and the muscular response is measured. When applied at a frequency of 1.0 Hz (1 stimulus per 1 s), changes in muscular response after neuromuscular blockade can be appreciated [67]. This makes single twitch monitoring an option when initiating neuromuscular blockade. However, it is not possible to measure adequate recovery with single twitch monitoring.

Train-of-four (TOF) stimulation is when four identical single twitch stimuli are delivered at a frequency of 2 Hz. The amplitude of muscular response of the fourth twitch is compared to the first twitch to produce a train-of-four ratio. The train-of-four is the gold standard for measurement of neuromuscular blockade and reversal of blockade prior to endotracheal extubation [64, 68]. Without administration of a neuromuscular blocking agent, all four twitches should produce the same muscular response. This produces a ratio between the first twitch (T1) and fourth twitch (T4) of 1.0 or 100%. With administration of a nondepolarizing agent, the muscular response of subsequent twitches will decrease, a phenomenon referred to as "fade." The ratio of blockade, or degree of "fade," corresponds with a percentage of acetylcholine receptor blockade. Approximately 70% of acetylcholine receptors can be blocked before there is any visual appreciation of fade [67]. This is why quantitative measurement of muscular response, instead of visual or tactile monitoring, is required to prevent residual weakness after reversal of neuromuscular blockade [69]. With deepening nondepolarizing blockade, eventually all four twitches will become undetectable. This corresponds with approximately 95% acetylcholine receptor blockade [67]. Unlike with nondepolarizing agents, there is usually no fade response to depolarizing agents. Administration of succinylcholine will result in an equal degree of twitch suppression in all four twitches, termed a phase 1 block. Supratherapeutic doses of succinylcholine or pseudocholinesterase deficiency can result in fade, referred to as phase 2 block. While not fully understood, presynaptic acetylcholine receptor binding preventing acetylcholine release or postsynaptic receptor desensitization may play a role in the development of phase 2 block [70].

In patients with profound neuromuscular block resulting in no detectable muscular activity, tetanic or post-tetanic stimulation may be required to assess the degree of deep blockade. Tetanic stimulation is produced by repetitive stimulation fusing together to form the appearance of one sustained contraction. This requires stimulation at a frequency of at least 30 Hz [67]. The rapid nerve impulses lead to large quantities of acetylcholine production in the axon terminal. This amplifies acetylcholine release and muscle contraction for approximately 3–5 min after tetany. In patients without detectable twitches with traditional train-of-four stimulation, further assessing the degree of blockade can be done by quantifying post-tetany twitches, more commonly known as a post-tetanic count. This is done by producing a 50 Hz tetany for 5 s followed by twenty 1 Hz twitches. The lack of post-tetanic twitches is associated with profound neuromuscular blockade. This is useful when deciding the timing and dosage of reversal of deep blockade [71].

Many studies have shown that subjective monitoring by visual or tactile methods can significantly underestimate the degree of neuromuscular blockade. The human eye is unable to detect significant variations in fade [64, 69, 72, 73]. Quantitative monitoring can be done by acceleromyography, mechanomyography, or electromyography. In acceleromyography, an accelerometer is placed on the muscle group and acceleration of the muscle is measured after stimulation of the corresponding nerve. Acceleromyograph is the most widely used technique given the convenience of measurement in the clinical setting [67, 74]. Careful attention should be given to prevent movement of the surrounding muscle groups to avoid artifacts in measurements. Mechanomyography is similar in concept to acceleromyography. Instead of measuring muscle movement, the muscle is kept under constant tension and the change in tension is measured and transformed into an elective signal. In this case, no subjective movement of the muscle is witnessed. Furthermore, since the muscle must be stabilized and kept under constant tension, its clinical application in the operating room or intensive care unit is limited. Electromyography measures action potentials that occur in the muscle during nerve stimulation. Like acceleromyography, with electromyography the limb does not need to be under constant restraint. Nonetheless, it is prone to significant artifact from movement and temperature changes.

Sensitivities of muscle groups to neuromuscular blockade varies. Central muscles such as the diaphragm and larynx have faster onset of blockade due to their large volume of blood supply. Similarly, the diaphragm has quick recovery from blockade. This concept is important when deciding where to place the nerve stimulator and explains why the ulnar nerve and adductor pollicis muscle is the most used site [67]. One can assume that once adductor pollicis activity has fully recovered, the diaphragm has done so as well. Unfortunately, the wrist and hand are often unable to be accessed due to other monitors, restraints, or surgical positioning. In this case, the posterior tibial nerve and flexor hallucis muscle can be used by detection of toe movement. Another common, albeit not widely recommended, site of monitoring is the orbicularis oculi or corrugator supercilii facial muscles. Unfortunately, these muscles recover quicker than laryngeal and upper airway muscles. Monitoring of this site may lead to premature extubation and subsequent respiratory compromise. Furthermore, direct muscle stimulation can lead to wildly inaccurate measurements of orbicularis oculi or corrugator supercilii blockade [75, 76].

47.3.2　Subjective Measurement of Neuromuscular Blockade

Since the introduction of neuromuscular blocking agents, clinical evaluation has been used to guide depth of blockade. This includes measurement of respiratory parameters (tidal volume, minute ventilation) and muscular function (5-s head lift, grip strength, and the tongue depressor test) [68, 69, 73]. However, multiple studies have shown that clinical evaluations are incapable of predicting adequate reversal from neuromuscular blockade. Unfortunately, despite the magnitude of evidence supporting quantitative monitoring, it is still not routinely utilized to monitor neuromuscular blockade and recovery in the ICU [65]. Nonetheless, international organizations continue to recommend the mandatory use of quantitative monitoring in patients receiving neuromuscular blocking agents [64, 66].

47.4 Reversal Agents

Residual neuromuscular blockade is a well-described phenomenon in the postoperative setting. Patients with residual neuromuscular blockade may develop respiratory failure, unplanned reintubation, unintended ICU admission, and psychological distress [77]. Reversing the effects of NMBDs decreases the risk of residual blockade and its potential complications [64]. Reversal agents are commonly administered in the operating room; however, their use in the ICU is not as routine [53]. Unfortunately, as many as 40% of patients have unidentified residual neuromuscular blockade in the post-anesthesia care unit (PACU) when appropriate reversal is not confirmed with quantitative monitoring, highlighting the possibility of this complication in the ICU. This is especially concerning with the lack of routine quantitative monitoring in the ICU [78].

Acetylcholinesterase inhibitors have historically been the agent of choice for reversal of nondepolarizing neuromuscular blockade. Inhibition of acetylcholinesterase increases acetylcholine in the synaptic cleft. With adequate dose and timing of administration, acetylcholine will outcompete neuromuscular blocking agents for binding sites on the acetylcholine receptors. Neostigmine is the primary medication of this class used for reversal. The onset time of reversal is dependent on the duration of action of the nondepolarizing agent (short vs. intermediate vs. long-acting) and degree of blockade at administration (TOF count) [79]. Shorter acting agents will undergo spontaneous recovery more quickly and will be reversed more quickly after administration of an acetylcholinesterase inhibitor. For deeper levels of blockade (TOF <2), reversal is unreliable and can take over 10 min [80]. For this reason, current recommendations reserve neostigmine reversal for minimal blockade detected with quantitative monitoring (TOF >40%) [64]. Dosing of neostigmine ranges from 0.015 mg/kg for shallow block (TOF 4) to 0.05 mg/kg for deeper block (TOF <2) [12]. Larger doses should be avoided due to the risk of weakness from increased acetylcholine levels and potential cholinergic crisis. Neostigmine increases systemic acetylcholine, requiring concomitant administration of an antimuscarinic medication such as glycopyrrolate or atropine. This prevents potentially serious complications including bradycardia, hypotension, and bronchospasm. Acetylcholinesterase inhibitors also inhibit the action of pseudocholinesterase, increasing duration of action of subsequent doses of succinylcholine.

In the last two decades, sugammadex has gained increasing popularity for blockade reversal. Sugammadex is a gamma-cyclodextrin that chelates aminosteroid nondepolarizing NMBDs, specifically rocuronium and vecuronium [81]. Eight hydroxyl chains are bound together to form a hydrophobic core with a hydrophilic exterior. Non-covalent hydrophobic attractions at the core form a near-irreversible bond between sugammadex and rocuronium. Affinity between sugammadex and vecuronium is approximately threefold lower [82]. Binding occurs in the plasma, decreasing the blood concentration of the blocking agent. This mobilizes the NMBD down a concentration gradient from the synaptic cleft to the plasma, decreasing its clinical effect. Sugammadex does not affect acetylcholine binding at muscarinic receptors, negating the need for antimuscarinic medications. Speed of reversal is dependent on dose and depth of blockade at time of administration [83, 84]. For minimal and moderate blockade (TOF $\geq$ 2), 2 mg/kg is recommended. For deep block (TOF <1), 4 mg/kg is recommended. Sugammadex works more reliably and rapidly than neostigmine, with an average of 3 min for reversal [85]. Furthermore, perhaps its most noteworthy advantage, at high doses (16 mg/kg) sugammadex is capable of reversing rapid sequence intubation doses of rocuronium. This can be life-saving when airway management is impossible and requires the return of spontaneous ventilation [86].

Comparisons of sugammadex to neostigmine in reversal of blockade in the ICU is lacking. On the contrary, data in the perioperative environment is extensive. In 2023, the American Society of Anesthesiologists released guidelines supporting the use of sugammadex over neostigmine in deep, moderate, and shallow depths of blockade, guided using quantitative monitoring [64]. Use with neostigmine was only recommended with a train-of-four ratio above 40%. The sparse use of quantitative monitoring in the ICU supports the use of sugammadex given its more reliable reversal and less residual blockade [87].

Concern for adverse reactions has limited adaptation of sugammadex [88]. Although sugammadex does not interact with muscarinic receptors, severe, life-threatening bradycardia has been reported. Incidence varies but remains extremely rare. While the mechanism is not yet understood, patients with cardiac comorbidities or perioperative use of beta blockers may be at higher risk [89]. Allergic reactions including anaphylaxis have also been documented with sugammadex use [90]. The sugammadex-rocuronium complex is excreted entirely via the kidneys. Theoretically, patients with renal failure may be at risk of recurrence of neuromuscular blockade with dissociation of the sugammadex-rocuronium bond [91]. However, studies have shown safe administration in patients with end-stage renal failure [92, 93]. Furthermore, the complex can be eliminated via dialysis if there is significant concern for recurrence of paralysis [94]. In vitro studies have suggested that sugammadex may bind with progesterone, potentially limiting the efficacy of oral contraceptives. Any patient of childbearing age should be counseled about this potential adverse effect and recommended to use an additional form of anticontraceptive for at least 7 days [95].

47.5 Medication Interactions

Certain medications can amplify or attenuate the effects of neuromuscular blocking agents. The mechanism of these interactions can involve the spinal nerve roots, acetylcholine synthesis and release, acetylcholine receptor sensitivity, and action potential propagation [96].

High doses of local anesthetics prolong nondepolarizing neuromuscular blockade by decreased nerve conduction, acetylcholine synthesis and release, and acetylcholine receptor channel opening. This is particularly important in the era of opioid sparing pain management, where lidocaine infusions have shown potential benefit [97]. Aminoglycoside antibiotics, more specially gentamicin, and clindamycin can prolong blockade by decreasing acetylcholine release and decreasing acetylcholine receptor sensitivity to acetylcholine [98]. More commonly used antimicrobials such as penicillins and cephalosporins are not thought to have a significant effect on blockade. Antiseizure medications can have varying effects depending on the chronicity of their use [99]. Patients with chronic antiseizure use can develop resistance to NMBD by increased acetylcholine receptor expression, increased protein binding of NMBDs, and increase hepatic elimination of NMBDs. Given the intrinsic neuromuscular blocking effects of antiseizure medications, their acute use can potentiate blockade by both pre- and post-junctional receptor antagonism. Magnesium can potentiate NMBD via calcium-antagonizing properties, leading to decrease release of acetylcholine [100]. Lithium may potentiate NMBD by blocking sodium influx in the motor endplate [101].

47.6 Indications for Neuromuscular Blockade

Neuromuscular blocking agents provide the intensivist with a unique tool to manage their patients' increasingly challenging needs. While there may be many proposed indications for neuromuscular blockade, supporting evidence greatly varies. Currently, facilitation of endotracheal intubation remains the most widely accepted indication for neuromuscular blockade in the ICU. Other indications such as acute respiratory distress syndrome, status asthmaticus, therapeutic hypothermia, and elevated intracranial pressures are practiced with varying degrees of acceptance [53].

47.6.1 Facilitation of Intubation

Endotracheal intubation is one of the most common procedures performed in the hospital, making it one of the most common indications for neuromuscular blockade in the ICU. Studies have shown approximately 17–69% of ICU patients require intubation at some point during their hospital stay [102]. Intubations in the ICU are also more difficult and prone to complications compared to those performed in the operating room. Patient comorbidities, body habitus, hemodynamic instability, and hypoxemia are common occurrences that can complicate airway management. Complication rates are as high as 40%, with severe complications including severe hypotension and hypoxemia occurring in roughly 28% of patients [103, 104]. Furthermore, while rates of obesity in the ICU compare with that in the operating room, intubation in obese patients is more difficult and associated with a significant increase in complications when taking place in the ICU [22]. Regardless of body habitus, intubation requiring greater than three attempts occurs in over 10% of patients in the ICU [105].

Despite advancements in technologies to facilitate intubation (video laryngoscopy, fiberoptic bronchoscope), improvements in hemodynamic monitoring (arterial catheters, pulmonary arterial catheters), and a better understanding of hemodynamically stable induction agents, ICU intubation remains dangerous and requires reliable, fast-acting neuromuscular blockade [53, 106]. In the many ICU patients at high risk for aspiration and require emergent intubation, rapid sequence intubation is the preferred technique [39]. This requires intubating conditions to be achieved as fast as possible, necessitating the use of neuromuscular blocking agents. The use of neuromuscular blockade has been shown to decrease rates of complications and increase success rates, even in patients with assumed difficult airways [107, 108].

To avoid manipulating a potentially difficult airway, awake intubation is an option that maintains spontaneous ventilation and avoids use of NMBDs. Unfortunately, this is not without the risk of hemodynamic instability, aspiration, and elevated intracranial pressures [109].

47.6.2 *Acute Respiratory Distress Syndrome*

Acute Respiratory Distress Syndrome (ARDS) is a state of severe lung inflammation that occurs most often because of lung injury or critical illness. This includes pneumonia, aspiration pneumonitis, non-pulmonary sepsis, trauma, and many others. Severe inflammation increases permeability of the lung-capillary barrier and leakage of blood and fluid in the lung, significantly impacting oxygenation and ventilation. Patients routinely require intubation, mechanical ventilation, hemodynamic support, and management of multiorgan failure.

ARDS occurs in as many as 10–15% of ICU patients, including nearly 25% of mechanically ventilated patients [110]. Severity is described as mild, moderate, or severe, depending on the patient's oxygenation. Approximately 75% of cases are classified as moderate or severe. Patients with severe disease have a mortality rate of over 40% [111].

No single medication or treatment modality has been proven to "cure" ARDS. Care is mostly supportive, focused on preventing further lung injury and treating the presumed underlying cause. For decades, significant academic interest has been placed in developing treatments and protocols for ARDS. This includes the well-established NIH-NHLBI ARDS Network (ARDSnet), a research network formed to conduct large, multi-center clinical trials of ARDS treatments. In addition to the use of neuromuscular blocking drugs, this includes mechanical ventilatory parameters for intubated patients (lung protective ventilation, LPV), noninvasive ventilation for patients with mild disease, optimizing nutrition and volume status, glucocorticoid administration, prone positioning, and mechanical circulatory support (extracorporeal membrane oxygenation, ECMO).

Lung protective ventilation (LPV) with lower tidal volumes has been a staple of ARDS treatment for over two decades [112]. LPV reduces mortality and decreases the number of days spent on mechanical ventilation. Neuromuscular blockade may help facilitate mechanical ventilation in patients with severe disease in which ventilation of poorly compliant lung is unable to be achieved with sedation alone. These patients may need blocking agents to suppress their own respiratory effort to avoid barotrauma and overdistension of alveoli. Neuromuscular blockade may also help decrease the metabolic rate of oxygen consumption, improving the oxygen supply-demand relationship in the peripheral tissue and decrease organ failure. Prone positioning of intubated patients is also deployed to help optimize ventilation-perfusion matching in the diseased lung. Neuromuscular blockade can be deployed to facilitate the act of proning and improve ventilator synchrony while proning.

Multiple randomized control trials have shown conflicting results of NMBD in patients with ARDS. Earlier trials showed evidence that continuous infusion of cisatracurium may improve mortality, oxygenation, ventilator-free days, organ failure, and markers of inflammation [54, 113]. Unfortunately, some of these studies were underpowered to detect mortality benefit. Furthermore, the mortality benefit that was observed occurred more than 2 weeks after cessation of cisatracurium. Nonetheless, a meta-analysis of these trials suggested improvement in oxygenation, mortality, ventilator-free days, and barotrauma [114]. More recently, a large, randomized trial showed no benefit in mortality in patients with moderate-to-severe ARDS treated with neuromuscular blockade and deep sedation versus patients treated with light sedation and no neuromuscular blockade [55].

It is difficult to determine the overall utility of neuromuscular blockade in ARDS given the large degree of confounding therapies utilized for ARDS. This includes ventilator management, depth of sedation, glucocorticoid use, prone positioning, and fluid volume management. That said, a panel of international experts recently produced evidence-based recommendations to help guide clinical decision-making. It was recommended that in patients unable to achieve ventilator synchrony or prone positioning after optimization of ventilator settings and deep sedation, it is reasonable to use a 48-h infusion of neuromuscular blockade in patients with moderate-to-severe ARDS [53, 115].

47.6.3 Severe Asthma Exacerbation

Asthma is a chronic airway disease marked by recurrent inflammation and airway hyperreactivity affecting nearly 300 million people worldwide [116]. Severe asthma exacerbation, or status asthmaticus, is a potentially fatal form of severe bronchoconstriction refractory to most standard therapies. As many as 16% of patients admitted with asthma exacerbation progress to respiratory failure requiring ICU admission and mechanical ventilation. Outcomes vary, with studies reporting ICU mortality as high as 10% [117]. Others report that although 61% of ICU admissions required intubation, mortality was less than 1% [118].

While an exact, agreed upon definition for severe asthma exacerbation does not exist, it is commonly accepted that these patients fail multiple standard therapies. Mainstay therapies of asthma exacerbation include bronchodilators (albuterol), corticosteroids, and noninvasive mechanical ventilation. More severe disease may require mechanical ventilation with special attention to prevent alveolar overdistension secondary to expiratory airflow obstruction. Like patients with ARDS, the requirements of mechanical ventilation for severe asthma exacerbation may not be tolerated by lightly sedated patients, thus requiring deep sedation or neuromuscular blockade.

Neuromuscular blockade for mechanical ventilation in patients with severe asthma exacerbation remains a point of contention. Given the concern for significant barotrauma, alveolar distension, and the accompanied hemodynamic instability, patients require a prolonged expiratory time, decreased respiratory rate, and may need to tolerate significant hypercapnia. To fulfill these requirements, complete control of ventilation by the intensivist is required. While certain organizations recommend against the routine use of neuromuscular blocking drugs for these patients, it is not unreasonable to consider in severe cases of ventilator dyssynchrony, hypoxemia, acidosis, or hemodynamic instability [53, 116]. A common concern with neuromuscular blockade in the ICU is the risk of critical illness myopathy. This is especially concerning for asthmatics with chronic corticosteroid use [119–121].

47.6.4 Therapeutic Hypothermia After Cardiac Arrest

Therapeutic hypothermia is most often deployed for neuroprotection in the setting of post-cardiac arrest care. Other common uses for therapeutic hypothermia include increased intracranial pressure due to stroke or traumatic brain injury and severe anemia. Hypothermia aims to reduce cerebral metabolism and improve the oxygen supply-demand relationship. However, literature support for therapeutic hypothermia for cardiac arrest is inconsistent and application varies widely among institutions [122–126]. Neuromuscular blockade can treat and prevent shivering, which is associated with increased metabolic demand and delays in achieving the targeted hypothermia [127]. Unfortunately, mortality and neurological benefit from the use of neuromuscular blockade has not been well established [128–130]. Current recommendations support blockade in patients with overt shivering but do not comment on the routine use in therapeutic hypothermia [53].

47.6.5 *Intracranial Hypertension*

Patients with acute brain injury from stroke, trauma, mass-occupying lesions or post-surgical changes are at high risk of significantly elevated intracranial pressure (ICP). This can lead to life-threatening changes in cerebral perfusion pressure and brain herniation. Neuromuscular blockade in these patients may be useful in decreasing cerebral metabolism and preventing critical elevations in ICP during cough-stimulating procedures such as airway suctioning. Nonetheless, strong evidence supporting their use is lacking [131, 132]. The benefits of cough suppression, treating and preventing shivering during therapeutic hypothermia, and decreasing cerebral metabolism should be weighed against the harms of immobilization, deep sedation, and prolonged mechanical ventilation.

47.7 Complications of Neuromuscular Blockade

Neuromuscular blockade can provide the intensivist with an invaluable tool to facilitate care in some of their sickest patients. However, these medications have potential complications that limit their utility and are a source of hesitation for many critical care clinicians. This is especially true in an era of critical care that values ICU liberation [133, 134].

47.7.1 *ICU Associated Weakness*

With advancements in critical care, patients are surviving longer, more complicated ICU admissions. Unfortunately, ICU-associated weakness (ICU-AW) is a common and debilitating consequence of ICU admission. ICU-AW can be further classified into critical illness myopathy and critical illness polyneuropathy. While the pathophysiology is not completely understood, axonal nerve degeneration and myofiber necrosis occur due to multiple factors involving inflammatory, circulatory, and metabolic derangements [135, 136]. Patients with increased ICU length of admission, immobility, ARDS, sepsis, or coma have increased incidence and severity of ICU-AW [136]. ICU-AW may be present in as many as 70% of ICU patients who are admitted for 7 days and in 100% of patients with septic shock [136, 137]. These patients can suffer long-term debilitation, cognitive dysfunction, and chronic respiratory failure [138].

Despite the lack of strong, causal evidence, neuromuscular blocking agents have been implicated as a cause of ICU-AW for decades [139, 140]. However, it is likely these studies were affected by confounding factors. Furthermore, a vast majority of evidence is derived from case reports and observational studies, with very few randomized controlled studies. These studies often include heterogeneous populations, including patients with multiple risk factors for ICU-AW, such as steroid use, septic shock, and elder age [140–142]. ICU-AW is also associated with more critically ill patients, which are also the patients that most often require neuromuscular blockade.

The risk of awareness and its psychosocial consequences many sway clinicians to opt for deeper sedation protocols when treating patients with NMBDs [143]. Over-sedation, alone or in combination with neuromuscular blocking drugs, may lead to prolonged immobilization and ICU-AW [144, 145]. Early studies assessing the benefit of cisatracurium infusions in ARDS showed mortality benefit that more recent trials were unable to replicate. However, in more recent trials, control groups with lighter depths of sedation had a lower incidence of ICU-AW compared to those treated with neuromuscular blocking agents and deep sedation. In fact, even when controlled for degree of immobility, patients with sedation had higher rates of ICU-AW than those without sedation [146, 147].

47.7.2 Residual Neuromuscular Blockade

Inappropriate reversal or monitoring of the depth of neuromuscular blockade can lead to residual neuromuscular blockade (RNMB), airway obstruction, respiratory failure, and unplanned ICU admissions [77, 148]. While residual blockade is more commonly associated with postoperative complications, the incidence in the ICU is as high as 50% [149]. In some cases, RNMB has been documented up to 7 days after cessation of the infusion [45].

While the exact definition of RNMB is debated, persistent pharyngeal weakness and increased risk of aspiration can occur at train-of-four (TOF) ratios up to 0.9 [150, 151]. Furthermore, patients may exhibit signs of discomfort or distress even at TOF ratios as high as 0.9 [152]. This stresses the need for quantitative monitoring in addition to subjective clinical analysis to guide dosing and reversal [53, 153]. Ensuring full reversal of neuromuscular blockade is a requirement in determination of brain death. If residual neuromuscular blockade is suspected, confirmatory testing may be necessary.

47.7.3 Unintended Recall and Awareness

Awareness during neuromuscular blockade is a tragic complication that can lead to long- and short-term sequelae including post-traumatic stress disorder (PTSD) [154]. In contrast to the operating room, awareness in the ICU occurs to a much higher degree [155]. Underdosing sedatives in hemodynamically unstable patients, administration during emergencies, and lasting paralysis after rapid sequence intubation may increase the risk of recall. Furthermore, anesthetics performed strictly with intravenous medications, similar to how sedation is administered in the ICU, are associated with increased awareness in the operating room. This is because the clinician is unable to measure the concentration of intravenous sedative in the patient, as is typically done with end-tidal measurement with volatile anesthetics [156]. Monitors measuring the depth of anesthesia (electroencephalogram-EEG and BiSpectral Index-BIS) are widely used in the operating room and have shown benefit in reducing intraoperative awareness [157]. These monitors may also have a role in the ICU; however, this is controversial [158–160]. Because of inconsistent data regarding the utility of EEG and BIS in ICU patients, current guidelines make no recommendation about their use [53]. Nonetheless, BIS monitoring is used widely as a part of sedation protocols when administering NMBD. Additional strategies include deepening sedation prior to administering NMBD and allowing adequate time for metabolism and elimination of NMBD prior to lightening sedation, with the assistance of quantitative neuromuscular monitoring.

47.7.4 Ocular Injuries

Critically ill patients are at high risk of ocular injuries as a consequence of the loss of ocular protective mechanisms [161]. Injuries include corneal abrasions and infectious and noninfectious keratitis. Patients treated with NMBD may be at higher risk compared to other ICU patients and injuries can develop in as soon as 48 h [162, 163]. Possible therapies and preventative measures include lubricating medications and protective eye-closure mechanisms. Many protocols have been developed to maintain eye care in the ICU, without robust evidence supporting the most effective method. Nonetheless, it is strongly recommended that patients receiving NMBD should receive scheduled eye care with lubricating medications and eyelid closure [53]. It is important to note that neuromuscular blockade does not interfere with pupillary light reflexes.

47.7.5 Anaphylaxis/Tachyphylaxis

Neuromuscular blocking agents are one of the most implicated medications in allergic reactions in the perioperative environment [164]. The overall incidence of NMBD-induced allergic reactions is unknown [165, 166]. Rocuronium and succinylcholine are believed to be the main culprits among NMBDs, with a tenfold increase in incidence compared to atrucurium [167, 168]. Furthermore, in patients with confirmed allergic reaction, cisatracurium has the lowest rate of cross reactivity, making it a safe alternative for these patients [168]. However, given false-negative allergic testing, it is reasonable to withhold additional NMBD after suspected allergic reaction [90]. Although anaphylaxis is a rare occurrence, clinicians should practice vigilance and send appropriate laboratory and skin testing when any concern arises. There are some case reports of tachyphylaxis associated with prolonged infusions of NMBDs, predominantly with cisatracurium infusions [169].

47.8 Special Considerations

47.8.1 Myasthenia Gravis and Lambert Eaton Syndrome

Myasthenia Gravis (MG) and Lambert Eaton Syndrome (ELS) are disorders of skeletal muscle weakness due to antibodies in the neuromuscular junction. Both disorders can present with significant weakness and may be due to paraneoplastic syndrome or isolated autoimmune disorder.

MG is due to antibodies to nicotinic acetylcholine receptors. Weakness is most common in the extraocular and bulbar muscles, leading to visual and swallowing disturbances. In more severe cases, patients may present with significant respiratory failure requiring ICU admission. ELS is due to antibodies against the presynaptic calcium channels, leading to decreased acetylcholine release. Unlike patients with MG, ELS is more likely to present with extremity weakness, especially in the proximal muscle groups. Patients are commonly treated with acetylcholinesterase inhibitors to increase the presence of acetylcholine in the NMJ and reduce or prevent muscle weakness.

MG and ELS patients are severely sensitive to NMBD, requiring significant dose reductions compared to healthy individuals [170–173]. Unlike with ELS, patients with MG may require increased dosage of succinylcholine to overcome competitive inhibition of the nicotinic receptor [174]. These patients may also experience increased duration of action of succinylcholine if they received acetylcholinesterase inhibitors as treatment for their MG. Nonetheless, depending on severity of disease and use of acetylcholinesterase inhibitors, response to NMBD can be very unpredictable. Dosing should be administered with extreme caution and the assistance of train-of-four monitoring. While some studies suggest differences in monitoring at different neuromuscular sites in these patients, no formal recommendations on location of monitoring has been made [53].

Reversal of rocuronium and vecuronium induced-blockade with sugammadex is highly recommended on account of the increased risk of residual blockade in these patients [64, 175, 176]. Patients reversed with acetylcholinesterase inhibitors may be at risk of weakness and cholinergic crisis [177].

47.8.2 Burn Injury

Severe burn injury can cause widespread muscle damage and increased acetylcholine receptor expression. Increase immobility due severe thermal injury may further increase the degree of acetylcholine receptor exposure [10, 178]. These patients have an increased risk of life-threatening hyperkalemia with succinylcholine use, making nondepolarizing NMBDs the medication of choice. Unfortunately, immature receptors have decreased affinity to nondepolarizing medications, requiring an increase in dosage [179–181]. Increased risk of hyperkalemia is thought to begin approximately 48 h after injury and may persist for months [182–184].

47.8.3 Obstetrics

Obstetric patients are at remarkably high risk of mortality and fetal loss when in the ICU [185, 186]. This highlights the severity of disease these patients face when admitted to the ICU and the possible need for NMBDs. Obstetric patients have multiple considerations regarding administration of NMBDs, including placental transfer of medications, changes in maternal physiology, and interactions with peripartum medications.

Most medications will exhibit a degree of placental transfer, but with varying clinical significance. Placental drug transfer is influenced by multiple factors including molecule size, protein binding, electrical charge, and lipid solubility. It is generally accepted that succinylcholine and nondepolarizing agents do not cross the fetal-placental barrier, and do not induce adverse neonatal or fetal effects, making them widely used in pregnant patients [187, 188]. This is due to the highly ionized succinylcholine molecule and the large molecular weight of nondepolarizing drugs [157]. Neostigmine has a quaternary structure that should have little placental transfer, however case studies of fetal bradycardia suggest otherwise [189]. When using neostigmine, atropine has historically been the antimuscarinic of choice in pregnant patients because, unlike glycopyrrolate, it readily crosses the placenta [189, 190].

Sugammadex is routinely used to reverse neuromuscular blockade after cesarean section and, to a lesser extent, non-obstetric surgery in pregnant patients [191–193]. Nonetheless, major obstetric societies continue to recommend caution in its use due to concern for increased risk of preterm labor [194]. Recent case series and animal studies have disputed these findings [191, 195, 196]. Furthermore, its large molecular weight and negative charge should theoretically limit any significant placental transfer of sugammadex [197]. Nonetheless, the Federal Drug Administration (FDA) has not approved sugammadex in pregnant patients due to the lack of large randomized controlled trials, which rarely include pregnant patients.

Patients with preeclampsia and premature deliveries may receive magnesium for maternal and fetal neuroprotection, respectively. This may significantly exacerbate neuromuscular blockade [100]. Additionally, antibiotics administered during labor or the perioperative period may exhibit neuromuscular blocking properties and increase blockade in patients receiving NMBD [98]. Given that pregnant patients are already at increased risk of difficult airway and respiratory failure, this further supports the need for quantitative TOF monitoring in this population [198, 199].

47.8.4 Pediatrics

Indications and concerns for NMBD use in critically ill pediatric patients are similar to those in adults. Potential benefit in ventilator synchronization and decreased oxygen consumption must be weighted against the risks of immobilization and deep sedation [200]. Most formal recommendations are harm-reducing [200]. Evidence supporting the use of NMBD in this population is inconsistent, lacking large, randomized controlled trials, and mostly dependent on adult studies. Best practice is on a case-by-case basis and clinicians should use their best judgment [200]. Pediatric patients experience differences in pharmacokinetics due to underdeveloped organ systems which may affect metabolism, elimination, protein binding, and volume of distribution. For instance, increased volume of distribution of NMBD in neonates may necessitate a higher initial dose to achieve blockade [201]. Furthermore, compared to adults and older children, neonates have increased cardiac output in relation to their weight. This allows NMBD to be eliminated from their site of action more quickly, possibly requiring more frequent dosing [202]. Levels of pseudocholinesterase are also decreased in pediatric patients with underdeveloped hepatic function, leading to theoretical increases in duration of action of succinylcholine [201, 202].

Succinylcholine is used judiciously in pediatrics because of concern for significant bradycardia and fear of life-threatening hyperkalemia due to undiagnosed neuromuscular disorders such as Duchenne Muscular Dystrophy (DMD). Neonates and infants are at particularly high risk of bradycardia as a consequence of their parasympathetic-dominant autonomic nervous system [203]. Antimuscarinic medications should be readily available when administering succinylcholine. The unpredictability of bradycardia in these patients makes pretreatment with an antimuscarinic agent controversial [203–205]. Due to an increase in immature acetylcholine receptors, patients with DMD are at significantly higher risk of succinylcholine-induced hyperkalemia [10, 206]. Pediatric patients with underlying DMD may be without family history of myopathies and undiagnosed until later in childhood [207, 208]. This has led to black-box warnings and near-universal avoidance of elective use of succinylcholine in early childhood [209].

References

1. Nishimune H, Shigemoto K. Practical anatomy of the neuromuscular junction in health and disease. Neurol Clin. 2018;36(2):231–40. https://doi.org/10.1016/j.ncl.2018.01.009.
2. Ruff RL. Neurophysiology of the neuromuscular junction: overview. Ann N Y Acad Sci. 2003;998(1):1–10. https://doi.org/10.1196/annals.1254.002.
3. Akaike A, Izumi Y. Overview. In: Akaike A, Shimohama S, Misu Y, editors. Nicotinic acetylcholine receptor signaling in neuroprotection. Singapore: Springer; 2018. https://doi.org/10.1007/978-981-10-8488-1_1.
4. Smith SJ, Augustine GJ. Calcium ions, active zones and synaptic transmitter release. Trends Neurosci. 1988;11(10):458–64. https://doi.org/10.1016/0166-2236(88)90199-3.
5. Ramakrishnan NA, Drescher MJ, Drescher DG. The SNARE complex in neuronal and sensory cells. Mol Cell Neurosci. 2012;50(1):58–69. https://doi.org/10.1016/j.mcn.2012.03.009.
6. Lindstrom JM. Nicotinic acetylcholine receptors of muscles and nerves: comparison of their structures, functional roles, and vulnerability to pathology. Ann N Y Acad Sci. 2003;998(1):41–52. https://doi.org/10.1196/annals.1254.007.
7. Naguib M, Flood P, McArdle JJ, Brenner HR. Advances in neurobiology of the neuromuscular junction. Anesthesiology. 2002;96(1):202–31. https://doi.org/10.1097/00000542-200201000-00035.

8. Ruff RL, Whittlesey D. Na+ current densities and voltage dependence in human intercostal muscle fibres. J Physiol. 1992;458(1):85–97. https://doi.org/10.1113/jphysiol.1992.sp019407.

9. Mishina M, Takai T, Imoto K, et al. Molecular distinction between fetal and adult forms of muscle acetylcholine receptor. Nature. 1986;321(6068):406–11. https://doi.org/10.1038/321406a0.

10. Martyn JAJ, Richtsfeld M, Warner DO. Succinylcholine-induced hyperkalemia in acquired pathologic states. Anesthesiology. 2006;104(1):158–69. https://doi.org/10.1097/00000542-200601000-00022.

11. Caulfield MP, Birdsall NJM. International union of pharmacology. XVII. Classification of muscarinic acetylcholine receptors. Pharmacol Rev. 1998;50(2):279.

12. Lien CA, Eikermann M. Neuromuscular blockers and reversal drugs. In: Pharmacology and physiology for anesthesia. Elsevier; 2019. p. 428–54. https://doi.org/10.1016/B978-0-323-48110-6.00022-3.

13. Bowman WC, Rodger IW, Houston J, Marshall RJ, McIndewar I. Structure:action relationships among some desacetoxy analogues of pancuronium and vecuronium in the anesthetized cat. Anesthesiology. 1988;69(1):57–62.

14. Lien CA, Matteo RS, Omstein E, Schwartz AE, Diaz J. Distribution, elimination, and action of vecuronium in the elderly. Anesth Analg. 1991;73(1):39–42. https://doi.org/10.1213/00000539-199107000-00008.

15. Matteo RS, Ornstein E, Schwartz AE, Ostapkovich N, Stone JG. Pharmacokinetics and pharmacodynamics of rocuronium (Org 9426) in elderly surgical patients. Anesth Analg. 1993;77(6):1193–7. https://doi.org/10.1213/00000539-199312000-00019.

16. Sorooshian SS, Stafford MA, Eastwood NB, Boyd AH, Hull CJ, Wright PMC. Pharmacokinetics and pharmacodynamics of Cisatracurium in young and Elderly adult patients. Anesthesiology. 1996;84(5):1083–91. https://doi.org/10.1097/00000542-199605000-00010.

17. Ornstein E, Lien CA, Matteo RS, Ostapkovich ND, Diaz J, Wolf KB. Pharmacodynamics and pharmacokinetics of Cisatracurium in geriatric surgical patients. Anesthesiology. 1996;84(3):520–5. https://doi.org/10.1097/00000542-199603000-00005.

18. Kovesdy CP, Furth SL, Zoccali C, On behalf of the World Kidney Day Steering Committee. Obesity and kidney disease: hidden consequences of the epidemic. Can J Kidney Health Dis. 2017;4:205435811769866. https://doi.org/10.1177/2054358117698669.

19. Ingrande J, Lemmens HJM. Dose adjustment of anaesthetics in the morbidly obese. Br J Anaesth. 2010;105:i16–23. https://doi.org/10.1093/bja/aeq312.

20. Meyhoff CS, Lund J, Jenstrup MT, et al. Should dosing of rocuronium in obese patients be based on ideal or corrected body weight? Anesth Analg. 2009;109(3):787–92. https://doi.org/10.1213/ane.0b013e3181b0826a.

21. Lemmens HJM, Brodsky JB. The dose of succinylcholine in morbid obesity. Anesth Analg. 2006;102(2):438–42. https://doi.org/10.1213/01.ane.0000194876.00551.0e.

22. De Jong A, Molinari N, Pouzeratte Y, et al. Difficult intubation in obese patients: incidence, risk factors, and complications in the operating theatre and in intensive care units. Br J Anaesth. 2015;114(2):297–306. https://doi.org/10.1093/bja/aeu373.

23. Marsch SC, Steiner L, Bucher E, et al. Succinylcholine versus rocuronium for rapid sequence intubation in intensive care: a prospective, randomized controlled trial. Crit Care. 2011;15(4):R199. https://doi.org/10.1186/cc10367.

24. Ahmad M, Khan NA, Furqan A. Comparing the functional outcome of different dose regimes of succinylcholine when used for rapid induction and intubation. J Ayub Med Coll Abbottabad. 2018;30(3):401–4.

25. Szalados JE, Donati F, Bevan DR. Effect of d-tubocurarine pretreatment on succinylcholine twitch augmentation and neuromuscular blockade. Anesth Analg. 1990;71(1):55–9. https://doi.org/10.1213/00000539-199007000-00009.

26. Schreiber JU, Lysakowski C, Fuchs-Buder T, Tramèr MR. Prevention of succinylcholine-induced fasciculation and myalgia. Anesthesiology. 2005;103(4):877–84. https://doi.org/10.1097/00000542-200510000-00027.

27. Andersson ML, Møller AM, Wildgaard K. Butyrylcholinesterase deficiency and its clinical importance in anaesthesia: a systematic review. Anaesthesia. 2019;74(4):518–28. https://doi.org/10.1111/anae.14545.

28. Davis L, Britten JJ, Morgan M. Cholinesterase its significance in anaesthetic practice. Anaesthesia. 1997;52(3):244–60. https://doi.org/10.1111/j.1365-2044.1997.084-az0080.x.

29. Paul D, Atherton L, Hunter JM. Clinical pharmacokinetics of the newer neuromuscular blocking drugs. Clin Pharmacokinet. 1999;36(3):169–89. https://doi.org/10.2165/00003088-199936030-00001.

30. Gronert GA. Cardiac arrest after succinylcholine. Anesthesiology. 2001;94(3):523–9. https://doi.org/10.1097/00000542-200103000-00026.

31. Biebuyck JF, Martyn JAJ, White DA, Gronert GA, Jaffe RS, Ward JM. Up-and-down regulation of skeletal muscle acetylcholine receptors effects on neuromuscular blockers. Anesthesiology. 1992;76(5):822–43. https://doi.org/10.1097/00000542-199205000-00022.

32. Schuster F, Moegele S, Johannsen S, Roewer N. Malignant hyperthermia in the intensive care setting. Crit Care. 2014;18(1):411. https://doi.org/10.1186/cc13744.

33. O'Flynn RP, Shutack JG, Rosenberg H, Fletcher JE. Masseter muscle rigidity and malignant hyperthermia susceptibility in pediatric patients an update on management and diagnosis. Anesthesiology. 1994;80(6):1228–33. https://doi.org/10.1097/00000542-199406000-00009.

34. Hopkins PM. Malignant hyperthermia: advances in clinical management and diagnosis. Br J Anaesth. 2000;85(1):118–28. https://doi.org/10.1093/bja/85.1.118.

35. Kelly RE, Dinner M, Turner LS, Haik B, Abramson DH, Daines P. Succinylcholine increases intraocular pressure in the human eye with the extraocular muscles detached. Anesthesiology. 1993;79(5):948–52. https://doi.org/10.1097/00000542-199311000-00012.

36. Martyn JAJ, Fagerlund MJ, Eriksson LI. Basic principles of neuromuscular transmission. Anaesthesia. 2009;64(s1):1–9. https://doi.org/10.1111/j.1365-2044.2008.05865.x.

37. Goodner JA, Likar EJ, Hoff AL, Quedado JM, Kohli A, Ellison P. Clinical impact of sugammadex in the reversal of neuromuscular blockade. Cureus. 2021;3:e15413. https://doi.org/10.7759/cureus.15413.

38. Bash LD, Turzhitsky V, Black W, Urman RD. Neuromuscular blockade and reversal agent practice variability in the US inpatient surgical settings. Adv Ther. 2021;38(9):4736–55. https://doi.org/10.1007/s12325-021-01835-2.

39. Tran DT, Newton EK, Mount VA, Lee JS, Wells GA, Perry JJ. Rocuronium versus succinylcholine for rapid sequence induction intubation. Cochrane Database Syst Rev. 2015;2015(10):CD002788. https://doi.org/10.1002/14651858.CD002788.pub3.

40. Lennon RL, Olson RA, Gronert GA. Atracurium or Vecuronium for rapid sequence endotracheal intubation. Anesthesiology. 1986;64(4):510–2. https://doi.org/10.1097/00000542-198604000-00018.

41. Khuenl-Brady KS, Sparr H. Clinical pharmacokinetics of rocuronium bromide. Clin Pharmacokinet. 1996;31(3):174–83. https://doi.org/10.2165/00003088-199631030-00002.

42. Tarbeeh GA, Othman MM. The pharmacodynamics of vecuronium in chronic renal failure patients: the impact of different priming doses. Ren Fail. 2012;34(7):827–33. https://doi.org/10.3109/0886022X.2012.684552.

43. Khalil M, D'Honneur G, Duvaldestin P, Slavov V, Hys CD, Gomeni R. Pharmacokinetics and pharmacodynamics of rocuronium in patients with cirrhosis. Anesthesiology. 1994;80(6):1241–7. https://doi.org/10.1097/00000542-199406000-00011.

44. Szenohradszky J, Fisher DM, Segredo V, et al. Pharmacokinetics of rocuronium bromide (ORG 9426) in patients with normal renal function or patients undergoing cadaver renal transplantation. Anesthesiology. 1992;77(5):899–904. https://doi.org/10.1097/00000542-199211000-00010.

45. Segredo V, Caldwell JE, Matthay MA, Sharma ML, Gruenke LD, Miller RD. Persistent paralysis in critically ill patients after long-term administration of vecuronium. N Engl J Med. 1992;327(8):524–8. https://doi.org/10.1056/NEJM199208203270804.

46. Lynam DP, Cronnelly R, Castagnoli KP, et al. The pharmacodynamics and pharmacokinetics of vecuronium in patients anesthetized with isoflurane with normal renal function or with renal failure. Anesthesiology. 1988;69(2):227–31. https://doi.org/10.1097/00000542-198808000-00012.

47. Somogyi AA, Shanks CA, Triggs EJ. Clinical pharmacokinetics of pancuronium bromide. Eur J Clin Pharmacol. 1976;10(5):367–72. https://doi.org/10.1007/BF00565627.

48. Kopman AF. Pancuronium, gallamine, and d-tubocurarine compared: is speed of onset inversely related to drug potency? Anesthesiology. 1989;70(6):915–20.

49. Gursoy S, Bagcivan I, Durmus N, et al. Investigation of the cardiac effects of pancuronium, rocuronium, vecuronium, and mivacurium on the isolated rat atrium. Curr Ther Res. 2011;72(5):195–203. https://doi.org/10.1016/j.curtheres.2011.09.001.

50. Wastila WB, Maehr RB, Turner GL, Hill DA, Phil M, Savarese JJ. Comparative pharmacology of cisatracurium (51W89), atracurium, and five isomers in cats. Anesthesiology. 1996;85(1):169–77. https://doi.org/10.1097/00000542-199607000-00023.

51. Kisor DF, Schmith VD. Clinical pharmacokinetics of cisatracurium besilate. Clin Pharmacokinet. 1999;36(1):27–40. https://doi.org/10.2165/00003088-199936010-00003.

52. Caldwell JE, Heier T, Kitts JB, Lynam DP, Fahey MR, Miller RD. COMPARISON OF THE NEUROMUSCULAR BLOCK INDUCED BY MIVACURIUM, SUXAMETHONIUM OR ATRACURIUM DURING NITROUS OXIDE-FENTANYL ANAESTHESIA. Br J Anaesth. 1989;63(4):393–9. https://doi.org/10.1093/bja/63.4.393.

53. Murray MJ, DeBlock H, Erstad B, et al. Clinical practice guidelines for sustained neuromuscular blockade in the adult critically ill patient. Crit Care Med. 2016;44(11):2079–103. https://doi.org/10.1097/CCM.0000000000002027.

54. Papazian L, Forel JM, Gacouin A, et al. Neuromuscular blockers in early acute respiratory distress syndrome. N Engl J Med. 2010;363(12):1107–16. https://doi.org/10.1056/NEJMoa1005372.

55. National Heart, Lung, and Blood Institute PETAL Clinical Trials Network, Moss M, Huang DT, Brower RG, et al. Early neuromuscular blockade in the acute respiratory distress syndrome. N Engl J Med. 2019;381(8):785–8. https://doi.org/10.1056/NEJMc1908874.

56. Flannery AH, Moss M. Rescue neuromuscular blockade in acute respiratory distress syndrome should not be flat dose. Crit Care Med. 2020;48(4):588–90. https://doi.org/10.1097/CCM.0000000000004171.

57. Co I, Hyzy RC. Rescue neuromuscular blockade in acute respiratory distress syndrome should be flat dose. Crit Care Med. 2020;48(4):591–3. https://doi.org/10.1097/CCM.0000000000004198.

58. Hraiech S, Forel JM, Guervilly C, et al. How to reduce cisatracurium consumption in ARDS patients: the TOF-ARDS study. Ann Intensive Care. 2017;7(1):79. https://doi.org/10.1186/s13613-017-0305-2.

59. Tateishi A, Zornow MH, Scheller MS, Canfell PC. ELECTROENCEPHALOGRAPHIC EFFECTS OF LAUDANOSINE IN AN ANIMAL MODEL OF EPILEPSY. Br J Anaesth. 1989;62(5):548–52. https://doi.org/10.1093/bja/62.5.548.

60. Fodale V, Santamaria LB. Laudanosine, an atracurium and cisatracurium metabolite. EJA. 2002;19(07):466. https://doi.org/10.1017/S0265021502000777.

61. Cook DR, Stiller RL, Weakly JN, Chakravorti S, Brandom BW, Welch RM. In vitro metabolism of mivacurium chloride (BW B1090U) and succinylcholine. Anesth Analg. 1989;68(4):452–6.

62. Basta SJ. Clinical pharmacology of mivacurium chloride: a review salvatore. J Clin Anesth. 1992;4(2):153–63. https://doi.org/10.1016/0952-8180(92)90034-X.

63. Soto RG, Dunipace D. Mivacurium: return of a drug seeking an indication? ASA Monitor. 2017;81(5):30–1.

64. Thilen SR, Weigel WA, Todd MM, et al. 2023 American Society of Anesthesiologists Practice Guidelines for monitoring and antagonism of neuromuscular blockade: a report

by the American Society of Anesthesiologists Task Force on neuromuscular blockade. Anesthesiology. 2023;138(1):13–41. https://doi.org/10.1097/ALN.0000000000004379.

65. Phillips S, Slewarl PA, Bilgin AB. A survey of the management of neuromuscular blockade monitoring in Australia and New Zealand. Anaesth Intensive Care. 2013;41(3):374–9. https://doi.org/10.1177/0310057X1304100316.

66. Checketts MR, Alladi R, Ferguson K, et al. Recommendations for standards of monitoring during anaesthesia and recovery 2015: Association of Anaesthetists of Great Britain and Ireland. Anaesthesia. 2016;71(1):85–93. https://doi.org/10.1111/anae.13316.

67. Ortega R, Brull SJ, Prielipp R, Gutierrez A, De La Cruz R, Conley CM. Monitoring neuromuscular function. N Engl J Med. 2018;378(4):e6. https://doi.org/10.1056/NEJMvcm1603741.

68. Brull SJ, Kopman AF. Current status of neuromuscular reversal and monitoring. Anesthesiology. 2017;126(1):173–90. https://doi.org/10.1097/ALN.0000000000001409.

69. Pedersen T, Viby-Mogensen J, Bang U, Olsen NV, Jensen E, Engbæk J. Does perioperative tactile evaluation of the train-of-four response influence the frequency of postoperative residual neuromuscular blockade? Anesthesiology. 1990;73(5):835–9. https://doi.org/10.1097/00000542-199011000-00007.

70. Appiah-Ankam J, Hunter JM. Pharmacology of neuromuscular blocking drugs. Contin Educ Anaesth Crit Care Pain. 2004;4(1):2–7. https://doi.org/10.1093/bjaceaccp/mkh002.

71. El-Orbany MI, Joseph NJ, Salem MR. The relationship of posttetanic count and train-of-four responses during recovery from intense cisatracurium-induced neuromuscular blockade. Anesth Analg. 2003;97:80–4. https://doi.org/10.1213/01.ANE.0000063825.19503.49.

72. Cammu G, De Witte J, De Veylder J, et al. Postoperative residual paralysis in outpatients versus inpatients. Anesth Analg. 2006;102(2):426–9. https://doi.org/10.1213/01.ane.0000195543.61123.1f.

73. Murphy GS, Szokol JW, Marymont JH, Greenberg SB, Avram MJ, Vender JS. Residual neuromuscular blockade and critical respiratory events in the postanesthesia care unit. Anesth Analg. 2008;107(1):130–7. https://doi.org/10.1213/ane.0b013e31816d1268.

74. Eikermann M, Groeben H, Hüsing J, Peters J. Accelerometry of adductor pollicis muscle predicts recovery of neuromuscular blockade in anesthetized patients. Anesthesiology. 2003;98(6):1333–7. https://doi.org/10.1097/00000542-200306000-00006.

75. Lee HJ, Kim KS, Jeong JS, Cheong MA, Shim JC. Comparison of the adductor pollicis, orbicularis oculi, and corrugator supercilii as indicators of adequacy of muscle relaxation for tracheal intubation. Br J Anaesth. 2009;102(6):869–74. https://doi.org/10.1093/bja/aep064.

76. Itoh H, Shibata K, Yoshida M, Yamamoto K. Neuromuscular monitoring at the orbicularis oculi may overestimate the blockade in myasthenic patients. Anesthesiology. 2000;93(5):1194–7. https://doi.org/10.1097/00000542-200011000-00010.

77. Murphy GS, Brull SJ. Residual neuromuscular block: lessons unlearned. Part I definitions, incidence, and adverse physiologic effects of residual neuromuscular block. Anesth Analg. 2010;111(1):120–8. https://doi.org/10.1213/ANE.0b013e3181da832d.

78. Foster J, Kish G. A national survey of critical care nurses' practices related to administration of neuromuscular blocking agents. Am J Crit Care. 2001;10(3):139.

79. Beemer GH, Bjorksten AR, Dawson PJ, Dawson RJ, Heenan PJ, Robertson BA. DETERMINANTS OF THE REVERSAL TIME OF COMPETITIVE NEUROMUSCULAR BLOCK BY ANTICHOLINESTERASES. Br J Anaesth. 1991;66(4):469–75. https://doi.org/10.1093/bja/66.4.469.

80. Srivastava A, Hunter JM. Reversal of neuromuscular block. Br J Anaesth. 2009;103(1):115–29. https://doi.org/10.1093/bja/aep093.

81. Gijsenbergh F, Ramael S, Houwing N, Van Iersel T. First human exposure of org 25969, a novel agent to reverse the action of rocuronium bromide. Anesthesiology. 2005;103(4):695–703. https://doi.org/10.1097/00000542-200510000-00007.

82. Asztalos L, Szabó-Maák Z, Gajdos A, et al. Reversal of vecuronium-induced neuromuscular blockade with low-dose sugammadex at train-of-four count of four. Anesthesiology. 2017;127(3):441–9. https://doi.org/10.1097/ALN.0000000000001744.

83. Fink H, Schaller. Sugammadex as a reversal agent for neuromuscular block: an evidence-based review. Core Evid. 2013;8:57. https://doi.org/10.2147/CE.S35675.

84. Bowdle TA, Haththotuwegama KJ, Jelacic S, Nguyen ST, Togashi K, Michaelsen KE. A dose-finding study of sugammadex for reversal of rocuronium in cardiac surgery patients and postoperative monitoring for recurrent paralysis. Anesthesiology. 2023;139(1):6–15. https://doi.org/10.1097/ALN.0000000000004578.

85. Geldner G, Niskanen M, Laurila P, et al. A randomised controlled trial comparing sugammadex and neostigmine at different depths of neuromuscular blockade in patients undergoing laparoscopic surgery*. Anaesthesia. 2012;67(9):991–8. https://doi.org/10.1111/j.1365-2044.2012.07197.x.

86. Chambers D, Paulden M, Paton F, et al. Sugammadex for reversal of neuromuscular block after rapid sequence intubation: a systematic review and economic assessment. Br J Anaesth. 2010;105(5):568–75. https://doi.org/10.1093/bja/aeq270.

87. Carvalho H, Verdonck M, Cools W, Geerts L, Forget P, Poelaert J. Forty years of neuro-muscular monitoring and postoperative residual curarisation: a meta-analysis and evaluation of confidence in network meta-analysis. Br J Anaesth. 2020;125(4):466–82. https://doi.org/10.1016/j.bja.2020.05.063.

88. O'Reilly-Shah VN, Wolf FA, Jabaley CS, Lynde GC. Using a worldwide in-app survey to explore sugammadex usage patterns: a prospective observational study. Br J Anaesth. 2017;119(2):333–5. https://doi.org/10.1093/bja/aex171.

89. Hunter JM, Naguib M. Sugammadex-induced bradycardia and asystole: how great is the risk? Br J Anaesth. 2018;121(1):8–12. https://doi.org/10.1016/j.bja.2018.03.003.

90. Takazawa T, Mitsuhata H, Mertes PM. Sugammadex and rocuronium-induced anaphylaxis. J Anesth. 2016;30(2):290–7. https://doi.org/10.1007/s00540-015-2105-x.

91. Hunter JM. Reversal of neuromuscular block. BJA Educ. 2020;20(8):259–65. https://doi.org/10.1016/j.bjae.2020.03.008.

92. Staals LM, Snoeck MMJ, Driessen JJ, Flockton EA, Heeringa M, Hunter JM. Multicentre, parallel-group, comparative trial evaluating the efficacy and safety of sugammadex in patients with end-stage renal failure or normal renal function. Br J Anaesth. 2008;101(4):492–7. https://doi.org/10.1093/bja/aen216.

93. Kim YS, Lim BG, Won YJ, Oh SK, Oh JS, Cho SA. Efficacy and safety of sugammadex for the reversal of rocuronium-induced neuromuscular blockade in patients with end-stage renal disease: a systematic review and meta-analysis. Medicina. 2021;57(11):1259. https://doi.org/10.3390/medicina57111259.

94. Cammu G, Van Vlem B, Van Den Heuvel M, et al. Dialysability of sugammadex and its complex with rocuronium in intensive care patients with severe renal impairment. Br J Anaesth. 2012;109(3):382–90. https://doi.org/10.1093/bja/aes207.

95. Richardson MG, Raymond BL. Sugammadex administration in pregnant women and in women of reproductive potential: a narrative review. Anesth Analg. 2020;130(6):1628–37. https://doi.org/10.1213/ANE.0000000000004305.

96. Feldman S, Karalliedde L. Drug interactions with neuromuscular blockers. Drug Safety. 1996;15(4):261–73. https://doi.org/10.2165/00002018-199615040-00004.

97. Foo I, Macfarlane AJR, Srivastava D, et al. The use of intravenous lidocaine for postoperative pain and recovery: international consensus statement on efficacy and safety. Anaesthesia. 2021;76(2):238–50. https://doi.org/10.1111/anae.15270.

98. Kang JM. Antibiotics and muscle relaxation. Korean J Anesthesiol. 2013;64(2):103. https://doi.org/10.4097/kjae.2013.64.2.103.

99. Soriano SG, Martyn JAJ. Antiepileptic-induced resistance to neuromuscular blockers: mechanisms and clinical significance. Clin Pharmacokinet. 2004;43(2):71–81. https://doi.org/10.2165/00003088-200443020-00001.

100. Berdai MA, Labib S, Harandou M. Prolonged neuromuscular block in a preeclamptic patient induced by magnesium sulfate. Pan Afr Med J. 2016;25:25. https://doi.org/10.11604/pamj.2016.25.5.6616.

101. Kishimoto N, Yoshikawa H, Seo K. Potentiation of rocuronium bromide by lithium carbonate: a case report. Anesth Prog. 2020;67(3):146–50. https://doi.org/10.2344/anpr-66-04-04.

102. Siu BMK, Kwak GH, Ling L, Hui P. Predicting the need for intubation in the first 24 h after critical care admission using machine learning approaches. Sci Rep. 2020;10(1):20931. https://doi.org/10.1038/s41598-020-77893-3.

103. Jaber S, Amraoui J, Lefrant JY, et al. Clinical practice and risk factors for immediate complications of endotracheal intubation in the intensive care unit: a prospective, multiple-center study*. Crit Care Med. 2006;34(9):2355–61. https://doi.org/10.1097/01.CCM.0000233879.58720.87.

104. Simpson GD, Ross MJ, McKeown DW, Ray DC. Tracheal intubation in the critically ill: a multi-centre national study of practice and complications. Br J Anaesth. 2012;108(5):792–9. https://doi.org/10.1093/bja/aer504.

105. Divatia J, Khan P, Myatra S. Tracheal intubation in the ICU: life saving or life threatening? Indian J Anaesth. 2011;55(5):470. https://doi.org/10.4103/0019-5049.89872.

106. Wilcox SR, Bittner EA, Elmer J, et al. Neuromuscular blocking agent administration for emergent tracheal intubation is associated with decreased prevalence of procedure-related complications*. Crit Care Med. 2012;40(6):1808–13. https://doi.org/10.1097/CCM.0b013e31824e0e67.

107. Lundstrøm LH, Duez CH, Nørskov AK, et al. Avoidance versus use of neuromuscular blocking agents for improving conditions during tracheal intubation or direct laryngoscopy in adults and adolescents. Cochrane Database Syst Rev. 2017;5(5):CD009237. https://doi.org/10.1002/14651858.CD009237.pub2.

108. Lundstrøm LH, Møller AM, Rosenstock C, Astrup G, Gätke MR, Wetterslev J. Avoidance of neuromuscular blocking agents may increase the risk of difficult tracheal intubation: a cohort study of 103 812 consecutive adult patients recorded in the Danish Anaesthesia Database. Br J Anaesth. 2009;103(2):283–90. https://doi.org/10.1093/bja/aep124.

109. Fitzgerald E, Hodzovic I, Smith AF. 'From darkness into light': time to make awake intubation with videolaryngoscopy the primary technique for an anticipated difficult airway? Anaesthesia. 2015;70(4):387–92. https://doi.org/10.1111/anae.13042.

110. Bellani G, Laffey JG, Pham T, et al. Epidemiology, patterns of care, and mortality for patients with acute respiratory distress syndrome in intensive care units in 50 countries. JAMA. 2016;315(8):788. https://doi.org/10.1001/jama.2016.0291.

111. Zambon M, Vincent JL. Mortality rates for patients with acute lung injury/ARDS have decreased over time. Chest. 2008;133(5):1120–7. https://doi.org/10.1378/chest.07-2134.

112. Acute Respiratory Distress Syndrome Network, et al. Ventilation with lower tidal volumes as compared with traditional tidal volumes for acute lung injury and the acute respiratory distress syndrome. N Engl J Med. 2000;342(18):1301–8. https://doi.org/10.1056/NEJM200005043421801.

113. Gainnier M, Roch A, Forel JM, et al. Effect of neuromuscular blocking agents on gas exchange in patients presenting with acute respiratory distress syndrome*. Crit Care Med. 2004;32(1):113–9. https://doi.org/10.1097/01.CCM.0000104114.72614.BC.

114. Neto AS, Pereira VGM, Espósito DC, Damasceno MCT, Schultz MJ. Neuromuscular blocking agents in patients with acute respiratory distress syndrome: a summary of the current evidence from three randomized controlled trials. Ann Intensive Care. 2012;2(1):33. https://doi.org/10.1186/2110-5820-2-33.

115. Alhazzani W, Belley-Cote E, Møller MH, et al. Neuromuscular blockade in patients with ARDS: a rapid practice guideline. Intensive Care Med. 2020;46(11):1977–86. https://doi.org/10.1007/s00134-020-06227-8.

116. Le Conte P, Terzi N, Mortamet G, et al. Management of severe asthma exacerbation: guidelines from the Société Française de Médecine d'Urgence, the Société de Réanimation de Langue Française and the French Group for Pediatric Intensive Care and Emergencies. Ann Intensive Care. 2019;9(1):115. https://doi.org/10.1186/s13613-019-0584-x.

117. Afessa B, Morales I, Cury JD. Clinical course and outcome of patients admitted to an ICU for status asthmaticus. Chest. 2001;120(5):1616–21. https://doi.org/10.1378/chest.120.5.1616.
118. Peters JI, Stupka JE, Singh H, et al. Status asthmaticus in the medical intensive care unit: a 30-year experience. Respir Med. 2012;106(3):344–8. https://doi.org/10.1016/j.rmed.2011.11.015.
119. Awadh Behbehani N, Al-Mane F, D'yachkova Y, Paré P, Fitz Gerald JM. Myopathy following mechanical ventilation for acute severe asthma. Chest. 1999;115(6):1627–31. https://doi.org/10.1378/chest.115.6.1627.
120. Shapiro JM, Condos R, Cole RP. Myopathy in status asthmaticus: relation to neuromuscular blockade and corticosteroid administration. J Intensive Care Med. 1993;8(3):144–52. https://doi.org/10.1177/088506669300800305.
121. Kesler SM, Sprenkle MD, David WS, Leatherman JW. Severe weakness complicating status asthmaticus despite minimal duration of neuromuscular paralysis. Intensive Care Med. 2009;35(1):157–60. https://doi.org/10.1007/s00134-008-1267-5.
122. Khera R, Humbert A, Leroux B, et al. Hospital variation in the utilization and implementation of targeted temperature management in out-of-hospital cardiac arrest. Circ Cardiovasc Quality Outcomes. 2018;11(11):e004829. https://doi.org/10.1161/CIRCOUTCOMES.118.004829.
123. Dankiewicz J, Cronberg T, Lilja G, et al. Hypothermia versus normothermia after out-of-hospital cardiac arrest. N Engl J Med. 2021;384(24):2283–94. https://doi.org/10.1056/NEJMoa2100591.
124. Hypothermia after Cardiac Arrest Study Group. Mild therapeutic hypothermia to improve the neurologic outcome after cardiac arrest. N Engl J Med. 2002;346(8):549–56. https://doi.org/10.1056/NEJMoa012689.
125. Bernard SA, Gray TW, Buist MD, et al. Treatment of comatose survivors of out-of-hospital cardiac arrest with induced hypothermia. N Engl J Med. 2002;346(8):557–63. https://doi.org/10.1056/NEJMoa003289.
126. Lüsebrink E, Binzenhöfer L, Kellnar A, et al. Targeted temperature management in postresuscitation care after incorporating results of the TTM2 trial. JAHA. 2022;11(21):e026539. https://doi.org/10.1161/JAHA.122.026539.
127. Haman F, Blondin DP. Shivering thermogenesis in humans: origin, contribution and metabolic requirement. Temperature. 2017;4(3):217–26. https://doi.org/10.1080/23328940.2017.1328999.
128. Moskowitz A, Andersen LW, Rittenberger JC, et al. Continuous neuromuscular blockade following successful resuscitation from cardiac arrest: a randomized trial. JAHA. 2020;9(17):e017171. https://doi.org/10.1161/JAHA.120.017171.
129. Lin T, Yao Y, Xu Y, Huang HB. Neuromuscular blockade for cardiac arrest patients treated with targeted temperature management: a systematic review and meta-analysis. Front Pharmacol. 2022;13:780370. https://doi.org/10.3389/fphar.2022.780370.
130. Hifumi T, Inoue A, Arimoto H, et al. The association between neuromuscular blockade use during target temperature management and neurological outcomes. Am J Emerg Med. 2021;46:289–94. https://doi.org/10.1016/j.ajem.2020.07.078.
131. Sanfilippo F, Santonocito C, Veenith T, Astuto M, Maybauer MO. The role of neuromuscular blockade in patients with traumatic brain injury: a systematic review. Neurocrit Care. 2015;22(2):325–34. https://doi.org/10.1007/s12028-014-0061-1.
132. Lazaridis C, DeSantis SM, McLawhorn M, Krishna V. Liberation of neurosurgical patients from mechanical ventilation and tracheostomy in neurocritical care. J Crit Care. 2012;27(4):417.e1–8. https://doi.org/10.1016/j.jcrc.2011.08.018.
133. Ely EW. The ABCDEF bundle: science and philosophy of how ICU liberation serves patients and families. Crit Care Med. 2017;45(2):321–30. https://doi.org/10.1097/CCM.0000000000002175.
134. Mehta S, Burry L, Fischer S, et al. Canadian survey of the use of sedatives, analgesics, and neuromuscular blocking agents in critically ill patients*. Crit Care Med. 2006;34(2):374–80. https://doi.org/10.1097/01.CCM.0000196830.61965.F1.

135. Zhou C, Wu L, Ni F, Ji W, Wu J, Zhang H. Critical illness polyneuropathy and myopathy: a systematic review. Neural Regen Res. 2014;9(1):101. https://doi.org/10.4103/1673-5374.125337.
136. Latronico N, Bolton CF. Critical illness polyneuropathy and myopathy: a major cause of muscle weakness and paralysis. Lancet Neurol. 2011;10(10):931–41. https://doi.org/10.1016/S1474-4422(11)70178-8.
137. Coakley JH, Nagendran K, Yarwood GD, Honavar M, Hinds CJ. Patterns of neurophysiological abnormality in prolonged critical illness. Intensive Care Med. 1998;24(8):801–7. https://doi.org/10.1007/s001340050669.
138. Guarneri B, Bertolini G, Latronico N. Long-term outcome in patients with critical illness myopathy or neuropathy: the Italian multicentre CRIMYNE study. J Neurol Neurosurg Psychiatry. 2008;79(7):838–41. https://doi.org/10.1136/jnnp.2007.142430.
139. Barohn RJ, Jackson CE, Rogers SJ, Ridings LW, McVey AL. Prolonged paralysis due to nondepolarizing neuromuscular blocking agents and corticosteroids. Muscle Nerve. 1994;17(6):647–54. https://doi.org/10.1002/mus.880170613.
140. Puthucheary Z, Rawal J, Ratnayake G, Harridge S, Montgomery H, Hart N. Neuromuscular blockade and skeletal muscle weakness in critically ill patients: time to rethink the evidence? Am J Respir Crit Care Med. 2012;185(9):911–7. https://doi.org/10.1164/rccm.201107-1320OE.
141. Pereira RMR, Freire De Carvalho J. Glucocorticoid-induced myopathy. Joint Bone Spine. 2011;78(1):41–4. https://doi.org/10.1016/j.jbspin.2010.02.025.
142. O'Rourke KS. MYOPATHIES IN THE ELDERLY. Rheum Dis Clin North Am. 2000;26(3):647–72. https://doi.org/10.1016/S0889-857X(05)70160-5.
143. Wagner BK, Zavotsky KE, Sweeney JB, Palmeri BA, Hammond JS. Patient recall of therapeutic paralysis in a surgical critical care unit. Pharmacotherapy. 1998;18(2):358–63.
144. Strøm T, Martinussen T, Toft P. A protocol of no sedation for critically ill patients receiving mechanical ventilation: a randomised trial. Lancet. 2010;375(9713):475–80. https://doi.org/10.1016/S0140-6736(09)62072-9.
145. Girard TD, Kress JP, Fuchs BD, et al. Efficacy and safety of a paired sedation and ventilator weaning protocol for mechanically ventilated patients in intensive care (awakening and breathing controlled trial): a randomised controlled trial. Lancet. 2008;371(9607):126–34. https://doi.org/10.1016/S0140-6736(08)60105-1.
146. Parry SM, Puthucheary ZA. The impact of extended bed rest on the musculoskeletal system in the critical care environment. Extrem Physiol Med. 2015;4(1):16. https://doi.org/10.1186/s13728-015-0036-7.
147. Vanhorebeek I, Latronico N, Van Den Berghe G. ICU-acquired weakness. Intensive Care Med. 2020;46(4):637–53. https://doi.org/10.1007/s00134-020-05944-4.
148. Grabitz SD, Rajaratnam N, Chhagani K, et al. The effects of postoperative residual neuromuscular blockade on hospital costs and intensive care unit admission: a population-based cohort study. Anesth Analg. 2019;128(6):1129–36. https://doi.org/10.1213/ANE.0000000000004028.
149. Ross J, Ramsay DP, Sutton-Smith LJ, Willink RD, Moore JE. Residual neuromuscular blockade in the ICU: a prospective observational study and national survey. Anaesthesia. 2022;77(9):991–8. https://doi.org/10.1111/anae.15789.
150. Eriksson LI, Sundman E, Olsson R, et al. Functional assessment of the pharynx at rest and during swallowing in partially paralyzed humans. Anesthesiology. 1997;87(5):1035–43. https://doi.org/10.1097/00000542-199711000-00005.
151. Sundman E, Witt H, Olsson R, Ekberg O, Kuylenstierna R, Eriksson LI. The incidence and mechanisms of pharyngeal and upper esophageal dysfunction in partially paralyzed humans. Anesthesiology. 2000;92(4):977–84. https://doi.org/10.1097/00000542-200004000-00014.
152. Kopman AF, Yee PS, Neuman GG. Relationship of the train-of-four fade ratio to clinical signs and symptoms of residual paralysis in awake volunteers. Anesthesiology. 1997;86(4):765–71. https://doi.org/10.1097/00000542-199704000-00005.
153. Rosboch GL, Ceraolo E, Balzani E, Brazzi L. Neuromuscular blocking agents in the ICU: why work blindfolded? Anesth Analg. 2021;132(5):e73. https://doi.org/10.1213/ANE.0000000000005353.

154. Leslie K, Chan MTV, Myles PS, Forbes A, McCulloch TJ. Posttraumatic stress disorder in aware patients from the B-aware trial. Anesth Analg. 2010;110(3):823–8. https://doi.org/10.1213/ANE.0b013e3181b8b6ca.

155. Pappal RD, Roberts BW, Winkler W, Yaegar LH, Stephens RJ, Fuller BM. Awareness with paralysis in mechanically ventilated patients in the emergency department and ICU: a systematic review and meta-analysis*. Crit Care Med. 2021;49(3):e304–14. https://doi.org/10.1097/CCM.0000000000004824.

156. Parate L, Kaur N, Iyer S, Geetha C. The study of postoperative recall in patients under total intravenous anesthesia. Anesth Essays Res. 2021;15(2):233. https://doi.org/10.4103/aer.aer_126_21.

157. Punjasawadwong Y, Phongchiewboon A, Bunchungmongkol N. Bispectral index for improving anaesthetic delivery and postoperative recovery. Cochrane Database Syst Rev. 2014;2014(6):CD003843. https://doi.org/10.1002/14651858.CD003843.pub3.

158. Karamchandani K, Rewari V, Trikha A, Batra RK. Bispectral index correlates well with Richmond agitation sedation scale in mechanically ventilated critically ill patients. J Anesth. 2010;24(3):394–8. https://doi.org/10.1007/s00540-010-0915-4.

159. Schuller PJ, Newell S, Strickland PA, Barry JJ. Response of bispectral index to neuromuscular block in awake volunteers. Br J Anaesth. 2015;115:i95–i103. https://doi.org/10.1093/bja/aev072.

160. Messner M, Beese U, Romstöck J, Dinkel M, Tschaikowsky AK. The bispectral index declines during neuromuscular block in fully awake persons. Anesth Analg. 2003;97(2):488–91. https://doi.org/10.1213/01.ANE.0000072741.78244.C0.

161. Sivasankar S, Jasper S, Simon S, Jacob P, John G, Raju R. Eye care in ICU. Indian J Crit Care Med. 2006;10(1):11–4.

162. Sorce LR, Hamilton SM, Gauvreau K, et al. Preventing corneal abrasions in critically ill children receiving neuromuscular blockade: a randomized, controlled trial. Pediatr Crit Care Med. 2009;10(2):171–5. https://doi.org/10.1097/PCC.0b013e3181956ccf.

163. Ezra DG. Preventing exposure keratopathy in the critically ill: a prospective study comparing eye care regimes. Br J Ophthalmol. 2005;89(8):1068–9. https://doi.org/10.1136/bjo.2004.062406.

164. Dong SW, Mertes PM, Petitpain N, Hasdenteufel F, Malinovsky JM, GERAP. Hypersensitivity reactions during anesthesia. Results from the ninth French survey (2005-2007). Minerva Anestesiol. 2012;78(8):868–78.

165. Levy JH. Anaphylactic reactions to neuromuscular blocking drugs: are we making the correct diagnosis? Anesth Analg. 2004;98:881–3. https://doi.org/10.1213/01.ANE.0000115146.70209.4B.

166. Mertes PM, Guttormsen AB, Harboe T, et al. Can spontaneous adverse event reporting systems really be used to compare rates of adverse events between drugs? Anesth Analg. 2007;104(2):471–2. https://doi.org/10.1213/01.ane.0000253671.90500.0b.

167. Reddy JI, Cooke PJ, Van Schalkwyk JM, Hannam JA, Fitzharris P, Mitchell SJ. Anaphylaxis is more common with rocuronium and succinylcholine than with atracurium. Anesthesiology. 2015;122(1):39–45. https://doi.org/10.1097/ALN.0000000000000512.

168. Sadleir PHM, Clarke RC, Bunning DL, Platt PR. Anaphylaxis to neuromuscular blocking drugs: incidence and cross-reactivity in Western Australia from 2002 to 2011. Br J Anaesth. 2013;110(6):981–7. https://doi.org/10.1093/bja/aes506.

169. Haddad S. Tachyphylaxis to cisatracurium—case reports and literature review. Middle East J Anaesthesiol. 2008;19(5):1079–92.

170. Eisenkraft JB, Book WJ, Papatestas AE. Sensitivity to vecuronium in myasthenia gravis: a dose-response study. Can J Anaesth. 1990;37(3):301–6. https://doi.org/10.1007/BF03005579.

171. Paterson IG, Hood JR, Russell SH, Weston MD, Hirech NP. Mivacurium in the myasthenic patient. Br J Anaesth. 1994;73(4):494–8. https://doi.org/10.1093/bja/73.4.494.

172. Nilsson E, Meretoja OA. Vecuronium dose—response and maintenance requirements in patients with myasthenia gravis. Anesthesiology. 1990;73(1):28–32. https://doi.org/10.1097/00000542-199007000-00005.

173. Seigne RD, Scott RPF. Mivacurium chloride and myasthenia gravis. Br J Anaesth. 1994;72(4):468–9. https://doi.org/10.1093/bja/72.4.468.

174. Eisenkraft JB, Book WJ, Mann SM, Papatestas AE, Hubbard M. Resistance to succinylcholine in myasthenia gravis. Anesthesiology. 1988;69(5):760–2. https://doi.org/10.1097/00000542-198811000-00021.

175. Carron M, De Cassai A, Linassi F. Sugammadex in the management of myasthenic patients undergoing surgery: beyond expectations. Ann Transl Med. 2019;7(S8):S307. https://doi.org/10.21037/atm.2019.10.35.

176. De Boer HD, Shields MO, Booij LHDJ. Reversal of neuromuscular blockade with sugammadex in patients with myasthenia gravis: a case series of 21 patients and review of the literature. Eur J Anaesthesiol. 2014;31(12):715–21. https://doi.org/10.1097/EJA.0000000000000153.

177. Naguib M, Kopman AF. Neostigmine-induced weakness: what are the facts? Anaesthesia. 2018;73(9):1055–7. https://doi.org/10.1111/anae.14322.

178. Ibebunjo C, Martyn JAJ. Thermal injury induces greater resistance to d-tubocurarine in local rather than in distant muscles in the rat. Anesth Analg. 2000;91(5):1243–9. https://doi.org/10.1097/00000539-200011000-00036.

179. Dwersteg JF, Pavlin EG, Heimbach DM. Patients with burns are resistant to atracurium. Anesthesiology. 1986;65(5):517–20. https://doi.org/10.1097/00000542-198611000-00012.

180. Han T, Kim H, Bae J, Kim K, Martyn JAJ. Neuromuscular pharmacodynamics of rocuronium in patients with major burns. Anesth Analg. 2004;99:386–92. https://doi.org/10.1213/01.ANE.0000129992.07527.4B.

181. Marathe PH, Dwersteg JF, Pavlin EG, Haschke RH, Heimbach DM, Slattery JT. Effect of thermal injury on the pharmacokinetics and pharmacodynamics of atracurium in humans. Anesthesiology. 1989;70(5):752–5. https://doi.org/10.1097/00000542-198905000-00007.

182. MacLennan N, Heimbach DM, Cullen BF. Anesthesia for major thermal injury. Anesthesiology. 1998;89(3):749–70. https://doi.org/10.1097/00000542-199809000-00027.

183. Ward JM, Martyn JAJ. Burn injury—induced nicotinic acetylcholine receptor changes on muscle membrane. Muscle Nerve. 1993;16(4):348–54. https://doi.org/10.1002/mus.880160403.

184. Bittner EA, Shank E, Woodson L, Martyn JAJ. Acute and perioperative care of the burn-injured patient. Anesthesiology. 2015;122(2):448–64. https://doi.org/10.1097/ALN.0000000000000559.

185. Cartin-Ceba R, Gajic O, Iyer VN, Vlahakis NE. Fetal outcomes of critically ill pregnant women admitted to the intensive care unit for nonobstetric causes*. Crit Care Med. 2008;36(10):2746–51. https://doi.org/10.1097/CCM.0b013e318186b615.

186. Karnad DR, Guntupalli KK. Critical illness and pregnancy: review of a global problem. Crit Care Clin. 2004;20(4):555–76. https://doi.org/10.1016/j.ccc.2004.05.001.

187. Shin J. Anesthetic management of the pregnant patient: part 2. Anesth Prog. 2021;68(2):119–27. https://doi.org/10.2344/anpr-68-02-12.

188. Upadya M, Saneesh P. Anaesthesia for non-obstetric surgery during pregnancy. Indian J Anaesth. 2016;60(4):234. https://doi.org/10.4103/0019-5049.179445.

189. Clark RB, Brown MA, Lattin DL. Neostigmine, atropine, and glycopyrrolate. Anesthesiology. 1996;84(2):450–2. https://doi.org/10.1097/00000542-199602000-00026.

190. Murad SH, Conklin KA, Tabsh KM, Brinkman CR, Erkkola R, Nuwayhid B. Atropine and glycopyrrolate: hemodynamic effects and placental transfer in the pregnant ewe. Anesth Analg. 1981;60(10):710–4.

191. Torres SM, Duarte DF, Glória AS, et al. Sugammadex administration in pregnant patients undergoing non-obstetric surgery: a case series. Braz J Anesthesiol (English Edition). 2022;72(4):525–8. https://doi.org/10.1016/j.bjane.2021.07.034.

192. Stourac P, Adamus M, Seidlova D, et al. Low-dose or high-dose rocuronium reversed with neostigmine or sugammadex for cesarean delivery anesthesia: a randomized controlled noninferiority trial of time to tracheal intubation and extubation. Anesth Analg. 2016;122(5):1536–45. https://doi.org/10.1213/ANE.0000000000001197.

193. Shibusawa M, Ejima Y, Nishino R, Toyama H, Kurosawa S. Use of sugammadex in patients undergoing caesarean section using general anesthesia with rocuronium. Masui. 2012;61(8):805–9.

194. Gaston IN, Lange EMS, Farrer JR, Toledo P. Sugammadex use for reversal in nonobstetric surgery during pregnancy: a reexamination of the evidence. Anesth Analg. 2023;136(6):1217–9. https://doi.org/10.1213/ANE.0000000000006442.

195. Singh S, Klumpner TT, Pancaro C, Rajala B, Kountanis JA. Sugammadex administration in pregnant women: a case series of maternal and fetal outcomes. A&A Practice. 2021;15(2):e01407. https://doi.org/10.1213/XAA.0000000000001407.

196. Et T, Topal A, Erol A, Tavlan A, Kilicaslan A, Tuncer US. The effects of sugammadex on progesterone levels in pregnant rats. Balkan Med J. 2015;32(2):203–7. https://doi.org/10.5152/balkanmedj.2015.15502.

197. Nag K, Singh D, Shetti A, Kumar H, Sivashanmugam T, Parthasarathy S. Sugammadex: a revolutionary drug in neuromuscular pharmacology. Anesth Essays Res. 2013;7(3):302. https://doi.org/10.4103/0259-1162.123211.

198. Mushambi MC, Kinsella SM, Popat M, et al. Obstetric Anaesthetists' Association and Difficult Airway Society guidelines for the management of difficult and failed tracheal intubation in obstetrics. Anaesthesia. 2015;70(11):1286–306. https://doi.org/10.1111/anae.13260.

199. Rucklidge M, Hinton C. Difficult and failed intubation in obstetrics. Contin Educ Anaesth Crit Care Pain. 2012;12(2):86–91. https://doi.org/10.1093/bjaceaccp/mkr060.

200. Smith HAB, Besunder JB, Betters KA, et al. 2022 Society of Critical Care Medicine clinical practice guidelines on prevention and management of pain, agitation, neuromuscular blockade, and delirium in critically ill pediatric patients with consideration of the ICU environment and early mobility. Pediatr Crit Care Med. 2022;23(2):e74–e110. https://doi.org/10.1097/PCC.0000000000002873.

201. Maheshwari M, Sanwatsarkar S, Katakwar M. Pharmacology related to paediatric anaesthesia. Indian J Anaesth. 2019;63(9):698. https://doi.org/10.4103/ija.IJA_487_19.

202. Meakin GH. Neuromuscular blocking drugs in infants and children. Contin Educ Anaesth Crit Care Pain. 2007;7(5):143–7. https://doi.org/10.1093/bjaceaccp/mkm032.

203. Gupta B, Mishra P. A systematic review and meta-analysis of the use of succinylcholine to facilitate tracheal intubation in neonates. Ain-Shams J Anesthesiol. 2021;13(1):68. https://doi.org/10.1186/s42077-021-00185-z.

204. McAuliffe G, Bissonnette B, Boutin C. Should the routine use of atropine before succinylcholine in children be reconsidered? Can J Anaesth. 1995;42(8):724–9. https://doi.org/10.1007/BF03012672.

205. Kovacich NJ, Nelson AC, McCormick T, Kaucher KA. Incidence of bradycardia and the use of atropine in pediatric rapid sequence intubation in the emergency department. Pediatr Emer Care. 2022;38(2):e540–3. https://doi.org/10.1097/PEC.0000000000002382.

206. Segura LG, Lorenz JD, Weingarten TN, et al. Anesthesia and Duchenne or Becker muscular dystrophy: review of 117 anesthetic exposures. Pediatr Anesth. 2013;23(9):855–64. https://doi.org/10.1111/pan.12248.

207. Wong SH, McClaren BJ, Archibald AD, et al. A mixed methods study of age at diagnosis and diagnostic odyssey for Duchenne muscular dystrophy. Eur J Hum Genet. 2015;23(10):1294–300. https://doi.org/10.1038/ejhg.2014.301.

208. Birnkrant DJ, Bushby K, Bann CM, et al. Diagnosis and management of Duchenne muscular dystrophy, part 1: diagnosis, and neuromuscular, rehabilitation, endocrine, and gastrointestinal and nutritional management. Lancet Neurol. 2018;17(3):251–67. https://doi.org/10.1016/S1474-4422(18)30024-3.

209. Kumar A, Kumar A, Bharti AK, Choudhary A, Hussain M, Dhiraj S. A randomized double-blind comparative study of the intubating conditions and hemodynamic effects of Rocuronium and succinylcholine in pediatric patients. Cureus. 2023;15:e44631. https://doi.org/10.7759/cureus.44631.

Chapter 48
Rapid Sequence Intubation

Alyson M. Esteves

48.1 Introduction

Rapid sequence intubation (RSI) is generally considered the preferred pathway for tracheal intubation for patients who have evidence of respiratory failure, loss of airway protection, or impending airway compromise. RSI is conducted by a series of interventions to facilitate successful intubation and minimize the risk of aspiration. These interventions include equipment preparation, planning, pre-oxygenation, pretreatment medication therapy, induction, paralysis, intubation, confirmation of placement, adjustment of mechanical ventilation, and initiation of continuous sedation post-intubation [1]. RSI may not be the preferred intubation strategy for all patients (e.g., head and neck malignancy or upper airway obstruction) [2]. Intubation strategies and medication management for this select patient population are beyond the scope of this chapter. RSI in comparison to non-RSI intubation strategies results in higher first-pass rates of intubation, which is used a surrogate for quality and safety [3, 4]. The rate of first-pass intubation success with RSI is dependent on a number of factors including environment, patient anatomy, equipment, personnel, training, and more [4–6]. These factors make first-pass success rates extremely variable in literature, ranging from 54 to >80% [4–6]. As the number of intubation attempts rises, complications of RSI increase in frequency; however, there is not a direct correlation to increases in mortality [4]. Airway team members vary significantly based on the intubation environment including pre-hospital, emergency department, intensive care unit, operating room, or other locations. Pharmacists have the opportunity to play a pivotal role in the medication management of RSI in a variety of these settings.

A. M. Esteves (✉)
Dartmouth Hitchcock Medical Center, Lebanon, NH, USA
e-mail: alyson.m.esteves@hitchcock.org

© The Author(s), under exclusive license to Springer Nature
Switzerland AG 2025
Y. Alzaidi, M. A. Gebily (eds.), *The Pharmacist's Expanded Role in Critical
Care Medicine*, https://doi.org/10.1007/978-3-031-77335-8_48

48.2   Medication Management

The medication portion of RSI is divided into four sections: premedication, induction, paralysis, and post-intubation care.

48.2.1   Premedication

Premedications for RSI have been considered in a number of disease states; however, utilization is infrequent and controversial. The theory behind premedication is to blunt the sympathetic effects that can occur during the RSI process [7]. RSI has been attributed to hypertension, tachycardia, and rises in intracranial pressure (ICP). These effects are not firmly supported by data and many medications used in the RSI process can actually contribute to hypotension post-intubation [7–9]. Premedications are most commonly considered for RSI scenarios in patients presenting with active airway disease, elevated ICP, or those with cardiovascular presentations and/or comorbidities [7]. Lidocaine and opioids are agents that have the most robust data in this space. Other agents have been utilized, but consensus does not support routine administration. These agents include neuromuscular blockers, atropine, and β-blockers [7, 10, 11]. Timing of administration of premedications is essential to optimize pharmacokinetics in hopes of having the greatest impact toward a successful intubation attempt. Ideally, premedications are administered 3–5 min prior to induction [7]. Potential delays to the RSI process should be considered in this context. The urgent/emergent nature of RSI often doesn't lend itself to additional medications that require delays in therapy to yield optimal benefit. It is important to note that despite these agents being recommended, data is relatively sparse and outdated in this practice area. Furthermore, premedication administration is not covered in the Society of Critical Care Medicine (SCCM) Clinical Practice Guidelines for RSI in the Critically Ill Adult Patient [12].

48.2.2   Premedication: Lidocaine

Lidocaine has been proposed to be beneficial in patients with reactive airway disease, as well as patients with elevated ICP. Lidocaine has been shown in multiple studies to effectively suppress cough and reduce bronchospasm; however, mechanisms behind these benefits are not well understood [13]. Lidocaine should be avoided in patients with bradycardia or heart block, as administration may precipitate cardiac arrest [7, 14]. Literature surrounding lidocaine for cough suppression is diverse around the peri-intubation and post-extubation timeframe, making it generally recognized as a safe and effective therapy. Dosing is variable across literature, with 1.5 mg/kg intravenous (IV) once being the most common strategy [7, 13].

Despite robust cough suppression literature, lidocaine's benefit in bronchospasm is more controversial. A prospective randomized controlled trial (RCT) found that albuterol provided bronchospasm benefit as a pretreatment therapy, whereas lidocaine 1.5 mg/kg IV did not have any benefit [15]. Due to the sparseness of literature and conflicting data, utilization of lidocaine for bronchospasm should be limited. Additionally, literature supporting lidocaine's reduction in ICP is less current, limited in quantity, and conflicting [7, 16]. Some literature has demonstrated reductions or relative reductions in ICP when lidocaine 1.5 mg/kg IV was administered, albeit these studies were outside of the RSI environment [7, 16, 17]. In conclusion, the role of lidocaine for pretreatment of cough, bronchospasm, or prevention/further escalation of ICP increase should be weighed on an individual patient basis. Likely, lidocaine provides minimal benefit for the vast majority of RSI scenarios.

48.2.3   Premedication: Opioids

Short-acting opioids, such as fentanyl, may have a role in pretreatment for RSI. Their primary benefit is to mitigate the sympathetic response from RSI. Ideally short-acting agents are preferred, as longer acting agents may have greater impacts on respiratory depression, somnolence, and hypotension [7]. Fentanyl has been utilized as a pretreatment agent for RSI in doses ranging from 2 to 3 mcg/kg IV [7, 18]. Chest wall rigidity with fentanyl may be witnessed. Rigidity is typically dose dependent, with doses exceeding 500 mcg, but has been implicated with lower doses of 3–5 mcg/kg [7, 19]. Overall, studies have demonstrated favorable hemodynamic benefits with fentanyl as a pretreatment agent in RSI [18, 20]. A prospective RCT evaluated remifentanil (1 mcg/kg) in comparison to lidocaine (1.5 mg/kg) and found that remifentanil was more beneficial at improving hemodynamics during RSI in the setting of propofol induction [21]. In contrast, a subgroup analysis of a prospective multicenter study found fentanyl administration was associated with a higher rate of post-intubation hypotension (OR 1.73; 95% CI 1.01–2.97). Fentanyl was used in 37% of RSI cases in this study [22]. Conflicting literature makes it difficult to recommend pretreatment with fentanyl or other short-acting opiates. Individual patient risk/benefits should be weighed and delays in induction should not occur in order to administer pretreatment agents.

48.2.4   Induction

Administration of induction agents, or sedatives, is the most common initial medication step in RSI. Prevailing induction agents include ketamine, etomidate, fentanyl, midazolam, or propofol. The SCCM RSI guidelines do not recommend any singular agent, nor are there nationally recognized decision pathways for agent selection [12]. The lack of clear guidance makes pharmacists pivotal members of the RSI team by enhancing the knowledge surrounding these medications including aiding in agent selection, dosing, and timing.

Utility of induction agents has been questioned in patients with baseline reduced consciousness (e.g., severe traumatic brain injury). The SCCM RSI guidelines recommend induction in these cases despite the potential increased risk of agent-specific adverse events [12]. Minimal studies exist evaluating RSI in the absence of induction. One multicenter study found that neuromuscular blocker agent (NMBA) utilization in the absence of induction was infrequent (13%) and did not result in any differences in intubation success or hemodynamics [23]. This practice should be avoided due to concerns of awareness with paralysis which will be discussed later in this chapter. Furthermore, there is a small body of literature surrounding the timing of induction and NMBA administration. Concerningly, this literature demonstrated a high rate of NMBA administration (73%) prior to induction agent administration. Administration on NMBAs first was found to yield faster time to intubation (6 s); however, this time is not clinically significant [24]. Consequences of this practice will be discussed later; however, all RSI events should start with the administration of induction agents in order to induce deep sedation prior to NMBA administration [12].

48.2.5 Induction: Ketamine

Ketamine is a noncompetitive *N*-methyl-D-aspartic acid (NMDA) receptor antagonist. Ketamine is beneficial in RSI due to its rapid onset (~30 s) secondary to its high lipophilicity, as well as its amnestic, analgesic, and sedative properties [25, 26]. Ketamine can also provide a secondary benefit of bronchial smooth muscle relaxation. [25, 27] In contrast, administration of ketamine can cause hypertension and tachycardia which seemingly is dose dependent and degrees of rise are not predictable. Ketamine is administered as a 1–2 mg/kg IV bolus over 1 min [26].

The utilization of ketamine in patients with elevated ICP is controversial. Historically, given the sympathomimetic effects of ketamine, it was avoided due to the concern that its use would cause a further rise in ICP. In recent years, a number of publications and systematic reviews have evaluated the impact of ketamine on ICP elevation across a number of clinical scenarios. Cumulatively, these publications state that there is no evidence of harm secondary to ketamine administration when compared to opioids and there was no difference in ICP elevation [28–31]. Heterogeneity of the literature in these reviews should be considered; however, there is little evidence to support avoidance of ketamine in patients with elevated ICP.

Ketofol, or the combination of ketamine and propofol, has been an area of growing interest. The theory behind the medication combination is to mitigate hypotension after intubation. A proof-of-concept case series was conducted evaluating ketofol in RSI in critically ill patients. Ketofol was dosed as 0.5 mg/kg IV of ketamine and 0.5 mg/kg IV of propofol. No significant hemodynamic changes were witnessed and the combination led to successful intubations across all six patients presented [32]. Subsequently, a randomized controlled trial was conducted evaluating ketofol (0.5 mg/kg IV of ketamine and 0.5 mg/kg IV of propofol with one repeat dose available) in comparison to etomidate 0.15 mg/kg IV. The patient population was focused on critically ill patients, with a baseline mean arterial pressure (MAP) of 81 mmHg. There was no clinically significant difference in hemodynamic effects between the two treatment arms. It is worth noting, as will be discussed later, that adrenal insufficiency was more prevalent in the etomidate arm; however, there were no long-term outcomes evaluated in this trial [33]. Ketofol remains a promising medication combination in RSI for patients who may benefit from an improved hemodynamic medication profile.

Furthermore, ketamine can cause an increase in saliva production and tracheobronchial secretions. Although extremely unlikely given the singular dose nature in RSI, untoward complications may arise. Laryngospasm has been theorized in this setting. Anticholinergic agents such as atropine and glycopyrrolate have been evaluated in pediatric literature for management of this adverse effect; however, no literature supports routine utilization in adult patients undergoing RSI with ketamine [34, 35].

Lastly, delirium and dissociative reactions are also a consideration when administering ketamine. Dissociative effects of ketamine have been seen across a variety of publications with doses that are lower than those utilized for RSI [25]. Mitigation of dissociation with benzodiazepines is controversial in literature and opinions vary based on ketamine indication. Ketamine administration should likely be avoided in patients with a past medical history significant for mental health disorders.

48.2.6 Induction: Etomidate

Etomidate is a general anesthetic that has an onset of <1 min and a short duration of action (3–5 min) [36]. Etomidate for RSI is typically dosed as a 0.3 mg/kg IV bolus [36]. Etomidate has been preferred in RSI scenarios due to its favorable pharmacokinetic profile, hemodynamic stability, and reduction in ICP [37]. The largest concern with utilization of etomidate is subsequent adrenal suppression. Through direct enzyme inhibition, etomidate reduces cortisol secretion and production, thus causing relative adrenal insufficiency [38, 39]. This effect is thought to be dose dependent [39]. Literature on this subject is robust and often conflicting based on the patient population studied and evaluated outcomes. It is estimated that the average duration of adrenal insufficiency after a standard intubation dose of etomidate is 48 h [40]. In critically ill patients, etomidate administration during RSI has not been found to have a consistent impact on ICU length of stay, hospital length of stay, duration of mechanical ventilation, increased need for catecholamine support, or mortality [41–44]. One meta-analysis showed a trend towards worsening mortality in patients with higher severity of illness scores who received etomidate. It is worth noting that the severity of illness score classifications differed amongst the included trials [43]. Overall, the SCCM RSI guidelines continue to recommend etomidate as an induction agent in critically ill patients [12].

Evaluation of etomidate in sepsis or septic shock patients is more controversial. One meta-analysis of septic patients showed that patients who received etomidate had a higher mortality (pooled relative risk 1.2). Mortality outcomes included 28-day mortality and in-hospital mortality depending on the included studies [45]. A single center review sought to identify additional patient specific risk factors in septic patients who received etomidate and died during their hospital admission. Abdominal infections (OR 4.55; 95% CI, 2.33–6.25) and multiple vasopressors (OR 7.09; 95% CI, 4.54–16.7) were further attributed to increases in mortality in the setting of etomidate use in sepsis [46]. In contrast, numerous studies and meta-analysis/reviews have demonstrated that use of etomidate in sepsis or septic shock patients does not contribute to longer ICU length of stay, hospital length of stay, duration of mechanical ventilation, or increased mortality [39, 47, 48]. One of these studies demonstrated an increase in post-RSI hypotension; however, that has not been demonstrated across other head-to-head RSI induction trials [33, 39]. Given other favorable RSI induction agents, etomidate should be avoided in the setting of sepsis or septic shock given the mixed results related to long-term outcomes in this patient population.

Minimal studies have evaluated the use of steroids after etomidate initiation to mitigate adrenal insufficiency. The SCCM RSI guidelines recommend against utilization of steroids in this setting [12]. A randomized controlled trial evaluated 48 h of hydrocortisone, administered as a continuous infusion of 200 mg/day, after induction with etomidate. Norepinephrine administration was lower in the hydrocortisone arm; however, long-term outcomes including duration of mechanical ventilation, ICU length of stay, and 28-day mortality did not differ between groups [49]. An additional study evaluated administration of steroids in the operating room (OR) after etomidate administration. Steroid administration included dexamethasone (57%), hydrocortisone (26%), and methylprednisolone (16%). Despite the variation of steroid agent's mineralocorticoid and glucocorticoid activity, there was no difference in in-hospital mortality or cardiovascular morbidity (e.g., hypotension, cardiac arrest, heart failure, shock) across the steroid group. In contrast to the prior study, this review found that steroid administration resulted in a reduction in-hospital length of stay by 1 day [50]. Given the limited amount of evidence for steroid utilization after etomidate, as well as the lack of impact on morbidity and mortality outcomes, steroids should be avoided unless otherwise clinically indicated post-RSI.

48.2.7 Induction: Fentanyl

As described previously, fentanyl is a short-acting opiate with a rapid onset of action. Fentanyl is not indicated as a monotherapy agent in RSI [51]. Minimal data exists discussing the role of fentanyl as a co-agent for RSI. A French study evaluated fentanyl (3 mcg/kg IV) with etomidate and succinylcholine for RSI. The trial noted successful intubation with the use of fentanyl and a deeper depth of sedation

10 min after intubation in the absence of hemodynamic compromise [52]. Another trial evaluated fentanyl (200 mcg IV, non-weight-based dose) in addition to ketamine and rocuronium. The primary outcome, deviation of systolic blood pressure outside of 100–150 mmHg, did not differ between groups. It was noted that the fentanyl group did experience more hypotension (systolic blood pressure [SBP] < 99 mmHg). There was no difference in first-pass success, mortality, or ventilator-free days [53]. In conclusion, the addition of fentanyl may represent a beneficial adjunct to traditional RSI agents; however, further review is warranted to determine what patient population would benefit the most from the addition especially when balancing the risk for hypotension witnessed in the premedication and induction literature.

48.2.8   Induction: Midazolam

Midazolam is a gamma-aminobutyric acid (GABA) agonist with an onset of 1–5 min and a variable duration of action, that is dependent on hepatic and renal function [54]. The SCCM RSI guidelines state that midazolam may be less desirable in the RSI setting due to its longer onset of action in comparison to other induction agents [12]. Despite this, midazolam has demonstrated a high intubation success rate in published literature [55]. Midazolam for induction is dosed as a range of 0.1–0.3 mg/kg IV; however, some studies have evaluated flat dose strategies [54]. A registry review evaluated midazolam dosing strategies and found that adults received on average 3.7 ± 2.5 mg IV (0.08 ± 0.04 mg/kg) of midazolam for RSI, with flat doses of 2, 4, or 5 mg being common strategies [56]. One additional consideration when utilizing midazolam is the risk of hypotension. A single center prospective observational study found a 10% reduction in systolic blood pressure with the utilization of midazolam (2–4 mg) for RSI, resulting in the need for supplemental fluid administration, but not vasopressor therapy [57]. Additionally, a retrospective chart review found no difference in hypotension between midazolam and etomidate [55]. In contrast, a retrospective chart review evaluated midazolam 0.1 mg/kg versus a dose cap strategy (0.1 mg/kg, max of 5 mg) and the incidence of hypotension (SBP <90 mmHg). This study revealed a statistically significant risk of hypotension with escalating doses of midazolam (mean 3.5 mg) [58]. Given these factors, midazolam's role in RSI is limited. If utilized, consideration for the smallest effective dose should be given to avoid hypotension.

48.2.9   Induction: Propofol

Propofol is a GABA-A receptor agonist and also has some NMDA receptor blockade. Propofol has an extremely rapid onset of action (~30 s) due to its high degree of lipophilicity and has a short duration of action (3–10 min). Propofol induction doses range from 1.5 to 3 mg/kg IV [59]. A single center retrospective cohort study evaluated ketamine, propofol, and etomidate in critically ill patients with the goal of assessing long-term outcomes. Propofol demonstrated improved hospital mortality, hospital-free days, ICU mortality, and ICU-free days in comparison to the other studied agents [60]. However, there are conflicting findings in the trauma population related to long-term morbidity and mortality outcomes [61, 62]. Hemodynamic compromise is the largest concern when using propofol for RSI. A multinational prospective observational study evaluating adverse events after intubation found that propofol, although administered at the highest frequency (41.5%), was attributed to the highest rate of cardiovascular instability (63.7%) [SBP <65 mmHg, SBP <90 mmHg for >30 min, new or increase need of vasopressors or fluid bolus >15 mL/kg, severe hypoxemia, or cardiac arrest] [63]. Additional studies have demonstrated similar findings with high rates of post-intubation hypotension [64]. As discussed previously, ketofol may be a beneficial agent combination to ameliorate post-intubation hypotension. Propofol is a favorable and commonly used induction agent, but hypotension risks should be evaluated prior to use.

48.2.10   Paralytics

In RSI, NMBA administration follows induction. NMBA utilization yields more favorable intubation conditions by allowing for ease of ventilation and relaxation of the vocal cords resulting in a higher percentage of first-pass intubation success [12]. A systematic review conducted an analysis of NMBA utilization versus no paralysis during intubation. Lack of paralysis was associated with increased risk of difficult laryngoscopy [risk ratio 2.54, 95% CI 1.53–4.21), as well as upper airway discomfort or injury [65]. As the number of failed intubation attempts rises, the risk of aspiration, desaturation, incorrect tube placement, hypotension, and cardiac arrest increases [66]. Another publication noted increased complications of aspiration, airway trauma, and death in intubations without the utilization of NMBAs [67]. Two paralytics predominate current RSI literature and practice: succinylcholine and rocuronium. The SCCM RSI guidelines recommend either succinylcholine or rocuronium in the absence of contraindications [12]. Despite this recommendation, certain clinical scenarios may benefit from sedation-facilitated intubation (also referred to as awake intubation), or intubation that is conducted in the absence of a paralytic. Clinical scenarios that have been recognized to benefit from the absence of NMBAs include patients with anticipated difficult airways, specifically: patients with head and neck pathology (e.g., malignancy), morbid obesity, and progressive airway compromise [2]. The intubation process and medication utilization differs from that of RSI and is beyond the scope of this chapter.

48.2.11   Succinylcholine

Succinylcholine is a depolarizing NMBA that mimics the action of acetylcholine causing paralysis, as well as muscle fasciculations after administration. Succinylcholine has a rapid onset of <1 min and a duration of paralysis lasting 4–6 min [68]. RSI dosing ranges from 1 to 1.5 mg/kg IV. A meta-analysis compared the efficacy of various dosing strategies of succinylcholine in RSI. The study found that doses ≤0.5 mg/kg were ineffective when compared to 1 mg/kg. There were no differences in intubation conditions when comparing 1 and 1.5 mg/kg. Higher doses were studied (2 mg/kg); however, there is limited safety and efficacy data to support this practice [69].

Succinylcholine has been attributed to rises in serum potassium levels of 0.5–1 mEq/L in the absence renal dysfunction or other conditions that predispose patients to hyperkalemia [70]. Succinylcholine induces rises in potassium, by binding to the acetylcholine receptor longer than acetylcholine, allowing for greater potassium efflux [71]. Specific patient populations are more vulnerable to increases in potassium as they already have an underlying predisposition to hyperkalemia. These populations include patients with crush injuries, burn injuries, rhabdomyolysis, immobility, or demyelinating diseases [70]. Mixed data exists surrounding the risk of hyperkalemia in the setting of renal dysfunction (e.g., hemodialysis or chronic kidney disease) [72]. If patients are deemed to be at an increased risk, alternative NMBAs should be investigated.

Bradycardia is another potential adverse effect of succinylcholine. Atropine has some literature to support its use in ameliorating this effect in the pediatric population, but as described previously this is an uncommon practice in adults [73]. Bradycardia is likely transient and dose related. Minimal data exists in the adult patient population surrounding further management or prevention of bradycardia.

A rare adverse effect of succinylcholine is malignant hyperthermia. The Malignant Hyperthermia Association of the United States (MHAUS) notes that prevalence of malignant hyperthermia with succinylcholine is increased when used in combination with volatile anesthetics, which is predominantly in the OR setting [74]. Despite rare incidence outside of the OR, providers and pharmacists should be aware of the presenting symptoms, as malignant hyperthermia is a medical emergency. Symptoms include masseter tightness, muscle rigidity, tachycardia, hypercapnia, hypoxia, and subsequent acidosis. If identified, immediate administration of dantrolene 2.5 mg/kg IV should occur [75].

48.2.12   Rocuronium

Rocuronium is a non-depolarizing NMBA with an onset of action of ~1 min and a long duration of 20–70 min [76]. Rocuronium dosing varies from 0.6 to 1.5 mg/kg IV. A registry study found that rocuronium doses >1.4 mg/kg were associated with higher first-pass intubation success rates in RSI without an increase in adverse events [77]. Overall, rocuronium has a favorable safety profile, thus making it a commonly used agent in RSI. The largest consideration with its utilization is the prolonged duration, making post-RSI sedation and reversal need important topics.

Rocuronium versus succinylcholine has become a source of debate and has led many providers and pharmacists to have anecdotal preferences. An emergency department (ED) RSI registry review found no difference in the rate of first-pass intubation success between the two medications [78]. Similar findings were confirmed in a prior prospective randomized controlled trial which demonstrated equal efficacy and safety with both agents [79]. Some older literature suggests that rocuronium does not offer as favorable of intubation conditions as succinylcholine, but often these studies used lower rocuronium doses than current practice [80]. Overall patient-specific risk factors for hyperkalemia in contrast to prolonged paralysis should be weighed when selecting an NMBA agent.

48.2.13   Reversal

Reversal of NMBA is rare in the setting of RSI. Typically, reversal is only considered in a "cannot intubate, cannot ventilate" scenario. Sugammadex or neostigmine can be utilized for NMBA reversal. Sugammadex is only effective for reversing rocuronium or vecuronium. It acts by forming a complex around these agents, inhibiting further binding at the nicotinic cholinergic receptors [81]. Sugammadex does not have immediate reversal dosing for vecuronium. Rocuronium reversal doses are higher than traditional reversal doses in this setting (16 mg/kg versus 2–4 mg/kg) [81]. Sugammadex has a rapid onset of action (<3 min), making it an effective reversal agent in an emergency setting. Bradycardia, hypotension, and hypersensitivity reactions have been reported with sugammadex use. Co-administration with other medications has not been studied nor is recommended at this time. In contrast, neostigmine causes elevations in acetylcholine by inhibiting acetylcholinesterase resulting in more competition at the receptor sites with the present NMBA [82]. Neostigmine is effective for all non-depolarizing NMBAs with doses ranging from 0.02 to 0.07 mg/kg (max 5 mg) IV. Neostigmine has a longer onset than sugammadex (~10 min), making it less ideal in an emergent administration scenario. Additionally, bradycardia is a common side effect; therefore, neostigmine should always be administered with glycopyrrolate (0.2 mg IV for each 1 mg of neostigmine) or atropine (15–20 mcg/kg IV) [82]. A small retrospective cohort study evaluated hemodynamic differences between sugammadex versus neostigmine-glycopyrrolate when reversing rocuronium in RSI. This study, albeit 37 patients, did not find any hemodynamic difference between groups [83]. A randomized controlled trial evaluated administration of rocuronium-sugammadex in comparison to succinylcholine and time to spontaneous ventilation. The time to spontaneous ventilation was significantly faster in the NMBA reversal arm (216 s versus 406 s, $P = 0.002$) [84]. Despite the statistical significance, this is likely not clinically significant. The British Difficult Airway Society guidelines state that having sugammadex as a reversal agent for rocuronium is advantageous; however, it does not guarantee clinical improvement in the "cannot intubate, cannot ventilate" scenario. These guidelines do not make recommendations surrounding the utilization of sugammadex in this clinical scenario and defer to individual facility plans [85]. The American Society of Anesthesiologists Management of Difficult Airway Guidelines have less emphasis on sugammadex utilization and state that literature is not robust enough to recommend its use [86]. One proposed published difficult airway pathway focused on airway management alone, specifically emergent cricothyroidotomy, which appears to align with both society guideline recommendations. NMBA reversal was not included in the pathway [87]. Overall, there is limited to no evidence for NMBA reversal in a "cannot intubate, cannot ventilate" scenario, despite reversal being a common discussion.

Additionally, there is a small body of literature focused on NMBA reversal after intubation in patients with neurologic injuries, with the goal of facilitating rapid neurologic exams. A retrospective case series evaluated a small number of patients with traumatic brain injury ($n = 12$ sugammadex administrations). Utilization of sugammadex was associated with changes in neurologic assessments that ultimately changed interventions [88]. A case report of rocuronium reversal in a dialysis-dependent traumatic brain injury patient found similar findings of more rapid assessment and deployment of interventions [89]. An additional retrospective case series ($n = 9$) found similar results in their population [90]. At this time, due to the limited quantity of data, small sample size, and potential for bias within the literature, there is an unclear role of sugammadex in paralytic reversal to expedite neurologic assessments.

48.2.14   Post-intubation Sedation and Analgesia

Immediately following successful intubation, long-term sedation and analgesia plans should be implemented. Depending on the paralytic used during intubation, deep sedation (Richmond Agitation Sedation Scale [RASS]-5) should be continued until the duration of the paralytic action has subsided. The duration is typically <10 min for succinylcholine and ~60 min for rocuronium. Pharmacists should be involved in the discussions surrounding sedation and analgesic choices. While paralytic effects are present, preferred sedatives include continuous infusion propofol or benzodiazepines in combination with an opiate [91]. Specifics surrounding agent selection is beyond the scope of this chapter, but guiding principles should follow suggestions outlined in the SCCM Clinical Practice Guidelines for the Prevention and Management of Pain, Agitation/Sedation, Delirium, Immobility, and Sleep Disruption in Adult Patients in the ICU [91].

A growing body of clinical literature, as well as patient-specific reports, is being published surrounding the concept of awareness with paralysis (i.e., patients that are not deeply sedated and receive paralytic agents). Awareness with paralysis has been linked to post-traumatic stress disorder in patients who encountered this in the OR setting [92]. Incidence in the OR setting has been demonstrated to be 0.13% [93]. Two ED studies sought to evaluate awareness with paralysis incidence in patients who received NMBAs for any indication in the ED (i.e., RSI or post-RSI). These studies found a higher incidence of awareness with paralysis in this setting (2.6–3.4%). Both of these studies attributed higher rates of awareness with paralysis to patients who received rocuronium (OR 5.1–8.64) [94, 95]. The incidence was further supported by a systematic review and meta-analysis of awareness with paralysis in both the ED and ICU environments, which demonstrated an incidence of 3.4% [96]. A recent prospective observational trial of patients who underwent RSI in the ED evaluated the incidence of awareness with paralysis in specifically the RSI setting. Concerningly, the incidence was significantly greater than previously described at 7.4% [97]. Definitions of awareness varied across studies and included possible and definite awareness with paralysis patients. Notably, this publication did not find a difference in rates of awareness with paralysis between NMBAs, induction agent selection, or post-intubation sedation. It is important to recognize that deeper sedation from induction was shown to reduce awareness with paralysis (adjusted OR 0.39; 95% CI 0.22–0.69) [97].

48.2.15 Hemodynamic Support in RSI

Hypotension post-intubation is well described across numerous environments including the ED and ICU. A retrospective cohort study of RSI in the ED found a 23% incidence of post-intubation hypotension (SBP <90 mmHg within 60 min from intubation). Post-intubation hypotension was correlated with an increase in in-hospital mortality (OR 1.9; 95% CI 1.1–3.5), increased ICU length of stay, and increased hospital length of stay. Etomidate and succinylcholine represented the most common induction/paralytic combination [98]. In contrast, an international observational study evaluated RSI in a variety of clinical environments and subsequent complications. The rate of cardiovascular instability (SBP <65 mmHg once or SBP <90 mmHg for >30 min; new or increase in vasopressors; fluid bolus >15 mL/kg to maintain blood pressure) was 42.6%. Notably, propofol and rocuronium were the most commonly used agents [63]. Based on these findings, it is likely that induction and paralytic agent selection influences the rate of post-intubation hypotension.

Further studies evaluated the rate of cardiac arrest post-intubation and factors that increase the likelihood of this occurrence. The incidence of cardiac arrest post-intubation ranges from 2.7 to 4.2% [63, 99, 100]. Cardiac arrest most commonly occurs within 10 min after administration of induction agents [100]. In the ED, a matched case-control study demonstrated that hypotension (SBP ≤ 90 mmHg) prior to intubation was a predictor of cardiac arrest post-intubation (OR 3.67; 95% CI 1.58–8.55) [101]. A multicenter retrospective review of RSI in ICU patients found that pre-intubation hypotension (SBP <90 mmHg), pre-intubation hypoxemia, absence of pre-oxygenation, overweight/obesity, and age >75 to be predictors of post-intubation cardiac arrest [99]. Furthermore, studies have evaluated shock index as a predictor of post-intubation hypotension and cardiac arrest [98, 100]. Shock index is determined by heart rate divided by SBP [102]. Generally, 0.5–0.7 is considered a normal shock index range, with values exceeding 1 predicting an increase in morbidity and mortality [102]. A retrospective cohort study found that a pre-intubation shock index of ≥0.8 predicted post-intubation hypotension (67% sensitivity; 80% specificity) [98]. In a different study, a multivariate regression analysis found that for every 0.1 increase in shock index, the odds of cardiac arrest increased 1.16 times [100]. Due to the ease of calculation and potential impact on morbidity and mortality outcomes, pre-intubation shock index should be evaluated and used as an influential data point when selecting induction and paralytic medication therapy. In patients with a high risk of post-intubation hypotension, ketamine and etomidate should be considered preferential induction agents [103–105]. Propofol and midazolam should generally be avoided in these patients [57, 63, 64].

Evaluation of pre-intubation therapies to resolve pre-existing hypotension is a common discussion. The SCCM RSI guidelines state that there is not enough evidence available at this time to make a recommendation on fluid administration, continuous infusion vasopressors, or push dose vasopressors [12]. Minimal data exists to show outcome benefits when implementing these strategies in patients with pre-intubation hypotension.

Volume resuscitation with blood, if clinically appropriate, or fluid, could be an initial consideration when managing a patient with pre-intubation hypotension. A multicenter, randomized, unblinded trial evaluated prevention of cardiovascular collapse (SBP <60 mmHg; new or increased vasopressor use; cardiac arrest within 1 h; death within 1 h) with a 500 mL IV crystalloid bolus. Cardiovascular collapse occurred in 20% of the crystalloid group versus 18% in the no-fluid group ($P = 0.76$). Individual components of the composite outcome did not differ with fluid administration [106]. Additionally, in a previously mentioned trial, a post-hoc analysis evaluated utilization of a 15 mL/kg IV fluid bolus pre-intubation and was found to not have an influence on hypotension (OR 1.17; 95% CI 0.96–1.44) [107]. Although often a consideration, it appears that fluid boluses have no impact on post-intubation hypotension or the subsequent progression of cardiac arrest.

Vasopressor therapy is a common class of agents used to prevent and treat hypotension in this setting. Push dose vasopressors have become a popular treatment modality. Phenylephrine and epinephrine are most commonly considered; however, there are no standards as to how products should be prepared, standard concentrations, administration strategies, or dosing regimens. Push dose phenylephrine is commonly described using preparations from phenylephrine syringes or vials, yielding a goal concentration of 100 mcg/mL. Generally, recommended doses range from 50 to 200 mcg every 1–5 min [108]. Phenylephrine is advantageous in this setting due to its alpha-2 agonism allowing for vasoconstriction in the absence of increased heart rate. Epinephrine is administered in a 10 mcg/mL concentration. Caution should be exercised if institutional push dose protocols call for dilution of 0.1 mg/mL epinephrine syringes that are used in cardiac arrest. Doses range from 2 to 20 mcg every 1–5 min [108]. Epinephrine is preferred in patients that would benefit from increased inotropy secondary to beta-2 agonism.

The efficacy of push dose vasopressors has been evaluated in several studies. One analysis of two multicenter clinical trials looked at prophylactic vasopressor utilization (bolus or infusion dose increase) and subsequent impact on outcomes. Prophylactic vasopressors were administered in 10% of patients. Vasopressor administration was not associated with a reduction in the rate of post-intubation hypotension or a change in baseline SBP [109]. Similar results were found in a multicenter cohort study, where vasopressors were not found to reduce cardiovascular instability (OR 1.14, 95% CI 0.96–1.44) [107]. In contrast, some studies have found benefits to push dose vasopressor administration when using phenylephrine or epinephrine [110–112]. It is worth noting that two of these studies highlight the need for improved medication safety practices surrounding push dose vasopressors. One study highlighted a medication error rate of 11.2% secondary to doses exceeding the upper recommended limits [110]. The second study highlights the extreme variability in practice patterns surrounding push dose vasopressors, including determination of conditions that warrant administration, timing, and co-administration with other medications [111]. An additional retrospective chart review found a push dose pressor medication error rate of 19%, with 3% of patients receiving overdoses. It was noted that only 1 of these errors happened in the presence of a pharmacist [113]. The contrasting literature and extreme practice variability makes definitive recommendations surrounding push dose vasopressors difficult.

48.2.16 Expanded Role of the Pharmacist

Critical care pharmacists are often at the forefront of patient stabilization across various hospital environments. Practice sites often dictate the overlapping roles of emergency medicine and critical care pharmacists in RSI; however, pharmacists in general can have a significant impact on RSI. To date, there is no emphasis on the role of the critical care pharmacist as it relates to RSI participation [114]. In contrast, emergency medicine pharmacist literature continues to highlight the benefit of pharmacists in this clinical scenario. The American Society of Health-System Pharmacists (ASHP) guideline on emergency medicine pharmacist services recommends a few specific roles pertaining to RSI: intubation, post-intubation care, and medication kit management for RSI [115]. The role of the pharmacist within the RSI preparation and intubation portion is expansive. Pharmacists can aid in risk/benefit discussions surrounding premedication administration, induction agent selection and dosing, paralytic administration selection and dosing, and mitigation strategies for post-intubation hypotension. Using the knowledge of medication's mechanism of action, pharmacokinetics, and pharmacodynamics discussed throughout this chapter, pharmacists can make informed decisions based on patient specific factors to recommend an ideal intubation medication regimen. Furthermore, when intubation conditions deviate (e.g., discussion surrounding awake intubation), pharmacists are primed with the knowledge to extrapolate medication regimens to these scenarios. These roles are emphasized in an emergency medicine position paper [116].

The area with the most evidence surrounding the benefit of a pharmacist in RSI management involves timely initiation of analgesic and sedative medications after intubation. One retrospective cohort study found that after implementation of a pharmacist education intervention, rates of post-intubation analgesia initiation increased. Percentages varied based on pharmacist hours, with higher rates when a pharmacist was present; however, overall rates increased from 20 to 49% [117]. Another retrospective cohort study found that pharmacist presence at RSIs reduced the time to sedation initiation from 28 min to 9 min ($P = 0.007$) and reduced time to analgesia initiation from 44 min to 21 min ($P = 0.057$) [118]. A third retrospective review also demonstrated similar findings with a reduction in average time to sedation initiation from 49 min to 20 min ($P < 0.001$). This study also evaluated long-term outcomes such as duration of mechanical ventilation, hospital length of stay, and ICU length of stay; however, no differences were observed [119]. Despite there being a lack of impact on long-term outcomes in this study, it is likely that rapid initiation of sedation and analgesia post-intubation contributes to reductions in rates of awareness with paralysis and subsequently reduces rates of post-traumatic stress disorder.

Lastly, pharmacists are essential members of the team when it comes to medication preparation. As highlighted earlier, medication safety events are notable in this environment. Medication shortages have also plagued many of the medications involved in the RSI process. Shortages have increased the prevalence of alternative concentrations within care areas, as well as increased reliance on less frequently used agents. Some medications, such as push dose vasopressors, require dilutions, which increases the rate of errors. Pharmacists should be considered the expert when preparing these complex dosing strategies. Additionally, ASHP recommends pharmacist involvement in RSI kit preparation and maintenance. While the critical care environment is not as notorious for emergency kits as the ED, pharmacists should be primed with the knowledge of medications within the kit and ensure that available kits contain medications that are appropriate for the vast majority of patients. Specialized medications (e.g., premedications) should be reserved outside of the kit to help inform decision-making in these urgent/emergent scenarios. Lastly, there is no data surrounding pharmacist training for RSI management. Institutions should consider internal training programs to ensure that pharmacists are well informed of all of the steps in the RSI process to enhance their role and influence on medication management, successful intubation, and subsequent post-intubation care.

References

1. Tintinalli JE, Ma OJ, Yealy DM, Meckler GD, Stapczynski JS, Cline DM, et al. Tintinalli's emergency medicine: a comprehensive study guide, 9e. New York, NY: McGraw-Hill Education; 2020.
2. Ahmad I, El-Boghdadly K, Bhagrath R, Hodzovic I, McNarry AF, Mir F, et al. Difficult airway society guidelines for awake tracheal intubation (ATI) in adults. Anaesthesia. 2020;75(4):509–28.
3. Okubo M, Gibo K, Hagiwara Y, Nakayama Y, Hasegawa K, On behalf of the Japanese Emergency Medicine Network Investigators. The effectiveness of rapid sequence intubation (RSI) versus non-RSI in emergency department: an analysis of multicenter prospective observational study. Int J Emerg Med. 2017;10(1):1.

4. Ljungqvist H, Pirneskoski J, Saviluoto A, Setälä P, Tommila M, Nurmi J. Intubation first-pass success in a high performing pre-hospital critical care system is not associated with 30-day mortality: a registry study of 4496 intubation attempts. Scand J Trauma Resusc Emerg Med. 2022;30:61.

5. Jung W, Kim J. Factors associated with first-pass success of emergency endotracheal intubation. Am J Emerg Med. 2020;38(1):109–13.

6. Nauka PC, Moskowitz A, Fein DG. Appraising first-pass success: during emergency airway management, what does it mean to be successful? Ann Am Thorac Soc. 2023;20(1):21–3.

7. Caro D, Bush S. Pretreatment agents. In: Manual of emergency airway management. 4th ed. Lippincott Williams &Wilkins; 2012. p. 234–9.

8. Kihara S, Brimacombe J, Yaguchi Y, Watanabe S, Taguchi N, Komatsuzaki AT. Hemodynamic responses among three tracheal intubation devices in normotensive and hypertensive patients. Anesth Analg. 2003;96:890–5.

9. Xue FS, Zhang GH, Sun HY, Li CW, Li P, Sun HT, et al. Blood pressure and heart rate changes during intubation: a comparison of direct laryngoscopy and a fibreoptic method. Anaesthesia. 2006;61(5):444–8.

10. Clancy M, Halford S, Walls R, Murphy M. In patients with head injuries who undergo rapid sequence intubation using succinylcholine, does pretreatment with a competitive neuromuscular blocking agent improve outcome? A literature review. Emerg Med J EMJ. 2001;18(5):373–5.

11. Bean A, Jones J. Atropine: re-evaluating its use during paediatric RSI. Emerg Med J. 2007;24(5):361–2.

12. Acquisto NM, Mosier JM, Bittner EA, Patanwala AE, Hirsch KG, Hargwood P, et al. Society of Critical Care Medicine clinical practice guidelines for rapid sequence intubation in the critically ill adult patient. Crit Care Med. 2023;51(10):1411–30.

13. Yang SS, Wang NN, Postonogova T, Yang GJ, McGillion M, Beique F, et al. Intravenous lidocaine to prevent postoperative airway complications in adults: a systematic review and meta-analysis. Br J Anaesth. 2020;124(3):314–23.

14. Lidocaine. https://www.accessdata.fda.gov/drugsatfda_docs/label/2017/018461s058lbl.pdf.

15. Maslow AD, Regan MM, Israel E, Darvish A, Mehrez M, Boughton R, et al. Inhaled albuterol, but not intravenous lidocaine, protects against intubation-induced bronchoconstriction in asthma. Anesthesiology. 2000;93(5):1198–204.

16. Robinson N, Clancy M. In patients with head injury undergoing rapid sequence intubation, does pretreatment with intravenous lignocaine/lidocaine lead to an improved neurological outcome? A review of the literature. Emerg Med J. 2001;18(6):453–7.

17. Salhi B, Stettner E. In defense of the use of lidocaine in rapid sequence intubation. Ann Emerg Med. 2007;49(1):84–6.

18. Adachi YU, Satomoto M, Higuchi H, Watanabe K. Fentanyl attenuates the hemodynamic response to endotracheal intubation more than the response to laryngoscopy. Anesth Analg. 2002;95(1):233–7.

19. Çoruh B, Tonelli MR, Park DR. Fentanyl-induced Chest Wall rigidity. Chest. 2013;143(4):1145–6.

20. Chung KS, Sinatra RS, Halevy JD, Paige D, Silverman DG. A comparison of fentanyl, esmolol, and their combination for blunting the haemodynamic responses during rapid-sequence induction. Can J Anaesth. 1992;39(8):774–9.

21. Kim JT, Shim JK, Kim SH, Ryu HG, Yoon SZ, Jeon YS, et al. Remifentanil vs. lignocaine for attenuating the haemodynamic response during rapid sequence induction using Propofol: double-blind randomised clinical trial. Anaesth Intensive Care. 2007;35(1):20–3.

22. Takahashi J, Goto T, Okamoto H, Hagiwara Y, Watase H, Shiga T, et al. Association of fentanyl use in rapid sequence intubation with post-intubation hypotension. Am J Emerg Med. 2018;36(11):2044–9.

23. Sato N, Hagiwara Y, Watase H, Hasegawa K. A comparison of emergency airway management between neuromuscular blockades alone and rapid sequence intubation: an analysis of multicenter prospective study. BMC Res Notes. 2017;10(1):6.

24. Driver BE, Klein LR, Prekker ME, Cole JB, Satpathy R, Kartha G, et al. Drug order in rapid sequence intubation. Acad Emerg Med. 2019;26(9):1014–21.
25. Zanos P, Moaddel R, Morris PJ, Riggs LM, Highland JN, Georgiou P, et al. Ketamine and ketamine metabolite pharmacology: insights into therapeutic mechanisms. Pharmacol Rev. 2018;70(3):621–60.
26. Ketamine. https://www.accessdata.fda.gov/drugsatfda_docs/label/2017/016812s043lbl.pdf.
27. Goyal S, Agrawal A. Ketamine in status asthmaticus: a review. Indian J Crit Care Med Peer-Rev Off Publ Indian Soc Crit Care Med. 2013;17(3):154–61.
28. Gregers MCT, Mikkelsen S, Lindvig KP, Brøchner AC. Ketamine as an anesthetic for patients with acute brain injury: a systematic review. Neurocrit Care. 2020;33(1):273–82.
29. Cohen L, Athaide V, Wickham ME, Doyle-Waters MM, Rose NGW, Hohl CM. The effect of ketamine on intracranial and cerebral perfusion pressure and health outcomes: a systematic review. Ann Emerg Med. 2015;65(1):43–51.e2.
30. Wang X, Ding X, Tong Y, Zong J, Zhao X, Ren H, et al. Ketamine does not increase intracranial pressure compared with opioids: meta-analysis of randomized controlled trials. J Anesth. 2014;28(6):821–7.
31. Loflin R, Koyfman A. When used for sedation, does ketamine increase intracranial pressure more than fentanyl or sufentanil? Ann Emerg Med. 2015;65(1):55–6.
32. Smischney NJ. Ketamine and propofol combination ("Ketofol") for endotracheal intubations in critically ill patients: a case series. Am J Case Rep. 2015;16:81–6.
33. Smischney NJ, Nicholson WT, Brown DR, Gallo De Moraes A, Hoskote SS, Pickering B, et al. Ketamine/propofol admixture vs etomidate for intubation in the critically ill: KEEP PACE randomized clinical trial. J Trauma Acute Care Surg. 2019;87(4):883–91.
34. Heinz P, Geelhoed GC, Wee C, Pascoe EM. Is atropine needed with ketamine sedation? A prospective, randomised, double blind study. Emerg Med J EMJ. 2006;23(3):206–9.
35. Green SM, Roback MG, Krauss B, for the Emergency Department Ketamine Meta-analysis Study Group. Anticholinergics and ketamine sedation in children: a secondary analysis of atropine versus glycopyrrolate. Acad Emerg Med. 2010;17(2):157–62.
36. Etomidate. https://www.accessdata.fda.gov/drugsatfda_docs/label/2017/018227s032lbl.pdf.
37. Oglesby AJ. Should etomidate be the induction agent of choice for rapid sequence intubation in the emergency department? Emerg Med J. 2004;21(6):655–9.
38. De Jong FH, Mallios C, Jansen C, Scheck PAE, Lamberts SWJ. Etomidate suppresses adrenocortical function by inhibition of 1 1β-hydroxylation. J Clin Endocrinol Metab. 1984;59(6):1143–7.
39. Thompson Bastin ML, Baker SN, Weant KA. Effects of etomidate on adrenal suppression: a review of intubated septic patients. Hosp Pharm. 2014;49(2):177–83.
40. Vinclair M, Broux C, Faure P, Brun J, Genty C, Jacquot C, et al. Duration of adrenal inhibition following a single dose of etomidate in critically ill patients. Intensive Care Med. 2008;34(4):714–9.
41. Hildreth AN, Mejia VA, Maxwell RA, Smith PW, Dart BW, Barker DE. Adrenal suppression following a single dose of etomidate for rapid sequence induction: a prospective randomized study. J Trauma Inj Infect Crit Care. 2008;65(3):573–9.
42. Jabre P, Combes X, Lapostolle F, Dhaouadi M, Ricard-Hibon A, Vivien B, et al. Etomidate versus ketamine for rapid sequence intubation in acutely ill patients: a multicentre randomised controlled trial. Lancet. 2009;374(9686):293–300.
43. Albert SG, Sitaula S. Etomidate, adrenal insufficiency and mortality associated with severity of illness: a meta-analysis. J Intensive Care Med. 2021;36(10):1124–9.
44. Cagliani JA, Ruhemann A, Molmenti E, Smith C, Coppa G, Barrera R. Association between etomidate use for rapid sequence intubation and adrenal insufficiency in sepsis. Cureus. 2021;13:e13445. https://www.cureus.com/articles/46596-association-between-etomidate-use-for-rapid-sequence-intubation-and-adrenal-insufficiency-in-sepsis.
45. Chan CM, Mitchell AL, Shorr AF. Etomidate is associated with mortality and adrenal insufficiency in sepsis: a meta-analysis*. Crit Care Med. 2012;40(11):2945–53.

46. Rech MA, Bennett S, Chaney W, Sterk E. Risk factors for mortality in septic patients who received etomidate. Am J Emerg Med. 2015;33(10):1340–3.

47. Ehrman R, Wira C, Lomax A, Hayward A, Marcelin J, Ellis T, et al. Etomidate use in severe sepsis and septic shock patients does not contribute to mortality. Intern Emerg Med. 2011;6(3):253–7.

48. McPhee LC, Badawi O, Fraser GL, Lerwick PA, Riker RR, Zuckerman IH, et al. Single-dose etomidate is not associated with increased mortality in ICU patients with sepsis: analysis of a large electronic ICU database*. Crit Care Med. 2013;41(3):774–83.

49. Payen JF, Dupuis C, Trouve-Buisson T, Vinclair M, Broux C, Bouzat P, et al. Corticosteroid after etomidate in critically ill patients: a randomized controlled trial*. Crit Care Med. 2012;40(1):29–35.

50. Komatsu R, You J, Rajan S, Kasuya Y, Sessler DI, Turan A. Steroid administration after anaesthetic induction with etomidate does not reduce in-hospital mortality or cardiovascular morbidity after non-cardiac surgery. Br J Anaesth. 2018;120(3):501–8.

51. Taylor I, Marsh DF. Fentanyl is not best anaesthetic induction agent in rapid sequence intubation. BMJ. 1998;317(7169):1386.

52. Gindre S, Ciais JF, Levraut J, Dellamonica J, Guerin JP, Grimaud D. Induction à séquence rapide en urgence: quelle est la place du fentanyl ? Ann Fr Anesth Réanimation. 2002;21(10):760–6.

53. Ferguson I, Buttfield A, Burns B, Reid C, Shepherd S, Milligan J, et al. Fentanyl versus placebo with ketamine and rocuronium for patients undergoing rapid sequence intubation in the emergency department: the FAKT study—a randomized clinical trial. Acad Emerg Med. 2022;29(6):719–28.

54. Midazolam. https://www.accessdata.fda.gov/drugsatfda_docs/label/2017/208878Orig1s000lbl.pdf.

55. Swanson E. Comparison of etomidate and midazolam for prehospital rapid-sequence intubation. Prehosp Emerg Care. 2004;8(3):273–9.

56. Sagarin MJ, Barton ED, Sakles JC, Vissers RJ, Chiang V, Walls RM, et al. Underdosing of midazolam in emergency endotracheal intubation. Acad Emerg Med Off J Soc Acad Emerg Med. 2003;10(4):329–38.

57. Choi YF. Midazolam is more likely to cause hypotension than etomidate in emergency department rapid sequence intubation. Emerg Med J. 2004;21(6):700–2.

58. Davis D, Kimbro U, Vilke G. The Use of Midazolam For Prehospital Rapid Sequence Intubation May be Associated with a Dose-Related Increase in Hypotension. Prehosp Emerg Care. 2001;5(2):163–8. https://doi.org/10.1080/10903120190940065.

59. Propofol. https://www.accessdata.fda.gov/drugsatfda_docs/label/2014/019627s062lbl.pdf.

60. Wan C, Hanson AC, Schulte PJ, Dong Y, Bauer PR. Propofol, ketamine, and etomidate as induction agents for intubation and outcomes in critically ill patients: a retrospective cohort study. Crit Care Explor. 2021;3(5):e0435.

61. Breindahl N, Baekgaard J, Christensen RE, Jensen AH, Creutzburg A, Steinmetz J, et al. Ketamine versus propofol for rapid sequence induction in trauma patients: a retrospective study. Scand J Trauma Resusc Emerg Med. 2021;29(1):136.

62. Kuza CM, To J, Chang A, Mert M, Yau A, Singh M, et al. A retrospective data analysis on the induction medications used in trauma rapid sequence intubations and their effects on outcomes. Eur J Trauma Emerg Surg. 2022;48(3):2275–86.

63. Russotto V, Myatra SN, Laffey JG, Tassistro E, Antolini L, Bauer P, et al. Intubation practices and adverse peri-intubation events in critically ill patients from 29 countries. JAMA. 2021;325(12):1164–72.

64. Dietrich SK, Mixon MA, Rogoszewski RJ, Delgado SD, Knapp VE, Floren M, et al. Hemodynamic effects of propofol for induction of rapid sequence intubation in traumatically injured patients. Am Surg. 2018;84(9):1504–8.

65. Lundstrøm LH, Duez CHV, Nørskov AK, Rosenstock CV, Thomsen JL, Møller AM, et al. Effects of avoidance or use of neuromuscular blocking agents on outcomes in tracheal intubation: a Cochrane systematic review. Br J Anaesth. 2018;120(6):1381–93.

66. Sakles JC, Chiu S, Mosier J, Walker C, Stolz U. The importance of first pass success when performing orotracheal intubation in the emergency department. Acad Emerg Med. 2013;20(1):71–8.

67. Li J, Murphy-Lavoie H, Bugas C, Martinez J, Preston C. Complications of emergency intubation with and without paralysis. Am J Emerg Med. 1999;17(2):141–3.

68. Succinylcholine. https://www.accessdata.fda.gov/drugsatfda_docs/label/2010/008453s027lbl.pdf.

69. Putzu A, Tramèr MR, Giffa M, Czarnetzki C. The optimal dose of succinylcholine for rapid sequence induction: a systematic review and meta-analysis of randomized trials. BMC Anesthesiol. 2020;20(1):54.

70. Martyn JAJ, Richtsfeld M, Warner DO. Succinylcholine-induced hyperkalemia in acquired pathologic states. Anesthesiology. 2006;104(1):158–69.

71. Hovgaard HL, Juhl-Olsen P. Suxamethonium-induced hyperkalemia: a short review of causes and recommendations for clinical applications. Crit Care Res Pract. 2021;2021:1–6.

72. Thapa S, Brull SJ. Succinylcholine-induced hyperkalemia in patients with renal failure: an old question revisited. Anesth Analg. 2000;91(1):237–41.

73. Fleming B, McCollough M, Henderson SO. Myth: atropine should be administered before succinylcholine for neonatal and pediatric intubation. CJEM. 2005;7(02):114–7.

74. Dexter F, Epstein R, Wachtel R, Rosenberg H. Succinylcholine for Triggering Malignant Hyperthermia—MHAUS. https://www.mhaus.org/blog/succinylcholine-for-triggering-malignant-hyperthermia/.

75. Rosenberg H, Davis M, James D, Pollock N, Stowell K. Malignant hyperthermia. Orphanet J Rare Dis. 2007;2(1):21.

76. Rocuronium. https://www.accessdata.fda.gov/drugsatfda_docs/label/2008/078717s000lbl.pdf.

77. Levin NM, Fix ML, April MD, Arana AA, Brown CA, on behalf of the NEAR Investigators. The association of rocuronium dosing and first-attempt intubation success in adult emergency department patients. Can J Emerg Med. 2021;23(4):518–27.

78. April MD, Arana A, Pallin DJ, Schauer SG, Fantegrossi A, Fernandez J, et al. Emergency department intubation success with succinylcholine versus rocuronium: a National Emergency Airway Registry Study. Ann Emerg Med. 2018;72(6):645–53.

79. Marsch SC, Steiner L, Bucher E, Pargger H, Schumann M, Aebi T, et al. Succinylcholine versus rocuronium for rapid sequence intubation in intensive care: a prospective, randomized controlled trial. Crit Care. 2011;15(4):R199.

80. Tran DT, Newton EK, Mount VA, Lee JS, Wells GA, Perry JJ. Rocuronium versus succinylcholine for rapid sequence induction intubation. Cochrane Database Syst Rev. 2015;2015:CD002788. https://doi.org/10.1002/14651858.CD002788.pub3.

81. Sugammadex. https://www.accessdata.fda.gov/drugsatfda_docs/label/2015/022225lbl.pdf.

82. Neostigmine. https://www.accessdata.fda.gov/drugsatfda_docs/label/2021/203629s003lbl.pdf.

83. Hile GB, Healy KJ, Almassalkhi LR. Rocuronium reversal in the emergency department: retrospective evaluation of hemodynamic instability following administration of sugammadex versus neostigmine with glycopyrrolate. J Pharm Pract. 2023;36(2):336–41.

84. Sørensen MK, Bretlau C, Gätke MR, Sørensen AM, Rasmussen LS. Rapid sequence induction and intubation with rocuronium–sugammadex compared with succinylcholine: a randomized trial. Br J Anaesth. 2012;108(4):682–9.

85. Frerk C, Mitchell VS, McNarry AF, Mendonca C, Bhagrath R, Patel A, et al. Difficult airway society 2015 guidelines for management of unanticipated difficult intubation in adults. Br J Anaesth. 2015;115(6):827–48.

86. Apfelbaum JL, Hagberg CA, Connis RT, Abdelmalak BB, Agarkar M, Dutton RP, et al. 2022 American Society of Anesthesiologists practice guidelines for management of the difficult airway. Anesthesiology. 2022;136(1):31–81.

87. Heard AMB, Green RJ, Eakins P. The formulation and introduction of a 'can't intubate, can't ventilate' algorithm into clinical practice. Anaesthesia. 2009;64(6):601–8.
88. Hyland SJ, Pandya PA, Mei CJ, Yehsakul DC. Sugammadex to facilitate neurologic assessment in severely brain-injured patients: retrospective analysis and practical guidance. Cureus. 2022;14:e30466. https://www.cureus.com/articles/113935-sugammadex-to-facilitate-neurologic-assessment-in-severely-brain-injured-patients-retrospective-analysis-and-practical-guidance.
89. Curley JM, Ciceri DP, Culp WC. Sugammadex administration to facilitate timely neurologic examination in the traumatic brain injury patient. Neurocrit Care. 2020;32(3):880–2.
90. Christodoulides A, Palma S, Zaazoue MA, Huh A, Tobin MK, Dine SA, et al. Utility of neuromuscular blockade reversal in the evaluation of acute neurosurgical patients: a retrospective case-series. J Clin Neurosci. 2022;104:82–7.
91. Devlin JW, Skrobik Y, Gélinas C, Needham DM, Slooter AJC, Pandharipande PP, et al. Clinical practice guidelines for the prevention and management of pain, agitation/sedation, delirium, immobility, and sleep disruption in adult patients in the ICU. Crit Care Med. 2018;46(9):e825–73.
92. Leslie K, Chan MTV, Myles PS, Forbes A, McCulloch TJ. Posttraumatic stress disorder in aware patients from the B-aware trial. Anesth Analg. 2010;110(3):823–8.
93. Sebel PS, Bowdle TA, Ghoneim MM, Rampil IJ, Padilla RE, Gan TJ, et al. The incidence of awareness during anesthesia: a multicenter United States study. Anesth Analg. 2004;99(3):833–9.
94. Fuller BM, Roberts BW, Mohr NM, Faine B, Drewry AM, Wessman BT, et al. The feasibility of implementing targeted SEDation in mechanically ventilated emergency department patients: the ED-SED pilot trial*. Crit Care Med. 2022;50(8):1224–35.
95. Pappal RD, Roberts BW, Mohr NM, Ablordeppey E, Wessman BT, Drewry AM, et al. The ED-AWARENESS study: a prospective, observational cohort study of awareness with paralysis in mechanically ventilated patients admitted from the emergency department. Ann Emerg Med. 2021;77(5):532–44.
96. Pappal RD, Roberts BW, Winkler W, Yaegar LH, Stephens RJ, Fuller BM. Awareness with paralysis in mechanically ventilated patients in the emergency department and ICU: a systematic review and meta-analysis*. Crit Care Med. 2021;49(3):e304.
97. Driver BE, Prekker ME, Wagner E, Cole JB, Puskarich MA, Stang J, et al. Recall of awareness during paralysis among ED patients undergoing tracheal intubation. Chest. 2023;163(2):313–23.
98. Heffner AC, Swords D, Kline JA, Jones AE. The frequency and significance of postintubation hypotension during emergency airway management. J Crit Care. 2012;27(4):417.e9–417.e13.
99. De Jong A, Rolle A, Molinari N, Paugam-Burtz C, Constantin JM, Lefrant JY, et al. Cardiac arrest and mortality related to intubation procedure in critically ill adult patients: a multicenter cohort study. Crit Care Med. 2018;46(4):532–9.
100. Heffner AC, Swords DS, Neale MN, Jones AE. Incidence and factors associated with cardiac arrest complicating emergency airway management. Resuscitation. 2013;84(11):1500–4.
101. Kim WY, Kwak MK, Ko BS, Yoon JC, Sohn CH, Lim KS, et al. Factors associated with the occurrence of cardiac arrest after emergency tracheal intubation in the Emergency Department. PLoS ONE. 2014;9(11):e112779.
102. Koch E, Lovett S, Nghiem T, Riggs RA, Rech MA. Shock index in the emergency department: utility and limitations. Open Access Emerg Med OAEM. 2019;11:179–99.
103. Zed PJ, Abu-Laban RB, Harrison DW. Intubating conditions and hemodynamic effects of etomidate for rapid sequence intubation in the emergency department: an observational cohort study. Acad Emerg Med. 2006;13(4):378–83.
104. Miller M, Kruit N, Heldreich C, Ware S, Habig K, Reid C, et al. Hemodynamic response after rapid sequence induction with ketamine in out-of-hospital patients at risk of shock as defined by the shock index. Ann Emerg Med. 2016;68(2):181–188.e2.

105. Foster M, Self M, Gelber A, Kennis B, Lasoff DR, Hayden SR, et al. Ketamine is not associated with more post-intubation hypotension than etomidate in patients undergoing endotracheal intubation. Am J Emerg Med. 2022;61:131–6.
106. Janz DR, Casey JD, Semler MW, Russell DW, Dargin J, Vonderhaar DJ, et al. Effect of a fluid bolus on cardiovascular collapse among critically ill adults undergoing tracheal intubation (PrePARE): a randomised controlled trial. Lancet Respir Med. 2019;7(12):1039–47.
107. Russotto V, Tassistro E, Myatra SN, Parotto M, Antolini L, Bauer P, et al. Peri-intubation cardiovascular collapse in patients who are critically ill: insights from the INTUBE study. Am J Respir Crit Care Med. 2022;206(4):449–58.
108. Weingart S. Push-dose pressors for immediate blood pressure control. Clin Exp Emerg Med. 2015;2(2):131–2.
109. Fuchita M, Pattee J, Russell DW, Driver BE, Prekker ME, Barnes CR, et al. Prophylactic administration of vasopressors prior to emergency intubation in critically ill patients: a secondary analysis of two multicenter clinical trials. Crit Care Explor. 2023;5(7):e0946.
110. Rotando A, Picard L, Delibert S, Chase K, Jones CMC, Acquisto NM. Push dose pressors: experience in critically ill patients outside of the operating room. Am J Emerg Med. 2019;37(3):494–8.
111. Panchal AR, Satyanarayan A, Bahadir JD, Hays D, Mosier J. Efficacy of bolus-dose phenylephrine for peri-intubation hypotension. J Emerg Med. 2015;49(4):488–94.
112. Davis DP, Olvera D, Selde W, Wilmas J, Stuhlmiller D. Bolus vasopressor use for air medical rapid sequence intubation: the vasopressor intravenous push to enhance resuscitation trial. Air Med J. 2023;42(1):36–41.
113. Cole JB, Knack SK, Karl ER, Horton GB, Satpathy R, Driver BE. Human errors and adverse hemodynamic events related to "push dose pressors" in the emergency department. J Med Toxicol. 2019;15(4):276–86.
114. Lat I, Paciullo C, Daley MJ, MacLaren R, Bolesta S, McCann J, et al. Position paper on critical care pharmacy services (executive summary): 2020 update. Am J Health Syst Pharm. 2020;77(19):1619–24.
115. Ortmann MJ, Johnson EG, Jarrell DH, Bilhimer M, Hayes BD, Mishler A, et al. ASHP guidelines on emergency medicine pharmacist services. Am J Health Syst Pharm. 2021;78(3):261–75.
116. Hampton JP, Hommer K, Musselman M, Bilhimer M. Rapid sequence intubation and the role of the emergency medicine pharmacist: 2022 update. Am J Health Syst Pharm. 2023;80(4):182–95.
117. Robey-Gavin E, Abuakar L. Impact of clinical pharmacists on initiation of postintubation analgesia in the emergency department. J Emerg Med. 2016;50(2):308–14.
118. Amini A, Faucett EA, Watt JM, Amini R, Sakles JC, Rhee P, et al. Effect of a pharmacist on timing of postintubation sedative and analgesic use in trauma resuscitations. Am J Health Syst Pharm. 2013;70(17):1513–7.
119. Johnson EG, Meier A, Shirakbari A, Weant K, Baker Justice S. Impact of rocuronium and succinylcholine on sedation initiation after rapid sequence intubation. J Emerg Med. 2015;49(1):43–9.

Chapter 49
Anticoagulation in the Intensive Care Unit

Natasha D. Lopez, Kristine N. Schwietz, and Christine S. Ji

49.1 Hemostasis in the Critically Ill Patient

Hemostasis is the process by which bleeding is stopped after vascular injury. It involves a complex interplay between the vasculature, platelets, coagulation factors and proteins, and fibrinolysis. Displayed in Fig. 49.1 are the components of normal hemostasis [1]. After blood vessel wall injury, vasoconstriction and platelet activation occur. Activated platelets recruit additional platelets and express surface receptors allowing the cross-linking resulting in platelet aggregation and formation of a platelet plug [2]. This process is known as primary hemostasis. Concurrently, the coagulation cascade is initiated, whereby sequential activation of clotting factors culminates in thrombin generation. Thrombin in turn cleaves fibrinogen into fibrin strands, reinforcing the platelet plug; this stabilization phase is referred to as secondary hemostasis [2]. Simultaneously to prevent unchecked clot propagation, innate anticoagulant mechanisms like antithrombin (AT), protein C and S, and tissue factor inhibitor are activated [1]. Plasmin also forms to begin controlled fibrin degradation. The balance between clot formation and regulation determines hemostatic success. Defects in these pathways can lead to hemorrhage or thrombosis.

In the context of critical illness, the process of hemostasis can undergo profound alterations, giving rise to both prothrombotic and anticoagulant states. Activation of the coagulation cascade may ensue in response to pronounced inflammation and vascular injury stemming from conditions such as trauma, surgical procedures, or

N. D. Lopez (✉) · K. N. Schwietz
Department of Pharmacy, Massachusetts General Hospital, Boston, MA, USA
e-mail: nlopez3@mgh.harvard.edu

C. S. Ji
Department of Pharmacy, Beth Israel Deaconess Medical Center, Boston, MA, USA

© The Author(s), under exclusive license to Springer Nature Switzerland AG 2025

Y. Alzaidi, M. A. Gebily (eds.), *The Pharmacist's Expanded Role in Critical Care Medicine*, https://doi.org/10.1007/978-3-031-77335-8_49

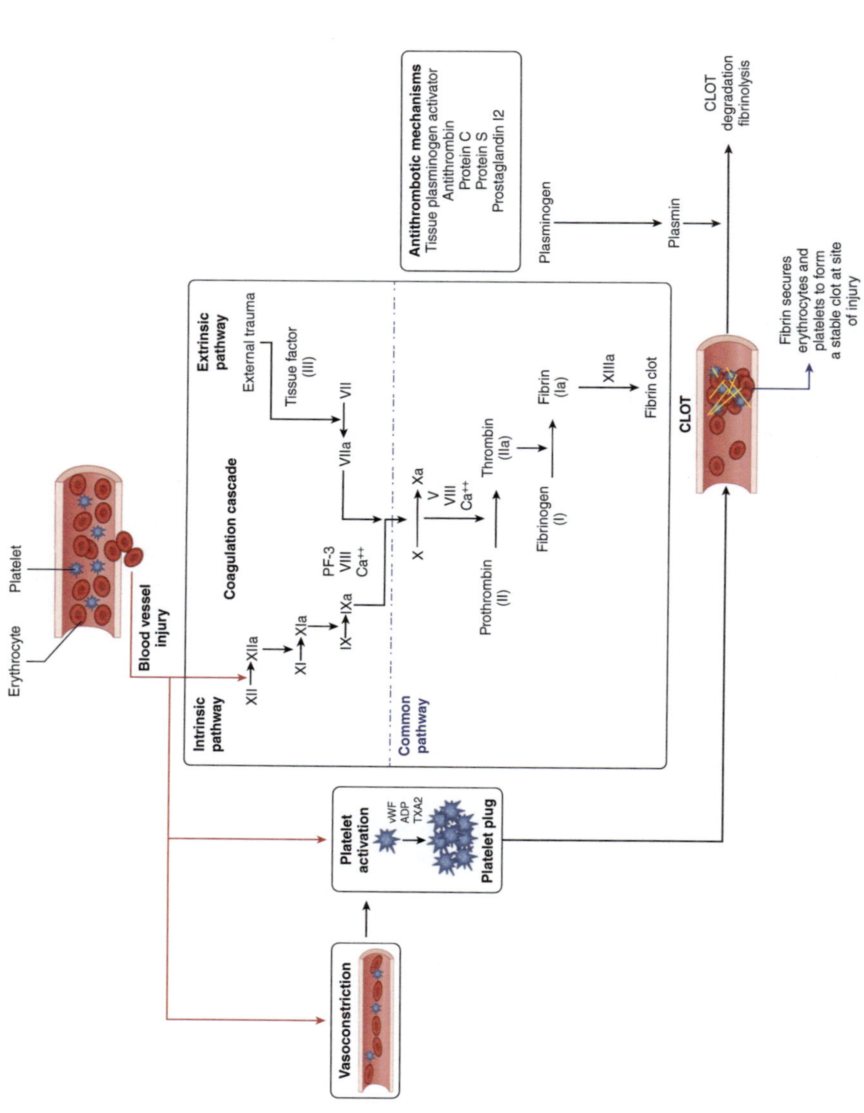

Fig. 49.1 Hemostasis overview. Abbreviations: *ADP* adenosine diphosphate; *PF-3* platelet factor 3; *TXA2* thromboxane; *vWF* von Willebrand factor

sepsis [3]. Suppression of anticoagulant pathways in such scenarios elevates the predisposition to thrombotic events. Critically ill patients may also present with thrombocytopenia attributable to heightened platelet consumption and compromised production. Thrombopoietin, responsible for regulating platelet production, is synthesized in both the liver and kidney, and its deficiency is evident in these pathological conditions [4]. In patients with renal disease, uremic toxins hinder platelet aggregation by inducing dysfunctional von Willebrand factor, reducing thromboxane production, and altering platelet activation [4]. Furthermore, depletion of coagulation factor levels can transpire due to ongoing thrombus formation, hemodilution, impaired hepatic synthetic function, or deficiencies in vitamin K. Additionally, an upsurge in tissue plasminogen activator release can precipitate accelerated fibrinolysis. In liver disease, hyperfibrinolysis may occur as a result of the liver's inability to metabolize tissue plasminogen activator [5].

These abnormalities may be further complicated by the necessity for anticoagulation therapy in instances of thrombotic complications, administration of procoagulant agents, or anticoagulant reversal strategies in the management of hemorrhagic events.

49.2 Coagulation Laboratory Monitoring

Coagulation assays are useful for identifying coagulopathies and monitoring antithrombotic therapies in critically ill patients. Assays such as prothrombin time (PT), activated partial thromboplastin time (aPTT), and thrombin time/dilute thrombin time (TT/dTT) are fibrin clot-based assays and can be used to identify problems within the different hemostatic pathways. Thromboelastography (TEG) and rotational thromboelastometry (ROTEM) are global functional assays that measure clot initiation, amplification, and resolution and can be useful in the identification of both hypo- and hypercoagulable states. Other assays, such as chromogenic anti-factor Xa (AFXa) and chromogenic factor X activity, can only be used to measure the anticoagulant effect of certain drug therapies.

Accurate assessment and interpretation of coagulation assays are reliant on minimization of pre-analytical and analytical issues. Appropriate sample collection, handling, storage, reagent and instrument use, quality control, and calibration are imperative for accurate lab results. Blood samples for coagulation assays should be collected in citrate-containing tubes to prevent activation of clotting factors. Tubes should be adequately filled as under-filling can lead to falsely prolonged clotting times via excess citrate concentrations or clotting factor consumption if a clot develops in the sampling tube [6]. Samples should be transported and stored at room temperature and tested as soon as possible. Common biological factors that can interfere with coagulation assays are shown in Table 49.1.

Table 49.1 Common biological interferences on coagulation labs [6]

Biological interference	Lab assay	Expected effect on lab assay
Hypertriglyceridemia[a]	AFXa	Decreased
Hyperbilirubinemia[a]	AFXa	Decreased
Elevated hematocrit >55%	PT/INR	Prolonged
	aPTT	Prolonged
Lupus anticoagulant	aPTT	Prolonged
Elevated factor VIII and fibrinogen	aPTT	Shortened
Antithrombin deficiency	aPTT	Shortened
	AFXa	Decreased
Hemolyzed sample	AFXa	Decreased
End-stage liver disease	PT/INR	Prolonged
	aPTT	Prolonged

Abbreviations: *AFXa* anti-factor Xa; *aPTT* activated partial thromboplastin time; *INR* international normalized ratio; *PT* prothrombin time

[a] The levels at which triglycerides and bilirubin interfere with labs may vary institutionally based on the reagents used. Refer to specific reagent package insert for possible lab interferences and thresholds

49.2.1 Clot-Based Assays

aPTT, PT, TT, and dTT are assays that assess the time to fibrin clot formation via clotting factor activation. Assay results are dependent on the sensitivity of reagents used and the concentration or activity of clotting factor in the patient sample. Clotting factor activity of about 30% is required to achieve hemostasis, and functional assay times may be prolonged when clotting factor activity is less than 50%. aPTT and PT assays may be helpful tools to screen for clotting factor deficiencies in patients not receiving anticoagulation.

49.2.1.1 Activated Partial Thromboplastin Time

The aPTT is used to assess the functionality of factors I, II, V, VIII, IX, X, and XII and contact activators in fibrin clot formation via activation of the intrinsic clotting pathway. This assay can be prolonged in patients with coagulation factor deficiency or presence of inhibitors or lupus anticoagulant. Anticoagulants such as unfractionated heparin (UFH) and direct thrombin inhibitors (DTIs) will prolong aPTT. The assay may also be prolonged in patients on direct oral anticoagulants (DOACs) and is not a reliable method to monitor therapy. High concentrations of factors VIII or II may result in shortened aPTT and be indicative of a hypercoagulable state. The reference range for aPTT varies across populations and test reagents utilized in the lab. Institutions will calibrate a reference range based on their local patient demographic and lab assay availability.

49.2.1.2 Prothrombin Time

PT/INR is used to assess the functionality of factor VII in fibrin clot formation via activation of the extrinsic clotting pathway. PT/INR can be prolonged in patients on warfarin or IV DTI and patients who have decreased clotting factor synthesis due to vitamin K deficiency or liver disease. PT/INR may be prolonged in patients receiving DOACs, but it is not a reliable measure to assess anticoagulation status. Prolonged PT/INR results in patients not receiving anticoagulation should be interpreted cautiously as prolonged PT/INR is not indicative of anticoagulation status or hemorrhagic risk. INR is the ratio of the PT to a normal value and standardizes PT variability when using different lab reagents.

49.2.1.3 Thrombin Time and Dilute Thrombin Time

TT and dTT are used to assess conversion of fibrinogen to fibrin in the presence of exogenous thrombin. These assays can be prolonged in patients on unfractionated heparin or direct thrombin inhibitor therapy and in patients with dysfibrinogenemia. TT and dTT are not widely available assays, making aPTT the assay of choice for monitoring UFH, argatroban, or bivalirudin therapy. TT is highly sensitive to subtherapeutic concentrations of dabigatran below 30 ng/mL, making dTT the preferred monitoring strategy for dabigatran therapy. A normal dTT can effectively rule out the presence of dabigatran in a patient's plasma sample.

49.2.2 Chromogenic Assays

Chromogenic assays utilize light spectrophotometry to indirectly measure anticoagulant effect via residual uninhibited clotting factor (anti-factor Xa) or directly measure clotting factor activity (factor X activity).

49.2.2.1 Anti-factor Xa

The chromogenic anti-factor Xa or anti-Xa (AFXa) assay is utilized to measure anticoagulant effects of FXa inhibitors (e.g., UFH, enoxaparin, fondaparinux, apixaban, edoxaban, rivaroxaban). A chromogenic substrate is added to a patient plasma sample. Uninhibited residual factor Xa cleaves the chromogenic substrate to produce color change measured via spectrophotometry. The amount of light absorbance is inversely proportional to the concentration of FXa inhibitor in the plasma sample. Drug-specific calibration curves should be utilized whenever possible to accurately determine FXa inhibitor concentrations.

While aPTT is the most widely used lab to monitor UFH, the chromogenic AFXa assay may be preferred given less laboratory interference as AFXa is not impacted by clotting factor deficiencies or the presence of lupus anticoagulant. Anti-factor Xa monitoring has been shown to achieve therapeutic anticoagulation quicker and decrease the number of lab draws and dose adjustments compared to aPTT monitoring [7, 8]. Importantly, no differences in bleeding or thrombosis have been observed when comparing AFXa and aPTT monitoring strategies for UFH [9].

Anti-factor Xa monitoring for oral FXa inhibitors (apixaban, edoxaban, and rivaroxaban) is not routinely required; however, it may be necessary to evaluate in patients who are bleeding or undergoing emergent or invasive procedures and requiring anticoagulation reversal. Suggested thresholds for reversal are levels greater than 50 ng/mL for life-threatening bleeding and 30–50 ng/mL for invasive procedures [10]. Important to note is that FXa inhibitor levels have not been associated with clinical outcomes and should be interpreted cautiously. Peak and trough values were collected during FXa inhibitor clinical trials to establish reference ranges but were not intended to be considered therapeutic ranges.

49.2.2.2 Factor X Activity

The chromogenic factor X activity assay is used to quantify factor X levels and can be used to detect factor X deficiency and, more commonly, measure anticoagulant effects of warfarin therapy in patients that have lupus anticoagulant PT/INR interference or patients on DTIs being transitioned to warfarin. This assay should not be used to monitor UFH or other FXa inhibitors (e.g., apixaban, edoxaban, rivaroxaban). A chromogenic substrate is added to a patient plasma sample. Patient factor X is activated in the presence of added reagents and hydrolyzes the chromogenic substrate to produce color change. The amount of light absorbance is directly proportional to the amount of factor X. The reference range for factor X activity is 60–140%. Factor X activity of 20–40% corresponds to the INR range of 2–3 [11].

49.2.3 Global Hemostasis Assays

Thromboelastography (TEG) and rotational thromboelastometry (ROTEM) are point-of-care, viscoelastic assays that provide a comprehensive assessment of clot formation rather than solely assessing time to clot formation. TEG measures tension on a torsion wire, and ROTEM measures rotational resistance of a pin during clot formation. These assays measure clot initiation, amplification, and fibrinolysis. Their utility lies in the ability to quickly identify coagulopathies and guide clinicians on tailored blood component transfusion based on abnormalities detected, thereby reducing the risk of over-transfusion or inadequate correction of coagulopathy. See Fig. 49.2 and Table 49.2 for viscoelastic assay components and associated transfusion recommendations when results are abnormal.

Fig. 49.2 Viscoelastic assay components [12]. Abbreviations: *a* alpha angle; *CFT* clot formation time; *CL30* clot lysis at 30 min; *CL60* clot lysis at 60 min; *CT* clotting time; *K* kinetic time; *LY30* lysis at 30 min; *LY60* lysis at 60 min; *MA* maximum amplitude; *MCF* maximum clot firmness

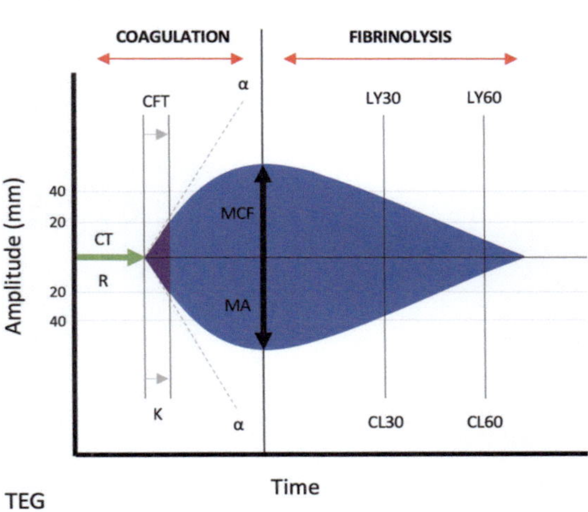

49.2.4 Platelet Function Testing

Platelet function assays provide insight into platelet activation, aggregation, and overall hemostatic function. Light transmission aggregometry (LTA) is the gold standard for evaluating platelet function and can be used as a screening test for bleeding disorders and monitoring antiplatelet drugs. LTA measures changes in light transmission through platelet-rich plasma as platelets aggregate in response to an agonist. The agonist panel includes collagen, adenosine diphosphate (ADP), epinephrine, and arachidonic acid, which are all physiologic platelet activators, and ristocetin, an antibiotic which causes platelets to agglutinate. Antiplatelet agents including aspirin, nonsteroidal anti-inflammatory drugs (e.g., naproxen, ibuprofen), glycoprotein IIb/IIIa inhibitors, and P2Y12 inhibitors (e.g., clopidogrel, prasugrel, ticagrelor) will all impact the results of the LTA, but due to the variable response, it is not recommend to monitor antiplatelet therapy [14]. LTA is not routinely used in clinical practice due to lack of technique standardization.

Similar to LTA, rapid platelet function analyzer (RPFA) is a point-of-care assay that utilizes a cartridge-based system to measure light transmission through platelet aggregation in whole blood and assess P2Y12-mediated platelet inhibition. In critically ill patients, RPFA can be used as a surrogate measure to assess gut absorption and can aid in the decision of timing for urgent or invasive procedures when awaiting antiplatelet washout. Additionally, if genotype testing is not available to determine metabolizer status for clopidogrel, RPFA can be used to indirectly confirm sufficient activation of clopidogrel. According to the manufacturer of VerifyNow, results between 180 and 376 PRU [P2Y12 reaction units] are normal and results below 180 PRU indicate P2Y12 inhibition. It is important to note that the reference ranges to determine P2Y12 responsiveness have only been evaluated in patients who underwent percutaneous coronary intervention [15]. The American College of Cardiology suggests that values greater than 208 PRU [P2Y12 reaction units] are indicative of normal platelet reactivity or insufficient platelet inhibition and values below 85 PRU may be associated with increased bleeding.

Table 49.2 Viscoelastic assay components and directed transfusion recommendations [13]

Phase of hemostasis	Coagulation parameter	TEG parameter	ROTEM parameter	Expected result in hypocoagulable state	Transfusion/treatment recommendation
Initial clot formation	Time to reach 2 mm	Reaction time (R), min	Clotting time (CT), sec	Increased = clotting factor deficiency	FFP PCC
Clot amplification (fibrin polymerization)	Speed of clot development	Alpha angle (a), degrees	Alpha angle (a), degrees	Decreased = fibrin deficiency	Cryoprecipitate Fibrinogen concentrate
Clot amplification	Time to clot amplification from 2 to 20 mm	Kinetic time (K), min	Clot formation time (CFT), sec	Increased = fibrin deficiency	Cryoprecipitate Fibrinogen concentrate
Clot strength (fibrinogen and PLT activation)	Maximum clot strength	Max amplitude (MA), mm	Max clot firmness (MCF), mm	Decreased = fibrin or platelet deficiency	Cryoprecipitate Fibrinogen concentrate Platelets Desmopressin
Clot resolution	% reduction in AUC at 30/60 min after reaching MA/MCF	CL30/CL60	LY30/LY60	Increased = clot instability	Tranexamic acid Aminocaproic acid

Abbreviations: *AUC* area under curve; *CT* clotting time; *FFP* fresh frozen plasma; *PCC* prothrombin complex concentrate; *PLT* platelet

49.2.5 Application of Coagulation Assays in the Intensive Care Unit

Coagulation assays are useful for drug therapy monitoring, identifying issues within the different phases of hemostasis and monitoring of transfusion therapy in critically ill patients.

49.2.5.1 Therapeutic Drug Monitoring

Ensuring that appropriate coagulation assays and labs are ordered to monitor drug therapies in the intensive care unit is essential to safe and effective management of antithrombotic agents. Pharmacists should interpret assay and lab results cautiously, taking into consideration any variables that may lead to interference or abnormal results, and recommend therapy or monitoring adjustments as necessary. Table 49.3 is a summary table of coagulation assays, their intended drug monitoring, and causes for abnormal assays.

Table 49.3 Summary of coagulation assays

Coagulation assay	Therapeutic drug monitoring	Causes for abnormal assay	
		Prolonged	Shortened
aPTT	– UFH – Argatroban – Bivalirudin	– Factor deficiency: I, II, V, VIII, IX, X, XI, XII – VWD with associated low FVIII – Presence of lupus anticoagulant – UFH, argatroban, bivalirudin – Unreliably, DOACs may prolong aPTT	– Elevated FVIII or II levels – Emicizumab
PT/INR	– Warfarin	– Factor deficiency: I, II, V, VII, X – Warfarin – Argatroban, bivalirudin – Unreliably, DOACs may prolong PT/INR	
TT/dTT	– UFH – Argatroban – Bivalirudin – Dabigatran	– Factor deficiency: I – UFH, argatroban, bivalirudin, dabigatran	
Anti-Xa (AFXa)	– UFH – Enoxaparin – Fondaparinux – Apixaban, edoxaban, rivaroxaban	**Increased AFXa** – FXa inhibitors (UFH, LMWH, fondaparinux, apixaban, edoxaban, rivaroxaban)	**Decreased AFXa** – Hemolyzed sample, hyperbilirubinemia, hypertriglyceridemia

49.2.5.2 Evaluation of Coagulopathy

Pharmacists can play an essential role in ordering and interpretation of labs and coagulation assays and evaluating for medication causes of coagulopathy. See the stepwise approach below for evaluating coagulopathy:

1. Send CBC, fibrinogen, aPTT, and PT.
2. Evaluate for medication causes (e.g., anticoagulants, antiplatelets, fibrinolytics, drug-induced thrombocytopenia).
3. Interpretation of aPTT/PT screen:

    (a) aPTT prolonged: factor deficiency or inhibitor, UFH, DTI, lupus anticoagulant
    (b) PT prolonged: factor deficiency or inhibitor, severe liver disease, vitamin K deficiency/antagonist, lupus anticoagulant
    (c) Both aPTT and PT prolonged: factor deficiency or inhibitor, severe liver disease, vitamin K deficiency/antagonist, DIC, lupus anticoagulant

        (i) Additional lab results indicative of DIC: low fibrinogen, low platelet count, elevated d-dimer, schistocytes on smear
    (d) Both aPTT and PT normal: platelet dysfunction, VWD, FXIII deficiency, dysfibrinogenemia

4. If aPTT or PT is prolonged, send mixing studies:

Mixing Study Interpretation			
	PT Mixing Study Result	aPTT Mixing Study Result	Causes for Abnormal Results
Baseline aPTT prolonged		Corrected aPTT	Factor deficiency
		Prolonged/uncorrected aPTT	Factor inhibitor, UFH, dabigatran, lupus anticoagulant
Baseline PT prolonged	Corrected PT		Factor deficiency, VKA, vitamin K deficiency
	Prolonged/uncorrected PT		Factor VII inhibitor, DOAC
Baseline aPTT and PT prolonged	Corrected PT	Corrected aPTT	Factor deficiency
	Corrected PT	Prolonged/uncorrected aPTT	UFH
	Prolonged/uncorrected PT	Prolonged/uncorrected	Factor inhibitor, DOAC, UFH

5. If the cause of coagulopathy cannot be adequately assessed with aPTT/PT, consider global hemostasis tests (TEG/ROTEM) to assess overall coagulation status and/or assist with targeted transfusion therapy.
6. After identification of the cause(s) for coagulopathy, transfusion and coagulopathy reversal strategies can be implemented.

49.2.6 Monitoring of Transfusion Therapy

Pharmacists may be involved in the development of viscoelastic-based transfusion protocols and provide recommendations for tailored transfusion or clotting factor concentrates based on viscoelastic results in a variety of patient populations. The use of viscoelastic testing to guide transfusion therapy has been studied in several patient populations including cardiac surgery, cirrhosis and liver transplantation, trauma, and extracorporeal membrane oxygenation [16–18]. Monitoring with TEG or ROTEM has been shown to reliably predict coagulopathy, massive transfusion requirement, and mortality and lead to cost savings by reducing the number of transfusions [13]. TEG-guided transfusion methods may improve all-cause mortality in both trauma and surgical patients compared to transfusion guided by any method (RR 0.52; 95% CI, 0.28–0.95), but it is important to note that the quality of evidence remains low due to study heterogeneity included for analysis [19]. Examples of TEG-guided transfusion protocols are shown below:

Rapid TEG-based massive transfusion protocol for trauma [20]

TEG parameter	TEG results	Treatment
ACT (s)	>128	2 units FFP
Alpha angle (degrees)	<65	10 units cryoprecipitate
MA (mm)	<55	1 unit platelets
LY30	≥5%	1 g TXA

TEG-based transfusion protocol in cardiac surgery [21]

TEG parameter	TEG result	Treatment
R (min)	11–14	2 units FFP
	>14	4 units FFP
MA (mm)	46–54	0.3 mcg/kg DDAVP
	41–45	1 unit platelets
	<40	2 units platelets
Alpha angle (degrees)	<45	0.06 units/kg cryoprecipitate

TEG-based transfusion protocol in non-variceal bleeding in patients with advanced liver cirrhosis [22]

TEG parameter	TEG results	Treatment
R (min)	>10	10 mL/kg IBW FFP
MA (mm)	<55	1 unit platelets
Alpha angle (degrees)	<45	5 units cryoprecipitate

49.3 Anticoagulants

Critically ill patients often receive anticoagulation during their intensive care unit (ICU) admission for various indications ranging from venous thromboembolic prophylaxis to treatment of an acute thrombotic event. Some patients may be admitted to the ICU with preexisting hemostatic disorders or already receiving anticoagulation, necessitating further management. The use of anticoagulants in the ICU must be balanced in their efficacy with the inherent risk of bleeding. This requires careful consideration of factors including indication, anticoagulant pharmacokinetics and pharmacodynamics, monitoring, reversibility, and available evidence [23]. These considerations must be tailored to the critically ill patient by assessing their underlying thrombotic and bleeding risk, organ function, and comorbidities. The following section will focus on the current anticoagulants encountered in the ICU, parenteral and oral, and details regarding the pharmacology, pharmacokinetics, dosing, monitoring, and special population considerations.

49.3.1 Parenteral Anticoagulants

49.3.1.1 Unfractionated Heparin

Mechanism of Action

Unfractionated heparin (UFH) is a sulfated glycosaminoglycan that binds to antithrombin III, i.e., antithrombin (AT), through a unique pentasaccharide sequence, converting AT from a slow to a rapid inhibitor of coagulation proteases like thrombin and factor Xa. Only about one-third of UFH molecules contain this key sequence; the rest have minimal activity. For thrombin (factor IIa) inhibition to occur, UFH must bridge AT and thrombin. In addition to thrombin inactivation, UFH and AT complex catalyzes the inhibition of factors Xa, IXa, and XIIa; this is considered its primary mechanism of anticoagulation. Secondary to the reduction in thrombin generation and activity, UFH inhibits fibrin formation, platelet activation, and coagulation factors V, VIII, and XI. Beyond anticoagulation, UFH also modulates platelet function, vascular permeability, smooth muscle proliferation, and bone metabolism.

Pharmacokinetics

Heparin is administered intravenously by continuous infusion or subcutaneously by injection. Intravenous UFH has an immediate action, whereas subcutaneous absorption is delayed 1–2 h. UFH binds extensively to plasma proteins like factor VIII, contributing to variable anticoagulant responses. It undergoes both saturable renal clearance and slower non-saturable clearance, being degraded by the reticuloendo-thelial system. Due to its complex clearance, UFH exhibits nonlinear pharmacoki-netics in which both the intensity and duration of anticoagulation increase disproportionately with higher doses [24]. These factors make precise anticoagula-tion dosing of intravenous UFH challenging.

Dosing

Therapeutic Unfractionated heparin can be used for both therapeutic and prophy-laxis anticoagulation. Dosing for therapeutic anticoagulation is variable based on indication and requires no adjustment for renal impairment. Therapeutic heparin is administered as a 60–80 unit/kg bolus followed by a continuous infusion of 12–18 units/kg/h titrated to an appropriate anticoagulation target. Therapeutic sub-cutaneous UFH has historically been an option for the initial management of VTE; applicability to patients admitted to the ICU is limited and should be reserved as a long-term or bridging option therapy for patients in whom low-molecular-weight heparin or direct oral anticoagulants are contraindicated. Therapeutic subcutaneous dosing is 333 units/kg loading dose followed by 250 units/kg twice daily using con-centrated heparin 10,000–20,000 units/mL.

Prophylaxis Thromboprophylaxis dosing of UFH is standardly 5000 units subcu-taneously twice or three times daily. The optimal frequency is controversial; in a multicenter retrospective study evaluating critically ill patients on mechanical ven-tilation, efficacy at venous thromboembolism prevention did not differ between heparin twice daily and three times daily [25]. Opposed to those findings, in the surgical and trauma patient population, both excluded from the previous study, three times daily is recommended [26, 27]. Evaluating the patient's risk of VTE, altered pharmacokinetics, bleeding risk, and literature in specific patient populations should factor into dosing.

Monitoring

At therapeutic doses, heparin can be monitored by measuring the aPTT or AFXa. A therapeutic aPTT range for heparin is equivalent to a plasma heparin level of 0.3–0.7 units/mL determined by the AFXa assay. It is assumed that an aPTT 1.5–2.5× the normal mean aPTT is therapeutic. In patients undergoing cardiopul-monary bypass or percutaneous coronary intervention, where high doses of heparin are administered, the ACT is employed due to the heightened sensitivity of aPTT and AFXa. The strengths and limitations of these assays and use in critically ill patients can be referred to in the coagulation monitoring Sect. 49.2; aPTT or AFXa is monitored initially at baseline followed by every 4–6 h to determine dose adjustments.

Heparin-Induced Thrombocytopenia

The development of heparin-induced thrombocytopenia (HIT) is one of the major nonhemorrhagic effects of heparin agents. Although UFH exposure is more likely to cause HIT than low-molecular-weight heparin agents, both agents should be considered. Due to its high morbidity and mortality from thrombosis development, early recognition and treatment are paramount. The condition results from the production of platelet-activating IgG antibodies against heparin-platelet glycosaminoglycan and platelet factor 4 (PF4) complexes. Further details on the diagnosis, testing, and management of HIT are in Sect. 49.7.2.

Heparin Resistance

Heparin resistance can be simply defined as the inability to achieve therapeutic anticoagulation despite an adequate heparin dose [28]. Despite a referenced dose greater than 35,000 units UFH per day to achieve a therapeutic aPTT, consensus on the specific heparin dose is controversial as this value does not account for the patient's weight. Heparin resistance can be related to both patient factors, such as antithrombin deficiency, and UFH drug properties, such as nonspecific binding to AT. Details on testing for patients with suspected heparin resistance are detailed in Sect. 49.4. Treatment can include the administration of fresh frozen plasma or AT, if AT deficiency is the culprit, or changing to an alternative anticoagulant which bypasses the need for AT such as direct thrombin inhibitors or fondaparinux.

Special Populations

Low body weight For VTE prophylaxis in patients less than 50 kg, heparin 5000 units subcutaneously twice daily in comparison to three times daily demonstrated reduced risk of bleeding and similar rates of venous thromboembolism in critically ill patients [29]. Underweight patients with elevated aPTTs receiving standard-dosed heparin prophylaxis should prompt further evaluation to rule out heparin accumulation and if dose adjustments are needed. A heparin weight-based dosing nomogram should be utilized for therapeutic indications.

High body weight For obese patients with a BMI >30 kg/m^2, heparin prophylaxis with 5000–7500 units subcutaneously three times daily has been suggested [30]. The high dose regimen, 7500 units three times daily, has not demonstrated decreased incidence of VTE but potentially has an increased bleeding for patients with a BMI $\geq$30 kg/m^2 or weight >100 kg [31–33]. Based on the limited data, it is reasonable for patients with a BMI 30–49 mg/kg^2 to use 5000 units three times daily, and for patients with a BMI $\geq$50 mg/kg^2 and at high VTE risk, 7500 units three times daily can be considered. For treatment indications, weight-based heparin regimens have demonstrated significantly lower recurrent thromboembolism when compared to fixed dosing [34]. The appropriate weight to dose heparin infusions, total versus adjusted body weight, in patients with BMI $\geq$40 kg/m^2 is not clearly defined in previous and current guidelines for the treatment of VTE [35–37]. Retrospective studies have demonstrated that patients with a BMI $\geq$40 kg/m^2 may require lower heparin dose, but using an adjusted body weight or dosing capping may lead to subtherapeutic anticoagulation and no difference in safety outcomes [38]. Additionally, the use of various weights for different continuous infusion may result in a medication error if the incorrect weight is used. Based on the current literature, it is reasonable to use actual body weight for therapeutic heparin dosing, especially in the setting of acute VTE management. Another option in patients at lower risk thrombotic risk, for example patients transitioning to heparin infusion from oral therapy or patients with atrial fibrillation with low CHA$_2$DS$_2$-VASc score with no plan for immediate cardioversion, utilizing a lower maintenance infusion rate such as 12–14 units/kg/h using total body weight in patients with a BMI $\geq$40 kg/m^2 has demonstrated similar time to therapeutic anticoagulation in critically ill patients [39].

Despite UFH limitations, it remains the most utilized parenteral anticoagulant in the intensive care unit. Provider familiarity, low cost, rapid onset of action, short half-life, lack of renal elimination, and full reversibility with protamine are key factors contributing to its ongoing use.

49.3.1.2 Low-Molecular-Weight Heparin

Mechanism of Action

Low-molecular-weight heparins (LMWHs) are derived from unfractionated heparin through chemical or enzymatic depolymerization processes. As a result, they are about one-third the size with an average molecular weight of 4000–5000 daltons compared to unfractionated heparin's 12,000–15,000 daltons. Similar to UFH, LMWHs provide anticoagulation by catalyzing antithrombin-mediated inhibition of coagulation factors, especially factor Xa. The lower molecular weight does reduce LMWHs' ability to bridge antithrombin and thrombin, resulting in being less effective at inactivation of thrombin. However, reduced thrombin binding also leads to less platelet activation by LMWH and nearly tenfold lower rates of heparin-induced thrombocytopenia. Additionally, there is reduced binding to plasma proteins and cells, which provides a more predictable pharmacokinetics and dose-response relationships.

Pharmacokinetics

Low-molecular-weight heparins can be administered subcutaneously, which is the standard route, or intravenously in settings like acute myocardial infarction. The bioavailability after subcutaneous administration is ~90%, with peak AFXa activity occurring after 3–5 h. Depending on the specific LMWH, the half-life ranges from 3 to 6 h. The longer plasma half-life allows for once- or twice-daily dosing. These agents are primarily eliminated by the kidney, in which drug clearance is highly correlated with creatinine clearance. Therefore, dosing adjustments or an alternative anticoagulation agent may be required in the setting of renal impairment.

Dosing

Indications for LMWH include both therapeutic and prophylactic anticoagulation. Dosing regimens are listed in Table 49.4, and dose reductions are required for a creatinine clearance less than 30 mL/min.

Monitoring

Monitoring LMWH is generally not recommended due to unestablished risk associated and therapeutic outcomes with specific AFXa levels [43]. However, variations in critically ill patient's pharmacokinetics and pharmacodynamics are less predictable and may warrant monitoring. Examples of patient populations or clinical factors which may benefit in monitoring AFXa to ensure adequate exposure are listed in Table 49.5. Anti-factor Xa should be measured at steady state, after the third or fourth dose, as a peak concentration ~4 h after subcutaneous administration. Assays should be calibrated to the specific LMWH agent and consideration if exogenous antithrombin is added when interpreting results in critically ill patients. Specific goals are dependent on the LMWH; examples of target AFXa levels for enoxaparin are listed in Table 49.4. Although trough AFXa levels are not usual practice, these may be warranted for specific scenarios (i.e., assess accumulation in renal dysfunction or adequate prophylaxis in trauma patients).

Special Populations

Low body weight Limited evidence in this patient population, including one study in critically ill patients ≤50 kg, has demonstrated that standard LMWH prophylaxis dosing (enoxaparin 40 mg daily or 30 mg twice daily) resulted in supratherapeutic AFXa levels, higher bleeding rates, and no difference in VTE events when compared to 30 mg once daily [29, 44–46]. In patients ≤55 kg or BMI <18 kg/m^2, it is reasonable to adjust dosing to enoxaparin 30 mg once daily, especially in elderly patients or those with high bleeding risk; in underweight patients at a high thrombotic risk (i.e., trauma, surgical) or patients with augmented renal clearance, weight-based dosing 0.5 mg/kg twice daily with AFXa monitoring can be utilized [26]. Therapeutic enoxaparin weight-based dosing using total body weight is recommended, with close monitoring of signs and symptoms of bleeding and consideration for AFXa monitoring [41].

Table 49.4 Low-molecular-weight heparin dosing and target anti-factor Xa levels [40, 41]

Indication	Low-molecular-weight heparin	Dosing[a]	Target AFXa (IU/mL)
VTE prevention	Enoxaparin	30 mg twice daily or 40 mg once daily *CrCl < 30 mL/min:* 30 mg once daily *BMI ≥ 40 kg/m²:* 40 mg twice daily or 0.5 mg/kg twice daily *BMI ≥ 50 kg/m²:* 60 mg twice daily or 0.5 mg/kg twice daily	Peak: 0.2–0.4 Trough: 0.1–0.2
	Dalteparin	5000 units once daily *CrCL < 30 mL/min:* not recommended *BMI ≥ 40 kg/m²:* 7500 units once daily	Peak 0.2–0.2
VTE treatment	Enoxaparin	1 mg/kg twice daily *CrCl < 30 mL/min:* 1 mg/kg once daily *BMI ≥ 40 kg/m²:* standard dosing ABW *BMI ≥ 50 kg/m²:* 0.7–1 mg/kg ABW	Peak 0.6–1
		1.5 mg/kg once daily *CrCl < 30 mL/min:* not recommended *BMI ≥ 30 kg/m²:* recommend twice-daily regimen	Peak 1–2
	Dalteparin	100 units/kg twice daily *CrCl < 30 mL/min:* not recommended *BMI ≥ 30 kg/m²:* standard dosing ABW (max 190 kg)	Peak: 0.6–1
		200 units/kg once daily *CrCl < 30 mL/min:* not recommended *BMI ≥ 30 kg/m²:* standard dosing ABW, twice-daily regimen preferred (max 190 kg)	Peak: 0.5–1.5

Abbreviations: *AFXa* anti-factor Xa; *BMI* body mass index; *CrCl* creatinine clearance; *VTE* venous thromboembolism

[a] Administered subcutaneously

High body weight The optimal dosing, weight based or fixed, for VTE prophylaxis in patients with high body weight or high BMI remains undetermined. Prophylaxis regimens include either a fixed dosing based on BMI or weight-based dosing approach for patients with a BMI ≥40 kg/m². Fixed-dose regimen of enoxaparin 40 mg subcutaneously twice daily for a BMI of 40–49 kg/m² and 60 mg subcutaneously twice daily for a BMI ≥50 kg/m² has been suggested and has been used in patient populations including bariatric or gastric bypass surgery. Enoxaparin weight-based dosing regimens in the literature have ranged from 0.4 to 0.6 mg/kg every 12–24 h, but most often cited dose is 0.5 mg/kg subcutaneously every 12 h in patients with a creatinine clearance >30 mL/min [41]. Due to the lack of data comparing these regimens and outcomes such as incidence of VTE and bleeding complications, either regimen is considered acceptable prophylaxis [47–49]. It is reasonable in patients at high risk of VTE, including the surgical and trauma ICU patient population, to utilize weight-based prophylaxis dosing with AFXa monitoring [50, 51]. In patients with a BMI ≥50 kg/m² receiving fixed prophylaxis dosing and at high risk of VTE or bleeding, AFXa levels should be monitored to ensure

Table 49.5 Patient factors impacting anti-factor Xa levels [40, 42]

Patient factors	Pharmacokinetic or pharmacodynamic impact	Anti-factor Xa (AFXa)
Peripheral edema Hypotension requiring vasopressor therapy Obesity (weight >150 kg, BMI >40)	↓ Bioavailability ↓ Subcutaneous absorption	↓ Peak AFXa
Pregnancy Obesity (weight >150 kg, BMI >40)	↑ Volume of distribution	↓ Peak AFXa
Augmented renal function (i.e., trauma, burn, sepsis)	↑ Elimination	↓ Peak AFXa ↓ Trough AFXa
Renal impairment (CrCl <30 mL/min, AKI) Unreliable renal function assessed by CrCl (i.e., elderly, low body mass <55 kg, obesity)	↓ Elimination	↑ Peak AFXa ↑ Trough AFXa
Trauma Mechanical devices Cirrhosis	Acquired antithrombin (AT) deficiency	↓ Peak AFXa[a]

Abbreviations: *AKI* acute kidney injury; *BMI* body mass index; *CrCl* creatinine clearance; ↓ decreased or low; ↑ increased or high

[a] Impact will be dependent on the method of anti-factor Xa testing and if exogenous antithrombin (AT) is added to plasma samples. If AT added to the plasma sample during anti-factor Xa testing, results may overestimate the in vivo level of anticoagulation in a patient with AT deficiency

adequate exposure. For treatment of VTE, current guidelines recommend that obese patients be dosed by actual body weight with no dosing capping [36]. Despite these recommendations, retrospective studies have demonstrated that in patients with BMI >40, enoxaparin dose adjustment of 0.75–0.8 mg/kg every 12 h achieved therapeutic AFXa concentration. Despite supratherapeutic AFXa levels using 1 mg/kg q12h dosing regimen, this did not transpire to bleeding complications [52, 53]. In patients with a high thrombotic risk including new venous thromboembolism, the risk of underdosing outweighs the risk of bleeding; therefore, actual body weight should be used without dose capping. Reduced dosing could be considered in patients with high bleeding risk or low thrombotic risk.

49.3.1.3 Fondaparinux

Mechanism of Action

Fondaparinux is a synthetic pentasaccharide derived from the minimal antithrombin-binding region of heparin and modified to bind to AT with a higher affinity. Binding to AT causes a confirmational change that increases AT activity to inactivate factor Xa indirectly. Opposed to UFH and LMWH, fondaparinux cannot form a complete ternary with AT and thrombin; therefore, it cannot inactivate thrombin (factor IIa). Due to the binding specificity, there is no interaction with platelet factor 4 (PF4) removing the risk of developing HIT, and it is considered a therapeutic option for the treatment of HIT or prophylaxis in patients with a remote history of HIT.

Pharmacokinetics

Fondaparinux is 95% bound to AT in the plasma with minimal nonspecific binding to other plasma proteins. Hepatic metabolism is minimal and requires no dose adjustment for hepatic impairment. Elimination is highly dependent on renal function with up to 77% unchanged drug excreted by the kidneys requiring dose adjustments.

Dosing

Fondaparinux is administered subcutaneously for both prophylaxis and treatment of VTE including HIT. Therapeutic anticoagulation is based on weight categories: 5 mg daily for patients <50 kg, 7.5 mg daily for weight 50–100 kg, and 10 mg daily for weight >100 kg. Standard prophylactic dosing is 2.5 mg daily. Considerations for low body weight and renal impairment are discussed in special population section.

Monitoring

Routine monitoring of fondaparinux AFXa levels is not standard but should be considered in patients with a BMI >40 kg/m^2, in those with a weight <50 kg or >150 kg, in elderly (>75 years old), or in those with renal impairment (CrCl less than 30 mL/min or receiving RRT). These factors have been identified to increase the risk of hemorrhagic complications and subtherapeutic or supratherapeutic AFXa requiring dose adjustments. Fondaparinux AFXa peak concentrations should occur 3 h after subcutaneous administration and trough concentrations at least 1 h prior to the next dose. Although therapeutic AFXa levels and dose adjustments based on these levels are not established, concentrations reported by the manufacturer have been used as a surrogate in studies. Fondaparinux thromboprophylaxis peak steady-state concentrations of 0.39–0.5 mg/L and trough of 0.14–0.19 mg/L, and therapeutic peak concentration of 1.2–1.26 mg/L and trough of 0.46–0.62 mg/L, have been reported.

Special Populations

Renal Impairment Fondaparinux for all indications should be considered contraindicated in the setting of acute kidney injury, doubling of serum creatinine, or urine output less than 0.5 mL/kg/h, due to the unpredictable elimination. According to the manufacturer labeling, renal impairment with a CrCl less than 30 mL/min or receiving renal replacement therapy (RRT) is contraindicated, and an alternative anticoagulant should be recommended. In the setting of acute HIT treatment in the critically ill patient with renal impairment, the risk of under- or overdosing, feasibility of monitoring, and long half-life of fondaparinux warrant the use of direct thrombin inhibitor infusion as the primary anticoagulant. Although data is limited, in patients with a history of HIT and renal impairment or receiving RRT, fondaparinux thromboprophylaxis could be considered. In patients with a CrCl 20–50 mL/min, a 50% dose reduction or 1.5 mg daily is recommended for thromboprophylaxis [24, 54]. Alternatively, in critically ill patients with CrCl <30 mL/min or on hemodialysis receiving 2.5 mg every 48 h and patients on CVVH receiving 1.25 mg daily or 2.5 mg every 48 h demonstrated similar peak and trough AFXa as standard 2.5 mg daily dosing [55, 56]. In North America, the lowest commercially available syringe dose is 2.5 mg without graduated markings; therefore, the product would require manipulation into another syringe to administer a 1.25–1.5 mg dose. In patients with a history of HIT at high risk of VTE, it is reasonable to use 2.5 mg every 48-h dosing for prophylaxis with further dose adjustment according to AFXa peak and trough levels.

Low body weight Patients weighing <50 kg have demonstrated a 30% decrease in total clearance of fondaparinux; therefore, when used for treatment, AFXa levels should be monitored. According to the manufacturer labeling, in patients <50 kg, fondaparinux is contraindicated for the indication of thromboprophylaxis. To date, there is no literature evaluating prophylaxis with fondaparinux in this patient population; therefore, an alternative agent should be considered; in the setting where no other option is available, reduced dosing of 1.25–1.5 mg daily could be considered with AFXa monitoring but should be used with caution due to the increased bleeding risk. Similar to prophylaxis, data on the use of fondaparinux for VTE treatment in patients <50 kg is limited. In cases of extreme low body weight <30 kg, although not validated in the adult patient population, 0.1 mg/kg once daily in the pediatric population aged 1–18 years has demonstrated therapeutic AFXa [57]. Due to limited data, in patients with low body weight, an alternative agent should be considered if available.

High body weight Patients with a BMI $\geq$40 kg/m^2 receiving standard prophylaxis dosing of fondaparinux have the risk of subtherapeutic AFXa levels. In a study evaluating standard prophylaxis dosing in a population with a mean BMI of 51.2 kg/m^2, 43% of patients had subtherapeutic AFXa levels, but no differences in VTE or bleeding episodes were noted [58]. When fondaparinux 5 mg daily dosing was compared to enoxaparin 40 mg twice daily in patients with a mean BMI of 45 kg/m^2 after bariatric surgery, there were similar VTE and bleeding rates, but fondaparinux was more likely to result in a prophylactic AFXa level [59]. Based on this data, fondaparinux 5 mg daily could be considered in patients with BMI $\geq$45 kg/m^2, but due to the limited duration of 2–3 days in which patients received this dosing, AFXa monitoring should occur if used for prolonged prophylaxis to ensure no accumulation. When fondaparinux was evaluated for acute VTE treatment in patients with a BMI < or >30 kg/m^2 or weight < or >100 kg, there was no difference in the incidence of VTE reoccurrence or bleeding deeming 10 mg daily dosing of fondaparinux safe and effective in obese patients [60]. Due to the limited patients included with a BMI $\geq$50 kg/m^2, use in this patient population should include AFXa monitoring.

Overall, due to the long half-life and risk of accumulation with renal dysfunction, fondaparinux use in the ICU is limited but could be considered in patients with remote HIT requiring prophylaxis, as a transition therapy for patients with HIT, or in patients with a porcine allergy or avoidance of animal-based product. Refer to Table 49.6 that shows parenteral anticoagulation.

Table 49.6 Parenteral anticoagulants [24]

	Unfractionated heparin	Low-molecular-weight heparin[a]	Fondaparinux	Argatroban	Bivalirudin
Product source[b]	Biologic	Biologic	Synthetic	Synthetic	Synthetic
Mechanism of action	AT-mediated indirect inhibition of FXa and IIa	AT-mediated indirect inhibition of FXa and FIIa	Selective AT-mediated indirect inhibition of FXa	Direct binding of thrombin (reversible)	Direct binding of thrombin (reversible)
Factor target	FXa, FIIa (thrombin)	FXa, some FIIa	FXa	FIIa	FIIa
Route	Intravenous or subcutaneous	Subcutaneous[c]	Subcutaneous[c]	Intravenous	Intravenous
Time to peak	IV: Immediate SC: 2–4 h	3–5 h	2–3 h	Immediate	Immediate
Half-life	1–2 h (dose dependent)	4.5–7 h (normal renal function)	17–21 h (normal renal function)	39–51 min Hepatic impairment: 181 min	25 min CrCl <30 mL/min: 57 min Dialysis: 3.5 h
Metabolism	No enzymatic degradation	Minimal hepatic by desulfation and/or depolymerization	Minimal; majority eliminated unchanged	Hepatic via CYP3A4/5 hydroxylation, aromatization	Proteolytic cleavage
Elimination	Reticuloendothelial primarily in the liver and spleen	Renal	Renal (77% unchanged)	Feces (14% unchanged) Urine (16% unchanged)	Proteolysis 20% renal via glomerular filtration
Renal impairment	No dose adjustment	CrCl <30 mL/min: adjust frequency q24h	CrCl 30–50 mL/min: use with caution, consider 50% reduction when used for prophylaxis CrCl <30 mL/min: contraindicated	No dose adjustment	CrCl <60 mL/min requires lower initial rate CrCl <30 mL/min: Lower initial rate 0.04–0.07 mg/kg/h

(continued)

Table 49.6 (continued)

	Unfractionated heparin	Low-molecular-weight heparin[a]	Fondaparinux	Argatroban	Bivalirudin
Renal replacement	No dose adjustment	Alternative recommended limited data	Alternative recommended limited data	HD/CRRT: No dose adjustment	Dialyzable (25% over 4 h) HD/CRRT: Lower initial rate 0.03–0.07 mg/kg/h[d]
Hepatic impairment	No dose adjustment	No dose adjustment	No dose adjustment	Child Pugh B: lower initial rate 0.5 mcg/kg/min Child Pugh C: Lower initial rate 0.25 mcg/kg/min	No dose adjustment
Monitoring	aPTT AFXa	AFXa	AFXa	aPTT dTT	aPTT dTT
Reversal agent	Protamine	Protamine (partial neutralization ~60% AFXa activity)	Potentially Andexanet alfa but unclear specific dosing	None	None
Adverse effects	HIT Allergic reaction Hyperkalemia Bleeding	HIT Allergic reaction Hyperkalemia Bleeding	Bleeding	Bleeding (no reversal)	Bleeding (no reversal)
Considerations	Heparin resistance		Can be used in the setting of HIT or remote HIT	Dose reductions suggested for: Critical illness: 0.25–1 mcg/kg/min Heart failure: 0.25–0.5 mcg/kg/min False prolonging of the PT/INR	False prolonging of the PT/INR but less than argatroban

Abbreviations: *aPTT* activated partial thromboplastin time; *AFXa* anti-factor Xa; *AT* antithrombin; *dTT* dilute thromboplastin time; *HIT* heparin-induced thrombocytopenia; *HD* hemodialysis; *CRRT* continuous renal replacement therapy

[a] Low-molecular-weight heparin products include enoxaparin and dalteparin

[b] Synthetic formulations can be administered to patients with allergies to animal products or in those who have religious preferences to avoid select animal-derived products

[c] Enoxaparin can be administered intravenously in the setting of acute arterial thrombosis and to protect dialysis circuit from thrombosis. Fondaparinux can be administered intravenously in the setting of acute arterial thrombosis

[d] Drug clearance will be dependent on the method and mode of RRT, effluent rate, and filter type

49.3.1.4 Direct Thrombin Inhibitors

Mechanism of Action

Opposed to requiring a plasma cofactor to exert their activity, direct thrombin inhibitors (DTIs) have intrinsic activity because they reversibly bind and block the enzymatic activity of both circulating and clot-bound thrombin. The inhibition of thrombin thereby blocks the conversion of fibrinogen to fibrin and thrombin platelet activation. Direct thrombin inhibitors include argatroban and bivalirudin; despite similar mechanism of action, differences in metabolism and elimination can be a reason for selecting one DTI over the other. Their use in the ICU is primarily for HIT or suspected HIT, but can be considered for patients demonstrating heparin resistance, anticoagulation for extracorporeal membrane oxygenation, or as adjunctive anticoagulation for percutaneous coronary intervention.

Pharmacokinetics and Dosing

Specific differences in pharmacokinetics and dosing adjustments are listed in Table 49.6 that shows parenteral anticoagulants and discussed in drug-specific sections. Minimal plasma protein binding provides stable and predictable anticoagulation.

Argatroban Dosing for HIT in patients with normal hepatic function is 2 mcg/kg/min. Predominantly hepatically metabolized and excreted through the biliary system, dose adjustments are necessary in patients with hepatic but not renal impairment; hepatic dose reductions are according to the Child-Pugh classification system. Recommended starting doses for patients with Child-Pugh class B (moderate hepatic impairment) and Child-Pugh class C (severe hepatic impairment) are 0.5 and 0.25 mcg/kg/min, respectively. Additionally, dose reductions in patients with heart failure and critical illness in the setting of multiorgan dysfunction are recommended. With minimal removal from high-flux membranes during hemodialysis and continuous renal replacement therapy, argatroban may be preferred in patients on renal replacement therapy [61, 62]. In patients with a BMI $\geq$30 kg/m^2, dosing based on total body weight is suggested [63, 64].

Bivalirudin Although bivalirudin does not have FDA indication for the treatment of HIT, it can be used as an alternative to argatroban with similar to faster times to achieve therapeutic aPTT range and provide similar outcomes [65]. The initial dosing for HIT in patients with a creatinine clearance >60 mL/min is 0.15–0.2 mg/kg/h. Opposed to argatroban, bivalirudin is metabolized via proteolytic cleavage with renal elimination via glomerular filtration, tubular secretion, and tubular reabsorption. There is an inverse relationship with renal function and elimination half-life; therefore, dose adjustments in renal impairment or renal replacement therapy are recommended. In patients with a BMI $\geq$30 kg/m^2, dosing based on total body weight is suggested [66].

Monitoring

Typical monitoring and titration of DTIs are according to the aPTT assessing every 2 h. When designing a hospital protocol, it is important to consider for patients on argatroban with hepatic impairment, heart failure, or bivalirudin with renal impairment that the longer half-life may warrant additional aPTT checks beyond two consecutive 2-h aPTT within range. In patients with an elevated aPTT at baseline, dilute thrombin time (dTT) can be used as an alternative monitoring; refer to coagulation monitoring Sect. 49.2. Both DTIs can falsely prolong the PT/INR; this is secondary to their interaction with thromboplastin and tissue factor in the PT assay, and the high molar plasma concentrations necessary to achieve effective thrombin inhibition. Argatroban has a more pronounced effect on PT/INR due to its lower affinity to thrombin requiring higher molar concentrations when compared to bivalirudin. Vitamin K should not be administered to try to reverse this INR elevation.

Transitioning to Vitamin K Antagonist

The interaction with the PT/INR makes transitioning from a DTI a challenge, and premature discontinuation of the DTI may result in recurrent thrombosis [67]. The optimal method to transition has not been identified, but chromogenic factor X monitoring or overlapping until INR >4 for agatroban or INR >2 for bivalirudin can be considered. Institutional protocols for the management of anticoagulants should include a protocol for transitioning due to the complexity.

Transitioning argatroban to warfarin using chromogenic factor:

1. Overlap argatroban and warfarin for no less than 5 days in the setting of acute HIT management.
2. Start warfarin therapy at expected daily dose (dose varies).

    (a) In patients with HIT, warfarin should not be initiated until platelets are >150,000/μL.

3. On day 3, obtain a chromogenic factor X

    (a) Chromogenic factor X level of 40% corresponds to an INR of 2.
    (b) Chromogenic factor X level of 20% corresponds to an INR of 3.

4. Warfarin dose is adjusted by chromogenic factor X levels.
5. Discontinuing argatroban:

    (a) Once chromogenic factor X therapeutic, discontinue argatroban.
    (b) Obtain an INR 4–6 h after discontinuing argatroban to ensure that INR is within therapeutic range. If INR <2, argatroban should be resumed.

If chromogenic factor X is not available, the combined warfarin and argatroban INR threshold >4 can be used.

1. Overlap argatroban and warfarin for no less than 5 days in the setting of acute HIT management.
2. Start warfarin therapy at expected daily dose (dose varies):

    (a) In patients with HIT, warfarin should not be initiated until platelets are >150,000/μL.

3. Discontinuing argatroban:

    (a) If argatroban dose is ≤2 mcg/kg/min, once INR is >4, hold argatroban and repeat an INR at 4–6 h. If INR is less than the therapeutic goal, argatroban should be resumed.

    (b) If argatroban is >2 mcg/kg/min, lower the dose to 2 mcg/kg/min and obtain INR 4–6 h after the dose is lowered. If INR is >4, hold argatroban and repeat an INR at 4–6 h. If INR is less than the therapeutic goal, argatroban should be resumed.

49.3.2 Oral Anticoagulants

49.3.2.1 Vitamin K Antagonist (VKA)

The use of warfarin in the ICU is limited. Warfarin exhibits nonlinear pharmacokinetics; therefore, small changes in dose, enteral nutrition, organ perfusion, acute infection, protein binding, or drug interactions can result in large changes in the level of anticoagulation. Additionally, the long duration of action often requires preemptive planning to hold days prior to invasive procedures, and the prolonged onset of vitamin K for acute reversal makes warfarin not optimal for anticoagulation in the ICU.

Mechanism of Action

Warfarin is an oral VKA which produces an anticoagulant effect by inhibiting vitamin K epoxide reductase, the key enzyme responsible for converting vitamin K-dependent coagulation factors (II, VII, IX, X) and anticoagulant proteins C and S into their active form. The onset and duration of action are based on both the pharmacokinetic half-life of the drug, 36–42 h, and half-life of the vitamin k-dependent factors and proteins [68]. Synthesis of clotting factors is depleted according to their elimination half-lives (Table 49.7); since warfarin has no impact on functional clotting factors, the onset of action is often delayed. The antithrombotic effect is dependent on the depletion of prothrombin and factor X, which is delayed at least 5–7 days into therapy. Depletion of natural anticoagulants protein C and S results in a hypercoagulable state in the first few days of therapy. For these reasons, a minimum 5-day overlap with parenteral anticoagulation is required until warfarin reaches full antithrombotic effect [36]. Rapid achievement of a therapeutic INR prior to 5 minimum

Table 49.7 Vitamin
K-dependent factor and
protein half-lives

Vitamin K-dependent factor/protein	Plasma half-life
Factor II (prothrombin)	42–72 h
Factor VII	4–6 h
Factor IX	21–30 h
Factor X	27–48 h
Protein C	8 h
Protein S	30 h

is reflecting FVII depletion and should not be considered adequate anticoagulation overlap during warfarin initiation.

Pharmacokinetics

Warfarin is absorbed in the upper gastrointestinal tract with 100% bioavailability and can be crushed for feeding tube administration. The high protein binding (99%), primarily to albumin, can result in increased free fraction of unbound (active) drug in ICU patients with hypoalbuminemia. Additionally, medications with higher protein binding affinity can displace warfarin creating more unbound drug. Metabolism is dependent on hepatic function and occurs through the cytochrome P450 (CYP450) system including isoenzymes CYP2C9, CYP3A4, CYP1A2, and CYP2C19. Warfarin is subject to multiple drug interactions; CYP2C9 is a primarily responsible metabolism of the more potent enantiomer; drug interactions inducing or inhibiting this pathway can have a larger impact.

Common medications used in the ICU which *inhibit* warfarin metabolism are listed below based on the class of medication [69, 70]:

Antimicrobials: clarithromycin, erythromycin, fluconazole, fluoroquinolones (ciprofloxacin, levofloxacin), isoniazid, itraconazole, ketoconazole (systemic), metronidazole, posaconazole, ritonavir, sulfamethoxazole/trimethoprim, voriconazole

Cardiac medications: amiodarone, mexiletine, propafenone, verapamil, diltiazem

Immunosuppressants: cyclosporine

Common medications used in the ICU which *induce* warfarin metabolism are listed below based on the class of medication [69, 70]:

Antimicrobials: rifampin

Cardiac medications: bosentan

Antiepileptic medications: carbamazepine, phenobarbital, phenytoin

Although renal function will not impact the elimination of warfarin, decreased expression of CYP2C9 observed in chronic kidney disease can indirectly alter warfarin metabolism. Dietary intake of vitamin K will impact warfarin requirements; enteral nutrition formulas can contain vitamin K at various amounts; therefore, alterations in nutrition orders (holding, advancement, formula change) could affect dosing.

Monitoring

Vitamin K is a fat-soluble vitamin that is an essential cofactor in the conversion of clotting factors II, VII, IX, and X into their active form. The best coagulation test to monitor warfarin is prothrombin time (PT), which is then standardized to an international normalized ratio (INR). There are multiple interferences with monitoring PT/INR that can occur in the ICU patient, including acute or chronic liver failure, which creates difficulty in assessing the therapeutic effect of warfarin. Details on interferences of testing can be found in the coagulation monitoring Sect. 49.2.

49.3.2.2 Direct Oral Anticoagulants

Direct oral anticoagulants (DOACs) include direct FXa inhibitors (apixaban, rivaroxaban, edoxaban) and direct thrombin inhibitor dabigatran. The use of DOACs remains an attractive option due to rapid onset allowing therapeutic anticoagulation within hours of administration, predictable pharmacokinetics and pharmacodynamics, and no required routine monitoring. Additionally, DOACs have demonstrated a better safety profile and noninferiority to VKAs for VTE treatment or prophylaxis and stroke prevention in patients with nonvalvular atrial fibrillation. However, there are few studies evaluating these outcomes and safety in critically ill patients. Initiation of DOACs in the ICU is typically limited to clinically stable patients, but it is not uncommon to encounter patients receiving DOACs prior to admission for indications either related or unrelated to their current admission [71].

Pharmacokinetics and Dosing

Physiological changes in the critically ill patients including gastric perfusion or motility, impaired hepatic and/or renal function, and changes in volume of distribution can lead to unpredictable anticoagulation and increased risk of adverse effects. The different amounts of renal and hepatic elimination of the various DOACs are included in Table 49.8. All DOACs are substrates to P-glycoprotein; rivaroxaban and apixaban are additionally metabolized by CYP450 3a4; therefore, these drugs are subject to drug interactions with both inducers and inhibitors. Examples of medications used in the ICU that are inhibitors and inducers of P-glycoprotein and CYP3A4 are listed in Table 49.9. Specific considerations for patients with hepatic and renal impairment are included in each specific DOAC section and the special population section. A comparison of the DOAC dosing is included in Table 49.8.

Table 49.8 Direct oral anticoagulants [72]

	Dabigatran	Apixaban	Edoxaban	Rivaroxaban
Mechanism	Direct IIa inhibitor	Direct Xa inhibitor	Direct Xa inhibitor	Direct Xa inhibitor
Bioavailability	3–7%	50%	62%	66% without food 80–100% with food
Site of absorption	Proximal small intestine	Upper GI tract ↓ along distal GI tract	Upper GI tract	Primarily stomach Minimal small intestine ↓ along distal GI tract
Feeding tube administration	No	Yes	Yes	Yes
Onset	1.5–3 h	2–3 h	1–2 h	2–4 h
Half-life	12–17 h	12 h	9–10 h	9–13 h
Protein binding	35%	87%	55%	90%
Metabolism	P-gp transporter	P-gp transporter and CYP3A4	P-gp transporter	P-gp transporter and CYP3A4
Hepatic metabolism	20%	75%	50%	65%
Renal excretion	80%	25%	50%	35%
Dialysis removal	Yes	No	No	No
Dosing AF	150 mg twice daily 75 mg twice daily • CrCl 15–30 mL/min/1.73 m^2 • CrCl 30–50 mL/min/1.73 m^2 with ketoconazole or dronedarone	5 mg twice daily 2.5 mg twice daily • Two of the three criteria (age ≥80 years, weight ≤60 kg, or SCr ≥1.5 mg/dL) • Use with strong CYP3A4 and P-gp inhibitors (e.g., protease inhibitors, itraconazole, ketoconazole, conivaptan)	60 mg daily 30 mg once daily • CrCl 15–50 mL/min/1.73 m^2 • Potent P-gp inhibitor (verapamil, dronedarone, or quinidine) • Weight ≤60 kg	20 mg daily with food 15 mg daily with food • CrCl 15–50 mL/min/1.73 m^2
Dosing DVT/PE	150 mg twice daily after 5–10 days of parenteral anticoagulant	10 mg twice daily for 7 days, then 5 mg twice daily	60 mg once daily after 5–10 days of parenteral anticoagulant	15 mg twice daily for 21 days, then 20 mg daily with food

Abbreviation: *AF* atrial fibrillation; *DVT* deep vein thrombosis; *PE* pulmonary embolism
Note: Upper gastrointestinal tract includes the duodenum, jejunum, and ileum

Table 49.9 Common medication inhibitors and inducers of DOAC metabolism in the ICU [73]

	P-Glycoprotein inducers	P-Glycoprotein inhibitors	CYP3A4 inducers	CYP3A4 inhibitors
Medications	Carbamazepine Dexamethasone Fosphenytoin Phenytoin Rifampin	Amiodarone Azithromycin Clarithromycin Cobicistat Cyclosporine Diltiazem Dronedarone Erythromycin Isavuconazole Ketoconazole (systemic) Posaconazole Propafenone Ritonavir Tacrolimus Ticagrelor Tolvaptan Verapamil Voriconazole	Dexamethasone Fosphenytoin Phenytoin Phenobarbital	Amiodarone Clarithromycin Cyclosporine Diltiazem Erythromycin Fluconazole Itraconazole Ketoconazole (systemic) Posaconazole Ritonavir Tacrolimus Verapamil Voriconazole

Inhibitors of P-glycoprotein efflux pump may increase serum concentration of DOAC substrates
Inducers of P-glycoprotein efflux pump may increase serum concentration of DOAC substrates
Inhibitors of CYP450 3a4 may increase serum concentration of DOAC substrates
Inducers of CYP450 3a4 may decrease serum concentrations of DOAC substrates
Note: This list does not include all medication interactions, and each medication should be evaluated with all new medications to determine if an interaction exists. Each medication can have a varying degree of induction/inhibition (mild, moderate, severe). When evaluating drug interactions, the degree interaction, administration of multiple interacting medications, medications which interact with both p-glycoprotein and CYP450, and risk of adverse effects should be evaluated on an individual basis to determine if co-administration is contraindicated, and alternative agent should be used or can be co-administered with caution and monitoring

Dabigatran etexilate It is an oral direct thrombin inhibitor currently approved to reduce the risk of stroke and systemic embolism in patients with nonvalvular atrial fibrillation and is used for the treatment of VTE after receiving 5–10 days of parenteral anticoagulation. Dabigatran etexilate is a prodrug converted by the liver to dabigatran, the active form. The capsule cannot be opened or crushed for feeding tube administration; administration of the powder without the capsule shell results in a 75% increase in bioavailability. Dose adjustments are required for renal dysfunction and should be avoided in patients with CrCl <15–30 mL/h or on hemodialysis and with severe hepatic impairment. As a substrate for p-glycoprotein, drug interactions can impact dosing in the setting of concomitant renal impairment and may require changing to an alternative therapy in the setting of a strong p-glycoprotein inhibitor [74, 75].

Apixaban This is an oral factor Xa inhibitor approved to reduce the risk of stroke and systemic embolism in patients with nonvalvular atrial fibrillation and is used as VTE prophylaxis after orthopedic procedures, as initial therapy for acute treatment of VTE, and as secondary prophylaxis to reduce the risk of recurrent VTE. A dose reduction is required for atrial fibrillation with specific criteria (Table 49.8). Apixaban has the least dependence on renal elimination and is the only DOAC with labeling for administration in patients with renal impairment and patients receiving hemodialysis [75–77]. Apixaban is contraindicated in severe hepatic impairment, Child-Pugh class C. Apixaban is a substrate of CYP450 3a4, and p-glycoprotein therefore is subject to drug interactions. The formulation can be crushed for feeding tube administration, and absorption is unaffected by food. In the clinically stable patients, transitioning to oral therapy apixaban can be used for the initial management of VTE without a minimum 5 days on parenteral anticoagulation.

Rivaroxaban It is an oral factor Xa inhibitor approved to reduce the risk of stroke and systemic embolism in patients with nonvalvular atrial fibrillation; it is used as initial therapy for acute treatment of VTE and secondary prophylaxis to reduce reoccurrence of VTE and for the prevention of VTE in acutely ill medical patients and orthopedic surgery and for ischemic heart disease. Dosing varies based on indication and renal function. In patients with renal impairment, CrCl <30 mL/min, an alternative agent is recommended. Rivaroxaban is contraindicated in patients with a CrCl <15 mL/min or on hemodialysis and moderate and severe hepatic impairment (Child-Pugh classes B and C) [78]. Similar to apixaban, it is a substrate of CYP450 3a4 and p-glycoprotein. The formulation can be crushed for feeding tube administration. Doses 15 mg or more should be administered with food to increase the bioavailability [79]. Rivaroxaban can be considered in the clinically stable patient transitioning to oral therapy for the initial management of VTE without a minimum 5 days on parenteral anticoagulation.

Edoxaban It is an oral direct thrombin inhibitor currently approved to reduce the risk of stroke and systemic embolism in patients with nonvalvular atrial fibrillation and is used for the treatment of VTE after receiving 5–10 days of parenteral anticoagulation. Dosing varies based on indication and renal function. Edoxaban for nonvalvular atrial fibrillation should be avoided in patients with a CrCl >95 mL/min due to the increased risk of ischemic stroke. For all indications, edoxaban should be avoided in patients with a CrCl <15 mL/min or on hemodialysis and patients with severe hepatic impairment (Child-Pugh class C) [80]. Edoxaban is a substrate of p-glycoprotein. The formulation can be crushed for feeding tube administration, and absorption is unaffected by food.

Monitoring

The need of routine coagulation monitoring is not required with DOACs, but clinical scenarios in the ICU including acute bleeding, acute hepatic or renal impairment, drug interactions, unclear compliance, potential therapeutic failure, and need for an emergent procedure warrant further laboratory evaluation of coagulation parameters. Details regarding anticoagulation monitoring for DOACs are in coagulation monitoring Sect. 49.2.

Transitioning from DOAC to Parenteral Anticoagulation

In the setting of critical illness, oral anticoagulation is often transitioned to a parenteral anticoagulant with a shorter half-life. The standard package insert recommendation, to initiate parenteral anticoagulation at the time of the next scheduled DOAC, may not be applicable to patients with acute end-organ dysfunction and can result in dual anticoagulation due to decreased DOAC elimination. Patients presenting with acute kidney injury or on renal replacement therapy, severe hepatic impairment (Child-Pugh class C) or acute liver failure, and critical illness are at higher risk of major bleeding. The ideal method to transition patients in this setting has not been determined, but a delayed initiation or DOAC-calibrated AFXa monitoring approach versus standard package insert recommendations has been suggested [81, 82]. Even with DOAC AFXa monitoring, the optimal level which results in decreased bleeding without increased thrombosis has not been determined. Based on limited retrospective evidence, an AFXa concentration <100 ng/mL is a reasonable safe cutoff for transition, an AFXa between 100 and 200 ng/mL requires clinical evaluation of risk versus benefits, and an AFXa >200 ng/mL parenteral anticoagulation can be held with repeat AFXa monitoring in 12–24 h unless clinically warranted [81].

Special Patient Populations

Heparin- induced thrombocytopenia Direct oral anticoagulation agents do not complex with PF4; therefore, they do not stimulate an antibody response allowing their use as a therapeutic option for the management of HIT. In critically ill patients, a parenteral non-heparin anticoagulant may be preferred in the setting of increased bleeding risk, potential for urgent procedures or HIT complicated by life- or limb-threatening thromboembolism, such as massive pulmonary embolism or venous limb gangrene. In clinically stable patients, DOACs provide an ideal agent in transitioning from intravenous to oral therapy due to the rapid onset of action and unlike VKA do not cause reductions in protein C; therefore, in comparison, it could decrease the length of hospital stay and cost associated with awaiting platelet recovery, monitoring, and reaching a therapeutic INR [83]. Additional information on the management and therapeutic options for HIT are discussed in the heparin-induced thrombocytopenia Sect. 49.7.2.

Hepatic impairment Hepatic function affects all DOACs' drug metabolism to varying extents. Apixaban is the most dependent on hepatic metabolism, followed by rivaroxaban, edoxaban, and dabigatran (Table 49.8). Hepatic clearance of DOACs can be compromised in patients with hepatic impairment (acute and chronic) in the setting of decreased hepatic perfusion and decreased hepatocyte function, and the development of hepatorenal syndrome can further increase the risk of DOAC accumulation. Highly protein-bound DOACs, apixaban and rivaroxaban, in patients with impaired hepatic synthesis of albumin can result in an increase of unbound active drug in the blood, which can result in toxicity. Apixaban and rivaroxaban require cytochrome P450 (CYP) enzymes for metabolism compared to dabigatran and edoxaban. Progression of cirrhosis is known to reduce CYP3A4 levels and therefore would be expected to impact metabolize and increase serum concentrations [84, 85]. Restrictions for the use of DOACs in patients with hepatic impairment are based on the Child-Pugh classification, which accounts for both clinical (ascites, encephalopathy) and laboratory abnormalities (bilirubin, albumin, INR) to assess the severity and predicted mortality in cirrhosis patients. Metabolism of drugs involving CYP3A4 has demonstrated an inverse relationship in drug concentration with severity of liver failure categorized by Child-Pugh classification [84]. Summarized in Table 49.10 are DOAC recommendations based on the Child-Pugh class. Exclusion criteria of large, randomized trials evaluating DOACs in atrial fibrillation or VTE often included acute or chronic hepatitis, cirrhosis, liver function test two to three times upper limit of normal (ULN), total bilirubin 1.5 times ULN, and thrombocytopenia; therefore, the applicability in patients with hepatic impairment in the ICU is limited [87]. Overall, all DOACs should be held from initiation or transitioned to an alternative anticoagulant in patients with acute liver failure or progression from Child-Pugh class B to class C.

Renal impairment All DOACs have some extent of renal elimination. Currently, the FDA has approved apixaban, rivaroxaban, dabigatran, and edoxaban in patients with a creatinine clearance as low as 15 mL/min; refer to Table 49.8 for specific DOAC dosing. The Cockcroft-Gault equation was used in clinical trials to determine CrCl and should be used for dosing DOAC [75]. Dabigatran is the most reliant on renal function with 80% of unchanged drug eliminated in the urine and is the only DOAC significantly removed by hemodialysis. Apixaban elimination is the least dependent on renal function and requires no dose adjustment for end-stage renal impairment, including hemodialysis, alone. This is based on single-dose studies in patients with severe renal impairment, with creatinine clearance <30 mL/min, and on hemodialysis [76, 77]. Literature evaluating apixaban pharmacokinetics in hemodialysis patients after 8 days of therapy demonstrated significant accumulation, but when translated into clinical practice compared to warfarin, there was no

Table 49.10 Direct oral anticoagulant (DOAC) recommendations based on hepatic impairment [86]

DOAC	Child-Pugh class A	Child-Pugh class B	Child-Pugh class C
Dabigatran	No dose reduction	Use with caution	Contraindication
Apixaban	No dose reduction	Use with caution	Contraindication
Edoxaban	No dose reduction	Use with caution	Contraindication
Rivaroxaban	No dose reduction	Contraindication	Contraindication

Child-Pugh score of <7 is class A (well-compensated disease, mild impairment), 7–9 is class B (significant functional compromise, moderate impairment), and 10–15 is class C (decompensated disease, severe impairment)

difference in major bleeding events in chronic kidney disease and dialysis-dependent patients [88, 89].

Opposed to chronic kidney disease or hemodialysis, acute kidney injury (AKI) results in dynamic physiological changes which may impact DOAC pharmacokinetics including alterations in nonrenal clearance, increased volume of distribution, changes in protein binding, and reduction in hepatic metabolizing enzymes including CYP3A4 [90]. A study evaluating apixaban continuation in AKI, when compared to patients without an AKI, found no difference in major bleeding events. The patient population was primarily in general floor patients and not critically ill; majority had prerenal etiology, stage 1 AKI, and the duration of AKI while on apixaban was a median of 72 h [91]. Another study evaluating apixaban and rivaroxaban continuation in the setting of AKI found a median time to major bleeding event of 72 h, and major bleeding events were more likely in patients with AKI stages 2 and 3; therefore, it is possible that differences in severity of AKI and duration could impact major bleeding events [92]. Given the changes in pharmacokinetics and inability to quantify DOAC clearance due to the dynamic changes in renal function, DOACs including apixaban should be avoided in AKI. Data on the use of DOACs in CRRT is also limited. An in vitro pharmacokinetic evaluation of apixaban concentrations during various CRRT modalities, filters, flow rates, and point of replacement fluid dilution demonstrated that key factors impacting apixaban dosing included CRRT modality, filter, and flow rate, which would impact the clearance of apixaban. Simulated dosing recommendations based on CRRT flow rate and type of filter ranged from 2.5 to 7.5 mg twice daily [93]. Extrapolating this into clinical practice warrants in vivo data evaluating the impact of nonrenal clearance and alterations in protein binding, safety, and efficacy. Lastly, in vitro modeling does not account for CRRT circuit downtime which often occurs in ICU patients and could significantly impact the total clearance [94].

49.4 Heparin Resistance in the ICU

49.4.1 Pathophysiology

Decreased heparin response may be seen in patients with elevated heparin-binding proteins, antithrombin deficiency, increased heparin clearance, or elevated factor VIII levels. Heparin is a strong, negatively charged molecule that can bind proteins like PF4, lipoproteins, von Willebrand factor, factor VIII, fibrinogen, endothelial cells, as well as surfaces of IV tubing and circuit components for continuous renal replacement therapy (CRRT) and extracorporeal membrane oxygenation (ECMO) [95]. Antithrombin (AT) deficiency can be inherited or acquired and is the most common cause of heparin resistance. Inherited AT deficiency can be due to a genetic mutation resulting in decreased synthesis or functional defect [96]. Etiologies of acquired AT deficiency can include acute thrombosis, asparaginase therapy, disseminated intravascular coagulation (DIC), extracorporeal membrane oxygenation (ECMO), hemodialysis, liver disease, surgery or trauma, and ongoing heparin use [96]. The AT level necessary for adequate anticoagulation with heparin remains to be elucidated. There may also be a perceived lack of heparin response in patients with elevated factor VIII and fibrinogen levels if using aPTT monitoring. Elevated coagulation factors in response to acute inflammatory states, especially COVID-19, may result in shortened baseline aPTT and higher doses of heparin to achieve target aPTT. Switching to AFXa monitoring in these cases may be most appropriate as the AFXa assay is unaffected by elevated coagulation factor levels.

49.4.2 Diagnosis and Management

Heparin resistance may be suspected when a perceived adequate dose of heparin fails to achieve a target level of anticoagulation by either aPTT or AFXa. Identification and workup of heparin resistance can be difficult in the absence of specific thresholds that define it. The most commonly reported definitions for heparin resistance were >35,000 units/day and >30 units/kg/h on a recent ISTH survey [97]. The approach to managing suspected heparin resistance involves checking UFH AFXa and administration of higher heparin doses. If therapeutic anticoagulation cannot be achieved after escalating heparin doses or if patients require urgent therapeutic anticoagulation, switching to a direct thrombin inhibitor (argatroban or bivalirudin) may be warranted. Alternatively, if therapeutic targets cannot be achieved with heparin, antithrombin repletion may be considered. The 2022 ELSO guidelines suggest antithrombin supplementation to a goal antithrombin level of 50–80% in ECMO patients who are unable to achieve therapeutic targets on maximum doses of heparin [98]. However, data to support antithrombin administration outside of the cardiac surgery setting is very limited. Future studies are needed to guide antithrombin monitoring and supplementation in critically ill patients. Figure 49.3 outlines the approach to diagnosis and management of heparin resistance.

49.4.3 Role of the Pharmacist

The critical care pharmacist can play a key role in the identification and management of heparin resistance through interpretation of coagulation assays and assessment of cumulative heparin therapy. From an antithrombotic stewardship perspective, the pharmacist can guide safe and appropriate administration of direct thrombin inhibitors and antithrombin III, agents that typically carry a formulary restriction, as clinically appropriate. Additionally, pharmacists may be involved in the development of an institutional guideline or protocol for evaluating and managing suspected heparin resistance patients.

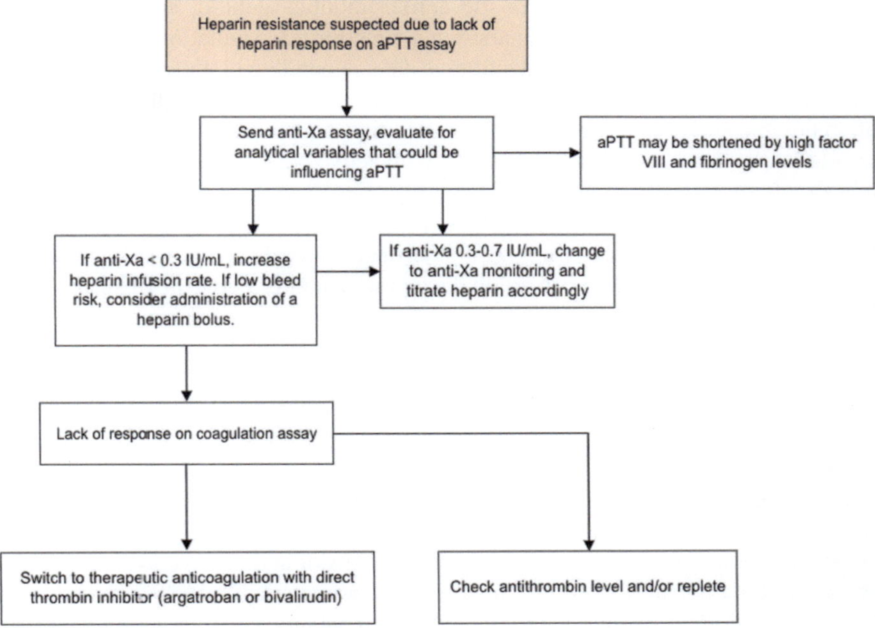

Fig. 49.3 Approach to diagnosis and management of heparin resistance [28]

49.5 Antithrombotic Reversal

Per the International Society on Thrombosis and Haemostasis, major bleeding refers to bleeding that results in hemodynamic compromise and/or bleeding in a critical site (intracranial, intraspinal, intraocular, retroperitoneal, pericardial, intra-articular, or intramuscular with compartment syndrome) and/or an acute hemoglobin decrease by more than 2 g/dL or requirement of more than 2 units of whole blood or red blood cells. All nonmajor bleeds are classified as minor but are still clinically relevant if they lead to a hospital admission, require medical or surgical treatment, or require a change to antithrombotic therapy, including interruption or discontinuation [99].

49.5.1 Indications for Antithrombotic Reversal

Antithrombotic reversal in critically ill patients may be warranted in various clinical scenarios to manage bleeding complications or prepare for emergent procedures when the benefit of restoring hemostasis outweighs the risks associated with reversal and interruption of antithrombotic therapy. It is imperative to discontinue the antithrombotic agent(s) immediately and assess the time of last dose administered, the pharmacokinetic properties of the antithrombotic agent(s), and the patient's ability to eliminate the drug (hepatic/renal function). Coagulation assays can be used to provide qualitative and quantitative data, depending on the available institutional assays, and aid in the decision to provide reversal (Table 49.11). In the case of major bleeding, fluid and blood resuscitation and local hemostatic measures should be provided, as indicated. Patients with active bleeding or symptomatic anemia should receive RBC to maintain a hemoglobin >7 g/dL, PLT to maintain platelet count >50 × 10^9/L, and cryoprecipitate to maintain fibrinogen >100 mg/dL [101, 102]. Additionally, maintaining normothermia, ionized calcium concentrations >1.1 mmol/L, and pH >7.25 can aid in the attainment of effective hemostasis [103].

49.5.2 Reversal of Anticoagulants

Reversal of anticoagulation is detailed based on the specific anticoagulant agent. Details regarding the pharmacokinetics and therapeutic monitoring targets of each antithrombotic agent can be found in coagulation monitoring Sect. 49.2. Table 49.12 displays a summary of reversal agents, mechanisms of action, reversal indications, onset and duration of action, and monitoring parameters. Table 49.13 displays a summary of clotting factor content in blood components.

Table 49.11 Anticoagulant effects on clotting assays [100]

Agent	aPTT	PT/INR	Other	Half-life	Dialyzable
IV UFH	Increase	Neutral	Increase AFXa	30 min	No
LMWH	Increase/ neutral	Neutral	Increase AFXa	4.5–5 h	No
Argatroban	Increase	Increase	Increase TT/dTT	30–50 min	Poorly
Bivalirudin	Increase	Increase	Increase TT/dTT	20–25 min	Poorly
Fondaparinux	Increase/ neutral	Increase/ neutral	Increase AFXa	17–21 h	Poorly
Warfarin	Increase/ neutral	Increase	Decrease chromogenic FX	5–7 days	No
Apixaban	Increase/ neutral	Increase/ neutral	Increase AFXa	12 h	Poorly
Rivaroxaban	Increase/ neutral	Increase/ neutral	Increase AFXa	5–9 h	No
Edoxaban	Neutral	Increase/ neutral	Increase AFXa	10–14 h	No
Dabigatran	Increase	Increase/ neutral	Increase TT/dTT	12–17 h	Yes

Abbreviations: *AFXa* anti-factor Xa; *dTT* dilute thrombin time; *FX* factor X; *TT* thrombin time
For patients experiencing minor bleeding, local and supportive measures in combination with temporary discontinuation of antithrombotic therapy should be sufficient in achieving hemostasis. Likewise, temporary discontinuation or dose reduction of antithrombotic therapies should be recommended prior to planned and nonurgent procedures, and full reversal is generally unnecessary

Table 49.12 Summary of reversal agents [104–110]

Reversal agent	Mechanism	Reversal indication	Onset	Duration	Coagulation assay monitoring	Warnings/pearls
Andexanet alfa	Recombinant modified human factor Xa decoy that targets and sequesters factor Xa inhibitors	Oral FXa inhibitors	Rapid	~1 h	AFXa	– Boxed warning for thromboembolic risks, ischemic risks, cardiac arrest, and sudden death
Idarucizumab	Humanized monoclonal antibody that binds dabigatran and metabolites	Dabigatran	Effects observed within min	12–24 h	aPTT TT/dTT	
Phytonadione (vitamin K)	Promotes hepatic biosynthesis of vitamin K-dependent clotting factors	Warfarin	IV: 1–2 h PO: 6–10 h	IV: 12–24 h PO: 24–48 h	INR	– Boxed warning for hypersensitivity reactions with IV and IM use (max infusion rate 1 mg/min)
Protamine	UFH antagonist that forms protamine-heparin complex and disrupts heparin-antithrombin III complex	Complete reversal of UFH Incomplete reversal of LMWH	5 min	Up to 2 h	ACT aPTT AFXa	– Boxed warning for hypersensitivity reactions (increased risk with high protamine doses or rapid administration; max infusion rate 5 mg/min) – Test dose recommended for the following patients if receiving more than 10 mg dose: previous exposure to protamine, treatment with insulin NPH, history of fish allergy – Cardiac and blood pressure monitoring recommended

(continued)

Table 49.12 (continued)

Reversal agent	Mechanism	Reversal indication	Onset	Duration	Coagulation assay monitoring	Warnings/pearls
4F PCC	Concentrate of nonactivated coagulation factors II, VII, IX, X and proteins C and S	Warfarin Factor Xa inhibitors	Rapid, within 30 min	6–24 h	INR (warfarin)	– Boxed warning for arterial and venous thromboembolic complications – Potency defined by factor IX content – Contraindications: DIC, HIT within previous 100 days (contains ~500 units of heparin/vial)
aPCC	Concentrate of activated coagulation factor VII and nonactivated coagulation factors II, IX, X	Fondaparinux Alternative to 4F PCC if heparin contraindicated	15–30 min	8–12 h	No reliable assays to measure efficacy	– Boxed warning for thromboembolic events – Contraindications: DIC
rFVIIa	Recombinant activated factor VII	Refractory reversal cases Fondaparinux	10–20 min	2–4 h	No reliable assays to measure efficacy	– Boxed warning for thrombosis (arterial and venous)
Fibrinogen concentrate	Increase available fibrinogen to be converted to fibrin	Alteplase, tenecteplase	Within 1 h	100 h	Fibrinogen level	

Abbreviations: *4F PCC* four-factor prothrombin complex concentrate, *aPCC* activated prothrombin complex concentrate; *rFVIIa* recombinant activated factor VII; *AFXa* anti-factor Xa; *aPTT* activated partial thromboplastin time; *dTT* dilute thrombin time; *INR* international normalized ratio; *TT* thrombin time; *IV* intravenous; *IM* intramuscular; *DIC* disseminated intravascular coagulation; *HIT* heparin-induced thrombocytopenia

Table 49.13 Summary of blood components [111, 112]

Blood component	Content	Dosing	Pearls	Warnings
Cryoprecipitate	Fibrinogen Factor VIII VWF	10 units (150–200 mL)	Administration of 10 units of cryo is expected to increase fibrinogen levels by 50–70 mg/dL	Transfusion reactions: hemolytic, anaphylactic, bacterial/viral contamination, transfusion-related acute lung injury, transfusion-associated circulatory overload
Fresh frozen plasma (FFP)	Fibrinogen (lower concentration than cryoprecipitate) Factors V, VII, VIII, IX, X, XI, XIII VWF	10–20 mL/kg (4–6 units)	Administration of 4–6 units of FFP is expected to raise clotting factor levels by about 20%	

49.5.2.1 Unfractionated Heparin

Unfractionated heparin is a common parenteral anticoagulant in the intensive care unit used for both treatment and prophylaxis of thromboembolism. For patients experiencing minor bleeding or undergoing planned procedures, unfractionated heparin administration can be discontinued to allow for clearance. For patients who require reversal, protamine should be administered. When administered alone, protamine has weak but clinically insignificant anticoagulant effects. The protamine dose required to neutralize heparin activity depends on the amount administered within about 3 h before reversal. Generally, 1 mg of protamine is required to neutralize 100 units of heparin administered within the past 1 h of administration, and less protamine is required for heparin administered greater than 1 h previously.

Time since UFH administration	Dose per 100 units of UFH
<1 h	1 mg
1–2 h	0.5 mg
>2 h	0.25 mg
Example calculation: TG is a 50 kg female who experiences major bleeding related to UFH. She received a 4000 unit bolus (80 units/kg) 3 h ago and has been on an infusion running at 18 units/kg/h. How much protamine is needed to neutralize the heparin administered within the last 3 h?	
• <1 h: 18 units/kg/h × 50 kg = 900 units × 1 mg/100 units	9 mg
• 1–2 h: 18 units/kg/h × 50 kg = 900 units × 0.5 mg/100 units	4.5 mg
• >2 h: 18 units/kg/h × 50 kg = 900 units + 4000 units × 0.25 mg/100 units	12.25 mg
Total	25.75 mg
TG should receive 26 mg of protamine to reverse the UFH she has received in the last 3 h	

The maximum recommended dose of protamine at a single time is 50 mg infused over 10 min to reduce the risk of bradycardia, severe hypotension, cardiovascular collapse, and anaphylactic reactions. Successful reversal of heparin can be assessed by normalization and/or reduction of ACT, aPTT, or anti-factor Xa (AFXa) concentration.

49.5.2.2 Low-Molecular-Weight Heparin (LMWH)

LMWHs (enoxaparin) are also common parenteral anticoagulants used for thromboembolism treatment and prevention in the intensive care unit. Like UFH, patients experiencing minor bleeding or undergoing planned procedures should have LMWH discontinued to allow for clearance, taking into consideration the potential need for earlier discontinuation in patients with renal dysfunction prior to procedures. Unlike UFH, there are currently no agents available that can completely reverse LMWH. Administration of protamine will result in about 60% reversal of anticoagulant effects. Protamine dosing is dependent on the amount of LMWH administered within the previous 8–12 h. If the last dose of LMWH was administered within the previous 8 h, 1 mg of protamine should be administered for every 1 mg of enoxaparin. If the last dose of LMWH was administered between 8 and 12 h previously, 0.5 mg of protamine should be administered for every 1 mg of enoxaparin. Reversal of LMWH can be assessed through reduction in aPTT (if prolonged prior to reversal) and AFXa concentration.

49.5.2.3 Direct Thrombin Inhibitors (DTIs)

Intravenous direct thrombin inhibitors, argatroban and bivalirudin, have no specific reversal agent; however, given their short half-lives, a combination of drug discontinuation, supportive care, and local hemostatic methods can be utilized in the case of major and minor bleeding. Clearance of intravenous direct thrombin inhibitors can be monitored with aPTT or TT/dTT.

Reversal of oral dabigatran may be necessary in the setting of bleeding or emergent procedure. Idarucizumab is the FDA-approved, first-line therapy for reversal of dabigatran. The REVERSE-AD trial evaluated idarucizumab 5 g administered as two 2.5 g bolus infusions in 503 patients and found 100% median maximal coagulation assay reversal at 4 h. Hemostasis was confirmed within 24 h in 68% of 203 patients evaluated for bleeding, and periprocedural hemostasis was deemed normal in 93% of 197 patients [113]. Thromboembolic events were reported in 4.8% of patients within 30 days and 6.8% of patients within 90 days [113]. If idarucizumab is unavailable, current guidelines recommend 4F PCC 25–50 units/kg for dabigatran reversal [114]. Renal replacement therapy may be considered to facilitate additional clearance of dabigatran.

Patients with elevated pre-reversal dabigatran levels (e.g., renal failure with drug accumulation) may experience incomplete reversal or rebound of coagulation parameters within 1–4 h after idarucizumab administration [113, 115]. If incomplete reversal is suspected or coagulation parameters rebound in the setting of ongoing or recurrent bleeding, repeat administration of idarucizumab 5 g may be warranted [114]. Successful reversal of dabigatran can be assessed by normalization of aPTT (if initially prolonged) or confirmed with normalization of TT/dTT.

49.5.2.4 Fondaparinux

Fondaparinux has a half-life of about 16 h, but anticoagulant activity can persist for 48–96 h after the last dose in patients with normal renal function, and longer in patients with renal impairment. No specific reversal agents are available for fondaparinux. rFVIIa and aPCC may partially reverse fondaparinux based on very limited clinical data [116, 117]. Reversal of fondaparinux may be assessed through reduction of aPTT or INR, if prolonged prior to reversal [118].

49.5.2.5 Warfarin

Patients admitted to the intensive care unit with minor bleeding or prior to planned procedure may require holding or decreasing warfarin doses and/or administration of vitamin K, with appropriate bridging strategies as necessary for planned procedures (refer to Sect. 49.9). Patients requiring urgent reversal of INR should have their warfarin discontinued, and vitamin K-dependent clotting factors should be administered, either by 4-factor prothrombin complex concentrate (4F PCC) or fresh frozen plasma (FFP). Vitamin K should also be administered to allow for clotting factor synthesis and sustained INR reversal. Reversal of warfarin with activated products such as aPCC or recombinant activated factor VII (rFVIIa) has been associated with increased thrombotic risk, and therefore, it is generally not recommended. INR can be used to assess successful reversal of warfarin therapy. One can expect an INR decrease within 30 min after PCC administration, within 2–4 h after FFP and IV vitamin K administration and within 8 h after oral vitamin K administration.

4F PCC contains clotting factors FIX, FII, FVII, and FX at concentrations nearly 25 times that of blood, as well as proteins C and S. 4F PCC is dosed in FIX units and has similar INR reduction with standard INR-based dosing and fixed-dose strategies [119–123]. Fixed 4F PCC dosing strategies include 1500–2000 units for intracranial hemorrhage (ICH) and 1000 units for non-ICH bleeding. Fixed dosing with 1000 units may not provide sufficient INR reversal, and supplemental 4F PCC administration may be required [123]. Refer to Table 49.14 for standard INR-based dosing with a maximum dose of 5000 units.

FFP is a nonspecific reversal agent that contains clotting factors, fibrinogen (400–900 mg/unit), proteins C and S, albumin and other plasma proteins, antithrombin, and tissue factor pathway inhibitor [111]. Conventional dosing for INR reversal with FFP is 10–20 mL/kg (approximately 4–6 units in adults) which will increase

Table 49.14 INR and weight-based dosing for PCC [114, 124]

Pretreatment INR	PCC dose
1.3–1.9	10–20 units/kg
2–3.9	25 units/kg
4–6	35 units/kg
>6	50 units/kg

clotting factor levels by approximately 20% [111]. FFP is no longer recommended for warfarin reversal, unless PCC is unavailable, given the risk for transfusion-related reactions, significant volume required for efficacy, and prolonged administration time. PCC has also been shown to achieve higher rates of hemostasis, shorter time to INR correction, and significant reduction in all-cause mortality compared to FFP [125].

Vitamin K is a necessary cofactor for the synthesis of clotting factors II, VII, IX, and X. Dosing and route of administration of vitamin K are dependent on the severity of bleeding and INR resulted prior to reversal. For major bleeding, vitamin K 10 mg IV should be administered in combination with PCC (or FFP if PCC unavailable) to allow for delayed and sustained INR reversal after clearance of PCC. Subcutaneous and intramuscular vitamin K administration is not recommended due to variable absorption and lower efficacy in lowering the INR. In minor bleeding or nonurgent warfarin reversal, oral or IV vitamin K can be administered with doses between 0.5 and 10 mg depending on the INR and when warfarin therapy is to be reinitiated. It is important to note that vitamin K itself is not prothrombotic; however, it can precipitate thromboembolism by returning patients to baseline prothrombotic states (e.g., atrial fibrillation, mechanical heart valves, antiphospholipid antibody syndrome) in the setting of subtherapeutic INR.

49.5.2.6 FXa Inhibitors (Apixaban, Rivaroxaban, Edoxaban)

Patients on oral FXa inhibitors who are undergoing planned procedure should have their anticoagulant held for 24–48 h prior to procedure to allow sufficient clearance. Critically ill patients with organ dysfunction may require additional time to clear anticoagulant effects. In patients undergoing emergent procedures or experiencing major bleeding, reversal of FXa inhibitors with andexanet alfa or PCC may be necessary. DOAC-specific calibrated AFXa levels can aid in the decision to provide reversal. Suggested thresholds for reversal are levels greater than 50 ng/mL for life-threatening bleeding and 30–50 ng/mL for invasive procedures [10]. If DOAC-calibrated AFXa is unavailable, AFXa calibrated to LMWH/UFH can provide qualitative information to assess the presence (>0.1 IU/mL) or absence of FXa inhibitor. Andexanet alfa is the only FDA-approved agent for the reversal of apixaban and rivaroxaban and is recommended as the first-line agent for reversal in patients experiencing life-threatening major bleeding [114, 124]. PCC is a reasonable alternative for FXa inhibitor reversal for patients experiencing life-threatening bleeding or requiring invasive procedures. Institutions and health organizations

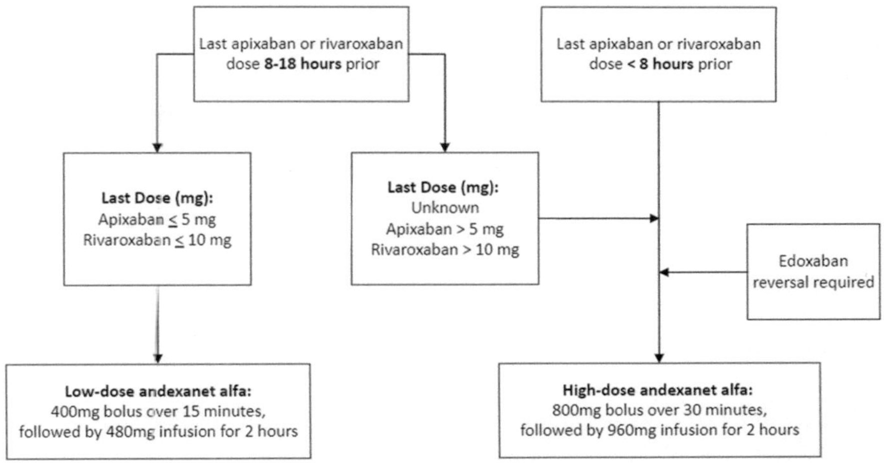

Fig. 49.4 Andexanet alfa dosing strategy [104, 126]

must consider access and cost-effectiveness of both reversal approaches given the lack of studies directly comparing the two reversal strategies.

Andexanet alfa dosing is based on dose and time since the last dose of oral FXa (Fig. 49.4). Andexanet alfa is not FDA approved for reversal of edoxaban; however, it is recommended to use the high-dose strategy for reversal in these patients [126]. The ANNEXA-4 trial evaluated andexanet alfa for the reversal of apixaban- and rivaroxaban-associated major bleeding and found that although andexanet alfa decreased median AFXa by 92%, the relationship between hemostatic efficacy and AFXa reduction was not significant [127]. Excellent or good hemostatic efficacy was achieved in 82% of patients with confirmed bleeding and a baseline AFXa of at least 75 ng/mL [127]. Thirty-day events were reported at 10% for thrombotic events and 14% for mortality. Reversal of FXa inhibitors with andexanet alfa may be assessed with AFXa. It is important to note that AFXa levels may return to baseline within 2 h of completing andexanet alfa infusion.

Reversal of FXa inhibitors with PCC is an off-label indication, and the optimal dosing strategy is not well defined. PCC reversal strategies may include fixed dose 2000 units or weight-based 25–50 units/kg [114]. A systematic review including 25 studies and 1760 patients found no differences in hemostatic efficacy, thromboembolic events, or mortality between fixed and variable dosing strategies [128]. Anti-factor Xa will not be affected by PCC administration and cannot be used to assess successful FXa inhibitor reversal.

The largest study to date ($n = 4395$) comparing andexanet alfa and 4F PCC for the treatment of apixaban- or rivaroxaban-associated major bleeding events found a 50% reduction in the odds of in-hospital mortality for andexanet alfa compared to 4F PCC on multivariate analysis adjusted for various factors, including bleed location and type [129]. Several other studies have compared andexanet alfa and 4F PCC and shown similar hemostatic efficacy outcomes between the two reversal strategies; however, the studies were limited by small sample size [130, 131]. Additionally, a meta-analysis evaluating reversal of oral FXa inhibitors in ICH with andexanet alfa (17 trials, $n = 525$) and majority weight-based PCC (22 trials, $n = 967$) found similar results for successful reversal, mortality, and thromboembolic events, although limited by study heterogeneity [132]. Most recently, the ANNEXA-I trial was terminated early after andexanet alfa showed superior hemostatic efficacy compared to usual care in patients with ICH, but the full study report has yet to be published.

49.5.3 Reversal of Thrombolytics

Major bleeding after administration of thrombolytic therapies is affected by several patient factors including baseline National Institutes of Health Stroke Scale (NIHSS) score, age, weight, systolic blood pressure, serum glucose, history of hypertension, concomitant antiplatelet therapy, and symptom onset to treatment time [133]. Patients who develop ICH and experience decreased neurologic function after administration of thrombolytic therapy should receive treatment. The plasma half-life of alteplase is 4 min and tenecteplase is 20 min; however, effects on fibrinogen concentrations extend beyond 24 h [134]. Reversal of thrombolytic therapy includes fibrinogen replacement to a goal of greater than 150 mg/dL with cryoprecipitate, fibrinogen-concentrate, or FFP, based on limited evidence.

The Neurocritical Care Society/Society of Critical Care Medicine recommend using 10 units of cryoprecipitate for patients who experience symptomatic ICH within 24 h of thrombolytic administration [135]. Fibrinogen concentrate is a reasonable alternative to cryoprecipitate for fibrinogen repletion in the setting of thrombolytic-associated ICH [134]. Fibrinogen concentrate can be more easily stored and prepared at the bedside compared to cryoprecipitate. Each vial of fibrinogen concentrate contains 900–1300 mg of fibrinogen per vial, and a dose of 70 mg/ kg is expected to increase fibrinogen concentration by approximately 125 mg/dL [107]. FFP contains less fibrinogen per unit than cryoprecipitate and is generally not recommended due to the substantial volume required to sufficiently replete fibrinogen in thrombolytic-associated ICH.

There is very little evidence to support the use of antifibrinolytics in thrombolytic-associated ICH; however, administration may be recommended when cryoprecipitate is unavailable or contraindicated. Antifibrinolytics (aminocaproic acid, tranexamic acid) prevent fibrin degradation by inhibiting conversion of plasminogen to plasmin. Dosing strategies are as follows: aminocaproic acid 4–5 g IV bolus, followed by 1 g/h infusion over 8 h or tranexamic acid 1 g (or 10–15 mg/kg) IV over 20 min [135].

49.5.4 Reversal of Antiplatelets

Antiplatelet therapy is common in the intensive care unit, especially for cardiology and vascular indications. Refer to Table 49.15 for pharmacokinetic data on antiplatelet agents (include reversible vs. irreversible, timing of platelet recovery). There are currently no reversal agents available for antiplatelet therapies, and limited evidence exists to support reversal, except in patients with ICH [135]. Nonspecific reversal strategies include platelet transfusion, desmopressin (DDAVP), and tranexamic acid.

Table 49.15 Pharmacokinetics of antiplatelets and reversal strategies [135]

Mechanism of platelet inhibition	Antiplatelet	Reversibility	Half-life	Time to platelet recovery	Reversal options
COX-1 and COX-2 inhibitor	Aspirin	Irreversible	20 min	3 days	– If ICH + neurosurgical intervention, PLT transfusion – DDAVP
Adenosine reuptake inhibitor	Dipyridamole	Reversible	10 h	3 days	
P2Y12 ADP receptor antagonist	Cangrelor	Reversible	3–6 min	60 min	
	Clopidogrel	Irreversible	6–8 h	7 days	– If ICH + neurosurgical intervention, PLT transfusion may be considered – DDAVP
	Prasugrel	Irreversible	2–15 h	7 days	
	Ticagrelor	Reversible	7 h (metabolite 9 h)	5 days	– Albumin – Bentracimab (investigational) – DDAVP (limited efficacy)
PDE III inhibitor	Cilostazol	Reversible	10 h	3 days	
Glycoprotein IIb/IIIa antagonist	Eptifibatide	Reversible	20–40 min	4 h	– If ICH, cryoprecipitate or FFP – If emergency surgery, PLT transfusion may be considered
	Tirofiban	Reversible	20–45 min	4 h	
PAR-1 thrombin receptor antagonist	Vorapaxar		3–4 days (terminal half-life 8 days)	>4 weeks	– PLT transfusion may be considered

49.5.4.1 Platelet Transfusion

Platelet transfusion is recommended for aspirin- or P2Y12 inhibitor-associated ICH in patients who are undergoing a neurosurgical procedure [135]. The Neurocritical Care Society/Society of Critical Care Medicine guidelines do not recommend platelet transfusion in all other clinical scenarios involving antiplatelet-associated ICH. Mixed outcomes have been reported for platelet transfusion in the setting of aspirin and P2Y12 inhibitor reversal [136–138]. There may be higher rates of platelet restoration from platelet transfusion with lower potency P2Y12 inhibitors than high-potency P2Y12 inhibitors [137]. Overall, there is a lack of evidence to support platelet transfusion for antiplatelet-associated bleeding at sites other than intracranial.

49.5.4.2 Desmopressin (DDAVP)

Desmopressin is a vasopressin analog that has been shown to increase von Willebrand factor and factor VIII, leading to improved platelet adhesion. Administration of desmopressin prior to elective or emergent procedures in patients taking antiplatelet agents may be reasonable. Desmopressin 0.3–0.4 mcg/kg has been shown to decrease red blood cell transfusion, volume of blood loss, and risk of bleeding-related reoperation in cardiac surgery patients with platelet dysfunction due to antiplatelet agents and cardiopulmonary bypass [139]. The Neurocritical Care Society/Society of Critical Care Medicine guidelines recommend a single dose of DDAVP 0.4 mcg/kg IV in COX- or ADP inhibitor-related ICH [135]. Patients who also require neurosurgical intervention may receive DDAVP in combination with platelet transfusion.

49.5.4.3 Tranexamic Acid

Tranexamic acid is an antifibrinolytic agent that inhibits conversion of plasminogen to plasmin. It is theorized that tranexamic acid may improve platelet function by inhibiting plasmin degradation of glycoprotein receptors, a common target for antiplatelet agents, thereby allowing the interaction of glycoprotein receptors and VWF [140]. Tranexamic acid administration in patients on mono- or dual-antiplatelet therapy undergoing surgery has been shown to reduce red blood cell and platelet transfusion, volume of blood loss, and incidence of reoperation due to bleeding [140]. Tranexamic acid is unlikely to make a difference in bleeding and transfusion requirements in patients that stopped taking their antiplatelet agents more than a week prior to surgery [141]. It may be reasonable to follow the dosing strategy for thrombolytic-associated ICH: tranexamic acid 1 g (or 10–15 mg/kg) IV over 20 min.

49.5.5 Role of the Pharmacist

Determining how and who to provide antithrombotic reversal can be particularly challenging, especially in high-acuity settings like life-threatening bleeding or emergent surgical procedures. Pharmacists play a crucial role in evaluating clinical scenarios, interpreting laboratory data, and working with the multidisciplinary team to ensure administration of appropriate and optimized reversal strategies. Pharmacists may be involved in the development of institutional protocols or guidelines for antithrombotic reversal. Additionally, institutions may implement pharmacist-driven anticoagulation reversal programs or pharmacist-run antithrombotic stewardship programs to guide appropriate reversal, which have been shown to produce favorable clinical outcomes and economic benefit [142].

In any instance of emergent reversal or cessation of antithrombotic therapy, the management plan should prioritize halting the bleeding event while also continuously evaluating the optimal timing for resuming anticoagulation. Once bleeding has been addressed, it is essential to reintroduce anticoagulation as soon as possible while prioritizing safety. This is especially crucial considering the potential procoagulant state in critically ill patients and the effects of reversing DOACs. The reintroduction strategy should involve considering a lower intensity target range for parameters like aPTT or AFXa, or beginning without a bolus for heparin to minimize the risks of both bleeding and thrombosis simultaneously.

49.6 Anticoagulation of Devices in the Intensive Care Unit

49.6.1 Mechanical Circulatory Support Devices

49.6.1.1 Intra-aortic Balloon Pump

The intra-aortic balloon pump (IABP) is a temporary mechanical circulatory support (MCS) device indicated in myocardial ischemia and cardiogenic shock that is inserted into the descending aorta via the femoral, axillary, or subclavian arteries. The balloon inflates and deflates in synchronization with the cardiac cycle to reduce afterload and enhance coronary perfusion. Both bleeding and ischemic complications may occur while the device is inserted, although bleeding complications seem to predominate [143]. Bleeding events may result from vascular injury during insertion, anticoagulation therapy, or platelet dysfunction. Thrombocytopenia secondary to IABP is a frequent complication and has been associated with an increased risk for major bleeding and increased ICU and hospital length of stays [144]. Inflation and deflation of the balloon result in mechanical trauma and destruction of platelets by force of shear stress and turbulent blood flow.

Use of anticoagulation with IABP is variable depending on institutional practices, indication for IABP, and presence of comorbidities requiring systemic anticoagulation. No specific recommendations exist for anticoagulation or monitoring of antithrombotic therapies. Most small studies have compared unfractionated heparin (UFH) with no anticoagulation or selective anticoagulation for patients with concomitant indications for anticoagulation. No differences have been observed in thrombotic outcomes, while lower rates of bleeding were seen in the groups not receiving anticoagulation [145]. If starting anticoagulation without a concomitant indication, it is reasonable to start lower doses of UFH and target a lower PTT goal (e.g., 50–70 s). Limited data exist regarding the use of alternative parenteral anticoagulants while IABP is inserted. Case report evidence suggests that IV direct thrombin inhibitors may be reasonable alternatives to UFH if heparin-induced thrombocytopenia is suspected or confirmed [146].

49.6.1.2 Percutaneous Ventricular Assist Device (Impella)

The Impella is a temporary, microaxial, continuous-flow MCS device approved for use in high-risk percutaneous coronary interventions and cardiogenic shock. The device is a catheter-based Impella pump that propels blood from the left ventricle or aorta or inferior vena cava into the ascending aorta or pulmonary artery. Foreign surfaces and shear force stress result in activation of the coagulation system making anticoagulation necessary in most patients supported with Impella devices. Higher bleeding complications have been reported in head-to-head comparisons between IABP and Impella; however, anticoagulation management strategies were not evaluated as a possible risk factor [147, 148]. Similar to IABP, thrombocytopenia is a common complication in patients supported with Impella.

Per the Impella manufacturer, systemic anticoagulation with UFH is recommended to prevent or decrease the risk of developing a device thrombus. Manufacturer recommendations are to target an ACT range of 160–180 s, although other studies have shown safe outcomes with targeting aPTT in 55–80 s or AFXa in 0.3–0.5 s [149–151].

The Impella device is unique from other MCS devices in that it requires a purge solution that flows in the opposite direction of the blood to prevent blood and proteins from disrupting the motor. Heparin- and sodium bicarbonate-based purge solutions have been shown to protect the motor. Heparin-based purge solutions may have a concentration of 25 or 50 U/mL. In patients with small body surface area, therapeutic anticoagulation may be achieved through heparin in the purge solution alone. Extra caution to not overdose anticoagulation is warranted with monitoring in patients receiving systemic UFH in addition to heparin-based purge solution. To simplify anticoagulation administration or for patients who are unable to tolerate anticoagulation or UFH, bicarbonate-based (25 mEq per 1000 mL of 5% dextrose) purge solution is a safe alternative [152, 153]. Direct thrombin inhibitors and normal saline should not be used in Impella purge solution due to lack of ionic charge and increased risk for motor malfunction [149].

Role of the Pharmacist

Pharmacists play an essential role in the optimization of anticoagulation strategies for patients being supported with IABP or Impella MCS devices given the high risk of bleeding and vascular complications. Anticoagulation, usually with UFH, is required to prevent clotting of the circuit and mitigate device-related thrombus. They may assist in evaluating bleeding risk and concomitant indications for therapeutic anticoagulation in patients with IABPs. For patients with Impella devices on heparin-based purge solution and systemic UFH, pharmacists may be responsible for calculating the total doses of UFH being administered and recommending dose adjustments based on PTT or AFXa results. To provide safe anticoagulation practices across institutions and health organizations, standardization of monitoring strategies, anticoagulation practices, and purge solutions may be beneficial. Pharmacists may be involved in protocol or guideline development that aids in the standardization process. Evaluation of internal practices and safety outcomes (bleeding, thrombosis, time in therapeutic range) may help guide practice change.

49.6.2 Extracorporeal Membrane Oxygenation

Extracorporeal membrane oxygenation (ECMO) is a type of mechanical support which provides temporary life support in patients with severe cardiac or pulmonary failure. Patients undergoing ECMO are at a delicate coagulation balance between thrombosis and bleeding. In addition to the underlying physiology requiring ECMO such as sepsis or cardiogenic shock contributing to coagulopathies, the ECMO circuit itself can further alter the coagulation process. The ECMO circuit consists of a mechanical blood pump, heat exchanger, oxygenator, tubing set, and cannulas. The interaction between circulating blood and the ECMO circuit, vessel wall injury, and blood flow stasis can all activate the coagulation cascade placing patients at risk for thrombotic complications and bleeding complications [154]. Thrombotic complications in patients on ECMO support range from 10 to 46% and include circuit or oxygenator thrombosis, hemolysis, VTE, and ischemic stroke [155, 156]. To offset the risk of clot formation in the ECMO circuit and oxygenator systemic anticoagulation is required. Anticoagulation inherently increases the risk of bleeding, which has been reported in 10–30% of patients undergoing ECMO [155, 157]. Developed coagulopathies on the ECMO circuit can result from high shearing forces in the pump and membrane oxygenator along with reduced glycoprotein levels causing platelet dysfunction, acquired von Willebrand syndrome, and hyperfibrinolysis; all of these factors place the patient at risk of bleeding, which has been associated with a higher mortality [156]. Bleeding complications can range from superficial mucosal and surgical or cannula site to major bleeding including intracranial or intrapulmonary hemorrhage.

49.6.2.1 Anticoagulant Agents in ECMO

Unfractionated Heparin (UFH) This is the most commonly used anticoagulant during ECMO support and is currently recommend by the International Society of Thrombosis and Haemostasis guidance document for anticoagulation in adult patients supported with ECMO [158]. Advantages of UFH during ECMO support include clinician familiarity, reversibility with protamine, and short half-life of 60–90 min. Despite these advantages, nonspecific binding to plasma proteins and endothelial cells can result in a variable anticoagulant response and difficulty remaining within the therapeutic range. Acquired antithrombin (AT) deficiency during ECMO support is an additional etiology of heparin resistance. One of the most concerning risks with UFH is heparin-induced thrombocytopenia (HIT). Diagnosis of HIT is less than 5% in ECMO patients and is not more common compared to critically ill patients not on ECMO support [158].The diagnosis of HIT in the ECMO patient population remains a challenge; standard predictive tools are often confounded and were not studied in this patient population. Further discussion on the diagnosis and management of HIT in the ICU is given in Sect. 49.7.2 [159]. Institutions utilizing UFH as the primary anticoagulant for ECMO should include routine monitoring for AT and platelets to evaluate UFH complications. Dosing and considerations in ECMO are summarized in Table 49.16. Cannulation bolus dose ranges from 50 to 100 units/kg, followed by a maintenance infusion ranging from 7.5 to 20 units/kg/h [161].

The integration of heparin covalently bound to circuit components including tubing, cannula, and oxygenator was designed to minimize the coagulation and

Table 49.16 Anticoagulants in extracorporeal membrane oxygenation support [160]

Anticoagulant	Dosing	Monitoring parameter	Considerations
Unfractionated heparin	Bolus: 50–100 units/kg Infusion starting rate: 7.5–18 units/kg/h	aPTT AFXa ACT	HIT Heparin resistance ATIII deficiency High protein binding results in less predictable anticoagulation
Argatroban	Bolus: 100–200 mcg/kg – Typically, no bolus administered Infusion starting rate: 0.2–0.5 mcg/kg/min	aPTT ACT dTT	False elevation of INR Reduce dose in hepatic impairment Child-Pugh classes B and C Reduce dose in acute decompensated heart failure or postcardiac surgery Reduce dose in critical illness with multiorgan dysfunction
Bivalirudin	Bolus: 0.04–0.5 mg/kg – Typically, no bolus administered Infusion starting rate: 0.02–0.15 mg/kg/h CRRT: 0.05 mg/kg/h	aPTT ACT dTT	False elevation of INR (<argatroban) Reduce dose in renal impairment or renal replacement therapy Low-flow states and risk of spontaneous thrombosis

Abbreviations: *ACT* activated clotting time; *aPTT* activated partial thromboplastin clotting time; *ATIII* antithrombin; *dTT* dilute thrombin time; *HIT* heparin-induced thrombocytopenia; *INR* international ratio; *CRRT* continuous renal replacement therapy inflammatory response when blood contacts these foreign surfaces. The decrease in thrombotic complications yet similar bleeding rates throughout the years of ECMO practices could be related to the increased use of heparin-coated circuits but similar levels of systemic anticoagulation. Although these coated surfaces release an insignificant amount of heparin systemically, their use should be avoided or exchanged for a heparin-free system in patients with confirmed HIT [154].

Direct thrombin inhibitors (DTIs) Historically DTIs, argatroban and bivalirudin, have been reserved for patients with HIT, suspected HIT, or heparin resistance [98, 158]. Emerging evidence for using a DTI as a primary anticoagulant in the ECMO patient population is increasing, but data on DTI efficacy and safety compared to UFH remains limited to small retrospective studies. Both DTIs have demonstrated both safety and efficacy when compared to UFH in ECMO patients [162–165]. Opposed to heparin, DTIs provide a more predicable effect due to their decreased protein binding and their independence of ATIII to exert their anticoagulation. Direct thrombin inhibitors inhibit both thrombin and fibrin-bound thrombin increasing their efficacy compared to UFH. Additionally, use of a DTI removes HIT as a potential etiology for thrombocytopenia. One disadvantage is the lack of a reversal agent. Since DTIs are monitored using aPTT, patients with an unreliable aPTT, such as antiphospholipid syndrome or acute liver failure causing a prolonged baseline aPTT, can result in having underdosing. The availability of alternative monitoring, such as acute clotting time (ACT) or dilute thrombin time (dTT), should be considered if DTIs are commonly used for ECMO. Determining the specific DTI agent will be based on institutional availability, cost, and concomitant end-organ dysfunction as discussed in anticoagulant DTI Sect. 49.3.1.4.

A comparison of anticoagulant dosing and considerations are summarized in Table 49.16. There is limited reporting on DTI bolus dosing in ECMO; the short half-life of DTIs allows therapeutic concentrations to be quickly achieved with every 2- to 4-h titration and monitoring. Bolus doses should be considered for cannulation of a documented HIT-positive patient and low-flow states. Low-flow states, such as during weaning trials where circuit flows are decreased, can create blood to stagnate in the cardiac chambers. Rapid local cleavage by proteolytic enzymes can predispose patients to spontaneous thrombosis with bivalirudin therapy. Argatroban dosing is often lower in patients on ECMO support with initial dosing recommendations of 0.2–0.5 mcg/kg/h, similar to patients with hepatic impairment or critical illness with multiorgan dysfunction [162, 163, 166]. Bivalirudin dosing ranges from 0.02 to 0.15 mg/kg/h has been required for patients on ECMO support with adjustments required for renal dysfunction or renal replacement therapy [167–169].

49.6.2.2 Anticoagulation Monitoring in ECMO

Finding the correct balance between bleeding and thrombosis is critical in patients on ECMO support. Along with the standard advantages and limitations for each monitoring parameter referenced in coagulation monitoring Sect. 49.2, additional considerations of these testing methods in the ECMO patient population are included in Table 49.17. There is controversy on the optimal method to assess

Table 49.17 Anticoagulation monitoring parameters in extracorporeal membrane oxygenation [98, 158]

Laboratory	Anticoagulants	Frequency	Goal range[a]	Advantages	Interferences and considerations in ECMO

Activated clotting time (ACT)	UFH and DTI	1–2 h	180–220	– Whole blood test
				– Point-of-care test
				– Widely available
					– Least correlated with heparin dosing
					– Factors influencing assay include[b]:
					  Platelet dysfunction, thrombocytopenia
					  ↑ d-dimers
					  ↓ fibrinogen
					  Hypo/hyperthermia
					  Hemodilution

Activated partial thromboplastin time (aPTT)	UFH and DTI	6–12 h	50–70 s or 1.5–2.5× baseline PTT *Conservative goal*: 40–60 s	– Widely available – User familiarity	– Less reliable in critical illness – Prolonged baseline aPTT could result in underdosing – Interpatient and intrapatient variability – No standardization between aPTT reagents – ↑ Factor VIII, ↑fibrinogen can ↓ aPTT

Anti-factor Xa (AFXa)	UFH	6–12 h	0.3–0.7 IU/mL
			Alternative goal: 0.3–0.5 IU/mL
				– Highest correlation to UFH dosing
				– Less variability compared to aPTT
					– Exogenous AT added to assay could overestimate true heparin effect in AT-deficient patients
					– Cannot use to monitor DTI
					– Chromogenic assay interferences[b]:
					  ↑ Bilirubin = falsely ↓ AFXa
					  ↑ Triglycerides = falsely ↓ AFXa
					  ↑ Plasma free Hgb (≥50 mg/dL) = falsely ↓ AFXa

Dilute thrombin time (dTT)	DTI	6–12 h	No established target in ECMO	Not affected by antiphospholipid antibodies	– Limited availability – Limited data on specific target level in ECMO
Viscoelastic coagulation (TEG, ROTEM)	UFH DTI	Daily As needed		– Whole blood test – Point of care – Evaluates clot strength and fibrinolysis	– Limited availability – Expensive – Limited data correlating UFH and clinical outcomes

Abbreviations: *AT* antithrombin; *DTI* direct thrombin inhibitor; *ROTEM* rotational thromboelastometry; *TEG* thromboelastography; *UFH* unfractionated heparin; ↓ decreased or low; ↑ increased or high

[a] Goals are generalized recommendations; assessment of institution-specific reagent should be evaluated

[b] The threshold laboratory value interference that occurs should be referenced based on institution-specific reagent

anticoagulation in this patient population, and level of anticoagulation using these parameters is also debatable and a subject of ongoing research. At an institution level, availability of specific monitoring test, turnaround time frame, and coagulation reagent sensitivity should be accounted for when determining standard monitoring requirements and method to titrate anticoagulation. Although the current International Society on Thrombosis and Haemostasis (ISTH) guidance document recommends AFXa with a goal of 0.3–0.5 IU/mL for UFH, the Extracorporeal Life Support (ELSO) anticoagulation guidelines make no specific recommendation on one anticoagulation monitoring parameter [98, 158]. The ELSO guidelines suggest a tailored strategy for each patient and potentially utilizing multiple tests to allow multimodal interpretation in the setting of correlation discrepancy. An example is using both AFXa with aPTT or AFXa with ACT to assess anticoagulation and dosing titrations [98]. Additional laboratory monitoring to assess hemostasis and need for transfusion include complete blood count to evaluate hemoglobin and platelets, fibrinogen, international normalized ratio (INR), plasma free hemoglobin to assess hemolysis, and AT in the setting of heparin anticoagulation.

Viscoelastic hemostatic assays The two validated viscoelastic hemostatic assays include thromboelastogram (TEG) and rotational thromboelastometry (ROTEM). These tests are whole-blood point-of-care coagulation tests, which provide evaluation of a clot initiation, strength, and stability including breakdown of the fibrin clot and fibrinolysis in real time. Further details on viscoelastic testing are detailed in coagulation monitoring Sect. 49.2. The availability of these assays is limited, but when available, they can be used to guide administration of blood products and coagulation factors [98].

49.6.2.3   Antithrombin Deficiency

Acquired antithrombin (AT) deficiency can occur during ECMO support, which decreases the anticoagulant effect of UFH. Mechanisms of AT deficiency can include high UFH exposure during cardiac surgery, liver dysfunction, disseminated intravascular coagulation (DIC), exposure to the ECMO circuit, and prolonged UFH exposure during ECMO support [170]. Antithrombin levels measure the ability of AT to inhibit thrombin when UFH is present, and although it is assumed that low levels of AT reduce UFH anticoagulation effects, the threshold that is observed is variable. The management is variable among ECMO centers but can consist of AT supplementation by transfusing fresh frozen plasma (FFP), administration of AT concentrate (human derived or recombinant), or transition to a direct thrombin inhibitor for anticoagulation. In comparison to FFP, AT concentrate offers less volume and decreased transfusion-related complications such as transfusion-related acute lung injury or infection. To illustrate the difference in volume, to give a supplement of 500 IU of AT, this would require either 500 mL or 2 units of FFP compared to 10 mL of AT concentrate [171]. The ELSO guidelines suggest that in the setting of maximum dose of UFH with subtherapeutic coagulation levels, AT supplementation could be considered with a target AT >50–80% [98]. Despite the rationale of AT supplementation decreasing UFH requirements, clinical outcomes including decreased bleeding and thrombosis have not been observed [172]. In a prospective randomized controlled trial in VV-ECMO patients evaluating AT supplementation for a goal level, 80–120% found no difference in UFH dosing requirements, blood transfusion, bleeding, and thrombosis between groups randomized to supplementation versus none [173]. Based on these findings, the routine use of AT repletion is controversial and not recommended by the ISTH guidelines [158]. Despite the controversy of the best treatment of AT deficiency resulting in heparin resistance, institutions with UFH as their primary anticoagulant should include routine AT monitoring, especially in the setting of thrombosis development or high heparin dosing with subtherapeutic anticoagulation levels. Developing an algorithm of treatment options and dosing based on institutional preference would allow standardized management.

49.6.2.4 Topical Hemostatic Agents

The most commonly cited sites of bleeding are the cannulation, mucosal, and surgical sites. These types of bleeding events can benefit from localized hemostasis through the administration of topical hemostatic agents; examples of agents used are listed in Table 49.18.

49.6.2.5 Role of the Pharmacist

Extracorporeal membrane oxygenation programs can benefit from including clinical pharmacists as members of the multidisciplinary ECMO team. Pharmacists can optimize patient-specific anticoagulation management through evaluating discordant laboratory values and assess appropriate anticoagulant intensity based on thrombosis or bleeding risk and how to modify anticoagulation therapy plan accordingly [174]. Including the emergency response pharmacist or unit pharmacist for bedside cannulation can assist with initial anticoagulation bolus dosing and follow-up monitoring for ongoing anticoagulation. Pharmacist can be an asset for evaluating adjunctive coagulation management including coagulation factors, antithrombin, anticoagulation reversal, and agents for refractory bleeding. Pharmacist stewardship of these products can result in cost savings [175]. At an institutional level, pharmacist can assist with integrating institution-specific practices into standardized guidelines or protocols. Standardized practice can limit variability across different units or services in which ECMO is performed and can be especially helpful for a unit provider to rotate through such as medical residents. To provide safe anticoagulation practices in this patient population, programs should develop guidelines or protocols including the preferred anticoagulant agent, dosing, monitoring, standard anticoagulation intensity, and titration algorithms. In the setting where UFH is the primary anticoagulant, standard monitoring for heparin resistance and HIT should

Table 49.18 Topical hemostatic agents in extracorporeal membrane oxygenation [98]

Classification	Agent	Examples	Description
Physical[a]	Oxidized regenerated cellulose	Surgicel	Plant-based agent that promotes clot formation by providing a mesh-like structure for platelet aggregation and activation of the intrinsic coagulation cascade. The acidic pH provides for bactericidal activity. Primarily for minimal bleeding
Physical[a]	Gelatin matrix	Gelfoam, Surgifoam	Porcine-derived collagen that provides a matrix for platelet adhesion and activation of the coagulation cascade. The neutral pH allows it to be used concomitantly with topical thrombin
Biologically active[b]	Thrombin	Thrombin-JMI, Recothrom	Bovine or human derived, thrombin promotes clot formation by catalyzing the conversion of fibrinogen to fibrin
Biologically active[b]	Antifibrinolytics	Aminocaproic acid, tranexamic acid	Inhibits fibrinolysis resulting in clot stabilizing via preventing the binding of plasminogen to fibrin and activation of plasminogen to plasmin. The intravenous formulations can be used to soak gauze or dressings. Tranexamic acid can be nebulized for the management of hemoptysis or pulmonary bleeding

[a] Physical agents promote hemostasis by activation of the extrinsic cascade using a substrate (cellulose, gelatin) by forming a matrix at the site of bleeding
[b] Biologic agents promote hemostasis by enhancing coagulation at the site of bleeding

be incorporated into guidance documents. Additional monitoring standards to assess for bleeding or thrombotic complications and need for product transfusions should be included. Data to guide optimal anticoagulation management is sparse, often limited to retrospective study design in which large variability in patient population and anticoagulation intensity and anticoagulant reagent differences make external validity challenging. Evaluating outcomes including major bleeding and thrombosis, time within therapeutic range including sub- and supratherapeutic, changes in guideline recommendations, or changes in circuit technology can assist in providing evidence for practice changes within the institution.

49.6.3 Continuous Renal Replacement Therapy

Continuous renal replacement therapy (CRRT) is recommended for patients with hemodynamic instability, increased intracranial pressure or cerebral edema, and acute brain injury due to potential blood pressure shifts with rapid volume removal during intermittent modes [176]. Clotting of the renal replacement circuit is a common complication which can result in decreased time on renal replacement, decreased effective surface area of the filter, blood loss with filter replacement, and increased hospital resources [177, 178].

Methods to reduce the need for circuit anticoagulation include the following:

– Large-bore double-lumen central venous catheter with access in the right jugular or femoral veins can minimize blood flow interruptions [179].
– Higher blood flow rates [179].
– Delivery of replacement fluids prefilter compared to postfilter. Prefilter administration decreases clotting by diluting the blood first, preventing hemoconcentration [180].

Despite these methods, anticoagulation is often needed in continuous methods of renal replacement to maintain circuit patency.

49.6.3.1 Anticoagulation Agents in CRRT

Deciding to start anticoagulation is based on evaluating patient risk for bleeding with the benefits for anticoagulation, such as circuit blood loss and treatment interruption. A summary of therapeutic options is listed in Table 49.19.

Table 49.19 Methods of anticoagulation for continuous renal replacement therapy

Method	Medication	Dosing	Titration parameters	Monitoring
Regional citrate (RCA)	Citrate infusion (hypertonic) or Citrate replacement fluid (isotonic)	Based on the CRRT blood flow rate and citrate concentration	Citrate delivery titrated to postfilter iCa target <0.35 mmol/L (between 0.8 and 1.3 mg/dL) Calcium infusion titrated to systemic Ca	Ca (total + ionized) Na (for hypertonic citrate) Acid-base (pH, bicarbonate) Lactate
Unfractionated heparin (UFH)	Regional heparin prefilter + protamine postfilter	Initial ratio 100 units prefilter heparin: 1 mg postfilter protamine	UFH titrated to circuit aPTT 1.5–2 times normal (therapeutic) Protamine titrated to systemic aPTT <40 s (subtherapeutic)	aPTT (circuit + systemic) Platelets Hgb/Hct
	Systemic heparin prefilter	+/– Bolus 30–40 unit/kg Infusion: 5–10 units/kg/h	UFH titrated to systemic aPTT or AFXa Goals vary from undetectable to therapeutic (aPTT 1.5–2 times normal or AFXa 0.3–0.7)	aPTT or AFXa (systemic) Platelets Hgb/Hct

(continued)

Table 49.19 (continued)

Method	Medication	Dosing	Titration parameters	Monitoring
Low-molecular-weight heparin	Enoxaparin	Bolus 0.15 mg/kg Infusion: 0.05 mg/kg/h	AFXa level <1 (0.5–1 considered therapeutic)	AFXa (systemic) Platelets Hgb/Hct
Direct thrombin inhibitors	Argatroban	+/− Bolus 100 mcg/kg Infusion: 0.25–1 mcg/kg/min	Titrated to systemic aPTT aPTT goals vary (therapeutic aPTT 1.5–2 times normal)	aPTT Hgb/Hct
	Bivalirudin	Infusion: 0.03–0.07 mg/kg/h	Titrated to systemic aPTT aPTT goals vary (therapeutic aPTT 1.5–2 times normal)	

Method	Medication	Advantages	Disadvantages
Regional citrate (RCA)	Citrate infusion prefilter (hypertonic) or Citrate replacement fluid (isotonic)	Preferred for CRRT Prolonged filter duration vs. UFH ↓ Bleeding risk	Requires standard protocol to avoid adverse events Requires Ca repletion, risk of hyper/hypocalcemia Risk of hypernatremia with hypertonic citrate Citrate toxicity (↑ lactate predictor of toxicity) Metabolic acidosis/alkalosis Hepatic failure, hypoperfusion impair citrate metabolism ↑ risk of citrate toxicity High effluent rates with isotonic citrate can result in citrate overload or accumulation
Unfractionated heparin (UFH)	Regional heparin prefilter + protamine postfilter Systemic heparin prefilter	UFH preferred for iHD Low cost Short half-life Reversible via protamine ↓ Bleeding risk with regional method	Regional method not recommended as standard of practice → risk of adverse effects and protamine dosing variability to reverse UFH ↑ Bleeding with systemic method Heparin resistance Risk of HIT High-risk medication requires standard protocol for dosing and monitoring
Low-molecular-weight heparin	Enoxaparin	Reliable anticoagulant response compared to UFH	Accumulation risk due to impaired elimination AFXa monitoring recommended; increased cost and availability should be considered Less predictable reversal with protamine

(continued)

Table 49.19 (continued)

Method	Medication	Advantages	Disadvantages
Direct thrombin inhibitors	Argatroban Bivalirudin	Preferred agents for HIT Short half-life	Argatroban requires dose adjustment for hepatic dysfunction (Child-Pugh class B/C), heart failure, hypoperfusion Bivalirudin clearance may be impacted by effluent rate and mode of CRRT No reversal agent Can falsely ↑ INR (argatroban > bivalirudin)

Abbreviations: *AFXa* anti-factor Xa; *aPTT* activated partial thromboplastin clotting time; *Ca* calcium; *CRRT* continuous renal replacement therapy; *Hct* hematocrit; *HIT* heparin-induced thrombocytopenia; *Hgb* hemoglobin; *iCa* ionized calcium; intermittent hemodialysis; *Na* sodium; *UFH* unfractionated heparin; ↓ decreased or low; ↑ increased or high

Regional Citrate

Regional citrate anticoagulation (RCA) is recommended by the Kidney Disease Improving Global Outcomes (KDIGO) Clinical Guidelines for patients receiving CRRT without a contraindication for citrate [176]. These recommendations are based on clinical trials demonstrating the decreased bleeding profile and prolonged circuit duration compared to UFH.

Sodium citrate acts as an anticoagulant by chelating ionized calcium, an essential cofactor in the coagulation cascade. Additionally, citrate acts as a buffer from its metabolism, primarily by the liver, into bicarbonate and is a source of carbohydrate energy providing 0.59 kcal/mmol. There are various RCA administration, dosing, and titration protocols cited in the literature [181, 182]. Citrate dosing will be dependent on the blood flow, to target citrate concentration (3–4 mmol/L) within the circuit, and citrate solution concentration. Postfilter ionized calcium is monitored for a target <0.35 mmol/L (between 0.8 and 1.3 mg/dL). Refer to Fig. 49.5 for additional details on administration and monitoring.

Citrate solution can be either high-concentration citrate solutions, also known as hypertonic due to the high sodium content, or low concentration, also known as isotonic solutions, with citrate containing replacement fluid. Hypertonic citrate solutions, such as 2.2% anticoagulant citrate dextrose (ACD) solution or 4% trisodium citrate solution, are used as both the anticoagulant and buffer solution. It is delivered as a separate prefilter solution allowing for separate titration of citrate for anticoagulation and delivered CRRT dose. Isotonic citrate solutions are used as both the anticoagulant and predilution replacement fluid. Providing citrate within the replacement fluid can complicate acid-base management as the dose of CRRT will impact the citrate dose. Higher CRRT effluent rates can therefore increase the risk of citrate accumulation or citrate overload.

The primary disadvantages are the metabolic complications including metabolic alkalosis or acidosis, hypocalcemia, hypercalcemia, and hypernatremia from hypertonic citrate solutions. Metabolic complications from RCA are detailed in Table 49.20. Citrate accumulation, due to impaired metabolism, is the most critical

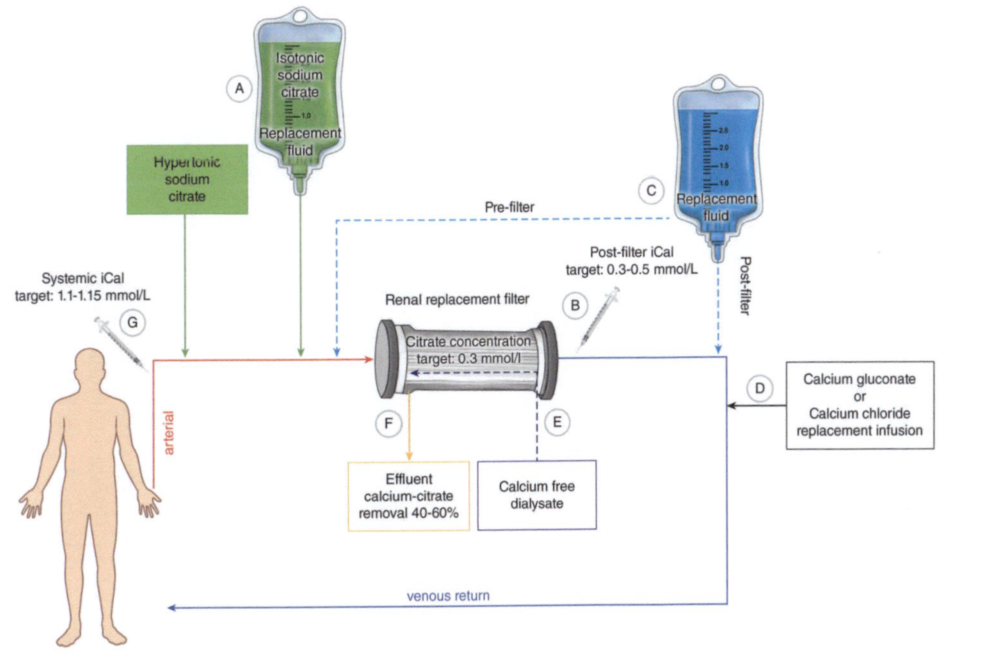

Fig. 49.5 Citrate anticoagulation during continuous renal replacement therapy (CRRT) [182, 183]. (**a**) Sodium citrate is administered prefilter as either hypertonic sodium citrate or isotonic sodium citrate replacement fluid. Hypertonic citrate solutions are delivered as a separate infusion allowing for titration of desired citrate exposure independent of the prescribed dose of CRRT. With isotonic sodium citrate replacement fluid, the amount of citrate delivered is dependent on the dose of CRRT in which higher effluent rates can increase the risk of citrate accumulation or overload. (**b**) Hypertonic sodium citrate is titrated to a postfilter ionized calcium (iCa) to provide a desired citrate concentration within the renal replacement filter. (**c**) For CRRT convection modes, replacement fluids composed of low sodium and minimal to no bicarbonate or lactate buffering agents can be administered pre/postfilter. (**d**) Calcium infusions are delivered postfilter to counteract systemic hypocalcemia induced by calcium-citrate complexes. (**e**) For CRRT diffusion modes, calcium-free dialysate is administered. (**f**) Removal of calcium-citrate complexes by convection or diffusion ranges from 40 to 60%; the remainder primarily undergoes hepatic metabolism. (**g**) Systemic iCa is monitored to titrate calcium replacement infusion, and concomitant total calcium levels in relation to iCa are obtained to assess for citrate toxicity

Table 49.20 Metabolic complications of regional citrate anticoagulation (RCA) [181, 183]

Metabolic complication	RCA etiology	Mechanism	Methods to correct
Metabolic alkalosis	Citrate overload	↑Bicarbonate generated from citrate > base deficient	↓ Blood flow rate or citrate concentration = ↓ Citrate delivered to patient ↑ Dialysate or replacement rate = ↑ Citrate removal
Metabolic acidosis	Inadequate buffering	Buffering from citrate < base deficient/metabolic demand ↓ Bicarbonate ↔ Lactate ↔ Serum tCa and iCa ↔ tCa/iCa ratio	↑ Blood flow rate or citrate concentration = ↑ Citrate returned to patient ↓ Dialysate or replacement flow = ↓ Citrate-Ca complex filtration
	Citrate accumulation	↓ Citrate metabolism ↓ Bicarbonate ↑ Lactate ↑ Serum tCa ↓ Serum iCa ↑ tCa/iCa ratio[a]	Terminate RCA Change to alternative anticoagulation option

Abbreviations: *Ca* calcium; *tCa* total calcium; *iCa* ionized calcium; ↓ decreased or low; ↑ increased or high; ↔ no change
[a] Accumulation can be assumed when the total calcium-ionized calcium ratio is >2.5:1 mmol/L or >10:1 mg/dL [184]

of these complications. Hepatic clearance is the primary method of citrate metabolism; therefore, clinical conditions including liver failure or decreased hepatic perfusion may impair the conversion of citrate to bicarbonate. Opposed to liver function test, predictors of citrate accumulation include prothrombin time ≥33 s and a lactic acid >3.4 mmol/L. Additionally, impaired lactate clearance due to hypoperfusion during shock or underlying mitochondria dysfunction (e.g., metformin overdose) can be used to predict metabolic complications [185, 186]. Although current KDIGO guidelines list liver failure as a contraindication to citrate anticoagulation, a meta-analysis concluded that with close monitoring of the patient's acid-base status and electrolytes, it can be used in liver failure [187, 188]. Prior to profound metabolic acidosis, the first sign of citrate toxicity is a fall in ionized calcium and increased calcium supplementation. Citrate accumulation can be assumed when the total calcium-ionized calcium ratio is >2.1–2.5:1 mmol/L or >10:1 mg/dL [184].

Unfractionated Heparin (UFH)

Unfractionated heparin is an alternative method of anticoagulation for renal replacement therapy in patients unable to receive RCA or when there is inability to administer and monitor RCA therapy without an increased bleeding risk [176]. Methods of anticoagulation with UFH include regional and systemic.

Regional anticoagulation with UFH allows therapeutic anticoagulation within the filter by administering heparin prefilter, which is reversed with postfilter protamine before entering systemic circulation. This method requires both circuit and systemic aPTT to be monitored with a goal of therapeutic aPTT in the circuit and subtherapeutic systemic aPTT. Determining the accurate dosing regimen can be difficult due to interpatient variability and significantly different half-lives of heparin and protamine. Due to the lack of superiority to other methods of anticoagulation and risk of adverse effects of protamine (i.e., anaphylaxis, hypotension, thrombocytopenia, right-sided heart failure), it is not recommended in practice [189, 190].

Systemic anticoagulation with UFH is provided through prefilter UFH administration with monitoring of anticoagulation effect through systemic aPTT or AFXa values. Various dosing regimens have been reported in literature but often include a bolus dose ranging from 2000 to 5000 units (30–40 units/kg) followed by a continuous infusion of 5–10 units/kg/h titrated to an aPTT 1.5–2 times normal or AFXa 0.3–0.7 [190, 191]. In patients with high bleeding risk, low-dose heparin administration without systemic effects or a stepwise approach of increasing anticoagulation intensity based on effect has been reported [192, 193]. Disadvantages of UFH for CRRT are similar to systemic heparin for other anticoagulation indications including heparin resistance and heparin-induced thrombocytopenia.

Low-Molecular-Weight Heparin (LMWH)

Even with the advantages of LMWH, including more predictable anticoagulant response and lower incidence of HIT compared to UFH, its use in CRRT is limited. In a small crossover study, 37 patients were treated with UFH continuous infusion titrated to an aPTT of 40–50 s and enoxaparin 0.15 mg/kg bolus followed by a continuous infusion of 0.05 mg/kg/h titrated to an AFXa of 0.25–0.3 IU/mL. The filter life was significantly longer with enoxaparin compared to UFH, and no difference in bleeding was observed [194]. Despite these findings, the risk of accumulation and ability to monitor AFXa have limited LMWH use for CRRT filter clotting.

Direct Thrombin Inhibitors (DTIs)

For patients with acute HIT or history of HIT, direct thrombin inhibitors, argatroban and bivalirudin, can be used. The specific agent will be dependent on concomitant organ dysfunction. Argatroban primarily undergoes hepatic metabolism compared to bivalirudin, which is 80% eliminated by organ-independent proteolysis and 20% excreted by the kidney unchanged. It would be reasonable based on the pharmacokinetics to utilize argatroban for patients with renal dysfunction without hepatic dysfunction and bivalirudin for patients with hepatic dysfunction with or without renal dysfunction [195–197]. In patients with acute HIT on RRT, DIT anticoagulants should be administered and titrated to a therapeutic aPTT [65].

Role of the Pharmacist

Due to the high risk of metabolic derangements, bleeding risk, specific administration methods, and monitoring during the various anticoagulation methods for CRRT, the critical care pharmacist should collaborate with multidisciplinary teams (i.e., nephrology, hematology, nursing, intensivist) to standardize these methods at your institution. Creation of a policy, protocol, guideline, or decision support algorithm can assist with ensuring that appropriate medication, administration, monitoring, titration, and therapeutic goals are outlined [191]. Additionally, considering who the ordering provider will be (e.g., specialty services such as the nephrologist versus primary team such as medical interns) and/or the complexity of these orders (e.g., multiple agents with specific titration instructions, specific laboratory monitoring frequency, and various laboratory draw locations), the creation of a standardized order set can assist with avoiding entry or omission errors. Factors the critical care pharmacist should consider include the following: methods of CRRT (hemofiltration, hemodialysis, both), CRRT technology, citrate concentration and administration method, dialysate and replacement fluid composition, calcium product and replacement scale for RCA methods, and required laboratory and monitoring frequency. Periodic review to assess anticoagulation practices for both safety and efficacy, safety events or errors, and institution compliance with the set policy, protocol, or guideline should occur [192].

49.7 Thrombocytopenia in the Intensive Care Unit

Thrombocytopenia defined as a platelet count below the lower limit of the reference range <150,000/μL (<150 × 10^9/L) in adults may be related to a variety of clinical conditions and symptoms ranging from bleeding to thrombosis. Severity of thrombocytopenia can be further subsided into mild (100–149 × 10^9/L), moderate (59–99 × 10^9/L), and severe (<50 × 10^9/L) [198].

In the critically ill patient population, thrombocytopenia is a common complication with an incidence ranging from 14 to 44% and a reported 5–20% developing severe thrombocytopenia during their ICU admission [199, 200]. Thrombocytopenia has been associated with increased length of stay and increased risk of bleeding and identified as an independent risk factor for mortality in the ICU. Risk factors in the development of thrombocytopenia include severity of illness, sepsis, and organ dysfunction [4, 199–201].

The major mechanisms of thrombocytopenia in the ICU include the following: hemodilution, pseudothrombocytopenia, increased platelet consumption, increased platelet destruction, increased sequestration of platelet, and decreased platelet production. Table 49.21 lists the mechanisms of thrombocytopenia and associated etiologies. Although often multifactorial, identifying the etiology and understanding the mechanism of thrombocytopenia are crucial for management.

Table 49.21 Mechanisms and associated etiologies of thrombocytopenia in the intensive care unit [4, 12]

Mechanism	Etiology/clinical scenario
Hemodilution	Fluid resuscitation Massive transfusion for major bleeding
Pseudothrombocytopenia	GPIIb/IIIa receptor antagonist EDTA platelet clumping (sample clotting)

Platelet consumption	Major blood loss
	Disseminated intravascular coagulation
	Sepsis < septic shock
	Extracorporeal devices:
	  – Extracorporeal membrane oxygenation
	  – Continuous renal replacement therapy
	Intravascular devices (IABP, cardiac assist devices)
	Hyperfibrinolysis (cirrhosis)
	Severe thrombosis/pulmonary embolism

Platelet destruction	Drug-induced immune thrombocytopenia (DITP)
	Heparin-induced thrombocytopenia (HIT)
	Thrombotic microangiopathies:
	  – Thrombotic thrombocytopenic purpura
	  – Hemolytic uremic syndrome
	  – HELLP syndrome
	Sepsis
	Immune thrombocytopenia:
	  – Systemic lupus erythematosus
	  – HCV

Platelet sequestration	Cirrhosis Hypersplenism Hypothermia

Decreased platelet production	Bone marrow toxicity:
	  – Drugs
	  – Chemotherapy
	  – Intoxication
	Cancer bone marrow infiltration
	Chronic liver disease
	Alcohol abuse (folate deficiency)
	Radiation
	Viral infection:
	  – HIV, HCV, EBV, CMV

Abbreviations: *CMV* cytomegalovirus; *EBV* Epstein-Barr virus; *HCV* hepatitis C virus; *HELLP* hemolysis elevated liver enzymes and low platelets; *HIV* human immunodeficiency virus; *IABP* intra-aortic balloon pump; *EDTA* ethylenediaminetetraacetic acid

The threshold for platelet transfusion is typically less than 10,000/µL in non-bleeding patients due to the increased risk of spontaneous bleeding and less than 50,000/µL who are actively bleeding or undergoing invasive procedures [202].

49.7.1 Drug-Induced Thrombocytopenia (DTP)

Hundreds of drugs have been reported to cause thrombocytopenia, including antibiotics, antiplatelet agents like GP IIb/IIa inhibitors, chemotherapy drugs, and most notoriously heparin. The risk of developing drug-induced thrombocytopenia (DTP) is up to 25% in critically ill patients. Risk factors for developing DTP include prior drug exposure, inflammatory states that increase antibody production, higher drug/metabolite levels, and greater immunogenic potential.

49.7.1.1 Pathophysiology

Drug-induced thrombocytopenia can be classified based on if the mechanism is through platelet destruction or bone marrow suppression/megakaryocyte. Details of mechanisms of DTP, common medications, and expected timing of thrombocytopenia are included in Table 49.22.

Drug-induced thrombocytopenia due to accelerated platelet destruction can be subdivided into the following immune or nonimmune mechanisms. Drug-induced immune thrombocytopenia (DITP) typically occurs within days of drug exposure and can be further categorized based on the immune-mediated mechanism. (1) Hapten-dependent type occurs when the drug molecule covalently links to a larger

Table 49.22 Mechanisms of drug-induced thrombocytopenia [12, 203]

Platelet destruction		
Mechanism	Drugs	Timing of platelet decrease
Immune		
Hapten-induced antibody	Antibacterial: – Cephalosporins – Penicillins	7 days 7 days
	Anticonvulsants: – Carbamazepine – Phenytoin – Valproate	7 days 7 days 7 days
Quinine type	Anticonvulsants Ceftriaxone Nonsteroidal anti-inflammatory drugs Quinidine/quinine Rifampin Sulfamethoxazole Vancomycin	Rapid onset (recovery 7–10 days)
GPIIb/IIIa inhibitors	Eptifibatide Tirofiban Abciximab	Hours after exposure (recovery 2–6 days) Abciximab can have a delayed reaction 2 weeks after exposure

Platelet destruction		
Mechanism	Drugs	Timing of platelet decrease
Drug-induced autoantibodies	Heparin > low-molecular-weight heparin	5–10 days' initial exposure ≤1-day re-exposure in 30–100 days
	Vaccine (COVID-19)	14 days, range 5–30 days
	Humanized monoclonal antibodies: – Adalimumab – Bevacizumab – Infliximab – Ipilimumab – Natalizumab – Nivolumab – Pembrolizumab – Rituximab	Within days of exposure
Nonimmune		
	Cyclosporine Mitomycin C Tacrolimus	21 days, if drug taken daily 1 day, if drug taken intermittently
Bone marrow suppression or megakaryocyte impairment		
Myelosuppression	Antibacterial: – Linezolid – Vancomycin – Beta-lactams Trimethoprim/sulfamethoxazole	10–14 days 6–12 days 10 days 9 days
	Antiviral agents: – Ganciclovir/valganciclovir Foscarnet	10–20 days 10–20 days
	Chemotherapy: – Cyclophosphamide – Gemcitabine Azathioprine/6-mercaptopurine Methotrexate	14–28 days Months Months
Megakaryopoiesis ↓	Antiparasitic: – Quinine	5–10 days
	GPIIb/IIIa inhibitors: – Eptifibatide – Tirofiban	Hours
	Histone deacetylase inhibitors: – Panobinostat – Romidepsin – Vorinostat	15–30 days
Megakaryocyte apoptosis	BH3 mimetic class: – Navitoclax – Venetoclax	14–28 days

Abbreviations: *GPIIb/IIIa* glycoprotein IIIb/IIa; *BH3* Bcl-2 homology 3 carrier protein, which triggers the generation of drug-dependent antibodies (DDAbs) that bind to the drug-protein complex resulting in platelet destruction. These are usually small drugs, <5000 Da, such as antibacterial or anticonvulsant medications. (2) Quinine type occurs by the culprit drug binding to platelet glycoproteins, which allows platelet-reactive antibodies to bind when the drug is present. For example, quinine has demonstrated binding directly to the antibody complementarity-determining region (CDR) of the DDAb creating a modified antigen-binding region, thereby increasing antibody-binding affinity to platelet surface antigens marking the platelets for destruction [204]. (3) GPIIb/IIIa inhibitor-induced type can result from drugs, such as tirofiban and eptifibatide, binding to the arginine-glycine-aspartic acid recognition site on GPIIb/IIa creating a target for antibodies. Specifically abciximab, which is a modified monoclonal antibody to the GP IIb/IIIa receptor, occurs through naturally occurring antibodies that recognize the murine structure [205]. (4) Autoantibody occurs through the formation of drug-independent platelet autoantibodies, which can bind to platelet antigens in the absence of the drug. In heparin-induced thrombocytopenia (HIT), antibodies form against the heparin-platelet factor 4 complex, which can result in thrombogenesis or in HIT with thrombosis; further details regarding HIT diagnosis, testing, and management are included in Sect. 49.7.2. Nonimmune drug-induced platelet destruction can develop in cases of thrombotic microangiopathy and hemolytic uremic syndrome caused by dose-related toxicity on platelets from medications such as cyclosporine, tacrolimus, or mitomycin C.

Bone marrow suppression or interference with cell maturation is the other classification of DTP. Opposed to DITP, thrombocytopenia typically occurs within weeks to months. Chemotherapy-induced thrombocytopenia is one of the common etiologies, and although most induced myelosuppression occurs in all hematopoietic cell lineages, some medications result in isolated thrombocytopenia due to their selective megakaryocyte effects. An understanding of the type of cancer, specific agent, and typical timing of when platelets nadir will assist in assessing risk and development of DTP associated with chemotherapy [203, 206].

49.7.1.2 Diagnosis and Management

Diagnosis of DTP can be difficult in the intensive care unit as patients often have underlying predisposing comorbidities and multiple drug exposures, and it is not uncommon for a combination of etiologies to be involved with the development of thrombocytopenia. The clinical pharmacist can play an essential role in the diagnosis of DTP through their knowledge of common culprit medications, mechanism causing thrombocytopenia, and associated timing of onset and recovery of thrombocytopenia [203, 205, 207, 208].

The following steps will assist in the assessment of DTP:

1. Obtaining complete blood cell count (CBC) and peripheral blood smear:

(a) If available, historical CBC should be reviewed to determine if the onset is acute or chronic, and associated timing with drug exposure (refer to Table 49.22).

(b) Platelet counts less than 20,000/mm^3 may be related to a drug-induced immune thrombocytopenia (DITP).

(c) On peripheral smear, due to decreased mature platelets being released, larger sized platelets often occur with DITP.

2. Clinical exam:

(a) Petechiae, oral, nasal, mucosal, gastrointestinal, and genitourinary bleeding are likely to occur with DITP.

3. Medication review of patient's drug exposure prior to admission (home medications, herbal supplements, recent vaccines, medications administered at outside facilities) and during hospital admission (refer to Table 49.22).

4. Review other etiologies of thrombocytopenia in the ICU (refer to Table 49.21).

5. For the assessment of suspected drug, determine if testing using enzyme immunoassays and flow cytometry can be sent to identify drug-dependent antibodies. Although these may not be effective for the immediate treatment due to the accessibility and turnaround time, testing can assist with confirming the suspected drug.

6. Diagnosis of DITP is further supported if the suspected drug is rechallenged with rapid reoccurrence of the thrombocytopenia.

Management involves reviewing the suspected medication risk and benefits of continuing therapy; if risk outweighs benefit of the medication and/or an alternative agent can be used, the suspected medication should be discontinued. In clinical practice, it is not uncommon that more than one drug is on the differential for DTP. In this setting, discontinuing the medications should occur in a stepwise process and evaluating the typical platelet recovery to assess response. If the clinical suspicion of DITP is high, platelet transfusions will likely be ineffective until four to five half-lives of the culprit drug and/or metabolite have passed [207]. If a drug is confirmed as the etiology of thrombocytopenia, the medication should be reported using the MedWatch, the FDA Adverse Event Reporting System, https://www.fda.gov/safety/medwatch, and if no or limited data is available, a case report write-up should be considered.

49.7.2 Heparin-Induced Thrombocytopenia

Despite the high incidence of thrombocytopenia in the critically ill, the incidence of HIT ranges in 0.02–0.45% in the medical-surgical ICU patients and 1–3% in cardiac ICU patients [209, 210]. Risk factors associated with the development of HIT include exposure to UFH and to a lesser extent LMWH, being female, undergoing surgery, and an elevated body mass index (BMI) [209].

Thrombocytopenia presents as a >50% decrease in baseline platelet count with a typical nadir of $\geq 20 \times 10^9$/L. Platelet counts less than this will have other etiologies such as marrow suppression and drug-induced or autoimmune disorders [211].

49.7.2.1   Pathophysiology

Heparin-induced thrombocytopenia is a prothrombotic, immune-mediated adverse response in which IgG antibodies formed against the heparin-platelet factor 4 (PF4) complex bind the FC receptor on platelets and cause platelet activation. Activated platelets release additional PF4 and other prothrombotic particles, leading to more heparin-PF4 complexes and IgG-mediated platelet activation. If heparin exposure is not discontinued, the cycle of platelet activation in response to PF4 release will continue resulting in thrombocytopenia and a severely hypercoagulable state.

49.7.2.2   Diagnosis and Management

Clinical evaluation for HIT is warranted when there is an otherwise unexplained platelet count decrease after 5–14 days of heparin or LMWH exposure, or within 1 day of heparin exposure in patients who received heparin products in the previous 30–100 days. Pharmacists can play an essential role in identifying patients with thrombocytopenia who have been exposed to heparin products and initiate evaluation for HIT utilizing the 4T score risk assessment tool. Refer to Table 49.23 for the 4T score risk assessment measure and associated positive predictive values for the incidence of HIT. In critically ill patients, there may be many other causes for thrombocytopenia (see etiologies for TCP in the ICU Table 49.21), and pharmacists are crucial in identifying other drugs that may cause thrombocytopenia. Patients with 4T scores greater than or equal to 4 should have all forms of heparin products discontinued and PF4 antibody immunoassay and serotonin release assay (SRA) tests sent to confirm the diagnosis of HIT. Patients with 4T scores below 4 are very unlikely to have HIT [212] and should not be tested for HIT given the high sensitivity and low specificity of PF4 antibody immunoassays and frequent false-positive results [65]. Frequent reassessment of the 4T score may be necessary due to ever-changing clinical statuses of critically ill patients.

Management of HIT should be started as soon as possible in patients whose 4T score is 4 or higher. The initial step is to discontinue all heparin products, including heparin IV flushes, heparinized dialysate, and heparin-coated catheters. Therapeutic anticoagulation with alternative agents should be initiated in patients with active thrombosis, all patients with 4T scores of 6–8, and patients with 4T scores of 4–5; an additional indication for therapeutic anticoagulation is low bleeding risk [65]. IV direct thrombin inhibitors, argatroban and bivalirudin, are generally preferred in critically ill patients given that they have short duration of effect and can be quickly discontinued in cases of bleeding or prior to procedures. Caution should be used in patients with liver and renal dysfunction for argatroban and bivalirudin, respectively. Institutional aPTT goals for DTI monitoring may vary but should be titrated

Table 49.23 4T scoring system [12] and probability of HIT [12, 212]

Category	2 points	1 point	0 points
Thrombocytopenia	Platelet count fall >50% *and* nadir ≥20 × 10⁹/L	Platelet count fall 30–50% *or* nadir 10–19 × 10⁹/L	Platelet count fall <30% *or* nadir <10 × 10⁹/L
Timing of platelet count fall	Clear onset 5–10 days or ≤1 day + prior heparin exposure within 30 days	Unclear onset 5–10 days, onset after day 10, or <1 day + prior heparin exposure within 30–100 days	≤4 days without recent heparin exposure
Thrombosis or other sequelae	Confirmed new thrombosis, skin necrosis acute systemic reaction after bolus of UFH	Progressive or recurrent thrombosis, non-necrotizing (erythematous) skin lesions, suspected thrombosis	None
Other causes of thrombocytopenia	None apparent	Possible	Definite

Interpretation

4T score	**Risk category**	**Probability of HIT**	**Lab testing**
≥6	High	64%	Send PF4 and SRA
4–5	Intermediate	14%	Send PF4 and SRA
≤3	Low	0.2%	Do not send labs

to an aPTT 1.5–3 times baseline for argatroban and 1.5–2.5 times baseline for bivalirudin. In critically ill patients with prolonged baseline aPTT, custom aPTT goals may be necessary following the same principles for 1.5–3 times and 1.5–2.5 times baseline, respectively. If available, dilute thrombin time may be utilized and titrated to institutional therapeutic ranges. For patients with adequate renal function who are clinically stable or not undergoing procedures, fondaparinux or DOACs may be suitable alternatives to IV DTIs.

If the PF4 immunoassay results return negative, HIT is unlikely, and heparin may be resumed if indicated. Non-heparin anticoagulation should be continued if PF4 immunoassay results are positive until SRA results are received. According to the American Society of Hematology, patients without thrombotic complications of HIT should continue non-heparin anticoagulation until platelet count recovery is >150 K, and patients with thrombotic complications should be treated for a 3- to 6-month course; however, the optimal duration of treatment for HIT is unknown [65]. Heparin-PF4 antibodies may remain in the body for up to 100 days, and heparin products may be cautiously reintroduced if necessary.

49.7.2.3 Role of the Pharmacist

Clinical pharmacist can assist the appropriate testing for diagnosis, interpretation of results, and therapeutic management. For example, clinical pharmacist can create diagnosis (clinical scoring, initial testing based on sensitivity and specificity) and treatment algorithms for the management of HIT.

For additional information on this topic, refer to Chap. 44, Approach to Thrombocytopenia.

49.8 Transfusion Replacement Strategies in Patients Declining Blood Products

Patients who cannot accept blood products due to religious beliefs, medical conditions, or personal preferences require careful consideration in the management of anemia and acute bleeding. Bloodless Medicine and Surgery Programs have been developed to provide a multidisciplinary approach to providing optimal care without allogeneic or autologous blood transfusion. To avoid treatment delays and create individualized care plans, it is imperative to have early discussions with patients and/or healthcare proxies on which blood products or blood fraction products may be accepted, if any. Pharmacists can provide crucial information regarding which pharmacologic and hemostatic agents contain blood components.

In general, whole blood or any major component (red blood cells, platelets, fresh frozen plasma, white blood cells) is not acceptable. Products considered accepted include hemostatic drug products [antifibrinolytics (aminocaproic acid, tranexamic acid), desmopressin, conjugated estrogens, and recombinant factor VIIa] and hematopoietic growth factors [thrombopoietin receptor agonist (avatrombopag, eltrombopag, romiplostim), granulocyte colony-stimulating factor, recombinant erythropoietin albumin-free formulations] [213]. Non-blood volume expanders such as lactated ringers, normal saline (0.9% NaCl), and hydroxyethyl starch can be used as in the setting of hypovolemia. Products which should be determined acceptable on an individual basis include plasma-derived fraction products (albumin, cryoprecipitate, immunoglobulins), stimulating factors buffered in albumin (recombinant human erythropoietin), plasma-derived clotting factors (von Willebrand factor concentrate, prothrombin complex concentrates), autologous blood recovery and reinfusion (cell saver), and topical hemostatic agents (fibrin and thrombin sealant) [213].

The following are key strategies in managing critically ill patients unable to accept blood products: minimize blood loss, correct coagulopathies, and optimize oxygen delivery and consumption.

Minimize Blood Loss and Correct Coagulopathies

1. Pharmacists should evaluate the medication list and notify the team regarding any medications that may increase the patient's risk of bleeding (e.g., anticoagulants, antiplatelet, nonsteroidal anti-inflammatory drugs, SSRI/SNRIs, other medications that can cause thrombocytopenia). A risk-benefit discussion regarding continuing these medications is warranted.
2. In critically ill patients, venous thromboembolism (VTE) prophylaxis with intermittent pneumatic compression devices and graduated compression stockings is

a reasonable alternative to chemical VTE prophylaxis in patients where the risk of anticoagulation outweighs the benefits [214].

3. Obtain only essential lab tests, conduct multiple tests per sample, and utilize pediatric (small volume) phlebotomy tubes for adult patients.

4. If bleeding occurs, determine the likely causes (e.g., surgery/trauma vs. antithrombotic agents vs. coagulation defects) and intervene as quickly as possible. Pharmacologic agents and topical hemostatic agents can aid in temporizing patients until definitive hemostasis can be achieved (refer to Table 49.18 for topical hemostatic agents). Despite limited evidence, antifibrinolytics and recombinant activated factor VII are the agents most accepted and used in this patient population. Etiology-targeted pharmacologic intervention should also be provided (e.g., proton pump inhibitor for upper GI bleed). Refer to the antithrombotic reversal Sect. 49.5 for additional information if antithrombotic-related hemorrhage is suspected.

Antifibrinolytics

The use of antifibrinolytics to reduce perioperative blood loss and/or transfusion has been well established across a variety of surgical procedures [215–217]. Additionally, administration of tranexamic acid in trauma patients may reduce all-cause and bleeding-related mortality [218]. The benefit of tranexamic in other settings of bleeding, however, is not well defined. In the setting of GI bleeding, tranexamic acid did not reduce the incidence of mortality and increased the risk for VTE events [219]. Tranexamic acid in patients who are unable to accept blood products may be considered when the benefits outweigh the risks. The optimal dose of tranexamic acid in this setting is unknown, but it may be reasonable to follow the dosing strategy used in trauma patients: 1 g IV over 10 min, followed by 1 g infused over 8 h.

Recombinant Activated Factor VII

Recombinant activated factor VII (rFVIIa) is approved for use in patients with factor VII deficiency and hemophilia with inhibitors. Off-label use of rFVIIa has been evaluated in several different bleeding populations including intracranial hemorrhage, cardiac surgery, body trauma, and liver transplantation. When compared with usual care in off-label indications, rFVIIa has failed to show any mortality benefit [220]. Administration of rFVIIa in cardiac surgery and intracranial hemorrhage populations increased the rate of thromboembolic events [220]. Studied doses of rFVIIa have ranged from 30 to 200 mcg/kg, and the optimal dosing strategy for off-label use is unknown. It is reasonable to follow package insert recommendations and administer 90 mcg/kg every 3–6 h until bleeding has resolved.

Optimize Oxygen Delivery and Consumption

1. Adequate delivery of oxygen is dependent on sufficient cardiac output. Management of volume status and vasoactive/inotropic drugs may be necessary to maintain cardiac output. Intravenous fluids should be cautiously administered to maintain cardiac output as aggressive fluid resuscitation may disrupt clots and cause dilutional coagulopathy, further contributing to the problem in a bleeding

patient. Additionally, permissive hypotension with systolic blood pressures between 80 and 90 mmgHg may be beneficial until definitive hemostasis is achieved. In trauma patients, restrictive fluid resuscitation to maintain systolic blood pressure less than 90 mmHg has been associated with lower mortality rates [221].

2. Management of anemia with erythropoiesis-stimulating agents (ESAs) and iron, B12, and folate supplementation should be implemented, as appropriate.

Erythropoiesis-Stimulating Agents

ESAs induce erythropoiesis via stimulation of division and differentiation of erythroid progenitor cells, which results in increased erythrocytes and subsequent elevations in hemoglobin and hematocrit. The onset of increased reticulocyte count is about 10 days, and peak hemoglobin effect is seen between 2 and 6 weeks [222]. Epoetin alfa-epbx and darbepoetin alfa are albumin-free products and generally accepted in this patient population, whereas epoetin alfa is not. Preoperative administration of ESAs has been shown to reduce transfusion incidence in elective surgeries, but the role in anemia related to acute blood loss is less established [223]. Dosing strategies and route of administration (IV or subcutaneous) for ESAs vary across available published literature. Doses range from 500 to 20,000 units with frequencies between daily and weekly administration. The highest daily dose identified was IV epoetin alfa 40,000 units twice daily in combination with iron, B12, and folate [224].

Vitamin and Mineral Supplementation

Iron, vitamin B12, and folate supplementation in addition to ESAs should be given in patients with anemia. The combination of daily ESA and iron supplementation has been shown to increase hemoglobin levels and prevent transfusion in patients with burn injury, GI bleeding, and exsanguinating trauma [225–227]. An anemia management protocol for Jehovah's Witness patients published by the University of Michigan's Division of Acute Care Surgery recommends supplementation with IV iron sucrose 100 mg daily for at least 10 days in combination with epoetin alfa 40,000 units daily until hemoglobin is greater than 7 g/dL [228]. Additionally, their protocol recommends folate 1 mg daily (IV or PO), vitamin B12 supplementation, and vitamin C 500 mg three times daily (once daily in renal failure) [228].

3. Pain, agitation, and shivering can lead to increased oxygen consumption [229]. Adequate analgesia and sedation should be provided to keep patients comfortable and aid in ventilator compliance. Oxygen consumption may also be decreased with hypothermia and paralysis with neuromuscular blockade, although outcomes related to these strategies in this patient population have not been evaluated at a large scale [230].

4. Hemoglobin-based oxygen carriers (glutaraldehyde-polymerized bovine hemoglobin) are only available in the United States for clinical trial or through the FDA Expanded Access program for compassionate use due to increased risk for mortality and myocardial ischemia [231, 232]. The utility of glutaraldehyde-polymerized bovine hemoglobin for acute anemia management is limited by the

FDA and institutional review board approval process where turnaround time may be more than 24 h.

Role of the Pharmacist

The critical care pharmacist is responsible for safe medication review and selection, ensuring that patients do not receive products that contain blood products. Additionally, they should discuss any medications that may increase bleeding risk with the interdisciplinary team to determine if the benefit of administering these medications outweighs the risk. Determining which labs are essential for monitoring medications and limiting the frequency of nonessential labs can aid in reducing iatrogenic blood loss. Many of the hemostatic agents reviewed in this chapter do not have optimal dosing strategies. The critical care pharmacist should provide prescribers with sufficient information and available study data to dose these medications for off-label indications. Additionally, pharmacists may be involved in the bloodless medicine multidisciplinary team and assist with institutional protocol or guideline development.

For additional information on this topic, please refer to Chap. 54, Rational Use of Blood Products.

49.9 Periprocedural Management of Antithrombotic Therapy

Managing antithrombotic and antiplatelet therapy before and after invasive procedures or surgeries poses a frequent challenge for healthcare providers. Achieving the optimal patient outcome involves carefully weighing the risks of bleeding and thrombosis. To devise an effective antithrombotic management strategy before procedures, one can systematically evaluate factors such as the procedure's bleeding risk, potential consequences of bleeding, patient-specific thromboembolic risk factors, and particular oral anticoagulant or antiplatelet medication in use. The following steps can assist with the process of accessing each aspect.

49.9.1 Step 1: Procedure or Surgical Bleeding Risk

The assessment of procedural or surgical bleeding risk forms the cornerstone of developing a periprocedural anticoagulant management strategy. While various professional bodies have issued guidelines for evaluating this risk, a common approach involves categorizing bleeding risk into three tiers based on the frequency of major bleeding events. Recent guidelines from the International Society on Thrombosis and Haemostasis (ISTH) categorize procedural/surgical bleeding risk based on the 30-day probability of major bleeding events: high risk involves a major bleeding rate exceeding 2% or the potential for catastrophic consequences, while low/

Table 49.24 Procedural bleeding risk [233, 234]

Procedural/surgery risk assessment	
Risk category	Examples
High	Major operation >45 min Neuraxial anesthesia Cardiac surgery (CABG, aortic aneurysm repair, heart valve replacement) Neurosurgery (intracranial, spinal surgery) Surgery of a high vascular organ (liver, kidney, spleen) Urologic surgery (including nephrectomy, biopsy) Major orthopedic surgery PEG or ERCP
Low/moderate	Bronchoscopy including biopsy Coronary angiography, femoral Central venous catheter removal Paracentesis Thoracentesis Abdominal hernia repair, hysterectomy Gastrointestinal endoscopy including biopsy Cholecystectomy
Minimal	Minor cutaneous procedures Minor dental procedures Cataract procedure Pacemaker or defibrillator implantation

Abbreviations: *AVR* aortic valve replacement; *CABG* coronary artery bypass; *TIA* transient ischemic attack; *VTE* venous thromboembolism, *PEG* percutaneous endoscopic gastrostomy; *ERCP* endoscopic retrograde cholangiopancreatography

moderate risk encompasses a 0–2% major bleeding rate, and minimal risk indicates a major bleeding rate of approximately 0%. Table 49.24 provides examples of procedures falling within each category; it is important to acknowledge that bleed risk classification may vary among different professional organizations, and there are procedures for which bleeding risk has not yet been standardized.

49.9.2 Step 2: Thromboembolic Risk

Evaluating the patient's thromboembolic risk provides valuable insight into the necessity of minimizing interruptions in anticoagulant therapy. For patients receiving vitamin K antagonist (VKA) therapy, this assessment guides healthcare providers in determining whether parenteral anticoagulation is required as a bridging measure. Thromboembolism risk frequently serves as the underlying condition necessitating anticoagulation therapy. These conditions include atrial fibrillation, mechanical valve replacement, venous thromboembolism (VTE), thrombophilia disorders (protein C, protein S, antithrombin deficiency, antiphospholipid antibodies), and cerebral vascular disease. Each of these factors can be classified according to their annual stroke risk or monthly risk of VTE, with high-risk scenarios representing probabilities exceeding 10%, moderate-risk scenarios ranging from 4 to 10%, and low-risk scenarios indicating probabilities below 4% [234].

The thromboembolic risk associated with nonvalvular atrial fibrillation is assessed using the patient's individual CHA_2DS_2VASc score (congestive heart failure +1, hypertension +1, age ≥ 75 + 2, diabetes +1, history of stroke or transient ischemic attack +2, vascular disease +1, age 65–74 + 1, female sex category +1). A CHA_2DS_2VASc score greater than 7 indicates high risk, while scores of 5–6 and 1–4 (without a history of stroke or TIA) represent moderate and low risk, respectively.

For patients with mechanical valves, an understanding of the type of valve, placement location, and other thromboembolic risk factors is required to determine the level of thrombotic risk. High-risk patients are considered those with a mechanical mitral valve or a caged ball or tilting disc aortic valve replacement (AVR). Moderate risk includes mechanical AVR with stroke risk factors, and low risk is a mechanical AVR without stroke risk factors.

Patients with a history of VTE can be stratified based on the time elapsed since the VTE event occurred: high risk being a VTE less than 3 months ago, moderate risk a VTE within 3–12 months or recurrent VTE, and low risk a VTE greater than 12 months ago. Additional high thrombotic risk factors include a history of stroke or TIA within the past 3 months and specific thrombophilia disorders such as protein C or S, antithrombin deficiency, or antiphospholipid antibodies.

These risk factors are outlined and can be further reviewed in both ISTH guidance document and the perioperative management of antithrombotic therapy guideline by the American College of Chest Physicians (ACCP) [233, 234].

49.9.3 Step 3: Anticoagulant Management

49.9.3.1 Perioperative Interruption

The timing of anticoagulant interruption will be dependent on the specific anticoagulant agent, the half-life of the drug, and the risk of the procedure. High-risk procedures require complete elimination, four to five half-lives of the drug, and low/moderate-risk procedures can have partial drug elimination, two to three half-lives of the drug. Minimal risk procedures often do not require holding but the day of procedure.

In patients undergoing treatment with DOACs, it is crucial to assess renal function via creatinine clearance calculated (CrCl) by the Cockcroft-Gault equation, as it can significantly influence the drug's half-life. Unlike warfarin, DOACs exhibit a shorter half-life and faster onset, eliminating the necessity for bridging with parenteral anticoagulants. The PAUSE (Perioperative Anticoagulant Use for Surgery Evaluation) study was specifically designed to establish a standardized protocol for managing anticoagulation in patients with atrial fibrillation who are scheduled to undergo elective procedures or surgeries. The objective was to devise a protocol that could effectively mitigate thrombotic events and minimize bleeding complications without the need for anticoagulation testing or bridging with heparin [235]. The successful outcomes of the PAUSE study have led to widespread adoption of its protocol in clinical practice for the perioperative management of DOACs [233]. A schematic of the study protocol is in Table 49.25; one exception is categories with the CrCl less than 30 mL/min or hemodialysis, which were excluded from the study. While the PAUSE trial focused specifically on patients with atrial fibrillation, the

Table 49.25 Management of direct oral anticoagulants for planned or elective procedures [235, 236]

Low/moderate-bleed-risk procedure/surgery

Creatinine clearance[a]	Direct oral anticoagulant	Day −5	Day −4	Day −3	Day −2	Day −1	Procedure/ surgery	Day 1	Day 2	Day 3
>50 mL/min	Apixaban Edoxaban Rivaroxaban Dabigatran	+	+	+	+	−	−	−/+	+	+
30–50 mL/min	Apixaban Edoxaban Rivaroxaban	+	+	+	+	−	−	−/+	+	+
	Dabigatran	+	+	+	−	−	−	−/+	+	+
15–29 mL/min[2]	Apixaban Edoxaban Rivaroxaban	+	+	+	−	−	−	−/+	+	+
	Dabigatran	+	+	−	−	−	−	−/+	+	+
<15 mL/min or dialysis[b]	Apixaban Edoxaban Rivaroxaban	+	+	−	−	−	−	−/+	+	+
	Dabigatran	+	−	−	−	−	−	−/+	+	+

High-bleed-risk procedure/surgery

Creatinine clearance[a]	Direct oral anticoagulant	Day −6	Day −5	Day −4	Day −3	Day −2	Day −1	Procedure/ surgery	Day 1	Day 2	Day 3
>50 mL/min	Apixaban Edoxaban Rivaroxaban Dabigatran	+	+	+	+	−	−	−	−	−/+	+
30–50 mL/min	Apixaban Edoxaban Rivaroxaban	+	+	+	+	−	−	−	−	−/+	+
	Dabigatran	+	+	−	−	−	−	−	−	−/+	+
15–29 mL/min[2]	Apixaban Edoxaban Rivaroxaban	+	+	+	−	−	−	−	−	−/+	+
	Dabigatran	+	−	−	−	−	−	−	−	−/+	+
<15 mL/min or dialysis[b]	Apixaban Edoxaban Rivaroxaban	+	+	+	−	−	−	−	−	−/+	+
	Dabigatran	+	−	−	−	−	−	−	−	−/+	+

+ Continue regular dose of direct oral anticoagulant; − Hold dose of direct oral anticoagulant; −/+ Assessment based on postprocedural bleeding can resume or hold based on clinical judgment
[a] Creatinine clearance calculated via Cockcroft and Gault formula
[b] No data; hold period is based on estimated half-life of the drug; consider anticoagulation monitoring

cessation strategy for DOACs outlined in the study can also be applied to patients with VTE [233]. Routine monitoring of specific DOAC levels, such as AFXa or dTT, prior to procedures is generally unnecessary. The optimal DOAC AFXa level deemed adequate for a procedure has not been established; a level less than 30 ng/mL for high-risk procedures or a level of 50 ng/mL has been suggested [235, 237]. The PAUSE study protocol demonstrated less than 10% of all patients having residual anticoagulant ($\geq$50 ng/mL) periprocedural, and in 1.8% of patients with a high bleed risk procedure. To further support this practice, a prospective study evaluating preprocedural DOAC levels found that DOAC discontinuation 49–72 h prior to the procedure resulted in minimal residual anticoagulant ($\leq$30 ng/mL) in 95% of patients [237]. Factors including age, weight, renal function, and DOAC dosing could influence residual anticoagulant levels following the PAUSE protocol. However, it is worth considering monitoring in specific patient populations, such as those with acute kidney injury and hepatic impairment or in emergent procedural settings. Vitamin K antagonists (VKAs), like warfarin, necessitate an extended period of anticoagulation interruption owing to the drug's half-life and vitamin K-dependent coagulation factors. Patients undergoing minimal risk procedures may continue anticoagulation, while all other procedural risk categories require temporary discontinuation [233]. To ascertain the appropriate timing for discontinuation, determining the periprocedural INR threshold and obtaining an INR measurement 7–10 days before the procedure are recommended. Generally, a cessation period of at least 5 days is sufficient to achieve near elimination of warfarin. However, certain patient factors, such as advanced age, reduced metabolism, or a supratherapeutic INR exceeding 3.5, may necessitate an extended discontinuation period of over 6 days. Assessing the patient's thrombotic risk profile can inform decisions regarding the necessity of therapeutic bridging with a parenteral anticoagulant.

49.9.3.2 Procedural Bridging

The term "bridging" denotes the utilization of short-acting parenteral anticoagulants such as LMWH or UFH at therapeutic doses while withholding VKA and maintaining a subtherapeutic INR. Bridging is generally not recommended for most patients, as evidence indicates a heightened risk of major bleeding with no discernible difference in thromboembolic events [238, 239]. Notably, the BRIDGE (Bridging Anticoagulation in Patients who Require Temporary Interruption of Warfarin Therapy for an Elective Invasive Procedure or Surgery) trial highlights that patients with atrial fibrillation requiring warfarin interruption for elective procedures showed comparable arterial thrombotic event rates, but higher rates of major bleeding when bridged with LMWH compared to those who were not [238]. It is crucial to recognize that this study primarily encompassed patients with low to intermediate thrombotic risk undergoing low-risk procedures, excluding high-risk procedures prone to both thrombotic and bleeding complications (e.g., major cancer surgery, cardiac surgery, neurosurgery). This study underscores that anticoagulation bridging may not be necessary for all patients with atrial fibrillation. While the general recommendation is to avoid bridging for patients with low to moderate thromboembolic risk (refer to step 2 section), certain factors such as high-risk surgeries (e.g., cardiovascular surgery, carotid endarterectomy) or specific patient histories (e.g., prior perioperative stroke) may influence the decision to bridge despite their thrombotic risk category. Patients classified as high thrombotic risk should receive bridging during VKA interruption. A schematic depicting the timing of VKA interruption and bridging with LMWH is illustrated in Table 49.26. Postprocedural bridging is typically initiated within 24 h for procedures associated with low to moderate bleeding risk, and within 48–72 h for those with high bleeding risk, continuing until the patient achieves a therapeutic INR. Early postprocedural bridging with therapeutic anticoagulation is associated with a higher risk of major bleeding [240]. For patients at high thrombotic risk but also facing a high postprocedural bleeding risk, prophylactic dosing of LMWH or UFH may be considered until therapeutic anticoagulation is reestablished.

49.9.4 Step 4: Antiplatelet Management

Antiplatelet therapies can include aspirin (ASA), P2Y12 inhibitors (e.g., clopidogrel, prasugrel, ticagrelor, cangrelor), reversible inhibitors (e.g. cilostazol, dipyridamole), and nonsteroidal anti-inflammatory drugs (NSAIDs) (e.g., ibuprofen, indomethacin, meloxicam, naproxen). Management of antiplatelet therapy will be dependent on bleeding risk of the procedure and thrombotic risk of the patients. Timing of antiplatelet interruption will be dependent on the mechanism of platelet inhibition. For antiplatelet agents that irreversibly inhibit platelet function, 7–10 days, which is the lifespan of the platelet, are required. This includes ASA, clopidogrel, and prasugrel. Reversible inhibitors such as ticagrelor, cangrelor, cilostazol, dipyridamole, and NSAIDs are dependent on the half-life of the drug. Unless the patient is at high risk (e.g., coronary stent in a critical location within 3 months), bridging with P2Y12 cangrelor is deemed unnecessary. Resumption of antiplatelet therapy will depend on the onset of antiplatelet onset and postprocedural bleeding risk. Further details on the timing of antiplatelet therapy and risk consideration based on the timing of coronary stent placement can be referred to in the ACCP clinical practice guideline on perioperative management of antithrombotic therapy [233].

49.9.5 Step 5: Antithrombotic Resumption

Determining the appropriate timing to resume antithrombotic therapy should include an evaluation of procedural site hemostasis, intraprocedural bleeding complications, postprocedural risk of bleeding complication, and patient-specific bleeding risk factors (e.g., concomitant antiplatelet, platelet dysfunction, renal or liver dysfunction) [236]. A schematic for resumption of therapeutic anticoagulation with either a DOAC or a VKA based on procedural bleeding risk is demonstrated in Tables 49.25 and 49.26. Due to the longer time to onset, patients on VKA are

Table 49.26 Management of vitamin K antagonist requiring bridging for planned or elective procedures [233, 238, 239]

Procedural bleeding risk	Anticoagulant	Day −6	Day −5	Day −4	Day −3	Day −2	Day −1	Procedure/surgery	Day 1	Day 2	Day 3
Low/moderate bleeding risk	Warfarin	+	−	−	−	−	−	−/+[a]	+	+	+
	LMWH	−	−	−	+	+	+/−[b]	−	+	+	+[c]
High bleeding risk	Warfarin	+	−	−	−	−	−	−/+[a]	+	+	+
	LMWH	−	−	−	+	+	+/−[b]	−	−[d]	+[d]	+[c]

Abbreviations: *LMWH* low-molecular-weight heparin

+ Administer full dose; − Hold dose; −/+ Administer the evening dose; omit morning dose; +/− Administer the morning dose; omit evening dose

[a] Warfarin can be restarted either the evening of or the day after the procedure at usual dose

[b] Last preprocedural dose 24 h prior to procedure at half dose the total daily dose

[c] Continue until INR within therapeutic range

[d] Prophylaxis dose LMWH can be used in patients with high VTE risk postprocedural for 24–72 h until full dose is resumed

typically restarted either the evening of the procedure or within 24 h. Postprocedural bridging to a VKA is discussed in the procedural bridging section. Patients on DOACs can be resumed within 24–72 h depending on the bleed risk of the procedure. As mentioned previously, in patients at high thrombotic risk but also facing a high postprocedural bleeding risk, prophylactic dosing of LMWH or UFH may be considered until therapeutic anticoagulation is deemed appropriate.

49.9.5.1 Neuraxial Anesthesia

The consequences of bleeding into the spinal or epidural space although rare can have catastrophic complications including paralysis. Neuraxial procedures for anesthesia, including both catheter placement and removal, are therefore classified as a high-bleed-risk procedure in which antiplatelet and anticoagulant therapy should be evaluated. Anticoagulation, while an epidural catheter is in place, should be limited to therapeutic UFH at the lowest possible dose, UFH prophylaxis twice to three times daily, or LMWH prophylaxis once-daily dosing [241]. Therapeutic LMWH and twice-daily LMWH prophylaxis should wait until catheter removal. All DOAC agents have a US Food and Drug Administration (FDA)-issued black box warning regarding the risk of spinal and epidural hematomas in patients undergoing neuraxial interventions and should be avoided until after catheter removal. The American Society of Regional Anesthesia and Pain Medicine provides evidence-based guidelines on antithrombotic and antiplatelet management before and after neuraxial procedures; these guidelines should be consulted for further details [241].

49.9.5.2 Urgent or Emergent Procedures

The previously discussed steps are typically for planned or elective procedures. For urgent or emergent procedures, anticoagulant reversal may be required; refer to the anticoagulation reversal Sect. 49.5 for agent-specific reversal options.

49.9.5.3 Role of the Pharmacist

Clinical pharmacist can be involved in multiple phases of care regarding procedural management of antithrombotic therapy. Pharmacist can assist by evaluating patient thromboembolic, procedural bleeding risk, and outpatient oral anticoagulant regimen to determine the optimal periprocedural plan. Additionally, they can provide guidance on urgent/emergent procedures requiring reversal, product or factor supplementation, need for parenteral anticoagulant bridging, and resumption of therapeutic or prophylaxis anticoagulation [242].

Reducing the likelihood of anticoagulant-related harm to patients is a national patient safety goal set by the Joint Commission; this includes the development of evidence-based practice guidelines on the perioperative management of oral anticoagulants such as the use of bridging medications and timing of anticoagulant interruption and resumption [243]. When involved in surgical quality committees, the pharmacist can be a pivotal interdisciplinary team member in the development of institutional guidance documents addressing antithrombotic management across diverse clinical settings such as cardiac surgery, interventional radiology, and neuraxial antithrombotic protocols. The education of pharmacists regarding new evidence and updates to periprocedural guidelines can influence the anticoagulation practices adopted by healthcare providers [244].

Pharmacists possess valuable insights into medication utilization and management systems, serving as a crucial information source for medication practices tied to specific quality metrics and facilitating the implementation of process improvement initiatives. These may involve establishing protocols for selecting VTE prophylaxis through evidence-based thrombotic assessment scales and consideration of patient-specific factors such as weight and renal function. Furthermore, optimizing surgical or procedural order sets can ensure timely initiation of VTE prophylaxis, while implementing alerts for ordering neuraxial anesthesia epidurals in patients with active prescriptions for antithrombotic therapy enhances safety measures.

References

1. LaPelusa A, Dave HD. Physiology, hemostasis. In: StatPearls. Treasure Island, FL: StatPearls Publishing; 2024. http://www.ncbi.nlm.nih.gov/books/NBK545263/. Accessed 18 Apr 2024.
2. Gale AJ. Current understanding of hemostasis. Toxicol Pathol. 2011;39(1):273–80. https://doi.org/10.1177/0192623310389474.
3. Levi M, Schultz M. Coagulopathy and platelet disorders in critically ill patients. Minerva Anestesiol. 2010;76(10):851–9.
4. Hunt BJ. Bleeding and coagulopathies in critical care. N Engl J Med. 2014;370(9):847–59. https://doi.org/10.1056/NEJMra1208626.
5. Armando T, Mannuccio MP. The coagulopathy of chronic liver disease. N Engl J Med. 2011;365(2):147–56.
6. Favaloro EJ, Funk DM, Lippi G. Pre-analytical variables in coagulation testing associated with diagnostic errors in hemostasis. Lab Med. 2012;43(2):1.2-10. https://doi.org/10.1309/LM749BQETKYPYPVM.
7. Guervil DJ, et al. Activated partial thromboplastin time versus Antifactor Xa heparin assay in monitoring unfractionated heparin by continuous intravenous infusion. Ann Pharmacother. 2011;45(7–8):861–8. https://doi.org/10.1345/aph.1Q161.
8. Zaki HV, Elbeialy MAK, Soliman AM. The use of activated partial thromboplastin time versus antifactor Xa assay in monitoring continuous unfractionated heparin infusion therapy in obstetric intensive care unit. Ain-Shams J Anesthesiol. 2019;11(1):3. https://doi.org/10.1186/s42077-019-0021-2.
9. Swayngim R, et al. Comparison of clinical outcomes using activated partial thromboplastin time versus antifactor-Xa for monitoring therapeutic unfractionated heparin: a systematic review and meta-analysis. Thromb Res. 2021;208:18–25. https://doi.org/10.1016/j.thromres.2021.10.010.
10. Levy JH, et al. When and how to use antidotes for the reversal of direct oral anticoagulants: guidance from the SSC of the ISTH. J Thromb Haemost. 2016;14(3):623–7. https://doi.org/10.1111/jth.13227.

11. McGlasson DL, Romick BG, Rubal BJ. Comparison of a chromogenic factor X assay with international normalized ratio for monitoring oral anticoagulation therapy. Blood Coagul Fibrinolysis. 2008;19(6):513–7. https://doi.org/10.1097/MBC.0b013e328304e066.

12. Santoshi RK, et al. A comprehensive review of thrombocytopenia with a spotlight on intensive care patients. Cureus. 2022;14:e27718. https://doi.org/10.7759/cureus.27718.

13. Brill JB, et al. The role of TEG and ROTEM in damage control resuscitation. Shock. 2021;56(1S):52–61. https://doi.org/10.1097/SHK.0000000000001686.

14. Cuker A. Light transmission aggregometry. Hematologist. 2014;11(2) https://doi.org/10.1182/hem.V11.2.2555.

15. Sibbing D, et al. Updated expert consensus statement on platelet function and genetic testing for guiding P2Y12 receptor inhibitor treatment in percutaneous coronary intervention. J Am Coll Cardiol Intv. 2019;12(16):1521–37. https://doi.org/10.1016/j.jcin.2019.03.034.

16. Riehl K, et al. Is ROTEM diagnostic in trauma care associated with lower mortality rates in bleeding patients?—a retrospective analysis of 7461 patients derived from the TraumaRegister DGU®. J Clin Med. 2022;11(20):6150. https://doi.org/10.3390/jcm11206150.

17. Rodriguez Martin I. VISCOELASTIC TESTING IN CARDIAC SURGERY. Chest. 2022;161(6):A38. https://doi.org/10.1016/j.chest.2021.12.070.

18. Wei H, Child LJ. Clinical utility of viscoelastic testing in chronic liver disease: a systematic review. World J Hepatol. 2020;12(11):1115–27. https://doi.org/10.4254/wjh.v12.i11.1115.

19. Wikkelsø A, et al. Thromboelastography (TEG) or thromboelastometry (ROTEM) to monitor haemostatic treatment versus usual care in adults or children with bleeding. Cochrane Database Syst Rev. 2016;2018(12):CD007871. https://doi.org/10.1002/14651858.CD007871.pub3.

20. Gonzalez E, Moore EE, Moore HB. Management of trauma-induced coagulopathy with thrombelastography. Crit Care Clin. 2017;33(1):119–34. https://doi.org/10.1016/j.ccc.2016.09.002.

21. Fleming K, et al. TEG-directed transfusion in complex cardiac surgery: impact on blood product usage. J Extra Corpor Technol. 2017;49(4):283–90.

22. Kumar M, et al. Thromboelastography-guided blood component use in patients with cirrhosis with nonvariceal bleeding: a randomized controlled trial. Hepatology. 2020;71(1):235–46. https://doi.org/10.1002/hep.30794.

23. Dager WE, Trujillo TC, Gilbert BW. Approaches to precision-based anticoagulation management in the critically ill. Pharmacotherapy. 2023;43(11):1221–36. https://doi.org/10.1002/phar.2868.

24. Garcia DA, et al. Parenteral anticoagulants. Chest. 2012;141(2 Suppl):e24S–43S. https://doi.org/10.1378/chest.11-2291.

25. Reynolds PM, et al. Evaluation of prophylactic heparin dosage strategies and risk factors for venous thromboembolism in the critically ill patient. Pharmacotherapy. 2019;39(3):232–41. https://doi.org/10.1002/phar.2212.

26. Ley EJ, et al. Updated guidelines to reduce venous thromboembolism in trauma patients: a Western trauma association critical decisions algorithm. J Trauma Acute Care Surg. 2020;89(5):971–81. https://doi.org/10.1097/TA.0000000000002830.

27. Yorkgitis BK, et al. American Association for the Surgery of Trauma/American College of Surgeons-Committee on Trauma Clinical Protocol for inpatient venous thromboembolism prophylaxis after trauma. J Trauma Acute Care Surg. 2022;92(3):597–604. https://doi.org/10.1097/TA.0000000000003475.

28. Levy JH, Frere C, Koster A. Resistance to unfractionated heparin in the ICU: evaluation and management options. Intensive Care Med. 2023b;49(8):1005–7. https://doi.org/10.1007/s00134-023-07103-x.

29. Knox H, et al. Venous thromboembolism prophylaxis in low body weight critically ill patients. J Intensive Care Med. 2023;39:08850666231217693. https://doi.org/10.1177/08850666231217693.

30. Shaikh S, et al. Venous thromboembolism chemoprophylaxis regimens in trauma and surgery patients with obesity: a systematic review. J Trauma Acute Care Surg. 2020;88(4):522–35. https://doi.org/10.1097/TA.0000000000002538.

31. Samuel S, et al. High dose subcutaneous unfractionated heparin for prevention of venous thromboembolism in overweight neurocritical care patients. J Thromb Thrombolysis. 2015;40(3):302–7. https://doi.org/10.1007/s11239-015-1202-x.
32. Joy M, et al. Safety and efficacy of high-dose unfractionated heparin for prevention of venous thromboembolism in overweight and obese patients. Pharmacotherapy. 2016;36(7):740–8. https://doi.org/10.1002/phar.1775.
33. Regis T, Goriacko P, Ferguson N. Safety of high-dose unfractionated heparin for prophylaxis of venous thromboembolism in hospitalized obese patients. Ann Pharmacother. 2021;55(8):963–9. https://doi.org/10.1177/1060028020974569.
34. Raschke RA. The weight-based heparin dosing nomogram compared with a standard care nomogram: a randomized controlled trial. Ann Intern Med. 1993;119(9):874. https://doi.org/10.7326/0003-4819-119-9-199311010-00002.
35. Kearon C, et al. Antithrombotic therapy for VTE disease. Chest. 2016;149(2):315–52. https://doi.org/10.1016/j.chest.2015.11.026.
36. Ortel TL, et al. American Society of Hematology 2020 guidelines for management of venous thromboembolism: treatment of deep vein thrombosis and pulmonary embolism. Blood Adv. 2020;4(19):4693–738. https://doi.org/10.1182/bloodadvances.2020001830.
37. Stevens SM, et al. Antithrombotic therapy for VTE disease. Chest. 2021;160(6):e545–608. https://doi.org/10.1016/j.chest.2021.07.055.
38. Barletta JF, et al. Limitations of a standardized weight-based nomogram for heparin dosing in patients with morbid obesity. Surg Obes Relat Dis. 2008;4(6):748–53. https://doi.org/10.1016/j.soard.2008.03.005.
39. Gerlach AT, et al. Comparison of heparin dosing based on actual body weight in non-obese, obese and morbidly obese critically ill patients. Int J Crit Illn Inj Sci. 2013;3(3):195–9. https://doi.org/10.4103/2229-5151.119200.
40. Boneu B, De Moerloose P. How and when to monitor a patient treated with low molecular weight heparin. Semin Thromb Hemost. 2001;27(05):519–22. https://doi.org/10.1055/s-2001-17961.
41. Sebaaly J, Covert K. Enoxaparin dosing at extremes of weight: literature review and dosing recommendations. Ann Pharmacother. 2018;52(9):898–909. https://doi.org/10.1177/1060028018768449.
42. Sikes L, et al. Anti-factor Xa level monitoring for enoxaparin prophylaxis and treatment in high-risk patient groups. HCA Healthcare J Med. 2023;4(2):105. https://doi.org/10.36518/2689-0216.1464.
43. Witt DM, et al. American society of hematology 2018 guidelines for management of venous thromboembolism: optimal management of anticoagulation therapy. Blood Advances. 2018;2(22): pp. 3257–3291. Available at: https://doi.org/10.1182/bloodadvances.2018024893.
44. Kaylor DM, et al. Venous thromboembolism prophylaxis with enoxaparin versus unfractionated heparin in patients with low body weight. Plasmatology. 2023;17:26348535231156848. https://doi.org/10.1177/26348535231156848.
45. Rojas L, et al. Anti-Xa activity after enoxaparin prophylaxis in hospitalized patients weighing less than fifty-five kilograms. Thromb Res. 2013;132(6):761–4. https://doi.org/10.1016/j.thromres.2013.10.005.
46. Yam L, et al. Enoxaparin thromboprophylaxis dosing and anti–factor xa levels in low-weight patients. Pharmacotherapy. 2019;39(7):749–55. https://doi.org/10.1002/phar.2295.
47. Schünemann HJ, et al. American Society of Hematology 2018 guidelines for management of venous thromboembolism: prophylaxis for hospitalized and nonhospitalized medical patients. Blood Adv. 2018;2(22):3198–225. https://doi.org/10.1182/bloodadvances.2018022954.
48. Andersen DR, et al. American Society of Hematology 2019 guidelines for management of venous thromboembolism: prevention of venous thromboembolism in surgical hospitalized patients. Blood Adv. 2019;3(23):3898–944. https://doi.org/10.1182/bloodadvances.2019000975.
49. Ceccato D, et al. Weight-adjusted versus fixed dose heparin thromboprophylaxis in hospitalized obese patients: a systematic review and meta-analysis. Eur J Intern Med. 2021;88:73–80. https://doi.org/10.1016/j.ejim.2021.03.030.

50. Ludwig KP, et al. Implementation of an enoxaparin protocol for venous thromboembolism prophylaxis in obese surgical intensive care unit patients. Ann Pharmacother. 2011;45(11):1356–62. https://doi.org/10.1345/aph.1Q313.
51. Bickford A, et al. Weight-based enoxaparin dosing for venous thromboembolism prophylaxis in the obese trauma patient. Am J Surg. 2013;206(6):847–52. https://doi.org/10.1016/j.amjsurg.2013.07.020.
52. Lee YR, et al. Monitoring enoxaparin with Antifactor Xa levels in obese patients. Pharmacotherapy. 2015;35(11):1007–15. https://doi.org/10.1002/phar.1658.
53. Curry MA, et al. Evaluation of treatment-dose enoxaparin in acutely ill morbidly obese patients at an Academic Medical Center: a randomized clinical trial. Ann Pharmacother. 2019;53(6):567–73. https://doi.org/10.1177/1060028018821149.
54. Turpie AG, et al. Pharmacokinetic and clinical data supporting the use of fondaparinux 1.5 mg once daily in the prevention of venous thromboembolism in renally impaired patients. Blood Coagul Fibrinolysis. 2009;20(2):114–21. https://doi.org/10.1097/MBC.0b013e328323da86.
55. Cope J, et al. Clinical experience with prophylactic Fondaparinux in critically ill patients with moderate to severe renal impairment or renal failure requiring renal replacement therapy. Ann Pharmacother. 2015;49(3):270–7. https://doi.org/10.1177/1060028014563325.
56. Wahby KA, Riley LK, Tennenberg SD. Assessment of an extended interval Fondaparinux dosing regimen for venous thromboembolism prophylaxis in critically ill patients with severe renal dysfunction using Antifactor Xa levels. Pharmacotherapy. 2017;37(10):1241–8. https://doi.org/10.1002/phar.2014.
57. Young G, et al. FondaKIDS: a prospective pharmacokinetic and safety study of fondaparinux in children between 1 and 18 years of age. Pediatr Blood Cancer. 2011;57(6):1049–54. https://doi.org/10.1002/pbc.23011.
58. Martinez L, et al. Effect of fondaparinux prophylaxis on anti-factor Xa concentrations in patients with morbid obesity. Am J Health Syst Pharm. 2011;68(18):1716–22. https://doi.org/10.2146/ajhp110010.
59. Steele KE, et al. The EFFORT trial: preoperative enoxaparin versus postoperative fondaparinux for thromboprophylaxis in bariatric surgical patients: a randomized double-blind pilot trial. Surg Obes Relat Dis. 2015;11(3):672–83. https://doi.org/10.1016/j.soard.2014.10.003.
60. Davidson BL, et al. Effect of obesity on outcomes after fondaparinux, enoxaparin, or heparin treatment for acute venous thromboembolism in the Matisse trials. J Thromb Haemost. 2007;5(6):1191–4. https://doi.org/10.1111/j.1538-7836.2007.02565.x.
61. Tang IY, et al. Argatroban and renal replacement therapy in patients with heparin-induced thrombocytopenia. Ann Pharmacother. 2005;39(2):231–6. https://doi.org/10.1345/aph.1E480.
62. Linkins L-A, et al. Treatment and prevention of heparin-induced thrombocytopenia. Chest. 2012;141(2):e495S–530S. https://doi.org/10.1378/chest.11-2303.
63. Rice L, et al. Argatroban anticoagulation in obese versus nonobese patients: implications for treating heparin-induced thrombocytopenia. J Clin Pharmacol. 2007;47(8):1028–34. https://doi.org/10.1177/0091270007302951.
64. Elagizi S, Davis K. Argatroban dosing in obesity. Thromb Res. 2018;163:60–3. https://doi.org/10.1016/j.thromres.2018.01.011.
65. Cuker A, et al. American Society of Hematology 2018 guidelines for management of venous thromboembolism: heparin-induced thrombocytopenia. Blood Adv. 2018a;2(22):3360–92. https://doi.org/10.1182/bloodadvances.2018024489.
66. Tsu LV, Dager WE. Comparison of Bivalirudin dosing strategies using total, adjusted, and ideal body weights in obese patients with heparin-induced thrombocytopenia. Pharmacotherapy. 2012;32(1):20–6. https://doi.org/10.1002/PHAR.1016.
67. Hursting MJ, Lewis BE, Macfarlane DE. Transitioning from Argatroban to warfarin therapy in patients with heparin-induced thrombocytopenia. Clin Appl Thromb Hemost. 2005;11(3):279–87. https://doi.org/10.1177/107602960501100306.

68. Ansell J, et al. Pharmacology and Management of the Vitamin K Antagonists. Chest. 2008;133(6):160S–98S. https://doi.org/10.1378/chest.08-0670.
69. Nutescu E, Chuatrisorn I, Hellenbart E. Drug and dietary interactions of warfarin and novel oral anticoagulants: an update. J Thromb Thrombolysis. 2011;31(3):326–43. https://doi.org/10.1007/s11239-011-0561-1.
70. Vega AJ, et al. Warfarin and antibiotics: drug interactions and clinical considerations. Life. 2023;13(8):1661. https://doi.org/10.3390/life13081661.
71. Lal A, et al. Anticoagulation prescribing patterns in intensive care unit patients admitted with prehospital direct Oral anticoagulant therapy: a single academic center experience. Hosp Pharm. 2023;58(1):84–91. https://doi.org/10.1177/00185787221122656.
72. Wahab A, Patnaik R, Gurjar M. Use of direct oral anticoagulants in ICU patients. Part I—applied pharmacology. Anaesthesiol Intensive Ther. 2021;53(5):429–39. https://doi.org/10.5114/ait.2021.110607.
73. Rali P, et al. Direct-acting oral anticoagulants in critically ill patients. Chest. 2019;156(3):604–18. https://doi.org/10.1016/j.chest.2019.05.025.
74. Stangier J, et al. Influence of renal impairment on the pharmacokinetics and pharmacodynamics of oral dabigatran Etexilate: an open-label, parallel-group, single-Centre study. Clin Pharmacokinet. 2010;49(4):259–68. https://doi.org/10.2165/11318170-000000000-00000.
75. Chan KE, et al. Nonvitamin K anticoagulant agents in patients with advanced chronic kidney disease or on dialysis with AF. J Am Coll Cardiol. 2016;67(24):2888–99. https://doi.org/10.1016/j.jacc.2016.02.082.
76. Chang M, et al. Effect of renal impairment on the pharmacokinetics, pharmacodynamics, and safety of apixaban. J Clin Pharmacol. 2016;56(5):637–45. https://doi.org/10.1002/jcph.633.
77. Wang X, et al. Pharmacokinetics, pharmacodynamics, and safety of apixaban in subjects with end-stage renal disease on hemodialysis. J Clin Pharmacol. 2016;56(5):628–36. https://doi.org/10.1002/jcph.628.
78. Kubitza D, et al. Effects of renal impairment on the pharmacokinetics, pharmacodynamics and safety of rivaroxaban, an oral, direct factor Xa inhibitor. Br J Clin Pharmacol. 2010;70(5):703–12. https://doi.org/10.1111/j.1365-2125.2010.03753.x.
79. Stampfuss J, et al. The effect of food on the absorption and pharmacokinetics of rivaroxaban. Int J Clin Pharmacol Therapeut. 2013;51(07):549–61. https://doi.org/10.5414/CP201812.
80. Stacy ZA, et al. Edoxaban: a comprehensive review of the pharmacology and clinical data for the management of atrial fibrillation and venous thromboembolism. Cardiol Therapy. 2016;5(1):1–18. https://doi.org/10.1007/s40119-016-0058-2.
81. Dinunno CV, et al. Direct oral to parenteral anticoagulant transitions: role of factor Xa inhibitor-specific anti-Xa concentrations. Pharmacotherapy. 2022;42(10):768–79. https://doi.org/10.1002/phar.2726.
82. Lopez CN, et al. Direct Oral to parenteral anticoagulants: strategies for inpatient transition. J Clin Pharmacol. 2021;61(1):32–40. https://doi.org/10.1002/jcph.1694.
83. Aljabri A, et al. Cost-effectiveness of anticoagulants for suspected heparin-induced thrombocytopenia in the United States. Blood. 2016;128(26):3043–51. https://doi.org/10.1182/blood-2016-07-728030.
84. Rodighiero V. Effects of liver disease on pharmacokinetics: an update. Clin Pharmacokinet. 1999;37(5):399–431. https://doi.org/10.2165/00003088-199937050-00004.
85. Armani S, et al. Effect of changes in metabolic enzymes and transporters on drug metabolism in the context of liver disease: impact on pharmacokinetics and drug–drug interactions. Br J Clin Pharmacol. 2024;90:bcp.15990. https://doi.org/10.1111/bcp.15990.
86. Costache RS, et al. Oral anticoagulation in patients with chronic liver disease. Medicina. 2023;59(2):346. https://doi.org/10.3390/medicina59020346.
87. Graff J, Harder S. Anticoagulant therapy with the oral direct factor xa inhibitors rivaroxaban, apixaban and edoxaban and the thrombin inhibitor dabigatran etexilate in patients with hepatic impairment. Clin Pharmacokinet. 2013;52(4):243–54. https://doi.org/10.1007/s40262-013-0034-0.

88. Mavrakanas TA, et al. Apixaban pharmacokinetics at steady state in hemodialysis patients. J Am Soc Nephrol. 2017;28(7):2241–8. https://doi.org/10.1681/ASN.2016090980.

89. Feldberg J, et al. A systematic review of direct oral anticoagulant use in chronic kidney disease and dialysis patients with atrial fibrillation. Nephrol Dialysis Transpl. 2019;34(2):265–77. https://doi.org/10.1093/ndt/gfy031.

90. Blanco V, et al. Acute kidney injury pharmacokinetic changes and its impact on drug prescription. Healthcare. 2019;7(1):10. https://doi.org/10.3390/healthcare7010010.

91. Givens G, Neu D, Marler J. The risk of major bleeding with apixaban administration in patients with acute kidney injury. Ann Pharmacother. 2023;57(7):795–802. https://doi.org/10.1177/10600280221129831.

92. Towers W, et al. Apixaban and rivaroxaban anti-Xa level monitoring versus standard monitoring in hospitalized patients with acute kidney injury. Ann Pharmacother. 2022;56(6):656–63. https://doi.org/10.1177/10600280211046087.

93. Andrews L, et al. Pharmacokinetics and dialytic clearance of apixaban during in vitro continuous renal replacement therapy. BMC Nephrol. 2021;22(1):45. https://doi.org/10.1186/s12882-021-02248-7.

94. Lyndon WD, Wille KM, Tolwani AJ. Solute clearance in CRRT: prescribed dose versus actual delivered dose. Nephrol Dial Transplant. 2012;27(3):952–6. https://doi.org/10.1093/ndt/gfr480.

95. Levy JH, Connors JM. Heparin resistance—clinical perspectives and management strategies. New England J Med. 2021;385(9):826–32. https://doi.org/10.1056/NEJMra2104091.

96. Durrani J, et al. To be or not to be a case of heparin resistance. J Community Hosp Intern Med Perspect. 2018;8(3):145–8. https://doi.org/10.1080/20009666.2018.1466599.

97. Levy JH, et al. Defining heparin resistance: communication from the ISTH SSC Subcommittee of Perioperative and Critical Care Thrombosis and Hemostasis. J Thromb Haemost. 2023a;21(12):3649–57. https://doi.org/10.1016/j.jtha.2023.08.013.

98. McMichael ABV, et al. 2021 ELSO adult and pediatric anticoagulation guidelines. ASAIO J. 2022;68(3):303–10. https://doi.org/10.1097/MAT.0000000000001652.

99. Schulman S, Kearon C. Definition of major bleeding in clinical investigations of antihemostatic medicinal products in non-surgical patients. J Thromb Haemost. 2005;3(4):692–4. https://doi.org/10.1111/j.1538-7836.2005.01204.x.

100. Aldhaeefi M, et al. Practical guide for anticoagulant and antiplatelet reversal in clinical practice. Pharmacy. 2023;11(1):34. https://doi.org/10.3390/pharmacy11010034.

101. Carson JL, et al. Clinical practice guidelines from the AABB: red blood cell transfusion thresholds and storage. JAMA. 2016;316(19):2025. https://doi.org/10.1001/jama.2016.9185.

102. Contreras M. Final statement from the consensus conference on platelet transfusion. Transfusion. 1998;38(8):796–7. https://doi.org/10.1046/j.1537-2995.1998.38898375520.x.

103. Singh. Approach to the coagulopathic patient in the intensive care unit. Indian J Crit Care Med. 2019;23(S3):S215. https://doi.org/10.5005/jp-journals-10071-23256.

104. Andexanet alfa. Alexion Pharmaceuticals, Inc. 2021. https://dailymed.nlm.nih.gov/dailymed/drugInfo.cfm?setid=ae7f0c50-ff2d-49e5-8e10-4efa861556e6. Accessed 25 Mar 2024.

105. Anti-inhibitor coagulant complex. Takeda Pharmaceuticals America, Inc. 2023. https://dailymed.nlm.nih.gov/dailymed/drugInfo.cfm?setid=752604e5-4ea2-44f4-83ed-1569373f6412. Accessed 9 Apr 2024.

106. Coagulation factor VIIA (recombinant). Novo Nordisk; 2020. https://www.fda.gov/media/70442/download. Accessed 9 Apr 2024.

107. Fibrinogen (Human). Octapharma USA Inc.; 2022. https://dailymed.nlm.nih.gov/dailymed/drugInfo.cfm?setid=007a93f4-d84b-1fa9-51ed-32f6140bf423. Accessed 9 Apr 2024.

108. Idarucizumab injection. Boehringer Ingelheim Pharmaceuticals, Inc.; 2024. https://dailymed.nlm.nih.gov/dailymed/drugInfo.cfm?setid=c7400f8a-dcf4-a6df-6d07-983081b1bf34. Accessed 9 Apr 2024.

109. Phytonadione. Merck & Co., Inc.; 2002. https://www.accessdata.fda.gov/drugsatfda_docs/label/2003/012223orig1s039lbl.pdf. Accessed 9 Apr 2024.

110. Prothrombin Complex Concentrate (Human). CSL Behring GmbH; 2023. https://dailymed. nlm.nih.gov/dailymed/drugInfo.cfm?setid=eee1afb8-324c-42e4-8bf0-f0c9da5e6d42. Accessed 9 Apr 2024.
111. Khawar H, et al. Fresh frozen plasma (FFP). In: StatPearls. Treasure Island, FL: StatPearls Publishing; 2024. http://www.ncbi.nlm.nih.gov/books/NBK513347/. Accessed 9 Apr 2024.
112. Yaghi S, et al. Treatment and outcome of hemorrhagic transformation after intravenous alteplase in acute ischemic stroke: a scientific statement for healthcare professionals from the American Heart Association/American Stroke Association. Stroke. 2017;48(12):e343. https://doi.org/10.1161/STR.0000000000000152.
113. Pollack CV, et al. Idarucizumab for dabigatran reversal—full cohort analysis. N Engl J Med. 2017;377(5):431–41. https://doi.org/10.1056/NEJMoa1707278.
114. Tomaselli GF, et al. 2020 ACC expert consensus decision pathway on management of bleeding in patients on oral anticoagulants. J Am Coll Cardiol. 2020;76(5):594–622. https://doi.org/10.1016/j.jacc.2020.04.053.
115. Steele AP, Lee JA, Dager WE. Incomplete dabigatran reversal with idarucizumab. Clin Toxicol. 2018;56(3):216–8. https://doi.org/10.1080/15563650.2017.1349911.
116. Desmurs-Clavel H, et al. Reversal of the inhibitory effect of Fondaparinux on thrombin generation by rFVIIa, aCCP and PCC. Thromb Res. 2009;123(5):796–8. https://doi.org/10.1016/j.thromres.2008.07.007.
117. Young G, et al. Recombinant activated factor VII effectively reverses the anticoagulant effects of heparin, enoxaparin, fondaparinux, argatroban, and bivalirudin ex vivo as measured using thromboelastography. Blood Coagul Fibrinolysis. 2007;18(6):547–53. https://doi.org/10.1097/MBC.0b013e328201c9a9.
118. Bijsterveld NR, et al. Ability of recombinant factor VIIa to reverse the anticoagulant effect of the Pentasaccharide Fondaparinux in healthy volunteers. Circulation. 2002;106(20):2550–4. https://doi.org/10.1161/01.CIR.0000038501.87442.02.
119. Bitonti MT, et al. Prospective evaluation of a fixed-dose 4-factor prothrombin complex concentrate protocol for urgent vitamin K antagonist reversal. J Emerg Med. 2020;58(2):324–9. https://doi.org/10.1016/j.jemermed.2019.10.013.
120. Dietrich SK, et al. Multi-centered evaluation of a novel fixed-dose four-factor prothrombin complex concentrate protocol for warfarin reversal. Am J Emerg Med. 2020;38(10):2096–100. https://doi.org/10.1016/j.ajem.2020.06.017.
121. Dietrich SK, et al. Comparison of 3 different prothrombin complex concentrate regimens for emergent warfarin reversal: PCCWaR study. Ann Pharmacother. 2021;55(8):980–7. https://doi.org/10.1177/1060028020978568.
122. Gilbert BW, et al. Modified version of the American College of Cardiology's recommendation for low-dose prothrombin complex concentrate is effective for warfarin reversal. Am J Emerg Med. 2020;38(4):806–9. https://doi.org/10.1016/j.ajem.2019.12.005.
123. McMahon C, et al. Evaluation of a fixed-dose regimen of 4-factor prothrombin complex concentrate for warfarin reversal. Ann Pharmacother. 2021;55(10):1230–5. https://doi.org/10.1177/1060028021992142.
124. Greenberg SM, et al. 2022 guideline for the Management of Patients with Spontaneous Intracerebral Hemorrhage: a guideline from the American Heart Association/American Stroke Association. Stroke. 2022;53(7):e282. https://doi.org/10.1161/STR.0000000000000407.
125. Chai-Adisaksopha C, et al. Prothrombin complex concentrates versus fresh frozen plasma for warfarin reversal a systematic review and meta-analysis. Thromb Haemost. 2016;116(11):879–90. https://doi.org/10.1160/TH16-04-0266.
126. Cuker A, et al. Reversal of direct oral anticoagulants: guidance from the anticoagulation forum. Am J Hematol. 2019;94(6):697–709. https://doi.org/10.1002/ajh.25475.
127. Connolly SJ, et al. Full study report of Andexanet alfa for bleeding associated with factor Xa inhibitors. N Engl J Med. 2019;380(14):1326–35. https://doi.org/10.1056/NEJMoa1814051.
128. Chiasakul T, Crowther M, Cuker A. Four-factor prothrombin complex concentrate for the treatment of oral factor Xa inhibitor-associated bleeding: a meta-analysis of fixed versus

variable dosing. Res Pract Thromb Haemost. 2023;7(2):100107. https://doi.org/10.1016/j. rpth.2023.100107.

129. Dobesh PP, et al. Lower mortality with andexanet alfa vs 4-factor prothrombin complex concentrate for factor Xa inhibitor-related major bleeding in a U.S. hospital-based observational study. Res Pract Thromb Haemost. 2023;7(6):102192. https://doi.org/10.1016/j. rpth.2023.102192.

130. Barra ME, Das AS, et al. Evaluation of andexanet alfa and four-factor prothrombin complex concentrate (4F-PCC) for reversal of rivaroxaban- and apixaban-associated intracranial hemorrhages. J Thromb Haemost. 2020a;18(7):1637–47. https://doi.org/10.1111/jth.14838.

131. Vestal ML, et al. Andexanet alfa and four-factor prothrombin complex concentrate for reversal of apixaban and rivaroxaban in patients diagnosed with intracranial hemorrhage. J Thromb Thrombolysis. 2022;53(1):167–75. https://doi.org/10.1007/s11239-021-02495-3.

132. Chaudhary R, et al. Evaluation of direct Oral anticoagulant reversal agents in intracranial hemorrhage: a systematic review and meta-analysis. JAMA Netw Open. 2022;5(11):e2240145. https://doi.org/10.1001/jamanetworkopen.2022.40145.

133. Mazya M, et al. Predicting the risk of symptomatic intracerebral hemorrhage in ischemic stroke treated with intravenous Alteplase: safe implementation of treatments in stroke (SITS) symptomatic intracerebral hemorrhage risk score. Stroke. 2012;43(6):1524–31. https://doi. org/10.1161/STROKEAHA.111.644815.

134. Barra ME, Feske SK, et al. Fibrinogen concentrate for the treatment of thrombolysis-associated hemorrhage in adult ischemic stroke patients. Clin Appl Thromb Hemost. 2020b;26:107602962095186. https://doi.org/10.1177/1076029620951867.

135. Frontera JA, et al. Guideline for reversal of antithrombotics in intracranial hemorrhage: executive summary. A statement for healthcare professionals from the Neurocritical care society and the Society of Critical Care Medicine. Crit Care Med. 2016;44(12):2251–7. https://doi. org/10.1097/CCM.0000000000002057.

136. Baharoglu MI, et al. Platelet transfusion versus standard care after acute stroke due to spontaneous cerebral haemorrhage associated with antiplatelet therapy (PATCH): a randomised, open-label, phase 3 trial. Lancet. 2016;387(10038):2605–13. https://doi.org/10.1016/ S0140-6736(16)30392-0.

137. O'Connor SA, et al. Efficacy of ex vivo autologous and in vivo platelet transfusion in the reversal of P2Y $_{12}$ inhibition by clopidogrel, prasugrel, and ticagrelor: the APTITUDE study. Circ Cardiovasc Interv. 2015;8(11):e002786. https://doi.org/10.1161/ CIRCINTERVENTIONS.115.002786.

138. Zakko L, et al. No benefit from platelet transfusion for gastrointestinal bleeding in patients taking antiplatelet agents. Clin Gastroenterol Hepatol. 2017;15(1):46–52. https://doi. org/10.1016/j.cgh.2016.07.017.

139. Desborough MJR, et al. Desmopressin for treatment of platelet dysfunction and reversal of antiplatelet agents: a systematic review and meta-analysis of randomized controlled trials. J Thromb Haemost. 2017;15(2):263–72. https://doi.org/10.1111/jth.13576.

140. Fischer K, et al. Reversing bleeding associated with antiplatelet use: the role of tranexamic acid. Cureus. 2020;12:e10290. https://doi.org/10.7759/cureus.10290.

141. Weber CF, et al. Tranexamic acid partially improves platelet function in patients treated with dual antiplatelet therapy. Eur J Anaesthesiol. 2011;28(1):57–62. https://doi.org/10.1097/ EJA.0b013e32834050ab.

142. Procopio GL, et al. Impact of a pharmacist driven anticoagulation reversal program at a large academic medical center. J Thromb Thrombolysis. 2022;53(1):158–66. https://doi. org/10.1007/s11239-021-02491-7.

143. Stone GW, et al. Contemporary utilization and outcomes of intra-aortic balloon counterpulsation in acute myocardial infarction. J Am Coll Cardiol. 2003;41(11):1940–5. https://doi. org/10.1016/S0735-1097(03)00400-5.

144. Tong W, et al. Incidence, predictors, and prognosis of thrombocytopenia among patients undergoing intra-aortic balloon pumping in the intensive care unit: a propensity score analysis. J Geriatr Cardiol. 2021;18(2):123–34. https://doi.org/10.11909/j.issn.1671-5411.2021.02.003.

145. Pucher PH, et al. Is heparin needed for patients with an intra-aortic balloon pump? Interact Cardiovasc Thorac Surg. 2012;15(1):136–9. https://doi.org/10.1093/icvts/ivs017.

146. Tabata N, et al. Management of intra-aortic balloon counterpulsation by argatroban anticoagulation in a patient with a history of heparin-induced thrombocytopenia. J Cardiol Cases. 2012;6(5):e154–7. https://doi.org/10.1016/j.jccase.2012.08.001.

147. Amin AP, et al. The evolving landscape of impella use in the United States among patients undergoing percutaneous coronary intervention with mechanical circulatory support. Circulation. 2020;141(4):273–84. https://doi.org/10.1161/CIRCULATIONAHA.119.044007.

148. Dhruva SS, et al. Association of use of an intravascular microaxial left ventricular assist device vs intra-aortic balloon pump with in-hospital mortality and major bleeding among patients with acute myocardial infarction complicated by cardiogenic shock. JAMA. 2020;323(8):734. https://doi.org/10.1001/jama.2020.0254.

149. Abiomed. FAQ: Anticoagulation. 2021. https://www.heartrecovery.com/education/education-library/faq-anticoagulation#:~:text=What%20is%20the%20recommended%20heparin. Accessed 25 Mar 2024.

150. Burzotta F, et al. Impella ventricular support in clinical practice: collaborative viewpoint from a European expert user group. Int J Cardiol. 2015;201:684–91. https://doi.org/10.1016/j.ijcard.2015.07.065.

151. Jennings DL, Nemerovski CW, Kalus JS. Effective anticoagulation for a percutaneous ventricular assist device using a heparin-based purge solution. Ann Pharmacother. 2013;47(10):1364–7. https://doi.org/10.1177/1060028013503623.

152. Bashline M, et al. Outcomes of systemic bivalirudin and sodium bicarbonate purge solution for Impella 5.5. Artif Organs. 2023;47(2):361–9. https://doi.org/10.1111/aor.14428.

153. Beavers CJ, et al. Optimizing anticoagulation for patients receiving Impella support. Pharmacotherapy. 2021;41(11):932–42. https://doi.org/10.1002/phar.2629.

154. Doyle AJ, Hunt BJ. Current understanding of how extracorporeal membrane oxygenators activate Haemostasis and other blood components. Front Med. 2018;5:352. https://doi.org/10.3389/fmed.2018.00352.

155. Brokmeier HM, et al. Hemostatic management in extracorporeal membrane oxygenation. Crit Care Nurs Q. 2022;45(2):132–43.

156. Nunez JI, et al. Bleeding and thrombotic events in adults supported with venovenous extracorporeal membrane oxygenation: an ELSO registry analysis. Intensive Care Med. 2022;48(2):213–24. https://doi.org/10.1007/s00134-021-06593-x.

157. Willers A, et al. HEROES V-V—HEmorRhagic cOmplications in veno-venous extracorporeal life support—development and internal validation of multivariable prediction model in adult patients. Artif Organs. 2022;46(5):932–52. https://doi.org/10.1111/aor.14148.

158. Helms J, et al. Anticoagulation in adult patients supported with extracorporeal membrane oxygenation: guidance from the Scientific and Standardization Committees on Perioperative and Critical Care Haemostasis and Thrombosis of the International Society on Thrombosis and Haemostasis. J Thromb Haemost. 2023;21(2):373–96. https://doi.org/10.1016/j.jtha.2022.11.014.

159. Zaaqoq AM, et al. Heparin-induced thrombocytopenia in extra-corporeal membrane oxygenation: epidemiology, outcomes, and diagnostic challenges. J Thromb Thrombolysis. 2022;53(2):499–505. https://doi.org/10.1007/s11239-021-02546-9.

160. Zeibi Shirejini S, et al. Current and future strategies to monitor and manage coagulation in ECMO patients. Thromb J. 2023;21(1):11. https://doi.org/10.1186/s12959-023-00452-z.

161. Rajsic S, et al. Anticoagulation strategies during extracorporeal membrane oxygenation: a narrative review. J Clin Med. 2022;11(17):5147. https://doi.org/10.3390/jcm11175147.

162. Menk M. Efficacy and safety of argatroban in patients with acute respiratory distress syndrome and extracorporeal lung support. Ann Intensive Care. 2017;7(1):82.

163. Fisser C. Argatroban versus heparin in patients without heparin-induced thrombocytopenia during venovenous extracorporeal membrane oxygenation: a propensity-score matched study. Crit Care. 2021;25(1):160.

164. Rivosecchi RM, et al. Comparison of anticoagulation strategies in patients requiring venovenous extracorporeal membrane oxygenation: heparin versus bivalirudin*. Crit Care Med. 2021;49(7):1129–36. https://doi.org/10.1097/CCM.0000000000004944.

165. Sheridan EA, et al. Comparison of Bivalirudin versus unfractionated heparin for anticoagulation in adult patients on extracorporeal membrane oxygenation. ASAIO J. 2022;68(7):920–4. https://doi.org/10.1097/MAT.0000000000001598.

166. Sin JH, Lopez ND. Argatroban for heparin-induced thrombocytopenia during venovenous extracorporeal membrane oxygenation with continuous venovenous hemofiltration. J Extracorpor Technol. 2017;49(2):115–20. https://doi.org/10.1051/ject/201749115.

167. Lopez ND, et al. Evaluation of Bivalirudin during adult extracorporeal membrane oxygenation: a retrospective characterization of dosing, efficacy and bleeding. Hosp Pharm. 2024;59(1):77–85. https://doi.org/10.1177/00185787231188924.

168. Netley J, et al. Bivalirudin anticoagulation dosing protocol for extracorporeal membrane oxygenation: a retrospective review. J Extra Corpor Technol. 2018;50(3):161–6.

169. Walker EA, et al. Bivalirudin dosing requirements in adult patients on extracorporeal life support with or without continuous renal replacement therapy. ASAIO J. 2019;65(2):134–8. https://doi.org/10.1097/MAT.0000000000000780.

170. Kumar G, Maskey A. Anticoagulation in ECMO patients: an overview. Indian J Thoracic Cardiovasc Surg. 2021;37(S2):241–7. https://doi.org/10.1007/s12055-021-01176-3.

171. Spiess BD. Treating heparin resistance with antithrombin or fresh frozen plasma. Ann Thorac Surg. 2008;85(6):2153–60. https://doi.org/10.1016/j.athoracsur.2008.02.037.

172. Morrisette MJ, et al. Antithrombin supplementation in adult patients receiving extracorporeal membrane oxygenation. Perfusion. 2020;35(1):66–72. https://doi.org/10.1177/0267659119856229.

173. Panigada M, et al. A randomized controlled trial of antithrombin supplementation during extracorporeal membrane oxygenation. Crit Care Med. 2020;48(11):1636–44. https://doi.org/10.1097/CCM.0000000000004590.

174. Dzierba AL, et al. Optimizing pharmacotherapy regimens in adult patients receiving extracorporeal membrane oxygenation: a narrative review for clinical pharmacists. JACCP. 2023;6(6):621–31. https://doi.org/10.1002/jac5.1780.

175. Ciolek A, et al. Identification of cost-saving opportunities for the use of Antithrombin III in adult and pediatric patients. Clin Appl Thromb Hemost. 2018;24(1):186–91. https://doi.org/10.1177/1076029617693941.

176. Khwaja A. KDIGO clinical practice guidelines for acute kidney injury. Nephron Clin Pract. 2012;120(4):c179–84. https://doi.org/10.1159/000339789.

177. Gaudry S, Palevsky PM, Dreyfuss D. Extracorporeal kidney-replacement therapy for acute kidney injury. New England J Med. 2022;386(10):964–75. https://doi.org/10.1056/NEJMra2104090.

178. Singh S. Anticoagulation during renal replacement therapy. Indian J Crit Care Med. 2020;24(S3):112–6. https://doi.org/10.5005/jp-journals-10071-23412.

179. Joannidis M, Oudemans-van Straaten HM. Clinical review: patency of the circuit in continuous renal replacement therapy. Crit Care. 2007;11(4):218. https://doi.org/10.1186/cc5937.

180. Uchino S, et al. Pre-dilution vs. post-dilution during continuous Veno-venous hemofiltration: impact on filter life and Azotemic control. Nephron Clin Pract. 2004;94(4):c94–8. https://doi.org/10.1159/000072492.

181. Fiaccadori E, et al. Regional citrate anticoagulation for renal replacement therapies in patients with acute kidney injury: a position statement of the work group "renal replacement therapies in critically ill patients" of the Italian Society of Nephrology. J Nephrol. 2015;28(2):151–64. https://doi.org/10.1007/s40620-014-0160-2.

182. Morabito S, et al. Regional citrate anticoagulation for RRTs in critically ill patients with AKI. Clin J Am Soc Nephrol. 2014;9(12):2173–88. https://doi.org/10.2215/CJN.01280214.
183. Boyaci Dundar N. Regional citrate anticoagulation: basic principles and clinical applications. J Crit Intensive Care. 2023;14:28–32. https://doi.org/10.37678/dcybd.2023.2324.
184. Meier-Kriesche H-U, et al. Increased total to ionized calcium ratio during continuous venovenous hemodialysis with regional citrate anticoagulation. Crit Care Med. 2001;29(4):748–52. https://doi.org/10.1097/00003246-200104000-00010.
185. Schultheiß C, et al. Continuous venovenous hemodialysis with regional citrate anticoagulation in patients with liver failure: a prospective observational study. Crit Care. 2012;16(4):R162. https://doi.org/10.1186/cc11485.
186. Tan J-N, et al. Hyperlactatemia predicts citrate intolerance with regional citrate anticoagulation during continuous renal replacement therapy. J Intensive Care Med. 2019;34(5):418–25. https://doi.org/10.1177/0885066617701068.
187. Kramer L, et al. Citrate pharmacokinetics and metabolism in cirrhotic and noncirrhotic critically ill patients. Crit Care Med. 2003;31(10):2450–5. https://doi.org/10.1097/01.CCM.0000084871.76568.E6.
188. Zhang W, et al. Safety and efficacy of regional citrate anticoagulation for continuous renal replacement therapy in liver failure patients: a systematic review and meta-analysis. Crit Care. 2019;23(1):22. https://doi.org/10.1186/s13054-019-2317-9.
189. Gattas DJ, et al. A randomized controlled trial of regional citrate versus regional heparin anticoagulation for continuous renal replacement therapy in critically ill adults*. Crit Care Med. 2015;43(8):1622–9. https://doi.org/10.1097/CCM.0000000000001004.
190. Tolwani AJ, Wille KM. THE CLINICAL APPLICATION OF CRRT—CURRENT STATUS: anticoagulation for continuous renal replacement therapy. Semin Dial. 2009;22(2):141–5. https://doi.org/10.1111/j.1525-139X.2008.00545.x.
191. Ostermann M, et al. Heparin algorithm for anticoagulation during continuous renal replacement therapy. Crit Care. 2010;14(3):419. https://doi.org/10.1186/cc9003.
192. Endres P, et al. Filter clotting with continuous renal replacement therapy in COVID-19. J Thromb Thrombolysis. 2021;51(4):966–70. https://doi.org/10.1007/s11239-020-02301-6.
193. Rabbani A, et al. Continuous renal replacement therapy with low dose systemic heparin in liver transplant recipients. Iran J Kidney Dis. 2021;15(3):229–34.
194. Joannidis M, et al. Enoxaparin vs. unfractionated heparin for anticoagulation during continuous veno-venous hemofiltration: a randomized controlled crossover study. Intensive Care Med. 2007;33(9):1571–9. https://doi.org/10.1007/s00134-007-0719-7.
195. Chanas T, et al. Evaluation of the use of argatroban or bivalirudin for the management of suspected heparin-induced thrombocytopenia in the setting of continuous renal replacement therapy. Clin Med Insights Trauma Intensive Med. 2019;10:117956031984645. https://doi.org/10.1177/1179560319846452.
196. Link A, et al. Argatroban for anticoagulation in continuous renal replacement therapy*. Crit Care Med. 2009;37(1):105–10. https://doi.org/10.1097/CCM.0b013e3181932394.
197. Mueller SW, et al. Prefilter bivalirudin for preventing hemofilter occlusion in continuous renal replacement therapy. Ann Pharmacother. 2009;43(7–8):1360–5. https://doi.org/10.1345/aph.1M179.
198. Williamson DR, et al. Thrombocytopenia in critically ill patients receiving thromboprophylaxis. Chest. 2013;144(4):1207–15. https://doi.org/10.1378/chest.13-0121.
199. Greinacher A, Selleng K. Thrombocytopenia in the intensive care unit patient. Hematology. 2010;1:135–43. https://doi.org/10.1182/asheducation-2010.1.135.
200. Hui P, et al. The frequency and clinical significance of thrombocytopenia complicating critical illness. Chest. 2011;139(2):271–8. https://doi.org/10.1378/chest.10-2243.
201. Akca S, et al. Time course of platelet counts in critically ill patients. Crit Care Med. 2002;30(4):753–6. https://doi.org/10.1097/00003246-200204000-00005.
202. Kaufman RM, et al. Platelet transfusion: a clinical practice guideline from the AABB. Ann Intern Med. 2015;162(3):205–13. https://doi.org/10.7326/M14-1589.

203. Danese E, et al. Drug-induced thrombocytopenia: mechanisms and laboratory diagnostics. Semin Thromb Hemost. 2020;46(03):264–74. https://doi.org/10.1055/s-0039-1697930.

204. Zhu J, et al. Structural basis for quinine-dependent antibody binding to platelet integrin αIIbβ3. Blood. 2015;126(18):2138–45. https://doi.org/10.1182/blood-2015-04-639351.

205. Arnold DM, et al. Approach to the diagnosis and Management of Drug-Induced Immune Thrombocytopenia. Transfus Med Rev. 2013;27(3):137–45. https://doi.org/10.1016/j.tmrv.2013.05.005.

206. Priziola JL, Smythe MA, Dager WE. Drug-induced thrombocytopenia in critically ill patients. Crit Care Med. 2010;38:S145–54. https://doi.org/10.1097/CCM.0b013e3181de0b88.

207. Bakchoul T, Marini I. Drug-associated thrombocytopenia. Hematology. 2018;1:576–83. https://doi.org/10.1182/asheducation-2018.1.576.

208. George JN, Aster RH. Drug-induced thrombocytopenia: pathogenesis, evaluation, and management. Hematology. 2009;1:153–8. https://doi.org/10.1182/asheducation-2009.1.153.

209. East JM, Cserti-Gazdewich CM, Granton JT. Heparin-induced thrombocytopenia in the critically ill patient. Chest. 2018;154(3):678–90. https://doi.org/10.1016/j.chest.2017.11.039.

210. Selleng K, Warkentin TE, Greinacher A. Heparin-induced thrombocytopenia in intensive care patients. Crit Care Med. 2007;35(4):1165–76. https://doi.org/10.1097/01.CCM.0000259538.02375.A5.

211. Warkentin T. Heparin-induced thrombocytopenia in critically ill patients. Semin Thromb Hemost. 2015;41(01):049–60. https://doi.org/10.1055/s-0034-1398381.

212. Cuker A, et al. Predictive value of the 4Ts scoring system for heparin-induced thrombocytopenia: a systematic review and meta-analysis. Blood. 2012;120(20):4160–7. https://doi.org/10.1182/blood-2012-07-443051.

213. Scharman CD, et al. Treatment of individuals who cannot receive blood products for religious or other reasons. Am J Hematol. 2017;92(12):1370–81. https://doi.org/10.1002/ajh.24889.

214. Nicolaides AN, et al. Prevention and management of venous thromboembolism. International Consensus Statement. Guidelines according to scientific evidence. Int Angiol. 2024;43(1):1. https://doi.org/10.23736/S0392-9590.23.05177-5.

215. Crescenti A, et al. Intraoperative use of tranexamic acid to reduce transfusion rate in patients undergoing radical retropubic prostatectomy: double blind, randomised, placebo controlled trial. BMJ. 2011;343(oct19 3):d5701. https://doi.org/10.1136/bmj.d5701.

216. Ngaage DL, Bland JM. Lessons from aprotinin: is the routine use and inconsistent dosing of tranexamic acid prudent? Meta-analysis of randomised and large matched observational studies. Eur J Cardiothorac Surg. 2010;37(6):1375–83. https://doi.org/10.1016/j.ejcts.2009.11.055.

217. Weng K, et al. The effectiveness and safety of tranexamic acid in bilateral total knee arthroplasty: a meta-analysis. Medicine. 2016;95(39):e4960. https://doi.org/10.1097/MD.0000000000004960.

218. Roberts I, et al. The CRASH-2 trial: a randomised controlled trial and economic evaluation of the effects of tranexamic acid on death, vascular occlusive events and transfusion requirement in bleeding trauma patients. Health Technol Assess. 2013;17(10):1. https://doi.org/10.3310/hta17100.

219. Roberts I, et al. Effects of a high-dose 24-h infusion of tranexamic acid on death and thromboembolic events in patients with acute gastrointestinal bleeding (HALT-IT): an international randomised, double-blind, placebo-controlled trial. Lancet. 2020;395(10241):1927–36. https://doi.org/10.1016/S0140-6736(20)30848-5.

220. Yank V, et al. Systematic review: benefits and harms of in-hospital use of recombinant factor VIIa for off-label indications. Ann Intern Med. 2011;154(8):529. https://doi.org/10.7326/0003-4819-154-8-201104190-00004.

221. Albreiki M, Voegeli D. Permissive hypotensive resuscitation in adult patients with traumatic haemorrhagic shock: a systematic review. Eur J Trauma Emerg Surg. 2018;44(2):191–202. https://doi.org/10.1007/s00068-017-0862-y.

222. Epoetin alfa-epbx. Pfizer Laboratories Div Pfizer Inc.; 2023. https://dailymed.nlm.nih. gov/dailymed/drugInfo.cfm?setid=3af26b0d-8ad0-44e1-a538-8bdb5ab39374. Accessed 8 Apr 2024.

223. Warner MA, et al. Perioperative anemia: prevention, diagnosis, and management throughout the spectrum of perioperative care. Anesth Analg. 2020;130(5):1364–80. https://doi.org/10.1213/ANE.0000000000004727.

224. Asiedu JO, et al. Management and clinical outcomes for patients with gastrointestinal bleeding who decline transfusion. PLOS ONE. 2023;18(8):e0290351. https://doi.org/10.1371/journal.pone.0290351.

225. Barsun A, et al. Reducing Postburn injury anemia in a Jehovah's witness patient. J Burn Care Res. 2014;35(4):e258–61. https://doi.org/10.1097/BCR.0b013e3182a366c5.

226. Gannon CJ, Napolitano LM. Severe anemia after gastrointestinal hemorrhage in a Jehovah's witness: new treatment strategies*. Crit Care Med. 2002;30(8):1893–5. https://doi.org/10.1097/00003246-200208000-00036.

227. Lorentzen K, Kjær B, Jørgensen J. Supportive treatment of severe anaemia in a Jehovah's witness with severe trauma. Blood Transfus. 2013;11:452. https://doi.org/10.2450/2013.0263-12.

228. Posluszny JA, Napolitano LM. How do we treat life-threatening anemia in a J ehovah's W itness patient? Transfusion. 2014;54(12):3026–34. https://doi.org/10.1111/trf.12888.

229. Dunn J-O, Mythen M, Grocott M. Physiology of oxygen transport. BJA Educ. 2016;16(10):341–8. https://doi.org/10.1093/bjaed/mkw012.

230. Klein MJ, et al. Prophylactic hypothermia and neuromuscular blockade to limit myocardial oxygen demand in a critically anemic Jehovah's Witness after emergency surgery. J Surg Case Rep. 2014;2014(12):rju135. https://doi.org/10.1093/jscr/rju135.

231. Chen L, Yang Z, Liu H. Hemoglobin-based oxygen carriers: where are we now in 2023? Medicina (Kaunas). 2023;59(2):396. https://doi.org/10.3390/medicina59020396.

232. Natanson C, et al. Cell-free hemoglobin-based blood substitutes and risk of myocardial infarction and death: a meta-analysis. JAMA. 2008;299(19):2304. https://doi.org/10.1001/jama.299.19.jrv80007.

233. Douketis JD, et al. Perioperative management of antithrombotic therapy. Chest. 2022;162(5):e207–43. https://doi.org/10.1016/j.chest.2022.07.025.

234. Spyropoulos AC, et al. Scientific and standardization committee communication: guidance document on the periprocedural management of patients on chronic oral anticoagulant therapy: recommendations for standardized reporting of procedural/surgical bleed risk and patient-specific thromboembolic risk. J Thromb Haemost. 2019;17(11):1966–72. https://doi.org/10.1111/jth.14598.

235. Douketis JD, et al. Perioperative management of patients with atrial fibrillation receiving a direct oral anticoagulant. JAMA Intern Med. 2019;179(11):1469–78. https://doi.org/10.1001/jamainternmed.2019.2431.

236. Doherty JU, et al. 2017 ACC expert consensus decision pathway for Periprocedural Management of Anticoagulation in patients with Nonvalvular atrial fibrillation. J Am Coll Cardiol. 2017;69(7):871–98. https://doi.org/10.1016/j.jacc.2016.11.024.

237. Godier A, et al. Predictors of pre-procedural concentrations of direct oral anticoagulants: a prospective multicentre study. Eur Heart J. 2017;38(31):2431–9. https://doi.org/10.1093/eurheartj/ehx403.

238. Douketis JD, et al. Perioperative bridging anticoagulation in patients with atrial fibrillation. N Engl J Med. 2015;373(9):823–33. https://doi.org/10.1056/NEJMoa1501035.

239. Kovacs MJ, et al. Postoperative low molecular weight heparin bridging treatment for patients at high risk of arterial thromboembolism (PERIOP2): double blind randomised controlled trial. BMJ. 2021;373:n1205. https://doi.org/10.1136/bmj.n1205.

240. Dunn AS, Spyropoulos AC, Turpie AGG. Bridging therapy in patients on long-term oral anticoagulants who require surgery: the prospective Peri-operative enoxaparin cohort trial

(PROSPECT). J Thromb Haemost. 2007;5(11):2211–8. https://doi.org/10.1111/j.1538-783
6.2007.02729.x.
241. Horlocker TT, et al. Regional anesthesia in the patient receiving antithrombotic or thrombolytic therapy: American Society of Regional Anesthesia and Pain Medicine evidence-based guidelines (fourth edition). Reg Anesth Pain Med. 2018;43(3):263–309. https://doi.org/10.1097/AAP.0000000000000763.
242. Patel GP, et al. Perioperative clinical pharmacy practice: responsibilities and scope within the surgical care continuum. JACCP. 2020;3(2):501–19. https://doi.org/10.1002/jac5.1185.
243. Dager WE, et al. "Reduce the likelihood of patient harm associated with the use of anticoagulant therapy": commentary from the anticoagulation forum on the updated joint commission NPSG.03.05.01 elements of performance. Jt Comm J Qual Patient Saf. 2020;46(3):173–80. https://doi.org/10.1016/j.jcjq.2019.12.004.
244. Awker AL, et al. Impact of educational intervention on management of periprocedural anticoagulation. Am J Health Syst Pharm. 2017;74(23_Supplement_4):S95–S101. https://doi.org/10.2146/ajhp160726.

Chapter 50
Vasopressor Therapy in the Intensive Care Unit

Fanny Li and Dexter Wimer

50.1 Introduction

Understanding how to select and manage vasopressor agents is essential for pharmacists working in critical care settings. This knowledge enables them to optimize patient care and contribute to positive outcomes. Pharmacists should have a solid grasp of how these medications function and their anticipated effects. Equally important is an understanding of the targets for monitoring hemodynamic goals and the devices used to obtain this information.

Pharmacists should be familiar with various monitoring devices outlined in Table 50.1, which play a crucial role in assessing hemodynamic parameters. Additionally, they should comprehend how receptor effects translate to hemodynamic changes. For example, the $\alpha 1$ stimulation induced by norepinephrine (an $\alpha 1$ agonist) typically leads to an increase in mean arterial pressure (MAP).

In this chapter, we will delve into the physiologic mechanisms of blood pressure regulation and the methods for measuring and calculating hemodynamic parameters. We will then review the therapeutic agents used to achieve these goals and provide practical insights. Finally, we will address some of the ongoing debates surrounding the use of vasopressor agents and adjuncts in the intensive care unit (ICU), including pertinent ordering and administration considerations.

F. Li (✉) · D. Wimer
Departments of Clinical Pharmacy and Pharmaceutical Services, University of California, San Francisco Health, San Francisco, CA, USA
e-mail: fanny.li@ucsf.edu

© The Author(s), under exclusive license to Springer Nature Switzerland AG 2025

Y. Alzaidi, M. A. Gebily (eds.), *The Pharmacist's Expanded Role in Critical Care Medicine*, https://doi.org/10.1007/978-3-031-77335-8_50

Table 50.1 Hemodynamic parameters

Parameter	Measurement device	Normal range	Receptor effects
Mean Arterial Pressure (MAP)	Non-invasive Cuff Arterial line	65–80 mmHg	↑ by α_1 ↓ by α_2 ↑ by β_1
Cardiac Output (CO)	Swan-Ganz Catheter	5–6 L/min	↑ by β_1
Cardiac Index (CI)	Swan-Ganz Catheter	2.5–4.2 L/min/m^2	↑ by β_1
Stroke Volume (SV)	Swan-Ganz Catheter	50–100 mL	Potentially ↓ by β_1
Central Venous Pressure (CVP)	Central line Swan-Ganz Catheter	8–12 mmHg 12–16 mmHg (mechanical ventilation)	↑ by V_2
Pulmonary Vascular Resistance (PVR)	Calculated value; Swan-Ganz Catheter	37–250 dynes/s/cm^{-5}	↑ by α_1 ↓ by β_2
Systemic Vascular Resistance (SVR)	Calculated value; Swan-Ganz Catheter	900–1440 dynes/s/cm^{-5}	
Central Venous Oxygen Saturation (ScvO$_2$)	Central line	>70%	↑ by β_1

α_1 =alpha 1, α_2 =alpha 2, β_1 =beta 1, β_2 =beta2, V_2 =vasopressin 2

50.2 Pathophysiology and Measurement

To begin, let's consider blood pressure (BP), calculated as cardiac output (CO) multiplied by system vascular resistance (SVR).

$$BP = CO \times SVR$$

Mean arterial pressure (MAP) is the most common assessment of blood pressure in the critically ill patient. It can be summarized mathematically most commonly as the relatonship of Diastolic Blood Pressure (DBP) and Systolic Blood Pressure (SBP) in the following equation:

$$MAP = DBP + \frac{1}{3}(SBP - DBP)$$

This simplified version leaves out a lot of other pathophysiologic determinants such as central venous pressure (CVP) or Cardiac Output/Index (CO or CI). We do not want to forget about CO, particularly in the cardiogenic shock population. CO can be defined as the product of heart rate (HR) and stroke volume (SV).

$$CO = HR \times SV$$

Affecting the response of all of these homeostatic mechanisms is volume status which can be assessed at the bedside by point-of-care ultrasound (POCUS) or via a centrally inserted catheter measuring CVP or more accurately a pulmonary artery catheter (PAC). We typically think of volume status in terms of preload or the amount of blood flow returning to the right ventricle through the Inferior Vena Cava (IVC).

Based on a relationship referred to as the Frank-Starling Curve, preload augments stroke volume until the right heart is not able to accommodate more volume, at which time the stroke volume is decreased and cardiac output declines with more preload.

50.2.1 *Physiologic Regulation*

A full discussion on the balance of vasoconstriction and vasodilation and the various counter-regulatory mechanisms is outside the scope of this chapter; however, it is worthwhile to briefly discuss the pharmacologic pathways that affect MAP as these will be important therapeutic targets [1]. Namely, there are three main pathways that regulate blood pressure, as illustrated in Fig. 50.1; these pathways are the catecholamine (adrenal), the renin-angiotensin-aldosterone system (RASS), and the vasopressin pathway.

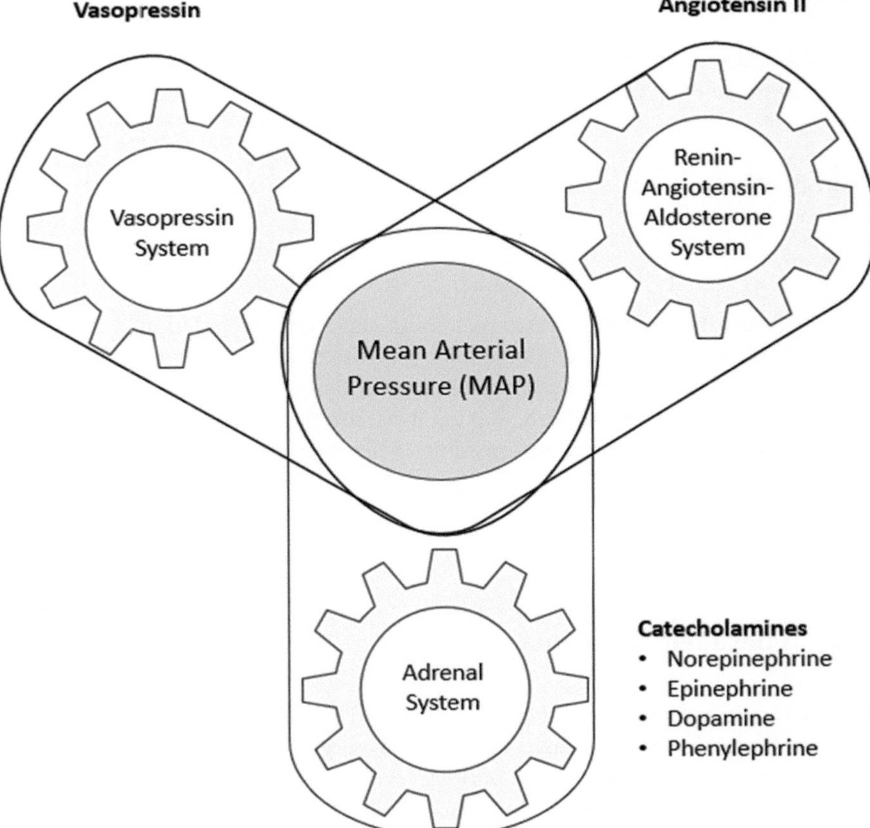

Fig. 50.1 Pathways impacting mean arterial pressure

50.2.1.1 Catecholamine (Adrenal)

Composed of alpha and beta receptors, alpha receptors have two subclasses that are important in the regulation of MAP and can be found throughout the peripheral circulation and in the pulmonary vasculature. Alpha 1 agonism is primarily responsible for vasoconstriction, whereas alpha 2 agonism serves the opposite function and leads to vasodilation and a decrease in MAP.

50.2.1.2 Renin-Angiotensin-Aldosterone System (RAAS)

The renin-angiotensin-aldosterone system is a complex neurohormonal pathway that regulates blood pressure in response to changes in glomerular function. This is thought to be triggered by changes in sodium delivery, reduced flow or perfusion pressure to the kidney, or beta receptor stimulation. The result is a release of renin which ultimately is responsible for the conversion of angiotensinogen to its final form of angiotensin II (with the assistance of angiotensin-converting enzyme), leading to a direct arterial vasoconstrictive effect. Angiotensin II also stimulates the release of aldosterone leading to water and solute retention. All effects of angiotensin II culminate in an increase in blood pressure.

50.2.1.3 Vasopressin

50.2.2   Primarily working through regulation and counter-regulation of antidiuretic hormone, vasopressin receptor subclasses exist in two types, V_1 and V_2. One clinical advantage of vasopressin and its analogs is lack of existence within the pulmonary vasculature, making these receptors an attractive target for patients with pulmonary hypertension or other restrictive pulmonary diseases.

50.3 Therapeutics agents

Pharmacologic vasopressor agents are indicated for hypotension and primarily work by increasing SVR. Some vasopressors may also increase cardiac output through their inotropic effect. The various receptor profiles and dosing ranges of common agents may be seen in Table 50.2. Agent selection is guided by their pharmacologic properties matching with disease states and lesser extent per specific treatment syndrome since literature in therapy may be limited.

Table 50.2 Therapeutic agents

Vasopressor	Dopamine	Alpha	Beta$_1$	Beta$_2$	Other mechanism	Usual dose range
Epinephrine		++++	++++	+++		0–0.5 mcg/kg/min
Norepinephrine		+++++	+++	+++		0–0.4 mcg/kg/min 0–40 mcg/min
Phenylephrine		+++++				0–5 mcg/kg/min 0–400 mcg/min
Dopamine[a]	+++++	+++	++++	++		0–20 mcg/kg/min
Vasopressin	N/A				V$_1$ and V$_2$ agonism	0–0.04 units/min
Angiotensin II	N/A				AT$_1$ and AT$_2$ agonism	0–40 ng/kg/min

[a]Dose-dependent receptor effects, *V* vasopressin, *AT* angiotensin

50.3.1 *Adrenergic/Catecholamine-Based Vasopressors*

50.3.1.1 Epinephrine

Epinephrine has dose-dependent receptor affinities for α and β adrenergic receptors. At low-to-moderate doses, β effects predominate, leading to inotropic support in addition to vasoconstriction. Epinephrine will increase heart rate and blood pressure as a result. Historically, this mechanism makes epinephrine a preferred agent in the treatment of cardiogenic shock syndromes, particularly when inotropy or cardiac "squeeze" is needed in addition to blood pressure support or in the treatment of symptomatic bradycardia. Additionally, because epinephrine affects β-1 and β-2, it is the drug of choice for anaphylactic shock. Some adverse effects unique to epinephrine include induction of a type B lactic acidosis, increased insulin resistance, and tachycardia.

50.3.1.2 Norepinephrine

Norepinephrine is a potent agonist of α-1 and β-1 adrenergic receptors commonly used in distributive shock to induce vasoconstriction and increase MAP, with minimal impact on heart rate. It is recommended as the first-line vasopressor in septic shock according to the 2021 Surviving Sepsis Guidelines [2]. Studies comparing norepinephrine with dopamine and epinephrine for shock reversal have demonstrated similar outcomes in terms of shock reversal, with norepinephrine potentially with fewer adverse side effects [3, 4]. Thus making a case for its use as first-line vasoactive medication of choice in all shock types.

50.3.1.3 Phenylephrine

Phenylephrine acts as a selective agonist of α-1 receptors, exerting minimal or no activity on β receptors. This pharmacological profile makes it an optimal choice for elevating MAP through venous vasoconstriction. Phenylephrine has demonstrated effectiveness in mitigating hypotension commonly encountered with both general and neuraxial anesthesia. Additionally, its rapid onset of action and short half-life render it particularly suitable for use during surgical procedures when there are transient periods of hypotension from decreases in MAP.

50.3.1.4 Dopamine

Dopamine is likely the most promiscuous vasopressor in terms of receptor activity and associated effects. At lower doses of 0–5 mcg/kg/min, dopamine mostly exerts its action via the dopamine receptors which leads primarily to inotropy and renal vasodilation as well as bloodflow [5]. This property led to a historic belief that low-dose dopamine might help improve perfusion to the kidneys; however, this has been unsubstantiated in subsequent literature. At moderate doses of 5–10 mcg/kg/min, dopamine becomes more similar to epinephrine, exerting its action on dopamine and primarily beta-adrenergic receptors, shifting its hemodynamic effects to inotropy. At doses >10 mcg/kg/min, dopamine has alpha receptor properties leading to vasoconstriction. Dopamine is less favored as a vasopressor due to the results of the SOAP II study with higher incidence of arrhythmia compared to norepinephrine [4]. Its niche in therapy is an initial vasopressor in resource poor areas as it is readily available as a premix infusion with a long shelf life, it can be easily stocked by emergency medical responders and can be used in the initial treatment of symptomatic bradycardia.

50.3.2 Non-adrenergic Vasopressors

50.3.2.1 Vasopressin

Vasopressin stands out among the other vasopressor agents via a unique mechanism of action. Vasopressin works via two mechanisms to increase blood pressure. One is via vasoconstriction by action at the V_1 vasopressin receptors in the peripheral artery system. The other is via its secondary action similar to antidiuretic hormone whereby blood pressure is increased as a result of free water retention, via the V_2 receptor. Vasopressin receptors are not located within the pulmonary vasculature, making vasopressin an attractive vasopressor in patients with right heart dysfunction or those with pulmonary hypertension [6]. Vasopressin was initially studied in the septic shock population at a dose of up to 0.03 units/min which was thought to provide physiologic levels in a depleted septic condition [7]. Since then, many studies have used alternative fixed dosing and even titratable doses. While these strategies vary, there is no established difference in outcomes with any one strategy [8–10]. Additionally, patients who are post-cardiopulmonary bypass are relatively vasopressin depleted and can benefit from supraphysiologic vasopressin doses up to 1 unit/min. Our practice has been in septic shock to initiate at a fixed dose of 0.03 units/min with no titration. In the cardiac surgery and pulmonary hypertension populations, higher doses and titratable doses are allowed. These strategies have been built into our electronic medical record orders such that when sepsis is the indication for vasopressin, fixed dosing with nursing instructions on when to start and wean are added automatically. Side effect concerns with vasopressin include hyponatremia and slightly higher rates of bowel ischemia that may be dose dependent when compared with other vasopressors in clinical trials. These dose dependent side effects may support the decision to limit doses in septic shock in the future.

Timing of the initiation of vasopressin in septic shock is a debated topic. In previous iterations of the surviving sepsis campaign, there were references of considering addition of vasopressin when norepinephrine reached doses of 35–90 mcg/min (or about 0.5 mcg/kg/min in a 70 kg patient). Most would agree this is a large dose of norepinephrine. However, the VASST trial found benefit in an exploratory subgroup analysis in patients who were receiving a much lower threshold of <15 mcg/min or 0.2 mcg/kg/min of norepinephrine [11]. Subsequent studies have shown a similar trend toward early initiation with lower norepinephrine doses leading to improved MAP achievement, lower lactate levels, and even mortality. Given the data, our practice has been to start recommending vasopressin when norepinephrine dose reaches a threshold of 0.2 mcg/kg/min or when norepinephrine dose is rapidly escalating.

50.3.2.2   Angiotensin II

Angiotensin II is a hormone naturally produced in the body, known for its potent vasoconstrictive effects. These effects are mediated by the stimulation of AT_1 and AT_2 receptors within the renin-angiotensin system. Angiotensin II is primarily utilized in the management of catecholamine-resistant vasodilatory shock (CRVS).

Only available as a continuous IV infusion for central line administration, the starting dose of angiotensin II is 10–20 ng/kg/min, with a recommended maximum maintenance dose of 40 ng/kg/min. Drug interaction includes increased effect with the use of angiotensin-converting enzyme inhibitors (ACEI) and decreased effect with angiotensin receptor blockers (ARB). The most commonly reported adverse effects during clinical trials were thromboembolic event (12.9% vs 5%), including deep vein thrombosis (DVT) (4.3% vs 0%) when compared to placebo [12]. Thus all treated patients should receive the appropriate DVT prophylaxis, unless contraindicated. Monitoring includes hypertension during medication titration to effect and kidney function tests with blood urea nitrogen and serum creatinine.

The ATHOS III clinical trial showed an increase in MAP (>75 mmHg or increase of 10 mmHg from baseline) with angiotensin II compared to placebo (70% vs 23%, $p < 0.0001$). However, there were no mortality benefits [12]. The drug is currently branded and is approximately ~8x more costly than norepinephrine.

At our institution, it was added to formulary with the following use criteria (1) confirmed distributive shock, (2) refractory hypotension (MAP </=65 mmHg) despite adequate fluid resuscitation and norepinephrine dose of >/= 20 mcg/min and vasopressin, (3) eligible for VTE prophylaxis, and (4) the above criteria met for at least 6 h. Medication use evaluation after one and half year of use showed no difference in MAP changes and angiotensin II was removed from drug formulary in 2020.

Newer studies of angiotensin II explore measurement of patient's serum renin concentration to guide those with deficiency to allow for better predictability of response or earlier initiation of drug therapy [13]. However, renin level is not typically included as a routine lab drawn upon hospital admission, which limits its availability for acute decision-making later on if needed. Additionally, renin concentration is not commonly supported by laboratories for quick turnaround time. Therefore, the use of renin level to guide therapy warrants further study and validation.

Other ongoing areas of research include the investigation of optimal timing of angiotensin II initiation in relation to the administration of other vasopressors. One study suggests earlier initiation of angiotensin II (4.9 h vs. 9.9 h) may have a positive correlation with 28-day mortality [14]. Also, angiotensin II has been reported in use as adjunct vasopressor in treating shock secondary to drug poisoning (e.g., calcium channel blockers and psychotropic) [15, 16].

50.3.3 *Vasopressor Sparing Agents*

50.3.3.1 Steroids

Over the years, corticosteroids have been used and studied for shock reversal, especially in the setting of septic shock. In sepsis, the theory of relative adrenal insufficiency or critical illness-related corticosteroid insufficiency (CIRCI) is based on cortisol metabolism alteration, tissue resistance to glucocorticoid, and dysregulation of hypothalamic-pituitary axis. Administering hydrocortisone, which closely mimics endogenous corticosteroid and mineralocorticoid receptor activation, aims to restore this balance. The goal is to improve hemodynamics and achieve meaningful outcomes such as reduced mortality.

Bollaert et al. in 1998 reported that a dose of hydrocortisone (100 mg IV three times a day for 5 days) resulted in improvement in hemodynamics and mortality benefit in patients with septic shock [17]. This finding then led to a series of studies on corticosteroids in septic shock over the last few decades as mentioned in Table 50.3.

The 2021 Surviving Sepsis Guideline and 2024 Focused Update on Guidelines on Use of Corticosteroids in Sepsis suggest administering hydrocortisone 200 mg IV per day (continuous infusion or intermittent push every 6 h) with or without fludrocortisone 50 mcg enteral daily for 7 days or until ICU discharge to adult patients with septic shock [2, 23]. In clinical practice, intermittent IV push dosing is commonly used due to limited line access and IV compatibilities. Fludrocortisone is often excluded because of the lack of oral access at the time of shock presentation or because some believe that hydrocortisone already has adequate mineralocorticoid activity. Overall, corticosteroids may lead to increased neuromuscular weakness, hypernatremia, and hyperglycemia. However, there is uncertainty regarding their potential effects on gastrointestinal bleeding, superinfection, stroke, and myocardial infarction [23].

Table 50.3 Critical illness-related corticosteroid insufficiency (CIRCI) studies

Study	Study size	Study arms (treatment vs placebo)	Results
Annane 2002 [18]	$n = 300$	HC 50 mg IV q6h + fludrocortisone 50 mcg PO qday × 7d	**Improved 28-day mortality** benefits in relative adrenal insufficiency pts with HC (53% vs. 63%, $p = 0.02$)
Corticus 2008 [19]	$n = 499$	HC 50 mg IV q6h × 5d, then 6d taper	**No difference** in shock reversal or 28-day mortality overall or those non-responsive to corticotropin test (39.2% vs. 36.1%, $p = 0.69$)
HYPRESS 2016 [20]	$n = 340$	HC 200 mg/d continuous infusion × 5d, then 6d taper	**No significant difference** in septic shock development within 14 days of HC (21.1% vs. 22.9%, $p = 0.7$)
ADRENAL 2018 [21]	$n = 3658$	HC 200 mg/d continuous infusion × 7d	**No significant difference** in 90-day mortality (27.9% vs. 28.8%, $p = 0.5$).
			Improved shock reversal with HC (3d vs. 4d, $p < 0.001$)
APROCCHSS 2018 [22]	$n = 1241$	HC 50 mg IV q6h + fludrocortisone 50 mcg PO qday × 7d	**Improved 90-day mortality** benefits with HC (43% vs. 49.1%, $p = 0.03$).
			Improved pressor-free days with HC (17d vs. 15d, $p < 0.001$).

HC hydrocortisone

During intermittent shortages of IV hydrocortisone, alternative pharmacotherapy options include methylprednisolone or dexamethasone, combined with fludrocortisone [24].

50.3.3.2 Methylene Blue and Hydroxocobalamin

Methylene blue and hydroxocobalamin are both nitric oxide scavenging agents with chief difference of methylene blue inhibiting production through nitric oxide synthase inhibition and also scavenges free nitric oxide while hydroxocobalamin only scavenges nitric oxide. Both agents have the most robust body of evidence is post-cardiopulmonary bypass vasoplegia, with some varying evidence in other shock states [25–28]. However, neither has been shown in a robust data set, or in our own experience to affect outcomes measures such as mortality [29, 30].

Methylene blue is dosed as 0.5–1.5 mg/kg IV piggyback up a total dose of 3 mg/kg. More severe adverse events such as serotonin syndrome and induced methemoglobinemia are seen in doses beyond 3 mg/kg. Methylene blue has a relatively quick time to peak effect at 30 min to 1 hour to allow for reassessment and redosing, but also has a relatively short half-life of about 5 hours. Due to the short half-life, many have recommended methylene blue as a continuous infusion. However, stability data is lacking and most of the practice evidence comes from anesthesia literature in the operating room where stability may also be lacking.

Hydroxocobalamin is typically used as an antidote for cyanide poisoning; however, its ability to scavenge nitric oxide makes it an attractive agent for use in shock states where this may be a primary driving factor. Hydroxocobalamin is given as an IV piggyback of 5 g, or one equivalent vial. Its stability of 6 hours per package insert allows some to advocate for a slow continuous infusion, with some profound vasopressor effect sometimes observed. Similar to methylene blue, hydroxocobalamin's effect can be seen within 30 min to 1 hour, but unlike methylene blue, hydroxocobalamin has a very long half-life, bordering on 24 hours and thus should not be redosed unless the source of excessive nitric oxide production is ongoing, such as the case of ongoing extracorporeal membrane oxygenation (ECMO) therapy. No data supports the redosing of hydroxocobalamin, but if redosed, waiting until 3–5 half-lives have passed, would make sense.

Both therapies should be considered in cases where patients are within 96 hours of being on cardiopulmonary bypass or continuing to undergo ECMO therapy. Cornerstone therapies of norepinephrine and vasopressin should be initiated prior to a trial of either agent or consideration given to adjunctive therapies such as corticosteroids. The criteria to use at our institution are threshold of vasopressin and norepinephrine of 0.2 mcg/kg/min or escalating doses and within 96 hours of cardiopulmonary bypass or ongoing extracorporeal life support (ECLS). Our preferred agent is methylene blue given the more robust published evidence surrounding its usage.

50.3.3.3 Intravenous Vitamin C

Vitamin C has been considered as an adjunctive therapy in the treatment of septic shock based on relative depletion of ascorbate levels in septic shock and its importance for many cellular processes related to immune system function. The initial excitement of intravenous vitamin C in the treatment of septic shock was derived from an observational, non-blinded, pre-post study showing an absolute risk reduction in mortality exceeding 30% [31]. However, all subsequent randomized trials and investigations have been unable to replicate this finding, and some even showed an increased risk of mortality [32–34]. As such the latest edition of the surviving sepsis campaign guidelines recommend against the administration of vitamin C in the treatment of sepsis [2]. Any new development in the treatment of shock is met with much excitement in the critical care community. While this is warranted in such a morbid and high mortality condition, we must also remember the lessons of caution warranted in past promising therapies, such as Xigris (Drotrecogin alfa), which seemed promising at first, but actually increased mortality upon further studies.

50.3.4 *Oral Vasopressor Therapies*

Oral agents with vasopressor properties have become an attractive option to help wean IV vasopressors and increase ICU throughput, particularly in patients prolonging their ICU stay due to only being on low doses of IV vasopressors. These oral agents mimic the physiologic effects of IV vasopressor agents. We will focus on the review of the two most popular agents, midodrine and droxidopa.

50.3.4.1 Midodrine

Midodrine is an oral α-1 agonist and is used commonly in the dialysis population to help mitigate intradialytic hypotension. The largest and best designed trial to date is the MIDAS trial [35]. Patients were included in this randomized controlled trial if vasopressor doses were less than norepinephrine 8 mcg/min (~0.06 mcg/kg/min in the trial) and unable to wean vasopressors for >24 hours after all causes for hypotension were addressed. Midodrine was given at a dose of 20 mg orally every 8 hours. There was no significant differences in any meaningful outcome including ICU length of stay and time to weaning off of vasopressors. There was a higher rate of bradycardia in the midodrine group. Until there is more robust data, midodrine for weaning off of a persistent vasopressor requirement cannot be recommended based on the best available evidence. As highlighted in the MIDAS trial, reflex bradycardia can happen with midodrine and we have seen this in our practice. Our current practice mirrors the MIDAS trial. However, we have used doses exceeding that of the MIDAS trial (up to 40 mg every 8 hours or 20 mg every 6 hours) and have not seen much meaningful benefit. One caution is to avoid midodrine in the pulmonary hypertension patient who has a persistent vasopressor need as it may further constrict pulmonary vessels.

50.3.4.2 Droxidopa

Droxidopa is an oral precursor drug of norepinephrine. It is provided in a capsule dosage form which has very little data in administration via feeding tube. Droxidopa has an FDA-labeled indication for the treatment of neurogenic orthostatic hypotension, but has found a niche in potentially providing a replacement for low-dose norepinephrine to liberate patients from the ICU. While most of the data supporting this use exists in the spinal cord injury population, there is emerging observational data in other populations. Lessing et al. investigated droxidopa in the cardiothoracic ICU in patients who had refractory hypotension on midodrine [36]. While the study overall found no difference in droxidopa, there was a signal of a shortened time to vasopressor discontinuation. Our current practice is not to use droxidopa, mostly due to cost considerations. Droxidopa is typically well tolerated. Dosing range is 100–600 mg three times daily, with 200 mg three times daily as the most common dose we have used.

50.3.5 Controversies in Vasopressor Administration

50.3.5.1 Peripheral Administration of Vasopressors

Administering vasopressors through central venous access is crucial to minimize the risk of extravasation and tissue necrosis. However, it is important to note that central venous catheter (CVC) placement can be time-consuming and associated

Table 50.4 Peripheral IV Vasopressor Studies

Tian et al. (2020) [39]	7 studies $n = 1382$	• Mean duration of PIV vasopressor infusion = 22 hours • Top three vasopressors: norepinephrine, phenylephrine, and dopamine • Extravasation occurred in 3.4% of patients • No reported episodes of tissue necrosis or limb ischemia
Tran et al. (2020) [40]	9 studies $n = 1835$	• 7% complications • Studies with PIV vasopressor safety guidelines in place were associated with significant lower prevalence of complications
Owens et al. (2021) [41]	32 studies $n = 16,443$	• Adverse effects of PIV vasopressor administration: 1.8% adults and 3.3% in pediatrics

with potential complications such as vascular injury, pneumothorax, and even death [37]. Recent data suggests that infusing vasopressors through a peripheral IV (PIV) line may be safe. A single-center study showed an average duration of PIV vasopressor use of 49 hours, with a 2% extravasation rate and no tissue injury following antidote treatment [38]. This evidence has led to a new recommendation in the 2021 Surviving Sepsis Guideline, which suggests initiating vasopressors peripherally rather than delaying initiation until central venous access is secured [2].

Several meta-analyses in recent years suggest low incidence of adverse effects such as extravasation with PIV vasopressor administration in both the adult and pediatric population. Table 50.4 outlines meta-analyses performed in peripheral IV pressors in the recent years.

Infusing vasopressors peripherally may obviate the need for CVC placement. A small pilot study involving 87 patients demonstrated that peripheral administration of norepinephrine is safe and may reduce the necessity for CVC placement [42]. Yerke et al.'s prospective observational study found that implementing a protocol for peripheral administration of norepinephrine safely avoided an average of 1 CVC day per patient, with 52% of patients not requiring CVC insertion [43].

Additional research is needed to investigate the effects of factors such as PIV location and size, vasopressor type and dose, and patient characteristics on the safety of PIV vasopressor administration. However, successful implementation of a PIV vasopressor workflow will require a robust monitoring and antidote protocol.

Standardizing the concentration of continuous medication infusions is an additional helpful step toward safer administration of pressors. Initiatives like Standardize 4 Safety, a national and interprofessional effort sponsored by the Food and Drug Administration (FDA) and the American Society of Health-System Pharmacists, publish standard concentrations for common IV infusions to reduce errors, particularly during transitions of care.

50.3.5.2 Vasopressor Extravasation Management

Management of PIV vasopressor extravasation involves recognizing early signs and symptoms, halting the vesicant infusion immediately, disconnecting the IV line, gently aspirating the extravasated solution from the IV line, and elevating the extremity. While most accidental vasopressor extravasations can be managed without pharmacologic treatment, the stage of injury and the vesicant's mechanism of tissue injury will dictate the appropriate treatment [44].

IV extravasation of vasopressor leads to localized vasoconstriction and reduced blood flow in the exposed tissue, resulting in ischemia and necrosis. Phentolamine, a non-selective alpha-adrenoceptor antagonist, serves as an antidote and is injected subcutaneously at doses of 5–10 mg around the extravasated area of IV vasopressors with alpha-adrenoceptor agonist activity (e.g., norepinephrine, epinephrine, dopamine, phenylephrine). The antidote should be administered as soon as possible or within 12 hours of extravasation. Applying warm compresses to the area is also recommended to increase circulation for IV vasopressor extravasation [45]. Antidotes for IV vasopressin infusion extravasation are less well studied compared to other vasopressors. However, topical nitroglycerin 2% ointment has been reported as a potential option [44, 45]. Additionally, hyaluronidase injection at a dose of 150 units has been reported for extravasation of other vasoactive agents, such as esmolol [44].

Overall, morbidity and mortality from extravasation of IV vasopressors are relatively small [46]. Being knowledgeable about the risk factors, early detection, and having quick access to standardized care protocols are key elements for timely prevention and treatment. At our institution, pharmacists and critical care nursing have partnered to launch an electronic health record order set for "Non-Chemotherapy Extravasation/Infiltrate," which provides direct nursing instructions on documentation and care, as well as speedy and concise ordering of extravasation antidotes.

50.3.5.3 Enteral Nutrition in Patients on Vasopressors

Providing enteral nutrition (EN) during shock is a subject of debate due to the potential risk of developing non-occlusive mesenteric ischemia (NOMI) in the setting of low tissue perfusion and increased gut oxygen demand exceeding delivery. Vasopressors can decrease gastrointestinal (GI) blood flow while inotropes can increase cardiac index and GI blood flow.

The incidence of bowel ischemia and NOMI is low (~1%), but with a high mortality rate ranging from 46% to 100% [47]. It is generally accepted that initiating low-rate, trophic EN for a patient with stable or decreasing pressor dose is safe. Tolerability of EN is likely related to the maximum cumulative vasopressor dose and may be related to the specific vasopressor administered [48].

The Vasoactive-Inotropic Score (VIS) has been studied to quantify the amount of cardiovascular support received in cardiac surgery patients [49]. This score was initially published in the pediatric critical care literature [50]. Given that inotropes can *increase* cardiac index and GI blood flow, dobutamine is likely unnecessary to be included in the vasopressor scoring. Thus, the American Society for Parenteral and Enteral Nutrition (ASPEN) guideline uses another score called the "Vasopressor Dose Equivalent (VDE)," which does not include inotropes, as a guide for patients on vasopressors who are being considered for enteral nutrition initiation [47, 51].

Table 50.5 Enteral nutrition and vasopressors dose equivalent score

Vasopressor dose equivalent (VDE) score
Sum of:
  Dopamine dose (mcg/kg/min) × 1
  Epinephrine dose (mcg/kg/min) × 100
  Norepinephrine dose (mcg/kg/min) × 100
  Phenylephrine dose (mcg/kg/min) × 10
  Vasopressin dose (units/min) × 250
  Angiotensin II dose (mcg/kg/min) × 1000
  Metaraminol dose (mcg/kg/min) × 12.5
	Recommendation [47]:
	• EN may be administered to patients with MAPs >60, should be held with MAP <50 mmHg
	• Holding EN if VDE >12; or give only trophic feed if VDE >12

Table 50.5 outlines the VDE score and recommendation on EN during vasopressor use.

Overall, when contemplating the initiation of EN for patients on vasopressors, it's crucial to not only assess vasopressor dose burden, but patient's overall clinical status. Resuscitation markers and suggestions for EN delivery safety include: lactate normalized or falling rapidly, vasopressor dose decreasing or stable, mixed venous oxygen within normal limits, fluid requirements stabling or no ongoing active bleeding, and limit fluid over-resuscitation to reduce bowel edema [52].

50.3.5.4 Weight-Based vs. Non-Weight-Based Dosing

Vasopressor medications are dosed in two main methods, either a weight-based or a non-weight-based strategy. Hospital systems may use different dosing methods for different medications, for example, at our hospital we use a non-weight-based strategy, mcg/min, for phenylephrine, but a weight-based strategy, mcg/kg/min, for norepinephrine. It is not advised for a drug to have more than one available dosing strategy at a single institution (e.g., phenylephrine allowed to be dosed in both mcg/min and mcg/kg/min). These differences between dosing strategies have led to errors and confusion among providers, nursing, and pharmacists. As a result, the Standardize 4 Safety campaign was launched by the American Society of Health-System Pharmacists. This campaign recommends standardized dosing units across all locations of care and standardized concentration options such that potential for error is minimized [53]. To take it a step further, it would be ideal for institutions to attempt to use the same strategy for all continuous infusions, for example, weight-based dosing or non-weight-based dosing for all. However, it can be challenging to know which is more appropriate, particularly with drugs that have wide dosing ranges and variable volumes of distribution. Fortunately, continuous infusions are generally titrated to effect, so either strategy should be acceptable, and no strategy has shown clinically meaningful differences [54–56]. At our institution, we standardized many of our infusions to a weight-based approach and on admission, a single "drug dosing weight" is chosen and used for all titratable infusions in that admission. This strategy works in most cases, however in our more complex patients like those with severe volume overload, heart failure, or morbidly obese, these weight-based doses can be quite large and may lead to a higher than initial intended dose. Pharmacists should consider this when starting new infusions that may have variable volumes of distribution. Furthermore, dosing weights should be readdressed when large changes occur and the pharmacist should be involved in converting the dose based on the newly selected weight, or when all infusions are held, a newer and appropriate dosing weight could be reassessed and established.

50.3.5.5 Weaning Order of Vasopressors

Just as critical as initiating vasopressors is the de-escalation of vasopressor therapies as underlying disease processes resolve. Often, the default strategy is to remove vasopressors in the reverse order they were added (e.g. vasopressin was added last and it will be removed first). One pharmacokinetic drug property of vasopressors to consider is their half-life. Most catecholamine-based vasopressors have similar half-lives around 2–5 min, making these typically fast on and fast off agents. In contrast, vasopressin has a longer half-life of around 10–20 min, making it more likely to exert some level of effect on the blood pressure potentially for up to an hour after discontinuation [57]. Catecholamine-based vasopressors are likely the agents we would want to titrate off last to allow for quick response to positive and negative hemodynamic changes. In general, the sensible approach might be to remove each non-catecholamine vasopressor, one at a time. Start with titration off of the longest acting first, wait 3–5 half-lives for that agent's effect to clear and then titrate the next longest acting agent. If only short-acting agents are being utilized (i.e., two catecholamine-based vasopressors), then the order is likely dependent upon other patient-specific factors (e.g., weaning dopamine after norepinephrine due to the need for inotropy). Clinically, the effects of weaning one agent first over the other remain equivocal [58, 59].

References

1. Shahoud JS, Sanvictores T, Aeddula NR. Physiology, arterial pressure regulation. In: StatPearls. StatPearls Publishing; 2024 [cited 2024 Mar 31]. Available from: http://www.ncbi.nlm.nih.gov/books/NBK538509/
2. Evans L, Rhodes A, Alhazzani W, et al. Surviving sepsis campaign: international guidelines for management of sepsis and septic shock 2021. Crit Care Med. 2021;49(11):e1063–143. https://doi.org/10.1097/CCM.0000000000005337.
3. Myburgh JA, Higgins A, Jovanovska A, et al. A comparison of epinephrine and norepinephrine in critically ill patients. Intensive Care Med. 2008;34(12):2226–34. https://doi.org/10.1007/s00134-008-1219-0.

4. De Backer D, Biston P, Devriendt J, et al. Comparison of dopamine and norepinephrine in the treatment of shock. N Engl J Med. 2010;362(9):779–89. https://doi.org/10.1056/NEJMoa0907118.

5. Choi MR, Kouyoumdzian NM, Mikusic NLR, et al. Renal dopaminergic system: pathophysiological implications and clinical perspectives. World J Nephrol. 2015;4(2):196. https://doi.org/10.5527/wjn.v4.i2.196.

6. Augoustides JGT, Savino JS. Vasopressin: the perioperative gift that keeps on giving. Anesthesiology. 2014;121(5):914–5. https://doi.org/10.1097/ALN.0000000000000431.

7. Holmes CL, Patel BM, Russell JA, Walley KR. Physiology of vasopressin relevant to management of septic shock. Chest. 2001;120(3):989–1002. https://doi.org/10.1378/chest.120.3.989.

8. Bauer SR, Sacha GL, Lam SW, et al. Hemodynamic response to vasopressin dosage of 0.03 units/min vs. 0.04 units/min in patients with septic shock. J Intensive Care Med. 2022;37(1):92–9. https://doi.org/10.1177/0885066620977181.

9. Gordon AC, Mason AJ, Thirunavukkarasu N, et al. Effect of early vasopressin vs norepinephrine on kidney failure in patients with septic shock: the VANISH randomized clinical trial. JAMA. 2016;316(5):509–18. https://doi.org/10.1001/jama.2016.10485.

10. Torgersen C, Dünser MW, Wenzel V, et al. Comparing two different arginine vasopressin doses in advanced vasodilatory shock: a randomized, controlled, open-label trial. Intensive Care Med. 2010;36(1):57–65. https://doi.org/10.1007/s00134-009-1630-1.

11. Russell JA, Walley KR, Joel S, et al. Vasopressin versus norepinephrine infusion in patients with septic shock. N Engl J Med. 2008;358(9):877–87. https://doi.org/10.1056/NEJMoa067373.

12. Khanna A, English SW, Wang XS, et al. Angiotensin II for the treatment of vasodilatory shock. N Engl J Med. 2017;377(5):419–30. https://doi.org/10.1056/NEJMoa1704154.

13. Bellomo R, Forni LG, Busse LW, et al. Renin and survival in patients given angiotensin II for catecholamine-resistant vasodilatory shock. A clinical trial. Am J Respir Crit Care Med. 2020;202(9):1253–61. https://doi.org/10.1164/rccm.201911-2172OC.

14. Roberts M, Cahoon W, Baker C. 191: Correlation of clinical outcomes with timing of angiotensin II initiation. Crit Care Med. 2024;52(1):S71. https://doi.org/10.1097/01.ccm.0000998956.83684.12.

15. Chen A, Wong A. The role of angiotensin II in poisoning-induced shock—a review. J Med Toxicol. 2022;18(2):145–54. https://doi.org/10.1007/s13181-022-00885-4.

16. Laws J, Bridges B, Bruccoleri R, King J. 869: The use of angiotensin II for severe vasodilatory shock after verapamil poisoning. Crit Care Med. 2024;52(1):S407. https://doi.org/10.1097/01.ccm.0001001648.24248.da.

17. Bollaert PE, Charpentier C, Levy B, Debouverie M, Audibert G, Larcan A. Reversal of late septic shock with supraphysiologic doses of hydrocortisone. Crit Care Med. 1998;26(4):645–50. https://doi.org/10.1097/00003246-199804000-00010.

18. Annane D. Effect of treatment with low doses of hydrocortisone and fludrocortisone on mortality in patients with septic shock. JAMA. 2002;288(7):862. https://doi.org/10.1001/jama.288.7.862.

19. Sprung CL, Annane D, Keh D, et al. Hydrocortisone therapy for patients with septic shock. N Engl J Med. 2008;358(2):111–24. https://doi.org/10.1056/NEJMoa071366.

20. Keh D, Trips E, Marx G, et al. Effect of hydrocortisone on development of shock among patients with severe sepsis: the HYPRESS randomized clinical trial. JAMA. 2016;316(17):1775. https://doi.org/10.1001/jama.2016.14799.

21. Venkatesh B, Finfer S, Cohen J, et al. Adjunctive glucocorticoid therapy in patients with septic shock. N Engl J Med. 2018;378(9):797–808. https://doi.org/10.1056/NEJMoa1705835.

22. Annane D, Renault A, Brun-Buisson C, et al. Hydrocortisone plus fludrocortisone for adults with septic shock. N Engl J Med. 2018;378(9):809–18. https://doi.org/10.1056/NEJMoa1705716.

23. Chaudhuri D, Nei AM, Rochwerg B, et al. 2024 Focused update: guidelines on use of corticosteroids in sepsis, acute respiratory distress syndrome, and community-acquired pneumonia. Crit Care Med. 2024;52(5):e219–33. https://doi.org/10.1097/CCM.0000000000006172.

24. Aldhaeefi M, Alshaya A, Belrhiti S, Rungkitwattanakul D. Alternatives to hydrocortisone for hemodynamic support in septic shock management due to medication shortage. Crit Care Explor. 2023;5(7):e0940. https://doi.org/10.1097/CCE.0000000000000940.

25. Levin RL, Degrange MA, Bruno GF, et al. Methylene blue reduces mortality and morbidity in vasoplegic patients after cardiac surgery. Ann Thorac Surg. 2004;77(2):496–9. https://doi.org/10.1016/S0003-4975(03)01510-8.

26. Özal E, Kuralay E, Yildirim V, et al. Preoperative methylene blue administration in patients at high risk for vasoplegic syndrome during cardiac surgery. Ann Thorac Surg. 2005;79(5):1615–9. https://doi.org/10.1016/j.athoracsur.2004.10.038.

27. Mehaffey JH, Johnston LE, Hawkins RB, et al. Methylene blue for vasoplegic syndrome after cardiac operation: early administration improves survival. Ann Thorac Surg. 2017;104(1):36–41. https://doi.org/10.1016/j.athoracsur.2017.02.057.

28. Habib AM, Elsherbeny AG, Almehizia RA. Methylene blue for vasoplegic syndrome post-cardiac surgery. Indian J Crit Care Med. 2018;22(3):168–73. https://doi.org/10.4103/ijccm.IJCCM_494_17.

29. Feih JT, Rinka JRG, Zundel MT. Methylene blue monotherapy compared with combination therapy with hydroxocobalamin for the treatment of refractory vasoplegic syndrome: a retrospective cohort study. J Cardiothorac Vasc Anesth. 2019;33(5):1301–7. https://doi.org/10.1053/j.jvca.2018.11.020.

30. Shah PR, Reynolds PS, Pal N, Tang D, McCarthy H, Spiess BD. Hydroxocobalamin for the treatment of cardiac surgery-associated vasoplegia: a case series. Can J Anesth. 2018;65(5):560–8. https://doi.org/10.1007/s12630-017-1029-3.

31. Marik PE, Khangoora V, Rivera R, Hooper MH, Catravas J. Hydrocortisone, vitamin C, and thiamine for the treatment of severe sepsis and septic shock: a retrospective before-after study. Chest. 2017;151(6):1229–38. https://doi.org/10.1016/j.chest.2016.11.036.

32. Iglesias J, Vassallo AV, Patel VV, Sullivan JB, Cavanaugh J, Elbaga Y. Outcomes of metabolic resuscitation using ascorbic acid, thiamine, and glucocorticoids in the early treatment of sepsis: the ORANGES trial. Chest. 2020;158(1):164–73. https://doi.org/10.1016/j.chest.2020.02.049.

33. François L, Marie-Hélène M, Julie M, et al. Intravenous vitamin C in adults with sepsis in the intensive care unit. N Engl J Med. 2022;386(25):2387–98. https://doi.org/10.1056/NEJMoa2200644.

34. Wacker DA, Burton SL, Berger JP, et al. Evaluating vitamin C in septic shock: a randomized controlled trial of vitamin C monotherapy. Crit Care Med. 2022;50(5):e458. https://doi.org/10.1097/CCM.0000000000005427.

35. Santer P, Anstey MH, Patrocínio MD, et al. Effect of midodrine versus placebo on time to vasopressor discontinuation in patients with persistent hypotension in the intensive care unit (MIDAS): an international randomised clinical trial. Intensive Care Med. 2020;46(10):1884–93. https://doi.org/10.1007/s00134-020-06216-x.

36. Lessing JK, Kram SJ, Levy JH, Grecu LM, Katz JN. Droxidopa or atomoxetine for refractory hypotension in critically ill cardiothoracic surgery patients. J Cardiothorac Vasc Anesth. 2024;38(1):155–61. https://doi.org/10.1053/j.jvca.2023.09.023.

37. Heidemann L, Nathani N, Sagana R, Chopra V, Heung M. A contemporary assessment of mechanical complication rates and trainee perceptions of central venous catheter insertion. J Hosp Med. 2017;12(8):646–51. https://doi.org/10.12788/jhm.2784.

38. Cardenas-Garcia J, Schaub KF, Belchikov YG, Narasimhan M, Koenig SJ, Mayo PH. Safety of peripheral intravenous administration of vasoactive medication. J Hosp Med. 2015;10(9):581–5. https://doi.org/10.1002/jhm.2394.

39. Tian DH, Smyth C, Keijzers G, et al. Safety of peripheral administration of vasopressor medications: a systematic review. Emerg Med Australas. 2020;32(2):220–7. https://doi.org/10.1111/1742-6723.13406.

40. Tran QK, Mester G, Bzhilyanskaya V, et al. Complication of vasopressor infusion through peripheral venous catheter: a systematic review and meta-analysis. Am J Emerg Med. 2020;38(11):2434–43. https://doi.org/10.1016/j.ajem.2020.09.047.

41. Owen VS, Rosgen BK, Cherak SJ, et al. Adverse events associated with administration of vasopressor medications through a peripheral intravenous catheter: a systematic review and meta-analysis. Crit Care. 2021;25(1):146. https://doi.org/10.1186/s13054-021-03553-1.

42. Groetzinger LM, Williams J, Svec S, Donahoe MP, Lamberty PE, Barbash IJ. Peripherally infused norepinephrine to avoid central venous catheter placement in a medical intensive care unit: a pilot study. Ann Pharmacother. 2022;56(7):773–81. https://doi.org/10.1177/10600280211053318.

43. Yerke JR, Mireles-Cabodevila E, Chen AY, et al. Peripheral administration of norepinephrine: a prospective observational study. Chest. 2024;165(2):348–55. https://doi.org/10.1016/j.chest.2023.08.019.

44. Ong J, Van Gerpen R. Recommendations for management of noncytotoxic vesicant extravasations. J Infus Nurs. 2020;43(6):319–43. https://doi.org/10.1097/NAN.0000000000000392.

45. Reynolds PM, MacLaren R, Mueller SW, Fish DN, Kiser TH. Management of extravasation injuries: a focused evaluation of noncytotoxic medications. Pharmacotherapy. 2014;34(6):617–32. https://doi.org/10.1002/phar.1396.

46. David V, Christou N, Etienne P, et al. Extravasation of noncytotoxic drugs. Ann Pharmacother. 2020;54(8):804–14. https://doi.org/10.1177/1060028020903406.

47. Bechtold ML, Brown PM, Escuro A, et al. When is enteral nutrition indicated? J Parenter Enter Nutr. 2022;46(7):1470–96. https://doi.org/10.1002/jpen.2364.

48. Mancl EE, Muzevich KM. Tolerability and safety of enteral nutrition in critically ill patients receiving intravenous vasopressor therapy. J Parenter Enter Nutr. 2013;37(5):641–51. https://doi.org/10.1177/0148607112470460.

49. Ong CS, Brown PM, Yesantharao P, et al. Vasoactive and inotropic support, tube feeding, and ischemic gut complications after cardiac surgery. J Parenter Enter Nutr. 2020;44(8):1461–7. https://doi.org/10.1002/jpen.1769.

50. Gaies MG, Gurney JG, Yen AH, et al. Vasoactive–inotropic score as a predictor of morbidity and mortality in infants after cardiopulmonary bypass. Pediatr Crit Care Med. 2010;11(2):234–8. https://doi.org/10.1097/PCC.0b013e3181b806fc.

51. Goradia S, Sardaneh AA, Narayan SW, Penm J, Patanwala AE. Vasopressor dose equivalence: a scoping review and suggested formula. J Crit Care. 2021;61:233–40. https://doi.org/10.1016/j.jcrc.2020.11.002.

52. Wischmeyer PE. Enteral nutrition can be given to patients on vasopressors. Crit Care Med. 2020;48(1):122–5. https://doi.org/10.1097/CCM.0000000000003965.

53. Standardize 4 safety initiative - ASHP [cited 2024 Mar 31]. Available from: https://www.ashp.org/Pharmacy-Practice/Standardize-4-Safety-Initiative

54. DeMillard L, Thuyns M. Implementation and evaluation of weight-based vasopressors in intensive care units. J Pharm Technol. 2024;40(1):23–9. https://doi.org/10.1177/87551225231217905.

55. Selby AR, Khan NS, Dadashian T, Hall RG 2nd. Evaluation of dose requirements using weight-based versus non-weight-based dosing of norepinephrine to achieve a goal mean arterial pressure in patients with septic shock. J Clin Med. 2023;12(4):1344. https://doi.org/10.3390/jcm12041344.

56. Vadiei N, Daley MJ, Murthy MS, Shuman CS. Impact of norepinephrine weight-based dosing compared with non-weight-based dosing in achieving time to goal mean arterial pressure in obese patients with septic shock. Ann Pharmacother. 2017;51(3):194–202. https://doi.org/10.1177/1060028016682030.

57. Bhattacharjee S, Maitra S. Vasopressor weaning in sepsis: debate is being continued! J Anaesthesiol Clin Pharmacol. 2023;39(3):497–8. https://doi.org/10.4103/joacp.joacp_538_21.

58. Jeon K, Song JU, Chung CR, Yang JH, Suh GY. Incidence of hypotension according to the discontinuation order of vasopressors in the management of septic shock: a prospective randomized trial (DOVSS). Crit Care. 2018;22:131. https://doi.org/10.1186/s13054-018-2034-9.

59. Musallam N, Altshuler D, Merchan C, Zakhary B, Aberle C, Papadopoulos J. Evaluating vasopressor discontinuation strategies in patients with septic shock on concomitant norepinephrine and vasopressin infusions. Ann Pharmacother. 2018;52(8):733–9.

Chapter 51
Antimicrobial Management in the Intensive Care Unit

Gabrielle Gibson, Lauren Kolodziej, Sarah Matuszak, and Lauren Sutton

51.1 Antimicrobial Timing

Rapid administration of appropriate antimicrobials is imperative to reduce mortality and improve patient outcomes. In 2006, Kumar and colleagues demonstrated a decrease in survival of 7.6% per hour delay of initiation of effective antimicrobial therapy in patients with septic shock [1]. Since that time, additional studies have been published examining the impact that time-to-antimicrobial therapy has on clinical outcomes [2–4]. These studies have redemonstrated the importance of early initiation of appropriate antimicrobial therapy to decrease mortality in patients with shock.

Based on these results, patients with shock secondary to presumed sepsis or infection should have appropriate antimicrobials targeting the most likely pathogens for the presumed infection type administered within 1 h of shock onset/recognition to improve outcomes [5]. Broad antimicrobial coverage should be utilized initially, followed by prompt de-escalation when culture data is available.

In patients with a possible infection without shock, a more targeted work-up can be completed prior to initiation of antimicrobials to rule out non-infectious causes of illness [5]. This work-up may include additional imaging, laboratory tests, and treatment of infection mimics. When possible, cultures should be obtained prior to administration of antimicrobials, but obtaining cultures should not inappropriately delay antimicrobial administration. In this subset of patients with sepsis but without

G. Gibson (✉) · L. Kolodziej · S. Matuszak
Barnes-Jewish Hospital Plaza, St Louis, MO, USA
e-mail: gabrielle.gibson@bjc.org

L. Sutton
Barnes-Jewish Hospital Plaza, St Louis, MO, USA

University Medical Center New Orleans, New Orleans, USA

© The Author(s), under exclusive license to Springer Nature Switzerland AG 2025

Y. Alzaidi, M. A. Gebily (eds.), *The Pharmacist's Expanded Role in Critical Care Medicine*, https://doi.org/10.1007/978-3-031-77335-8_51

shock, antimicrobials should ideally be administered within 3 h of patient presentation or sepsis onset.

51.2 Pharmacokinetics

Critically ill patients often have altered pharmacokinetic (PK) and pharmacodynamic (PD) variables, leading to challenging treatment decisions. Pharmacokinetic parameters such as absorption, distribution, metabolism, and excretion are often variable in the critically ill patient population compared to non-critically ill patients. This can lead to inadequate dosing of antimicrobials and poor treatment outcomes. As such, this section will focus on PK/PD changes including increased volume of distribution (Vd), acute kidney injury (AKI), and augmented renal clearance (ARC) which can lead to unpredictable antimicrobial exposure in critically ill patients.

51.2.1 Volume of Distribution

Volume of distribution (Vd) is one of the most important PK properties affecting antimicrobial dosing in critically ill patients. Inaccurate assessments may lead to potential over- or under dosing of antimicrobials which may have serious clinical consequences.

Drugs that distribute into the extracellular fluid (i.e., hydrophilic, high water solubility) have a lower Vd, while those that have rapid cellular intake (i.e., lipophilic, high lipid solubility) have a higher Vd (Table 51.1). Hydrophilic drugs usually distribute in the plasma volume, and distribution into the tissue requires adequate tissue perfusion from the blood volume. Higher doses of hydrophilic drugs than recommended in package labeling may be required to reach therapeutic concentrations in certain tissues [6]. To rapidly achieve therapeutic levels, a loading dose, or an intentionally larger initial dose, may be administered. However, lipophilic drugs have adequate Vd to penetrate tissue independently of perfusion. Serum concentrations of lipophilic drugs are typically not affected by volume resuscitation or fluid shifts due to capillary leakage, which are common in critically ill patients.

Table 51.1 Classification of antimicrobials according to pharmacokinetic (PK) principles

	Hydrophilic antimicrobials	Lipophilic antimicrobials
Properties	Limited volume of distribution High water solubility	Large volume of distribution High lipid solubility
Antimicrobials	Beta-lactams Vancomycin Aminoglycosides Linezolid Colistin	Macrolides Fluoroquinolones Tetracyclines

Sepsis commonly occurs in critically ill patients and leads to the development of endothelial leakage, which causes an increase in capillary permeability. This capillary leak syndrome results in redistribution of fluid into the extravascular compartment, which leads to an increase in Vd of hydrophilic drugs. The increased Vd results in a subsequent decrease in drug concentrations and potentially subtherapeutic levels. This can be further perpetuated by volume resuscitation, the presence of mechanical ventilation, extracorporeal circuits, post-surgical drains, or burn injuries.

Protein binding is a factor that may influence the Vd and clearance (CL) of many antibiotic agents. The PK of highly protein bound drugs is altered in conditions such as sepsis and can result in higher unbound concentrations of drug that are then subject to greater clearance. Hypoalbuminemia is a common condition in critically ill patients due to increased capillary permeability. There is increased albumin escape through the leaky endothelium, which results in loss of oncotic pressure and leakage of fluid into the interstitial space. This albumin escape is one factor that influences the Vd and CL of many antibiotic agents. The decrease in plasma albumin in critical illness leads to an increase in the free fraction of a drug that is ordinarily highly bound to protein [6]. Unbound fractions of antibiotic agents are available not only for elimination, but also for distribution. Highly protein bound antibiotic agents that likely develop altered PK from hypoalbuminemia include oxacillin, ceftriaxone, ertapenem, and daptomycin [7].

51.2.2 Elimination/Clearance

For many drugs, the kidneys are the primary site for excretion. Critical illness can profoundly affect renal function and drug CL. Both increases and decreases in drug CL have been observed in critically ill patients. Urinary excretion of a drug is dependent on filtration, secretion, and re-absorption. It is crucial to understand that AKI in situations such as sepsis, not only alters renal excretion, but also affects the process of tubular secretion and re-absorption. Critically ill patients may experience increased, decreased, or normal renal excretion of drugs. The state of renal excretion depends on many factors and can change rapidly depending on how the clinical condition progresses. The frequency of AKI in critically ill patients is estimated to be 50–65% and while in one third of the cases, it occurs as a late complication, in approximately two thirds, it is diagnosed within the first 24 h after admission to the ICU [8, 9].

Sepsis-induced AKI is not only associated with decreased glomerular filtration, but also with impairment of tubular secretion and re-absorption [10]. As a result, there is decreased antibiotic clearance of hydrophilic antibiotic agents, prolonged half-life, potential toxicity from elevated antibiotic plasma concentrations, and accumulation of metabolites. Antibiotic agents that undergo post-filtration re-absorption, such as fluconazole, have a CL that is increased in patients with AKI and anuria undergoing continuous renal replacement therapy (CRRT), necessitating an increase, or even doubling of the amount of administered drug [11, 12]. When AKI is present or the patient requires renal replacement therapy (RRT), individualized therapy is required, and dose adjustments should be made to reflect these changes.

Although standard practice is to reduce antibiotic doses in the presence of AKI to avoid toxic effects, in some critically ill patients, ARC can develop where glomerular filtration is increased. Augmented renal clearance refers to enhanced renal elimination of drug, and its diagnosis relies on a urine creatinine clearance (CrCl) greater than normal values of 130 mL/min/1.73 m^2 in males and 120 mL/min/1.73 m^2 in females [13]. It is driven by the pathophysiologic responses to infection and treatment interventions (volume resuscitation and the use of vasopressors) that are also associated with an early increase in cardiac output and enhanced blood flow to major organs. Increased perfusion to the kidneys enhances drug delivery and, therefore, increases glomerular filtration and clearance of renally eliminated solutes, leading to under-dosing of hydrophilic antibiotics. Two scoring systems have been developed to assess the likelihood of ARC: the augmented renal clearance scoring system (ARC score) and the augmented renal clearance in trauma intensive care scoring system (ARTIC score). The ARC scoring system assigns points based on age <50 years (6 points), post-trauma admission (3 points), and a modified sequential organ failure assessment (SOFA) score <4 (1 point). The ARTIC score assigns points based on age <56 years (4 points), patients aged 56–75 years (3 points), a serum creatinine <0.7 mg/dL (3 points), and male sex (2 points). Cutoff scores of >7 for ARC score and >6 for the ARTIC score suggest a high risk for the occurrence of ARC and an appropriate cutoff at which antimicrobial adjustments may be considered [14, 15].

Augmented renal clearance is a common condition observed in critically ill patients and is crucial to identify before subtherapeutic antibiotics concentrations cause clinical failure. To optimize PK of antibiotics in patients with ARC, clinicians should aim to use the maximum approved dosing regimen, consider extended or continuous infusions, utilize therapeutic drug monitoring (TDM) when available, or switch to an alternative agent that is not primarily renally eliminated [16].

51.2.2.1 Organ Support

Critically ill patients with severe renal dysfunction necessitating CRRT also have altered PK. The three main modalities of CRRT are continuous venovenous hemodialysis (CVVHD), continuous venovenous hemofiltration (CVVH), and continuous venovenous hemodiafiltration (CVVHDF). To administer proper antibiotic doses to these patients, knowledge of PK changes and CL obtained by the specific type of CRRT is needed [17]. Drug properties that affect CL by CRRT include molecular weight, protein binding, Vd, and drug charge [18]. CVVH removes solute by convection allowing larger molecules to be removed, while in CVVHD, drug clearance occurs by passive diffusion allowing a higher CL of smaller molecules with a low molecular weight. CVVHDF removes molecules by both diffusion and convection [19]. It has been recommended that the initial dose of antimicrobial agents be based on the published Vd and subsequent doses be based on an estimate of total CL or the sum of the residual renal CL, non-renal non-CRRT CL, and CRRT

CL [17, 20, 21]. It is also important to note that when patients transition to intermittent hemodialysis, the rate of solute removal will change, and dosing should be adjusted accordingly.

Patients who are critically ill with cardiac and/or respiratory failure may undergo extracorporeal membrane oxygenation (ECMO), during which a cardiopulmonary bypass device circuit is used for temporary support. This circuit causes alterations in PK that can lead to therapeutic failure of antimicrobials or drug toxicity. Studies have demonstrated that the ECMO circuit sequesters certain antibiotics, especially lipophilic drugs, which lead to a decreased amount of drug reaching the patient [22, 23]. In addition to sequestration, there is an increased Vd and decreased drug elimination, which can lead to suboptimal antimicrobial concentrations in the patient [24, 25]. The PK parameters vary based on the individual antibiotic agents. For example, the PK of vancomycin, piperacillin-tazobactam, meropenem, and amikacin are not significantly altered in patients on ECMO; however, the PK parameters of many antifungal agents suggest that significant changes may occur that require alternate dosing and monitoring strategies [22]. Further, large PK studies are needed to provide optimal dosing guidelines for patients receiving antimicrobial agents on ECMO [26].

51.3 Pharmacodynamics

The relationship between drug serum concentrations and pharmacologic/toxicologic properties is termed *pharmacodynamics* (PD). The main interest for antimicrobial agents is the relationship between drug concentration and the antimicrobial effect [27]. Successful antimicrobial therapy requires sufficient drug concentrations to kill or suppress bacterial growth at the site of infection. Critical illness can severely alter antimicrobial PD. For example, decreased end-organ perfusion may lead to treatment failure due to inadequate drug concentrations at the site of infection, or exposure-related toxicity [15].

To provide optimal doses of antimicrobial agents in critically ill patients, the clinician must understand the exposure-effect relation of the drug and pathogen. There are three categories that define this relationship: time-dependent, concentration-dependent, and concentration-dependent with time-dependence (Table 51.2) [28]. The PD parameters used to characterize this antimicrobial activity of bacteria are the minimum inhibitory concentration (MIC) and minimum bactericidal concentration (MBC). The MBC is the level at which bacterial lysis begins to occur and determines the drug's potency against a pathogen. The MIC is the lowest concentration of an antibiotic at which bacterial growth is completely inhibited [29].

Maximal bacterial killing for time-dependent antimicrobial agents is based on the time the unbound fraction of antibiotic is above the MIC, known as $fT > \text{MIC}$ [28]. Beta-lactam $fT > \text{MIC}$ varies with near-maximal bactericidal effect observed with an $fT > \text{MIC}$ of 40–70% for cephalosporins, 30–50% for penicillins, and 20–40% for carbapenems with concentrations 4–5 times the MIC required [30].

Table 51.2 Classification of antimicrobials according to pharmacodynamic (PD) principle

Pharmacodynamic principle	Antimicrobial
Time-dependent ($fT > \mathrm{MIC}$)	Beta-lactams Macrolides Clindamycin Linezolid
Concentration-dependent (C_{max}/MIC)	Aminoglycosides
Concentration and time-dependent (AUC/MIC)	Vancomycin Fluoroquinolones Daptomycin Polymyxins

AUC area under the curve, C_{max} maximum concentration, *fT > MIC* fraction of antibiotic above the MIC, *MIC* minimum inhibitory concentration

Drug exposure can be affected by changes in Vd and increased drug CL in the critically ill. Time-dependent antimicrobial agents should be dosed more frequently, rather than administered in higher doses, to optimize bacterial killing.

Antimicrobials that demonstrate concentration-dependent killing require a higher peak concentration over the MIC of the bacterial pathogen (C_{max}/MIC). Higher doses and thus, higher concentrations lead to a greater rate and extent of bactericidal activity compared to more frequent dosing. Maximal antibacterial killing with aminoglycosides is thought to occur when the C_{max}/MIC is 8–10 times greater than the MIC [31]. In critically ill patients, it may be challenging to achieve these concentrations using standard dosing; therefore, higher daily doses may be required [31, 35].

Concentration and time-dependent bacterial killing is the last PD variable. For these antibiotic agents, the area under the concentration-time curve during a 24-h period to the MIC ratio (AUC/MIC) is used to guide dosing [28].

51.3.1 Therapeutic Drug Monitoring

Therapeutic drug monitoring measures individual drug exposure based on validated PK parameters that better reflect drug effect than drug dosage [36]. Although routine TDM is not recommended for all antimicrobials or for every critically ill patient, it may be useful in several circumstances. Therapeutic drug monitoring is useful when the antimicrobial has significant inter- or intrapatient PK variability [33]. In order to conduct TDM, specific criteria must be met. First, the antimicrobial must have a well-established therapeutic range where there is a higher probability of treatment success and lower/acceptable toxicity [33]. Second, there should be defined sampling times that enable accurate estimation of PK parameters. Finally, a routinely available assay must be available to ensure results are acquired in a timely fashion (turnaround time of <8 h) [33]. Therapeutic drug monitoring may also be useful if toxicity, subtherapeutic concentrations, or resistance is suspected;

adherence is questionable; new drug–drug interactions are present; a slow clinical response is evident; and/or there is a change in the patient's clinical status.

Antibiotics and antifungals are usually administered at repeated doses with a constant dosage interval, either enterally or intravenously (IV). Blood/plasma concentrations rise and fall in each dosing interval, from peak to trough. Antibiotic and antifungal TDM may be based on different parameters: trough concentration (i.e., just before drug administration, C_{min}), peak concentration (i.e., just after drug administration, C_{max}), or AUC. In most cases, TDM should be performed when steady state is reached; however, it can be performed earlier if toxicity is suspected or in the case of potential drug interactions, especially if the drug has a long half-life [34]. For drugs with linear PK administered at a fixed-dose regimen, drug concentrations reach steady state after 4–5 half-lives [34]. Therapeutic concentrations may be reached earlier if loading doses are used. This estimation does not apply to drugs with nonlinear PK; in such cases, drug concentrations increase disproportionately. During a continuous infusion, no fluctuations are expected in blood/plasma concentrations at steady state. Once steady state is reached, the plasma sample is generally measured in the elimination phase, which usually correlates with the C_{min}. However, some antibiotics, such as aminoglycosides, require C_{max} monitoring. Of note, plasma sampling should not occur during the distribution phase because there is disequilibrium between the plasma and tissue concentrations.

Therapeutic drug monitoring is commonly performed in the ICU because critically ill patients have severe infections requiring prompt treatment and optimization of the antimicrobial regimen. As explained above, critically ill patients may also have significant changes in organ function related to their illness. Therapeutic drug monitoring is typically performed for patients receiving drugs such as vancomycin and aminoglycosides because the benefits for optimizing efficacy and toxicity have been established [33, 35]. The 2016 Infectious Diseases Society of America (IDSA) guidelines on implementing an antibiotic stewardship program endorse PK monitoring and adjustment programs for aminoglycosides and vancomycin, mentioning that training, assessment of competencies, and integration into routine pharmacy activities should be pursued [36].

Although TDM implementation is a rational approach to optimizing antimicrobial dosing, few randomized controlled studies have been conducted, and most data supporting TDM are observational [37]. Observational data are limited by selection bias because TDM was only performed after clinical failure or toxicity was observed.

51.3.1.1 Aminoglycosides

Aminoglycosides are commonly used as part of combination regimens directed against Gram-negative bacteria as well as for synergy in combination with penicillins or cephalosporins against Gram-positive organisms. Empiric short-term use of aminoglycosides ("double coverage") can potentially be lifesaving, but prolonged or inappropriate use can cause harm, including ototoxicity and nephrotoxicity [38]. In some circumstances, aminoglycoside therapy is warranted for directed therapy, including infections with complex resistance patterns, synergistic treatment for endocarditis, and use of amikacin for mycobacterial infections.

Gentamicin, tobramycin, and amikacin have similar PK properties, with peak serum concentrations at 30–60 min after an intravenous infusion and a terminal half-life of 1.5–3.5 h in adult patients with normal renal function [38]. These agents are hydrophilic, have a low Vd (which can lead to decreased concentrations in septic shock), are minimally protein bound, and are renally eliminated. Aminoglycosides induce bacterial killing through concentration-dependent PD, meaning the extent of the bacterial killing increases as the ratio between the C_{max} and the MIC increases.

Two dosing strategies exist for aminoglycosides, traditional dosing and extended-interval dosing (Table 51.3). Traditional aminoglycoside dosing uses small doses administered several times per day. Extended-interval dosing employs higher doses administered at an extended interval [38]. Use of traditional dosing regimens has resulted in lower than the targeted amikacin peak concentrations in 30–40% of critically ill patients [39]. High-dose, extended-interval dosing allows for achievement of AUC values similar to traditional dosing. An added benefit may be the reduced incidence of nephrotoxicity when administered once daily versus several times a day. In addition, extended-interval dosing allows for optimization of concentration-dependent killing and the post-antibiotic effect.

Extended-interval dosing of aminoglycosides has traditionally used a population-based dosing nomogram (e.g., Hartford nomogram). The Hartford nomogram was designed to target peak serum concentrations 10 times the MIC of the specific institution's most serious Gram-negative pathogen, typically *Pseudomonas aeruginosa* (median gentamicin MIC 2 mg/L, median amikacin MIC 4 mg/L). When using the Hartford nomogram, patients are administered a 7 mg/kg dose of gentamicin or tobramycin (15 mg/kg of amikacin), and a random serum concentration is obtained 6–10 h after the first dose. This value is plotted to determine the patient's optimal dosing interval. The goal when using this nomogram is to achieve maximal killing by achieving high peaks and to minimize the risk of nephrotoxicity by achieving undetectable serum trough concentrations. Of note, patients with variable amino-glycoside kinetics (i.e., pediatric patients, pregnant women, patients with burns and

Table 51.3 Aminoglycoside dosing and therapeutic drug monitoring [36] targets

	Traditional dosing		Extended-interval dosing	
	Dose[a]	TDM target for serious Gram-negative infections	Dose[a]	TDM target for serious Gram-negative infections
Gentamicin Tobramycin	1–2 mg/kg every 8–12 h	Peak: 8–10 mg/L Trough: <1 mg/L	5–7 mg/kg every 24–48 h[b]	Peak: C_{max}/MIC >10–20 mg/L Trough: Undetectable
Amikacin	5–8 mg/kg every 8–12 h	Peak: 30–40 mg/L trough: <5 mg/L	15–20 mg/kg every 24–28 h[b]	Peak: C_{max}/MIC >40–60 mg/L Trough: Undetectable

[a]Actual body weight utilized unless actual body weight is great than 1.2 times ideal body weight, then adjusted body weight used
[b]Frequency based on nomogram information or patient-specific kinetics

ascites, and patients undergoing dialysis) were excluded during the development of this nomogram.

Individualized PK dosing and monitoring is an alternative approach to nomogram-based dosing. Individualized PK dosing and monitoring typically uses the initial doses suggested for extended-interval dosing but obtains two or more serum concentrations in the post-distributive phase (usually 2–10 h after the end of infusion) to calculate patient-specific PK (including Vd and half-life). Because of the large degree of interpatient PK variability in the ICU, this approach is becoming desired for dosing and monitoring extended-interval therapy in critically ill patients.

Regardless of the dosing strategy utilized, TDM of aminoglycosides is essential, not only to assess efficacy but also to prevent toxicity. Aminoglycoside TDM is recommended for critically ill patients after the first dose if more than 48 h of therapy is anticipated, the patient's renal function is rapidly changing, or the patient has variable PK [40]. One study of critically ill patients has shown that TDM can significantly reduce the duration of aminoglycoside therapy, hospital length of stay, and nephrotoxicity [41].

Of note, in 2023, the Clinical and Laboratory Standards Institute (CLSI) lowered aminoglycoside susceptibility breakpoints for *P. aeruginosa* and Enterobacterales which has resulted in more bacterial isolates demonstrating resistance to aminoglycosides [42]. Amikacin susceptibility breakpoints for *P. aeruginosa* have been changed to urine only (i.e., it should only be used to treat *P. aeruginosa* urinary tract infections); however, it may still be used for non-*Pseudomonas* Gram-negative infections outside the urinary tract. Susceptibility breakpoints for gentamicin have been removed for *P. aeruginosa*; therefore, gentamicin should not be used as empiric or targeted therapy against *P. aeruginosa*; however, it still may be used for non-*Pseudomonas* Gram-negative infections. Tobramycin still maintains activity against *P. aeruginosa*. These breakpoints are based on gentamicin and tobramycin doses of 7 mg/kg and amikacin doses of 15 mg/kg.

51.3.1.2 Vancomycin

Vancomycin is commonly used to treat serious Gram-positive infections, such as those caused by methicillin-resistant *Staphylococcus aureus* (MRSA). Vancomycin is a hydrophilic antibiotic that is widely distributed through body tissues. Vancomycin has moderate protein binding and a low Vd and is predominantly cleared through renal elimination [43]. Therefore, drug exposure is highly variable with alterations in Vd and CL.

The efficacy and toxicity of vancomycin are related to drug exposure; however, substantial interindividual PK variability exists. Although patient factors such as renal function, body weight, and age influence vancomycin disposition, variability in drug exposure between patients remains even after accounting for these factors. As a result, dose adjustment based on renal function, age, and body weight alone may result in sub- or supratherapeutic drug concentrations. Therefore, TDM is warranted in patients receiving vancomycin for serious MRSA infections, at high risk of nephrotoxicity, with fluctuating renal function, and receiving prolonged courses of vancomycin [35]. Vancomycin TDM should be frequent in hemodynamically unstable patients and those with end-stage renal disease but may be extended up to once weekly in those who are hemodynamically stable with stable renal function. The PK/PD parameter targeted to maximize bacterial killing is an $AUC/MIC_{0-24\ h}$ ratio of 400 or greater; however, serum trough concentrations of 15–20 mg/L are often targeted as a surrogate marker for the optimal AUC/MIC ratio [35]. AUC concentrations of 600–800 mg × h/L appear to be associated with an increased risk of nephrotoxicity [35].

In 2020, the American Society of Health-System Pharmacists, the IDSA, the Pediatric Infectious Diseases Society, and the Society of Infectious Diseases Pharmacists released a consensus guideline for vancomycin monitoring in the treatment of MRSA infections [35]. The guideline recommends utilizing the AUC/MIC target strategy and dosing vancomycin to achieve an AUC/MIC of 400 or greater. It is important to note that this AUC/MIC target only applies to invasive *S. aureus* infections as estimates of AUC/MIC values were made on the basis of vancomycin MICs for only *S. aureus*.

If the AUC/MIC monitoring strategy is used, two parts to the target must be addressed. The first is the AUC of vancomycin, which represents the total vancomycin concentration in the blood over a time interval, typically 24 h. Vancomycin AUC can be determined using an equation-based method, such as a trapezoidal model or other first-order equations, or the Bayesian approach [44]. Although both approaches accurately predict AUC values, they have notable differences.

Equation-Based Method

When the AUC is calculated manually, many equation-based methods can be used. One commonly used method is the trapezoidal model. This approach uses two post-infusion serum concentrations from the same dosing interval after the drug has reached steady state to calculate the AUC: one at 1–2 h after administration (peak) and the other just before the next scheduled dose (trough) [45]. It cannot account for fluctuations in AUC because of continuing physiologic changes [46]. This method may underestimate the AUC compared with Bayesian estimates because it cannot account for the entirety of the distribution phase [44]. Other first-order equation-based methods have been proposed and validated with accuracy similar to Bayesian methods, but the same limitations that apply to the trapezoidal method also apply to these other methods [44, 46].

Bayesian-Based Methods

Bayesian-based methods are the most accurate way to estimate AUC but are also more complex. Bayesian-based methods combine known trends in population PK and an individual patient's data and laboratory results to accurately simulate the patient-specific vancomycin AUC exposure for a given dose [45]. The Bayesian approach allows for more flexibility, by using one or two concentrations obtained at any time point after the dose is administered. However, using two concentrations increases accuracy and may be more appropriate in critically ill patient populations. Advantages of

Bayesian dosing include earlier intervention to optimize vancomycin dosing, which contrasts with the trough-only approach requiring that steady state be achieved. The Bayesian approach is adaptive and allows for quick predictions and potential cost savings because it results in fewer required vancomycin concentrations. The primary drawback to the Bayesian approach is the cost of the commercially available software. If cost is prohibitive, equation-based approaches may be used.

The other crucial component of the AUC/MIC PD target is the MIC itself. The reference method for calculating MIC is broth microdilution (BMD). Broth microdilution is a highly accurate measurement of MIC but is not easily replicated in the clinical setting. Most institutions use automated methods of calculating the MIC, but these are highly variable compared with BMD [35]. Despite this variability, MICs are not differentiated in the 2020 guidelines. Of note, national surveillance data show that in most cases, the MIC_{BMD} can be assumed to be 1 mg/L or less [35]. The guidelines state that even if the MIC_{BMD} is <1 mg/L, the vancomycin dose should not be decreased to achieve the desired AUC/MIC target. When the MIC_{BMD} is >1 mg/L, the probability of achieving the AUC/MIC target of >400 is low with conventional vancomycin dosing. In these cases, alternatives to vancomycin may be considered.

Trough Monitoring

Historically, vancomycin TDM has focused on using dosing nomograms or PK parameters to maintain trough concentrations of 10–20 mg/L or 15–20 mg/L for serious infections. This higher trough goal was chosen because it was thought to more likely achieve an AUC/MIC of 400 or greater in most patients (assuming an MIC of 1 mg/L or less), but clinical data are limited to support this goal. Recent studies have suggested that trough values are not as accurate in estimating AUC and may underestimate actual vancomycin exposure [35]. In addition, many studies have associated trough concentrations >15 mg/L with increased nephrotoxicity rates [47, 48].

Ultimately, despite the convenience and comfort of trough-only monitoring, it does have significant limitations and a study published in 2018 showed that AUC compared with trough-based vancomycin TDM was superior at reducing nephrotoxicity rates (<1% vs. 8%, $p = 0.01$) and had a shorter therapy duration (4.7–5.4 days vs. 8.2 days, $p = 0.03$) [49].

51.3.1.3   Future of TDM

Linezolid

Linezolid is a synthetic lipophilic antibacterial agent used for the treatment of severe Gram-positive infections, such as MRSA and vancomycin-resistant *Enterococcus faecium/faecalis* [36]. Linezolid is lipophilic and has low protein binding, low Vd, and low penetration into the adipose tissue [36]. Around 65% of linezolid is cleared non-renally, and around 30% of the dose appears unchanged in the urine of patients with normal renal function. Elimination occurs through renal excretion or enzymatic pathways. Elimination has been associated with nonlinear PK; therefore, PK is difficult to predict and presents a challenge to linezolid dosing [50].

Linezolid has time-dependent antibiotic activity with a modest concentration-dependent kill characteristic [33]. Maximum efficacy has been shown at $fT > $ MIC and AUC/MIC ratio of 85% and 80–120, respectively. As with most other antibiotics, linezolid efficacy is determined by exposure. Suboptimal exposure may result in treatment failure because of inefficacy, emergence of resistance, and increased mortality. Linezolid underexposure and lack of efficacy are often observed in obesity, critical illness, burns, or cystic fibrosis. Furthermore, traditional linezolid regimens (600 mg twice daily) may fail in up 10–30% of critically ill patients with linezolid-susceptible pathogens [51]. In addition, clinical evidence suggests that the recommended linezolid dose of 600 mg twice daily is suboptimal in up to 30% of critically ill patients undergoing RRT for treatment against a pathogen with a linezolid MIC of 2 mg/L; however, no alternative dosing recommendations have been suggested for this population, which suggests an opportunity to perform TDM.

In addition, linezolid toxicity depends on exposure. Monitoring C_{min} has been suggested as a means of monitoring linezolid toxicity. Linezolid-induced thrombocytopenia has been reported at a C_{min} and AUC of >7–10 mg/L and >300–350 mg×h/L, respectively [33]. To balance linezolid efficacy and toxicity, clinical studies have suggested various target trough concentrations, with the most common being 2–7 mg/L [50, 52].

An ideal TDM plan involves obtaining peak (C_{max}) and trough (C_{min}) linezolid samples. Together, these samples can be used to estimate the AUC. Peak plasma concentrations should be obtained 30 min after the end of the 1-h IV infusion or 2 h after oral dose administration [36]. However, the trough concentration has a stronger correlation with AUC and exposure than the peak concentration, which makes it acceptable for TDM if two samples cannot be obtained [36]. The C_{min} and C_{max} concentrations should be collected at steady state to reflect the PK response to a dosing regimen. Steady state usually occurs by the third day of therapy [36].

Although current linezolid dosing recommendations do not include TDM, traditional doses result in over- and underexposure in some critically ill patients. Therapeutic drug monitoring can be used, particularly in high-risk patients or those requiring prolonged treatment courses; however, widespread use may be limited by availability of the assay.

β-Lactams

β-Lactams generally have low to moderate protein binding though some agents have high protein binding (e.g., ceftriaxone). These agents are often categorized into three groups: penicillins, cephalosporins, and carbapenems. They are commonly administered using a traditional fixed-dosing scheme. Because of the hydrophilic nature and predominant renal elimination, total body drug clearance, and, to a lesser extent, Vd of β-lactam antibiotics may be altered in patients with sepsis and septic shock [53]. Under-dosing of β-lactams has been linked to therapeutic failure and the emergence of resistance, whereas overdosing has been linked to β-lactam antibiotic toxicity, most commonly neurotoxicity and nephrotoxicity.

β-Lactams have time-dependent bactericidal activity, and the PK/PD index associated with optimal bactericidal killing is the $fT > $ MIC [33]. As noted above, the $fT > $ MIC required is 40–70% for cephalosporins, 30–50% for penicillins, and 20–40% for carbapenems. However, data in immunocompromised and critically ill patients suggest they will benefit from longer (100% $fT > $ MIC) and higher (2–5 times the MIC) β-lactam exposures than previously described [54, 55].

β-Lactam TDM can be useful to maximize efficacy and reduce toxicity in critically ill patients who have altered PK (e.g., patients with obesity, sepsis, trauma, burn, or hematologic emergency) or in patients where there is a suspicion for treatment failure and/or toxicity [50, 53]. For example, one study determined that in patients with augmented renal clearance, β-lactam trough concentrations were less than the MIC 82% of the time ($p < 0.001$) and <4 times the MIC in 72% of patients ($p < 0.001$) [56]. The DALI trial examined the implications of failure to achieve $fT > $ MIC and showed that patients who failed to meet their $fT > $ MIC goals were less likely to have positive clinical outcomes [7, 9]. A retrospective review evaluated TDM results from 378 patients treated with piperacillin, meropenem, or flucloxacillin to define the thresholds above which toxicity would be more likely [57]. Patients who developed neurotoxicity while taking these antibiotics had significantly higher mean trough concentrations. This was similarly seen in a single-center retrospective cohort study of patients undergoing cefepime TDM where elevated trough concentrations led to neurologic adverse effects [58]. These studies highlight the need for specific PD targets in the critically ill patient population.

Therapeutic drug monitoring of β-lactams is only applied in specific cases and only in a few hospitals due to the lack of a method to determine antibiotic concentrations, limited availability of commercially available β-lactam assays, and limited knowledge about optimal doses for individual patients [50, 53]. There are also practical concerns that must be overcome, such as the instability of β-lactams at room temperature meaning samples should ideally be maintained on ice or frozen until processed to limit degradation [59]. Additionally, published protein binding percentages for β-lactams vary widely. Therefore, once a β-lactam concentration is obtained and reported, it should be corrected for protein binding to estimate free exposure before integration with the given target MIC. The most critical PK variable to define exposure for β-lactams is CL; thus, at least two sampling time points are recommended: the midpoint (at the halfway point of the dosing interval, i.e., 4 h after dose administration for a every 8 h regimen) and the trough. It is also recommended that a third sample be collected shortly after the infusion has been completed (peak). The samples must be evaluated using population PK software and Bayesian modeling. Although a subtherapeutic β-lactam concentration would clearly warrant an intervention, it is less obvious what to do with a β-lactam concentration that is well above the defined PD target [59].

Use of Extended Infusions

Since β-lactam antibiotics demonstrate time-dependent killing, it has been assumed that prolonged infusions will attain PD targets more effectively than intermittent infusions. Therefore, extended (over 2–4 h) or continuous (over the entire dosing interval) infusion strategies may improve microbiologic and clinical cure, especially when a pathogen demonstrates a higher MIC. Clinical data suggest that prolonged infusions of β-lactams may be effective in specific clinical scenarios, such as critical illness. However, high-quality, randomized controlled trials to support the use of prolonged infusions are lacking and rationale continues to be based on PD principles and evidence of clinical benefit demonstrated in observational trials. Despite the PD rationale for prolonged infusions of β-lactam antibiotics, there are barriers to be aware of including the need for continued intravenous access and issues with compatibility with concomitant medications. The 2023 international consensus recommendations for the use of prolonged-infusion β-lactam antibiotics suggest prolonged β-lactam infusions over intermittent infusions to reduce mortality or increase clinical cure in critically ill adults with Gram-negative infections [60].

Observational trials have demonstrated efficacy of prolonged infusions of piperacillin-tazobactam for Gram-negative infections. A single-center, retrospective study of critically ill adult patients with *P. aeruginosa* infection compared patients treated with extended infusion piperacillin-tazobactam to a historical control group [61]. Patients with higher APACHE II scores at presentation receiving extended infusion piperacillin-tazobactam had lower 14-day mortality and shorter length of stay. Likewise, a multicenter study of adult patients with Gram-negative bacterial infections evaluated patients receiving extended infusion piperacillin-tazobactam versus patients receiving intermittent infusions [62]. Extended infusion piperacillin-tazobactam was associated with lower mortality; however, differences in patient characteristics may have explained the findings. Conversely, two retrospective cohort studies evaluating extended infusion piperacillin-tazobactam failed to demonstrate improved clinical outcomes, including mortality, when compared to intermittent infusions [63, 64].

Prolonged infusions of carbapenems have been associated with similar mortality rates as intermittent infusions; however, other benefits, such as microbiologic cure, have been observed. A double-blind, randomized controlled trial of critically ill patients with sepsis or septic shock who received equal doses of meropenem by either continuous or intermittent administration, showed that 47% of patients experienced all-cause mortality and emergence of drug resistant bacteria on day 28 (RR 0.96, 95% CI 0.81–1.13, $p = 0.60$) [65]. Notably, baseline rates of carbapenem resistance were high; therefore, the choice of meropenem was not optimal.

Prolonged infusions of cephalosporins are also associated with similar outcomes as intermittent infusions. A meta-analysis of ten randomized controlled trials and one non-randomized controlled trial did not demonstrate a mortality difference or difference in clinical cure when comparing third- and fourth-generation cephalosporins administered as a prolonged infusion vs intermittent infusion [66].

β-lactam antibiotics demonstrate time-dependent PD effects on bacterial killing therefore infusing the antibiotic over a prolonged time period may effectively attain PD targets compared with intermittent infusions. Current data suggests that extended infusions are at least equally effective as intermittent infusions.

51.4 Unique Routes of Administration

Systemic administration of antimicrobials is generally appropriate for the treatment of standard infections. In limited cases, alternative routes may be required to ensure sufficient antimicrobial concentrations are present at the site of infection. As such, this section will focus on unique routes of administration including intracerebroventricular, intrathecal, intraperitoneal, intravitreal, inhalation, and lock therapy.

51.4.1 Intracerebroventricular or Intrathecal Antimicrobials

Due to the blood-brain barrier (BBB) and blood-cerebrospinal-fluid barrier (BCSFB), medication access to the central nervous system (CNS) and brain parenchyma may be limited when systemic administration is utilized [67]. To overcome this challenge, medications may be directly administered into the CNS via the intracerebroventricular (IVT) or intrathecal (IT) routes. These routes of administration have been studied for a variety of medications including antimicrobials, thrombolytics, vasoactive agents, opioids, and non-opioid pain medications [68–73]. IVT or IT antimicrobial administration should be considered when there is failure to eliminate bacteria from the CSF after an appropriate course of systemic therapy. Additionally, potentially seeded hardware should be removed either prior to or with the use of IVT or IT therapy [74].

When assessing a medication for IVT or IT administration, the physiochemical properties of the medication must be carefully assessed to maintain medication efficacy while increasing safety and tolerability. First, drug volume is important as an increase in cerebrospinal fluid (CSF) volume caused by direct injection of medication can cause an elevation in intracranial pressure (ICP) and decrease tolerability. In general, small volumes of <3 mL injected slowly appear to be safe [75]. If larger volumes are required or if there is a concern for increased ICP, an equal volume of CSF may be removed prior to medication administration. Next, pH should be examined as CSF does not have the ability to buffer exogenous substances. Medications with a pH similar to the CSF, 7.27–7.37, may be better tolerated and reduce neuronal injury [75]. Osmolarity should also be considered with isotonic medications (230–330 mOsm/L) preferentially utilized to minimize adverse effects [75]. Finally, preservatives present in medication formulations and intrinsic toxicity must be assessed. Ideally, preservative-free medication formulations should be utilized, however if preservative-free formulations are not available, neurotoxicity and CNS adverse effects must be considered (Table 51.4) [75, 76]. CNS adverse effects from the medication compound themselves must also be reviewed. For example, IVT and IT administration of beta-lactams, including carbapenems and cephalosporins, should not be pursued due to the epileptogenic risk of the compound itself [73, 75].

Once an appropriate medication is secured, access to administer the medication must be obtained. Various routes and methods of administration include direct injection or placement of a temporary or permanent catheter [75]. If repeated doses are required, a temporary or permanent device may be beneficial to minimize complications from repeated direct injection into the cerebral space. A common temporary catheter for administration into the lateral ventricles is an external ventricular device (EVD). After administration of a medication into an EVD, the drain should be clamped for at least 15 min, but ideally 30 min, to ensure appropriate medication exposure [74].

A variety of antimicrobial medications have been studied for administration via the IVT or IT route. Common medications and doses can be found in Table 51.5. Of these medications, the most utilized are vancomycin and aminoglycosides due to the poor CNS penetration from systemic therapy [75]. IVT or IT vancomycin has a reported efficacy of 66–95% for the treatment of Gram-positive infections with limited adverse effects [77–79]. In studies, mild reactions included CSF eosinophilia, headache, and CSF leukocytosis. However, it is difficult to determine if these are due to the underlying disease process or medication administration [77, 80–82]. Administration of systemic vancomycin, in combination with IVT or IT therapy, should be utilized to slow vancomycin diffusion out of the CSF [81]. For severe Gram-negative infections, aminoglycosides may be necessary. Systemic administration of gentamicin, tobramycin, and amikacin results in limited CSF concentrations leading to a lack of efficacy in treating CNS infections [75, 83]. IVT therapy has a reported efficacy of 31–86% for the treatment of Gram-negative meningitis or ventriculitis [83, 84]. When IVT or IT therapy is utilized, it is important to monitor for seizures, as aminoglycosides have a high epileptogenic potential [85]. Of note, tobramycin may be less epileptogenic than gentamicin. Other adverse effects common with systemic administration, including nephrotoxicity and ototoxicity, are not present [83]. Other antimicrobials, including colistin and daptomycin, may be

Table 51.4 Common preservatives/additives and associated CNS adverse effects [75]

Preservative/additive	Potential CNS adverse effects
Benzethonium chloride	None reported
Benzyl alcohol	Metabolic acidosis, cerebral palsy
Chlorobutanol	Neurotoxicity
Ethylenediaminetetraacetic acid (EDTA)	Seizures
Propylene glycol	None reported
Sodium metabisulfite	Seizures

Table 51.5 Recommended dosages of common IT or IVT antimicrobials per Infectious Diseases Society of America [74]

Medication	Common adult IT/IVT doses
Amikacin	5–50 mg, usual 30 mg every 24 h
Amphotericin B deoxycholate	0.5 mg every 24 h
Colistin	10 mg every 24 h
Daptomycin	5–10 mg every 24–72 h[a]
Gentamicin	1–8 mg every 24 h[b,c]
Tobramycin	5–20 mg every 24 h
Vancomycin	5–20 mg every 24 h[b,c]

[a]Various dosing recommendations available including daptomycin 5 mg every 24 h, daptomycin 10 mg every 24 h for 48 h followed by daptomycin 10 mg every 72 h, and daptomycin 5–10 mg every 72 h. After 72 h, accumulation in the CSF can occur when utilizing every 24-h regimens, which may increase toxicity. Recommend infectious diseases consultation for patient-specific dosing recommendations

[b]Dose may vary based on ventricle size: Slit ventricles—vancomycin 5 mg OR gentamicin 2 mg, normal ventricles—vancomycin 10 mg OR gentamicin 3 mg, enlarged ventricles—vancomycin 15–20 mg OR gentamicin 4–5 mg

[c]If EVD present, frequency may vary based on EVD output over 24 h: <50 mL/24 h—every 72 h, 50–100 mL/24 h—every 48 h, 100–150 mL/24 h—every 24 h, 150–200 mL/24 h—every 24 h and increase the dose of vancomycin by 5 mg OR increase the dose of gentamicin by 1 mg, >200 mL/24 h—every 24 h and increase the dose of vancomycin by 10 mg OR increase the dose of gentamicin by 2 mg

administered IVT or IT for multi-drug-resistant organisms due to poor CSF penetration when administered systemically [73–75].

When administering systemic vancomycin or aminoglycosides, TDM is utilized to ensure the safety and efficacy of the therapy. Unfortunately, there are not well-defined monitoring parameters for IVT or IT administration of these medications. When systemic therapy is administered, standard TDM should be utilized. Duration of therapy is overall dependent on infection type. The patient should be carefully monitored for clinical response, CSF improvement, and bacteriologic response. In general, a treatment duration of at least 7–21 days is utilized [74, 79]. Infectious diseases specialist consultation is recommended for assistance with determining a treatment duration in severe or refractory cases.

51.4.2 *Intraperitoneal Antibiotics*

Intraperitoneal (IP) antibiotics are administered directly into the peritoneal cavity, the space between the walls of the abdominopelvic cavity and the abdominal organs. By administration into the peritoneum through a peritoneal dialysis (PD) catheter, antibiotics are delivered directly to the site of infection. The IP route of administration has been associated with reduced treatment failure compared to IV antibiotics for PD catheter-associated peritonitis, likely due to higher concentrations in the peritoneal fluid [86]. IP administration has also been associated with trends towards fewer adverse effects compared to IV administration, likely due to lower systemic antibiotic concentrations [86, 87]. Practically, IP antibiotics allow for administration outside of the hospital, allowing for potential discharge prior to completion of an antibiotic course [88]. Due to these advantages, the International Society for Peritoneal Dialysis (ISPD) Peritonitis Guidelines recommend IP administration as the preferred route of antibiotics for PD catheter-associated peritonitis [89].

IP antibiotics can be administered intermittently (with one exchange daily and at least 6 h of dwell time) or continuously with each exchange of dialysis solution [90]. It is important to note that IP antibiotics are not recommended for other types of peritonitis including spontaneous bacterial peritonitis (SBP) and secondary peritonitis [91, 92]. Additionally, if the IP route or drug preparation is not readily accessible, IV antibiotics should be given temporarily to avoid delays in antibiotic administration [89].

When administering antibiotics intraperitoneally, consideration should be given to the compatibility and stability of the antimicrobial in the dialysate solution [90]. Traditional dextrose-based and icodextrin-based PD solutions have compatibility data with common antibiotics published in the ISPD Guidelines [89]. However, newer PD solutions like neutral-pH and low-glucose degradation products (GDP) have less information published regarding compatibility with specific antimicrobials. Compatibility data cannot be extrapolated between antibiotics or between PD solutions, so it is important to verify that the desired antibiotic is stable in the desired PD solution [88, 93]. It is also important to consider the type of PD being performed. Antibiotic dosing recommendations are primarily based upon use in continuous ambulatory peritoneal dialysis (CAPD). There are a paucity of data on dosing in Automated Peritoneal Dialysis (APD) and recommendations should not be extrapolated from CAPD literature [89]. Patients on APD may have greater clearance of antibiotics, so there is a risk of under-dosing if CAPD dosing is used while on APD. If data for APD dosing for the desired antibiotic is not available, it is recommended to temporarily switch to CAPD for the duration of antibiotic treatment [89]. If converting peritoneal dialysis strategies is not feasible, it is critical to use antibiotics and dosing that have been studied with APD such as cefazolin, ceftazidime, meropenem, and vancomycin [94, 95].

The most common pathogens causing PD-catheter-associated peritonitis worldwide are *Staphylococcus epidermidis*, other coagulase-negative staphylococci, and *Staphylococcus aureus* [96]. The incidence of Gram-negative PD-catheter-associated peritonitis is significantly lower but may be rising in certain parts of the world [97]. The ISPD Guidelines recommend empiric antibiotic coverage for both Gram-positive and Gram-negative organisms with a first-generation cephalosporin or vancomycin and a third-generation cephalosporin or an aminoglycoside, respectively [89]. The choice of antibiotic should consider patient-specific factors like allergies and PD type, as well as antibiotic-specific properties. For example, IP vancomycin is recommended to be given only once every 5–7 days due to slow clearance in patients on CAPD. Finally, certain antibiotics necessitate specific administration strategies to optimize their PK and safety profiles. ISPD recommends intermittent administration of aminoglycosides instead of continuous administration to optimize the concentration-dependent bactericidal properties and to minimize adverse effects like ototoxicity [89].

51.4.3   Intravitreal Antibiotics

Intravitreal antibiotics are administered by injection into the vitreous body in the eye. The vitreous body is a clear, gelatinous substance that fills the space between the retina and the lens [98]. Bacteria may invade this substance and cause endophthalmitis through exogenous sources like trauma and surgery, or less commonly endogenously through hematogenous spread from other sources in the body [98, 99]. Intravitreal administration of antibiotics is one of the mainstays of treatment for endophthalmitis due to improved penetration of the eye compared to systemic or topical antibiotics [98].

There are many physical and chemical barriers that prevent systemic and topical antibiotics from reaching the site of action in the eye [98]. Topical antibiotics are diluted in the intraocular space by the tear film, while systemic antibiotics are absorbed by the conjunctival capillaries and nasolacrimal mucosal surface resulting in lower concentrations at the site of action. Tight junctions of the corneal and retinal epithelium also limit topical drug absorption across these barriers. Intravitreal administration allows antibiotics to bypass these barriers by administration directly into the intravitreal body allowing free diffusion to the retinal surface [98].

While administration directly into the vitreous allows for improved bioavailability, there are several important considerations specific to both the eye and the antibiotic itself that may affect the PK. First, the hydrophilicity, the ionic nature, and the size of the antibiotic affect distribution and CL from the vitreous [98]. Cationic drugs (e.g., aminoglycosides and vancomycin) are cleared from the eye via passive diffusion. Anionic drugs (e.g., β-lactams) are cleared more rapidly via active transport resulting in shorter half-lives [100]. Similarly, lipophilic drugs are transported by passive diffusion while hydrophilic drugs are cleared more quickly via active transport (Table 51.1). Taken together, hydrophilic, anionic drugs are cleared from the vitreous quicker and often require repeat injections. Next, it is important to consider factors related to the eye itself. For example, antibiotics eliminated via passive diffusion across the anterior route are removed faster in an inflamed eye compared to a non-inflamed eye [101].

Empiric regimens typically consist of a Gram-negative agent like ceftazidime combined with a Gram-positive agent like vancomycin until a pathogen or source is identified. Gram-positive organisms are the most common cause of postoperative endophthalmitis and post-injection endophthalmitis [102]. In the Endophthalmitis Vitrectomy Study, a large randomized controlled trial performed in the United States including patients with post-cataract endophthalmitis, 70% of culture-positive infections were due to coagulase-negative staphylococci followed by 10% with *Staphylococcus aureus*, and 9% with *Streptococci* [103]. The bacterial etiologies of endogenous endophthalmitis vary by geographic location with Gram-positive organisms being the most common cause in developed countries and Gram-negative organisms being more common in Asian countries [99, 102]. Fungi also account for a significant number of cases of endogenous endophthalmitis necessitating intravitreal antifungals but are beyond the scope of this chapter [99].

Penicillin and aminoglycosides were the first antibiotics used for intraocular injection [98]. However, aminoglycosides increase the risk of macular infarction and retinal toxicity, so have fallen out of favor [104]. Since then, ceftazidime has been the preferred antibiotic for Gram-negative coverage; however, amikacin is still used in the setting of penicillin allergies. For Gram-positive coverage, vancomycin is the preferred option. While other agents active against resistant Gram-positive pathogens like daptomycin and linezolid have been studied, there is far less literature regarding the safety and efficacy of intravitreal administration [98, 105]. Dosing information for these agents can be found in Table 51.6.

The adjunctive use of systemic antibiotics is controversial and not well described in the literature. Concomitant systemic antibiotics should be used when the source of endophthalmitis is thought to be endogenous spread from other foci of infection [106]. However, the use of systemic antibiotics for exogenous sources of endophthalmitis is generally not recommended as there is no clear benefit and an increased risk of adverse effects [106].

In terms of frequency and administration, intravitreal antibiotics are typically given as one-time injections, which may be repeated if inflammation persists. Injections

Table 51.6 Recommended dosages of common intravitreal antibiotics[a]

Medication	Common adult intravitreal dose
Ceftazidime	2.25 mg/0.1 mL
Amikacin	0.4 mg/0.1 mL
Vancomycin	1.0 mg/0.1 mL

[a]Formal guidance on recommended dosing is lacking. Recommended dosing is based on primary literature and what is commonly used in practice [98]

are typically repeated at 48–72 h if the patient has not clinically improved, but the timeline for repeat doses varies by the antibiotic selected [98]. TDM to monitor systemic levels of medications in patients receiving intravitreal aminoglycosides or vancomycin is currently not recommended or part of usual practice. Preservative-free ingredients should be used to compound intravitreal injections as preservatives may be toxic to the eye [107]. Most intravitreal antibiotics are prepared immediately prior to use; however, extended stability and sterility up to 24 weeks has been documented in single-use polypropylene syringes [108]. Intravitreal antibiotics must be administered by trained personnel under sterile conditions [99, 109].

51.4.4   Inhaled Antibiotics

Inhaled antibiotics are delivered to the lungs via nebulizer or inhaler. Delivering antibiotics directly to the lower airways through inhalation results in higher concentrations at the site of action compared to systemically administered antibiotics [110]. Many systemic agents have poor penetration into the lungs resulting in low concentrations in the epithelial lining fluid compared to the serum [111]. Inhaled antibiotics not only maximize the concentration of the drug in the epithelial lining fluid, but also may spare adverse effects of systemic antibiotics since serum concentrations are reduced [112].

Inhaled antibiotics are used for several disease states including chronic infections in cystic fibrosis (CF), non-CF bronchiectasis, nontuberculous mycobacterial lung disease, treatment and prevention of ventilator-associated pneumonia (VAP), and chronic obstructive pulmonary disorder (COPD) [39, 113]. In patients with CF and persistent *P. aeruginosa* in respiratory cultures, inhaled tobramycin and amikacin are recommended to improve lung function and quality of life, and to reduce exacerbations [114]. While the literature is limited, inhaled antibiotics for non-CF bronchiectasis have been associated with a delay in exacerbations, a reduction in hospital admissions, and a reduction in the microbial count in sputum [115]. Practically, the use of inhaled antibiotics in place of systemic antibiotics for patients with chronic lung disease also allows for ease of administration in the outpatient setting. For patients with VAP, society guidelines recommend adding inhaled antibiotics as adjunct therapy for multi drug-resistant Gram-negative pathogens and to consider use in patients who are not responding to systemic treatment alone [116]. However, the use of inhaled antibiotics for VAP prevention in mechanically ventilated adults is controversial. Despite multiple meta-analyses showing a reduction in occurrence of VAP, they have not been associated with a reduction in mortality [117, 118]. Additionally, increasing antimicrobial resistance is a concern with the widespread use of prophylactic antibiotics. The recently published AMIKINHAL randomized controlled trial showed that 3 days of inhaled amikacin reduced rates of VAP in adults with prolonged ($\geq$72 h) mechanical ventilation courses [119]. These results may reignite the risk versus benefit conversation of prophylactic inhaled antibiotics for VAP. Finally, limited literature suggests that use of inhaled antibiotics in patients with COPD may decrease exacerbations, hospital admissions, and hospital length of stay [120].

Although inhaled antibiotics achieve significantly higher concentrations in the lungs compared to systemic antibiotics, they still face a variety of physical and chemical barriers to reaching the desired site of action [121]. The bronchial tree is a complex anatomical barrier lined with ciliary cells that make it difficult for the inhaled drug to reach the deep structures of the lungs. In addition, the mucus layer that lines the respiratory tract captures and removes foreign substances like inhaled antibiotics. The lungs also have proteolytic enzymes, surfactants, and alveolar macrophages that can inactivate or remove antibiotics from the lungs. Therefore, it is critical to optimize the delivery of inhaled antibiotics by proper use of nebulizers and inhalers. Vibrating mesh nebulizers are preferred over jet and ultrasonic nebulizers since they do not interfere with the ventilator, have low residual volumes, and are easiest to use [110]. Ideally, the heated humidifier would be turned off during inhaled antibiotic administration in mechanically ventilated patients to enhance drug delivery, and the ventilator would be set to low inspiratory flow and increased inspiratory time [110]. Some of the major studies of inhaled antibiotics for treatment of VAP did not modify ventilator settings during administration, which may have contributed to their negative findings [122, 123].

Reports of aerosolizing antibiotics were published as early as the 1940s [124]. However, early use of inhaled antibiotics was limited by the lack of advanced nebulizer delivery devices and patients' inability to tolerate the drugs. Early inhaled antibiotics were nebulized IV solutions designed for parenteral administration, so they were highly irritating to patients due to the preservatives and hyperosmolarity. In 1997, inhaled tobramycin was approved marking the first antibiotic solution specifically designed for inhalation [125]. Since then, several antibiotic inhalation solutions and dry powders have been approved including amikacin, colistin, aztreonam, levofloxacin, ciprofloxacin, amphotericin B, and combinations of fosfomycin and an aminoglycoside [113]. The most common adverse effects of inhaled antibiotics include bronchospasm, throat irritation, cough, abnormal taste, and changes in hearing. While systemic concentrations are minimized with inhaled antibiotic delivery, serum concentrations may still be detectable [126]. Therefore, it is critical to also monitor for systemic adverse effects in patients on inhaled antibiotics such as nephrotoxicity and ototoxicity in patients receiving aminoglycosides. Monitoring serum trough concentrations may be considered to assess for systemic accumulation in the setting of suspected toxicity or in patient groups with higher risks of accumulation such as those with renal dysfunction [126].

51.4.5 Antibiotic Lock Therapy

Long-term intravascular catheters pose several risks including thrombosis, placement-related complications (pneumothorax, air embolism, arrhythmias, arterial injuries), and infection; however, these catheters are often necessary for administration of medications, parenteral nutrition, or hemodialysis [127]. Antibiotic lock therapy (ALT) is a method utilized for the treatment and prevention of catheter-related blood stream infections (CRBSI), a significant contributor to morbidity and mortality in the critically ill [109, 128]. Though central venous catheter removal remains a mainstay of therapy in CRBSI, especially in *Staphylococcus aureus,* resistant Gram-negative, or fungal infections, line removal may result in loss of a patient's only reliable vascular access [129]. ALT involves the installation of an antimicrobial or antiseptic agent, typically combined with an anticoagulant, into the catheter lumen and allowing it to dwell to kill pathogens [130]. Utilizing this method, significantly higher concentrations of antibiotics may be used to sterilize the catheter while limiting the risks of systemic toxicity. Despite the potential benefits of lock therapy, there are several considerations pertaining to appropriate patient selection and the logistics behind its use.

Use of ALT is supported by available clinical practice guidelines for prophylactic and treatment purposes in select patient populations [129, 131]. The Center for Disease Control Guidelines for the Prevention of Intravascular Catheter-Related Infections endorse use of prophylactic ALT in patients with recurrent CRBSI despite optimal use of aseptic technique [131]. Available literature supporting prophylactic ALT primarily highlights use in hemodialysis patients, however, it also encompasses oncology and neonatal patients [132–135]. These studies compared ALT using various antimicrobial agents to controls or heparin lock solutions alone. Overall, these results largely support ALT as an effective method for CRBSI prevention. One of the largest available meta-analyses inclusive of multiple patient populations included 23 studies with 2896 patients and 383,710 catheter days [136]. Prophylactic ALT significantly reduced the rate of CRBSI (RR 0.31, 95% CI 0.24–0.4), and these results were demonstrated with both antimicrobial and non-antimicrobial lock solutions. Though data for ALT in the adult critically ill population are lacking, it may be reasonable to extrapolate these data as a CRBSI prevention measure in centers with the appropriate resources.

The IDSA Guidelines for the Diagnosis and Management of Intravascular Catheter-Related Infections endorse ALT for catheter salvage in uncomplicated CRBSI (defined as infection without metastatic seeding, endocarditis, osteomyelitis, or suppurative thrombophlebitis) caused by organisms other than *Staphylococcus aureus, P. aeruginosa, Micrococcus* species, *Bacillus* species, fungi, or mycobacteria without signs or symptoms of exit or tunnel infection [129]. ALT is administered for 7–14 days with concomitant systemic antibiotics. If ALT cannot be administered, it is recommended to attempt treatment with systemic antimicrobials and ensure they are administered through the catheter suspected to be colonized. Studies assessing the impact of ALT on the rates of catheter removal and treatment success are small, heterogeneous, and primarily observational with variable results [137–139]. However, a meta-analysis including eight studies and 396 patients comparing ALT with systemic antimicrobial therapy to systemic antimicrobial therapy alone or alternative catheter salvage methods, such as guidewire exchange, found reduced rates of catheter replacement with ALT use (OR 0.20, 95% CI 0.10–0.39) [137]. There was no statistically significant difference in the rate of infection relapse between groups. Despite a lack of large, randomized controlled trials evaluating the use of ALT, it remains a viable option for CRBSI prevention and treatment given the potential detriment posed by the loss of long-term intravascular access.

To successfully utilize ALT for the aforementioned indications, suitable lock solutions must be selected. As mentioned previously, significantly higher concentrations of antimicrobials may be safely utilized in lock solutions with the aim to penetrate biofilms formed on the catheter. Biofilm formation is an adaptive resistance mechanism for a variety of strains of bacteria and may increase the MIC of antimicrobials by up to 1000-fold [140]. Furthermore, different antimicrobial agents penetrate biofilms at varying degrees. Rifamycins and fluoroquinolones have excellent penetration, beta-lactams and vancomycin have variable penetration, and aminoglycosides weakly penetrate biofilms [140–144]. For adequate biofilm penetration, solutions are typically prepared at 100–1000 times the standard concentration. In addition to biofilm formation, other resistance mechanisms such as efflux pumps, β-lactamases, or other inducible resistance mechanisms may also impact antimicrobial susceptibility [140]. Given these considerations, the ALT agent utilized should be selected based on available individual or institutional susceptibility data. In addition to susceptibility, pharmacokinetic properties of certain antimicrobials may make them more favorable options for ALT. For example, aminoglycosides and fluoroquinolones possess concentration-dependent killing and post-antibiotic effect [145]. Because of these properties, they may not require extended dwell times to be efficacious. Conversely, β-lactams and vancomycin possess time-dependent killing and therefore may require extended dwell times at concentrations above the MIC to be efficacious [145].

Antimicrobial agents utilized in lock solutions are also typically compounded with an anticoagulant, such as heparin; therefore, compatibility must be considered [140]. It is thought that the addition of heparin, or another anticoagulant, to the lock solution prevents fibrin deposition on the catheter to which organisms may adhere [145]. Similarly, agents such as EDTA and citrate may also be added to lock solutions in an effort to maintain catheter patency and disrupt biofilm formation [140]. To successfully implement ALT protocols, institutions must consider prolonged stability of the solutions and the ability to prepare bulk solutions to facilitate continuation of care.

As with systemic antimicrobial therapy, the potential adverse effects of selected lock agents must also be considered. Practitioners should be aware of potential allergies and contraindications to medications included within the lock solution. For example, a patient with a history of heparin-induced thrombocytopenia likely should not receive a lock solution containing heparin [145]. Though the small volume of these agents instilled into the catheter lumen is unlikely to cause systemic toxicity, there have been reports of adverse effects. In 2002, a case report was published detailing an end-stage renal disease patient receiving an amikacin lock solution that was noted to develop irreversible hearing loss after several months of therapy, a side effect of high-dose aminoglycoside exposure [146]. Furthermore, the risk of inadvertent injection of a lock solution, rather than aspiration of the catheter lumen after the dwell time is complete, may expose patients to high concentrations of both antimicrobials and anticoagulants. In 2000, 46.7% citrate was voluntarily recalled in the United States due to a case of a patient experiencing cardiac arrest after inadvertently receiving it as an injection through a hemodialysis catheter [147]. The arrest was presumed to be secondary to hypocalcemia, a direct effect of the injection of concentrated citrate.

These reports demonstrate that education is crucial to successfully implementing an ALT protocol and avoiding inadvertent medication errors. Several hospitals have published their protocols, which outline the general steps for administration. If the volume of the catheter lumen is unknown, sterile saline may be flushed into the catheter then aspirated until blood return is noted. The volume of saline aspirated into the syringe corresponds to the volume of the lumen. Based on the volume of the catheter lumen, appropriate volumes of lock solution are then instilled into the catheter and the catheter is then clamped. Lumens are then labeled to indicate the presence of ALT and the date and time it was instilled and left to dwell for a pre-specified period. Dwell times are variable depending on stability of the instilled agents and need to access the catheter for other systemic therapies; however, the IDSA guidelines recommend a maximum dwell time of 48 h [129, 140]. Once the dwell is complete, the solution should be withdrawn from the catheter, the catheter should be flushed, and the label may be removed [148].

In addition to adverse effects, antimicrobial resistance is a common concern leading to hesitation with widespread implementation of ALT. Limited data exist detailing the impacts of long-term ALT use on antimicrobial resistance. A retrospective chart review of 1410 chronic hemodialysis patients who received ALT with gentamicin and heparin for CRBSI prophylaxis noted that 100% of *Staphylococcus epidermidis* strains colonizing catheter lumens were resistant to gentamicin, fluoroquinolones, and methicillin after 2 years of use [149]. Two years after discontinuing the gentamicin and heparin lock solution, the rates of resistance were significantly reduced. Another study compared 662 hemodialysis patients treated for CRBSI with gentamicin and vancomycin lock therapy, in addition to systemic antibiotics, to a historical control of 265 patients and did not find a difference in rates of resistance for Gram-positive organisms [150]. They did, however, observe increased rates of gentamicin resistance in *Enterobacter* species. Data describing the rates of resistance with ALT are limited; however, as with systemic therapy, overuse of antimicrobial agents may portend increased rates of resistance and therefore reduced efficacy.

To curtail the potential for resistance, some institutions have implemented the use of antiseptic lock solutions, such as ethanol. Ethanol possesses a broad antimicrobial spectrum and is not known to be affected by resistance [151]. Limitations with ethanol lock solutions mirror that of other lock solutions, including toxicity with inadvertent injection, especially in neonates [152, 153]. An additional consideration, however, is potential incompatibility with the materials the catheter is comprised of and may cause substances like polyurethane to leech from the catheter [154]. Given that this incompatibility may also compromise the catheter, it is pertinent to ensure that patients' catheters are made of material amenable to use with ethanol locks.

In summary, antimicrobials may be administered via many unique routes with the goal of optimizing both efficacy and safety through increasing exposure at the site of infection and decreasing systemic exposure and adverse effects. Each route requires careful consideration of drug properties and physiology, a role in which pharmacists are uniquely positioned to manage.

51.5 Antimicrobial Stewardship

Antimicrobial stewardship is defined as "a multidisciplinary and coordinated intervention designed to improve and measure the appropriate use of antimicrobial agents and to promote the selection of optimal antimicrobial drug regimen, including dosing, duration, and route of administration" [36]. The goal of antimicrobial stewardship is to optimize clinical outcomes while minimizing unintended consequences of antimicrobial use, which include the emergence of antimicrobial resistance and adverse drug reactions [36]. Minimizing antimicrobial resistance by optimizing therapy should lead to measurable benefits at the patient level because studies have shown the negative effects of antimicrobial resistance on several clinical outcomes. In addition, decreasing the costs associated with antimicrobial use should reduce the overall costs associated with treatment.

Core members of a multidisciplinary antimicrobial stewardship team are an infectious diseases physician, a clinical pharmacist, a clinical microbiologist, an information systems specialist, an infection control professional, and a hospital epidemiologist. The critical care pharmacist is well positioned to provide guidance on antimicrobial therapy, including expedited selection of appropriate initial agents, aggressive dosing to optimize PD, interpretation of microbiologic evidence, appropriate de-escalation of antimicrobials, monitoring of response and potential adverse effects, and determination of appropriate treatment duration. Critical care pharmacists could either have formal or informal roles on the antimicrobial stewardship team. They can complete core activities through official pathways or everyday clinical interventions including education with active intervention, guideline and clinical pathway development, streamlining or de-escalation of therapy, dose optimization, and parenteral to oral conversion [36].

Stewardship strategies include prospective audit with intervention and feedback (i.e., "back end" strategy) and formulary restriction and preauthorization (i.e., "front end" strategy). Prospective audit with intervention and feedback allows flexibility and minimizes delay in administering therapy. Formulary restriction and preauthorization may be resource intensive; however, initial choices of antimicrobials may be optimized through consultation with infectious diseases experts. Another formulary restriction method is antimicrobial cycling in which there is a scheduled removal and substitution of a specific antimicrobial or an antimicrobial class in an effort to reduce antimicrobial selection pressure. Evidence is insufficient to suggest that antimicrobial cycling strategies are effective and IDSA guidelines recommend against its use. Regardless of the strategies used, programmatic antimicrobial stewardship is not a substitute for clinical judgment. When assessing program success, process indicators such as days of therapy and time to effective therapy, as well as outcome measures such length of stay and mortality, should be utilized.

Studies evaluating antimicrobial stewardship in critically ill patients have been limited by poor study design; however, most studies have reported a decreased use in either antibiotics overall or a targeted class of antibiotics. Some studies have also reported a decrease in key resistance rates. Meta-analyses of before-after studies evaluating direct audit and feedback to ICU patients receiving antibiotics found no increase in mortality, suggesting this could be safely implemented in critically ill patients [155, 156].

51.6 Rapid Diagnostic Tests

Rapid diagnostic tests can be used as an antimicrobial stewardship tool by assisting with de-escalation efforts. In many cases, the implementation of rapid diagnostic tests may be cost neutral or even constitute a cost savings when decreased consumption of antibiotics occurs. Rapid diagnostic tests are recommended by the IDSA to be used in combination with stewardship teams to optimize antibiotic therapy and improve clinical outcomes.

Each of the tests that will be discussed attempts to shorten the time from blood culture positivity to species identification or susceptibility testing. Traditional pathogen identification and susceptibility testing can take 72–96 h. Early pathogen identification techniques seek to provide clinically actionable information within the first 24 h from the time of culture positivity. Most of these techniques, when combined with antibiotic stewardship efforts, lead to significant reductions in health care costs and improvement in clinical outcomes in relevant studies [157, 158]. Many of these studies were conducted in single centers, which make external validity questionable. The overall impact of the implementation of rapid diagnostic tests in a single institution is determined by several factors: epidemiology of targeted organism, presence and actions of existing antimicrobial stewardship teams, current clinical prescribing patterns, and patient populations.

Overall, the inability to detect polymicrobial infections is a common limitation to most of the tests described. Newer methods using whole blood have been developed which allow for identification of bacteria in patients with recent or current antibiotic exposure (i.e., LightCycler, SeptiFast, SepsiTest). Some technology has been developed for respiratory cultures, but the clinical adaption is considerably less than that for blood cultures. In the setting of sepsis, the ideal rapid diagnostic should provide quick and reliable results, have low detection limits, high-throughput testing, and identify organism and/or resistance directly from a clinical specimen [159]. This section will review the benefits and limitations of several rapid diagnostic tests that aim to improve clinical outcomes and reduce delay to appropriate antimicrobial therapy.

51.6.1   In Situ Hybridization-Based Methods

Peptic nucleic acid (PNA) fluorescent in situ hybridization.

PNA FISH targets species specific ribosomal RNA from positive blood cultures. It has a sensitivity and specificity of 96–100% [160, 161]. Currently available FISH products are only used for species identification. Clinically, PNA FISH could be utilized to separate *S. aureus* from possible skin flora contamination of coagulase-negative *Staphylococcus*, differentiate *Enterococcus faecium* from *Enterococcus faecalis*, identify fluconazole sensitive *Candida* species, and detect *Pseudomonas* from non-*Pseudomonas* Gram-negative species.

51.6.2   Mass Spectroscopy: Matrix-Assisted Desorption-Ionization/Time of Flight (MALDI-TOF)

This test serves to identify isolated colonies of bacteria and fungi. Mass spectroscopy is compared with library standards for identifying pathogen species and/or resistant mechanisms. It is an analytic technique whereby samples are ionized that produces a mass spectrogram for the sample [160–162]. Each sample has a unique mass spectrogram which can be matched to a library of reference standards for identification. It has a sensitivity and specificity of 98–100%. Similar to PNA FISH, no antimicrobial susceptibility is reported; however, this technology can detect genes that encode resistance. This method cannot be used for polymicrobial cultures, and no library is available for unusual organisms, although pathogen libraries are constantly being updated.

51.6.3   Magnetic Resonance Based-Methods

The T2 platform analyzes whole blood samples, mechanically lyses cells, and uses PCR primers to amplify target DNA sequences. Following hybridization, species level identification is possible, including *Candida* and bacterial detection [159]. It is important to note that blood cultures are still necessary to identify the specific organism. The bacterial panel identifies six pathogens, *Enterococcus faecium*,

S. aureus, Klebsiella pneumoniae, Acinetobacter baumannii, P. aeruginosa, and *E. coli*, and has displayed sensitivities and specificities >90%.

51.7   Future Directions

Antimicrobial resistance is a global threat that is continually evolving, necessitating continued innovation and development of new treatment strategies [163, 164]. Infections caused by antimicrobial-resistant infections have caused over 700,000 deaths worldwide, and it is predicted that this number could increase to over ten million deaths by 2050 [164]. In the critically ill, multi-drug-resistant organisms are known to be associated with increased mortality, primarily due to delays in appropriate therapy [165–168]. Given the imminent threat to public health worldwide, international organizations, including the World Health Organization, routinely monitor rates of antimicrobial resistance and the innovation of pipeline antimicrobial agents [169, 170]. Continued development of new antimicrobial agents and further research into more novel therapies, such as monoclonal antibodies, will prove to be necessary as resistance emerges to readily available therapies.

Several novel antibiotics have emerged in response to the ever-increasing prevalence of multi-drug resistant organisms, particularly Gram negatives [171, 172]. The World Health Organization continues to cite Gram-negative pathogens as a major concern, particularly carbapenem-resistant *Enterobacterales* and carbapenem and aminoglycoside-resistant strains of *Acinetobacter* species [170]. To combat resistance mechanisms, such as carbapenemases and metallo-β-lactamases (MBLs) [148], novel β-lactam and β-lactamase inhibitor (BLBI) combinations have been developed [172]. For example, the addition of zidebactam to cefepime, an agent routinely used in critically ill patients, extends the spectrum of activity to include extended spectrum β-lactamases, MBLs, *Klebsiella pneumoniae* carbapenemases, and OXA-48-like carbapenemases [172–174]. Currently, this agent is only available for compassionate use; however, it has demonstrated promising outcomes in case reports [175, 176].

Arbekacin, an aminoglycoside, is an additional example of a novel antimicrobial with an extended spectrum of activity encompassing both resistant Gram-negatives and MRSA [177]. This agent is not impacted by aminoglycoside-inactivating enzymes, therefore, conferring MRSA susceptibility and extending its spectrum to gentamicin-resistant *Enterococci,* and multi-drug-resistant strains of *P. aeruginosa and Acinetobacter baumannii* [177]. Furthermore, it has a longer post-antibiotic effect when compared to vancomycin [178]. Arbekacin has been available in Japan since 1990 and in Korea since 2000 [177]. Because arbekacin shares the adverse effect of nephrotoxicity with the rest of the aminoglycoside class, and there are many available anti-MRSA agents, arbekacin has yet to be widely adopted across other areas of the world [179, 180]. These agents, along with many other novel antimicrobials in the pipeline, highlight ongoing innovation as the world continues to fight the threat of antimicrobial resistance.

Monoclonal antibodies (mAbs) are routinely prescribed for a variety of conditions including rheumatologic conditions, malignancies, solid organ transplants, and many others. Given the variety of applications for mAbs, extending their role in the treatment or prevention of infections continues to be explored [172]. mABs may target multiple bacterial processes including binding to toxins or molecules released by the organism, cell-surface components, or interfering with the structure of encapsulated bacteria [172, 181]. There are currently three mAbs approved by the US Food and Drug Administration for use in bacterial infections: raxibacumab (Abthrax®), obiltoxaximab (Anthim®), and bezlotoxumab (Zinplava®) [182]. These agents exert their effects by neutralizing endotoxins produced by *Bacillus anthracis* (raxibacumab and obiltoxaximab) and *Clostridioides difficile* (bezlotoxumab). mAbs targeting commonly encountered nosocomial pathogens, including *Staphylococcus aureus* and *P. aeruginosa,* are currently being evaluated in clinical and pre-clinical research.

MRSA is a common nosocomial pathogen in critically ill patients with over 10% of patients in the ICU being colonized with the organism [183]. Given its propensity to cause a variety of infections, several mAbs have been developed with a variety of targets including toxins secreted by the organism, lipoteichoic acid (a cell wall component), microbial surface components recognizing adhesive matrix molecules (MSCRAMM), and quorum sensing peptide [184–187]. Suvratoxumab targets a toxin that causes pore formation leading to death of endothelial cells and leukocytes, bacterial spread, disruption tissues, and dysregulated the host immune response [188, 189]. Antibodies targeting MSCRAMM serve as a promising target for mAbs as these proteins are responsible for adhering to host tissues or artificial materials such as prosthetic joints or catheters [184, 187, 190, 191]. Once the MSCRAMM targeting mAb is bound to the cell wall of the *Staphylococci*, they also facilitate opsonophagocytosis, clearing the organism [107, 184, 192]. Though many mAbs targeting *Staphylococcus aureus* have been or are currently being studied, there are not currently any agents approved for use.

Like *Staphylococcus aureus, P. aeruginosa* is a common colonizer, cause of infection in critically ill patients, and potential target for mAb therapy [193, 194]. A unique target for *P. aeruginosa* is the PcrV protein, which is implicated in pore formation on host cell membranes [195, 196]. Because this gene has been demonstrated to be present on over 90% of isolates, PcrV-targeting therapies have potential to provide broad coverage against multiple *P. aeruginosa* strains [196]. The EVADE Trial recently evaluated gremubamab for the prevention of ventilator-associated pneumonia (VAP) caused by *P. aeruginosa* in colonized adults [197]. Gremubamab targets the PcrV protein as well as Psl, a key component of biofilm formation [197]. There was no difference in the incidence of *P. aeruginosa;* however, the study was terminated early due to slow enrollment and therefore, likely underpowered [197]. Though mAb therapy is an appealing treatment option for bacterial infections given they are less prone to resistance and have more specific targets, further clinical trial data are warranted before routine adoption of this strategy can occur [198].

Novel antimicrobials, including new antibiotic drugs and mAbs, are essential to continuing to combat antimicrobial resistance, a leading cause of death worldwide

[199]. If antimicrobial resistance is not contained, it is expected that high-income countries may sustain 2.4 million deaths between the years 2015 and 2050 [164]. Development of new antimicrobials, however, largely provides a reactive strategy. Without further infrastructure and incentives for development, innovation of new antimicrobial agents is likely to halt [200]. Therefore, it is essential for practitioners to make daily efforts to be good antimicrobial stewards and protect the efficacy of widely available agents.

51.8   Conclusion

Given the importance of appropriate antimicrobial therapy in the critically ill, pharmacists caring for these patients should be well equipped with strategies to facilitate optimal administration of these agents. Due to their alterations in PK/PD and severity of illness, this feat can often prove to be challenging. Furthermore, antimicrobial resistance is, and will continue to be, a threat to public health worldwide. Leveraging knowledge of individual drug properties, PK/PD, appropriate TDM, and other tools discussed within this chapter is pertinent to maximize efficacy and combat negative consequences of antibiotic misuse.

References

1. Kumar A, Roberts D, Wood KE, et al. Duration of hypotension before initiation of effective antimicrobial therapy is the critical determinant of survival in human septic shock. Crit Care Med. 2006;34(6):1589–96.
2. Ferrer R, Martin-Loeches I, Phillips G, et al. Empiric antibiotic treatment reduces mortality in severe sepsis and septic shock from the first hour: results from a guideline-based performance improvement program. Crit Care Med. 2014;42(8):1749–55.
3. Im Y, Kang D, Ko RE, et al. Time-to-antibiotics and clinical outcomes in patients with sepsis and septic shock: a prospective nationwide multicenter cohort study. Crit Care. 2022;26(1):19.
4. Liu VX, Fielding-Singh V, Greene JD, et al. The timing of early antibiotics and hospital mortality in sepsis. Am J Respir Crit Care Med. 2017;196(7):856–63.
5. Evans L, Rhodes A, Alhazzani W, et al. Surviving sepsis campaign: international guidelines for management of sepsis and septic shock 2021. Crit Care Med. 2021;49(11):e1063–143.
6. McKinnon PA, Yu VL. Pharmacologic considerations in antimicrobial therapy, with emphasis on pharmacokinetics and pharmacodynamics: reviews for the practicing clinician. Eur J Clin Microbiol Infect Dis. 2004;23(4):231–2.
7. Roberts JA, Lipman J. Pharmacokinetic issues for antibiotics in the critically ill patient. Crit Care Med. 2009;37(3):840–51.
8. Hoste EA, Kellum JA. RIFLE criteria provide robust assessment of kidney dysfunction and correlate with hospital mortality. Crit Care Med. 2006;34(7):2016–7.
9. Piccinni P, Cruz DN, Gramaticopolo S, et al. Prospective multicenter study on epidemiology of acute kidney injury in the ICU: a critical care nephrology Italian collaborative effort (NEFROINT). Minerva Anestesiol. 2011;77(11):1072–83.
10. Sun H, Frassetto L, Benet LZ. Effects of renal failure on drug transport and metabolism. Pharmacol Ther. 2006;109(1–2):1–11.

11. Muilwijk EW, de Lange DW, Schouten JA, et al. Suboptimal dosing of fluconazole in critically ill patients: time to rethink dosing. Antimicrob Agents Chemother. 2020;64(10):e00984–20.
12. Patel K, Roberts JA, Lipman J, et al. Population pharmacokinetics of fluconazole in critically ill patients receiving continuous venovenous hemodiafiltration: using Monte Carlo simulations to predict doses for specified pharmacodynamic targets. Antimicrob Agents Chemother. 2011;55(12):5868–73.
13. Cook AM, Hatton-Kolpek J. Augmented renal clearance. Pharmacotherapy. 2019;39(3):346–54.
14. Barletta JF, Mangram AJ, Byrne M, et al. Identifying augmented renal clearance in trauma patients: validation of the augmented renal clearance in trauma intensive care scoring system. J Trauma Acute Care Surg. 2017;82(4):665–71.
15. Udy AA, Roberts JA, Lipman J. Clinical implications of antibiotic pharmacokinetic principles in the critically ill. Intensive Care Med. 2013;39(12):2070–82.
16. Chen IH, Nicolau DP. Augmented renal clearance and how to augment antibiotic dosing. Antibiotics (Basel). 2020;9(7):393.
17. Wong WT, Choi G, Gomersall CD, et al. To increase or decrease dosage of antimicrobials in septic patients during continuous renal replacement therapy: the eternal doubt. Curr Opin Pharmacol. 2015;24:68–78.
18. Bugge JF. Pharmacokinetics and drug dosing adjustments during continuous venovenous hemofiltration or hemodiafiltration in critically ill patients. Acta Anaesthesiol Scand. 2001;45(8):929–34.
19. Awdishu L, Bouchard J. How to optimize drug delivery in renal replacement therapy. Semin Dial. 2011;24(2):176–82.
20. Bouman CS. Antimicrobial dosing strategies in critically ill patients with acute kidney injury and high-dose continuous veno-venous hemofiltration. Curr Opin Crit Care. 2008;14(6):654–9.
21. Choi G, Gomersall CD, Tian Q, et al. Principles of antibacterial dosing in continuous renal replacement therapy. Crit Care Med. 2009;37(7):2268–82.
22. Gomez F, Veita J, Laudanski K. Antibiotics and ECMO in the adult population-persistent challenges and practical guides. Antibiotics (Basel). 2022;11(3):338.
23. Sherwin J, Heath T, Watt K. Pharmacokinetics and dosing of anti-infective drugs in patients on extracorporeal membrane oxygenation: a review of the current literature. Clin Ther. 2016;38(9):1976–94.
24. Buck ML. Pharmacokinetic changes during extracorporeal membrane oxygenation: implications for drug therapy of neonates. Clin Pharmacokinet. 2003;42(5):403–17.
25. Shekar K, Fraser JF, Smith MT, et al. Pharmacokinetic changes in patients receiving extracorporeal membrane oxygenation. J Crit Care. 2012;27(6):741.e9–18.
26. Hahn J, Choi JH, Chang MJ. Pharmacokinetic changes of antibiotic, antiviral, antituberculosis and antifungal agents during extracorporeal membrane oxygenation in critically ill adult patients. J Clin Pharm Ther. 2017;42(6):661–71.
27. Craig WA. Pharmacokinetic/pharmacodynamic parameters: rationale for antibacterial dosing of mice and men. Clin Infect Dis. 1998;26(1):1–10.
28. Denny KJ, Cotta MO, Parker SL, et al. The use and risks of antibiotics in critically ill patients. Expert Opin Drug Saf. 2016;15(5):667–78.
29. Kowalska-Krochmal B, Dudek-Wicher R. The minimum inhibitory concentration of antibiotics: methods, interpretation, clinical relevance. Pathogens. 2021;10(2):165.
30. Droege ME, Van Fleet SL, Mueller EW. Application of antibiotic pharmacodynamics and dosing principles in patients with sepsis. Crit Care Nurse. 2016;36(2):22–32.
31. Roger C, Nucci B, Molinari N, et al. Standard dosing of amikacin and gentamicin in critically ill patients results in variable and subtherapeutic concentrations. Int J Antimicrob Agents. 2015;46(1):21–7.
32. Roger C, Muller L, Wallis SC, et al. Population pharmacokinetics of linezolid in critically ill patients on renal replacement therapy: comparison of equal doses in continuous venovenous

haemofiltration and continuous venovenous haemodiafiltration. J Antimicrob Chemother. 2016;71(2):464–70.

33. Abdul-Aziz MH, Alffenaar JC, Bassetti M, et al. Antimicrobial therapeutic drug monitoring in critically ill adult patients: a position paper. Intensive Care Med. 2020;46(6):1127–53.

34. Zhao W, Jacqz-Aigrain E. Principles of therapeutic drug monitoring. Handb Exp Pharmacol. 2011;205:77–90.

35. Rybak MJ, Le J, Lodise TP, et al. Therapeutic monitoring of vancomycin for serious methicillin-resistant Staphylococcus aureus infections: a revised consensus guideline and review by the American Society of Health-System Pharmacists, the Infectious Diseases Society of America, the Pediatric Infectious Diseases Society, and the Society of Infectious Diseases Pharmacists. Am J Health Syst Pharm. 2020;77(11):835–64.

36. Barlam TF, Cosgrove SE, Abbo LM, et al. Implementing an antibiotic stewardship program: guidelines by the Infectious Diseases Society of America and the Society for Healthcare Epidemiology of America. Clin Infect Dis. 2016;62(10):e51–77.

37. Kim HY, Byashalira KC, Heysell SK, et al. Therapeutic drug monitoring of anti-infective drugs: implementation strategies for 3 different scenarios. Ther Drug Monit. 2022;44(1):3–10.

38. Radigan EA, Gilchrist NA, Miller MA. Management of aminoglycosides in the intensive care unit. J Intensive Care Med. 2010;25(6):327–42.

39. de Montmollin E, Bouadma L, Gault N, et al. Predictors of insufficient amikacin peak concentration in critically ill patients receiving a 25 mg/kg total body weight regimen. Intensive Care Med. 2014;40(7):998–1005.

40. Hodiamont CJ, Janssen JM, de Jong MD, et al. Therapeutic drug monitoring of gentamicin peak concentrations in critically ill patients. Ther Drug Monit. 2017;39(5):522–30.

41. van Lent-Evers NA, Mathot RA, Geus WP, et al. Impact of goal-oriented and model-based clinical pharmacokinetic dosing of aminoglycosides on clinical outcome: a cost-effectiveness analysis. Ther Drug Monit. 1999;21:63–73.

42. Humphries R. AST news update June 2023: New! CLSI M100-Ed33: updated aminoglycoside breakpoints for Enterobacterales and *Pseudomonas aeruginosa*. Clinical Laboratory Standards Institute [cited 2024 Feb 26]. Available from: https://clsi.org/about/blog/ast-news-update-june-2023-new-clsi-m100-ed33-updated-aminoglycoside-breakpoints-for-enterobacterales-and-pseudomonas-aeruginosa

43. Cusumano JA, Klinker KP, Huttner A, et al. Towards precision medicine: therapeutic drug monitoring–guided dosing of vancomycin and beta-lactam antibiotics to maximize effectiveness and minimize toxicity. Am J Health Syst Pharm. 2020;77:1104–12.

44. Pai MP, Neely M, Rodvold KA, et al. Innovative approaches to optimizing the delivery of vancomycin in individual patients. Adv Drug Deliv Rev. 2014;77:50–7.

45. Biagi MJ, Butler DA, Wenzler E. AUC-based monitoring of vancomycin: closing the therapeutic window. J Appl Lab Med. 2019;3(4):743–6.

46. Turner RB, Kojiro K, Shephard EA, et al. Review and validation of bayesian dose-optimizing software and equations for calculation of the vancomycin area under the curve in critically ill patients. Pharmacotherapy. 2018;38(12):1174–83.

47. Bosso JA, Nappi J, Rudisill C, et al. Relationship between vancomycin trough concentrations and nephrotoxicity: a prospective multicenter trial. Antimicrob Agents Chemother. 2011;55(12):5475–9.

48. van Hal SJ, Paterson DL, Lodise TP. Systematic review and meta-analysis of vancomycin-induced nephrotoxicity associated with dosing schedules that maintain troughs between 15 and 20 milligrams per liter. Antimicrob Agents Chemother. 2013;57(2):734–44.

49. Neely MN, Kato L, Youn G, et al. Prospective trial on the use of trough concentration versus area under the curve to determine therapeutic vancomycin dosing. Antimicrob Agents Chemother. 2018;62(2):e02042–17.

50. Koch BCP, Muller AE, Hunfeld NGM, et al. Therapeutic drug monitoring of antibiotics in critically ill patients: current practice and future perspectives with a focus on clinical outcome. Ther Drug Monit. 2022;44(1):11–8.
51. Dong H, Xie J, Wang T, et al. Pharmacokinetic/pharmacodynamic evaluation of linezolid for the treatment of staphylococcal infections in critically ill patients. Int J Antimicrob Agents. 2016;48(3):259–64.
52. Cattaneo D, Gervasoni C, Cozzi V, et al. Therapeutic drug management of linezolid: a missed opportunity for clinicians? Int J Antimicrob Agents. 2016;48(6):728–31.
53. Dhaese S, Van Vooren S, Boelens J, et al. Therapeutic drug monitoring of beta-lactam antibiotics in the ICU. Expert Rev Anti-Infect Ther. 2020;18(11):1155–64.
54. Dulhunty JM, Roberts JA, Davis JS, et al. Continuous infusion of beta-lactam antibiotics in severe sepsis: a multicenter double-blind, randomized controlled trial. Clin Infect Dis. 2013;56:236–44.
55. Tam VH, McKinnon PS, Akins RL, et al. Pharmacodynamics of cefepime in patients with Gram-negative infections. J Antimicrob Chemother. 2002;50:425–8.
56. Udy AA, Varghese JM, Altukroni M, et al. Subtherapeutic initial beta-lactam concentrations in select critically ill patients: association between augmented renal clearance and low trough drug concentrations. Chest. 2012;142:30–9.
57. Imani S, Buscher H, Marriott D, et al. Too much of a good thing: a retrospective study of beta-lactam concentration-toxicity relationships. J Antimicrob Chemother. 2017;72(10):2891–7.
58. Boschung-Pasquier L, Atkinson A, Kastner LK, et al. Cefepime neurotoxicity: thresholds and risk factors. A retrospective cohort study. Clin Microbiol Infect. 2020;26(3):333–9.
59. Fratoni AJ, Nicolau DP, Kuti JL. A guide to therapeutic drug monitoring of beta-lactam antibiotics. Pharmacotherapy. 2021;41(2):220–33.
60. Hong LT, Downes KJ, FakhriRavari A, et al. International consensus recommendations for the use of prolonged-infusion beta-lactam antibiotics: endorsed by the American College of Clinical Pharmacy, British Society for Antimicrobial Chemotherapy, Cystic Fibrosis Foundation, European Society of Clinical Microbiology and Infectious Diseases Society of America, Society of Critical Care Medicine, and Society of Infectious Diseases Pharmacists. Pharmacotherapy. 2023;43:740–77.
61. Lodise TP Jr, Lomaestro B, Drusano GL. Piperacillin-tazobactam for *Pseudomonas aeruginosa* infection: clinical implications of an extended-infusion dosing strategy. Clin Infect Dis. 2007;44(3):357–63.
62. Yost RJ, Cappelletty DM, RECEIPT Study group. The retrospective cohort of extended-infusion piperacillin-tazobactam (RECEIPT) study: a multicenter study. Pharmacotherapy. 2011;31(8):767–75.
63. Chan JD, Dellit TH, Lynch JB. Hospital length of stay among patients receiving intermittent versus prolonged piperacillin/tazobactam infusion in the intensive care units. J Intensive Care Med. 2018;33(2):134–41.
64. Kaufman SE, Donnell RW, Hickey WS. Rationale and evidence for extended infusion of piperacillin-tazobactam. Am J Health Syst Pharm. 2011;68(16):1521–6.
65. Monti G, Bradic N, Marzaroli M, et al. Continuous vs intermittent meropenem administration in critically ill patients with sepsis: the MERCY randomized clinical trial. JAMA. 2023;330(2):141–51.
66. Korbila IP, Tansarli GS, Karageorgopoulos DE, et al. Extended or continuous versus short-term intravenous infusion of cephalosporins: a meta-analysis. Expert Rev Anti-Infect Ther. 2013;11(6):585–95.
67. de Boer AG, Gaillard PJ. Strategies to improve drug delivery across the blood-brain barrier. Clin Pharmacokinet. 2007;46(7):553–76.
68. Deer TR, Pope JE, Hanes MC, et al. Intrathecal therapy for chronic pain: a review of morphine and ziconotide as firstline options. Pain Med. 2019;20(4):784–98.

69. Dietz N, Wagers S, Harkema SJ, et al. Intrathecal and oral baclofen use in adults with spinal cord injury: a systematic review of efficacy in spasticity reduction, functional changes, dosing, and adverse events. Arch Phys Med Rehabil. 2023;104(1):119–31.
70. Gomez NAG, Warren N, Labko Y, et al. Intrathecal opioid dosing during spinal anesthesia for cesarean section: an integrative review. J Dr Nurs Pract. 2020;13(2):108–19.
71. Hafeez S, Grandhi R. Systematic review of intrathecal nicardipine for the treatment of cerebral vasospasm in aneurysmal subarachnoid hemorrhage. Neurocrit Care. 2019;31(2):399–405.
72. Hanley DF, Lane K, McBee N, et al. Thrombolytic removal of intraventricular haemorrhage in treatment of severe stroke: results of the randomised, multicentre, multiregion, placebo-controlled CLEAR III trial. Lancet. 2017;389(10069):603–11.
73. Nau R, Blei C, Eiffert H. Intrathecal antibacterial and antifungal therapies. Clin Microbiol Rev. 2020;33(3):e00190–19.
74. Tunkel AR, Hasbun R, Bhimraj A, et al. 2017 Infectious Diseases Society of America's clinical practice guidelines for healthcare-associated ventriculitis and meningitis. Clin Infect Dis. 2017;64(6):e34–65.
75. Cook AM, Mieure KD, Owen RD, et al. Intracerebroventricular administration of drugs. Pharmacotherapy. 2009;29(7):832–45.
76. Hodgson PS, Neal JM, Pollock JE, et al. The neurotoxicity of drugs given intrathecally (spinal). Anesth Analg. 1999;88(4):797–809.
77. Bayston R, Barnicoat M, Cudmore RE, et al. The use of intraventricular vancomycin in the treatment of CSF shunt-associated ventriculitis. Z Kinderchir. 1984;39(Suppl 2):111–3.
78. Lewin JJ 3rd, Cook AM, Gonzales A, et al. Current practices of intraventricular antibiotic therapy in the treatment of meningitis and ventriculitis: results from a multicenter retrospective cohort study. Neurocrit Care. 2019;30(3):609–16.
79. Ng K, Mabasa VH, Chow I, et al. Systematic review of efficacy, pharmacokinetics, and administration of intraventricular vancomycin in adults. Neurocrit Care. 2014;20(1):158–71.
80. Grabb PA, Albright AL. Intraventricular vancomycin-induced cerebrospinal fluid eosinophilia: report of two patients. Neurosurgery. 1992;30(4):630–4.
81. Luer MS, Hatton J. Vancomycin administration into the cerebrospinal fluid: a review. Ann Pharmacotherapy. 1993;27(7–8):912–21.
82. Wen DY, Bottini AG, Hall WA, et al. Infections in neurologic surgery. The intraventricular use of antibiotics. Neurosurg Clin N Am. 1992;3(2):343–54.
83. LeBras M, Chow I, Mabasa VH, et al. Systematic review of efficacy, pharmacokinetics, and administration of intraventricular aminoglycosides in adults. Neurocrit Care. 2016;25(3):492–507.
84. Wang JH, Lin PC, Chou CH, et al. Intraventricular antimicrobial therapy in postneurosurgical Gram-negative bacillary meningitis or ventriculitis: a hospital-based retrospective study. J Microbiol Immunol Infect. 2014;47(3):204–10.
85. Grondahl TO, Langmoen IA. Epileptogenic effect of antibiotic drugs. J Neurosurg. 1993;78(6):938–43.
86. Ballinger AE, Palmer SC, Wiggins KJ, et al. Treatment for peritoneal dialysis-associated peritonitis. Cochrane Database Syst Rev. 2014;2014(4):CD005284.
87. Morimoto K, Terawaki H, Washida N, et al. The impact of intraperitoneal antibiotic administration in patients with peritoneal dialysis-related peritonitis: systematic review and meta-analysis. Ren Replace Ther. 2020;6(1):19.
88. So SWY, Chen L, Woo AYH, et al. Stability and compatibility of antibiotics in peritoneal dialysis solutions. Clin Kidney J. 2022;15(6):1071–8.
89. Li PK, Chow KM, Cho Y, et al. ISPD peritonitis guideline recommendations: 2022 update on prevention and treatment. Perit Dial Int. 2022;42(2):110–53.
90. Porner D, Von Vietinghoff S, Nattermann J, et al. Advances in the pharmacological management of bacterial peritonitis. Expert Opin Pharmacother. 2021;22(12):1567–78.

91. Biggins SW, Angeli P, Garcia-Tsao G, et al. Diagnosis, evaluation, and management of ascites, spontaneous bacterial peritonitis and hepatorenal syndrome: 2021 practice guidance by the American Association for the Study of Liver Diseases. Hepatology. 2021;74(2):1014–48.

92. Mazuski JE, Tessier JM, May AK, et al. The Surgical Infection Society revised guidelines on the management of intra-abdominal infection. Surg Infect. 2017;18(1):1–76.

93. Ling CW, Sud K, Patel R, et al. Culture-directed antibiotics in peritoneal dialysis solutions: a systematic review focused on stability and compatibility. J Nephrol. 2023;36(7):1841–59.

94. Ling CW, Sud K, Van C, et al. Pharmacokinetics of culture-directed antibiotics for the treatment of peritonitis in automated peritoneal dialysis: a systematic narrative review. Perit Dial Int. 2021;41(3):261–72.

95. Mancini A, Piraino B. Review of antibiotic dosing with peritonitis in APD. Perit Dial Int. 2019;39(4):299–305.

96. Akoh JA. Peritoneal dialysis associated infections: an update on diagnosis and management. World J Nephrol. 2012;1(4):106–22.

97. Zeng Y, Jiang L, Lu Y, et al. Peritoneal dialysis-related peritonitis caused by Gram-negative organisms: ten-years experience in a single center. Ren Fail. 2021;43(1):993–1003.

98. Radhika M, Mithal K, Bawdekar A, et al. Pharmacokinetics of intravitreal antibiotics in endophthalmitis. J Ophthalmic Inflamm Infect. 2014;4:22.

99. Sadiq MA, Hassan M, Agarwal A, et al. Endogenous endophthalmitis: diagnosis, management, and prognosis. J Ophthalmic Inflamm Infect. 2015;5(1):32.

100. Barza M, Kane A, Baum J. Pharmacokinetics of intravitreal carbenicillin, cefazolin, and gentamicin in rhesus monkeys. Invest Opthalmol Vis Sci. 1983;24(12):1602–6.

101. Coco RM, Lopez MI, Pastor JC, et al. Pharmacokinetics of intravitreal vancomycin in normal and infected rabbit eyes. J Ocul Pharmacol Ther. 1998;14(6):555–63.

102. Kernt M, Kampik A. Endophthalmitis: pathogenesis, clinical presentation, management, and perspectives. Clin Ophthalmol. 2010;4:121–35.

103. Endophthalmitis Vitrectomy Study Group. Results of the endophthalmitis vitrectomy study. A randomized trial of immediate virectomy and of intravenous antibiotics for the treatment of postoperative bacterial endophthalmitis. Arch Opthalmol. 1995;113(12):1479–96.

104. Doft BH, Barza M. Ceftazidime or amikacin: choice of intravitreal antimicrobials in the treatment of postoperative endophthalmitis. Arch Ophthalmol. 1994;112(1):17–8.

105. Velez-Montoya R, Monroy-Esquivel L, Ortiz-Guevara R, et al. Alternative intravitreal antibiotics: a systematic review for consideration in recalcitrant or resistant endophthalmitis. Retina. 2023;43(9):1433–47.

106. Grzybowski A, Turczynowska M, Schwartz SG, et al. The role of systemic antimicrobials in the treatment of endophthalmitis: a review and an international perspective. Ophthalmol Ther. 2020;9(3):485–98.

107. Rozalska B, Wadstrom T. Protective opsonic activity of antibodies against fibronectin-binding proteins (FnBPs) of Staphylococcus aureus. Scand J Immunol. 1993;37(5):575–80.

108. Mehta S, Armstrong BK, Kim SJ, et al. Long-term potency, sterility, and stability of vancomycin, ceftazidime, and moxifloxacin for treatment of bacterial endophthalmitis. Retina. 2011;31(7):1316–22.

109. Fagan RP, Edwards JR, Park BJ, et al. Incidence trends in pathogen-specific central line-associated bloodstream infections in US intensive care units, 1990-2010. Infect Control Hosp Epidemiol. 2013;34(9):893–9.

110. Desgrouas M, Ehrmann S. Inhaled antibiotics during mechanical ventilation-why it will work. Ann Transl Med. 2021;9(7):598.

111. Rodvold KA, George JM, Yoo L. Penetration of anti-infective agents into pulmonary epithelial lining fluid: focus on antibacterial agents. Clin Pharmacokinet. 2011;50(10):637–64.

112. Maselli DJ, Keyt H, Restrepo MI. Inhaled antibiotic therapy in chronic respiratory diseases. Int J Mol Sci. 2017;18(5):1062.

113. Weers J. Inhaled antimicrobial therapy - barriers to effective treatment. Adv Drug Deliv Rev. 2015;85:24–43.

114. Mogayzel PJ Jr, Naureckas ET, Robinson KA, et al. Cystic fibrosis pulmonary guidelines. Chronic medications for maintenance of lung health. Am J Respir Crit Care Med. 2013;187(7):680–9.
115. Amjad Z, Abaza A, Vasavada AM, et al. Inhaled antibiotics in non-cystic fibrosis bronchiectasis (NCFB): a systematic review of efficacy and limitations in adult patients. Cureus. 2022;14(10):e30660.
116. Kalil AC, Metersky ML, Klompas M, et al. Management of adults with hospital-acquired and ventilator-associated pneumonia: 2016 clinical practice guidelines by the Infectious Diseases Society of America and the American Thoracic Society. Clin Infect Dis. 2016;63(5):e61–e111.
117. Povoa FCC, Cardinal-Fernandez P, Maia IS, et al. Effect of antibiotics administered via the respiratory tract in the prevention of ventilator-associated pneumonia: a systematic review and meta-analysis. J Crit Care. 2018;43:240–5.
118. Zha S, Niu J, He Z, et al. Prophylactic antibiotics for preventing ventilator-associated pneumonia: a pairwise and Bayesian network meta-analysis. Eur J Med Res. 2023;28(1):348.
119. Ehrmann S, Barbier F, Demiselle J, et al. Inhaled amikacin to prevent ventilator-associated pneumonia. N Engl J Med. 2023;389(22):2052–62.
120. Han Y, Hua J, He B, et al. Inhaled antibiotics and airway bacterial decolonization for patients with chronic obstructive pulmonary disease: the rationale and future. J Transl Int Med. 2022;10(3):181–4.
121. Tang J, Ouyang Q, Li Y, et al. Nanomaterials for delivering antibiotics in the therapy of pneumonia. Int J Mol Sci. 2022;23(24):15738.
122. Kollef MH, Ricard JD, Roux D, et al. A randomized trial of the amikacin fosfomycin inhalation system for the adjunctive therapy of Gram-negative ventilator-associated pneumonia: IASIS trial. Chest. 2017;151(6):1239–46.
123. Niederman MS, Alder J, Bassetti M, et al. Inhaled amikacin adjunctive to intravenous standard-of-care antibiotics in mechanically ventilated patients with Gram-negative pneumonia (INHALE): a double-blind, randomised, placebo-controlled, phase 3, superiority trial. Lancet Infect Dis. 2020;20(3):330–40.
124. Kuhn RJ. Formulation of aerosolized therapeutics. Chest. 2001;120(3 Suppl):94S–8S.
125. Rose LM, Neale R. Development of the first inhaled antibiotic for the treatment of cystic fibrosis. Sci Transl Med. 2010;2(63):63mr4.
126. Schultheis JM, Durham ME, Kram SJ, et al. Incidence and associated risk factors for systemic drug levels with inhaled aminoglycoside therapy. J Antimicrob Chemother. 2023;78(2):450–6.
127. Patel AR, Patel AR, Singh S, et al. Central line catheters and associated complications: a review. Cureus. 2019;11(5):e4717.
128. Ziegler MJ, Pellegrini DC, Safdar N. Attributable mortality of central line associated bloodstream infection: systematic review and meta-analysis. Infection. 2015;43(1):29–36.
129. Mermel LA, Allon M, Bouza E, et al. Clinical practice guidelines for the diagnosis and management of intravascular catheter-related infection: 2009 update by the Infectious Diseases Society of America. Clin Infect Dis. 2009;49(1):1–45.
130. Buetti N, Marschall J, Drees M, et al. Strategies to prevent central line-associated bloodstream infections in acute-care hospitals: 2022 update. Infect Control Hosp Epidemiol. 2022;43(5):553–69.
131. O'Grady NP, Alexander M, Burns LA, et al. Guidelines for the prevention of intravascular catheter-related infections. Am J Infect Control. 2011;39(4 Suppl 1):S1–34.
132. Abdul Salim S, Masoud AT, Thongprayoon C, et al. Systematic review and meta-analysis of antibiotic and antimicrobial lock solutions for prevention of hemodialysis catheter-related infections. ASAIO J. 2021;67(10):1079–86.
133. Dogra GK, Herson H, Hutchison B, et al. Prevention of tunneled hemodialysis catheter-related infections using catheter-restricted filling with gentamicin and citrate: a randomized controlled study. J Am Soc Nephrol. 2002;13(8):2133–9.
134. Elhassan NO, Stevens TP, Gigliotti F, et al. Vancomycin usage in central venous catheters in a neonatal intensive care unit. Pediatr Infect Dis J. 2004;23(3):201–6.

135. Norris LB, Kablaoui F, Brilhart MK, et al. Systematic review of antimicrobial lock therapy for prevention of central-line-associated bloodstream infections in adult and pediatric cancer patients. Int J Antimicrob Agents. 2017;50(3):308–17.
136. Zacharioudakis IM, Zervou FN, Arvanitis M, et al. Antimicrobial lock solutions as a method to prevent central line-associated bloodstream infections: a meta-analysis of randomzied controlled trials. Clin Infect Dis. 2014;59(12):1741–9.
137. O'Horo JC, Silva GL, Safdar N. Anti-infective locks for treatment of central line-associated bloodstream infection: a systematic review and meta-analysis. Am J Nephrol. 2011;34(5):415–22.
138. Raad I, Chaftari AM, Zakhour R, et al. Successful salvage of central venous catheters in patients with catheter-related or central line-associated bloodstream infections by using a catheter lock solution consisting of minocycline, EDTA, and 25% ethanol. Antimicrob Agents Chemother. 2016;60(6):3426–32.
139. Rijnders BJ, Van Wijngaerden E, Vandecasteele SJ, et al. Treatment of long-term intravascular catheter-related bacteraemia with antibiotic lock: randomized, placebo-controlled trial. J Antimicrob Chemother. 2005;55(1):90–4.
140. Justo JA, Bookstaver PB. Antibiotic lock therapy: review of technique and logistical challenges. Infect Drug Resist. 2014;7:343–63.
141. Anderl JN, Franklin MJ, Stewart PS. Role of antibiotic penetration limitation in Klebsiella pneumoniae biofilm resistance to ampicillin and ciprofloxacin. Antimicrob Agents Chemother. 2000;44(7):1818–24.
142. Araujo PA, Mergulhao F, Melo L, et al. The ability of an antimicrobial agent to penetrate a biofilm is not correlated with its killing or removal efficiency. Biofouling. 2014;30(6):675–83.
143. Shigeta M, Tanaka G, Komatsuzawa H, et al. Permeation of antimicrobial agents through *Pseudomonas aeruginosa* biofilms: a simple method. Chemotherapy. 1997;43(5):340–5.
144. Singh R, Ray P, Das A, et al. Penetration of antibiotics through Staphylococcus aureus and Staphylococcus epidermidis biofilms. J Antimicrob Chemother. 2010;65(9):1955–8.
145. Kim EY, Saunders P, Yousefzadeh N. Usefulness of anti-infective lock solutions for catheter-related bloodstream infections. Mt Sinai J Med. 2010;77(5):549–58.
146. Saxena AK, Panhotra BR, Naguib M. Sudden irreversible sensory-neural hearing loss in a patient with diabetes receiving amikacin as an antibiotic-heparin lock. Pharmacotherapy. 2002;22(1):105–8.
147. US Food and Drug Administration. Warning on tricitrasol dialysis catheter anticoagulant. FDA Talk Paper. 2000;16:4–14.
148. Zembles TN, Flannery LS, Huppler AR. Development and implementation of an antimicrobial lock therapy guideline in a pediatric hospital. Am J Health Syst Pharm. 2018;75(5):299–303.
149. Landry DL, Braden GL, Gobeille SL, et al. Emergence of gentamicin-resistant bacteremia in hemodialysis patients receiving gentamicin lock catheter prophylaxis. Clin J Am Soc Nephrol. 2010;5(10):1799–804.
150. Dixon JJ, Steele M, Makanjuola AD. Anti-microbial locks increase the prevalence of Staphylococcus aureus and antibiotic-resistant Enterobacter: observational retrospective cohort study. Nephrol Dial Transplant. 2012;27(9):3575–81.
151. Zhang J, Wang B, Wang J, et al. Ethanol locks for the prevention of catheter-related infection in patients with central venous catheter: a systematic review and meta-analysis of randomized controlled trials. PLoS One. 2019;14(9):e0222408.
152. Bookstaver PB, Rokas KE, Norris LB, et al. Stability and compatibility of antimicrobial lock solutions. Am J Health Syst Pharm. 2013;70(24):2185–98.
153. Takla TA, Zelenitsky SA, Vercaigne LM. Effect of ethanol/trisodium citrate lock on micro-organisms causing hemodialysis catheter-related infections. J Vasc Access. 2007;8(4):262–7.
154. Mermel LA, Alang N. Adverse effects associated with ethanol catheter lock solutions: a systematic review. J Antimicrob Chemother. 2014;69(10):2611–9.

155. Karanika S, Paudel S, Grigoras C, et al. Systematic review and meta-analysis of clinical and economic outcomes from the implementation of hospital-based antimicrobial stewardship programs. Antimicrob Agents Chemother. 2016;60(8):4840–52.
156. Lindsay PJ, Rohailla S, Taggart LR, et al. Antimicrobial stewardship and intensive care unit mortality: a systematic review. Clin Infect Dis 2019;68:748–56.
157. Beganovic M, McCreary EK, Mahoney MV, et al. Interplay between rapid diagnostic tests and antimicrobial stewardship programs among patients with bloodstream and other severe infections. J Appl Lab Med. 2019;3(4):601–16.
158. Timbrook TT, Morton JB, McConeghy KW, et al. The effect of molecular rapid diagnostic testing on clinical outcomes in bloodstream infections: a systematic review and meta-analysis. Clin Infect Dis. 2017;64(1):15–23.
159. Eubank TA, Long SW, Perez KK. Role of rapid diagnostics in diagnosis and management of patients with sepsis. J Infect Dis. 2020;222(Suppl 2):S103–9.
160. Bauer KA, Perez KK, Forrest GN, et al. Review of rapid diagnostic tests used by antimicrobial stewardship programs. Clin Infect Dis. 2014;59(Suppl 3):S134–45.
161. Lam SW, Bass SN. Advancing infectious diseases diagnostic testing and applications to antimicrobial therapy in the ICU. J Pharm Pract. 2019;32(3):327–38.
162. van Belkum A, Welker M, Pincus D, et al. Matrix-assisted laser desorption ionization time-of-flight mass spectrometry in clinical microbiology: what are the current issues? Ann Lab Med. 2017;37(6):475–83.
163. Magiorakos AP, Srinivasan A, Carey RB, et al. Multidrug-resistant, extensively drug-resistant and pandrug-resistant bacteria: an international expert proposal for interim standard definitions for acquired resistance. Clin Microbiol Infect. 2012;18(3):268–81.
164. World Health Organization. No time to wait: securing the future from drug-resistant infections. Report to the Secretary General of the United Nations. 2019 Apr [cited 2024 Feb 01]. Available from: https://www.who.int/publications/i/item/no-time-to-wait-securing-the-future-from-drug-resistant-infections
165. Kang CI, Kim SH, Park WB, et al. Bloodstream infections caused by antibiotic-resistant Gram-negative bacilli: risk factors for mortality and impact of inappropriate initial antimicrobial therapy on outcome. Antimicrob Agents Chemother. 2005;49(2):760–6.
166. Kollef MH, Sherman G, Ward S, et al. Inadequate antimicrobial treatment of infections: a risk factor for hospital mortality among critically ill patients. Chest. 1999;115(2):462–74.
167. Leibovici L, Shraga I, Drucker M, et al. The benefit of appropriate empirical antibiotic treatment in patients with bloodstream infection. J Intern Med. 1998;244(5):379–86.
168. Magira EE, Islam S, Niederman MS. Multi-drug resistant organism infections in a medical ICU: association to clinical features and impact upon outcome. Med Intensiva (Engl Ed). 2018;42(4):225–34.
169. World Health Organization. 2021 antibacterial agents in clinical and preclinical development: an overview and analysis. 2022 [cited 2024 Feb 01]. Available from: https://www.who.int/publications/i/item/9789240047655
170. World Health Organization. Global antimicrobial resistance and use surveillance system (GLASS) report: 2022. 2022 [cited 2024 Feb 01]. Available from: https://www.who.int/publications/i/item/9789240062702
171. Bassetti M, Garau J. Current and future perspectives in the treatment of multidrug-resistant Gram-negative infections. J Antimicrob Chemother. 2021;76(Suppl 4):iv23–37.
172. Reynolds D, Burnham JP, Vazquez Guillamet C, et al. The threat of multidrug-resistant/extensively drug-resistant Gram-negative respiratory infections: another pandemic. Eur Respir Rev. 2022;31(166):220068.
173. Isler B, Harris P, Stewart AG, et al. An update on cefepime and its future role in combination with novel beta-lactamase inhibitors for MDR Enterobacterales and *Pseudomonas aeruginosa*—authors' response. J Antimicrob Chemother. 2021;76(12):3327–8.

174. Mushtaq S, Garello P, Vickers A, et al. Activity of cefepime/zidebactam (WCK 5222) against 'problem' antibiotic-resistant Gram-negative bacteria sent to a national reference laboratory. J Antimicrob Chemother. 2021;76(6):1511–22.

175. Dubey D, Roy M, Shah TH, et al. Compassionate use of a novel beta-lactam enhancer-based investigational antibiotic cefepime/zidebactam (WCK 5222) for the treatment of extensively-drug-resistant NDM-expressing *Pseudomonas aeruginosa* infection in an intra-abdominal infection-induced sepsis patient: a case report. Ann Clin Microbiol Antimicrob. 2023;22(1):55.

176. Tirlangi PK, Wanve BS, Dubbudu RR, et al. Successful use of cefepime-zidebactam (WCK 5222) as a salvage therapy for the treatment of disseminated extensively drug-resistant New Delhi metallo-beta-lactamase-producing *Pseudomonas aeruginosa* infection in an adult patient with acute T-cell leukemia. Antimicrob Agents Chemother. 2023;67(8):e0050023.

177. Matsumoto T. Arbekacin: another novel agent for treating infections due to methicillin-resistant Staphylococcus aureus and multidrug-resistant Gram-negative pathogens. Clin Pharmacol. 2014;6:139–48.

178. Watanabe T, Ohashi K, Matsui K, et al. Comparative studies of the bactericidal, morphological and post-antibiotic effects of arbekacin and vancomycin against methicillin-resistant Staphylococcus aureus. J Antimicrob Chemother. 1997;39(4):471–6.

179. Lee JH, Lee CS. Clinical usefulness of arbekacin. Infect Chemother. 2016;48(1):1–11.

180. Sato R, Tanigawara Y, Kaku M, et al. Pharmacokinetic-pharmacodynamic relationship of arbekacin for treatment of patients infected with methicillin-resistant Staphylococcus aureus. Antimicrob Agents Chemother. 2006;50(11):3763–9.

181. Vacca F, Sala C, Rappuoli R. Monoclonal antibodies for bacterial pathogens: mechanisms of action and engineering approaches for enhanced effector functions. Biomedicines. 2022;10(9):2126.

182. Wang H, Chen D, Lu H. Anti-bacterial monoclonal antibodies: next generation therapy against superbugs. Appl Microbiol Biotechnol. 2022;106(11):3957–72.

183. Lin MY, Hayden MK, Lyles RD, et al. Regional epidemiology of methicillin-resistant staphylococcus aureus among adult intensive care unit patients following state-mandated active surveillance. Clin Infect Dis. 2018;66(10):1535–9.

184. Hall AE, Domanski PJ, Patel PR, et al. Characterization of a protective monoclonal antibody recognizing Staphylococcus aureus MSCRAMM protein clumping factor A. Infect Immun. 2003;71(12):6864–70.

185. Ragle BE, Bubeck WJ. Anti-alpha-hemolysin monoclonal antibodies mediate protection against Staphylococcus aureus pneumonia. Infect Immun. 2009;77(7):2712–8.

186. Weisman LE, Thackray HM, Garcia-Prats JA, et al. Phase 1/2 double-blind, placebo-controlled, dose escalation, safety, and pharmacokinetic study of pagibaximab (BSYX-A110), an antistaphylococcal monoclonal antibody for the prevention of staphylococcal bloodstream infections, in very-low-birth-weight neonates. Antimicrob Agents Chemother. 2009;53(7):2879–86.

187. Yang Y, Qian M, Yi S, et al. Monoclonal antibody targeting Staphylococcus aureus surface protein A (SasA) protect against Staphylococcus aureus sepsis and peritonitis in mice. PLoS One. 2016;11(2):e0149460.

188. Francois B, Jafri HS, Chastre J, et al. Efficacy and safety of suvratoxumab for prevention of Staphylococcus aureus ventilator-associated pneumonia (SAATELLITE): a multicentre, randomised, double-blind, placebo-controlled, parallel-group, phase 2 pilot trial. Lancet Infect Dis. 2021;21(9):1313–23.

189. Oganesyan V, Peng L, Damschroder MM, et al. Mechanisms of neutralization of a human anti-alpha-toxin antibody. J Biol Chem. 2014;289(43):29874–80.

190. Foster TG, Hook M. Surface protein adhesins of Staphylococcus aureus. Trends Microbiol. 1998;6(12):484–8.

191. Patti JM, Allen BL, McGavin MJ, et al. MSCRAMM-mediated adherence of microorganisms to host tissues. Ann Rev Microbiol. 1994;48:585–617.

192. Nilsson IM, Patti JM, Bremell T, et al. Vaccination with a recombinant fragment of collagen adhesin provides protection against Staphylococcus aureus-mediated septic death. J Clin Invest. 1998;101(12):2640–9.
193. Harris AD, Jackson SS, Robinson G, et al. *Pseudomonas aeruginosa* colonization in the intensive care unit: prevalence, risk factors, and clinical outcomes. Infect Control Hosp Epidemiol. 2016;37(5):544–8.
194. Magill SS, Edwards JR, Bamberg W, et al. Multistate point-prevalence survey of health care-associated infections. N Engl J Med. 2014;370(13):1198–208.
195. Hauser AR. The type III secretion system of *Pseudomonas aeruginosa*: infection by injection. Nat Rev Microbiol. 2009;7(9):654–65.
196. Tabor DE, Oganesyan V, Keller AE, et al. *Pseudomonas aeruginosa* PcrV and Psl, the molecular targets of bispecific antibody MEDI3902, are conserved among diverse global clinical isolates. J Infect Dis. 2018;218(12):1983–94.
197. Chastre J, Francois B, Bourgeois M, et al. Safety, efficacy, and pharmacokinetics of gremubamab (MEDI3902), an anti-*Pseudomonas aeruginosa* bispecific human monoclonal antibody, in *P. aeruginosa*-colonised, mechanically ventilated intensive care unit patients: a randomised controlled trial. Crit Care. 2022;26(1):355.
198. Motley MP, Banerjee K, Fries BC. Monoclonal antibody-based therapies for bacterial infections. Curr Opin Infect Dis. 2019;32(3):210–6.
199. Murray CJ, Ikuta KS, Sharara F, et al. Global burden of bacterial antimicrobial resistance in 2019: a systematic analysis. Lancet. 2022;399(10325):629–55.
200. Talbot GH, Jezek A, Murray BE, et al. The Infectious Diseases Society of America's 10 × '20 initiative (10 new systemic antibacterial agents US Food and Drug Administration approved by 2020): is 20 × '20 a possibility? Clin Infect Dis. 2019;69(1):1–11.

Chapter 52
Glycemic Control in the Intensive Care Unit

Traci M. Grucz, Michael A. DiCesare, and David Sugrue

52.1 Introduction

Glycemic control has been a consistent goal and therapeutic target within the intensive care unit (ICU) for the last several decades. This is due to the high prevalence of hyperglycemia seen in critically ill patients and its association with worse clinical outcomes [1]. The dysregulation of blood glucose (BG) levels seen in the ICU can arise from the patient's stress response to their acute illness, surgery, or trauma, which can lead to insulin resistance and impaired glucose utilization. Studies examining hyperglycemia in the ICU have demonstrated its association with increased mortality, increased infectious complications, prolonged hospital length of stay, and increased healthcare costs [1–3].

Glycemic control strategies have evolved since the late 1990s to the present day. This chapter explores the current understanding of glycemic control in the ICU, summarizing primary literature to date, guidelines and societal recommendations, challenges encountered in clinical practice, pragmatic management strategies, and innovative trends in therapy and monitoring. While this chapter is applicable to a wide variety of critically ill adult patients, please note that pediatric patients are not addressed.

T. M. Grucz (✉)
Department of Pharmacy, The Johns Hopkins Hospital, Baltimore, MD, USA
e-mail: tklotz1@jhmi.edu

M. A. DiCesare
Department of Pharmacy, Hospital of the University of Pennsylvania, Philadelphia, PA, USA

D. Sugrue
Department of Pharmacy, Duke Raleigh Hospital, A Campus of Duke University Hospital, Raleigh, NC, USA

© The Author(s), under exclusive license to Springer Nature Switzerland AG 2025
Y. Alzaidi, M. A. Gebily (eds.), *The Pharmacist's Expanded Role in Critical Care Medicine*, https://doi.org/10.1007/978-3-031-77335-8_52

52.1.1 Glucose Homeostasis and Stress Hyperglycemia

Glucose metabolism is a regulated process with the goal of maintaining stable BG, which provides energy to cells throughout the body. BG regulation is supported by a balance of glucose intestinal absorption, hepatic glucose production, and glucose utilization by muscle and adipose tissue. Insulin lowers BG by facilitating glucose uptake into cells, where it promotes glycogen synthesis and inhibits hepatic gluconeogenesis [4]. Glucagon serves as a counter-regulatory hormone in this process by stimulating glycogenolysis and gluconeogenesis in the liver during periods of hypoglycemia, increasing BG to maintain energy supply [5]. Insulin and glucagon work together to ensure glucose homeostasis, adapting to nutritional status and metabolic demands.

During acute illness, there are disruptions to BG regulation leading to elevations of BG which is known as stress hyperglycemia. In response to severe illness, injury, or trauma, there is a neuroendocrine release of stress hormones such as cortisol, endogenous catecholamines, and glucagon paired with decreased insulin sensitivity and secretion [6]. These hormonal changes promote hepatic glucose production and reduced glucose cellular uptake, with a net effect of elevated BG. In addition to the stress response, several other factors contribute to the development of stress hyperglycemia in critically ill patients (which are also discussed in more detail in the Factors Impacting Glycemic Control section):

- *Insulin Resistance*: As described above, release of stress hormones and cytokines such as TNF-alpha promotes insulin resistance in both peripheral tissue (skeletal muscle) and hepatic tissue. Peripheral insulin resistance decreases glucose uptake. Hepatic insulin resistance leads to increased glucose production and decreased glycogenolysis [6].
- *Medications*: Dextrose administration, provided as a component of intravenous (IV) fluid therapy or IV admixtures, contributes to hyperglycemia. Exogenous corticosteroid and catecholamine administration amplifies the effects of their endogenous release, which decreases insulin secretion and increases insulin resistance [7].
- *Nutrition Support*: Parenteral and enteral nutrition therapy can impact glucose metabolism and contribute to hyperglycemia. Inconsistent delivery of nutrition can lead to fluctuations in BG, making it challenging to maintain glycemic control.

If unmanaged, stress hyperglycemia can exacerbate systemic inflammation, prompt fluid depletion via osmotic diuresis, cause endothelial dysfunction, and increase infectious risk by impairing immune function [8]. These effects all contribute to an increase in patient morbidity and mortality.

52.1.2 Hypoglycemia and Associated Risks

In addition to hyperglycemia, critically ill patients may also be at risk for hypoglycemia. Commonly defined as BG ≤70 mg/dL, hypoglycemia may result in adverse neurologic and cardiac sequelae and is associated with increased mortality in critically ill patients [9]. Certain disease states such as significant liver dysfunction and severe adrenal insufficiency may predispose critically ill patients to hypoglycemia [10, 11]. Additional hypoglycemia risk factors in the ICU include increased severity of illness, mechanical ventilation, septic shock, diabetes history, and renal dysfunction [12]. The risk of iatrogenic hypoglycemia is increased with the use of insulin, a high-alert medication, with intensive insulin therapy targeting BG <140 mg/dL [13, 14]. Errors related to insulin administration and dosing may also contribute to hypoglycemia. Specifically, failure to account for changes in dynamic factors affecting glycemic control outlined in the section named as such below can increase this risk, such as failure to reduce insulin requirements despite a significant reduction in nutritional intake.

52.1.3   Historical Perspective

The concept of stress hyperglycemia and its potential complications in critically ill patients was identified and studied in the 1990s. Practitioners were recognizing the impact elevated BG had on morbidity and mortality in various patient populations including patients with diabetes, stroke and burn patients, and patients with coronary artery disease. IV insulin infusion therapy was explored as a therapeutic approach to managing BG and improving outcomes. The Diabetes Mellitus Insulin-Glucose in Acute Myocardial Infarction (DIGAMI) study randomized patients with diabetes with suspected acute myocardial infarction to a glucose management protocol or standard care. The glucose management protocol consisted of a continuous IV insulin infusion targeting BG of 126–196 mg/dL (7–10.9 mmol/L), followed by subcutaneous insulin therapy for at least 3 months. Mortality at 1 year was reduced in the insulin infusion group compared to the control group (18.6% vs. 26.1%, $p = 0.027$) and was also demonstrated during longer term follow-up of 3.4 years on average [15, 16]. This served as the impetus for further evaluation of tight glycemic control in later studies described below.

52.2   Blood Glucose (BG) Targets in Critically Ill Patients

This section evaluates landmark studies and clinical guideline recommendations assessing BG targets in the ICU in chronological order. Four landmark studies can also be compared in Table 52.1.

52.2.1   Leuven I (2001) and II (2006)

In the Leuven I study, approximately 1500 surgical ICU patients at a single center were randomized to an intensive glycemic control strategy (goal BG range of 80–110 mg/dL using an IV insulin infusion) or conventional treatment (initiation of

Table 52.1 Comparison of studies evaluating blood glucose (BG) targets in critically ill patients

	Leuven I (2001)	Leuven II (2006)	NICE-SUGAR (2009)	TGC-FAST (2023)
Patient population	1548 surgical ICU patients (62% cardiac surgery)	1200 medical ICU patients	6104 medical and surgical ICU patients (63% medical)	9230 ICU medical and surgical patients (45% cardiac surgery)
Intervention: Intensive therapy BG goal	80–110 mg/dL	80–110 mg/dL	81–108 mg/dL	80–110 mg/dL
Control: Conventional therapy BG goal	180–200 mg/dL	180–200 mg/dL	≤180 mg/dL	180–215 mg/dL
Outcomes: Intensive vs. conventional therapy	ICU mortality – 4.6% vs. 8.0%, $p < 0.04$ (adjusted) Hypoglycemia – 39 vs. 6 patients	In-hospital mortality – 37.3% vs. 40.0%, $p = 0.33$ Hypoglycemia – 18.7% vs. 3.1%; $p < 0.001$	90-day mortality – 27.5% vs. 24.9%, $p = 0.02$ Hypoglycemia – 6.8% vs. 0.5%; $p < 0.001$	ICU length of stay – HR 1.0 (95% CI, 0.96–1.04), $p = 0.94$ Hypoglycemia – 1% vs. 0.7% (HR 1.52 [95% CI, 0.97–2.39])

an IV insulin infusion if BG exceeded 215 mg/dL and then used to maintain BG between 180 and 200 mg/dL). All patients received 200–300 g of IV dextrose on ICU admission and were transitioned to parenteral, enteral, or parenteral plus enteral nutrition thereafter. ICU mortality was significantly lower in patients who received intensive glycemic control compared to conventional treatment (4.6% vs. 8.0%, $p < 0.04$ with adjustment for sequential analysis). This benefit was driven by a reduction in mortality in patients with ICU stays longer than 5 days (10.6% vs. 20.2%, $p = 0.005$). More patients experienced severe hypoglycemia (BG ≤40 mg/dL) in the intensive group compared to conventional treatment [17].

Five years later, the Leuven II study was replicated by the same author group in 1200 medical ICU patients. Unlike the Leuven I study, there was no difference in in-hospital mortality between the intensive glycemic control and conventional treatment groups (37.3% vs. 40.0%, $p = 0.33$). Severe hypoglycemia (BG ≤40 mg/dL) occurred more often in the intensive treatment group [18].

52.2.2 *NICE-SUGAR (2009) and Hypoglycemia Post Hoc Analysis (2012)*

Following these early studies, the landmark NICE-SUGAR trial was published in 2009. This study included over 6000 patients from both medical and surgical ICUs in 42 hospitals who were randomized to intensive BG control (goal BG range of 81–108 mg/dL) or conventional BG control (goal BG ≤180 mg/dL) utilizing an IV insulin infusion. The majority of patients were medically ill, and approximately 20% of patients in each group had a history of diabetes. Patients received similar nonprotein caloric intake between groups throughout the study. In contrast to the earlier studies, NICE-SUGAR found that patients in the intensive BG control group had higher mortality rates at 90 days compared to the conventional group (27.5% vs. 24.9%, $p = 0.02$), with a number needed to harm of 38. Hypoglycemia episodes (BG ≤ 40 mg/dL) were significantly higher in the intensive group compared to the conventional group (6.8% vs. 0.5%, $p < 0.001$) [14].

A post hoc analysis of NICE-SUGAR was published in 2012, evaluating patients with moderate (BG 41–70 mg/dL) or severe (BG ≤ 40 mg/dL) hypoglycemia and their risk of death. Of all patients included in the study, significantly more patients in the intensive BG control group experienced moderate hypoglycemia compared to the conventional group (74.2% vs. 15.8%). This trend was also observed with severe hypoglycemia (6.9% vs. 0.5%), with over 90% of episodes occurring in patients receiving intensive glycemic control. Hypoglycemia was associated with an increased risk of mortality (adjusted hazard ratio 1.41 [95% confidence interval 1.21–1.62, $p < 0.001$] and 2.10 [95% confidence interval 1.59–2.77, $p < 0.001$], respectively), which remained consistent after adjustment for baseline characteristics and post-randomization factors [9]. This analysis demonstrated the significant risks of even moderate hypoglycemia in critically ill patients and further advocated for the avoidance of intensive glycemic control strategies.

52.2.3   2012 American Diabetes Association (ADA) and Society of Critical Care Medicine (SCCM) Guidelines

After publication of the NICE-SUGAR trial, ADA and SCCM guidance in 2012 recommended conventional or non-intensive BG targets in critically ill patients. The ADA recommended that most critically ill patients should be initiated on insulin therapy for persistent hyperglycemia, stating a BG threshold of no >180 mg/dL, and to maintain BG between 140 and 180 mg/dL (which reflects the average BG attained in the conventional therapy group in NICE-SUGAR) [19]. SCCM suggested that BG >150 mg/dL should trigger the initiation of insulin therapy which should be titrated to BG <180 mg/dL for all patients using protocols that achieve low rates of hypoglycemia [20]. Both guidelines also comment on special populations, which will be discussed in the subsection titled as such below. Moving forward, targeting a goal BG of 140–180 mg/dL for most hyperglycemic critically ill patients became standard practice, with institutional protocols developed in alignment with this recommended range.

52.2.4   TGC-FAST (2023)

Despite its widespread clinical impact, questions related to NICE-SUGAR remained, particularly regarding the high rates of hypoglycemia observed which may have been attributed to aggressive IV insulin infusion titrations. Additionally, the earlier Leuven studies utilized early parenteral dextrose and/or nutrition which is no longer reflective of current nutrition support practices. Therefore, the TGC-FAST authors sought to re-evaluate BG targets and glycemic control in a contemporary trial.

TGC-FAST was a multicenter trial in Belgium that evaluated tight glycemic control (BG goal 80–110 mg/dL) compared to liberal glycemic control (initiation of an IV insulin infusion if BG exceeded 215 mg/dL on two occasions and then used to maintain BG between 180 and 215 mg/dL) in over 9000 ICU patients. The IV insulin infusion in the tight control group was adjusted using a high-performance computer algorithm, whereas titrations in the liberal control group were made by providers and nurses based on protocol alerts integrated into the electronic health record. Patients received enteral nutrition as soon as possible; if caloric intake targets were unable to be met, parenteral nutrition was initiated after 1 week in the ICU. Approximately 20% of patients in each group had a history of diabetes, and 45% of patients in each group were admitted after cardiac surgery or complications thereafter. This study demonstrated that tight glucose control did not affect the length of time in the ICU (hazard ratio 1.00 [95% CI, 0.96 to 1.04, $p = 0.94$]) or mortality within 90 days of randomization (10.5% vs. 10.1%, $p = 0.51$) compared to liberal control. Notably, the rates of severe hypoglycemia (BG <40 mg/dL) were low at 1% and 0.7%, respectively, as compared to previous trials which ranged from 5% to 18.7% in tight or intensive groups and 0.5% to 3.1% in conventional groups [13].

The TGC-FAST study suggests that even in the absence of hypoglycemia, no benefit has been seen with tight glucose control in the ICU.

52.2.5   2024 ADA and SCCM Guidelines

The ADA and SCCM released updated guidance in 2024 on glycemic control in the ICU, with BG target recommendations summarized in Table 52.2. The ADA's recommendation remained consistent with the 2012 iteration, suggesting a BG goal of 140–180 mg/dL for most critically ill patients. A more stringent approach was suggested for select ICU patients, particularly the cardiac surgery population, which is discussed in more detail in the Special Populations subsection [21].

The SCCM guidelines extended the upper threshold of the BG range from 180 mg/dL in the 2012 guidelines to 200 mg/dL in the 2024 guidelines [22]. It should be noted that while each study discussed in this chapter had an overall BG goal range, average BG in the conventional/liberal control groups was approximately 140–150 mg/dL in the NICE-SUGAR and TGC-FAST studies, which comprise the most robust data on glycemic control in the ICU. Since average BG did not appear to routinely exceed 180 mg/dL, let alone 200 mg/dL, the authors suggest continuing to target an upper BG threshold of 180 mg/dL for most patients so long as hypoglycemia may be avoided with that strategy, and such that current institutional insulin protocols targeting BG of 140–180 mg/dL may continue to be utilized at this time.

Table 52.2 2024 American Diabetes Association (ADA) and Society of Critical Care Medicine (SCCM) guidance on blood glucose targets in the ICU

Guideline	Recommendation	Level of evidence
2024 ADA standards of care in diabetes: diabetes care in the hospital	"Once therapy is initiated, a glycemic goal of 140–180 mg/dL is recommended for most critically ill (ICU) individuals with hyperglycemia."	A—Clear evidence from well-conducted, generalizable randomized controlled trials that are adequately powered
	"More stringent glycemic goals, such as 110–140 mg/dL, may be appropriate for selected critically ill individuals and are acceptable if they can be achieved without significant hypoglycemia."	B—Supportive evidence from well-conducted randomized controlled trials that are adequately powered
2024 SCCM guideline on glycemic control for critically ill children and adults	"In critically ill adults, we 'suggest against' titrating an insulin infusion to a lower BG target (80–139 mg/dL) as compared with a higher BG target range (BG 140–200 mg/dL) to reduce the risk of hypoglycemia."	Conditional recommendation, moderate certainty of evidence

52.2.6   Special Populations

Although a one-size-fits-all approach is often cautioned against in critical care medicine, the evidence to date has not warranted deviation from the generalized BG target recommendations in any specific patient population. A summary of various populations is described below.

52.2.6.1   Preexisting Diabetes

For the critically ill patient with a past medical history of diabetes, specific BG goals have not been well established. Specifically, concerns have been raised regarding lowering BG too aggressively compared to baseline in this population.

Patients with diabetes were included in the previous studies discussed, accounting for 13–20% of patients. Subgroup analyses of these patients demonstrated similar trends to the overall cohort, with no differences shown between intensive and conventional therapy groups in the primary outcomes of 90-day mortality or ICU length of stay in the NICE-SUGAR and TGC-FAST trials, respectively.

The LUCID trial evaluated a liberal approach to BG control (initiation of an IV insulin infusion if BG exceeded 252 mg/dL and then used to maintain BG between 180 and 252 mg/dL) compared to usual care (IV insulin initiation and titration as per existing institutional protocols, with insulin initiation at BG >180 mg/dL and titrated to a target range of 108–180 mg/dL) in ICU patients with type 2 diabetes. The liberal approach reduced hypoglycemia rates but did not improve any patient-centered outcomes such as 90-day mortality, ICU or hospital lengths of stay, or ICU-free survival days [23].

In similar fashion, the CONTROLLING study evaluated individualized BG goals, utilizing patients' baseline BG control via hemoglobin A1c prior to critical illness, compared to usual care (BG ≤180 mg/dL). History of diabetes was present in one-fourth of the patients included. There was no difference in 90-day survival utilizing individualized BG ranges compared to the usual care group (67.2% vs. 69.6%, $p = 0.23$), and severe hypoglycemia did not differ between groups [24].

The 2024 SCCM guidelines state that there is insufficient evidence to recommend personalized BG targets related to patients with preexisting diabetes or those with pre-admission hyperglycemia. It goes on to address that this is a particular area of need for further high-quality studies.

52.2.6.2 Cardiac Surgery

For patients undergoing cardiac surgery, BG targets have been a major point of emphasis to ensure appropriate wound healing. In the Leuven I trial, almost two-thirds of patients were admitted to ICU after cardiac surgery or due to related complications [17]. A pre-planned subgroup analysis and follow-up of the Leuven I trial found that of cardiac surgery patients, the intensive glucose control group had lower ICU and in-hospital mortality compared to the conventional group. Like many of the other trials evaluating intensive glucose control, higher rates of hypoglycemia were observed in the intensive glucose control group [25].

In 2009, the Society of Thoracic Surgeons published a practice guideline on BG management during adult cardiac surgery which recommended that patients with persistently elevated BG >180 mg/dL should receive an IV insulin infusion to maintain BG <180 mg/dL for the duration of their ICU care. An additional recommendation included maintenance of BG ≤150 mg/dL for patients requiring 3 or more days in the ICU due to mechanical ventilation, inotrope support, presence of intra-aortic balloon pump or left ventricular assist device, administration of anti-arrhythmic medications, or renal replacement therapy [26].

A single-center study in 2012 compared a strict BG strategy (BG 90–120 mg/dL) to a liberal BG strategy (BG 121–180 mg/dL) after coronary artery bypass graft (CABG) surgery using a software system for controlling BG. No difference in perioperative complications was demonstrated between groups. The liberal strategy group had more patients within BG goal range and less hypoglycemia events compared to the strict strategy group [27].

A similar but larger study, GLUCO-CABG, assessed differences in mortality in addition to perioperative complications such as sternal wound infections, bacteremia, and pneumonia with an intensive BG control strategy (BG 100–140 mg/dL) compared to a conservative BG control strategy (BG 141–180 mg/dL) in patients undergoing CABG surgery. Intensive BG control did not reduce mortality, perioperative complications, or hospital length of stay when compared to the conservative approach [28].

Based on these mixed data for post-cardiac surgery ICU patients, some institutions opted for more stringent BG control compared to noncardiac surgery patients. However, given the results from more contemporary and robust trials including TGC-FAST which included 45% of cardiac surgery patients, current evidence does not suggest clinical benefit with tighter glycemic control in this population. The 2024 SCCM guidelines recommend that cardiac surgery patients be managed like unselected patients [22].

52.2.6.3 Neurocritical Care

Traumatic brain injury (TBI) patients have been a specific group of interest within neurocritical care as it relates to glycemic control. In 2015, a subgroup analysis from the NICE-SUGAR trial was published evaluating intensive versus conventional BG control in TBI patients. There was no difference in the number of patients with a favorable neurologic outcome, though higher rates of hypoglycemia were observed in the intensive BG control group [29].

A meta-analysis from the 2024 SCCM guidelines demonstrated increased rates of severe hypoglycemia in neurologic ICU patients managed with intensive BG control, with no difference in other clinical outcomes of interest. The guidelines recommend that neurocritical care patients be managed like unselected patients when it comes to BG targets in the ICU [22].

52.3 Factors Impacting Glycemic Control

Prior to discussing hyper- and hypoglycemia management, it is important to note several significant factors that commonly impact glycemic control in the ICU so that clinicians may develop a systematic approach to assessing these factors. Many of these factors are dynamic and may fluctuate rapidly in critically ill patients, with concomitant factors contributing to additive or opposing effects. Critical care pharmacists play a key role in regularly identifying and evaluating these factors, subsequently optimizing the safety and efficacy of glycemic control management.

52.3.1 Nutrition-Related Factors

Nutrition support can greatly impact glycemic control in the ICU, with the expectation that an increase in the amount of carbohydrates given may lead to increased BG and that a decrease in carbohydrates may decrease BG. Therefore, careful consideration is warranted whenever nutrition is adjusted. Common situations in which carbohydrates are increased include advancing the patient's oral diet (e.g., clear liquid to regular), increasing the enteral tube feed rate to goal, and advancing dextrose in parenteral nutrition in a stepwise fashion. Common situations in which carbohydrates are decreased include making patients nil per os (NPO) in which an oral diet or enteral tube feeds are held (e.g., perioperatively) as well as intentional or inadvertent interruptions in parenteral nutrition. Diligence in confirming that diet orders are accurately reflective of the patient's actual nutritional intake is also key. For example, a patient may be ordered for a regular oral diet but may have minimal intake due to nausea; similarly, the intent may be to advance tube feeds to the goal rate by a certain timeframe, but gastrointestinal intolerance may preclude that. Frequent reassessment of nutrition support and carbohydrate intake and collaboration with nursing, dietitian, and provider colleagues are recommended when creating and modifying glycemic control plans for critically ill patients.

52.3.2 Medication-Related Factors

Several medication classes may impact BG through their metabolic effects over time; however, one medication class in particular is expected to have an impact on BG acutely. Corticosteroids can increase BG through several mechanisms including increased insulin resistance, increased gluconeogenesis, and insulin signaling interference [30]. Steroid-induced hyperglycemia typically manifests as a postprandial elevation in BG, with the extent and duration of hyperglycemia varying based on the medication and dose administered [31, 32]. Corticosteroid initiation, discontinuation, and dose adjustments should be considered when assessing glycemic control in critically ill patients.

Catecholamines such as epinephrine and somatostatin analogues such as octreotide mechanistically may increase BG, though there are limited data on the impact and significance of this effect in clinical practice [33–35]. Clinician discretion and consideration of additional patient-specific factors outlined below are advised when assessing these medication classes and their influence on BG.

A common question is the impact of dextrose-containing IV fluids on BG. The utility and indication for continuing dextrose-containing maintenance IV fluids in hyperglycemic patients should be reassessed. For dextrose-containing fluids used as medication diluents, such as dextrose 5% in water (D5W), the potential benefit of switching the diluent should be weighed against the feasibility with considerations related to compatibility, stability, and institutional policies or capabilities. To assist with determining the possible impact of a dextrose-containing medication diluent, the amount of dextrose per day being administered can be calculated by cross-multiplying the amount of dextrose per 100 mL of the diluent by the total volume of the diluent infused over a 24-h period. For example, the following equation could be used for an IV medication infusion in D5W running at 20 mL/h (or 480 mL/day):

$$\frac{5\,\mathrm{g\,dextrose}}{100\,\mathrm{mL}} \times \frac{x\,\mathrm{g\,dextrose}}{480\,\mathrm{mL}} = 24\,\mathrm{g\,dextrose\,per\,day}$$

The authors suggest that in the absence of high dextrose concentrations (e.g., dextrose 20% in water or higher) and/or volumes (e.g., ≥1000 mL/day), the dextrose content in most medication diluents is not expected to contribute significantly to hyperglycemia in the ICU.

52.3.3 Patient-Specific Factors

In addition to nutrition and medications, factors related to individual patients and their clinical status should also be considered when assessing glycemic control in the ICU. As described in the Glucose Homeostasis and Stress Hyperglycemia section, the stress response to illness and inflammation such as infection/sepsis, surgery, and trauma can cause an acute increase in BG and subsequent hyperglycemia [6]. Patients experiencing pro-inflammatory states may have higher BG during that acute period; alternatively, as inflammation subsides, so too may stress hyperglycemia resulting in lower BG. Additionally, certain disease states such as significant liver dysfunction and severe adrenal insufficiency may predispose critically ill patients to hypoglycemia [10, 11]. While factoring in these considerations is not an exact science, recognizing the potential impact inflammation or other disease states may have on BG and assessing general trends in clinical worsening or improvement can be helpful in evaluating glycemic control overall.

Patients with a history of diabetes should also be carefully evaluated. The type of diabetes can lend insight into the presence of preexisting insulin deficiency (such as with type 1 diabetes, for which all patients should receive insulin in the ICU) and/or insulin resistance (such as with type 2 diabetes) [21]. Evaluation of home medications along with hemoglobin A1c if known can also be useful in managing glycemic control in critically ill patients. A recent hemoglobin A1c <7% in most patients indicates adequate glycemic control on the current outpatient antihyperglycemic regimen, whereas higher A1cs indicate inadequate glycemic control prior to admission, which may warrant initiation of insulin in critically ill patients not receiving it prior to admission [36]. Prior-to-admission insulin regimens may be able to be resumed or modified in the ICU based on other factors outlined in this chapter.

52.4 Hyperglycemia Management

Despite ample evidence supporting BG targets in critically ill patients, optimal management strategies for achieving those targets are not solidly established. This section includes discussion on generalized treatment considerations. Institutional protocols or guidance tailored to specific patient populations and validated within specific institutions should be considered within the context of the following recommendations.

52.4.1 BG Threshold for Therapy Initiation

Recent guideline recommendations state that it is good practice to consider initiating antihyperglycemic pharmacotherapy at a BG trigger threshold of two consecutive readings ≥180 mg/dL [21, 22]. The authors suggest that initial evaluation of BG trends and consideration of therapy initiation may be warranted at a lower BG threshold of 140 mg/dL to mitigate the development of hyperglycemia, particularly through the initiation of correctional (or sliding scale) insulin.

52.4.2　Insulin vs. Non-insulin Antihyperglycemic Agents

Insulin is the preferred agent for hyperglycemia management in critically ill patients given its quick onset and titratability, safety, and overall evidence for use in the ICU setting [21, 22].

Despite their widespread use in the outpatient setting, oral and injectable non-insulin antihyperglycemic agents should be avoided for hyperglycemia management in critically ill patients [21]. Limited evidence has evaluated the safety and efficacy of these agents in hospitalized patients, including metformin, sulfonylureas, glucagon-like peptide receptor agonists, and sodium-glucose co-transporter 2 inhibitors [37]. Delayed onset and long durations of action pose challenges in initiating and titrating non-insulin agents in the acute setting. Additionally, risks of adverse effects such as hypoglycemia, lactic acidosis, infection, and euglycemic diabetic ketoacidosis are expected to outweigh benefits in critically ill patients, especially considering their dynamic clinical status, reduced physiologic reserve, and alterations in pharmacokinetics which may pose contraindications to non-insulin agents [38, 39].

Lastly, due to their variability of effect in the setting of dynamic factors affecting glycemic control in critically ill patients, the authors recommend against the use of mixed insulin products that combine long- or intermediate-acting and short-acting insulin, such as insulin 70% NPH/30% regular, in critically ill patients.

52.4.3　Intravenous (IV) Infusion vs. Subcutaneous Insulin

The 2024 SCCM Guidelines on Glycemic Control for Critically Ill Children and Adults suggest the use of continuous IV insulin infusions over intermittent subcutaneous insulin in critically ill patients, a conditional recommendation based on very-low-certainty evidence. In their meta-analysis of two randomized controlled trials and four observational studies, when compared to subcutaneous insulin, insulin infusions achieved target BG more frequently yet had more hypoglycemic events, with no differences in patient-centered outcomes such as mortality, ICU or hospital lengths of stay, or infection rate [22]. When considered as a whole, these results ultimately support tailoring the modality of insulin administration to individual patients and their current clinical status.

From a practical standpoint, benefits of intermittent subcutaneous insulin compared to an IV infusion include decreased resource utilization, such as monitoring and nursing workload, and ability to downgrade patients' level of care from ICU status as appropriate. Limitations of subcutaneous insulin include less titratability compared to an infusion, patient discomfort with repeated injections, and possible variability of effect due to factors that impact subcutaneous absorption, such as edema, vasopressor use, and poor perfusion [40].

Subcutaneous insulin can be a safe and effective hyperglycemia management strategy and is reasonable to consider for many critically ill patients at various times during their ICU admission. Given the paucity of high-quality studies comparing insulin administration modalities in this setting, the authors suggest avoiding subcutaneous insulin and considering an IV infusion in situations including, but not limited to (and barring hyperglycemic crises, which are discussed in a separate chapter):

1. High severity of illness in which frequent monitoring and titration are favorable.
2. Severe (e.g., BG >250 mg/dL) and/or persistent (e.g., BG >180–200 mg/dL for over 12–24 h) hyperglycemia.
3. Rapidly fluctuating or significantly opposing factors that impact BG (see the Factors Impacting Glycemic Control section).
4. When subcutaneous insulin pumps are interrupted or unable to be continued.

52.4.4 Intravenous (IV) Insulin Infusion Management Strategies

As described in the BG Targets in Critically Ill Patients section, continuous IV insulin infusions were used in all landmark glycemic control trials in critically ill patients due to their titratability and ability to maintain BG within target range; however, various algorithms and titrations were utilized. Numerous institutional protocols have been published and shared, with similar variability in guidance on initiation, dosing, and titration [41, 42]. Algorithms managed by nurses have demonstrated adequate BG control in hyperglycemic ICU patients and may be associated with improved glycemic control compared to algorithms managed by providers [43, 44]. Regardless of the specifics of the protocols used, quality improvement processes and regular reassessment of adherence, monitoring, and safety should be implemented [45].

Incorporating decision support tools into IV infusion algorithms, such as those that include explicit recommendations and an open-loop system to allow for agreement or disagreement with the output, is recommended. In a meta-analysis of 13 randomized controlled trials, decision support tools were associated with increased time within target BG range and fewer hypoglycemia episodes compared to conventional protocols [22].

Insulin adsorption to IV tubing could result in potential under-delivery of insulin and ongoing hyperglycemia, whereas eventual saturation of tubing could result in potential over-delivery and hypoglycemia. The clinical significance of this effect is not well studied and likely more impactful during the first hours of initiating an insulin infusion and at lower infusion rates; however, given the high-alert nature of insulin, consideration and consistency in management and handling should be applied [46]. Low-absorbency tubing is recommended; if unavailable, it is recommended to saturate binding sites in the tubing by flushing the tubing with 20–25 mL from the insulin infusion and discarding that volume prior to initiating the infusion [47].

52.4.5 Subcutaneous Insulin Management Strategies

52.4.5.1 General Subcutaneous Insulin Considerations

In addition to factors impacting subcutaneous absorption outlined in the IV infusion vs. subcutaneous insulin subsection, several other pharmacokinetic factors related to various subcutaneous insulin products should also be considered in critically ill patients. Knowledge of onset, duration, and elimination should be incorporated into the creation and modification of insulin therapy care plans. In general, compared to continuous IV insulin infusions, subcutaneous insulin is expected to have a slower onset and longer duration of action resulting in less titratability overall. Additionally, reduced insulin clearance in patients with renal impairment should also be considered [48, 49]. While the longer duration of subcutaneous insulin can often be appropriate and even desirable in many critically ill patients, a reminder of one of the pharmacists' golden rules is warranted—that additional medication may always be given but cannot be taken away.

52.4.5.2 Estimated Total Daily Dose (TDD) of Insulin

For hyperglycemic patients, estimating the total daily dose (TDD) of insulin, or the amount of insulin estimated to be required over a 24-h period, may be helpful in initiating and adjusting subcutaneous insulin regimens. An overview of TDD estimations is outlined as follows, with additional considerations related to nutritional (or bolus/postprandial) and long-acting (or basal) insulin outlined in the respective subsections below. Using multiple methods and comparing them as able are recommended to adjudicate these estimations in critically ill patients:

- *Weight based*: The estimated TDD of insulin based on weight in most insulin-naive patients can generally range from 0.3 to 0.6 units/kg based on factors such as weight, elderly age, renal impairment, and concomitant corticosteroid use [50]. For most critically ill patients, the authors recommend a conservative approach of 0.3 units/kg when initially estimating the TDD, with 30% attributed to basal (or long-acting) requirements and 70% attributed to bolus (or nutritional/ postprandial) requirements.
- *Home regimen based*: For patients with a history of diabetes receiving insulin, the total amount of insulin the patient receives per day prior to admission can be

calculated. This dose should be considered within the context of their outpatient glycemic control by assessing hemoglobin A1c outlined in the Patient-Specific Factors Impacting Glycemic Control subsection, as well as their current degree of hyperglycemia, carbohydrate intake, and overall clinical status.

- *Insulin requirement based*: Patients' current insulin requirements in the acute setting can also be considered, including correctional, nutritional, and long-acting insulin doses per day described in more detail in the subsections below:

  - For patients receiving an IV insulin infusion who are ready to be transitioned to subcutaneous insulin, the 24-h insulin utilization can be calculated by adding the amount of insulin received over a stable period of time (e.g., the last 6–24 h, with extrapolation over 24 h if the period is <24 h) [21]. The shorter the stable period being evaluated, the more caution should be used in extrapolating over a 24-h period—for example, if an 8-h period is evaluated when a patient receiving a regular oral diet was sleeping and therefore not receiving any nutritional intake, the 24-h insulin utilization may reflect basal insulin requirements but may not be indicative of bolus requirements. As a conservative approach in accounting for variability, many clinicians suggest utilizing 80% of this value to determine the estimated TDD on which to base subcutaneous insulin dosing [51].

52.4.5.3 Transitioning from Intravenous (IV) Infusion to Subcutaneous Insulin

Hyperglycemic patients receiving an IV insulin infusion may be transitioned to a subcutaneous insulin regimen once infusion rates have been steady (e.g., not varying by >2 units/h) and BG has been controlled at ≤180–200 mg/dL for at least 6 h. Nutrition and/or dextrose intake should also be consistent, and the patient should have a stable or non-worsening clinical status, ideally with hemodynamic stability without the need for vasoactive medications [51]. A premature transition when factors affecting glycemic control outlined above are still fluctuating significantly can predispose patients to risks of hyper- or hypoglycemia, depending on how insulin requirements are estimated and in which direction the factors continue to fluctuate.

The Estimated TDD of Insulin subsection describes how to extrapolate the estimated TDD based on the 24-h insulin utilization. When transitioning to subcutaneous insulin, the same general considerations outlined for correctional, nutritional, and long-acting insulin below may be applied:

- Transitioning from an IV infusion to correctional (or sliding scale) subcutaneous insulin alone is not recommended for most patients due to the risk of rebound hyperglycemia compared to long-acting (or basal) and/or nutritional (or bolus/postprandial) insulin regimens, unless the insulin infusion rate is consistently low (e.g., <2 units/h) and the patient does not have a history of diabetes [52, 53].

- For patients with minimal or no nutritional or carbohydrate intake during the period evaluated, institutional protocols may suggest that 80% of the 24-h insulin requirement (i.e., 100% of the estimated TDD) can be transitioned to long-acting insulin [51]. To account for the variability and influence of other dynamic factors impacting glycemic control, the authors suggest a more conservative approach of considering 50% of the 24-h insulin requirement as the initial long-acting insulin dose with the addition of correctional (or sliding scale) insulin as needed.

- For patients receiving relatively stable nutritional intake, the authors recommend a conservative split of 30% of the estimated TDD administered as long-acting insulin and 70% as nutritional insulin.

The IV insulin infusion may be discontinued within 2 h after administration of long-acting insulin based on its expected onset of action. Further modification of the subcutaneous insulin regimen should be based on the adequacy of glycemic control and any fluctuations in nutrition-, medication-, or patient-specific factors outlined in the Factors Impacting Glycemic Control section.

52.4.5.4 Correctional (or Sliding Scale) Subcutaneous Insulin

Correctional (or sliding scale) insulin refers to rapid-acting insulin such as aspart or lispro that is administered intermittently (e.g., 0–6 units every 4 h or with meals and nightly as needed) in response to elevated BG, with higher doses given for higher BG according to institutional nomograms. Because correctional insulin administration is reactive such that doses are only administered in response to already elevated BG, it does not need to be held in the setting of diminished nutrition or other factors. Correctional insulin can be ordered concomitantly with basal (or long-acting) and/ or bolus (or nutritional/postprandial) insulin regimens. When used on its own, it may be useful in mitigating hyperglycemia in patients with BG $\geq$140 mg/dL and/or in addressing very mild hyperglycemia (e.g., BG $\leq$200–220 mg/dL) in patients without ongoing and/or significant factors expected to elevate BG. There is limited utility of correctional insulin in adequately controlling moderate-to-severe hyperglycemia, with increased incidence of ongoing hyperglycemia compared to basal and/or bolus insulin regimens [52, 53].

Institutional correctional insulin nomograms often include various intensities, such as low-, medium-, and high-dose sliding scales, with a lower insulin dose generally given with the low-dose sliding scale compared to medium- and high-dose sliding scales at respective BG ranges. It should be noted, however, that nomograms may not always correlate linearly across intensities and/or as BG increases—for example, a BG of 210 mg/dL could result in 2 units of insulin on both the low- and medium-dose sliding scales and 4 units of insulin on the high-dose sliding scale. Therefore, there may be variable utility and impact in increasing the sliding scale intensity depending on the extent of hyperglycemia. Critical care pharmacists should familiarize themselves with their institutional correctional nomograms and consider specific nuances when selecting and adjusting sliding scale intensities for each patient.

52.4.5.5 Nutritional (or Bolus/Postprandial) Subcutaneous Insulin

Nutritional (or bolus/postprandial) insulin refers to rapid- or short-acting insulin such as aspart, lispro, or regular administered intermittently in a scheduled fashion around mealtime (e.g., 3 units every 4 h in patients receiving continuous tube feeds or parenteral nutrition, or three times daily with meals in patients tolerating an oral diet or bolus tube feeds). Since nutritional insulin is intended to cover insulin requirements from carbohydrates as the name implies, patients who are NPO or who have minimal nutritional intake should not be initiated or continued on nutritional insulin.

To determine the initial nutritional insulin dose and subsequent dose titrations, carbohydrate intake must be considered and frequently reassessed. For initial nutritional insulin dosing, the following practical approaches can be considered (with recommendation to consider multiple approaches and compare estimations for each patient as able):

- For most patients receiving full nutrition (e.g., tube feeds at goal rate), 50–70% of the estimated TDD of insulin (or approximately 0.2–0.3 units/kg) described above may be attributed to nutritional requirements.
- For patients receiving correctional (or sliding scale) insulin only, the amount of correctional insulin received during a period of relatively stable carbohydrate intake over the last 6–24 h can also be considered, then extrapolated to a 24-h estimated TDD if the period is <24 h, and divided into nutritional insulin doses. Patients with more severe hyperglycemia may also benefit from the initiation of long-acting (or basal) insulin, though some patients thought to be experiencing hyperglycemia primarily from nutrition may have adequate glycemic control on nutritional insulin alone (plus or minus correctional insulin).
- For patients receiving long-acting and correctional insulin, the amount of correctional insulin in addition to basal insulin received during a period of relatively stable carbohydrate intake over the last 6–24 h can be considered, with the estimated TDD of insulin split into long-acting and nutritional insulin doses (while continuing correctional insulin as needed). For most patients, due to the extended duration of long-acting insulin, the authors recommend a conservative split of 30% of the estimated TDD administered as long-acting insulin and 70% as nutritional insulin.
- For patients with diabetes receiving nutritional insulin prior to admission, their home nutritional insulin dose and current carbohydrate intake compared to that prior to admission can be considered.

The Hypoglycemia Management section below outlines examples of administration comments that can be considered within nutritional insulin orders that outline situations in which to hold the dose to mitigate the risk of hypoglycemia. Further modification of the nutritional insulin dose and/or frequency of administration should be based on the adequacy of glycemic control, modality of nutrition provision, and any fluctuations in nutritional factors outlined in the Factors Impacting Glycemic Control section.

Steroid-Induced Hyperglycemia

Given corticosteroids' propensity to elevate postprandial BG, steroid-induced hyperglycemia is another clinical scenario to consider within this subsection [32]. Due to the expected onset, peak, and duration of hyperglycemic effects particularly of short- and intermediate-acting steroids such as hydrocortisone and prednisone, insulin NPH has been studied in the setting of steroid-induced hyperglycemia [31, 54]. Insulin NPH is an intermediate-acting insulin with a peak effect of 4–10 h and duration of approximately 12–24 h, which may mimic the hyperglycemic effects of corticosteroids [55]. Small, prospective studies have demonstrated safety and efficacy of insulin NPH compared to long-acting insulin in managing steroid-induced hyperglycemia in non-critically ill patients, with variable dosing regimens stratified based on the steroid dose and/or presence of preexisting diabetes [56–58]. Due to its variable pharmacokinetics, insulin NPH may therefore have variable antihyperglycemic effects, especially in a critically ill population, so caution should be exercised. The authors suggest considering a conservative initial insulin NPH starting dose of 0.2 units/kg for most patients, dosed daily in the setting of daily steroid administration or twice daily with more frequent steroid administrations.

Insulin in Parenteral Nutrition

While not subcutaneous, it should also be noted that IV insulin administered in parenteral nutrition may also serve as a form of nutritional insulin, with initial doses generally ranging from 1 unit of insulin per 10–20 g of IV dextrose and titrated in response to dextrose adjustments and glycemic control. Potential advantages of this modality include stable IV administration, circumventing barriers to subcutaneous absorption, and patient discomfort, without the need for increased frequency of BG monitoring (e.g., every 1–2 h) such as with a continuous IV insulin infusion. The effect of insulin lasts as long as parenteral nutrition is continued which can be both an advantage and disadvantage—on the one hand, if parenteral nutrition is interrupted, the effect of insulin will not persist which may reduce the risk of hypoglycemia; on the other hand, titratability of insulin is limited (especially in the case of continuous parenteral nutrition administered over 24 h), and parenteral nutrition may have to be discontinued all together in the event that hypoglycemia does occur. A small, single-center, prospective study found similar rates of hyper- and hypoglycemia in stable ICU patients receiving insulin in parenteral nutrition compared to long-acting insulin; however, data on optimal timing of initiation, dosing and titration, concomitant subcutaneous insulin use, or efficacy and safety in less stable critically ill patients are currently lacking [59].

52.4.5.6   Long-Acting (or Basal) Subcutaneous Insulin

Long-acting (or basal) subcutaneous insulin refers to insulin with a long (e.g., 24 h) duration and peakless concentration such as insulin glargine, detemir, or degludec administered intermittently in a scheduled fashion (e.g., 15 units every 24 h). Long-acting insulin is intended to cover basal insulin requirements and therefore can be considered in patients regardless of their nutritional intake.

Before determining the initial long-acting insulin dose and subsequent dose titrations, it should be reiterated that due to the long duration, titratability is limited; therefore, the authors recommend a conservative dosing approach for most critically ill patients. For initial long-acting insulin dosing, the following practical approaches can be considered (with recommendation to consider multiple approaches and compare estimations for each patient as able):

- For most patients, 30–50% of the estimated TDD of insulin (or approximately 0.1–0.3 units/kg) described above may be attributed to basal requirements. The authors recommend a conservative approach of 0.1 units/kg for initial long-acting insulin dosing in ICU patients without a history of diabetes and/or receiving insulin prior to admission.
- For patients receiving correctional (or sliding scale) insulin only with minimal or no nutritional or carbohydrate intake, the amount of correctional insulin received over the last 6–24 h can also be considered, then extrapolated to a 24-h estimated TDD if the period is <24 h and considered as an initial long-acting insulin dose.
- For patients receiving nutritional and correctional insulin, the amount of nutritional insulin in addition to correctional insulin received during a period of relatively stable carbohydrate intake over the last 6–24 h can be considered, with the estimated TDD of insulin split into long-acting and nutritional insulin doses (while continuing correctional insulin as needed). For most patients, due to the extended duration of long-acting insulin, the authors recommend a conservative split of 30% of the estimated TDD administered as long-acting insulin and 70% as nutritional insulin.
- For patients with diabetes receiving long-acting insulin prior to admission, their home insulin dose and other factors affecting glycemic control compared to those prior to admission can be considered.

Further modification of the long-acting insulin regimen should be based on the adequacy of glycemic control and any fluctuations in nutrition-, medication-, or patient-specific factors outlined in the Factors Impacting Glycemic Control section.

52.5   Hypoglycemia Management

In addition to managing hyperglycemia, critical care pharmacists and teams must also be diligent about mitigating hypoglycemia risks as well as promptly recognizing and treating it, should it occur.

52.5.1 Hypoglycemia Recognition and Treatment

Timely recognition and treatment of hypoglycemia, along with reassessment of contributing factors, are key. It is important to note that many critically ill patients may be unable to endorse classic hypoglycemia symptoms such as lightheadedness, irritability, or hunger. Additionally, symptoms related to neuroglycopenia, including altered mentation, seizure, and coma, may be masked or confounded by other acute or chronic issues in ICU patients [60]. Therefore, accurate and frequent BG monitoring outlined in the BG Monitoring section is an important tool in identifying hypoglycemia in critically ill patients.

Implementation of a standardized, nurse-initiated hypoglycemia treatment protocol utilizing IV dextrose (or intramuscular glucagon in patients without IV access) to address any instance of BG ≤70 mg/dL is recommended for every institution. While specific protocols will vary based on patient- and hospital-specific factors, quality improvement processes should be implemented to re-evaluate protocol adherence and other safety measures [21]. Also, hypoglycemia episodes should be documented in the electronic health record and evaluated for a root cause in accordance with Joint Commission standards [61]. Critical care pharmacists can play an important role in mitigating future hypoglycemic episodes through real-time re-evaluation of insulin regimens and other medication- and nutrition-related factors affecting glycemic control.

An example of an inpatient hypoglycemia protocol is as follows [62, 63]:

A. For patients who are alert and able to take oral intake:

1. Discontinue all active insulin orders.
2. Give fast-acting carbohydrates:

   (a) If BG 50–70 mg/dL: give 15 g of fast-acting carbohydrates (e.g., 4 oz of juice).
   (b) If BG <50 mg/dL: give 30 g of fast-acting carbohydrates (e.g., 8 oz of juice).

3. Recheck BG in 15 min:

   (a) If BG >70 mg/dL, proceed to step 5.
   (b) If BG ≤70 mg/dL, repeat steps 2 and 3.

4. If BG on third check is >70 mg/dL, proceed to step 5:

   (a) If BG ≤70 mg/dL, hang 1 L of D5W at 42 mL/h and notify provider.

5. Reassess insulin regimen and dynamic factors affecting glycemic control.

B. For patients who are unalert and/or unable to take oral intake (with IV access):

1. Discontinue all active insulin orders.
2. Give dextrose IV push:

   (a) If BG 50–70 mg/dL: give dextrose 12.5 g IV push (e.g., 25 mL of D50W).

    (b) If BG <50 mg/dL: give dextrose 25 g IV push (e.g., 50 mL of D50W).

3. Recheck BG in 15 min:

    (a) If BG >70 mg/dL, proceed to step 5.
    (b) If BG ≤70 mg/dL, repeat steps 2 and 3.

4. If BG on third check is >70 mg/dL, proceed to step 5:

    (a) If BG ≤70 mg/dL, hang 1 L of D5W at 42 mL/h and notify provider.

5. Reassess insulin regimen and dynamic factors affecting glycemic control.

C. For patients who are unalert and/or unable to have oral intake (*without* IV access):

1. Give glucagon 1 mg IM.
2. Obtain IV access.
3. Recheck BG in 15 min, and follow the algorithm under "B" above.

For practical considerations related to hypoglycemia management, the authors suggest that most ICU patients, and all those ordered to receive insulin, should have active orders to implement the hypoglycemia treatment protocol, should BG fall to ≤70 mg/dL. To decrease the risk of inadvertent administration of insulin during undesired situations, standardized administration comments embedded in insulin orders can also be considered. For example, for patients receiving continuous tube feeds or parenteral nutrition, nutritional (or bolus/postprandial) insulin administration comments could instruct that the dose be held if nutrition is paused for more than 2 h or if BG is <100 mg/dL; alternatively, for patients receiving solid food or bolus tube feeds, administration comments could instruct the dose to be given only *after* 50% carbohydrate consumption or completion of bolus feeding.

52.6 Blood Glucose (BG) Monitoring

BG monitoring and its accuracy can be impacted by many factors, including device performance, sample site, and user interface. Point-of-care (POC) BG monitoring is commonly utilized in the ICU given its rapid result turnaround time. Capillary or finger-stick testing may lead to BG inaccuracies due to factors such as decreased perfusion, edema, and medication interference and can also cause patient discomfort. Therefore, vascular access sites with venous or arterial blood are preferred for POC testing when possible [22, 45]. Additionally, calibrated POC BG devices approved by the US Food and Drug Administration should be utilized, with implementation of quality improvement processes within individual institutions [21].

52.6.1 BG Monitoring Frequency

For patients receiving an IV insulin infusion, guideline recommendations for the frequency of BG monitoring range from every 30 min to every 2 h [21, 64]. More frequent (≤1 h) BG monitoring was associated with fewer hypoglycemia episodes and less time experiencing hyperglycemia compared to less frequent (>1 h) monitoring [22]. Hourly BG monitoring in patients receiving insulin infusions may be reasonable in balancing safety and efficacy with workload considerations compared to 30-min assessments.

For patients who are eating meals or receiving bolus tube feeds, BG can be monitored before meals and at bedtime. For patients who are receiving no or minimal nutrition (including an IV dextrose infusion or a clear liquid diet), continuous or cyclic tube feeds, or continuous or cyclic parenteral nutrition, BG should be monitored every 4–6 h [21]. The authors suggest monitoring every 4 h initially, with consideration of liberalizing to every 6 h in patients who demonstrate BG stability.

52.6.2 Continuous Glucose Monitoring (CGM)

Several studies have evaluated the use of CGM in the ICU given its potential to provide more data points with less workload compared to POC monitoring. Observational data characterizing CGM use during the COVID-19 pandemic demonstrated feasibility in a small number of critically ill patients [65, 66]. Other small, randomized studies have shown that CGM reduced hypoglycemic events, nursing workload, and daily costs in patients receiving an IV insulin infusion compared to standard-of-care monitoring [67, 68]. However, accuracy of CGM in critically ill patients may be impacted by clinical factors affecting subcutaneous measurements, and failure of CGM devices to meet mean absolute relative difference point accuracy standards should be considered [69]. Other barriers to routine CGM use in the ICU include cost, electronic health record and protocol integration, regulatory approval, and staff education and training. Additional research validating CGM accuracy and evaluating safety and efficacy in critically ill patients is needed [21, 22, 70].

52.7 Future Considerations and Research Areas

Despite existing research and current recommendations surrounding glycemic control in critically ill patients, additional questions remain. Future research areas include individualized BG targets in special populations (such as more liberal targets in patients with uncontrolled diabetes), use of personalized medicine, outcomes, and metrics related to glycemic control evaluation (such as time within goal

BG range or BG variability), and role of technology and informatics (such as CGM and advanced decision support tools or algorithms) [22].

52.8 Conclusion

Glycemic control consists of managing hyperglycemia, avoiding hypoglycemia, and reducing overall BG variability. Managing glycemic control in the ICU is a standard therapeutic goal to reduce adverse effects and improve morbidity and mortality. Critical care pharmacists can support managing BG in ICU adult patients by identifying risk factors for hyperglycemia and hypoglycemia, establishing appropriate therapeutic BG targets, evaluating and promoting the use of standardized insulin protocols, and optimizing insulin therapy regimens in critically ill patients.

References

1. Egi M, Bellomo R, Stachowski E, et al. Blood glucose concentration and outcome of critical illness: the impact of diabetes. Crit Care Med. 2008;36(8):2249–55.
2. Furnary AP, Zerr KJ, Grunkemeier GL, Starr A. Continuous intravenous insulin infusion reduces the incidence of deep sternal wound infection in diabetic patients after cardiac surgical procedures. Ann Thorac Surg. 1999;67(2):352–60; discussion 360–2.
3. Krinsley JS. Association between hyperglycemia and increased hospital mortality in a heterogeneous population of critically ill patients. Mayo Clin Proc. 2003;78(12):1471–8.
4. Saltiel AR, Kahn CR. Insulin signalling and the regulation of glucose and lipid metabolism. Nature. 2001;414(6865):799–806.
5. Habegger KM, Heppner KM, Geary N, Bartness TJ, DiMarchi R, Tschöp MH. The metabolic actions of glucagon revisited. Nat Rev Endocrinol. 2010;6(12):689–97.
6. McCowen KC, Malhotra A, Bistrian BR. Stress-induced hyperglycemia. Crit Care Clin. 2001;17(1):107–24.
7. Kavanagh BP, McCowen KC. Clinical practice. Glycemic control in the ICU. N Engl J Med. 2010;363(26):2540–6.
8. Godinjak A, Iglica A, Burekovic A, et al. Hyperglycemia in critically ill patients: management and prognosis. Med Arh. 2015;69(3):157–60.
9. NICE-SUGAR Study Investigators, Finfer S, Liu B, et al. Hypoglycemia and risk of death in critically ill patients. N Engl J Med. 2012;367(12):1108–18.
10. Arky RA. Hypoglycemia associated with liver disease and ethanol. Endocrinol Metab Clin N Am. 1989;18(1):75–90.
11. Lee SC, Baranowski ES, Sakremath R, Saraff V, Mohamed Z. Hypoglycaemia in adrenal insufficiency. Front Endocrinol (Lausanne). 2023;14:1198519.
12. Krinsley JS, Grover A. Severe hypoglycemia in critically ill patients: risk factors and outcomes. Crit Care Med. 2007;35(10):2262–7.
13. Gunst J, Debaveye Y, Güiza F, et al. Tight blood-glucose control without early parenteral nutrition in the ICU. N Engl J Med. 2023;389(13):1180–90.
14. NICE-SUGAR Study Investigators, Finfer S, Chittock DR, et al. Intensive versus conventional glucose control in critically ill patients. N Engl J Med. 2009;360(13):1283–97.

15. Malmberg K, Rydén L, Efendic S, et al. Randomized trial of insulin-glucose infusion followed by subcutaneous insulin treatment in diabetic patients with acute myocardial infarction (DIGAMI study): effects on mortality at 1 year. J Am Coll Cardiol. 1995;26(1):57–65.

16. Malmberg K. Prospective randomised study of intensive insulin treatment on long term survival after acute myocardial infarction in patients with diabetes mellitus. DIGAMI (Diabetes Mellitus, Insulin Glucose Infusion in Acute Myocardial Infarction) Study Group. BMJ. 1997;314(7093):1512–5.

17. van den Berghe G, Wouters P, Weekers F, et al. Intensive insulin therapy in critically ill patients. N Engl J Med. 2001;345(19):1359–67.

18. van den Berghe G, Wilmer A, Hermans G, et al. Intensive insulin therapy in the medical ICU. N Engl J Med. 2006;354(5):449–61.

19. American Diabetes Association. Standards of medical care in diabetes--2012. Diabetes Care. 2012;35(Suppl 1):S11–63.

20. Jacobi J, Bircher N, Krinsley J, et al. Guidelines for the use of an insulin infusion for the management of hyperglycemia in critically ill patients. Crit Care Med. 2012;40(12):3251–76.

21. American Diabetes Association. Diabetes care in the hospital: standards of care in diabetes—2024. Diabetes Care. 2024;47(Suppl 1):S295–306.

22. Honarmand K, Sirimaturos M, Hirshberg EL, et al. Society of critical care medicine guidelines on glycemic control for critically ill children and adults 2024. Crit Care Med. 2024;52(4):e161–81.

23. Poole AP, Finnis ME, Anstey J, et al. The effect of a liberal approach to glucose control in critically ill patients with type 2 diabetes: a multicenter, parallel-group, open-label randomized clinical trial. Am J Respir Crit Care Med. 2022;206(7):874–82.

24. Bohé J, Abidi H, Brunot V, et al. Individualised versus conventional glucose control in critically-ill patients: the CONTROLING study-a randomized clinical trial. Intensive Care Med. 2021;47(11):1271–83.

25. Ingels C, Debaveye Y, Milants I, et al. Strict blood glucose control with insulin during intensive care after cardiac surgery: impact on 4-years survival, dependency on medical care, and quality-of-life. Eur Heart J. 2006;27(22):2716–24.

26. Lazar HL, McDonnell M, Chipkin SR, et al. The Society of Thoracic Surgeons practice guideline series: blood glucose management during adult cardiac surgery. Ann Thorac Surg. 2009;87(2):663–9.

27. Desai SP, Henry LL, Holmes SD, et al. Strict versus liberal target range for perioperative glucose in patients undergoing coronary artery bypass grafting: a prospective randomized controlled trial. J Thorac Cardiovasc Surg. 2012;143(2):318–25.

28. Umpierrez G, Cardona S, Pasquel F, et al. Randomized controlled trial of intensive versus conservative glucose control in patients undergoing coronary artery bypass graft surgery: GLUCO-CABG trial. Diabetes Care. 2015;38(9):1665–72.

29. NICE-SUGAR Study Investigators for the Australian and New Zealand Intensive Care Society Clinical Trials Group and the Canadian Critical Care Trials Group, Finfer S, Chittock D, et al. Intensive versus conventional glucose control in critically ill patients with traumatic brain injury: long-term follow-up of a subgroup of patients from the NICE-SUGAR study. Intensive Care Med. 2015;41(6):1037–47.

30. van Raalte DH, Ouwens DM, Diamant M. Novel insights into glucocorticoid-mediated diabetogenic effects: towards expansion of therapeutic options? Eur J Clin Investig. 2009;39:81–93.

31. Clore JN, Thurby-Hay L. Glucocorticoid-induced hyperglycemia. Endocr Pract. 2009;15:469–74.

32. Yuen KC, McDaniel PA, Riddle MC. Twenty-four-hour profiles of plasma glucose, insulin, C-peptide and free fatty acid in subjects with varying degrees of glucose tolerance following short-term, medium-dose prednisone (20 mg/day) treatment: evidence for differing effects on insulin secretion and action. Clin Endocrinol. 2012;77:224–32.

33. Lunetta M, De Mauro M, Le Moli R, Nicoletti F. Effect of octreotide on blood glucose and counterregulatory hormones in insulin-dependent diabetic patients: the role of dose and route of administration. Eur J Clin Pharmacol. 1996;51(2):139–44.

34. McLaughlin SA, Crandall CS, McKinney PE. Octreotide: an antidote for sulfonylurea-induced hypoglycemia. Ann Emerg Med. 2000;36(2):133–8.
35. Phadke D, Beller JP, Tribble C. The disparate effects of epinephrine and norepinephrine on hyperglycemia in cardiovascular surgery. Heart Surg Forum. 2018;21(6):E522–6.
36. ElSayed NA, Aleppo G, Aroda VR, et al. 6. Glycemic targets: standards of care in diabetes-2023. Diabetes Care. 2023;46(Suppl 1):S97–S110.
37. Duan D, Mathioudakis NN, Pilla SJ. Treatment of diabetes in hospitals with noninsulin medications is a research priority. Diabetes Care. 2024;47(6):915–7.
38. Donihi AC, Moorman JM, Abla A, Hanania R, Carneal D, MacMaster HW. Pharmacists' role in glycemic management in the inpatient setting: an opinion of the endocrine and metabolism practice and research network of the American College of Clinical Pharmacy. J Am Coll Clin Pharm. 2019;2:167–76.
39. Moghissi ES, Korytkowski MT, DiNardo M, et al. American Association of Clinical Endocrinologists and American Diabetes Association consensus statement on inpatient glycemic control. Endocr Pract. 2009;15(4):353–69.
40. Gradel AKJ, Porsgaard T, Lykkesfeldt J, et al. Factors affecting the absorption of subcutaneously administered insulin: effect on variability. J Diabetes Res. 2018;2018:1205121.
41. Goldberg PA, Siegel MD, Sherwin RS, et al. Implementation of a safe and effective insulin infusion protocol in a medical intensive care unit. Diabetes Care. 2004;27:461–7.
42. Wilson M, Weinreb J, Hoo GW. Intensive insulin therapy in critical care: a review of 12 protocols. Diabetes Care. 2007;30(4):1005–11.
43. Passarelli AJ, Gibbs H, Rowden AM, Efird L, Zink E, Mathioudakis N. Evaluation of a nurse-managed insulin infusion protocol. Diabetes Technol Ther. 2016;18(2):93–9.
44. Quinn JA, Snyder SL, Berghoff JL, Colombo CS, Jacobi J. A practical approach to hyperglycemia management in the intensive care unit: evaluation of an intensive insulin infusion protocol. Pharmacotherapy. 2006;26(10):1410–20.
45. Kelly JL. Continuous insulin infusion: when, where, and how? Diabetes Spectr. 2014;27(3):218–23.
46. Knopp JL, Chase JG. Clinical recommendations for managing the impact of insulin adsorptive loss in hospital and diabetes care. J Diabetes Sci Technol. 2021;15(4):874–84.
47. Thompson CD, Vital-Carona J, Faustino EV. The effect of tubing dwell time on insulin adsorption during intravenous insulin infusions. Diabetes Technol Ther. 2012;14(10):912–6.
48. Park J, Lertdumrongluk P, Molnar MZ, Kovesdy CP, Kalantar-Zadeh K. Glycemic control in diabetic dialysis patients and the burnt-out diabetes phenomenon. Curr Diab Rep. 2012;12(4):432–9.
49. Sandler V, Misiasz MR, Jones J, Baldwin D. Reducing the risk of hypoglycemia associated with intravenous insulin: experience with a computerized insulin infusion program in 4 adult intensive care units. J Diabetes Sci Technol. 2014;8(5):923–9.
50. Magaji V, Johnston JM. Inpatient management of hyperglycemia and diabetes. Clin Diabetes. 2011;29(1):3–9.
51. Kreider KE, Lien LF. Transitioning safely from intravenous to subcutaneous insulin. Curr Diab Rep. 2015;15(5):23.
52. Datta S, Qaadir A, Villanueva G, et al. Once-daily insulin glargine versus 6-hour sliding scale regular insulin for control of hyperglycemia after a bariatric surgical procedure: a randomized clinical trial. Endocr Pract. 2007;13(3):225–31.
53. Umpierrez GE, Smiley D, Zisman A, et al. Randomized study of basal-bolus insulin therapy in the inpatient management of patients with type 2 diabetes (RABBIT 2 trial). Diabetes Care. 2007;30(9):2181–6.
54. Aberer F, Hochfellner DA, Sourij H, Mader JK. A practical guide for the management of steroid induced hyperglycaemia in the hospital. J Clin Med. 2021;10(10):2154.
55. Donnor T, Sarkar S. Insulin- pharmacology, therapeutic regimens and principles of intensive insulin therapy [updated 2023 Feb 15]. In: Feingold KR, Anawalt B, Blackman MR, et al., edi-

tors. Endotext [Internet]. South Dartmouth (MA): MDText.com, Inc.; 2000. Available from: https://www.ncbi.nlm.nih.gov/books/NBK278938/.

56. Khowaja A, Alkhaddo JB, Rana Z, Fish L. Glycemic control in hospitalized patients with diabetes receiving corticosteroids using a neutral protamine Hagedorn insulin protocol: a randomized clinical trial. Diabetes Ther. 2018;9(4):1647–55.

57. Radhakutty A, Stranks JL, Mangelsdorf BL, et al. Treatment of prednisolone-induced hyperglycaemia in hospitalized patients: insights from a randomized, controlled study. Diabetes Obes Metab. 2017;19(4):571–8.

58. Ruiz de Adana MS, Colomo N, Maldonado-Araque C, et al. Randomized clinical trial of the efficacy and safety of insulin glargine vs. NPH insulin as basal insulin for the treatment of glucocorticoid induced hyperglycemia using continuous glucose monitoring in hospitalized patients with type 2 diabetes and respiratory disease. Diabetes Res Clin Pract. 2015;110(2):158–65.

59. Oghazian MB, Javadi MR, Radfar M, et al. Effectiveness of regular versus glargine insulin in stable critical care patients receiving parenteral nutrition: a randomized controlled trial. Pharmacotherapy. 2015;35(2):148–57.

60. Lacherade JC, Jacqueminet S, Preiser JC. An overview of hypoglycemia in the critically ill. J Diabetes Sci Technol. 2009;3(6):1242–9.

61. Arnold P, Scheurer D, Dake AW, et al. Hospital Guidelines for Diabetes Management and the Joint Commission-American Diabetes Association Inpatient Diabetes Certification. Am J Med Sci. 2016;351(4):333–41.

62. Pasala S, Dendy JA, Chockalingam V, Meadows RY. An inpatient hypoglycemia committee: development, successful implementation, and impact on patient safety. Ochsner J. 2013;13(3):407–12.

63. Umpierrez GE, Hellman R, Korytkowski MT, et al. Management of hyperglycemia in hospitalized patients in non-critical care setting: an endocrine society clinical practice guideline. J Clin Endocrinol Metab. 2012;97(1):16–38.

64. Blonde L, Umpierrez GE, Reddy SS, et al. American Association of Clinical Endocrinology clinical practice guideline: developing a diabetes mellitus comprehensive care plan-2022 update. Endocr Pract. 2023;29(1):80–1.

65. Agarwal S, Mathew J, Davis GM, et al. Continuous glucose monitoring in the intensive care unit during the COVID-19 pandemic. Diabetes Care. 2021;44:847–9.

66. Faulds ER, Boutsicaris A, Sumner L, et al. Use of continuous glucose monitor in critically ill Covid-19 patients requiring insulin infusion: an observational study. J Clin Endocrinol Metab. 2021;106:e4007–16.

67. Boom DT, Sechterberger MK, Rijkenberg S, et al. Insulin treatment guided by subcutaneous continuous glucose monitoring compared to frequent point-of-care measurement in critically ill patients: a randomized controlled trial. Crit Care. 2014;18(4):453.

68. Holzinger U, Warszawska J, Kitzberger R, et al. Real-time continuous glucose monitoring in critically ill patients: a prospective randomized trial. Diabetes Care. 2010;33(3):467–72.

69. Krinsley JS, Chase JG, Gunst J, et al. Continuous glucose monitoring in the ICU: clinical considerations and consensus. Crit Care. 2017;21(1):197.

70. Stoudt K, Chawla S. Don't sugar coat it: glycemic control in the intensive care unit. J Intensive Care Med. 2019;34(11–12):889–96.

Chapter 53
Fluid Resuscitation in the Intensive Care Unit

Michael T. Kenes and Nicholas Farina

53.1 Introduction

Fluid management in critically ill patients is often complex. The unique needs of patients within an intensive care unit (ICU) setting often require a pharmacist to draw upon a strong foundation of chemistry and pathophysiology. While most fluid use in an ICU setting is for resuscitation, or the restoration of circulating intravascular volume to maintain adequate perfusion, other indications may be appropriate as well. Just as important, but beyond the scope of this chapter, replacement and maintenance fluids can also have an important role in the care of patients within an ICU. The rest of the chapter will cover intravenous (IV) fluid composition, choice of IV fluid, dose and monitoring, and, finally, de-resuscitation during the resolution of critical illness.

53.2 Fluid Composition

Fluids administered in the ICU setting can be broadly classified as crystalloids or colloids. Crystalloid fluids are aqueous solutions that contain salts, minerals, and/or sugar. Colloid fluids are sterile water solutions that contain macromolecules such as protein and electrolytes. Table 53.1 contains a comparison of components of common crystalloid solutions.

M. T. Kenes (✉) · N. Farina
Michigan Medicine, Ann Arbor, MI, USA

College of Pharmacy, University of Michigan, Ann Arbor, MI, USA
e-mail: mkenes@umich.edu; nfarina@med.umich.edu

© The Author(s), under exclusive license to Springer Nature Switzerland AG 2025
Y. Alzaidi, M. A. Gebily (eds.), *The Pharmacist's Expanded Role in Critical Care Medicine*, https://doi.org/10.1007/978-3-031-77335-8_53

Table 53.1 Composition of common crystalloid fluids

	Glucose (g/dL)	Sodium (mEq/L)	Chloride (mmol/L)	Potassium (mEq/L)	Buffer	Calcium (mg/dL)	Magnesium (mg/dL)	pH
Human plasma	0.07–0.11	135–145	95–105	3.5–5	23–30	8.8–10.4	1.6–2.4	7.35–7.45
5% Dextrose	5	0	0	0	0	0	0	3.5–6.5
Ringer's lactate	0	130	109	4	28	1.35	0	6–7.5
Ringer's acetate	0	130	112	5	27	1	1	8-Jun
0.9% Sodium chloride	0	154	154	0	0	0	0	4.5–7
Plasma-Lyte	0	140	98	4	50	0	1.5	4–6.5

Adapted from: Moritz and Ayus (2015) [1]

53.3 Crystalloids

Fluids were widely studied during the Indian blue cholera pandemic in 1831, where it was noted that injection of IV water temporarily improved symptoms in patients with fluid loss. Subsequently, William Brooke O'Shaughnessy proposed injecting oxygenated salts to treat cholera patients. Research throughout the nineteenth century culminated with the description of 0.9% sodium chloride by Hartog Jakob Hamburger, which he noted had a similar tonicity to human blood and, for the first time, did not result in the ultimate hemolysis of red blood cells when administered intravenously [2].

Crystalloid fluid can be further differentiated as isotonic, hypotonic, or hypertonic. The tonicity of blood is approximately 270–300 mOsm/kg. Administration of hypotonic or hypertonic fluids may cause shifts in fluid between intravascular and extravascular spaces. Thus, isotonic fluids are preferred for volume resuscitation in critically ill patients. Hypotonic solutions are more commonly utilized when providing maintenance fluids or IV free water to patients. Hypertonic solutions frequently contain high amounts of sodium chloride (>154 mEq/L) and are primarily used to treat sodium disorders or raise serum sodium levels to supraphysiologic concentrations.

Isotonic crystalloid solutions may be further differentiated as balanced or unbalanced. Balanced crystalloid solutions contain electrolyte solutions and buffers that make the composition similar to normal serum concentrations, whereas unbalanced crystalloids do not. The most used unbalanced crystalloid is 0.9% sodium chloride, often referred to as normal saline (NS). NS is profoundly hyperchloremic relative to normal serum concentrations. Hyperchloremia can be a cause of non-gap metabolic acidosis, and it may also alter tubuloglomerular feedback in the kidneys, leading to acute kidney injury via afferent arteriole vasoconstriction (AKI) [3]. Several randomized controlled trials in recent years have compared balanced to unbalanced crystalloids in critically ill adults. The SPLIT trial randomized medical ICU patients to receive either NS or Plasma-Lyte (PL) for all fluid administration and found no differences in AKI or mortality [4]. The SMART trial was a single-center crossover study that randomized all critically ill patients at an academic medical center to NS vs. PL or lactated Ringer's (LR) [5]. The SMART investigators found that hyperchloremia (35.6% vs. 24.5%) and AKI (15.4% vs. 14.3%) were more common in the NS group, but no differences in mortality were found. Patients in the balanced crystalloid arm of SMART primarily received LR. BaSICS was another randomized controlled trial that compared NS to PL and found no differences in mortality or new renal replacement therapy [6]. Finally, the PLUS trial randomized patients to either NS or PL, with no differences in mortality or renal replacement therapy found [7].

The results of the SPLIT and BaSICS trials are confounded by pre-enrollment fluid administration; however, a post hoc analysis of BaSICS that accounted for the type of pre-enrollment fluid administered indicated a mortality benefit in patients that received only balanced crystalloids [8]. Additionally, all of the trials are limited by the amount of study fluid administered post-enrollment. In some trials, patients only received a median of 1 L of fluid following enrollment, whereas median volume was closer to 4 L in others. SMART did find in subgroup analyses that differences in serum chloride levels were more substantial in patients who received larger amounts of fluids [5]. Secondary analyses of SMART and BaSICS also indicated that balanced crystalloids may be associated with slightly lower mortality when used in patients with sepsis [6, 9]. Additionally, balanced crystalloids are recommended for resuscitation of patients with large total body surface area burns or pancreatitis, where the dose exceeds usual (i.e., septic shock) indications [10]. Based on the available literature, balanced crystalloids seem most beneficial when they are prioritized for patients who have received large amounts of fluid volumes. In addition to sepsis and burns, other syndromes that may be encountered in critically ill patients requiring administration of large crystalloid volumes include rhabdomyolysis, tumor lysis syndrome, and diabetic ketoacidosis [3].

Crystalloid fluids, primarily NS and 5% dextrose (D5), are used in diluents for medications that are delivered to patients via IV piggyback or continuous infusions. Critically ill patients may easily receive over 1 L of fluid per day from medication diluents alone. Studies comparing composition of medication diluents have demonstrated that preferentially using D5 instead of NS may help to reduce the incidence of hyperchloremia [11]. One observational study even found that the preferential use of D5 diluents reduced the incidence of AKI [12]. IV medications may be limited to one diluent fluid due to stability reasons, but selection of D5 diluents may be an opportunity for pharmacists to help prevent hyperchloremia and AKI.

Colloid solutions contain higher oncotic pressure than crystalloid solutions and in theory should retain intravascular fluid volume better than crystalloids. Some literature suggests that highly concentrated colloids may even expand intravascular fluid volume by 250% of the fluid volume administered [13]. Synthetic colloids containing hydroxyethyl starch (HES) historically were preferred to albumin solutions due to lower cost. However, several randomized controlled trials have demonstrated the risks of HES compared to alternative fluids. The CHEST randomized controlled trial compares HES to NS for all fluid resuscitation in critically ill patients and found that new renal replacement therapy was more common (7.0% vs. 5.8%) in the HES group [14]. Another randomized controlled trial compared HES to Ringer's acetate in patients with severe sepsis. In that study, HES was found to have higher mortality (51% vs. 43%) and new-onset renal replacement therapy (22% vs. 16%) [15]. The results of these studies have largely pushed routine use of HES out of practice.

Use of albumin in critically ill patients is controversial due to the high cost of albumin relative to crystalloid. SAFE was a randomized controlled trial where critically ill patients were assigned to receive 4% albumin or NS for fluid resuscitation [16]. No differences were found in mortality, ICU length of stay, or days of renal replacement therapy. Notably, ratio of NS to 4% albumin volume administered during the first 4 days of the SAFE trial was essentially the same at 1:1.4, rather than the 1:4 ratio that was anticipated, questioning the real-world ability of colloid fluid to retain volume in intravascular space. Another randomized controlled trial compared 4% albumin to Ringer's acetate during cardiopulmonary bypass surgery and for the first 24 h postoperatively in the ICU [17]. The primary outcome of the study was major adverse events, which included mortality, myocardial injury, new-onset heart failure, re-sternotomy, stroke, arrhythmia, major bleeding, infection, or AKI. No differences in major adverse events were found. Broad use of albumin solutions for volume resuscitation in critically ill patients is not recommended.

Use of albumin solutions is more controversial in sepsis due to the high volumes of solution that may be required for fluid resuscitation and unique pathophysiology. In a subgroup analysis of the SAFE trial in patients with severe sepsis, use of albumin was associated with a lower odds ratio of death (OR 0.87, CI 0.74–1.02) [16]. This finding did not reach statistical significance, however. Subsequently, the ALBIOS trial randomized patients with severe sepsis or septic shock to receive albumin 20% daily if serum albumin levels were below 3 g/dL or placebo [18]. No difference in mortality was found when comparing the two study groups. However, a subgroup analysis of patients with septic shock found a lower risk ratio for mortality in the albumin arm of the study (OR 0.87, CI 0.77–0.99). The Surviving Sepsis Guidelines recommend that crystalloids should be utilized first but recommend using albumin in combination with crystalloids in patients receiving large volumes of resuscitation [19]. The guideline does not define a large volume of resuscitation. A recently published randomized controlled trial compared 5% albumin to balanced crystalloids for initial fluid resuscitation in patients with sepsis [20]. Patients in the trial were less acute, and most would not need ICU level of care and received a median of 1000–2000 mL of fluid following randomization. No differences in mortality were found. The results of this trial provide additional data to support the recommendations from Surviving Sepsis that crystalloids should be administered first.

The role of concentrated (20–25%) albumin solutions in the management of critically ill patients is more niche. Concentrated albumin solutions may expand intravascular volume by 200–250% of volume administered due to the oncotic pressure provided by concentrated albumin. However, less concentrated albumin solutions still provide volume expansion and are often more appropriate for volume resuscitation due to the larger fluid volume being administered. Surviving Sepsis does not recommend the use of either 4–5% albumin or 20–25% concentrations [19]. Concentrated albumin formulations are used to manage complications of acute liver failure. Albumin should be administered for patients receiving large-volume (>5 L) paracentesis, with recommendations to administer 6–8 g for every liter removed. For patients presenting with cirrhosis and spontaneous bacterial peritonitis, administration of albumin 1.5 g/kg on day one and 1 g/kg on day three has been shown to help prevent the development of hepatorenal syndrome [21]. Patients that do develop hepatorenal syndrome should also receive albumin for treatment. Dosing regimens vary, but one study strongly recommended the administration of 1 g/kg (to a maximum of 100 g) on each the first 2 days of therapy followed by 40 g/day for the duration of therapy after that [22]. Concentrated albumin may also help to augment diuresis in critically ill patients. One randomized controlled trial in patients with isolated acute lung injury with low serum protein (<6 g/dL) found that a combination of furosemide with 25% albumin 25 g every 8 h for 3 days compared to furosemide alone resulted in better oxygenation and greater net negative fluid balance at the end of 3 days [23]. It is unclear though if combining albumin with loop diuretic therapy is superior to other strategies to augment loop diuretics such as use of thiazide or carbonic anhydrase inhibitor diuretics.

53.4 Dose of Fluids

The dose of fluids administered for resuscitation remains controversial despite the ability to draw conclusions from several well-designed randomized clinical trials. Excluding hemorrhagic shock, where resuscitation with blood products is generally preferred to non-blood products, most literature within this realm applies to sepsis and septic shock. As discussed previously, special populations outside of sepsis have recommendations for large-volume fluid resuscitation that often exceed doses utilized in sepsis. For example, several formulas exist for the resuscitation of thermal burn injuries, with current guidelines recommending 2 mL/kg/percent total body surface area burn [10]. Additionally, in the treatment of hyperglycemic crises, guidelines recommend aggressive initial resuscitation (i.e., 500–1000 mL/h for 2–4 h), but do not specify a target other than "restoring intravascular volume." [24] The most recent Surviving Sepsis Campaign (SCC) Guidelines published in 2021 provide a weak recommendation for septic patients to receive a minimum of 30 mL/kg of IV crystalloid fluid within the first 3 h of resuscitation as part of the "3-hour sepsis bundle." [25] The guideline committee justified this recommendation due to the average receipt of 30 mL/kg in retrospective and observations from RCTs in sepsis, which they say suggests standard practice [26]. The three main RCTs (PROMISE, PROCESS, and ARISE) focused on bundled sepsis care as opposed to individual dose or timing of fluid; however, each of the three approached the now recommended 30 mL/kg dose [27–29].

The recommendation for fluid dose in the 2021 SSC Guideline is often viewed as more stringent and narrower than a previous iteration of the guideline, where the recommendation for larger volumes within the first 24 h was based primarily upon the landmark Early Goal Directed Therapy (EGDT) study where 4.9 L of crystalloid was given within the first 6 h and 13.4 L was given within the first 72 h [30]. This led to a large increase in recommended fluid doses compared to historical standards at that time. However, concerns for a standard 30 mL/kg fluid requirement were demonstrated with the publishing of the 2011 FEAST study, conducted in resource-scare setting for care of septic children, where mortality was decreased for children randomized to no fluid bolus administration [31]. More recently, the CLASSIC and CLOVERS trials attempted to evaluate fluid-restrictive (favoring more aggressive vasopressor therapy) versus fluid-liberal approaches to resuscitation in septic patients in the modern era of critical care practice [32, 33]. However, patients often received 2–3 L of IV crystalloids prior to enrollment, limiting the insight these trials are able to provide on initial resuscitative dose. Overall, concerns for over-administration of initial fluid therapy continue to exist, especially in special populations, which may or may not have been included in these large, randomized studies. Patients at perceived or actual risk of harm from fluid overload often include those with heart failure, cirrhosis, kidney disease, or obesity. To date, retrospective studies have failed to demonstrate harm with administering fixed 30 mL/kg volumes to these patient populations [34]. However, opponents of fixed volumes for these patients argue that patients not well enough to receive the full 30 mL/kg are at an unmeasurable risk of adverse effects at baseline [35]. Despite the robust trials in this area, the SCC guideline committee published a Research Priorities statement in 2023, identifying 13 gaps related to fluid therapy in sepsis, highlighting the many remaining questions in this realm [26].

Concerns over a "one-size-fits-all" approach to IV fluid resuscitation should prompt an evaluation of the purpose of initial fluid resuscitation and ongoing monitoring of resuscitation needs. Initial goals of fluid resuscitation include an increase in perfusion and oxygen delivery to end organs—by achieving either a goal mean arterial pressure (MAP, i.e., 65 mmHg) or an increase in cardiac output or stroke volume [36]. Patients with a stroke volume increase of 10–15% or MAP increase in 10 mm Hg after a fluid challenge (i.e., 250 mL or 4 mL/kg administered in <30 min) or passive leg raise (i.e., a "virtual" or reversible fluid challenge) are deemed to be "fluid responsive" and are thought to benefit from additional fluid resuscitation in order to increase cardiac output and oxygen delivery. Patients who are not fluid responsive are thought to derive no benefit from additional IV fluid therapy and only accumulate the harmful effects of volume overload. This may or may not be of concern initially, as institutional and national quality and reimbursement metrics specify a full 30 mL/kg for all sepsis patients, despite nearly half being found not to be fluid responsive [37].

In addition to the dose of IV fluid chosen, the rate of administration may be important for resuscitation. While early and prompt fluid administration has been well demonstrated, with delays of more than 2 h increasing mortality, the rate of infusing fluid has not been as well evaluated [37]. To date, only one RCT, the BaSICS trial, has compared the effect of fluid infusion rate on clinical outcomes [38]. When comparing a fast versus slow infusion rate (999 mL/h vs. 333 mL/h), there were no differences found in total fluid administered in the first 24 h, nor the primary outcome of 90-day mortality. Regardless, there exists biologic plausibility that a slower fluid infusion rate may lead to improved outcomes [39]. Some may argue that a slower rate may cause less degradation of the endothelial glycocalyx or perhaps lead to a more gradual change or improvement in hemodynamics and plasma concentrations. Further development of biomarkers for the endothelial glycocalyx or vascular integrity will likely prompt further investigation into both the volume and rate of fluid resuscitation.

53.5 Monitoring

Global markers of perfusion are commonly utilized to help to evaluate end-organ function and can be thought of as noninvasive (i.e., mental status, urine output, skin perfusion) or invasive (i.e., blood lactate concentration or venous oximetry [ScvO$_2$

and SvO_2]). While venous oximetry generally requires central venous access, blood lactate levels are easier to obtain and are a cornerstone of initial sepsis and septic shock care. Pharmacists should be familiar with medications and clinical scenarios that may interact with lactate concentrations [40]. Regional markers of tissue perfusion such as gastric tonometry may also be utilized but are less common in practice.

Guidelines suggest the use of dynamic measures of fluid responsiveness over the use of static measures [25]. Both static and dynamic hemodynamic variables are commonly assessed and are used often as surrogates for perfusion (Table 53.2). While critically ill patients may warrant placement of invasive devices and vascular access, there are trends towards minimizing their use and relying on noninvasive monitoring coupled with peripheral intravenous access [42]. As such, pharmacists should be familiar with the abilities and limitations of devices used in their clinical settings.

As above, the goal of resuscitative fluids is to increase preload and in turn increase SV, CO, and oxygen delivery [43]. Resuscitative fluids should be administered only if inadequate end-organ perfusion exists, resulting from inadequate CO and SV and only if the patient is fluid responsive. As previously stated, fluid responsiveness is generally defined as at least a 10–15% increase in CO after fluid administration (or passive leg raise). While clinicians often rely on changes in MAP or blood pressure to determine fluid responsiveness, this is often incorrect. As MAP is also a function of systemic vascular resistance (SVR) and CO, fluid administration to increase CO (and oxygen delivery) is often met with a resulting decrease in SVR as a result of hemodilution. While the MAP may also temporarily rise after a fluid

Table 53.2 Overview of hemodynamic monitoring

Device or device category	Obtainable hemodynamic parameters
Noninvasive blood pressure monitoring	SBP, DBP, MAP
Arterial blood pressure catheter	SBP, DBP, MAP
Central venous catheter	CVP or RAP, $ScvO_2$
Pulmonary artery catheter	CVP or RAP, PASP and PADP, mPAP, CO and CI, SvO_2, PVR, SVR
Echocardiography	Cardiac chamber sizes and functions, cardiac valve functions, pericardial appearance, IVC collapsibility/distensibility, ejection fraction, RVSP, LVOT VTI
Esophageal Doppler	CO, CI, SV, flow time
Arterial pulse pressure waveform analysis	CO, CI, SV, SVR, SVV, PPV
Bioimpedance or bioreactance	CO, CI, SV, SVR, SVV

Adapted from: Alhashemi et al. (2011) [41]
IVC inferior vena cava, *LV* left ventricular, *LVOT VTI* left ventricular outflow tract velocity time integral, *PAC* pulmonary artery catheter, *PPV* pulse pressure variation, *RVSP* right ventricular systolic pressure, *ScvO₂* central venous oxygen saturation, *SvO₂* mixed venous oxygen saturation, *SVR* systemic vascular resistance, *SVV* stroke volume variation

bolus, nearly any effect is gone within 30–60 min. Regardless of the goal of IV fluid administration, unfortunately <5% of a crystalloid bolus remains in the vasculature after 1 h in septic patients [44].

53.6 De-Resuscitation

While fluids are a key component of initial critical care resuscitation, the clinical effects are often transient due to shifts out of the intravascular space. It is well documented that a positive fluid balance is associated with an increased risk of poor outcomes, including mortality [45]. Alternatively, a positive fluid balance likely reflects a higher severity of illness, which may or may not be altered based upon increasing or decreasing fluid administration or net fluid balance. Regardless, there appears to be a dose-dependent increase in poor outcomes for a positive fluid balance, and many clinicians report emphasizing the importance of limiting fluid in their practice [46, 47].

In order to safely initiate de-resuscitation, two principles should initially be met [48]. First, patients should have and maintain adequate tissue perfusion. Second, patients should not be fluid responsive (i.e., have an increased preload from increasing intravascular fluid). As both of these principles are goals of initiating fluid resuscitation, they must be solidified prior to the decision to remove fluid. The two main modalities to achieve de-resuscitation are with diuretic agents or ultrafiltrate. Regardless of the strategy, one must allow for compensatory mechanisms to ensue, particularly capillary refill and redistribution of extravascular volume into the vascular space to facilitate removal. Debate remains as to the role of albumin in the de-resuscitative phase, even for patients demonstrating hypoalbuminemia.

Pharmacists are likely aware of the impact they may have upon ensuring adequate de-resuscitation after initial stabilization of critically ill patients. A single-center pre/post trial within a medical ICU demonstrated the clinical effectiveness of a multidisciplinary approach to de-resuscitation [49]. Pharmacists are also uniquely positioned to understand how to achieve pharmacologic diuresis in patients who may be resistant or refractory to standard diuretic strategies. A multimodal approach, often termed "sequential nephron blockade," can be effective for patients with minimal response to increasing diuretic doses [50].

While patients may transition out of the ICU prior to completing de-resuscitation, identification of stopping or safety limits is nevertheless important. Hypotension, often preceded by a decrease in perfusion, is often a common side effect during fluid removal, prompting cessation of therapy. Hypotension often serves as a decision point—either to continue with fluid removal, initiate or increase vasopressor therapy, or administer albumin or a fluid bolus. Unfortunately, limited data is available to guide clinicians in this area. An assessment of hemodynamic trends and clinical data often can help to guide further therapies. Vasopressors may increase not only the MAP, but also assist with the redistribution of fluids from the unstressed to stressed vasculature to facilitate effective removal. Albumin, while not well studied, may have theoretical benefit in limited setting, especially in patients with low serum albumin. Overall, an individualized approach is required to determine the safety and stopping points of fluid removal in patients recovering from critical illness.

53.7 Conclusion

As with the use of most medications in critically ill patients, IV fluid therapy is complex. Critical care clinicians can use their understanding of fluid composition to select the optimal fluid necessary for critically ill patients. Additionally, expertise in dosing of fluids is important to prevent volume overload. When fluid overload is present, clinicians should assess for the ability to pull back and de-resuscitate fluids.

References

1. Moritz ML, Ayus JC. Maintenance intravenous fluids in acutely ill patients. N Engl J Med. 2015;373(14):1350–60.
2. Awad S, Allison SP, Lobo DN. The history of 0.9% saline. Clin Nutr. 2008;27(2):179–88.
3. Most A, Nordbeck S, Farina N. Iatrogenic hyperchloremia: an overview in hospitalized patients for pharmacists. Am J Health Syst Pharm. 2024;81:e462.
4. Young P, Bailey M, Beasley R, et al. Effect of a buffered crystalloid solution vs saline on acute kidney injury among patients in the intensive care unit: the SPLIT randomized clinical trial. JAMA. 2015;314(16):1701–10.
5. Semler MW, Self WH, Wanderer JP, et al. Balanced crystalloids versus saline in critically ill adults. N Engl J Med. 2018;378(9):829–39.
6. Zampieri FG, Machado FR, Biondi RS, et al. Effect of intravenous fluid treatment with a balanced solution vs 0.9% saline solution on mortality in critically ill patients: the BaSICS randomized clinical trial. JAMA. 2021;326(9):1–12.
7. Finfer S, Micallef S, Hammond N, et al. Balanced multielectrolyte solution versus saline in critically ill adults. N Engl J Med. 2022;386(9):815–26.
8. Zampieri FG, Machado FR, Biondi RS, et al. Association between type of fluid received prior to enrollment, type of admission, and effect of balanced crystalloid in critically ill adults: a secondary exploratory analysis of the BaSICS clinical trial. Am J Respir Crit Care Med. 2022;205(12):1419–28.
9. Brown RM, Wang L, Coston TD, et al. Balanced crystalloids versus saline in sepsis. A secondary analysis of the SMART clinical trial. Am J Respir Crit Care Med. 2019;200(12):1487–95.
10. Pham TN, Cancio LC, Gibran NS, American Burn Association. American Burn Association practice guidelines burn shock resuscitation. J Burn Care Res. 2008;29(1):257–66.
11. Aoyagi Y, Yoshida T, Uchino S, Takinami M, Uezono S. Saline versus 5% dextrose in water as a drug diluent for critically ill patients: a retrospective cohort study. J Intensive Care. 2020;8:69.
12. Magee CA, Bastin MLT, Laine ME, et al. Insidious harm of medication diluents as a contributor to cumulative volume and hyperchloremia: a prospective, open-label, sequential period pilot study. Crit Care Med. 2018;46(8):1217–23.
13. Jacob M, Chappell D, Conzen P, Wilkes MM, Becker BF, Rehm M. Small-volume resuscitation with hyperoncotic albumin: a systematic review of randomized clinical trials. Crit Care. 2008;12(2):R34.

14. Myburgh JA, Finfer S, Bellomo R, et al. Hydroxyethyl starch or saline for fluid resuscitation in intensive care. N Engl J Med. 2012;367(20):1901–11.

15. Perner A, Haase N, Guttormsen AB, et al. Hydroxyethyl starch 130/0.42 versus Ringer's acetate in severe sepsis. N Engl J Med. 2012;367(2):124–34.

16. Finfer S, Bellomo R, Boyce N, et al. A comparison of albumin and saline for fluid resuscitation in the intensive care unit. N Engl J Med. 2004;350(22):2247–56.

17. Pesonen E, Vlasov H, Suojaranta R, et al. Effect of 4% albumin solution vs ringer acetate on major adverse events in patients undergoing cardiac surgery with cardiopulmonary bypass: a randomized clinical trial. JAMA. 2022;328(3):251–8.

18. Caironi P, Tognoni G, Masson S, et al. Albumin replacement in patients with severe sepsis or septic shock. N Engl J Med. 2014;370(15):1412–21.

19. Evans L, Rhodes A, Alhazzani W, et al. Executive summary: surviving sepsis campaign: international guidelines for the management of sepsis and septic shock 2021. Crit Care Med. 2021;49(11):1974–82.

20. Gray AJ, Oatey K, Grahamslaw J, et al. Albumin versus balanced crystalloid for the early resuscitation of sepsis: an open parallel-group randomized feasibility trial. The ABC-sepsis trial. Crit Care Med. 2024;52(10):1520–32.

21. Biggins SW, Angeli P, Garcia-Tsao G, et al. Diagnosis, evaluation, and management of ascites, spontaneous bacterial peritonitis and hepatorenal syndrome: 2021 practice guidance by the American Association for the Study of Liver Diseases. Hepatology. 2021;74(2):1014–48.

22. Wong F, Pappas SC, Curry MP, et al. Terlipressin plus albumin for the treatment of type 1 hepatorenal syndrome. N Engl J Med. 2021;384(9):818–28.

23. Martin GS, Moss M, Wheeler AP, Mealer M, Morris JA, Bernard GR. A randomized, controlled trial of furosemide with or without albumin in hypoproteinemic patients with acute lung injury. Crit Care Med. 2005;33(8):1681–7.

24. Umpierrez GE, Davis GM, ElSayed NA, et al. Hyperglycaemic crises in adults with diabetes: a consensus report. Diabetologia. 2024;67(8):1455–79.

25. Evans L, Rhodes A, Alhazzani W, et al. Surviving sepsis campaign: international guidelines for management of sepsis and septic shock 2021. Crit Care Med. 2021;49(11):e1063–143.

26. De Backer D, Deutschman CS, Hellman J, et al. Surviving sepsis campaign research priorities 2023. Crit Care Med. 2024;52(2):268–96.

27. ARISE Investigators, ACT Group, Peake SL, et al. Goal-directed resuscitation for patients with early septic shock. N Engl J Med. 2014;371(16):1496–506.

28. Mouncey PR, Osborn TM, Power GS, et al. Trial of early, goal-directed resuscitation for septic shock. N Engl J Med. 2015;372(14):1301–11.

29. Pro CI, Yealy DM, Kellum JA, et al. A randomized trial of protocol-based care for early septic shock. N Engl J Med. 2014;370(18):1683–93.

30. Rivers E, Nguyen B, Havstad S, et al. Early goal-directed therapy in the treatment of severe sepsis and septic shock. N Engl J Med. 2001;345(19):1368–77.

31. Maitland K, Kiguli S, Opoka RO, et al. Mortality after fluid bolus in African children with severe infection. N Engl J Med. 2011;364(26):2483–95.

32. Meyhoff TS, Hjortrup PB, Wetterslev J, et al. Restriction of intravenous fluid in ICU patients with septic shock. N Engl J Med. 2022;386(26):2459–70.

33. National Heart, Lung, Blood Institute Prevention and Early Treatment of Acute Lung Injury Clinical Trials Network, Shapiro NI, Douglas IS, et al. Early restrictive or liberal fluid management for sepsis-induced hypotension. N Engl J Med. 2023;388(6):499–510.

34. Khan RA, Khan NA, Bauer SR, et al. Association between volume of fluid resuscitation and intubation in high-risk patients with sepsis, heart failure, end-stage renal disease, and cirrhosis. Chest. 2020;157(2):286–92.

35. Kuttab HI, Lykins JD, Hughes MD, et al. Evaluation and predictors of fluid resuscitation in patients with severe sepsis and septic shock. Crit Care Med. 2019;47(11):1582–90.

36. Russell A, Rivers EP, Giri PC, Jaehne AK, Nguyen HB. A physiologic approach to hemodynamic monitoring and optimizing oxygen delivery in shock resuscitation. J Clin Med. 2020;9(7):2052.

37. Leisman DE, Doerfler ME, Schneider SM, Masick KD, D'Amore JA, D'Angelo JK. Predictors, prevalence, and outcomes of early crystalloid responsiveness among initially hypotensive patients with sepsis and septic shock. Crit Care Med. 2018;46(2):189–98.
38. Zampieri FG, Machado FR, Biondi RS, et al. Effect of slower vs faster intravenous fluid bolus rates on mortality in critically ill patients: the BaSICS randomized clinical trial. JAMA. 2021;326(9):830–8.
39. Alves JAM, Magalhaes MR, Zampieri FG, Veiga VC, Maia IS, Cavalcanti AB. Physiological and clinical effects of different infusion rates of intravenous fluids for volume expansion: a scoping review. J Crit Care. 2023;76:154295.
40. Reddy AJ, Lam SW, Bauer SR, Guzman JA. Lactic acidosis: clinical implications and management strategies. Cleve Clin J Med. 2015;82(9):615–24.
41. Alhashemi JA, Cecconi M, Hofer CK. Cardiac output monitoring: an integrative perspective. Crit Care. 2011;15:214.
42. Munroe ES, Heath ME, Eteer M, et al. Use and outcomes of peripheral vasopressors in early sepsis-induced hypotension across Michigan hospitals: a retrospective cohort study. Chest. 2024;165(4):847–57.
43. Ueyama H, Kiyonaka S. Predicting the need for fluid therapy-does fluid responsiveness work? J Intensive Care. 2017;5:34.
44. Sanchez M, Jimenez-Lendinez M, Cidoncha M, et al. Comparison of fluid compartments and fluid responsiveness in septic and non-septic patients. Anaesth Intensive Care. 2011;39(6):1022–9.
45. Sakr Y, Rubatto Birri PN, Kotfis K, et al. Higher fluid balance increases the risk of death from sepsis: results from a large international audit. Crit Care Med. 2017;45(3):386–94.
46. Messmer AS, Zingg C, Muller M, Gerber JL, Schefold JC, Pfortmueller CA. Fluid overload and mortality in adult critical care patients-a systematic review and meta-analysis of observational studies. Crit Care Med. 2020;48(12):1862–70.
47. Silversides JA, McAuley DF, Blackwood B, Fan E, Ferguson AJ, Marshall JC. Fluid management and deresuscitation practices: a survey of critical care physicians. J Intensive Care Soc. 2020;21(2):111–8.
48. De Backer D, Ostermann M, Monnet X. The nuts and bolts of fluid de-escalation. Intensive Care Med. 2023;49(9):1120–2.
49. Bissell BD, Laine ME, Thompson Bastin ML, et al. Impact of protocolized diuresis for deresuscitation in the intensive care unit. Crit Care. 2020;24(1):70.
50. Jentzer JC, DeWald TA, Hernandez AF. Combination of loop diuretics with thiazide-type diuretics in heart failure. J Am Coll Cardiol. 2010;56(19):1527–34.

Chapter 54
Rational Use of Blood Products in the Intensive Care Unit

Ethan Garrigan, Sachin Mehta, and Sharon L. McCartney

54.1 Introduction

Pharmacists are pivotal in ensuring safe, effective, and efficient blood transfusion practices. Their responsibilities span medication management, transfusion protocol development, patient consultation, management of transfusion reactions, education and training, and involvement in quality improvement and auditing processes. This chapter encapsulates the pharmacist's multifaceted role in managing blood transfusions in the ICU, emphasizing evidence-based practices, patient safety, and interdisciplinary collaboration.

54.2 Importance of Blood Transfusion in Critical Care Settings

Blood transfusion plays a crucial role in the management of critically ill patients, providing lifesaving support and optimizing outcomes in various clinical scenarios. The importance of blood transfusion in critical care settings stems from its ability to address acute blood loss, optimize oxygen delivery, and manage coagulopathies, thereby improving tissue perfusion and reducing mortality and morbidity. Below are key aspects highlighting the significance of blood transfusion in critical care:

E. Garrigan
Department of Anesthesiology, Duke University Medical Center, Durham, NC, USA

S. Mehta · S. L. McCartney (✉)
Department of Anesthesiology, Pain, and Perioperative Medicine, University of Kansas, Kansas City, USA
e-mail: sharon.mccartney@duke.edu

© The Author(s), under exclusive license to Springer Nature Switzerland AG 2025
Y. Alzaidi, M. A. Gebily (eds.), *The Pharmacist's Expanded Role in Critical Care Medicine*, https://doi.org/10.1007/978-3-031-77335-8_54

54.2.1 Management of Acute Hemorrhage

Blood transfusion is vital for restoring circulating blood volume and preventing hypovolemic shock in patients with acute hemorrhage due to trauma, surgery, or medical conditions such as gastrointestinal bleeding or ruptured aneurysms. Rapid administration of blood components, including red blood cells, plasma, and platelets, can stabilize hemodynamics, maintain tissue perfusion, and improve outcomes in critically ill patients with severe bleeding.

54.2.2 Optimization of Oxygen Delivery

Transfusion of red blood cells is essential for increasing oxygen-carrying capacity and improving tissue oxygenation in patients with anemia or impaired oxygen delivery. In critically ill patients with conditions such as sepsis, acute respiratory distress syndrome (ARDS), or cardiovascular collapse, maintaining adequate hemoglobin levels through transfusion therapy helps prevent tissue hypoxia, organ dysfunction, and mortality [1].

54.2.3 Correction of Coagulopathies

Blood transfusion plays a pivotal role in managing coagulopathies and preventing bleeding complications in critically ill patients. Transfusion of plasma, platelets, and clotting factors helps correct deficiencies in clotting function, enhances hemostasis, and reduces the risk of hemorrhage in patients with liver disease, disseminated intravascular coagulation (DIC), trauma, or massive transfusion requirements [2].

54.2.4 Support for Surgical and Interventional Procedures

Blood transfusion provides essential support during surgical procedures, trauma resuscitation, and interventional procedures in critical care settings. Transfusion of blood components before, during, or after procedures helps maintain hemostasis, replace blood loss, and minimize the risk of perioperative complications, ensuring optimal outcomes for critically ill patients undergoing invasive interventions.

54.2.5 Treatment of Specific Clinical Conditions

Blood transfusion is indicated in various specific clinical conditions encountered in critical care, including acute coronary syndromes, acute ischemic stroke, acute kidney injury, and septic shock. Tailored transfusion strategies based on patient characteristics, clinical context, and transfusion thresholds help address the unique challenges associated with these conditions and improve patient outcomes.

54.3 Pharmacists' Role in Blood Transfusion Management

Pharmacists are integral members of the interdisciplinary team involved in blood transfusion management in critical care settings. Their expertise in medication management, pharmacology, and patient safety contributes significantly to optimizing transfusion practices and ensuring patient outcomes. Several studies have shown that pharmacist intervention on anticoagulation leads to less drops in hemoglobin or lower overall utilization of blood component resources [3, 4].

Pharmacists play a critical role in ensuring safe, effective, and efficient blood transfusion practices in healthcare settings. Their expertise in medication management, pharmacotherapy, and healthcare systems uniquely positions them to contribute to various aspects of blood transfusion management. Pharmacists are increasingly asked to take on a more proactive and essential role in the clinical management of patients [5]. Below are key components of pharmacists' involvement in blood transfusion management [6].

54.3.1 Medication Management and Oversight

Pharmacists may be responsible for overseeing the procurement, storage, handling, and distribution of blood products within healthcare facilities. They ensure compliance with regulatory requirements, quality standards, and institutional protocols for blood transfusion, including appropriate documentation and tracking of blood products from donation to administration.

54.3.2 Transfusion Protocol Development and Implementation

Pharmacists collaborate with multidisciplinary teams to develop and implement evidence-based transfusion protocols and guidelines tailored to specific patient populations, clinical scenarios, and transfusion indications. They participate in transfusion committee meetings, conduct literature reviews, and provide recommendations for optimizing transfusion practices based on the latest evidence and best practices.

54.3.3　Patient Assessment and Consultation

Pharmacists contribute to patient care by participating in transfusion-related consultations, assessing patients' transfusion requirements, and identifying appropriate blood products based on clinical indications, laboratory parameters, and patient-specific factors. They collaborate with healthcare providers to ensure rational and individualized transfusion therapy that minimizes risks and maximizes benefits for patients.

54.3.4　Transfusion Reaction and Adverse Event Management

Pharmacists are trained to recognize and manage transfusion reactions and adverse events promptly. They play a vital role in assessing and documenting transfusion reactions, providing immediate interventions such as medication administration (e.g., antihistamines, corticosteroids), and coordinating follow-up care and reporting to regulatory agencies as required.

54.3.5　Education and Training

Pharmacists contribute to staff education and training on blood transfusion practices, transfusion safety, and adverse event management. They develop educational materials, conduct in-service training sessions, and provide ongoing support and guidance to healthcare providers, including nurses, physicians, and laboratory staff, to enhance their knowledge and skills in transfusion medicine.

54.3.6　Quality Improvement and Auditing

Pharmacists participate in quality improvement initiatives and auditing processes to monitor and evaluate transfusion practices, identify areas for improvement, and implement corrective actions to enhance patient safety and optimize resource utilization. They conduct audits of transfusion-related processes, review transfusion-related adverse events, and collaborate with stakeholders to implement quality improvement measures.

54.3.7 Interdisciplinary Collaboration

Pharmacists collaborate closely with members of the healthcare team, including transfusion medicine specialists, laboratory personnel, and critical care providers, to coordinate patient care and optimize transfusion outcomes. They actively participate in interdisciplinary rounds, case conferences, and transfusion committees to facilitate communication and decision-making regarding transfusion management.

54.4 Blood Components

54.4.1 Types of Blood Components

Blood transfusion in critical care settings involves the administration of various blood components to address specific clinical needs. Understanding the types of blood components and their indications is essential for optimizing transfusion therapy in critically ill patients (Fig. 54.1).

54.4.2 Red Blood Cells (RBCs)

Typically encountered as "packed red blood cells," they are processed by removing 200–250 mL of plasma from whole blood. The resultant volume is typically 250–300 mL per bag of packed red blood cells. Anticoagulant-preservative solutions with varying amounts of adenine are added to allow storage of up to 42 days. Packed RBCs can undergo further processing including leukocyte reduction, irradiation, or saline washing for various indications [7].

RBC transfusions are indicated to improve oxygen delivery in patients with anemia or acute blood loss. Packed RBCs contain concentrated RBCs with minimal plasma volume, making them suitable for rapidly increasing oxygen-carrying capacity. Anemia is the leading cause for allogeneic blood transfusion and a common independent predictor of mortality, morbidity, and diminished quality of life [8].

54.4.3 Plasma (FFP)

Plasma is the fluid portion of a unit of whole blood prepared by extracting the noncellular portion of blood and freezing it within 8 h of donation, hence the designation of fresh frozen plasma that it more commonly goes by. FFP contains all clotting

Blood Product	Indications for Use	Specific Considerations
Packed Red Blood Cells (PRBCs)	- Acute blood loss	- Monitor for transfusion reactions
	- Symptomatic anemia	- Adjust volume based on patient's cardiovascular status
	- Hemoglobin threshold management	
Platelets	- Thrombocytopenia with active bleeding	- Consider ABO compatibility
	- Prophylaxis in patients with critically low platelet counts	- Monitor for transfusion-associated sepsis and allergic reactions
Fresh Frozen Plasma (FFP)	- Correction of coagulopathy (INR >1.5 or active bleeding)	- Check for ABO compatibility
	- Massive transfusion protocol	- Risk of volume overload and TRALI
Cryoprecipitate	- Hypofibrinogenemia (<150 mg/dL)	- Contains fibrinogen, Factor VIII, XIII, vWF, and fibronectin
	- DIC with active bleeding	- Monitor for volume overload
	- Factor XIII deficiency	
Albumin	- Hypoalbuminemia with substantial edema or shock	- Monitor for allergic reactions
	- Volume expansion when crystalloids are insufficient	- Consider in liver disease and spontaneous bacterial peritonitis
Factor Concentrates	- Hemophilia A and B (Factor VIII and IX concentrates)	- Dose based on severity of deficiency and bleeding
	- Factor VII deficiency	- Monitor for development of inhibitors

Fig. 54.1 Commonly used blood and factor products in the ICU, primary indications, and key considerations for use

factors, fibrinogen, albumin, protein C, protein S, antithrombin, and tissue factor pathway inhibitor. It is absent of erythrocytes and leukocytes [9].

FFP transfusions can correct clotting abnormalities and improve hemostasis in patients with bleeding disorders or liver disease. One unit (~250–300 mL) contains roughly 400 mg of fibrinogen and will increase clotting factor levels by about 3% [10].

54.4.4   Platelets (Plt)

Platelets are obtained most often by centrifugation of whole blood with a single "pooled platelet" being obtained by the processing of 5–6 units of whole blood [11]. This is an alternative to "apheresis platelets," which is the result of a single patient's whole blood being separated into its components based on density while connected to the separation device, with the red blood cells being returned at the end of the process [12].

Platelet transfusions are indicated in patients with thrombocytopenia or platelet dysfunction to prevent or manage bleeding. Platelets play a crucial role in hemostasis and clot formation, making transfusions essential in patients at risk of bleeding complications.

54.4.5   Cryoprecipitate (Cryo)

Cryoprecipitate or "cryo," as it is more colloquially referred to, is a plasma-derived blood product rich in fibrinogen, factor VIII, factor XIII, von Willebrand factor (vWF), and fibronectin. To form cryo, FFP of the same ABO is slowly thawed at 1–6 °C until a precipitate begins to form, at which time it undergoes centrifugation and resuspension [13].

Cryo is indicated for patients with hypofibrinogenemia or specific clotting factor deficiencies. Cryoprecipitate transfusions can enhance clot formation and stability in patients with coagulopathies.

54.5   Blood Compatibility and Screening

54.5.1   ABO and Rh Blood Typing

ABO and Rh blood typing are fundamental aspects of blood transfusion compatibility assessment, ensuring safe and effective transfusion practices. The ABO Blood Group System classifies blood into four main groups: A, B, AB, and O. These classifications are based on the presence or absence of specific antigens on the surface of red blood cells. For example, individuals with blood group A have A antigens on their red blood cells, those with blood group B have B antigens, those with blood group AB have both A and B antigens, and those with blood group O have neither A nor B antigens [14].

The Rhesus D (RhD or Rh) blood group system is based on the presence or absence of the Rh antigen (D antigen) on the surface of red blood cells. Rh-positive individuals have the Rh antigen, while Rh-negative individuals lack this antigen. Rh compatibility is particularly crucial in preventing hemolytic transfusion reactions, especially in Rh-negative individuals receiving Rh-positive blood [15]. One of the primary reasons for Rh cross-matching is to prevent Rh hemolytic disease of the newborn (HDN) in Rh-negative mothers carrying Rh-positive fetuses. If an Rh-negative mother is exposed to Rh-positive blood during pregnancy or childbirth, her immune system may produce antibodies against Rh-positive red blood cells. Subsequent pregnancies with Rh-positive fetuses can lead to severe hemolytic disease of the newborn or hydrops fetalis, characterized by hemolytic anemia, jaundice, and potentially life-threatening complications in the newborn [16].

While ABO and RhD tend to be the most important antigens, occasionally several others have been found to be of significance and the cause of patient reactions. Kell, Duffy, and Kidd antigens have all been implicated in hemolytic reactions [17].

54.5.2 Crossmatching and Compatibility Testing

Crossmatching and compatibility testing are vital steps performed before blood transfusion to ensure compatibility between donor and recipient blood. To perform, there must be a collection of an appropriately labeled patient sample by the transfusion service, followed by testing of ABO and Rh D antigens, examining for the presence of unexpected antibodies and finally the crossmatching of red cell components with the patient sample [18].

Crossmatching itself involves mixing a sample of the recipient's serum (or plasma) with donor red blood cells and vice versa. The purpose is to detect any potential incompatibilities between donor and recipient blood, which could lead to adverse transfusion reactions. Major crossmatching involves testing recipient serum against donor red blood cells, while minor crossmatching involves testing donor serum against recipient red blood cells [19].

Compatibility testing evaluates the compatibility between donor and recipient blood based on ABO and Rh blood typing, as well as additional testing for other clinically significant blood group antigens. Various serological methods, such as gel column agglutination and solid-phase assays, are used to assess compatibility and ensure safe transfusion practices [20].

54.5.3 Screening for Infectious Diseases

Screening for infectious diseases is a critical component of blood safety protocols to prevent transfusion-transmitted infections (TTIs) and safeguard the health of recipients. Blood donors undergo thorough screening for infectious diseases, including HIV, hepatitis B and C, syphilis, and human T-cell lymphotropic virus (HTLV). Screening tests, such as enzyme immunoassays (EIAs) and nucleic acid testing (NAT), are used to detect viral antigens or nucleic acids with high sensitivity and specificity. With these recent testing advances, the per unit risks associated with transfusion are now <1 in 1,000,000 in the United States [21].

Blood establishments must implement robust quality assurance measures to ensure the accuracy and reliability of infectious disease screening tests. These measures include regular monitoring, proficiency testing, adherence to regulatory standards, and continuous improvement initiatives to enhance blood safety and minimize the risk of TTIs.

54.6 Transfusion Process and Best Practices

Ensuring safe transfusion practices is of paramount importance with multiple factors that must be accounted for and several safety checks in place to minimize any potential for patient harm. The following is recommended by the Association for the Advancement of Blood & Biotherapies [22]:

- **Proper Patient Identification:** Verify patient identity using two unique identifiers (e.g., name, date of birth, medical record number) before initiating any blood transfusion procedure.
- **Pre-transfusion Screening:** Conduct thorough pre-transfusion assessments to evaluate patient history, including prior transfusions, allergies, and risk factors for transfusion reactions.
- **Blood Product Verification:** Double-check the compatibility of blood products with the patient's blood type and any additional requirements (e.g., Rh factor, antibody screening) before administration.
- **Adequate Consent:** Ensure that patients or their authorized representatives provide informed consent for blood transfusion procedures, including potential risks and alternatives.
- **Monitoring During Transfusion:** Continuously monitor vital signs and assess for signs of transfusion reactions throughout the transfusion process.
- **Adherence to Transfusion Protocol:** Follow established transfusion protocols, including administration rates, monitoring intervals, and documentation requirements, to minimize errors and ensure consistency in practice.
- **Immediate Response to Adverse Events:** Promptly recognize and manage any transfusion reactions or complications, including allergic reactions, hemolytic reactions, and transfusion-associated circulatory overload (TACO).
- **Documentation and Reporting:** Accurately document all aspects of the transfusion process, including patient assessments, blood product administration, and any adverse events, and report any deviations from standard procedures according to institutional policies.
- **Posttransfusion Monitoring:** Monitor patients for delayed transfusion reactions and complications in the hours and days following blood product administration, as appropriate.

- **Continuous Quality Improvement:** Participate in ongoing quality improvement initiatives to identify areas for enhancement in transfusion practices and patient safety. Regularly review transfusion-related incidents, and implement corrective actions to prevent recurrence.

Patient blood management (PBM) has been defined as "the timely application of evidence-based medical and surgical concepts designed to maintain hemoglobin concentration, optimize hemostasis, and minimize blood loss in an effort to improve patient outcome" [23]. Key components of PBM typically include the following:

- **Preoperative Optimization:** Assessing and addressing modifiable factors such as anemia, nutritional deficiencies, and coagulopathies before surgery to reduce the likelihood of perioperative blood transfusions.
- **Minimally Invasive Techniques:** Utilizing minimally invasive surgical techniques, such as laparoscopic or robotic-assisted surgery, to reduce intraoperative blood loss and the need for transfusions.
- **Hemostatic Agents:** Employing pharmacological and mechanical hemostatic agents to control bleeding during surgery and minimize blood loss.
- **Blood Conservation Strategies:** Implementing strategies to conserve a patient's own blood, such as intraoperative cell salvage, acute normovolemic hemodilution, and autologous blood donation, to reduce reliance on allogeneic blood transfusions.
- **Rational Transfusion Practices:** Using evidence-based guidelines and protocols to guide transfusion decisions, including appropriate transfusion thresholds, blood component selection, and monitoring for transfusion reactions.
- **Postoperative Management:** Optimizing postoperative care to minimize complications, reduce the risk of anemia-related morbidity, and facilitate patient recovery without the need for additional transfusions.
- **Quality Improvement Initiatives:** Regular audits, quality assurance measures, and feedback mechanisms help identify areas for improvement in transfusion practices, leading to enhanced patient outcomes and reduced complications. With all these strategies in mind, it is easy to see how health-system pharmacists can become involved in multidisciplinary teams to help mitigate blood loss or reduce the need for transfusion in the hospital setting.

54.7 Indications for Blood Transfusion in Critical Care Patients

54.7.1 Acute Blood Loss

Transfusion may be necessary in patients with acute hemorrhage or trauma to restore circulating blood volume and prevent hypovolemic shock.

54.7.2 Anemia

Transfusion is indicated in patients with symptomatic anemia or impaired oxygen delivery due to low hemoglobin levels. Transfusion thresholds may vary based on individual patient factors and comorbidities.

54.7.3 Thrombocytopenia

Platelet transfusions are indicated in patients with thrombocytopenia or platelet dysfunction who are at risk of bleeding complications, such as those undergoing invasive procedures or with active bleeding.

54.7.4 Coagulopathy

Transfusion of plasma or cryoprecipitate may be indicated in patients with coagulopathies or clotting factor deficiencies to correct abnormal clotting parameters and prevent or manage bleeding.

54.8 Hemodynamic Parameters Guiding Transfusion Decisions

54.8.1 Hemoglobin Level

Hemoglobin concentration serves as a primary marker for oxygen-carrying capacity and is frequently used to establish transfusion thresholds in critically ill patients. While specific hemoglobin thresholds for transfusion may vary based on patient characteristics and clinical context, lower thresholds (e.g., 7–8 g/dL) are typically recommended for stable patients, while higher thresholds may be warranted in the presence of active bleeding, cardiovascular instability, or tissue hypoxia.

54.8.2 Hematocrit

Hematocrit, which represents the percentage of blood volume occupied by red blood cells, is closely related to hemoglobin levels and provides additional information about oxygen delivery. Changes in hematocrit levels may indicate alterations in blood viscosity, plasma volume, or red blood cell mass, all of which can impact tissue perfusion. Monitoring hematocrit levels alongside hemoglobin concentration allows clinicians to assess erythropoiesis, blood loss, and fluid balance more comprehensively.

54.8.3   Signs of Inadequate Tissue Perfusion

In addition to laboratory parameters, clinical signs of inadequate tissue perfusion play a crucial role in guiding transfusion decisions. These signs include hypotension, tachycardia, cool extremities, altered mental status, oliguria, and evidence of tissue hypoxia (e.g., lactic acidosis). Assessing these clinical indicators helps clinicians evaluate the severity of tissue hypoperfusion and determine the urgency of transfusion therapy to optimize oxygen delivery and tissue perfusion.

54.8.4   Ongoing Bleeding and Fluid Status

Continuous monitoring of ongoing bleeding and fluid status is essential in critically ill patients, as it influences transfusion decisions and overall hemodynamic management. Persistent bleeding requires prompt intervention, including transfusion of blood products to maintain hemostasis and prevent further blood loss. Moreover, assessing fluid balance and avoiding fluid overload are critical considerations in transfusion therapy, as excessive fluid administration may exacerbate tissue edema, impair oxygen delivery, and contribute to organ dysfunction.

In summary, hemodynamic parameters serve as valuable tools for guiding blood transfusion decisions in critically ill patients, allowing clinicians to assess oxygen delivery, tissue perfusion, and fluid status comprehensively. By integrating laboratory values, clinical signs, and ongoing assessments, clinicians can tailor transfusion therapy to individual patients' needs, optimizing outcomes in critical care settings.

54.9   Evidence-Based Transfusion Thresholds for Different Patient Populations

54.9.1   Critically Ill Adults

The Transfusion Requirements in Critical Care (TRICC) trial was a landmark randomized controlled trial conducted to evaluate the effects of a restrictive versus liberal transfusion strategy in critically ill patients. Published in the New England Journal of Medicine in 1999, the TRICC trial enrolled 838 critically ill patients from multiple centers across Canada and the United States.

In the trial, patients were randomized to receive either a restrictive transfusion strategy, with transfusions triggered by a hemoglobin threshold of 7.0 g/dL, or a liberal transfusion strategy, with transfusions triggered by a threshold of 10.0 g/dL. The primary outcome of the trial was 30-day mortality, with secondary outcomes including morbidity, length of stay, and resource utilization.

The TRICC trial found that there was no significant difference in 30-day mortality between the restrictive and liberal transfusion groups. Moreover, patients in the restrictive transfusion group received fewer transfusions overall and had similar rates of adverse events compared to those in the liberal transfusion group. These findings suggested that a restrictive transfusion strategy targeting a lower hemoglobin threshold could be as safe and effective as a liberal strategy in critically ill patients [24].

The TRICC trial results challenged the conventional practice of transfusing patients to maintain higher hemoglobin levels and contributed to a shift towards more conservative transfusion practices in critical care settings. Subsequent studies and meta-analyses have further supported the use of restrictive transfusion strategies in critically ill patients, highlighting the importance of individualized patient assessment and careful consideration of transfusion thresholds in clinical practice.

There have been several sub-analyses and follow-up studies conducted based on the primary TRICC trial. These sub-analyses aim to further explore specific aspects of transfusion strategies and their impact on various patient populations or outcomes. Some of these sub-analyses and follow-up studies include TRICS-3, TRIPICU, and TRISS.

54.9.2   Cardiac Surgery Patients

TRICS III specifically looked at cardiac surgery patients having on-pump procedures of all types and whether a restrictive strategy targeting a hemoglobin >7.5 g/dL was noninferior to a more liberal goal of >9.5 g/dL. Almost 5000 patients were examined for the composite outcome of death from any cause, MI, stroke, or new renal failure requiring hemodialysis. There was no significant difference between the two groups for the composite endpoint, and similar rates of adverse events between the two groups indicated noninferiority of a more restrictive transfusion strategy, even in cardiac surgery patients [25].

54.9.3   Acute Coronary Syndrome

Similarly, the REALITY trial looked at a population of patients with anemia and acute coronary syndrome, both with or without ST elevation. Groups included a liberal strategy with goal hemoglobin >10 g/dL or a more restrictive goal of >8 g/dL. The findings again demonstrated noninferiority of the restrictive group [26].

54.9.4   Sepsis

The Transfusion Requirements in Septic Shock or TRISS trial randomized 998 ICU patients with septic shock to a restrictive strategy of Hgb <7 g/dL or liberal strategy of Hgb ≤9 g/dL The primary outcome of the trial was 90-day mortality, with secondary outcomes including morbidity, length of stay, and resource utilization.

The findings of the TRISS trial indicated that there was no significant difference in 90-day mortality between patients managed with a restrictive transfusion strategy and those managed with a liberal strategy. Additionally, patients in the restrictive transfusion group received fewer transfusions overall and had similar rates of adverse events compared to those in the liberal transfusion group [27].

Another authority on care for patients with sepsis is the Surviving Sepsis Campaign. The most recent guidelines from 2021 included a strong recommendation for restrictive over liberal strategies for transfusion [28].

54.9.5   Pediatric

In the pediatric population, the Transfusion Strategies for Patients in Pediatric Intensive Care Units or TRIPICU study looked specifically at patients ranging in age from 3 days to 14 years old. Using either a restrictive strategy of goal hemoglobin <7 g/dL or a more liberal goal of 9.5 g/dL, this study again found the restrictive group to be noninferior to the more liberal group and mirrored the previous TRICC trials [29].

54.9.6   Guidelines for Specific Clinical Scenarios

54.9.6.1   Massive Hemorrhage

Guidelines for managing massive hemorrhage emphasize early recognition, aggressive resuscitation, and targeted transfusion therapy to optimize hemostasis and prevent coagulopathy. A balanced ratio of blood components (red blood cells, plasma, platelets, and occasionally cryoprecipitate) is recommended to maintain hemostasis and correct coagulopathy. Transfusion ratios such as 1:1:1 or 1:1:2 (red blood cells:plasma:platelets) have been proposed to guide transfusion therapy in the setting of massive hemorrhage, although individualized approaches based on ongoing bleeding, laboratory parameters, and patient response are crucial.

The PROPPR Randomized Clinical Trial showed that a 1:1:1 of FFP to Plt to RBCs to a 1:1:2 ratio did not result in significant differences in mortality at 24 h or at 30 days; however, the 1:1:1 group had more patients that achieved hemostasis and fewer that experienced death due to exsanguination by 24 h [30].

54.9.6.2 Perioperative Patients

In the perioperative period, several strategies can optimize patient outcomes, minimize complications, and improve recovery. The Society for the Advancement of Blood Management (SABM) Guidelines provide evidence-based recommendations on patient blood management, including managing perioperative patient anemia. These guidelines emphasize the importance of preoperative optimization of hemoglobin levels through iron supplementation, erythropoiesis-stimulating agents (ESAs), and other adjuvant therapies to reduce the need for allogeneic blood transfusions [31].

The American Society of Anesthesiology's (ASA) most recent Practice Guidelines for Perioperative Blood Management emphasizes several phases in the care of the perioperative patient. These encompass preoperative assessment of the patient, risk of transfusion related to comorbidities, and pending surgical procedure along with the use of adjunct medications to prevent and/or treat bleeding. The ASA guidelines differ from others in their reliance on pharmacologic therapies as adjuvants to optimize preoperative patients or minimize bleeding in high-risk surgical cases such as antifibrinolytics for cardiac surgeries. Additionally, greater emphasis is placed on the use of transfusion algorithms to aid in decision-making especially when coupled with real-time thromboelastographic testing such as thromboelastography (TEG) or rotational thromboelastometry (ROTEM). Most importantly, the guidelines strongly recommend restrictive transfusion strategies, in line with the majority of scientific literature [32].

Additional steps can be taken to aid in the care of perioperative patients including coordinating blood draws to minimize the number of blood draws and volume taken in the perioperative period and utilizing noninvasive hemodynamic monitoring techniques. As perioperative patients are at a higher risk of bleeding due to procedural complications or sequelae, a high index of suspicion must be maintained, and once bleeding occurs, prompt recognition and action are required.

Timely identification and management of perioperative bleeding are imperative to prevent severe complications like hemorrhagic or hypovolemic shock. It is essential to consider various factors such as patient comorbidities, preoperative condition, surgical procedure, and real-time clinical status. Correcting any coagulopathies or deficiencies promptly and efficiently, often guided by laboratory results, requires a balance of decisiveness and careful consideration, which may rely on clinical judgment in critical situations [33].

54.10 Risks and Complications

While the benefits of transfusion medicine are numerous, there are many potential pitfalls and complications that must be monitored. Transfusions are not to be taken lightly as each one is akin to a "transplant" of sorts and can have long-lasting implications to the patient [34].

54.10.1 Immediate Risks

Transfusion reactions can occur due to immune or nonimmune mechanisms and manifest as fever, chills, rash, dyspnea, hypotension, or hemolysis. Immediate cessation of transfusion, supportive care, and appropriate treatment based on the type of reaction (e.g., antihistamines, corticosteroids) are essential.

Hemolytic reactions result from the destruction of donor red blood cells due to ABO or Rh incompatibility, leading to intravascular or extravascular hemolysis. Management includes stopping the transfusion, supportive care, and ensuring adequate hydration. Severe cases may require additional interventions, such as diuresis or renal replacement therapy.

Transfusion-associated circulatory overload (TACO) occurs when the volume of transfused blood exceeds the recipient's circulatory capacity, leading to fluid overload and pulmonary edema. Prevention strategies include careful monitoring of fluid balance, transfusion rate, and patient hemodynamics. Management involves diuretics, oxygen therapy, and supportive care to alleviate symptoms and improve respiratory function. Based on the most recent United States Food and Drug Administration (FDA) report on transfusion fatalities, TACO remains the most common cause of death and thus a key complication to be aware of (reference: https://www.fda.gov/media/172382/download?attachment).

Transfusion-related acute lung injury (TRALI), while similar in presentation to TACO, is an entirely different entity and requires a considerably different treatment protocol. TRALI is characterized by an acute non-cardiogenic pulmonary edema associated with hypoxemia and thought to be immune mediated in nature [35].

54.10.2 Delayed Risks

Delayed risks of blood transfusion may manifest days to years after transfusion and require long-term monitoring and management:

Alloimmunization occurs when recipients develop antibodies against donor blood antigens, leading to immune-mediated hemolysis or refractoriness to future transfusions. Strategies for prevention include leukoreduction, extended antigen matching, and use of antigen-negative blood products. Management may involve selecting compatible blood components or immunosuppressive therapy in refractory cases [36].

Despite stringent screening measures, TTIs such as HIV, hepatitis B and C, syphilis, and cytomegalovirus (CMV) can rarely occur. Prevention strategies include donor screening, nucleic acid testing (NAT), pathogen inactivation technologies, and blood product irradiation. Management involves early detection, treatment of infections, and notification of affected recipients for further evaluation and monitoring [37].

54.10.3 Strategies for Prevention and Management of Complications

Prevention and management strategies for transfusion-related complications focus on optimizing blood product selection, transfusion practices, and patient monitoring [38]. Monitoring patients during and after blood transfusion is essential for early detection of adverse events and ensuring patient safety [39].

Regular assessment of vital signs, including blood pressure, heart rate, respiratory rate, and temperature, helps identify hemodynamic changes, fluid overload, or transfusion reactions. Vital signs should be monitored before, during, and after transfusion, with increased frequency during the initial stages of infusion.

Hemoglobin levels should be serially measured before and after transfusion allowing clinicians to evaluate the effectiveness of transfusion therapy in correcting anemia and optimizing oxygen delivery. Monitoring hemoglobin levels also helps guide transfusion decisions and assess the need for additional blood products.

Continuous observation for signs and symptoms of transfusion reactions, such as fever, chills, rash, dyspnea, hypotension, nausea, or back pain, is crucial for early detection and intervention. Prompt recognition and management of transfusion reactions minimize the risk of adverse outcomes and ensure patient safety.

Assessment of fluid balance, including intake and output, weight changes, and signs of fluid overload (e.g., peripheral edema, jugular venous distention), helps monitor for transfusion-associated circulatory overload (TACO) and prevent complications related to volume overload.

Urinalysis for hematuria or changes in urine color can indicate hemolysis or renal complications associated with transfusion reactions or transfusion-related acute lung injury (TRALI). Monitoring urine output and renal function parameters helps identify renal complications and guide management.

54.11 Pharmacologic Measures

Pharmacologic measures play a significant role in modern blood transfusion medicine by addressing various aspects of patient care, optimizing transfusion outcomes, and reducing the need for transfusions when possible. These measures are integrated into transfusion protocols and clinical practice guidelines to ensure safe and effective patient management.

54.11.1   Prothrombin Complex Concentrates and Factors

Prothrombin complex concentrates (PCCs) are synthetic products containing factors II, VII, IX, and X as well as proteins C and S, which play a crucial role in the coagulation cascade. PCCs are primarily used to rapidly correct coagulopathy or reverse anticoagulant effects in patients with bleeding or requiring urgent surgery.

PCCs are indicated for the urgent reversal of anticoagulation in patients receiving vitamin K antagonists (VKAs) who present with major bleeding or require emergency surgery (Fig. 54.2). PCCs have been found to be dramatic in their ability to rapidly correct coagulopathy associated with warfarin; however, the most optimal dosing strategy continues to be researched [40]. Most institutions have a protocol based on the available evidence.

Direct oral anticoagulants (DOACs) such as dabigatran, rivaroxaban, or apixaban are similarly amenable to PCC administration in cases of life-threatening bleeding or need for emergent surgery. PCCs may be considered as part of the reversal strategy, although specific reversal agents for DOACs such as andexanet alfa or idarucizumab may be preferred depending on the agent involved [41].

In the setting of massive hemorrhage, perioperative bleeding, or trauma, PCCs may be included as part of a comprehensive transfusion protocol to address coagulopathy and promote hemostasis alongside other blood products such as packed red blood cells, platelets, and fibrinogen concentrates.

In patients with congenital or acquired deficiencies of clotting factors (e.g., hemophilia, acquired coagulopathy), PCCs can provide rapid correction of coagulation abnormalities and control bleeding. Similarly, patients suffering from cirrhosis can have an acquired coagulopathy due to impaired clotting factor production. They too will benefit from PCCs as factor replacement to manage bleeding, especially since they are prone to volume overload associated with the administration of standard blood products [42].

Related to PCCs, which are made up of inactivated factors, recombinant factors are an emerging treatment option used in refractory bleeding or severe cases of hemorrhage. Most commonly used is recombinant factor VIIa, a crucial entity in the tissue factor pathway vital in converting factor X to Xa and forming hemostasis. Originally developed for use in patients with hemophilia and specific deficiencies, the acceptable applications for its use have been expanding to postcardiac surgery, intracranial bleeding, and more [43].

54.11.2   Antifibrinolytic Agents

Antifibrinolytic agents are medications that inhibit the breakdown of blood clots, thereby promoting hemostasis and reducing bleeding. They work by blocking the activity of plasmin, an enzyme that breaks down fibrin, the protein meshwork that forms the structure of blood clots. By inhibiting fibrinolysis (the process of fibrin

Anticoagulant	Mechanism of Action	Reversal Agent	Mechanism of Reversal Agent
Warfarin	Inhibits vitamin K-dependent synthesis of clotting factors II, VII, IX, and X.	Vitamin K	Promotes synthesis of clotting factors.
		Prothrombin Complex Concentrate (PCC)	Provides clotting factors to rapidly reverse anticoagulation.
		Fresh Frozen Plasma (FFP)	Supplies all coagulation factors to replenish deficient factors.
Heparin	Enhances activity of antithrombin, reducing action of thrombin and factor Xa.	Protamine Sulfate	Binds to heparin, neutralizing its anticoagulant effect.
Low Molecular Weight Heparin (LMWH)	Inhibits factor Xa and to a lesser extent, thrombin.	Protamine Sulfate	Partially reverses the effects of LMWH by binding to it.
Direct Oral Anticoagulants (DOACs) - Dabigatran	Direct thrombin inhibitor.	Idarucizumab	Specifically binds to dabigatran, neutralizing its effect.
DOACs - Rivaroxaban, Apixaban	Direct factor Xa inhibitors.	Andexanet Alfa	A decoy for factor Xa inhibitors, reversing their anticoagulant effects.
		Prothrombin Complex Concentrate (PCC)	Used off-label to reverse the effects by providing clotting factors.
Argatroban	Direct thrombin inhibitor, used especially in HIT.	No specific reversal agent	Supportive care and discontinuation of the drug for reversal.
Fondaparinux	Selective factor Xa inhibitor, does not inhibit thrombin.	No specific reversal agent	Supportive care and discontinuation of the drug for reversal.
Bivalirudin	Direct thrombin inhibitor, used in patients with or at risk for HIT.	No specific reversal agent	Primarily metabolized by proteolysis and has a short half-life. Discontinuation leads to rapid diminution of its effects.

Fig. 54.2 Common anticoagulants, their mechanisms of action, and associated reversal agents

breakdown), antifibrinolytic agents help stabilize blood clots and prevent excessive bleeding [44]. The most used antifibrinolytic agent is tranexamic acid (TXA), which is available in intravenous, oral, and inhaled formulations. Another common antifibrinolytic agent is aminocaproic acid.

Antifibrinolytics are often administered during surgical procedures to reduce intraoperative bleeding and minimize the need for blood transfusions. They are particularly useful in procedures associated with significant blood loss, such as cardiac surgery, orthopedic surgery, and trauma surgery. They may also be used to manage hemorrhage and prevent excessive bleeding in trauma patients, particularly in cases of severe injury or massive blood loss [45].

Antifibrinolytics are sometimes used to reduce bleeding during childbirth (postpartum hemorrhage) or in patients with bleeding disorders such as von Willebrand disease or hemophilia.

The CRASH-3 trial was a well-conducted large study that demonstrated that TXA not only is safe in TBI but may also be associated with reduced head injury-associated deaths [46].

54.11.3 *Vitamins and Minerals*

Vitamins and minerals play a crucial role in combating anemia and reducing the reliance on blood transfusions in clinical practice. Adequate intake of essential nutrients such as iron, vitamin B12, folate, and vitamin C is essential for optimal erythropoiesis and hemoglobin synthesis [47].

The INITIATE trial conducted by Kong et al. corroborates the importance of preoperative treatment with intravenous iron and erythropoiesis-stimulating agents in reducing perioperative blood transfusions, particularly in cardiac surgery patients. Compared to patients who received only oral iron, those treated with a single dose of intravenous iron and erythropoiesis-stimulating agents experienced a decreased likelihood of requiring blood transfusions during the perioperative period. These results underscore the potential role of preoperative iron supplementation and erythropoiesis-stimulating agents in optimizing hemoglobin levels and reducing transfusion-related risks in surgical patients [48]. Administering iron intravenously is preferred over oral supplementation in patients with severe anemia who are scheduled for surgery within 6 weeks. This preference arises from the relatively long period required for oral iron supplementation to take effect. Intravenous iron offers a more rapid and efficient means of replenishing iron stores in such cases. Notably, serious hypersensitivity reactions, once a concern with high-molecular-weight iron dextran formulations, are now rare with the current formulations available. The incidence of serious adverse events associated with iron infusion is estimated to be <1 in 250,000, which is ten times lower than the incidence of serious adverse events linked to allogeneic transfusions. This safety profile underscores the relative safety and efficacy of intravenous iron administration, making it a preferred option in the management of severe anemia, particularly in the preoperative period preceding imminent surgery [49].

Cobalamin-deficient or pernicious anemia is among the most common diagnoses in older populations and may be diagnosed in relation to a lack of intrinsic factor which is necessary for cobalamin absorption. Both oral and parenteral routes of vitamin B12 supplementation are effective in correcting vitamin B12 deficiency anemia. However, parenteral therapy, which involves direct injection of vitamin B12 into the muscle or under the skin, tends to achieve faster and more reliable results compared to oral therapy. This is particularly important in cases where patients have severe anemia or malabsorption issues that may impair the absorption of vitamin B12 from the gastrointestinal tract [50].

Folate deficiency can lead to megaloblastic or macrocytic anemia characterized by large red blood cells, a similar presentation to pernicious anemia. Inadequate dietary intake of folate-rich foods such as leafy greens, legumes, and fortified grains can induce deficiency. Malabsorption conditions like celiac disease and inflammatory bowel disease, alongside medications such as methotrexate, can hinder folate absorption. Increased folate demands, seen in pregnant women, those with hemolytic anemia or cancer, and excessive alcohol consumers, can lead to deficiency. Chronic diseases like liver disease and hereditary folate malabsorption can also disrupt folate metabolism. Addressing folate deficiency involves dietary changes, bolstering folate intake through foods or supplements like folic acid or folinic acid. Treating underlying conditions contributing to deficiency, such as malabsorption disorders or chronic diseases, is crucial. Regular monitoring of folate levels and red blood cell counts is essential for assessing treatment response and ensuring that optimal folate levels are maintained, sometimes necessitating ongoing supplementation [51].

Multimodal options have potential for the highest yield by aiding patients at several points in the hematologic pathway. The study by Rossler et al. highlights the effectiveness of an ultrashort combination treatment administered 1 day before surgery in reducing red blood cell transfusion requirements in patients undergoing elective cardiac surgery. This treatment regimen, consisting of intravenous iron, subcutaneous erythropoietin, vitamin B12, and oral folic acid, demonstrates the potential benefits of preoperative anemia management in minimizing the need for transfusions. These findings suggest that even a brief preoperative intervention can significantly impact transfusion outcomes and contribute to improved patient care in the perioperative period [52].

54.11.4 Erythropoietin-Stimulating Agents (ESAs)

ESAs are synthetic versions of erythropoietin, a hormone naturally produced by the kidneys in response to low oxygen levels in the blood. ESAs are created using recombinant DNA technology and mimic the action of endogenous erythropoietin. Their primary function is to stimulate the production of red blood cells (RBCs) in the bone marrow, leading to an increase in hemoglobin levels and improvement of anemia. ESAs have been widely used in the treatment of anemia associated with chronic kidney disease (CKD) and malignancy [53]. In patients with CKD, decreased kidney function leads to reduced production of erythropoietin, resulting in anemia. ESAs help alleviate anemia by stimulating RBC production, thereby improving symptoms and quality of life in these patients. Similarly, ESAs have shown efficacy in managing anemia associated with malignancies such as certain types of cancer. Cancer-related anemia can occur due to factors such as impaired erythropoietin production, chronic inflammation, or chemotherapy-induced bone marrow suppression. ESAs can help increase hemoglobin levels in cancer patients undergoing chemotherapy or experiencing anemia related to their disease, reducing the need for blood transfusions and improving overall well-being. Overall, ESAs play a valuable role in the management of anemia in patients with chronic kidney disease and cancer. Their ability to stimulate RBC production offers a targeted approach to addressing anemia and its associated symptoms, enhancing patient outcomes and quality of life in these clinical settings. Additionally, emerging evidence is supporting the use of ESAs perioperatively to optimize patients prior to surgery and is associated with reduced transfusion burdens [54].

54.12   Case Studies and Clinical Scenarios

54.12.1   Case Study #1: Managing a Complex ICU Patient on Warfarin with 4-Factor PCC Kcentra Administration

54.12.1.1   Background

A 68-year-old patient with a history of mechanical heart valve replacement was admitted to the ICU for an emergency abdominal surgery due to a suspected intestinal obstruction. The patient was on long-term warfarin therapy, which had to be urgently reversed due to the risk of bleeding during surgery.

54.12.1.2   Challenge

The patient's anticoagulation needed rapid reversal to reduce the risk of perioperative bleeding, yet the reversal had to be carefully balanced to avoid thrombotic complications, given the patient's mechanical heart valve. Additionally, the ICU team had to manage the patient's anticoagulation post-surgery to prevent valve thrombosis while ensuring adequate hemostasis.

54.12.1.3 Pharmacist's Role and Interventions

1. Warfarin Reversal:

   – The pharmacist recommended the administration of 4-factor prothrombin complex concentrate, a rapid-acting reversal agent, to normalize the patient's INR before surgery. The dose was calculated based on the patient's current INR and body weight.

2. Risk-Benefit Analysis:

   – Prior to 4-factor PCC administration, the pharmacist conducted a thorough risk-benefit analysis, considering the patient's history of mechanical heart valve and the potential for thromboembolic events post-reversal.

3. Collaborative Monitoring:

   – Throughout the reversal process, the pharmacist collaborated with the healthcare team to monitor the patient's INR, vital signs, and signs of bleeding or thrombosis, adjusting the treatment plan as necessary.

4. Postoperative Anticoagulation Management:

   – After surgery, the pharmacist played a crucial role in reinitiating anticoagulation therapy, carefully timing the reintroduction of warfarin, and bridging with low-molecular-weight heparin to ensure that the patient remained protected against thrombotic risks.

5. Education and Communication:

   – The pharmacist provided education to the nursing staff on monitoring for signs of bleeding or thromboembolic complications and communicated effectively with the surgical and medical teams to coordinate the patient's care.

54.12.1.4 Outcome

The patient's anticoagulation was successfully reversed with 4-factor PCC, allowing for a safe surgical intervention. Postoperatively, the pharmacist's involvement ensured a balanced approach to resuming anticoagulation, leading to the patient's stable recovery without bleeding or thrombotic complications.

54.12.1.5 Conclusion

This case illustrates the critical role of the pharmacist in managing complex ICU patients who require urgent reversal of warfarin anticoagulation with 4-factor PCC. Through meticulous planning, monitoring, and collaboration, the pharmacist ensured the patient's safe transition through surgery and effective management of anticoagulation postoperatively, highlighting the pharmacist's integral role in optimizing patient outcomes in high-risk clinical scenarios.

54.12.2 Case Study #2: Managing Hemorrhagic Shock in a Patient Who Refuses Blood Products

54.12.2.1 Background

A 60-year-old patient with a known history of gastrointestinal bleeding was admitted to the ICU in hemorrhagic shock. The patient, a Jehovah's Witness, firmly refused blood product transfusion, posing a significant ethical and clinical challenge in managing severe blood loss and maintaining hemodynamic stability.

54.12.2.2 Challenge

The primary challenge was to respect the patient's autonomy and religious beliefs while effectively managing hemorrhagic shock. The team needed to employ alternative strategies to blood transfusion to optimize the patient's oxygen-carrying capacity and clotting status without compromising the patient's wishes.

54.12.2.3 Pharmacist's Role and Interventions

1. Alternative Hemostatic Agents:

   - The pharmacist recommended the use of antifibrinolytic agents, such as tranexamic acid, to help reduce bleeding and enhance clot stability. They also reviewed the use of recombinant factor VIIa as a potential option to aid in hemostasis.

2. Volume Expanders:

   - To manage intravascular volume without blood products, the pharmacist suggested the use of crystalloids and colloids. They provided guidance on the judicious use of these fluids to maintain adequate perfusion while avoiding fluid overload.

3. Erythropoiesis-Stimulating Agents (ESAs):

   - Recognizing the need to enhance the patient's red blood cell production, the pharmacist discussed the potential use of ESAs to stimulate erythropoiesis, albeit acknowledging the delayed effect of such therapy.

4. Iron Supplementation:

   - Intravenous iron supplementation was recommended to support erythropoiesis and improve the patient's iron stores, critical for red blood cell production.

5. Nutritional Support:

   - The pharmacist advised on optimizing the patient's nutrition, particularly focusing on nutrients essential for hematopoiesis, such as vitamin B12 and folic acid.

6. Ethical Consultation and Patient Communication:

   - The pharmacist participated in ethical consultations and discussions with the healthcare team, ensuring that the patient's wishes were respected while exploring all viable medical interventions.

7. Monitoring and Adjustments:

   - They played a crucial role in monitoring the patient's response to the alternative therapies, ready to adjust the treatment plan based on clinical and laboratory indicators.

54.12.2.4 Outcome

Through the multidisciplinary efforts and alternative management strategies, the patient's condition stabilized over time. The patient appreciated the team's respect for their beliefs and their efforts to provide care within those constraints, leading to a trustful patient-healthcare provider relationship.

54.12.2.5 Conclusion

This case illustrates the pharmacist's integral role in managing a patient in hemorrhagic shock who refuses blood products. By employing a range of alternative strategies and maintaining a patient-centered approach, the pharmacist, alongside the healthcare team, successfully navigated the complex balance between respecting patient autonomy and delivering optimal critical care (Fig. 54.3).

Phase	Task	Details
Pre-Transfusion	Verification of Indications	Confirm clinical indications for transfusion, review medical history, lab values, and medications.
	Medication Reconciliation	Identify drug interactions affecting coagulation or bleeding risks; adjust medications as necessary.
	Crossmatch and Compatibility	Ensure proper blood type matching and compatibility testing; confirm correct product type and quantity.
	Pre-Transfusion Checks	Verify patient ID and blood product details; check for previous reactions or allergies.
	Dosage and Administration	Provide dosing recommendations and infusion rates; recommend pre-medication if needed.
During Transfusion	Monitoring Protocols	Establish monitoring protocols, including vital signs and adverse reaction signs; advise on documentation.
	Adverse Reaction Management	Have protocols for managing transfusion reactions; ensure availability of emergency medications.
	Communication with Healthcare Team	Maintain communication with the team; be available for consultations.
Post-Transfusion	Post-Transfusion Evaluation	Recommend post-transfusion lab tests; evaluate patient response in terms of symptom relief and lab improvements.
	Documentation and Reporting	Ensure comprehensive documentation; report any adverse reactions according to protocols.
	Follow-Up and Education	Provide follow-up care recommendations; offer educational resources to staff and patients.
	Quality Improvement	Participate in quality improvement initiatives; assess and enhance transfusion practices.
Continuing Education	Stay Informed	Keep updated with the latest research and guidelines; participate in educational opportunities.
	Interprofessional Collaboration	Collaborate with specialists and the ICU team; engage in multidisciplinary case reviews and meetings.

Fig. 54.3 Proposed pharmacist checklist for the use of blood products in the ICU

54.13 Conclusion

This chapter attempts to delineate the multifaceted and pivotal role pharmacists play in the use of blood products within the intensive care unit. Their involvement spans across various dimensions, including medication management, development and implementation of transfusion protocols, patient assessments, and management of transfusion reactions. The intricate responsibilities of pharmacists underscore their integral contribution to enhancing patient safety, optimizing clinical outcomes, and ensuring the rational use of blood products in critical care settings. The authors emphasize the significance of a collaborative approach, where pharmacists, alongside other healthcare professionals, engage in multidisciplinary efforts to ensure that blood transfusion practices are safe, effective, and aligned with the latest evidence-based guidelines. It highlights the importance of ongoing education and training programs, spearheaded by pharmacists, to keep the healthcare team updated on best practices in transfusion medicine. Furthermore, the critical role of pharmacists in quality improvement initiatives, auditing of transfusion practices, ensuring compliance with regulatory standards, and continuous enhancement of patient care protocols is self-evident. Through their expertise in pharmacology and therapeutics, pharmacists are uniquely positioned to contribute to the decision-making processes, optimizing transfusion strategies to address the complex needs of critically ill patients. Ultimately, healthcare leaders should have a heightened recognition of the pharmacist's role in blood transfusion management, advocating for their active participation in all aspects of patient care within the ICU. This holistic involvement is crucial for advancing patient blood management, reducing transfusion-related complications, and promoting a culture of safety and excellence in critical care medicine.

References

1. Russell A, Rivers EP, Giri PC, Jaehne AK, Nguyen HB. A physiologic approach to hemodynamic monitoring and optimizing oxygen delivery in shock resuscitation. J Clin Med. 2020;9(7):2052.
2. Spahn DR, Bouillon B, Cerny V, et al. The European guideline on management of major bleeding and coagulopathy following trauma: fifth edition. Crit Care. 2019;23(1):98.
3. Zhou L, Ma J, Bao J. Effect of pharmacist intervention on blood conservation therapy in total knee arthroplasty: a retrospective, observational study. Basic Clin Pharmacol Toxicol. 2019;124(6):681–90.
4. Shander A, Nemeth J, Cruz JE, Javidroozi M. Patient blood management: a role for pharmacists. Am J Health Syst Pharm. 2017;74(1):e83–9.
5. Pedersen CA, Schneider PJ, Ganio MC, Scheckelhoff DJ. ASHP national survey of pharmacy practice in hospital settings: prescribing and transcribing-2019. Am J Health Syst Pharm. 2020;77(13):1026–50.
6. Shander A, Hardy JF, Ozawa S, et al. A global definition of patient blood management. Anesth Analg. 2022;135(3):476–88.
7. Salyer SW. Essential emergency medicine: for the healthcare practitioner. Philadelphia: Saunders/Elsevier; 2007.
8. Groenveld HF, Januzzi JL, Damman K, et al. Anemia and mortality in heart failure patients a systematic review and meta-analysis. J Am Coll Cardiol. 2008;52(10):818–27.
9. Nascimento B, Callum J, Rubenfeld G, Neto JB, Lin Y, Rizoli S. Clinical review: fresh frozen plasma in massive bleedings - more questions than answers. Crit Care. 2010;14(1):202.
10. Quek J, Lee JJ, Lim FL, et al. Donor-type fresh frozen plasma is effective in preventing hemolytic reaction in major ABO incompatible allogeneic stem cell transplant. Transfusion. 2019;59(1):335–9.
11. Graham JM. Isolation of human platelets (thrombocytes). ScientificWorldJournal. 2002;2:1607–9.

12. Bock M, Rahrig S, Kunz D, Lutze G, Heim MU. Platelet concentrates derived from buffy coat and apheresis: biochemical and functional differences. Transfus Med. 2002;12(5):317–24.
13. Kovacic Krizanic K, Pruller F, Rosskopf K, Payrat JM, Andresen S, Schlenke P. Preparation and storage of cryoprecipitate derived from amotosalen and UVA-treated apheresis plasma and assessment of in vitro quality parameters. Pathogens. 2022;11(7):805.
14. Poole J, Daniels G. Blood group antibodies and their significance in transfusion medicine. Transfus Med Rev. 2007;21(1):58–71.
15. Avent ND, Reid ME. The Rh blood group system: a review. Blood. 2000;95(2):375–87.
16. Myle AK, Al-Khattabi GH. Hemolytic disease of the newborn: a review of current trends and prospects. Pediatric Health Med Ther. 2021;12:491–8.
17. Westhoff CM, Reid ME. Review: the Kell, Duffy, and Kidd blood group systems. Immunohematology. 2004;20(1):37–49.
18. Evanovitch D. A primer in pretransfusion testing. Transfus Apher Sci. 2012;46(3):281–6.
19. Swarup D, Dhot PS, Kotwal J, Verma AK. Comparative study of blood cross matching using conventional tube and gel method. Med J Armed Forces India. 2008;64(2):129–30.
20. Ekdahl KN, Hong J, Hamad OA, Larsson R, Nilsson B. Evaluation of the blood compatibility of materials, cells, and tissues: basic concepts, test models, and practical guidelines. Adv Exp Med Biol. 2013;735:257–70.
21. Busch MP, Bloch EM, Kleinman S. Prevention of transfusion-transmitted infections. Blood. 2019;133(17):1854–64.
22. Huestis DW. AABB guidelines and proposed standards. J Clin Apher. 1985;2(4):306–10.
23. Spahn DR, Munoz M, Klein AA, Levy JH, Zacharowski K. Patient blood management: effectiveness and future potential. Anesthesiology. 2020;133(1):212–22.
24. Hebert PC. Transfusion requirements in critical care (TRICC): a multicentre, randomized, controlled clinical study. Transfusion Requirements in Critical Care Investigators and the Canadian Critical care Trials Group. Br J Anaesth. 1998;81(Suppl 1):25–33.
25. Mazer CD, Whitlock RP, Fergusson DA, et al. Restrictive or liberal red-cell transfusion for cardiac surgery. N Engl J Med. 2017;377(22):2133–44.
26. Ducrocq G, Gonzalez-Juanatey JR, Puymirat E, et al. Effect of a restrictive vs liberal blood transfusion strategy on major cardiovascular events among patients with acute myocardial infarction and anemia: the REALITY randomized clinical trial. JAMA. 2021;325(6):552–60.
27. Holst LB, Haase N, Wetterslev J, et al. Lower versus higher hemoglobin threshold for transfusion in septic shock. N Engl J Med. 2014;371(15):1381–91.
28. Oczkowski S, Alshamsi F, Belley-Cote E, et al. Surviving sepsis campaign guidelines 2021: highlights for the practicing clinician. Pol Arch Intern Med. 2022;132(7–8):16290.
29. Lacroix J, Hebert PC, Hutchison JS, et al. Transfusion strategies for patients in pediatric intensive care units. N Engl J Med. 2007;356(16):1609–19.
30. Holcomb JB, Tilley BC, Baraniuk S, et al. Transfusion of plasma, platelets, and red blood cells in a 1:1:1 vs a 1:1:2 ratio and mortality in patients with severe trauma: the PROPPR randomized clinical trial. JAMA. 2015;313(5):471–82.
31. Tibi P, McClure RS, Huang J, et al. STS/SCA/AmSECT/SABM update to the clinical practice guidelines on patient blood management. J Cardiothorac Vasc Anesth. 2021;35(9):2569–91.
32. American Society of Anesthesiologists Task Force on Perioperative Blood Management. Practice guidelines for perioperative blood management: an updated report by the American Society of Anesthesiologists Task Force on Perioperative Blood Management. Anesthesiology. 2015;122(2):241–75.
33. Erdoes G, Faraoni D, Koster A, Steiner ME, Ghadimi K, Levy JH. Perioperative considerations in management of the severely bleeding coagulopathic patient. Anesthesiology. 2023;138(5):535–60.
34. Meier J, Muller MM, Lauscher P, Sireis W, Seifried E, Zacharowski K. Perioperative red blood cell transfusion: harmful or beneficial to the patient? Transfus Med Hemother. 2012;39(2):98–103.

35. Ackfeld T, Schmutz T, Guechi Y, Le Terrier C. Blood transfusion reactions-a comprehensive review of the literature including a Swiss perspective. J Clin Med. 2022;11(10):2859.
36. Hendrickson JE, Tormey CA. Understanding red blood cell alloimmunization triggers. Hematology Am Soc Hematol Educ Program. 2016;2016(1):446–51.
37. Dodd RY, Notari EP, Nelson D, et al. Development of a multisystem surveillance database for transfusion-transmitted infections among blood donors in the United States. Transfusion. 2016;56(11):2781–9.
38. Kleinman S, Busch MP, Murphy EL, et al. The National Heart, Lung, and Blood Institute Recipient Epidemiology and Donor Evaluation Study (REDS-III): a research program striving to improve blood donor and transfusion recipient outcomes. Transfusion. 2014;54(3 Pt 2):942–55.
39. Murphy MF, Stanworth SJ, Yazer M. Transfusion practice and safety: current status and possibilities for improvement. Vox Sang. 2011;100(1):46–59.
40. Dietrich SK, Rowe S, Cocchio CA, Harmon AJ, Nerenberg SF, Blankenship PS. Comparison of 3 different prothrombin complex concentrate regimens for emergent warfarin reversal: PCCWaR study. Ann Pharmacother. 2021;55(8):980–7.
41. Muller M, Eastline J, Nagler M, Exadaktylos AK, Sauter TC. Application of prothrombin complex concentrate for reversal of direct oral anticoagulants in clinical practice: indications, patient characteristics and clinical outcomes compared to reversal of vitamin K antagonists. Scand J Trauma Resusc Emerg Med. 2019;27(1):48.
42. Drebes A, de Vos M, Gill S, et al. Prothrombin complex concentrates for coagulopathy in liver disease: single-center, clinical experience in 105 patients. Hepatol Commun. 2019;3(4):513–24.
43. Roberts HR, Monroe DM, White GC. The use of recombinant factor VIIa in the treatment of bleeding disorders. Blood. 2004;104(13):3858–64.
44. Chapin JC, Hajjar KA. Fibrinolysis and the control of blood coagulation. Blood Rev. 2015;29(1):17–24.
45. Levy JH, Koster A, Quinones QJ, Milling TJ, Key NS. Antifibrinolytic therapy and perioperative considerations. Anesthesiology. 2018;128(3):657–70.
46. CRASH-3 Trial Collaborators. Effects of tranexamic acid on death, disability, vascular occlusive events and other morbidities in patients with acute traumatic brain injury (CRASH-3): a randomised, placebo-controlled trial. Lancet. 2019;394(10210):1713–23.
47. Fishman SM, Christian P, West KP. The role of vitamins in the prevention and control of anaemia. Public Health Nutr. 2000;3(2):125–50.
48. Kong R, Hutchinson N, Hill A, et al. Randomised open-label trial comparing intravenous iron and an erythropoiesis-stimulating agent versus oral iron to treat preoperative anaemia in cardiac surgery (INITIATE trial). Br J Anaesth. 2022;128(5):796–805.
49. Richards T, Baikady RR, Clevenger B, et al. Preoperative intravenous iron to treat anaemia before major abdominal surgery (PREVENTT): a randomised, double-blind, controlled trial. Lancet. 2020;396(10259):1353–61.
50. Lane LA, Rojas-Fernandez C. Treatment of vitamin b(12)-deficiency anemia: oral versus parenteral therapy. Ann Pharmacother. 2002;36(7–8):1268–72.
51. Chan YM, Bailey R, O'Connor DL. Folate. Adv Nutr. 2013;4(1):123–5.
52. Rossler J, Hegemann I, Schoenrath F, et al. Efficacy of quadruple treatment on different types of pre-operative anaemia: secondary analysis of a randomised controlled trial. Anaesthesia. 2020;75(8):1039–49.
53. Aapro M, Gascon P, Patel K, et al. Erythropoiesis-stimulating agents in the management of Anemia in chronic kidney disease or cancer: a historical perspective. Front Pharmacol. 2018;9:1498.
54. Weber EW, Slappendel R, Hemon Y, et al. Effects of epoetin alfa on blood transfusions and postoperative recovery in orthopaedic surgery: the European Epoetin Alfa Surgery Trial (EEST). Eur J Anaesthesiol. 2005;22(4):249–57.

Chapter 55
Clinical Nutrition in Critical Illness

Kathleen M. Gura

55.1 Introduction

Patients in intensive care have increased nutritional needs but are often incapable of sustaining themselves orally. Critical care nutrition is a rapidly evolving field. Specialized nutritional support is often used, but practice varies globally. The emphasis is tailoring a patient's nutritional regimen to the patient's characteristics, their medical requirements, their current therapies, and metabolic state [1]. This chapter addresses the role of nutritional support, both enteral and parenteral, in this complex patient population.

During critical illness, the body is in a hypercatabolic state in which muscle mass and energy stores are depleted, and nutrients are used at a high rate [2]. This catabolic state manifests clinically as weight loss, sarcopenia, and undernutrition. This has been shown to prolong length of stay within the intensive care unit, increase complications, postpone recovery, and, most disturbingly, increase mortality [3]. Optimizing nutritional support is of great importance for these patients, but many clinicians fail to appreciate, and malnutrition, either as undernutrition or overnutrition, may be critical in determining clinical outcomes. Special attention should be directed to those patients expected to remain longer than a week in the ICU [1].

Both the American Society for Parenteral and Enteral Nutrition (ASPEN) and the European Society for Clinical Nutrition and Metabolism (ESPEN) have recently updated their guidelines for the use of nutritional support in intensive care patients [4–7]. These differ on several key points from the previous versions. In comparison to the American guidelines, the European guidelines still recommend starting parenteral nutrition earlier and at higher macronutrient doses [5]. Moreover, these

K. M. Gura (✉)
Department of Pharmacy, Division of Gastroenterology, Hepatology, and Nutrition, Boston Children's Hospital, Boston, MA, USA
e-mail: Kathleen.Gura@childrens.harvard.edu

© The Author(s), under exclusive license to Springer Nature Switzerland AG 2025

Y. Alzaidi, M. A. Gebily (eds.), *The Pharmacist's Expanded Role in Critical Care Medicine*, https://doi.org/10.1007/978-3-031-77335-8_55

revised recommendations provide for more personal judgment, which assumes that the clinician has a solid foundation in basic nutrition knowledge and familiarity with these guidelines.

55.2   Metabolic Changes in the Critically Ill Patients

In the critically ill, the catabolism that occurs is a survival response. Stress hormones such as cortisol and inflammatory meditators trigger a series of complex metabolic changes [2]. In the liver, glucose is quickly consumed along with glycogen stores and converted into energy. Amino acids and other metabolites are released to replete glucose stores and to repair tissue damage and strengthen immune function. The nutritional needs of the glucose-dependent brain and central nervous system are prioritized over muscle tissue. Within the body, a strong insulin resistance develops, and a state of negative protein balance occurs. Often categorized as the metabolic acute phase, this occurs over the first 7 days, with the early acute phase happening during the first 48 h. The patient then enters a late phase where they transition to anabolic metabolism in which energy stores and tissues are built up. In more seriously ill patients, the catabolic phase may evolve into a chronic phase that can last for several weeks.

55.3   Assessing Nutritional Status

Upon admission to the ICU, while the patient is still in the early acute phase, nutritional screening should occur to determine the need for PN. In addition to weight and body mass, biochemical parameters (i.e., visceral proteins such as albumin) are used to determine the extent of disease severity. Since other methods are difficult to use in critically ill patients, several score sheets have been developed to assist in this process. Although not validated for use in the critically ill, ASPEN recommends patients be screened using the NRS-2002 tool, although European guidelines currently only suggest nutritional assessment without providing the use of a specific method [8].

Bedside body composition is increasingly being used to assess protein requirements, especially in obese and overweight individuals [7]. Although lean body mass (LBM) can best be assessed using MRI, CT scans, or dual-energy X-ray absorptiometry (DEXA), these are expensive and not practical to use at the bedside [9]. Bioelectric impedance (BIA) is a more practical alternative although fluid overload can result in LBM overestimates [9]. Furthermore, using multifrequency BIA can adjust for fluid excess [10].

In addition to the aforementioned tools, clinicians are attempting to validate biomarkers that may reflect metabolic responses at the organ or whole-body level [11]. These are being incorporated into risk stratification tools such as the Nutrition Risk in the Critically Ill (NUTRIC) score [12]. The most robust measures of whole-body nutrient utilization (absorption and metabolism) are those which address protein synthesis and breakdown [13]. Outside the critical care area, this is done using stable isotope tracer infusions. It has been considered impractical in the critically ill and pediatric populations [14]. In comparison to whole-body protein balance, estimates of nitrogen balance can be calculated by evaluating the net differences between protein synthesis and breakdown.

55.4 Determining Caloric Requirements

Identifying the most appropriate dosing weight for the provision of nutrition is an important consideration. Underweight patients (BMI <18.5 kg/m^2) should use actual body weight as using a calculated ideal body weight could result in caloric excess and predispose the patient to refeeding syndrome [15]. Once the patient is stable, then caloric advancement could be done. In contrast, patients with normal weight (BMI 18.5–24.9 kg/m^2) or overweight (BMI 25–29.9 kg/m^2) should also use actual weight, but adjustments should be made if peripheral edema is present. Obese patients (BMI >30 kg/m^2) should use the Penn State University 2010 predictive equation if more indirect calorimetry (described below) is not available. If expertise in using this equation did not exist, then a dosing weight should be used to account for the lack of metabolic requirements by fat tissues (Fig. 55.1).

To prevent the detrimental effects of over- and underfeeding, it is essential that accurate determination of energy requirements is performed. Energy expenditure and related requirements vary depending upon where in the phase of critical illness the patient is. In the initial phases, the resting energy expenditure (REE) will be close to total energy expenditure as the ICU patient has minimal physical activity. Indirect calorimetry (IC) is often used to determine energy needs and improve outcomes. Unlike predictive equations that can result in deviations as great as 1000 kcal/day in comparison to true energy expenditure, IC has been shown to

Examples of Dosing Weight Calculations

Dosing weight = IBW + 0.4 (ABW-IBW)

Dosing weight = 1.1 x IBW

IBW= ideal body weight

In patients with fluid overload (i.e.., hepatic failure), an estimate of dry weight is often used.

ABW = actual body weight

Fig. 55.1 Examples of dosing weight calculations

reduce short-term mortality by avoiding under- or overfeeding [16]. IC, however, does not account for endogenous energy production or use of insulin or exogenous feeding. Thus, it has been suggested that IC be utilized to assess energy requirements after the initial phase of high endogenous energy product has abated [17]. In the event that IC is not available, rather than using a predictive equation, VCO_2 measurements (kcal/24 h = VCO_2 × 8.19) should be utilized [5]. In comparison to IC, however, this approach may also overestimate actual energy expenditure [18].

55.5 Timing of Initiating Nutrition

An important consideration in managing the critically ill patient is when to start nutrition. Ideally, enteral nutrition should be started within 48 h of admission to the intensive care unit (ICU) in hopes of reducing the risk of infection. In contrast, no benefits are realized with the early initiation of parenteral nutrition [4–7]. Endogenous energy production is estimated to be 500–1400 kcal/day in the early phase of critical illness. To prevent overfeeding, current guidelines recommend that energy intake be gradually advanced over several days upward to 80–100% of the REE. In the early phase of critical illness, reducing caloric intake to 70–80% of the REE has been linked to a reduction in mortality [5]. During the first week of ICU admission, as soon as it is determined that the patient can safely tolerate them, feedings are initiated typically at 20–30% of estimated metabolic needs. Feeds should only be held in conditions such as septic shock, intestinal ischemia, or gastrointestinal hemorrhage.

55.6 Routes of Nutrition Administration

55.6.1 Enteral Nutrition

Upon admission to the ICU, oral nutrition should be attempted. Given that the majority of critically ill patients are unable to tolerate adequate amounts to meet their needs by the oral route, enteral nutrition, where a feeding tube is placed directly into the gastrointestinal tract, is often used. It is not without risk, however. Enteral feeding intolerance is associated with fewer ventilator-free days and greater mortality [19]. Complications such as bowel ischemia, bowel obstruction, and gastrointestinal bleeding can occur. Contraindications to using enteral nutrition include severe hemodynamic instability and high aspiration risk. In patients with high risk of aspiration, post-pyloric feedings, where the feeding tube enters the jejunum, should be considered before resorting to PN. In patients showing signs of feeding intolerance, prokinetic agents should be considered. If intolerance is observed in patients with nasogastric or gastrostomy tubes, switching to a post-pyloric feeding tube may be an alternative.

Advancement of enteral nutrition early in the ICU course should be done gradually over days to prevent overfeeding. Although enteral nutrition can be provided via continuous, intermittent, or bolus infusion schedules, most suggest continuous feeds over 24 h/day [5]. In one RCT, Lee et al. showed that critically ill patients fed continuously achieved >80% of their target nutritional goals in comparison to those fed intermittently [20]. Table 55.1 describes key differences between continuous versus intermittent feedings.

Regardless of the delivery method, feeding intolerance is a concern in the enterally fed patient. There is no uniform definition; however, high gastric residual volumes are often a basis for holding or advancing feeds. Reintam Blaser et al. suggest a definition of feeding intolerance in which 80% of goal feeds are not achieved in 72 h and the presence of at least one GI symptom [21]. In general, feeding intolerance is associated with worse clinical outcomes including extended length of ICU stay, longer time on the ventilator, and higher mortality rates [22]. Use of the post-pyloric route and administration of prokinetic agents may improve tolerance. The most common complications associated with enteral nutrition include diarrhea, aspiration, mechanical complications, and metabolic derangements.

55.6.2 Parenteral Nutrition

In patients unable to tolerate adequate enteral nutrition to meet needs (<50%), supplemental PN is often used in tandem with the tube feeding. Until recently, the ESPEN guidelines recommended PN be initiated within the first 48 h of admission to the ICU if it is not thought that the patient will be able to meet their needs enterally within 72 h. In contrast, ASPEN recommends waiting until the late phase, 8 days after admission to the ICU, unless the patient is already severely malnourished. This suggests that hypocaloric nutrition (i.e., permissive underfeeding) is preferred over the use of supplemental PN. In one trial evaluating early versus late initiation of PN, patients who were randomized to the late PN group experienced shorter lengths of stay and fewer infectious complications than those in the early PN

Table 55.1 Differences between continuous vs. intermittent feedings

	Continuous feeding	Intermittent feeding
Method	Slow release of nutrients into the stomach	
Benefits (theoretical)	Reduced feeding intolerance Reduced regurgitation Decreased incidence of respiratory complications (aspiration risk)	More physiologic Maintains normal GI hormone secretion and digestion Increases gut motility May attenuate muscle wasting May improve glucose control/insulin sensitivity

group. These findings have caused ESPEN to reevaluate their current guidelines and now suggest that PN not be started until the late acute phase, between days 3 and 7 of admission to the ICU [4–7].

Refeeding syndrome is a risk when specialized nutrition support is initiated, especially PN [15]. It is characterized by hypokalemia and hypophosphatemia. Preventing occurrence of symptoms by early identification of at-risk patients by correcting electrolyte, mineral, and vitamins prior to starting PN is essential. Patients at risk should receive supplemental thiamine prior to initiation to prevent Wernicke syndrome.

55.6.3 Which Route of Nutrient Provision Is Superior?

When direct comparisons of the enteral and parenteral nutrition routes of delivery in the critically ill are made, results from randomized trials suggest that patient outcomes using either route of delivery are comparable [6]. The most common complications associated with parenteral nutrition are catheter-related bloodstream infections (CLABSIs), metabolic derangements, and catheter-related complications (i.e., breakage, occlusion, thrombosis).

55.7 Macronutrient Requirements

55.7.1 Protein

The catabolism that occurs with critical illness involves the proteolysis of body proteins that results in rapid loss of muscle mass. Wasting of muscle mass leads to muscle weakness and impaired metabolism. This can result in decreased functional performance that can last for years after discharge from the ICU [23]. Protein anabolism is key in maintaining muscle mass. In healthy individuals, this is achieved through dietary protein which stimulates muscle protein anabolism. In times of critical illness, muscle wasting can be attenuated by augmenting protein intake. Observational studies have correlated increased protein intake with improved clinical outcomes, including reduced mortality [24]. Current guidelines recommend protein intakes of 1.2–2 g/kg/day [6, 7]. Interestingly, protein provision of 1.1 g/kg/day showed that despite a decline in skeletal muscle mass in the first 3 weeks of ICU stay, it was not associated with muscle loss as it was attenuated after weeks 5–7 [25]. A recent meta-analysis of 19 randomized clinical trials (RCTs) evaluated low- versus high-protein diets (0.9–2.6 g/kg/day) in critically patients showed that high intakes did not improve physical function or improve mortality [26]. However, when increased protein intake was combined with resistance training, muscle mass could be increased [27].

55.7.2 Fat

Lipids are biological substances that are soluble in organic solvents, but insoluble in water. Lipids include sterols, fats, triglycerides (TGs), various oils and waxes, as well as individual components known as fatty acids. Through the contribution of their fatty acid components, TGs serve as chief dietary sources of energy. Plus, selected lipids provide many of the structural and metabolically functional components of all biological membranes. Because of these properties, these lipids and fatty acids contribute substantially to the cellular functions necessary for the maintenance and biological activity of healthy living cells. For example, the structure of membrane lipids can include the fatty acids arachidonic acid (AA), docosahexaenoic acid (DHA), and eicosapentaenoic acid (EPA). These specific fatty acids are significantly important for proper development as well as inflammatory and other physiologic processes. For instance, the metabolic products of AA, EPA, and DHA include (1) gene regulators; (2) inflammatory mediators (eicosanoids such as prostaglandins, leukotrienes, and thromboxanes); (3) constituents that assist in the resolution of an inflammatory response (eicosanoids such as protectins, resolvins, and lipoxins); and (4) substances that regulate overall lipid metabolism [28–32].

Furthermore, the aforementioned fatty acids and others contribute to membrane fluidity, membrane and intracellular cell signals, and modulation of apoptotic pathways [33].

Fatty acids are composed of several carbon, hydrogen, and oxygen atoms. All fatty acids consist of a chain of carbon atoms linked together by covalent bonds. A methyl group is at one end of the chain, and at the opposite end of the chain is an acidic carboxyl group. Fatty acids are classified in a variety of ways. One classifies groups of fatty acids based on the number of carbon atoms within the hydrocarbon chain. A fatty acid may be classified as short chain (2–4 carbons), medium chain (6–12 carbons), long chain (14–18 carbons), or very long chain (20 or more carbons). The length of the hydrocarbon chain carries unique physical and chemical properties to fatty acids, and these properties are reflected in the lipids of which these fatty acids are a part. Humans can synthesize all fatty acids necessary for life except for linoleic acid (LA) and α-linolenic acid (ALA) and their downstream metabolites. Humans cannot synthesize these fatty acids because the specific desaturase enzymes that can insert a double bond past position 9–10 within a given fatty acid are absent, which prevents the de novo *synthesis* of LA and ALA fatty acids. Thus, the synthesis by elongation and subsequent desaturation of longer chained fatty acids necessary for life is barred. Absence of the necessary desaturase enzymes means that all human unsaturated fatty acids are synthesized from palmitoleic, oleic, LA, or ALA acids. Thus, both LA and ALA must be obtained via the diet, and each serves as a critical precursor for the synthesis of other necessary long-chain unsaturated fatty acids, such as AA and DHA. It is important to note that the efficiency of the conversion of LA to AA, and ALA to DHA, is suboptimal in the premature infant and the critically ill or malnourished patients [34].

55.7.3   Fat Supplementation in Critical Illness

The 2016 ASPEN/SCCM guidelines for nutrition support therapy in critical illness recommend that clinicians avoid the routine use of (1) all specialty formulas in critically ill patients in a medical ICU and (2) all disease-specific formulas in the surgical ICU [4]. In particular, the guidelines state that immune-modulating enteral formulations of arginine with other agents—including DHA, EPA, glutamine, and nucleic acid—should not be used routinely in the medical ICU; moreover, these formulations and other similar products (e.g., fish oil with or without arginine) should not be administered to severely septic patients [4]. Given the significant amount of conflicting data in patients with acute respiratory distress syndrome (ARDS) or severe acute lung injury, the ASPEN/SCCM guidelines state that no recommendation could be made concerning the routine use of enteral formulas considered to possess anti-inflammatory lipid profiles (e.g., ω-3 fish oils, borage oil) and antioxidants [4]. In contrast, the guidelines do recommend that formulas containing fish oil and arginine be considered in patients with severe trauma and recommend the use of either arginine-containing immune-modulating formulations or supplementing standard enteral formula with additional EPA/DHA in patients with traumatic brain injury (TBI) [4]. Similarly, in surgical ICU postoperative patients requiring EN, an immune-modulating formula (containing both arginine and fish oils) should routinely be used [4]. In summary, there is support for utilizing enteral regimens that incorporate immune-enhancing formulations in patients with severe trauma or TBI and those in the postoperative surgical ICU.

In 2021, ASPEN updated recommendations from the 2016 guidelines for five foundational questions central to critical care nutrition support [6]. In regard to the use of an intravenous lipid emulsion (ILE) in critically ill adults receiving PN, due to limited clinically/statistically significant differences in key outcomes, it was concluded that irrespective of the oil type (mixed oil or soybean oil monotherapy), ILE is a safe and effective energy source that can be included with the PN formulation at the time of initiation, including within the first week of admission to the ICU. Table 55.2 summarizes the composition of currently available products. Moreover, optimizing the ILE provision helps avoid complications associated with excessive dextrose intake such as hyperglycemia. The ability to clear lipids should be verified by monitoring serum triglyceride concentrations. For those requiring PN >10 days, adequate intake of essential fatty acids (EFAs) is required, and clinicians must remember that mixed oil ILE contains less EFAs in comparison to pure soybean oil ILE and limited restriction protocols should be avoided when using those products.

Table 55.2 Comparison of select intravenous lipid emulsions

Emulsion product	Lipid%	Energy kcal/L	Glycerol g/L	Omega 6:omega 3 ratio	Oil content, g/L			
					Soybean oil	Olive oil	MCT oil	Fish oil
Clinolipid	20	2000	22.5	9:1	40	160	–	–
Intralipid 30%	30	3000	17.0	7:1	300	–	–	–
Intralipid 20%	20	2000	22.5	7:1	200	–	–	–
Ivelip	20	2000	25	7:1	200	–	–	–
Lipofundin MCT	20	1908	25	7:1	100	–	100	–
Lipofundin N	20	2008	25	7:1	200	–	–	–
Lipoplus	20	1910	25	2.7:1	80	–	100	20
Lipovenoes	20	2000	25	7:1	200	–	–	–
Nutrilipid	20	2000	25	7:1	200	–	–	–
Omegaven	10	1120	25	1:8	–	–	–	100
Smoflipid	20	2000	25	2.5:1	60	50	60	30

LCT long-chain triglyceride, *MCT* medium-chain triglyceride

55.7.3.1 Specific Oils/Fatty Acids

ω-9 Fatty Acids

Diets containing oils rich in ω-9 fatty acids (principally, oleic acid found in olive oil) have been reported to possess health benefits as they lower cholesterol and TG levels without the negative effects of lipid peroxidation [35]. They are often used in enteral formulas because high-oleic oils are stable and have a favorable fatty acid profile (Table 55.3).

Medium-Chain Triglycerides (MCTs)

MCTs are saturated and are 6–12 carbons in length. These fatty acids were developed commercially in the 1950s and are among the first medical foods derived as an alternative to plant oils and other conventional fats. This oil source is isolated primarily from plants high in MCTs, such as coconut oils and palm kernel oils. Compared to short-chain triglycerides (SCTs), MCTs are significantly different with respect to absorption, metabolism, and physiological

Table 55.3 Fat composition of selected enteral formulas

Formula	Fat					
	% of Energy	Source	g/L	Linoleic acid, g/L	MCTs, g/L	Omega-3 fatty acids, g/L
Compleat	34	Canola oil	40	8.6	0	2.6
Diabetisource AC	44	Canola oil, refined fish oil (anchovy, sardine)	58.8	10	0	6.2
Fibersource HN	29	Canola oil, MCTs	40	6.6	8.0	2.7
Glucerna 1.0 Cal	49	High-oleic safflower and canola oils	54.5	7.8	0	0.7
Impact	25	Palm kernel oil, refined fish oil (anchovy, sardine), high-linoleic safflower oil, high-oleic sunflower oil	28.0	3.0	0	2.5
Impact Peptide 1.5	38	MCTs, refined fish oil (anchovy, sardine), canola oil, soybean oil	63.6	8.3	31.6	6.1
Isosource 1.5 Cal	35	Canola oil, MCTs	59.2	9.7	12.0	4.0
Isosource HN	29	Canola oil, MCTs	40.0	6.5	8.0	2.7
Jevity 1 Cal	29	Canola oil, corn oil, MCTs, soy lecithin	34.7	10.0	6.6	1.5
Nepro with carb steady	48	High-oleic safflower and canola oils	95.8	14.5	0.0	2.5
Nutren 1.0	30	Canola oil, MCTs	34.0	5.8	6.8	2.4
Nutren 1.0 fiber	30	Canola oil, MCTs	34.0	5.9	6.8	2.4
Osmolite 1 Cal	29	Canola oil, corn oil, MCTs, soy lecithin	34.7	9.5	6.9	1.8
Oxepa	55.2	Canola oil, MCTs, marine oil, borage oil, soy lecithin	93.8	15.9	23.5	11.7
Peptamen	33	MCTs, soybean oil	39.0	5.2	27.6	0.7
Peptamen with Prebio	35	MCTs, soybean oil	40	5.2	28	0.7
Peptamen 1.5	33	MCTs, soybean oil	56.0	6.6	40	0.8
Peptamen Af	40	MCTs, refined fish oil (anchovy, sardine), soybean oil	54	6.3	28	3.8
Promote	23	Soy oil, MCTs, safflower oil, soy lecithin	26.0	11.7	4.7	1.3
Promote with fiber	25	Soy oil, MCTs, safflower oil, soy lecithin	28.2	12.2	4.7	1.3
Pulmocare	55.1	Canola oil, MCTs, corn oil, high-oleic safflower oil, soy lecithin	93.3	18.4	18.7	4.8
RenalCal	36	MCTs, canola oil, corn oil	82	6.2	60	1.4

(continued)

Table 55.3 (continued)

Formula	Fat					
	% of Energy	Source	g/L	Linoleic acid, g/L	MCTs, g/L	Omega-3 fatty acids, g/L
Replete	30	Canola oil, MCTs	34.0	5.6	6.8	2.4
Replete fiber	30	Canola oil, MCTs	34.0	5.6	6.8	2.3
Suplena with carb steady	48	High-oleic safflower oil, canola oil	95.8	16.1	0.0	3.1
Tolerex	2	Safflower oil	2	1.2	0.0	0.0
TwoCal HN	40.1	High-oleic safflower oil, MCTs, canola oil, soy lecithin	90.5	10.1	16.9	1.1
Vital high protein	20	MCTs, marine oil, corn oil	23.2	0.95	11.6	4.2
Vivonex plus	6	Soybean oil	6.7	4	0.0	0.5
Vivonex RTf	10	Soybean oil, MCTs	11.6	3.6	4.8	0.5
Vivonex T.E.N.	3	Safflower oil	3	2.2	0.0	0.0

functions [36]. MCTs are smaller and more water soluble than LCTs. Release of fatty acids through hydrolysis of MCTs in the intestinal lumen is significantly faster relative to LCTs, and absorption of medium-chain fatty acids is more rapid in comparison to long-chain fatty acids. The rate of absorption of MCTs may be faster because they do not require the presence of bile or pancreatic lipases for absorption and are transported directly to the liver via the portal vein (thus bypassing the traditional LCT pathway). Once in the liver, MCTs are used mostly as an energy source. In comparison to LCTs, MCTs are not stored to any significant degree in adipose tissue, nor do they impact the reticuloendothelial system. Because MCTs are ketogenic, these TGs may provide a useful energy source for enterocytes, lymphocytes, and cells of other tissues in hypermetabolically stressed patients [37]. Oxidation of MCTs is less influenced by glucose and insulin than LCTs [38]. Additionally, oxidation of LCTs can be impaired by slow elimination rates from the plasma or by the requirement of carnitine for intracellular transport. In contrast, MCT metabolism is carnitine independent for transport into the mitochondria [39]. Thus, due to these metabolic differences, MCTs may be beneficial in decreasing inflammatory stress conditions. These metabolic properties may also increase the role of MCTs as an important lipid source for patients with impaired and dysfunctional gastrointestinal tracts. For example, MCTs may be advantageous for individuals who have impaired fat digestion and absorption (e.g., patients with pancreatitis), as well as those with malabsorption secondary to autoimmune enteropathies, intestinal resections, inflammatory bowel disease, or chylous ascites [40, 41].

Many enteral products have been formulated with MCTs serving as the major lipid component to maximize the absorption, metabolism, and tolerance of these products for use in various disease and metabolic conditions (Table 55.3).

55.7.3.2 Complications Associated with ILE

Hypertriglyceridemia/Dyslipidemia

The parenteral ILEs listed in Table 55.2 are each structurally designed to resemble natural with respect to size, core TGs, and a monolayer of phospholipid. Like natural chylomicrons, these spherical pseudo-chylomicrons are, on average, 200–500 nm in diameter and have a central TG core surrounded by a phospholipid (emulsifier) envelope [42]. Emulsifying agents, such as egg phosphatide, have a detergent-like action and are added to ILEs to provide a barrier that prevents the oil droplets from coalescing in the emulsion. However, this emulsifier can cause liposomes, a potentially undesirable structure, to form. Liposomes are <70 nm in diameter and consist primarily of a phospholipid bilayer that surrounds a trapped aqueous phase. Metabolism of each of these entities requires several stages, and the process begins immediately upon entrance into the bloodstream. These pseudo-chylomicrons behave very similarly to natural chylomicrons. Once in the circulation, they acquire apolipoproteins and endogenous cholesterol and, through cell membrane and other lipoprotein interactions, exchange phospholipids. Cellular interaction exposes the pseudo-chylomicron to lipoprotein lipase (LPL) activity, resulting in the release of fatty acids from the TG core and movement of free fatty acids into the cells. Remnants appear because of the degradation process. Like natural chylomicron remnants, pseudo-chylomicron remnants are hepatically removed. The activity of endothelial LPL is influenced by gestational age and stress. Its activity increases with gestational age but is inhibited in times of stress (i.e., surgery, sepsis), prematurity, and malnutrition [43]. Medications such as insulin and heparin appear to stimulate adipose tissue LPL activity, whereas theophylline can inhibit it [44].

Dysfunction of this process can lead to dyslipidemia. When TGs alone are involved, the condition is known as hypertriglyceridemia. For example, an abnormal lipoprotein known as lipoprotein-X can form from liposomes present in the circulation. Lipoprotein-X is comprised of a spherical bilayer of phospholipid and cholesterol. This abnormal protein inhibits lipase activity (both lipoprotein lipase and hepatic lipase) [45]. Consequently, a high concentration of lipoprotein-X in the circulation can inhibit lipid metabolism and lead to hypercholesterolemia or hypertriglyceridemia [46, 47]. The potential for lipoprotein-X to form depends on the oil content and the final concentration of the emulsion. Lower concentrations contain more liposomes. For example, a 10% (w/v) emulsion will contain a larger number of liposomes than a 20% (w/v) emulsion, because of the relative ratio of phospholipid emulsifier to oil. And although most commercial ILEs are available as 20% (w/v) formulations, ILEs used as vehicles for intravenous (IV) drug delivery (e.g., propofol) are usually 10% (w/v) ILE. Therefore, lipoprotein-X may still form under certain circumstances, and clinicians should consider this risk depending upon the duration of therapy or whenever high doses of ILEs are being used. Hypertriglyceridemia is a potential adverse effect of provision of lipids in PN. It occurs when the body cannot clear TGs from plasma lipids via oxidation and/or storage in adipose tissue, and it may be caused when the supply of lipids into the bloodstream exceeds LPL activity or whenever LPL activity is reduced [47, 48].

Hypertriglyceridemia is associated with various clinical and metabolic problems, such as sepsis, renal failure, and pancreatitis [48]. Patients with a type IV familial hypertriglyceridemia present a unique challenge as there is an overproduction of VLDL within the liver leading to hypertriglyceridemia that can result in acute pancreatitis; the use of ILE would be contraindicated [49]. Therefore, whenever ILEs are used, clinicians should routinely monitor patients for the threshold plasma TG level above which the exogenously administered lipids cannot be efficiently metabolized [50].

Essential Fatty Acid Deficiency

Burr and Burr first described essential fatty acid deficiency (EFAD) in animals in 1929, but it was not identified in humans receiving PN until four decades later [51]. Previously, case reports in humans were limited primarily to individuals with cystic fibrosis in which patterns of low EFAs were reported [52]. In the early 1970s and 1980s, biochemical and clinical manifestations of deficiencies of both LA and ALA were reported in patients requiring PN for extended periods of time (2–4 weeks) [53]. The most notable clinical change associated with LA deficiency is a dry, scaly skin rash. However, other clinical symptoms have been noted, including increased susceptibility to infection, impaired wound healing, and immune dysfunction (Table 55.4) [54].

In response to LA deficiency, the biochemical changes that occur include a decrease in LA and its metabolite AA (tetraenoic acid) levels and a corresponding increase in Mead acid (triene acid) level [55]. Mead acid is primarily produced in humans in the absence of EFAs. A triene:tetraene ratio >0.2 (i.e., the Holman index) has been used to identify the presence of EFAD [56]. The time required to exhibit an EFAD in adults varies depending on the individual's underlying nutritional status and disease state. Biochemical EFAD in the absence of clinical signs may occur rapidly in patients receiving prolonged courses of fat-free PN as adipose tissue lipolysis is prevented by elevated insulin levels. Similarly, clinical signs (Table 55.4)

Table 55.4 Essential fatty acid deficiency: biochemical signs and clinical characteristics

Biochemical signs	Clinical characteristics
Serum mead acid (20:3n-9)/arachidonic acid (20:4n-6) ratio >0.2	Coarse, sparse hair
Increased serum concentrations: Palmitoleic acid (16:1n-7) Oleic acid (18:1n-9) Mead acid (20:3n-9)	Decreased growth rate Dermatitis; dry, scaly skin Generalized erythema Impaired immune function
Decreased serum concentrations: Linoleic acid (18:2n-6) Dihomo-γ-linolenic acid (20:3n-6) Arachidonic acid (20:4n-6)	Slow wound healing Visual perturbations

may be detected earlier (e.g., between 10 and 20 days) in patients receiving fat-free PN [57].

In some cases, signs and symptoms of EFAD may be delayed. Hypocaloric fat-free PN or a cyclic feeding schedule of fat-free PN may postpone the onset of EFAD [58]. The rationale is that when hypocaloric PN is provided or PN is cycled, in response to a reduction in serum insulin concentration, EFAs are mobilized and enter the circulation as a result of increased lipolysis of endogenous fat stores. Furthermore, hypocaloric feeding decreases the risk of hepatic dysfunction that may occur if the energy deficit (caused by the reduction of fats) is corrected by replacing the loss in fat calories with additional dextrose or protein to maintain energy requirements. When ILEs are contraindicated, short-term hypocaloric, fat-free PN may be appropriate for the critically ill patient [59]. The dosing of ILEs depends on the ILE formulation used and the patient's clinical status, body weight, metabolic requirements, and tolerance. EFA requirements can be met by providing 2–4% of the energy requirement as LA [60].

Clinicians should base dose of the ILE on the amount of LA contained in the ILE to ensure adequate dosing of EFAs. Patients should be monitored for EFAD if all sources of fats are removed from the diet for more than 2–4 weeks. Starting low-dose or trophic enteral feedings may also be used to prevent EFAD. A polymeric enteral formula containing soybean oil and a mixture of other high-LA containing oils may be used. Normally, a polymeric enteral formula that provides 10–15% of the patient's total caloric needs will supply sufficient EFAs. Nevertheless, if an individual has fat malabsorption, or whenever enteral feedings are paused or stopped for a significant period of time (i.e., >14 days) with no other source of lipid, the risk of EFAD needs to be determined [61]. Moreover, malnourished adults may also be at risk for EFAD during refeeding [34]. Biochemical signs of EFAD have been shown to occur in malnourished adult patients upon initiation of PN [62]. Similar to what occurs with other nutrients in refeeding syndrome, severely malnourished adults, upon introduction of nutrition, may develop signs of biochemical EFAD without evidence of dermatologic findings. This may occur because baseline EFA tissue stores are low and supplementation with ILE may not be able to replete stores and prevent progression of EFAD. In such cases, higher doses of ILE may be needed to correct biochemical EFAD. Others have theorized that refeeding might have resulted in increased protein synthesis in the skin. This is reversed upon increasing the ILE dose [63].

55.7.4 Fat Overload Syndrome

Fat overload syndrome, a relatively rare complication of ILEs, may occur when the dose or rate of lipid infusion exceeds the body's ability to clear lipids. It is characterized by respiratory distress, fever, jaundice, hepatosplenomegaly, headache, and spontaneous hemorrhage [64].

Other symptoms include anemia, leukopenia, thrombocytopenia, coagulopathies, and a low fibrinogen level [65].

55.7.5 Carbohydrates (Dextrose)

Unlike protein and lipids, carbohydrates may not be considered an essential nutrient. In the liver and kidneys, carbohydrates can be synthesized from amino acids, glycerol, and lactate. However, its provision is also essential for stimulating the secretion of insulin and other anabolic hormones, which promotes protein synthesis and reduces lipolysis [66]. Given its convenience as source of energy, dextrose is a major component in PN. The suggested dose in PN is currently 3–3.5 g/kg/day [67]. However, in critically ill patients, including diabetics, those with sepsis, or those receiving corticosteroids, lower doses of dextrose should be administered (i.e., 1-2 g/kg/day) at a glucose infusion rate (GIR) not exceeding 6 mg/kg/day or 5 mg/kg/min [68, 69].

In times of critical illness, high intake of dextrose can result in physiologic stress rather than serving as macronutrient [70]. Sympathetic activity increases during dextrose infusions, which leads to a derangement of carbohydrate utilization and resulting in insulin resistance. Consequently, the hyperglycemia generated by exogenous glucose uptake can magnify the inflammatory response [71]. Furthermore, glucose utilization is decreased due to the enhanced activity of the sympathetic nervous system. This leads to an increase in lipolysis with subsequent liberation of free fatty acids [72].

55.7.6 Glycemic Control

Normoglycemia, through the use of insulin, has been shown to decrease morbidity and mortality among critically ill patients [73, 74]. It is theorized that in states of critical illness, insulin decreases blood glucose levels by increasing glucose uptake in skeletal muscle tissue as both skeletal muscle and adipose tissue remain insulin sensitive, while the liver becomes more insulin resistant [75]. The hyperglycemia that occurs in states of critical illness is thought to be necessary to maintain an adequate inflammatory response; aggressive reduction to euglycemia is not recommended [71]. Lowering glucose levels with the use of insulin has been shown to be beneficial [75]. In critically ill hospitalized patients, mortality rates have been shown to be the lowest in those whose blood glucose levels were between 80 and 110 mg/dL and greatest in individuals whose concentrations exceeded 300 mg/dL [76, 77]. The theoretical benefit of maintaining tight glycemic control is to prevent immune dysregulation and reduce systemic inflammation by reducing the concentration of C-reactive protein and adhesion molecules [74, 75].

In some critically ill patients, however, tight glycemic control may actually increase mortality [78]. This may be due to the high incidence of hypoglycemia whose complications may go undetected unless constant monitoring of blood glucose levels is performed [79]. Thus, maintaining blood glucose concentrations of 140–180 mg/dL may yield a better prognosis and reduce morbidity caused by hypoglycemia [4]. Given the high risk of hypoglycemia that may be fatal in critically ill patients, it is prudent to maintain blood glucose concentrations between 120 and 150 mg/dL [67].

55.7.7 Micronutrients

During times of critical illness, oxidative stress and inflammation occur as a response to different types of injury and stimuli [80]. In numerous studies, low micronutrient levels have been reported in critically ill patients. A deficiency in any of them may enhance oxidative stress and negatively impact patient outcomes. Thus, providing anti-inflammatory nutrients and antioxidants may be beneficial in helping to reduce the extent of oxidative stress and decrease complications in patients who are critically ill. Selenium, ascorbic acid, zinc, and vitamin D show the most promise in abating inflammation and oxidative stress.

Under healthy conditions, a certain level of oxidant production is needed to regulate physiologic mechanisms such as cell proliferation and differentiation, activation of immune cells (e.g., T cells, monocytes), stimulation of signaling pathways, and altering metabolism [81].

The balance between oxidants and reductants is preserved through the endogenous antioxidative processes, which are ensured with adequate intake of micronutrients per recommended for daily intakes [80]. In states of critical illness, the balance between oxidants and reductants is disrupted. There are increased losses of various antioxidants due to interventions such as medications, drains, extracorporeal membrane oxygenation, and renal replacement therapy. Similarly, there is an increase in oxidants due to an induction of prooxidant enzymes such as inducible nitric oxide and an increased production of reactive oxygen species and reactive nitrogen species by leukocytes and anaerobic cell metabolism [82]. Both are essential players in initiating, mediating, and regulating the cellular and biochemical complexity of oxidative stress.

55.8 Examples

55.8.1 Selenium

Selenium is an essential micronutrient, playing a key role in the synthesis of selenocysteine, which is necessary for the functionality of selenoproteins that are part of several endogenous antioxidant defense mechanisms [83]. Selenium is involved in activating several antioxidant enzymes and is responsible for the neutralization of reactive oxygen species and reactive nitrogen species. By binding to the selenoproteins, selenium acts as an antioxidant leading to the modulation of reactive oxygen species by inhibiting the nuclear factor-kappa B cascade and following the suppression of interleukins and TNF-α, therefore manipulating the inflammatory response [84]. Selenium status can be determined through serum/plasma levels using fluorometric methods as well as enzymatic measurement of glutathione peroxidase (GPx) activity in plasma, erythrocytes, thrombocytes, or whole blood. The concentration of selenoprotein P, the major selenoprotein in serum/plasma, accounts for about 60% of the total plasma selenium and serves as a surrogate biomarker of total selenium stores [85]. In healthy adults, the recommended levels of intake for selenium are 70 mcg/day (men) and 60 mcg/day (women) [86].

Critically ill patients are prone to developing significant selenium deficiency [87]. Several observational studies have shown a link between the systemic inflammatory response and selenium status, showing an inverse relationship between lower plasma selenium concentrations and plasma GPx activity and disease severity of illness and clinical outcomes [88]. Current nutrition guidelines recommend that EN should provide 50–150 mcg selenium/day/1500 kcal and PN 60–100 mcg/day. In patients with plasma selenium levels <0.4 mcmol/L (<32 mcg/L), 100 mcg selenium/day should be given until normal levels have been achieved [89]. Patients with burns, major trauma, and cardiac surgery, or those receiving renal replacement therapy, may need higher doses.

55.8.2 Zinc

Zinc is an essential trace element that is a cofactor for more than 300 enzymes and is necessary for maintaining immune system functions, metabolic control, and response to oxidative stress. Zinc is important for DNA synthesis, cell proliferation, protein synthesis, and cell membrane integrity [82]. Zinc status is measured in whole blood, plasma, serum, urine, and hair using ICP-MS or atomic absorption spectroscopy. Depending on the concomitant daily phytate intake, healthy adults have reference values set at 7–10 mg/day (females) and 11–16 mg/day (males) [90]. Low zinc levels have been observed in ICU patients from a multitude of factors, ranging across preexisting zinc deficiency, an acute-phase response, or disease-related losses/increased needs (e.g., through drains and exudates) [82, 91]. These low levels might be related with worse outcomes, including increased 28- and 90-day mortality [92]. Current nutrition guidelines suggest that in the case of normal losses, EN should provide ≥10 mg zinc/day/1500 kcal and PN 3–5 mg/day (in the case of normal losses). In patients with increased gastrointestinal losses due to diarrhea, fistula, and stomas, parenteral zinc administration can be increased up to 12 mg/day for as long as needed to achieve an adequate status [89]. Likewise, burn patients should receive 30–35 mg zinc/day intravenously over 2–3 weeks [89].

55.8.3   Vitamin C (Ascorbic Acid)

Ascorbic acid is an essential, water-soluble vitamin that serves as a cofactor in several enzymatic reactions and possesses antioxidative properties. Vitamin C is necessary for several physiological functions including the synthesis of catecholamines, immune cell function, collagen synthesis, maintenance of the endothelial barrier, and production of cortisol, neurotransmitters (e.g., norepinephrine, serotonin), and peptide hormones (e.g., vasopressin), as well as metabolism of folic acid and iron [82, 93]. Through its antioxidant properties, ascorbic acid limits the formation of reactive oxygen species by inhibiting the activity of inducible nitric oxide synthase and NADPH oxidase. In addition, vitamin C acts as a scavenger of radicals. It is involved in the regeneration of alpha-tocopherol from alpha-tocopheroxyl radicals, which are produced through the binding of lipid peroxyl radicals and, thus, inhibit the lipid peroxidation chain reaction. Vitamin C status can be assessed by the measurement of plasma or leukocyte levels using enzymatic and chromatographic assays or by the measurement of the oxidation-reduction potential [94].

Vitamin C is an essential vitamin and dietary intake from vegetables and fruits, which is necessary to preserve physiologic functions. In healthy adults, the recommended intake for vitamin C is 95–125 mg/day to maintain plasma levels within the adequate status of ≥50 mcmol/L [95]. Conversely, low vitamin C levels have been observed in critically ill septic or postoperative cardiac surgery patients [96]. Higher vitamin C intakes might be needed to offset disease-associated deficiencies. ESPEN recommends providing ≥100 mg vitamin C/day/1500 kcal EN and 100–200 mg/day in PN [89]. Additionally, in cases of chronic oxidative stress (e.g., dialysis, diabetes, heart failure), higher vitamin C dosages of 200–500 mg/day may be needed, while patients who are in the acute inflammatory phase may require intravenous doses as high as 2–3 g/day [89]. Evidence is still lacking as to the optimal dose and which patient populations would benefit most from supplementation.

55.8.4   Vitamin D

The essential fat-soluble vitamin D is primarily produced in the skin from cholesterol after exposure to sunlight. The primary dietary sources of vitamin D are fatty fish, mushrooms, eggs, milk, and cheese. Unfortunately, dietary intake cannot ensure that patient needs can be met. Acting more like a hormone than a vitamin, vitamin D plays an important role in bone metabolism by regulating calcium homeostasis. It also plays a major role in many endocrinologic and immunologic processes. Vitamin D impacts the immune system's response to acute systemic inflammation and infection through nuclear vitamin D receptors found within macrophages and B and T cells [97, 98]. Vitamin D levels are significantly decreased in critically ill patients due to lack of exposure to sunlight, which is necessary for the synthesis of cholecalciferol, i.e., vitamin D3, from 7-dehydrocholesterol in the skin.

Subsequently, a decrease in inactive (25-hydroxycholecalciferol, calcidiol) and active (1,25-dihydroxycholecalciferol, calcitriol) vitamin D occurs that further impairs the functions of several organs including muscles, lungs, kidney, heart, and immune system [99]. To determine if a patient is vitamin D sufficient, deficient, or toxic, 25(OH)D is the only vitamin D metabolite that is used [100]. This isomer is the major circulating form of vitamin D that has a half-life of approximately 2–3 weeks. 25(OH)D is the sum total of vitamin D dietary intake and the vitamin D that is produced in the skin from sun exposure [101]. The estimated value on adequate intake of vitamin D for a healthy adult is defined as 20 mcg/day to maintain a serum 25(OH)D level of at least 50 nmol/L [102]. In higher latitudes, where there is reduced exposure to sunlight, seasonal vitamin D hypovitaminosis can occur in an otherwise healthy population. In addition, low 25(OH)D levels have been reported in patients in the ICU, either preceding the ICU admission or developing during medical treatment because of lack of exposure to sunlight or due to the use of low vitamin D containing EN or PN [80]. During times of critical illness, vitamin D deficiency is associated with poor clinical outcomes (e.g., increased length of stay, prolonged courses of ventilatory support) [103].

Current nutrition guidelines recommend that EN provide $\geq$1000 IU vitamin D/day/1500 kcal (25 mcg) and PN $\geq$200 IU (5 mcg) [89]. In some instances, within the first week of admission to the ICU, high-dose vitamin D supplementation (500,000 IU) as bolus or administered as 50,000 IU/week over a period of 8 weeks is recommended in cases where 25(OH)D serum levels are <12.5 ng/mL (<50 nmol/L) [5]. In patients with recurrent 25(OH)D levels of 40–60 ng/mL, supplemental doses of vitamin D of 4000–5000 IU/day (100 mcg) over a 2-month period may be necessary [89].

55.9   Summary

Malnutrition is present in more than 50% of critically ill patients [67]. Hyperglycemia, loss of lean body mass, and inadequate utilization of nutrients are related with the inflammatory response seen in critical illness. It is imperative that adequate provision of each macronutrient is given to reduce morbidity and mortality in this population. The challenge is to determine the most appropriate dose of protein, fat, and carbohydrates, which will vary with each patient, given the heterogeneity of these individuals. Indirect calorimetry remains the gold standard for determining caloric and nutritional requirements. In general, EN is preferred over PN, and its initiation should occur as soon as possible after admission to the ICU. When to start PN remains controversial. To reduce catabolism, protein doses of 2–2.5 g/kg/day should be administered. When such doses are used in tandem with hypocaloric feedings (i.e., 10–20 kcal/kg/day), improved outcomes have been observed. Other factors that should be considered to reduce morbidity include maintaining blood glucose concentrations between 120 and 150 mg/dL through the use of insulin along with lower dextrose provision of 1–2 g/kg/day so as to prevent the risk of hypoglycemia and improve prognosis. ILEs should be used to meet energy requirements when dextrose intake must be reduced. ILEs have additional benefits such as being calorically dense and prevent complications associated with excessive glucose infusion rates.

References

1. Lambell KJ, Tatucu-Babet OA, Chapple LA, et al. Nutrition therapy in critical illness: a review of the literature for clinicians. Crit Care. 2020;24(1):35.
2. Preiser JC, Ichai C, Orban JC, et al. Metabolic response to the stress of critical illness. Br J Anaesth. 2014;113:945–54.
3. Casaer MP, Van den Berghe G. Nutrition in the acute phase of critical illness. N Engl J Med. 2014;370:1227–36.
4. McClave SA, Taylor BE, Martindale RG, et al. Guidelines for the provision and assessment of nutrition support therapy in the adult critically ill patient: SCCM and ASPEN. J Parenter Enter Nutr. 2016;40:159–211.
5. Singer P, Blaser AR, Berger MM, et al. ESPEN guideline on clinical nutrition in the intensive care unit. Clin Nutr. 2019;38:48–79.
6. Compher C, Bingham AL, McCall M, et al. Guidelines for the provision of nutrition support therapy in the adult critically ill patient: the American Society for Parenteral and Enteral Nutrition [published correction appears in JPEN J Parenter Enteral Nutr. 2022 Aug;46(6):1458–1459]. JPEN J Parenter Enteral Nutr. 2022;46(1):12–41.
7. Singer P, Blaser AR, Berger MM, et al. ESPEN practical and partially revised guideline: clinical nutrition in the intensive care unit. Clin Nutr. 2023;42(9):1671–89.
8. Kondrup J, Rasmussen HH, Hamberg O, Stanga Z, Ad Hoc ESPEN Working Group. Nutritional risk screening (NRS 2002): a new method based on an analysis of controlled clinical trials. Clin Nutr. 2003;22(3):321–36. https://doi.org/10.1016/s0261-5614(02)00214-5.
9. Moonen HPFX, Van Zanten ARH. Bioelectric impedance analysis for body composition measurement and other potential clinical applications in critical illness. Curr Opin Crit Care. 2021;27(4):344–53.
10. Moonen HPFX, van Zanten FJL, Driessen L, et al. Association of bioelectric impedance analysis body composition and disease severity in COVID-19 hospital ward and ICU patients: the BIAC-19 study. Clin Nutr. 2021;40(4):2328–36.
11. Stoppe C, Wendt S, Mehta N, et al. Biomarkers in critical care nutrition. Crit Care. 2020;24:499.
12. Heyland DK, Dhallwal R, Jiang X, Day AG. Identifying critically ill patients who benefit the most from nutrition therapy: the development and initial validation of a novel risk assessment tool. Crit Care. 2011;15:R268.
13. Milward DJ. Metabolic demands for amino acids and the human dietary requirement: Milward and Rivers (1988) revisited. J Nutr. 1998;128:25635–765.
14. Fullerton BS, Sparks EA, Khan FA, et al. Whole body protein turnover and net protein balance after pediatric thoracic surgery: a noninvasive single dose (15) N glycine stable isotope protocol with end-product enrichment. JPEN. 2018;42:361–70.
15. Kraft MD, Btaiche IF, Sacks GS. Review of the refeeding syndrome. NCP. 2005;20:625.
16. Duan JY, Zheng WH, Zhou H, Xu Y, Huang HB. Energy delivery guided by indirect calorimetry in critically ill patients: a systematic review and meta-analysis. Crit Care. 2021;25(1):88.
17. Alcantara JMA, Galgani JE, Jurado-Fasoli L, et al. Validity of four commercially available metabolic carts for assessing resting metabolic rate and respiratory exchange ratio in non-ventilated humans. Clin Nutr. 2022;41(3):746–54.

18. Koekkoek WAC, Xiaochen G, van Dijk D, van Zanten ARH. Resting energy expenditure by indirect calorimetry versus the ventilator-VCO_2 derived method in critically ill patients: the DREAM-VCO_2 prospective comparative study. Clin Nutr ESPEN. 2020;39:137–43.
19. Chapple LS, Plummer MP, Chapman MJ. Gut dysfunction in the ICU: diagnosis and management. Curr Opin Crit Care. 2021;27(2):141–6.
20. Lee HY, Lee JK, Kim HJ, et al. Continuous versus intermittent enteral tube feeding for critically ill patients: a prospective, randomized controlled trial. Nutrients. 2022;14(3):664.
21. Reintam Blaser A, Deane AM, Preiser JC, et al. Enteral feeding intolerance update in definitions and pathophysiology. Nutr Clin Pract. 2021;36:40–9.
22. Heyland DK, Orti A, Stoppe C, et al. Incidence, risk factors, and clinical consequence of enteral feeding intolerance in the mechanically ventilated critically ill: an analysis of a multicenter, multiyear database. Crit Care Med. 2021;49:49–59.
23. Boelens YFN, Melchers M, van Zanten ARH. Poor physical recovery after critical illness: incidence, features, risk factors, pathophysiology, and evidence-based therapies. Curr Opin Crit Care. 2022;28(4):409–16.
24. Wang D, Lin Z, Xie L, et al. Impact of early protein provision on the mortality of acute critically ill stroke patients. Nutr Clin Pract. 2022;37(4):861–8.
25. Lambell KJ, Goh GS, Tierney AC, et al. Marked losses of computed tomography-derived skeletal muscle area and density over the first month of a critical illness are not associated with energy and protein delivery. Nutrition. 2021;82:111061.
26. Lee ZY, Yap CSL, Hasan MS, et al. The effect of higher versus lower protein delivery in critically ill patients: a systematic review and meta-analysis of randomized controlled trials. Crit Care. 2021;25(1):260.
27. Heyland DK, Day A Clarke GJ, et al. Nutrition and Exercise in Critical Illness Trial (NEXIS Trial): a protocol of a multicentred, randomised controlled trial of combined cycle ergometry and amino acid supplementation commenced early during critical illness. BMJ Open. 2019;9(7):e027893.
28. Serhan CN. Resolvins and protectins: novel lipid mediators in anti-inflammation and resolution. Scand J Food Nutr. 2006;50(Suppl 2):68–78.
29. Le HD, Meisel JA, de Meijer VE, et al. The essentiality of arachidonic acid and docosahexaenoic acid. Prostaglandins Leukot Essent Fatty Acids. 2009;81:165–70.
30. Deckelbaum RJ, Worgall TS, Seo T. Fatty acids and gene expression. Am J Clin Nutr. 2006;83(6 Suppl):1520S–5S.
31. Kopecky J, Rossmeisl M, Flachs P, et al. Symposium on "Frontiers in adipose tissue biology" n-3 PUFA: bioavailability and modulation of adipose tissue function. Proc Nutr Soc. 2009;68:361–9.
32. Minihane AM. Nutrient gene interactions in lipid metabolism. Curr Opin Clin Nutr Metab Care. 2009;12:357–63.
33. Wanten GJA, Calder PC. Immune modulation by parenteral lipid emulsions. Am J Clin Nutr. 2007;85:1171–84.
34. Riedy M, DePaula B, Puder M, et al. Higher doses of fish oil-based lipid emulsions used to treat inadequate weight gain and rising triene:tetraene ratio in a severely malnourished infant with intestinal failure-associated liver disease. JPEN J Parenter Enteral Nutr. 2017;41(4):667–71.
35. Samieri C, Féart C, Proust-Lima C, et al. Olive oil consumption, plasma oleic acid, and stroke incidence: the Three-City study. Neurology. 2011;77:418–25.
36. Nimbkar S, Leena MM, Moses JA, Anandharamakrishnan C. Medium chain triglycerides (MCT): state-of-the-art on chemistry, synthesis, health benefits and applications in food industry. Compr Rev Food Sci Food Saf. 2022;21(2):843–67.
37. Ball MJ. Parenteral nutrition in the critically ill: use of a medium chain triglyceride emulsion. Intensive Care Med. 1993;19(2):89–95.

38. Bohles H, Akcetin Z, Lehnert W. The influence of intravenous medium and long-chain tri-glycerides and carnitine on the excretion of dicarboxylic acids. JPEN J Parenter Enteral Nutr. 1987;11:46–8.
39. Bach AC, Babayan VK. Medium-chain triglycerides: an update. Am J Clin Nutr. 1982;36:950–62.
40. Yadav SK, Bothra S, Chekavar AS, et al. A rare complication of left open adrenalectomy. Chirurgia (Bucur). 2016;111(5):432–4.
41. Kataoka M, Ohi Y, Sakanoue K, et al. Impact of dietary intake of medium-chain triacyl-glycerides on the intestinal absorption of poorly permeable compounds. Mol Pharm. 2020;17(1):212–8.
42. Ferezou J, Bach AC. Structure and metabolic fate of triacylglycerol and phospholipid-rich particles of commercial parenteral fat emulsions. Nutrition. 1999;15:44–50.
43. Salama GS, Kaabneh MA, Almasaeed MN, Alquran MIa. Intravenous lipids for preterm infants: a review. Clin Med Insights Pediatr. 2015;9:25–36.
44. Heird WC, Kashyap S, Gomez MR. Protein intake and energy requirements of the infant. Semin Perinatol. 1991;15(6):438–48.
45. Seidel D, Alaupovic P, Furman RH, et al. A lipoprotein characterizing obstructive jaundice 1. Method for quantitative separation and identification of lipoproteins in jaundiced subjects. J Clin Invest. 1969;48:1211–23.
46. Torsvik H, Berg K, Magnani HN, McConathy WJ, Alaupovic P, Gjone E. Identification of the abnormal cholestatic lipoprotein (LP-X) in familial lecithin:Cholesterol acyltransferase deficiency. FEBS Lett. 1972;24(2):165–68.
47. Miles JM, Park Y, Harris WS. Lipoprotein lipase and triglyceride rich lipoprotein metabo-lism. Nutr Clin Pract. 2001;16:273–9.
48. Rader DJ, Rosas S. Management of selected lipid abnormalities. Hypertriglyceridemia, low HDL cholesterol, lipoprotein(a), in thyroid and renal diseases, and post-transplantation. Med Clin North Am. 2000;84:43–61.
49. Rapp RP, Donaldson ES, Bivins BA. Parenteral nutrition in a patient with familial type IV hypertriglyceridemia: a dilemma. Drug Intell Clin Pharm. 1983 Jun;17(6):458–60.
50. Llop J, Sabin P, Garau M, et al. The importance of clinical factors in parenteral nutrition-associated hypertriglyceridemia. Clin Nutr. 2003;22:577–83.
51. Essential fatty acids: the work of George and Mildred Burr. J Biol Chem. 2012;287(42):35439–41.
52. Rivers JP, Hassam AG. Defective essential-fatty-acid metabolism in cystic fibrosis. Lancet. 1975;2(7936):642–3.
53. Wene JD, Connor WE, Den Besten L. The development of essential fatty acid deficiency in healthy men fed fat-free diets intravenously and orally. J Clin Invest. 1975;56:127–34.
54. Cederholm TE, Berg AB, Johansson EK, et al. Low levels of essential fatty acids are related to impaired delayed skin hypersensitivity in malnourished chronically ill elderly people. Eur J Clin Investig. 1994;24:615–20.
55. Gramlich L, Ireton-Jones C, Miles JM, et al. Essential fatty acid requirements and intrave-nous lipid emulsions. JPEN J Parenter Enteral Nutr. 2019;43(6):697–707.
56. Holman RT. The ratio of trienoic: tetraenoic acids in tissue lipids as a measure of essential fatty acid requirement. J Nutr. 1960;70(3):405–10.
57. Richardson TJ, Sgoutas D. Essential fatty acid deficiency in four adult patients during total parenteral nutrition. Am J Clin Nutr. 1975;28:258–63.
58. Dickerson RN, Rosato EF, Mullen JL. Net protein anabolism with hypocaloric parenteral nutrition in obese stressed patients. Am J Clin Nutr. 1986;44:747–55.
59. Petros S, Horbach M, Seidel F, Weidhase L. Hypocaloric vs normocaloric nutrition in critically ill patients: a prospective randomized pilot trial. JPEN J Parenter Enteral Nutr. 2016;40(2):242–9.

60. Mirtallo JM, Ayers P, Boullata J, et al. ASPEN lipid injectable emulsion safety recommendations, part 1: background and adult considerations [published correction appears in Nutr Clin Pract. 2022 Apr;37(2):482]. Nutr Clin Pract. 2020;35(5):769–82.
61. Gura KM, Parsons SK, Bechard LJ, et al. Use of a fish oil-based lipid emulsion to treat essential fatty acid deficiency in a soy allergic patient receiving parenteral nutrition. Clin Nutr. 2005;24(5):839–47.
62. Duerksen DR, Nehra V, Palombo JD, et al. Essential fatty acid deficiencies in patients with chronic liver disease are not reversed by short-term intravenous lipid supplementation. Dig Dis Sci. 1999;44(7):1342–8.
63. Duerksen D, McCurdy K. Essential fatty acid deficiency in a severely malnourished patient receiving parenteral nutrition. Dig Dis Sci. 2005;50(12):2386–8.
64. Gura KM, Puder M. Rapid infusion of fish oil-based emulsion in infants does not appear to be associated with fat overload syndrome. Nutr Clin Pract. 2010;25(4):399–402.
65. Hojsak I, Kolacek S. Fat overload syndrome after the rapid infusion of SMOFlipid emulsion. JPEN J Parenter Enteral Nutr. 2014;38:119–21.
66. Weissman C. Nutrition in the intensive care unit. Crit Care. 1999;3:R67–75.
67. Patkova A, Joskova V, Havel E, et al. Energy, protein, carbohydrate, and lipid intakes and their effects on morbidity and mortality in critically ill adult patients: a systematic review. Adv Nutr. 2017;8(4):624–34.
68. Bolder U, Ebener C, Hauner H, et al. Carbohydrates - guidelines on parenteral nutrition, Chapter 5. Ger Med Sci. 2009;7:Doc23.
69. Thibault R, Heidegger CP, Berger MM, Pichard C. Parenteral nutrition in the intensive care unit: cautious use improves outcome. Swiss Med Wkly. 2014;144:w13997.
70. Carlson GL. Insulin resistance and glucose-induced thermogenesis in critical illness. Proc Nutr Soc. 2001;60:381–8.
71. Losser MR, Damoisel C, Payen D. Bench-to-bedside review: glucose and stress conditions in the intensive care unit. Crit Care. 2010;14:231.
72. Ilias I, Vassiliadi DA, Theodorakopoulou M, et al. Adipose tissue lipolysis and circulating lipids in acute and subacute critical illness: effects of shock and treatment. J Crit Care. 2014;29(1130):e5–9.
73. Harper J. Glucose control in the intensive care unit: how it is done. Proc Nutr Soc. 2007;66:362–6.
74. Van den Berghe G, Wilmer A, Hermans G, et al. Intensive insulin therapy in the medical ICU. N Engl J Med. 2006;354:449–61.
75. Lazzeri C, Tarquini R, Giunta F, Gensini GF. Glucose dysmetabolism and prognosis in critical illness. Intern Emerg Med. 2009;4:147–56.
76. Krinsley JS. Association between hyperglycemia and increased hospital mortality in a heterogeneous population of critically ill patients. Mayo Clin Proc. 2003;78:1471–8.
77. Badawi O, Waite MD, Fuhrman SA, Zuckerman IH. Association between intensive care unit-acquired dysglycemia and in-hospital mortality. Crit Care Med. 2012;40:3180–8.
78. Treggiari MM, Karir V, Yanez ND, et al. Intensive insulin therapy and mortality in critically ill patients. Crit Care. 2008;12:R29.
79. Amrein K, Kachel N, Fries H, et al. Glucose control in intensive care: usability, efficacy and safety of Space Glucose Control in two medical European intensive care units. BMC Endocr Disord. 2014;14:62.
80. Dresen E, Pimiento JM, Patel JJ, et al. Overview of oxidative stress and the role of micronutrients in critical illness. JPEN J Parenter Enteral Nutr. 2023;47(Suppl 1):S38–49.
81. McClave SA, Wischmeyer PE, Miller KR, van Zanten ARH. Mitochondrial dysfunction in critical illness: implications for nutritional therapy. Curr Nutr Rep. 2019;8(4):363–73.
82. Koekkoek WACK, van Zanten ARH. Antioxidant vitamins and trace elements in critical illness. Nutr Clin Pract. 2016;31(4):457–74.
83. Holben DH, Smith AM. The diverse role of selenium within selenoproteins. J Am Diet Assoc. 1999;99(7):836–43.

84. Forman HJ, Torres M. Reactive oxygen species and cell signaling: respiratory burst in macrophage signaling. Am J Respir Crit Care Med. 2002;166(12 pt 2):S4–8.

85. Brodin O, Hackler J, Misra S, et al. Selenoprotein P as biomarker of selenium status in clinical trials with therapeutic dosages of selenite. Nutrients. 2020;12(4):1067.

86. Kipp AP, Strohm D, Brigelius-Flohé R, et al. Revised reference values for selenium intake. J Trace Elem Med Biol. 2015;32:195–9.

87. Stoppe C, McDonald B, Rex S, et al. Sodium Selenite Administration in Cardiac Surgery (SUSTAIN CSX-trial): study design of an international multicenter randomized double-blinded controlled trial of high dose sodium-selenite administration in high-risk cardiac surgical patients. Trials. 2014;15:339.

88. Manzanares W, Langlois PL, Heyland DK. Pharmaconutrition with selenium in critically ill patients: what do we know? Nutr Clin Pract. 2015;30(1):34–43.

89. Berger MM, Shenkin A, Schweinlin A, et al. ESPEN micronutrient guideline. Clin Nutr. 2022;41(6):1357–424.

90. Haase H, Ellinger S, Linseisen J, et al. German Nutrition Society (DGE). Revised D-A-CH-reference values for the intake of zinc. J Trace Elem Med Biol. 2020;61:126536.

91. Berger MM. Nutrition and micronutrient therapy in critical illness should be individualized. JPEN J Parenter Enteral Nutr. 2020;44(8):1380–7.

92. Hoeger J, Simon T-P, Beeker T, et al. Persistent low serum zinc is associated with recurrent sepsis in critically ill patients—a pilot study. PLoS One. 2017;12(5):e0176069.

93. Kressin C, Pandya K, Woodward BM, et al. Ascorbic acid in the acute care setting. JPEN J Parenter Enteral Nutr. 2021;45(5):874–81.

94. Rozemeijer S, van der Horst FAL, Man AMEde. Measuring vitamin C in critically ill patients: clinical importance and practical difficulties—is it time for a surrogate marker? Crit Care. 2021;25(1):310.

95. German Nutrition Society (DGE). New reference values for vitamin C intake. Ann Nutr Metab. 2015;67(1):13–20.

96. Koekkoek WAC, Hettinga K, Vries JHM, de van, Zanten ARH. Micronutrient deficiencies in critical illness. Clin Nutr. 2021;40(6):3780–6.

97. Patel JJ, McClave SA. Use of vitamin D in critical illness: a concept for whom the bell tolls. JPEN J Parenter Enteral Nutr. 2021;45(1):9–11.

98. Amrein K, Papinutti A, Mathew E, et al. Vitamin D and critical illness: what endocrinology can learn from intensive care and vice versa. Endocr Connect. 2018;7(12):R304–15.

99. Amrein K, Oudemans-van Straaten HM, Berger MM. Vitamin therapy in critically ill patients: focus on thiamine, vitamin C, and vitamin D. Intensive Care Med. 2018;44(11):1940–4.

100. Holick MF. High prevalence of vitamin D inadequacy and implications for health. Mayo Clin Proc. 2006;81(3):353–73.

101. Holick MF. Vitamin D status: measurement, interpretation, and clinical application. Ann Epidemiol. 2009;19(2):73–8.

102. German Nutrition Society. New reference values for vitamin D. Ann Nutr Metab. 2012;60(4):241–6.

103. McKinney TJ, Patel JJ, Benns MV, et al. Vitamin D status and supplementation in the critically ill. Curr Gastroenterol Rep. 2016;18(4):18.

Index

© The Editor(s) (if applicable) and The Author(s), under exclusive license to
Springer Nature Switzerland AG 2025
Y. Alzaidi, M. A. Gebily (eds.), *The Pharmacist's Expanded Role in Critical
Care Medicine*, https://doi.org/10.1007/978-3-031-77335-8

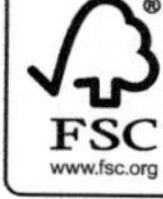

MIX
Papier aus verantwortungsvollen Quellen
Paper from responsible sources
FSC® C105338

FSC
www.fsc.org

If you have any concerns about our products,
you can contact us on
ProductSafety@springernature.com

In case Publisher is established outside the EU,
the EU authorized representative is:
Springer Nature Customer Service Center GmbH
Europaplatz 3, 69115 Heidelberg, Germany

Printed by Libri Plureos GmbH
in Hamburg, Germany